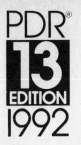

PDR®
13
EDITION
1992

PHYSICIANS' DESK REFERENCE

FOR NONPRESCRIPTION DRUGS®

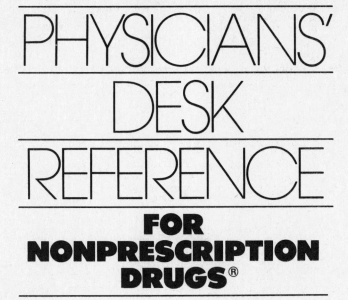

Director of Production:
MARJORIE A. DUFFY

Assistant Director of Production:
CARRIE WILLIAMS

Manager of Production Services:
ELIZABETH H. CARUSO
KIMBERLY V. HILLER

Format Editor:
MILDRED M. SCHUMACHER

Production Coordinator:
ELIZABETH A. KARST

Art Associate:
JOAN K. AKERLIND

Medical Consultant:
LOUIS V. NAPOLITANO, MD

Product Manager:
JOHN A. MALCZYNSKI

Sales Manager:
CHARLIE J. MEITNER

Account Managers:
CHAD E. ALCORN
MICHAEL S. SARAJIAN
JOANNE C. TERZIDES

Commercial Sales Manager:
ROBIN B. BARTLETT

Direct Marketing Manager:
ROBERT W. CHAPMAN

Manager, Professional Data:
MUKESH MEHTA, R.Ph.

Index Editor:
ADELE L. DOWD

Officers of Medical Economics Data, a division of Medical Economics Company Inc.: President and Chief Executive Officer: Norman R. Snesil; Senior Vice President and Chief Financial Officer: Joseph T. Deithorn; Senior Vice President of Business Development: Stephen J. Sorkenn; Senior Vice President of Operations: Mark L. Weinstein; Vice President, Data Sales and Acquisitions: Curtis Allen; Vice President, Sales and Marketing: Thomas F. Rice; Vice President of Circulation: Scott I. Rockman; Vice President of Information Systems Services: Edward J. Zecchini.

ISBN 1-56363-006-0

MEDICAL ECONOMICS DATA

Foreword to the Thirteenth Edition

Welcome to the thirteenth edition of the PHYSICIANS' DESK REFERENCE For NONPRESCRIPTION DRUGS®, the over-the-counter drug companion to the Physicians' Desk Reference. The shift of some drug ingredients and dosage forms from prescription to over-the-counter status is continuing. It is the goal of the PHYSICIANS' DESK REFERENCE For NONPRESCRIPTION DRUGS® to provide detailed labeling information to help ensure appropriate use of these products. Manufacturers of these nonprescription drug products have included inactive ingredients as well as active ingredients to alert those who may have sensitivity to certain ingredients.

The PHYSICIANS' DESK REFERENCE For NONPRESCRIPTION DRUGS® is published annually by Medical Economics Data, a division of Medical Economics Company, Inc., with the cooperation of the manufacturers whose products are described in the Product Information and Diagnostics, Devices and Medical Aids Sections. It is organized in a similar manner to the PHYSICIANS' DESK REFERENCE with a Manufacturers' Index, Product Name Index, Product Category Index, and Active Ingredients Index-all color coded for quick reference. Descriptive labeling appears in the Product Information Section and Diagnostics, Devices and Medical Aids Section.

The function of the publisher is the compilation, organization, and distribution of this information. Each product description has been prepared by the manufacturer, and edited and approved by the manufacturer's medical department, medical director, and/or medical consultant. In organizing and presenting the material in PHYSICIANS' DESK REFERENCE For NONPRESCRIPTION DRUGS®, the publisher does not warrant or guarantee any of the products described herein or perform any independent analysis in connection with any of the product information contained herein. PHYSICIANS' DESK REFERENCE For NONPRESCRIPTION DRUGS® does not assume, and expressly disclaims, any obligation to obtain and include information other than that provided to it by the manufacturer. In making this material available it should be understood that the publisher is not advocating the use of any product described herein. Besides the information given here, additional information on any product may be obtained through the manufacturer.

MEDICAL ECONOMICS DATA

Contents

Manufacturers' Index (White) **1**

The manufacturers appearing in this index have provided information concerning their products in the Product Information, Product Identification or Diagnostics, Devices and Medical Aids Sections. Included in this index are the names and addresses of manufacturers, individuals or departments to whom you may address inquiries, a partial list of products as well as emergency telephone numbers, wherever available.

Product Name Index (Pink) **101**

Products are listed in alphabetical order by brand or generic name. Page numbers have been included to assist you in locating additional information on described products.

Product Category Index (Blue) **201**

In this section described products are listed according to their appropriate product categories. The headings and sub-headings have been determined by the OTC Review process of the U.S. Food and Drug Administration.

Active Ingredients (Yellow) **301**

Products described in the Product Information Section are listed alphabetically in this section. The heading under which specific products are listed have been determined by the OTC Review process of the U.S. Food and Drug Administration.

Drug Information Centers **321**

An alphabetical listing by state of Drug Information Centers including address, telephone number and hours of operation.

Product Identification Section **401**

Capsules, tablets and packaging are shown in color as an aid to identification. Products are shown under company headings, and are not necessarily in alphabetical order since some manufacturers prefer to show their products in groups.

Product Information Section **501**

An alphabetical arrangement, by manufacturer, of nonprescription drugs which are described as to action, uses, administration and dosage, precautions, the form in which supplied and other information concerning their use, including common names and chemical names.

Diagnostics, Devices and Medical Aids **779**

This section contains product information on those product designed for home use. Items are listed alphabetically by manufacturer. Product descriptions supply essential information for appropriate understanding and use.

Poison Control Centers **784**

A list of centers and emergency telephone numbers.

SECTION 1

Manufacturers' Index

The manufacturers whose names appear in this index have provided information concerning their products in either the Product Information Section, Product Identification Section, or the Diagnostics, Devices and Medical Aids Section.

Included in this index are the names and addresses of manufacturers, individuals or departments to whom you may address inquiries, a partial list of products as well as emergency telephone numbers wherever available.

The symbol ◆ indicates that the product is shown in the Product Identification Section.

PAGE

ABBOTT LABORATORIES   403, 502
For Medical Information
  Pharmaceutical Products Division
                        (312) 937-7069
  Hospital Products Division
                        (312) 937-3806
Order Entry/Customer Service Inquiries
  Pharmaceutical Products Division
                        (800) 255-5162
  Hospital Products Division
                        (800) 222-6883
     OTC Products Available
Dayalets Filmtab
Dayalets Plus Iron Filmtab
◆Optilets-500 Filmtab
◆Optilets-M-500 Filmtab
Surbex
Surbex with C
◆Surbex-750 with Iron
◆Surbex-750 with Zinc
◆Surbex-T

ADRIA LABORATORIES   403, 503
  Division of Erbamont Inc.
     Administrative Offices
7001 Post Road
Dublin, OH 43017
     Mailing Address
P.O. Box 16529
Columbus, OH 43216-6529

     Address inquiries to:
Medical Dept.   (614) 764-8100
     OTC Products Available
◆Emetrol
Evac-Q-Kwik
Modane Plus Tablets
Modane Soft Capsules
Modane Tablets
Xylo-Pfan

PAGE

ALLERGAN PHARMACEUTICALS   504
A Division of Allergan, Inc.
2525 Dupont Drive
P.O. Box 19534
Irvine, CA 92713-9534
     Address Inquiries to:
Scientific Information/Medical
Compliance   (800) 433-8871
                  (714) 752-4500
   For Medical Emergencies Contact:
Scientific Information/Medical
Compliance   (714) 752-4500
     OTC Products Available
Cellufresh Lubricant Ophthalmic
  Solution
Celluvisc Lubricant Ophthalmic Solution
Lacri-Lube NP Lubricant Ophthalmic
  Ointment
Lacri-Lube S.O.P. Sterile Ophthalmic
  Ointment
Refresh P.M. Lubricant Ophthalmic
  Ointment
Tears Plus Lubricant Ophthalmic
  Solution

APOTHECON   403, 505
A Bristol-Myers Squibb Company
Princeton, NJ 08540
Mailing Address:
P.O. Box 4000
Princeton, NJ 08543-4000
                  (609) 987-6800
     Address inquiries to:
Apothecon Customer Service Dept.
P.O. Box 5250
Princeton, NJ 08543-5250
                  (800) 321-1335

PAGE

  Orders for Apothecon Products
     may be placed by:
1. Calling toll-free   (800) 631-5244
  Between 8:30 AM-6:00 PM EST
2. Mailing your purchase orders to:
  Apothecon
  Attn: Customer Service Dept.
  P.O. Box 5250
  Princeton, NJ 08543-5250
3. Orders may be telefaxed to:
  Customer Service Dept.
          FAX (800) 523-2965
     OTC Products Available
Naldecon CX Adult Liquid
Naldecon DX Adult Liquid
Naldecon DX Children's Syrup
Naldecon DX Pediatric Drops
Naldecon EX Children's Syrup
Naldecon EX Pediatric Drops
Naldecon Senior DX Cough/Cold Liquid
Naldecon Senior EX Cough/Cold Liquid
◆Theragran Liquid
◆Theragran Stress Formula
◆Theragran Tablets
◆Theragran-M Tablets

**B. F. ASCHER & COMPANY,   403, 509
INC.**
15501 West 109th Street
Lenexa, KS 66219
Mailing Address: P.O. Box 717
Shawnee Mission, KS 66201-0717
     Address inquiries to:
Joan F. Bowen   (913) 888-1880
  For Medical Emergencies Contact:
Dan Henry   (913) 888-1880
     OTC Products Available
◆Ayr Saline Nasal Drops
◆Ayr Saline Nasal Mist
◆Itch-X Gel

(◆ Shown in Product Identification Section)

◆Mobigesic Analgesic Tablets
◆Mobisyl Analgesic Creme
◆Pen•Kera Creme
Unilax Stool Softener/Laxative Softgel
Capsules

**ASTRA PHARMACEUTICAL   403, 510
PRODUCTS, INC.**
50 Otis Street
Westboro, MA 01581-4500
    Address inquiries to:
Roy E. Hayward, Jr.   (508) 366-1100
    For Medical Emergencies Contact:
Dr. William Gray   (508) 366-1100
    OTC Products Available
◆Xylocaine Ointment 2.5%

AU PHARMACEUTICALS, INC.   510
P.O. Box 476
Grand Saline, TX 75140
    Address inquiries to:
Michael Vick   (800) 232-2246
    For Medical Emergencies Contact:
Michael Vick   (800) 232-2246
    OTC Products Available
Aurum Analgesic Lotion
Feminine Gold Analgesic Lotion
Theragold Analgesic Lotion
Therapeutic Gold Analgesic Lotion

AYERST LABORATORIES   511
Division of American Home Products
Corporation
685 Third Avenue
New York, NY 10017-4071
For information for Ayerst's consumer
products, see product listings under
Whitehall Laboratories.
Please turn to Whitehall Laboratories,
page 761.

**BAKER CUMMINS   511
PHARMACEUTICALS, INC.**
8800 NW 36th Street
Miami, FL 33178-2404
    Address inquiries to:
        (305) 590-2282
    FAX (305) 590-2467
    For Medical Emergencies Contact:
Medical Department (305) 590-2451
        (305) 590-2218
    OTC Products Available
Acticort Lotion 100
Aqua-A Cream
Aquaderm Combination
Treatment/Moisturizer (SPF 15
Formula)
Aquaderm Cream
Aquaderm Lotion
Baker's Biopsy Punch (sizes 2, 3, 3.5,
4, 5 and 6 mm)
Baker's DTM
P & S Liquid
P & S Plus Tar Gel
P & S Shampoo
Panscol Medicated Lotion
Panscol Medicated Ointment
Phacid Shampoo
Snaplets (D, DM, EX, FR and Multi)
Ultra Mide 25
Ultraderm Bath Oil
Ultraderm Lotion
X-Seb Shampoo
X-Seb Plus Conditioning Shampoo
X-Seb T Shampoo
X-Seb T Plus Conditioning Shampoo

**BAUSCH & LOMB   403, 513
PERSONAL PRODUCTS
DIVISION**
1400 North Goodman Street
Rochester, NY 14692-0450
    OTC Products Available
◆Allergy Drops
◆Dry Eye Therapy Lubricating Eye Drops
◆Duolube Eye Ointment
◆Eye Wash
◆Moisture Drops

BEACH PHARMACEUTICALS   514
Division of Beach Products, Inc.
    Executive Office
5220 South Manhattan Avenue
Tampa, FL 33681   (813) 839-6565

Manufacturing and Distribution
Main Street at Perimeter Road
Conestee, SC 29605
    Toll Free 1-(800) 845-8210
    Address inquiries to:
Victor De Oreo, R Ph, V.P., Sales
        (803) 277-7282
Richard Stephen Jenkins, Exec. V.P.
        (813) 839-6565
    OTC Products Available
Beelith Tablets

BEIERSDORF INC.   404, 514
P.O. Box 5529
Norwalk, CT 06856-5529
    Address inquiries to:
Medical Division   (203) 853-8008
    FAX (203) 854-8180
    OTC Products Available
◆Aquaphor Antibiotic Ointment
◆Aquaphor Healing Ointment, Original
Formula
◆Aquaphor Natural Healing Ointment
Basis Facial Cleanser (Normal to Dry
Skin)
Basis Intensive Hydrating Oil
Basis Multi Protective Balm
Basis Over Night Recovery Creme
Basis Soap-Combination Skin
Basis Soap-Extra Dry Skin
Basis Soap-Normal to Dry Skin
Basis Soap-Sensitive Skin
◆Eucerin Cleansing Lotion Dry Skin Care
◆Eucerin Dry Skin Care Daily Facial
Lotion SPF 20
◆Eucerin Dry Skin Care Cleansing Bar
◆Eucerin Dry Skin Care Creme
◆Eucerin Lotion
◆Eucerin Dry Skin Care Lotion
(Fragrance-free)
Nivea Bath Silk Bath Oil
Nivea Bath Silk Bath & Shower Gel
(Extra-Dry Skin)
Nivea Bath Silk Bath & Shower Gel
(Normal-to-Dry Skin)
Nivea Moisturizing Creme
Nivea Moisturizing Lotion (Extra
Enriched)
Nivea Moisturizing Lotion (Original
Formula)
Nivea Moisturizing Oil
Nivea Skin Oil
Nivea Sun After Sun Lotion
Nivea Sun SPF 15
Nivea Visage Facial Nourishing Creme
Nivea Visage Facial Nourishing Lotion

BLAINE COMPANY, INC.   516
2700 Dixie Highway
Fort Mitchell, KY 41017
    Address inquiries to:
Mr. Alex M. Blaine   (606) 341-9437
    OTC Products Available
Mag-Ox 400
Uro-Mag

BLOCK DRUG COMPANY, INC.   516
257 Cornelison Avenue
Jersey City, NJ 07302
    Address inquiries to:
Steve Gattanella   (201) 434-3000
    For Medical Emergencies Contact:
James Gingold   (201) 434-3000
    OTC Products Available
Arthritis Strength BC Powder
BC Powder
BC Cold Powder Multi-Symptom
Formula
BC Cold Powder Multi-Symptom
Non-Drowsy Formula
Nytol Tablets
Promise Toothpaste
Mint Gel Sensodyne
Mint Sensodyne Toothpaste
Original Sensodyne Toothpaste
Tegrin Dandruff Shampoo
Tegrin for Psoriasis Lotion, Skin Cream
& Medicated Soap
Tegrin-HC with Hydrocortisone Anti-Itch
Ointment

BOIRON   404, 519
1208 Amosland Road
Norwood, PA 19074
    Address inquiries to:
Gina M. Casey
Assistant to the President
        (800) 258-8823
    For Medical Emergencies Contact:
Mark Land
Technical Services Department
        (800) 258-8823
    OTC Products Available
◆Oscillococcinum

BRISTOL LABORATORIES   519
A Bristol-Myers Squibb Company
2400 W. Lloyd Expressway
Evansville, IN 47721

Naldecon X-line is now being
distributed by Apothecon, page 505.

BRISTOL-MYERS PRODUCTS   404, 519
A Bristol-Myers Squibb Company
345 Park Avenue
New York, NY 10154
    Address inquiries to:
Bristol-Myers Products Division
Consumer Affairs Department
US Highway 202/206 North
P.O. Box 1279
Somerville, NJ 08876-1279
    In Emergencies Call:
        (800) 468-7746
    OTC Products Available
◆Alpha Keri Moisture Rich Body Oil
Alpha Keri Moisture Rich Cleansing Bar
Alpha Keri Moisturizing Body Lotion
Alpha Keri Moisturizing Spray Mist
Alpha Keri Shower & Bath Gelee
Ammens Medicated Powder
B.Q. Cold Tablets
BAN Antiperspirant Cream Deodorant
BAN Basic Non-Aerosol Antiperspirant
Spray
BAN Roll-On Antiperspirant Deodorant
BAN Solid Antiperspirant Deodorant
◆Arthritis Strength Bufferin Analgesic
Caplets
◆Extra Strength Bufferin Analgesic
Tablets
◆Bufferin Analgesic Tablets and Caplets
◆Bufferin A/F Nite Time
Analgesic/Sleeping Aid Caplets
◆Allergy-Sinus Comtrex Multi-Symptom
Allergy-Sinus Formula Tablets &
Caplets
◆Cough Formula Comtrex
◆Comtrex Multi-Symptom Cold Reliever
Tablets/Caplets/Liqui-Gels/Liquid
◆Comtrex Multi-Symptom Day-Night
Caplet-Tablet
◆Comtrex Multi-Symptom Non-Drowsy
Caplets
◆Congespirin For Children Aspirin Free
Chewable Cold Tablets
◆Datril Extra-Strength Analgesic Tablets
◆Aspirin Free Excedrin Analgesic Caplets
◆Excedrin Extra-Strength Analgesic
Tablets & Caplets
◆Excedrin P.M. Analgesic/Sleeping Aid
Tablets, Caplets and Liquid
◆Sinus Excedrin Analgesic, Decongestant
Tablets & Caplets
◆4-Way Cold Tablets
◆4-Way Fast Acting Nasal Spray (regular
& mentholated) & Metered Spray
Pump (regular)
◆4-Way Long Lasting Nasal Spray &
Metered Spray Pump
Fostex 10% Benzoyl Peroxide Bar
Fostex 10% Benzoyl Peroxide (Vanish)
Gel
Fostex 10% Benzoyl Peroxide Wash
Fostex Medicated Cleansing Bar
Fostex Medicated Cleansing Cream
Keri Facial Soap
◆Keri Lotion - Original Formula
◆Keri Lotion - Silky Smooth Formula

(◆ Shown in Product Identification Section)

◆Keri Lotion - Silky Smooth Fragrance
Free Formula
Minit-Rub Analgesic Ointment
Mum Antiperspirant Cream Deodorant
◆No Doz Fast Acting Alertness Aid
Tablets
◆No Doz Maximum Strength Caplets
◆Nuprin Ibuprofen/Analgesic Tablets &
Caplets
◆Pazo Hemorrhoid Ointment &
Suppositories
PreSun 15 Facial Sunscreen
PreSun 15 Lip Protector Sunscreen
PreSun Active 15 and 30 Clear Gel
Sunscreens
◆PreSun for Kids Lotion
◆PreSun 23 and For Kids, Spray Mist
Sunscreens
PreSun 8 and 15 Moisturizing
Sunscreens with KERI Moisturizers
PreSun 25 Moisturizing Sunscreen with
KERI Moisturizer
◆PreSun 15 and 29 Sensitive Skin
Sunscreens
◆PreSun 46 Moisturizing Sunscreen
◆Therapeutic Mineral Ice, Pain Relieving
Gel
◆Therapeutic Mineral Ice Exercise
Formula, Pain Relieving Gel
Tickle Roll-On
Antiperspirant/Deodorant

**BURROUGHS WELLCOME   406, 537
CO.**
3030 Cornwallis Road
Research Triangle Park, NC 27709
(800) 722-9292
For Medical or Drug Information:
Contact Drug Information Service
Business hours only
(8:15 AM to 4:15 PM EST)
(800) 443-6763
For 24-hour Medical Emergency
Information, call   (800) 443-6763
For Sales Information:
Contact Sales Distribution
Department
Address Other Inquiries to:
Consumer Products Division
OTC Products Available
◆Actifed Plus Caplets
◆Actifed Plus Tablets
◆Actifed Syrup
◆Actifed Tablets
Borofax Ointment
◆Empirin Aspirin
◆Filteray Broad Spectrum Sunscreen
Lotion
◆Marezine Tablets
◆Neosporin Cream
◆Neosporin Ointment
◆Neosporin Maximum Strength Ointment
◆Nix Creme Rinse
◆Polysporin Ointment
◆Polysporin Powder
◆Sudafed Children's Liquid
◆Sudafed Cough Syrup
◆Sudafed Plus Liquid
◆Sudafed Plus Tablets
◆Sudafed Severe Cold Formula Caplets
◆Sudafed Severe Cold Formula Tablets
◆Sudafed Sinus Caplets
◆Sudafed Sinus Tablets
◆Sudafed Tablets, 30 mg
◆Sudafed Tablets, Adult Strength, 60
mg
◆Sudafed 12 Hour Tablets
Wellcome Lanoline

CAMPBELL LABORATORIES INC.   544
Address Inquiries to:
Richard C. Zahn, President
P.O. Box 812, FDR Station
New York, NY 10150-0812
(212) 688-7684
OTC Products Available
Herpecin-L Cold Sore Lip Balm

**CARACO PHARMACEUTICAL   544
LABORATORIES, LTD.**
1150 Elijah McCoy Drive
Detroit, MI 48202

Address inquiries to:
C. Arnold Curry, M.D. (313) 871-8400
FAX (313) 871-8314
For Medical Emergencies Contact:
C. Arnold Curry, M.D. (313) 871-8400
OTC Products Available
Acetaminophen Tablets, 325 mg &
500 mg
Diphenhydramine Capsules, 25 mg
Docusate Calcium Softgels, 100 mg
Docusate Potassium Capsules, 100 mg
Docusate Sodium Softgels, 100 mg
Quinine Sulfate Capsules, 200 mg &
325 mg
Simethicone Tablets, 80 mg
Surelac Chewable Lactase Enzyme
Tablets

CARE-TECH LABORATORIES   544
3224 South Kingshighway Boulevard
St. Louis, MO 63139
Address inquiries to:
Sherry L. Brereton   (314) 772-4610
FAX (314) 772-4613
For Medical Emergencies Contact:
Customer Service   (800) 325-9681
Fax (314) 772-4613
OTC Products Available
Barri-Care Antimicrobial Barrier
Ointment
CC-500 Antibacterial Skin Cleanser
Care Creme
Clinical Care Dermal Wound Cleanser
Concept
Formula Magic Antibacterial Powder
Just Lotion - Highly Absorbent Aloe
Vera Based Skin Lotion
Loving Lather II Antibacterial Skin
Cleanser
Loving Lotion Antibacterial Skin & Body
Lotion
Orchid Fresh II Perineal/Ostomy
Cleanser
Satin Antimicrobial Skin Cleanser
Skin Magic - Antimicrobial Body Rub &
Emollient
Soft Skin Non-greasy Bath Oil with Rich
Emollients
Swirlsoft Whirlpool Emollient for Dry
Skin Conditions
Techni-Care Surgical Scrub
Velvet Fresh Non-irritating Cornstarch
Baby Powder

**CHATTEM INC., CONSUMER   545
PRODUCTS DIVISION**
Division of Chattem, Inc.
1715 West 38th Street
Chattanooga, TN 37409
Address Inquiries to:
David A. Robb, Jr.   (615) 821-4571
FAX (615) 821-5022
For Medical Emergencies Contact:
Walter Ludwig   (615) 821-4571
FAX (615) 821-5022
OTC Products Available
Black-Draught Granulated
Black-Draught Lax-Senna Tablets
Black-Draught Syrup
Blis-To-Sol Liquid
Blis-To-Sol Powder
Flex-all 454 Pain Relieving Gel
Icy Hot Balm
Icy Hot Cream
Icy Hot Stick
Norwich Maximum Strength Aspirin
Norwich Regular Strength Aspirin
Nullo Deodorant Tablets
Extra Strength Pamprin Multi-Symptom
Formula Tablets and Caplets
Maximum Strength Pamprin Cramp
Relief Formula Caplets
Pamprin-IB
Prēmsyn PMS Caplets
Soltice Quick-Rub

CHESEBROUGH-POND'S INC.   548
33 Benedict Place
Greenwich, CT 06830

Address inquiries to:
Consumer Affairs   (800) 243-5804
For Medical Emergencies Contact:
(800) 243-5804
OTC Products Available
Vaseline Intensive Care Moisturizing
Sunblock Lotion
Vaseline Intensive Care U.V. Daily
Defense Lotion for Hand and Body
Extra Strength Vaseline Intensive Care
Lotion
Vaseline Pure Petroleum Jelly Skin
Protectant/Lip Therapy

CHURCH & DWIGHT CO., INC.   548
469 North Harrison Street
Princeton, NJ 08540
Address inquiries to:
Mr. Stephen Lajoie   (609) 683-5900
For Medical Emergencies Contact:
Mr. Stephen Lajoie   (609) 683-5900
OTC Products Available
Arm & Hammer Pure Baking Soda

**CIBA CONSUMER   407, 549
PHARMACEUTICALS**
Division of CIBA-GEIGY Corporation
Mack Woodbridge II
Woodbridge, NJ 07095
Address inquiries to:
(908) 602-6600
For Medical Emergencies Contact:
(908) 277-5000
OTC Products Available
◆Acutrim 16 Hour Steady Control
Appetite Suppressant
◆Acutrim Late Day Strength Appetite
Suppressant
◆Acutrim II Maximum Strength Appetite
Suppressant
◆Doan's - Extra-Strength Analgesic
◆Extra Strength Doan's P.M.
◆Doan's - Regular Strength Analgesic
◆Dulcolax Suppositories
◆Dulcolax Tablets
◆Eucalyptamint 100% All Natural
Ointment
Fiberall Chewable Tablets, Lemon
Creme Flavor
◆Fiberall Fiber Wafers - Fruit & Nut
◆Fiberall Fiber Wafers - Oatmeal Raisin
◆Fiberall Powder Natural Flavor
◆Fiberall Powder Orange Flavor
◆Nõstril Nasal Decongestant
◆Nõstrilla Long Acting Nasal
Decongestant
◆Nupercainal Hemorrhoidal and
Anesthetic Ointment
◆Nupercainal Pain Relief Cream
◆Nupercainal Suppositories
◆Otrivin Nasal Drops
◆Otrivin Pediatric Nasal Drops
◆Privine Nasal Solution and Drops
◆Privine Nasal Spray
◆Q-vel Muscle Relaxant Pain Reliever
◆Slow Fe Tablets
◆Sunkist Children's Chewable
Multivitamins - Complete
◆Sunkist Children's Chewable
Multivitamins - Plus Extra C
◆Sunkist Children's Chewable
Multivitamins - Plus Iron
◆Sunkist Children's Chewable
Multivitamins - Regular
◆Sunkist Vitamin C - Chewable
◆Sunkist Vitamin C - Easy to Swallow

**COLUMBIA LABORATORIES,   408, 556
INC.**
4000 Hollywood Boulevard
Hollywood, FL 33021
Address inquiries to:
Professional Services Department
For Medical Emergencies Contact
(305) 964-6666
OTC Products Available
◆Diasorb Liquid
◆Diasorb Tablets
◆Legatrin Rub
◆Legatrin Tablets
Vaporizer in a Bottle Nasal
Decongestant

(◆ Shown in Product Identification Section)

**COPLEY PHARMACEUTICAL   408, 556
INC.**
25 John Road
Canton, MA 02021
Address inquiries to:
Copley Pharmaceutical Inc.
(617) 821-6111
For Medical Emergencies Contact:
Dr. Antoon   (617) 821-6111
OTC Products Available
Alum-Boro Effervescent Tablets and
Powder Packets
Bromatapp Extended Release Tablets
Brompheril Extended Release Tablets
Diphenhydramine Hydrochloride Spray
2%
Doxylamine Succinate 25 mg Tabs
Hydrocortisone 0.5% Aerosol and
1.0% Aerosol
◆Lice•Enz Foam
Miconazole Cream 2% and Spray
Powder
Saliv-Aid Oral Lubricant
Simethicone Drops
Tolnaftate 1% Liquid Aerosol
Tolnaftate 1% Powder Aerosol

DEL PHARMACEUTICALS   408, 557
A Subsidiary of Del Laboratories, Inc.
163 East Bethpage Road
Plainview, NY 11805
Addess inquiries to:
Peter Liman, V.P. Marketing
(516) 293-7070
FAX (516) 293-9018
For Medical Emergencies Contact:
Harry Gordon, Ph.D.
(516) 293-7070, Ext. 2068
OTC Products Available
Arthricare Pain Relieving Rubs
Auro-Dri Ear Drops
Boil-Ease Antiseptic Drawing Salve
Dermarest Gel
Diaper Guard Skin Rash Ointment
◆Baby Orajel
Baby Orajel Nighttime Formula
Baby Orajel Tooth & Gum Cleanser
Denture Orajel
◆Maximum Strength Orajel
◆Orajel Mouth-Aid
◆Pronto Lice Killing Shampoo Kit
◆Pronto Lice Killing Spray
Propa pH Astringent Cleansers
Propa pH Skin Cleanser
Stye Ophthalmic Ointment
Tanac Mouth and Lip Sore Medicines

**FISONS CONSUMER   408, 558
HEALTH**
Fisons Corporation
P.O. Box 1212
Rochester, NY 14603
Address inquiries to:
Product Service Department
P.O. Box 1212
Rochester, NY 14603
(716) 475-9000
FAX (716) 274-5304
For Medical Emergencies Contact
Fisons Corporation
(716) 475-9000
OTC Products Available
Allerest Children's Chewable Tablets
Allerest Eye Drops
Allerest Headache Strength Tablets
Allerest 12 Hour Caplets
Allerest 12 Hour Nasal Spray
◆Allerest Maximum Strength Tablets
◆Allerest No Drowsiness Tablets
Allerest Sinus Pain Formula
◆Americaine Hemorrhoidal Ointment
◆Americaine Topical Anesthetic First Aid
Ointment
◆Americaine Topical Anesthetic Spray
Bacid Capsules
◆Caldecort Anti-Itch Hydrocortisone
Cream
◆Caldecort Anti-Itch Hydrocortisone
Spray
◆Caldecort Light Cream
◆Caldesene Medicated Ointment
◆Caldesene Medicated Powder
Cholan HMB
◆Cruex Antifungal Cream

◆Cruex Antifungal Powder
◆Cruex Antifungal Spray Powder
Desenex Antifungal Cream
Desenex Antifungal Foam
◆Desenex Antifungal Ointment
◆Desenex Antifungal Powder
◆Desenex Antifungal Spray Liquid
◆Desenex Antifungal Spray Powder
◆Desenex Foot & Sneaker Powder &
Deodorant Spray Powder
Desenex Soap
Emul-O-Balm
Isoclor Liquid
Isoclor Tablets
◆Isoclor Timesule Capsules
Kondremul
Kondremul with Phenylphthalein
◆Myoflex Analgesic Creme
Neo-Cultol
Sinarest 12 Hour Nasal Spray
Sinarest No Drowsiness Tablets
Sinarest Tablets
Sinarest Extra Strength Tablets
◆Ting Antifungal Cream
◆Ting Antifungal Powder
◆Ting Antifungal Spray Liquid
◆Ting Antifungal Spray Powder
Vaponefrin
Vitron-C Tablets
Vitron-C Plus Tablets

**FISONS CORPORATION   562
PRESCRIPTION PRODUCTS**
755 Jefferson Road
Rochester, NY 14623
Address inquiries to:
Professional Services Department
(716) 475-9000
OTC Products Available
Delsym Cough Formula

FLEMING & COMPANY   563
1600 Fenpark Dr.
Fenton, MO 63026
Address inquiries to:
John J. Roth, M.D.   (314) 343-8200
For Medical Emergencies Contact:
John R. Roth, M.D.   (314) 343-8200
OTC Products Available
Chlor-3 Condiment
Impregon Concentrate
Magonate Tablets and Liquid
Marblen Suspension Peach/Apricot
Marblen Suspension Unflavored
Marblen Tablets
Nephrox Suspension
Nicotinex Elixir
Obegyn Powder
Ocean Nasal Mist
Purge Concentrate

GEBAUER COMPANY   564
9410 St. Catherine Avenue
Cleveland, OH 44104
Address inquiries to:
(800) 321-9348
FAX (216) 271-5335
For Medical Emergencies Contact:
(800) 321-9348
FAX (216) 271-5335
OTC Products Available
Dr. Caldwell Senna Laxative
Salivart Saliva Substitute

GLENBROOK LABORATORIES
See STERLING HEALTH, page 724.

HERALD PHARMACAL, INC.   564
6503 Warwick Road
Richmond, VA 23225
Address inquiries to:
Henry H. Kamps
(804) 745-3400
For Medical Emergencies Contact:
Henry H. Kamps
(804) 745-3400
OTC Products Available
Aqua Glycolic Lotion
Aqua Glycolic Shampoo
Aqua Glyde Cleanser
Aquaray 20 Sunscreen
Cam Lotion

**ICN PHARMACEUTICALS,   409, 564
INC.**
ICN Plaza
3300 Hyland Avenue
Costa Mesa, CA 92626
Address inquiries to:
Professional Service Department
(800) 556-1937
In CA (800) 331-2331
(714) 545-0100
For Medical Emergencies Contact:
Medical Department
(800) 548-5100
OTC Products Available
◆Insta-Glucose

INTER-CAL CORPORATION   564
421 Miller Valley Road
Prescott, AZ 86301
Address inquiries to:
Gerald W. Elders   (602) 445-8063
OTC Products Available
Ester-C Tablets

**JOHNSON & JOHNSON •   409, 565
MERCK CONSUMER
PHARMACEUTICALS CO.**
Camp Hill Road
Fort Washington, PA 19034
Address inquiries to:
Consumer Affairs Department
(215) 233-7000
For Medical Emergencies Contact:
(215) 233-7000
OTC Products Available
◆ALternaGEL Liquid
◆Dialose Tablets
◆Dialose Plus Tablets
◆Effer-Syllium Natural Fiber Bulking
Agent
Ferancee Chewable Tablets
◆Ferancee-HP Tablets
◆Mylanta Gas Tablets-40 mg
◆Mylanta Gas Tablets-80 mg
◆Mylanta Liquid
◆Mylanta Tablets
◆Mylanta Double Strength Liquid
◆Mylanta Double Strength Tablets
◆Maximum Strength Mylanta Gas
Tablets-125 mg
◆Mylicon Drops
◆The Stuart Formula Tablets
◆Stuartinic Tablets

KRAMER LABORATORIES   410, 570
8778 S.W. 8th Street
Miami, FL 33174
Address inquiries to:
Gloria Rodriguez   (800) 824-4894
FAX (305) 223-5510
OTC Products Available
Charcoal Plus Tablets
Fungi-Nail Tincture
◆Halfprin Low Strength Aspirin Tablets

LACTAID INC.   414, 571
Pleasantville, NJ 08232
Address inquiries to:
Alan E Kligerman   (609) 645-5100
OTC Products Available
◆Lactaid Caplets (Now marketed by
McNeil Consumer Products Co.)
◆Lactaid Drops (Now marketed by
McNeil Consumer Products Co.)

LAVOPTIK COMPANY, INC.   571, 781
661 Western Avenue North
St. Paul, MN 55103
Address inquiries to:
661 Western Avenue North
St. Paul, MN 55103   (612) 489-1351
For Medical Emergencies Contact:
B. C. Brainard   (612) 489-1351
OTC Products Available
Lavoptik Eye Cup
Lavoptik Eye Wash

LEDERLE LABORATORIES   410, 571
Division of American Cyanamid Co.
One Cyanamid Plaza
Wayne, NJ 07470

(◆ Shown in Product Identification Section)

*Address inquiries on
medical matters to:*
Professional Services Dept.
Lederle Laboratories
Pearl River, NY 10965
8 AM to 4:30 PM EST
(914) 735-2815
All other inquiries and
after hours emergencies
(914) 732-5000
Distribution Centers
ATLANTA
Contact EASTERN (Philadelphia)
Distribution Center
CHICAGO
Bulk Address
1100 East Business Center Drive
Mt. Prospect, IL 60056
Mail Address
P.O. Box 7614
Mt. Prospect, IL 60056-7614
(800) 533-3753
(708) 827-8871
DALLAS
Bulk Address
7611 Carpenter Freeway
Dallas, TX 75247
Mail Address
P.O. Box 655731
Dallas, TX 75265 (800) 533-3753
(214) 631-2130
LOS ANGELES
Bulk Address
2300 S. Eastern Avenue
Los Angeles, CA 90040
Mail Address
T.A. Box 2202
Los Angeles, CA 90051
(800) 533-3753
(213) 726-1016
EASTERN (Philadelphia)
Bulk Address
202 Precision Drive
Horsham, PA 19044
Mail Address
P.O. Box 993
Horsham, PA 19044 (800) 533-3753
(215) 672-5400
OTC Products Available
Acetaminophen Capsules, Tablets
Aureomycin Ointment 3%
◆Caltrate 600
◆Caltrate 600 + Iron & Vitamin D
◆Caltrate 600 + Vitamin D
◆Centrum
◆Centrum, Jr. (Children's Chewable) +
Extra C
◆Centrum, Jr. (Children's Chewable) +
Extra Calcium
◆Centrum, Jr. (Children's Chewable) +
Iron
◆Centrum Liquid
◆Centrum Silver
◆Ferro-Sequels
◆FiberCon
Filibon Prenatal Vitamin Tablets
Gevrabon Liquid
Gevral Protein Powder
Gevral T Tablets
Gevral Tablets
Incremin w/Iron Syrup
Lederplex Capsules and Liquid
Neoloid Emulsified Castor Oil
Stresscaps Capsules
◆Stresstabs
◆Stresstabs + Iron, Advanced Formula
◆Stresstabs + Zinc
◆Zincon Dandruff Shampoo

LEVER BROTHERS 578
390 Park Avenue
New York, NY 10022
Address inquiries to:
(212) 688-6000
OTC Products Available
Dove Bar
Liquid Dove Beauty Wash
Lever 2000

LUYTIES PHARMACAL COMPANY 578
P. O. Box 8080
St. Louis, MO 63156

Address Inquiries to:
Customer Service (800) 325-8080
OTC Products Available
Yellolax

MACSIL, INC. 579
1326 Frankford Avenue
Philadelphia, PA 19125
(215) 739-7300
OTC Products Available
Balmex Baby Powder
Balmex Emollient Lotion
Balmex Ointment

MARION MERRELL DOW 411, 579
INC.
Consumer Products Division
10123 Alliance Road
Mail: P.O. Box 429553
Cincinnati, OH 45242-9553
Address inquiries to:
Professional Information Department
Business hours only
(8:15 AM to 5:00 PM EST)
(800) 453-4865
*For Medical Emergency
Information Only after
hours or on weekends*
(513) 948-9111
OTC Products Available
◆Cēpacol Anesthetic Lozenges (Troches)
◆Cēpacol/Cēpacol Mint
Mouthwash/Gargle
◆Cēpacol Dry Throat Lozenges, Cherry
Flavor
◆Cēpacol Dry Throat Lozenges,
Honey-Lemon Flavor
◆Cēpacol Dry Throat Lozenges,
Menthol-Eucalyptus Flavor
◆Cēpacol Dry Throat Lozenges, Original
Flavor
◆CĒPASTAT Cherry Flavor Sore Throat
Lozenges
◆CĒPASTAT Extra Strength Sore Throat
Lozenges
◆CITRUCEL Orange Flavor
◆CITRUCEL Sugar Free Orange Flavor
◆Debrox Drops
◆Gaviscon Antacid Tablets
◆Gaviscon-2 Antacid Tablets
◆Gaviscon Extra Strength Relief Formula
Liquid Antacid
◆Gaviscon Extra Strength Relief Formula
Antacid Tablets
◆Gaviscon Liquid Antacid
◆Gly-Oxide Liquid
◆Novahistine DMX
◆Novahistine Elixir
◆Os-Cal 500 Chewable Tablets
◆Os-Cal 500 Tablets
◆Os-Cal 250+D Tablets
◆Os-Cal 500+D Tablets
◆Os-Cal Fortified Tablets
◆Os-Cal Plus Tablets
Simron Capsules
Simron Plus Capsules
Singlet Tablets
◆Throat Discs Throat Lozenges

MARLYN HEALTH CARE 586
14810 North 73rd Street
Scottsdale, AZ 85260
(800) 462-7596
OTC Products Available
4-Hair
4-Nails
Hep-Forte Capsules
Marlyn Formula 50
Marlyn Formula 50 Mega Forte
Marlyn PMS
Osteo Fem
Pro-Skin-E (Face Capsule)
Pro-Skin Nutribloxx

McNEIL CONSUMER 412, 587
PRODUCTS CO.
Division of McNeil-PPC, Inc.
Camp Hill Road
Fort Washington, PA 19034
(215) 233-7000
Address inquiries to:
Consumer Affairs Department
Fort Washington, PA 19034

Manufacturing Divisions
Fort Washington, PA 19034
Southwest Manufacturing Plant
4001 N. I-35
Round Rock, TX 78664
OTC Products Available
◆Imodium A-D Caplets and Liquid
◆Medipren ibuprofen Caplets and
Tablets
◆PediaCare Allergy Formula Liquid
◆PediaCare Cough-Cold Formula Liquid
and Chewable Tablets
◆PediaCare Decongestant Drops
◆PediaCare Night Rest Cough-Cold
Formula Liquid
◆PediaCare 6-12 Cough-Cold Formula
Chewable Tablets
◆Sine-Aid Maximum Strength Sinus
Headache Gelcaps, Caplets and
Tablets
◆Tylenol acetaminophen Children's
Chewable Tablets & Elixir
◆Tylenol Allergy Sinus Medication
Maximum Strength Gelcaps and
Caplets
◆Children's Tylenol Cold Multi Symptom
Liquid Formula and Chewable Tablets
◆Tylenol Cold & Flu Hot Medication,
Packets
◆Tylenol Cold & Flu No Drowsiness Hot
Medication, Packets
◆Tylenol Cold Multi Symptom Medication
Caplets and Tablets
◆Tylenol Cold Medication, Effervescent
Tablets
◆Tylenol Cold Medication No Drowsiness
Formula Caplets
◆Tylenol Cold Night Time Medication
Liquid
◆Tylenol Cough Medication Maximum
Strength Liquid
◆Tylenol Cough Medication Maximum
Strength Liquid with Decongestant
Tylenol, Extra Strength, acetaminophen
Adult Liquid Pain Reliever
◆Tylenol, Extra Strength, acetaminophen
Gelcaps, Caplets, Tablets
◆Tylenol, Infants' Drops
◆Tylenol, Junior Strength,
acetaminophen Coated Caplets,
Grape and Fruit Chewable Tablets
◆Tylenol, Maximum Strength, Sinus
Medication Gelcaps, Caplets and
Tablets
◆Tylenol, Regular Strength,
acetaminophen Caplets and Tablets
◆Tylenol PM Extra Strength Pain
Reliever/Sleep Aid Caplets and
Tablets

MEAD JOHNSON 414, 603
NUTRITIONALS
A Bristol-Myers Squibb Company
2400 W. Lloyd Expressway
Evansville, IN 47721
(812) 429-5000
Address inquiries to:
Scientific Information Section
Medical Department
OTC Products Available
Casec
Ce-Vi-Sol
Criticare HN
Enfamil Human Milk Fortifier
Enfamil Infant Formula
Enfamil Infant Formula Nursette
Enfamil With Iron Infant Formula
Enfamil Premature Formula
Enfamil Premature Formula With Iron
Fer-In-Sol
HIST 1
HIST 2
HOM 1
HOM 2
Isocal
Isocal HCN
Isocal HN
LYS 1
LYS 2
Lipisorb
Lofenalac Iron Fortified Low
Phenylalanine Diet Powder
Lonalac

(◆ Shown in Product Identification Section)

Low Methionine Diet Powder (Product 3200K)
Low PHE-TYR Diet Powder (Product 3200AB)
MCT Oil
MSUD Diet Powder
MSUD 1
MSUD 2
Moducal Dietary Carbohydrate
Mono- and Disaccharide-Free Diet Powder (Product 3232A)
Nutramigen Hypoallergenic Protein Hydrolysate Formula
OS 1
OS 2
PKU 1
PKU 2
PKU 3
Phenyl-Free Phenylalanine-Free Diet Powder
◆Poly-Vi-Sol Vitamins, Chewable Tablets and Drops (without Iron)
◆Poly-Vi-Sol Vitamins, Circus Shapes Chewable (without Iron)
◆Poly-Vi-Sol Vitamins with Iron, Chewable Tablets and Circus Shapes Chewable
◆Poly-Vi-Sol Vitamins with Iron, Drops
Portagen
Pregestimil Iron Fortified Protein Hydrolysate Formula with Medium Chain Triglycerides
ProSobee Soy Isolate Formula
ProSobee Soy Isolate Formula Nursette
Protein-Free Diet Powder (Product 80056)
◆Ricelyte, Rice-Based Oral Electrolyte Maintenance Solution
Special Metabolic Diets
Special Metabolic Modules
Sustacal Liquid, Powder, Pudding
Sustacal Plus
Sustacal with Fiber
Sustacal 8.8
Sustagen
TYR 1
TYR 2
◆Tempra 1 Acetaminophen Infant Drops
◆Tempra 2 Acetaminophen Toddlers Syrup
◆Tempra 3 Chewable Tablets, Regular or Double-Strength
TraumaCal
Trind
Trind-DM
◆Tri-Vi-Sol Vitamin Drops
◆Tri-Vi-Sol Vitamin Drops with Iron
UCD 1
UCD 2
Ultracal

MEAD JOHNSON   **415, 606**
PHARMACEUTICALS
A Bristol-Myers Squibb Company
2400 W. Lloyd Expressway
Evansville, IN 47721-0001
    (812) 429-5000
Address Inquiries to:
Scientific Information Section
Medical Department
OTC Products Available
◆Colace
◆Peri-Colace

MENLEY & JAMES   **415, 607**
LABORATORIES, INC.
Commonwealth Corporate Center
100 Tournament Drive, Suite 310
Horsham, PA 19044-3697
Address inquiries to:
Consumer Affairs Department
    (800) 321-1834
OTC Products Available
◆A.R.M. Allergy Relief Medicine Caplets
◆Acnomel Cream
◆Aqua Care Cream
◆Aqua Care Lotion
AsthmaHaler Mist Epinephrine Bitartrate Bronchodilator
AsthmaNefrin Solution "A" Bronchodilator
◆Benzedrex Inhaler
◆Congestac Caplets

◆Femlron Multi Vitamins and Iron
◆Hold Cough Suppressant Lozenge
◆Liquiprin Infants' Drops
◆Ornex Caplets
◆Maximum Strength Ornex Caplets
S.T.37 Antiseptic Solution
◆Serutan Toasted Granules Thermotabs
Troph-Iron Liquid
Trophite Liquid

MILES INC.   **416, 612**
CONSUMER HEALTHCARE DIVISION
1127 Myrtle Street
Elkhart, IN 46514
Address inquiries to:
Director, Consumer Relations
    (800) 800-4793
OTC Products Available
◆Alka-Mints Chewable Antacid
◆Alka-Seltzer Effervescent Antacid
◆Alka-Seltzer Effervescent Antacid and Pain Reliever
◆Alka-Seltzer Extra Strength Effervescent Antacid and Pain Reliever
◆Alka-Seltzer (Flavored) Effervescent Antacid and Pain Reliever
◆Alka-Seltzer Plus Cold Medicine
◆Alka-Seltzer Plus Cold & Cough Medicine
◆Alka-Seltzer Plus Night-Time Cold Medicine
◆Alka Seltzer Plus Sinus Allergy Medicine
◆Bactine Antiseptic/Anesthetic First Aid Liquid
◆Bactine First Aid Antibiotic Plus Anesthetic Ointment
◆Bactine Hydrocortisone Anti-Itch Cream
◆Bugs Bunny Children's Chewable Vitamins (Sugar Free)
◆Bugs Bunny Complete Children's Chewable Vitamins + Minerals with Iron and Calcium (Sugar Free)
◆Bugs Bunny With Extra C Children's Chewable Vitamins (Sugar Free)
◆Bugs Bunny Plus Iron Children's Chewable Vitamins (Sugar Free)
◆Domeboro Astringent Solution Effervescent Tablets
◆Domeboro Astringent Solution Powder Packets
◆Flintstones Children's Chewable Vitamins
◆Flintstones Children's Chewable Vitamins With Extra C
◆Flintstones Children's Chewable Vitamins Plus Iron
◆Flintstones Complete With Calcium, Iron & Minerals Children's Chewable Vitamins
◆Miles Nervine Nighttime Sleep-Aid
◆Mycelex OTC Cream Antifungal
◆Mycelex OTC Solution Antifungal
◆One-A-Day Essential Vitamins
◆One-A-Day Maximum Formula Vitamins and Minerals
◆One-A-Day Plus Extra C Vitamins
◆One-A-Day Stressgard Formula Vitamins
◆One-A-Day Women's Formula Multivitamins with Calcium, Extra Iron, Zinc and Beta Carotene

MURO PHARMACEUTICAL, INC.   **621**
890 East Street
Tewksbury, MA 01876-9987
Address inquiries to:
Professional Service Dept.
    (800) 225-0974
    (508) 851-5981
OTC Products Available
Bromfed Syrup
Guaifed Syrup
Guaitab Tablets
Salinex Nasal Mist and Drops

NATURE'S BOUNTY, INC.   **417, 622**
90 Orville Drive
Bohemia, NY 11716

Address inquiries to:
Professional Service Department
    (516) 567-9500
    (800) 645-5412
    FAX (516) 563-1623
OTC Products Available
ABC to Z
Acidophilus
B-Complex +C (Long Acting) Tablets
B-6 50 mg., 100 mg., 200 mg.
B-12 1000 mcg. Tablets
B-12 and B-12 Sublingual Tablets
B-50 Tablets
B-100 Tablets-Ultra B Complex
Beta-Carotene Capsules
Bounty Bears (Children's Chewables)
C-500 mg., C-1000 mg., C-1500 mg. & Time Release Formulas
Calcium Magnesium-Chelated Tablets
E-Oil 25,000 I.U.
◆Ener-B Vitamin B_{12} Nasal Gel Dietary Supplement
EnerVite (High Performance Nutrition)
Ferrous Sulfate
Garlic Oil 15 gr. & 77 gr.
KLB6 Capsules
l-Lysine 500 mg. Tablets & 1000 mg. Tablets
Lecithin 1200 mg. Capsules
M-KYA (For Leg Cramps)
Niacin 50 mg., 100 mg., & 250 mg.
Oat Bran 850 mg.
Oystercal-500 & Oystercal 500 + D
Ultra Vita-Time Tablets
Vitamin A 10,000 I.U. & 25,000 I.U.
Vitamin E (Natural d-alpha tocopheryl)
Water Pill (Natural Diuretic)
Zinc 10 mg., 25 mg., 50 mg. Tablets

NEUTRIN DRUG, INC.   **417, 622**
1800 North Charles Street
Baltimore, MD 21201
Address inquiries to:
    (301) 332-8484
    (800) 343-5729
For Medical Emergencies Contact:
Dr. Ha Yong Jung
President   (301) 332-8484
    (800) 343-5729
OTC Products Available
◆Anticon
Crown Royal Jelly 100 mg, 500 mg, 1000 mg
Natura Calcium
◆Natural Best Vitamin E 1000 I.U. and 400 I.U.
Norrhoid
Seleton

NEUTROGENA   **417, 622**
DERMATOLOGICS
Division of Neutrogena Corporation
5760 West 96th Street
Los Angeles, CA 90045
Address inquiries to:
Mitchell S. Wortzman, Ph D
    (213) 642-1150
    FAX (213) 337-5557
For Medical Emergencies Contact:
Mitchell S. Wortzman, Ph D
9:00AM to 5PM-PCT (213) 216-5345
    FAX (213) 337-5557
    After Hours (213) 641-8659
OTC Products Available
Neutrogena Acne Mask
Neutrogena Cleansing Bar for Acne-prone Skin
Neutrogena Cleansing Bar for Dry Skin (FF)
Neutrogena Cleansing Bar for Oily Skin
Neutrogena Cleansing Bar Original Formula (FF)
◆Neutrogena Cleansing Wash
Neutrogena Conditioner
Neutrogena Conditioner for Permed or Color-treated Hair
Neutrogena Lip Moisturizer (SPF 15)
◆Neutrogena Moisture
◆Neutrogena Moisture SPF 15 Untinted
◆Neutrogena Moisture SPF 15 with Sheer Tint

(◆ **Shown in Product Identification Section**)

◆Neutrogena Norwegian Formula
 Emulsion
◆Neutrogena Norwegian Formula Hand
 Cream
 Neutrogena Rainbath
 Neutrogena Shampoo
 Neutrogena Shampoo for Permed or
 Color-treated Hair
◆Neutrogena Sunblock
 Neutrogena T/Derm Tar Emollient
 Neutrogena T/Gel Therapeutic
 Conditioner
◆Neutrogena T/Gel Therapeutic
 Shampoo
◆Neutrogena T/Sal Therapeutic
 Shampoo
 Neutrogena Vehicle/N
 Neutrogena Vehicle/N Mild

NICHÉ PHARMACEUTICALS, INC.   624
 300 Trophy Club Drive, #400
 Roanoke, TX 76262
 Address inquiries to:
 Steve F. Brandon   (817) 491-2770
        FAX (817) 491-3533
 For Medical Emergencies Contact:
 Gerald L. Beckloff, M.D.
        (817) 491-2770
        FAX (817) 491-3533
 OTC Products Available
 MagTab SR Caplets

OHM LABORATORIES, INC.   418, 624
 P.O. Box 279
 Franklin Park, NJ 08823
 Address inquiries to:
 Arun Heble   (908) 297-3030
 For Medical Emergencies Contact:
        (908) 297-3030
 OTC Products Available
 Bisacodyl Tablets 5 mg.
◆Cramp End Tablets
 Docusate Potassium Capsules
 Docusate Potassium with Casanthranol
 Capsules and Caplets
◆Ibuprohm Ibuprofen Caplets
◆Ibuprohm Ibuprofen Tablets
 Ohmni-Scon Chewable Tablets, Extra
 Strength
 Pseudoephedrine Hydrochloride Tablets
 30mg and 60mg
 Senna Tablets
 Tribuffered Aspirin
 Trisudrine Tablets

ORTHO   418, 625, 781
 PHARMACEUTICAL
 CORPORATION
 Advanced Care Products
 Route #202 South
 Raritan, NJ 08869   (908) 524-0400
 For Medical Emergencies Contact:
 Dr. Carole Sampson-Landers
        (908) 524-1305
 OTC Products Available
◆Advance Pregnancy Test
◆Conceptrol Contraceptive Gel • Single
 Use Contraceptive
◆Conceptrol Contraceptive Inserts
◆Delfen Contraceptive Foam
◆Fact Plus Pregnancy Test
◆Gynol II Extra Strength Contraceptive
 Jelly
◆Gynol II Original Formula Contraceptive
 Jelly
◆Micatin Antifungal Cream
◆Micatin Antifungal Deodorant Spray
 Powder
◆Micatin Antifungal Powder
◆Micatin Antifungal Spray Liquid
◆Micatin Antifungal Spray Powder
 Micatin Jock Itch Cream
 Micatin Jock Itch Spray Powder
◆Monistat 7 Vaginal Cream
◆Monistat 7 Vaginal Suppositories
◆Ortho-Gynol Contraceptive Jelly

P & S LABORATORIES   628
 210 West 131st Street
 Los Angeles, CA 90061

 See STANDARD HOMEOPATHIC
 COMPANY

PADDOCK LABORATORIES, INC.   628
 3101 Louisiana Ave. North
 Minneapolis, MN 55427
 Address inquiries to:
 Patrick Johnson   (612) 546-4676
 Mary Beth Erstad   (800) 328-5113
 For Medical Emergencies Contact:
 Bruce G. Paddock   (800) 328-5113
 OTC Products Available
 Actidose with Sorbitol
 Actidose-Aqua, Activated Charcoal
 Glutose
 Ipecac Syrup, USP

PARKE-DAVIS   418, 628, 781
 Consumer Health Products Group
 Division of Warner-Lambert Company
 201 Tabor Road
 Morris Plains, New Jersey 07950
 See also Warner-Lambert Company
        (201) 540-2000
 For product information call:
        1-(800) 223-0432
 For medical information call:
        (201) 540-3950
 Regional Sales Offices
 Atlanta, GA 30328
  1140 Hammond Drive
        (404) 396-4080
 Baltimore (Hunt Valley), MD 21031
  11350 McCormick Road
        (301) 666-7810
 Chicago (Schaumburg), IL 60195
  1111 Plaza Drive   (312) 884-6990
 Dallas (Grand Prairie), TX 75234
  12200 Ford Road   (214) 484-5566
 Detroit (Troy), MI 48084
  500 Stephenson Highway
        (313) 589-3292
 Los Angeles (Tustin), CA 92680
  17822 East 17th Street
        (714) 731-3441
 Memphis, TN 38119
  1355 Lynnfield Road
        (901) 767-1921
 New York (Paramus, NJ) 07652
  12 Route 17 North
        (201) 368-0733
 Pittsburgh, PA 15220
  1910 Cochran Road
        (412) 343-9855
 Seattle (Bellevue), WA 98004
  301 116th Avenue, SE
        (206) 451-1119
 OTC Products Available
 Agoral, Marshmallow Flavor
 Agoral, Raspberry Flavor
 Alcohol, Rubbing (Lavacol)
◆Anusol Hemorrhoidal Suppositories
◆Anusol Ointment
◆Benadryl Anti-Itch Cream, Regular
 Strength 1% and Maximum Strength
 2%
◆Benadryl Cold Tablets
◆Benadryl Cold Nighttime Formula
◆Benadryl Decongestant Elixir
◆Benadryl Decongestant Kapseals
◆Benadryl Decongestant Tablets
◆Benadryl Elixir
◆Benadryl Spray, Maximum Strength 2%
◆Benadryl Spray, Regular Strength 1%
◆Benadryl 25 Kapseals
◆Benadryl 25 Tablets
◆Benylin Cough Syrup
◆Benylin Decongestant
◆Benylin DM Pediatric Cough Formula
◆Benylin Expectorant
◆Caladryl Clear Lotion
◆Caladryl Cream, Lotion, Spray
◆e.p.t. Early Pregnancy Test
◆Gelusil Liquid & Tablets
 Geriplex-FS Kapseals
 Geriplex-FS Liquid
 Lavacol (Rubbing Alcohol)
◆Medi-Flu Caplet, Liquid
◆Medi-Flu Without Drowsiness Caplets
◆Myadec
 Natabec Kapseals
 Proxacol-Hydrogen Peroxide Solution

 Siblin Granules
◆Sinutab Sinus Medication, Maximum
 Strength Caplets
◆Sinutab Sinus Allergy Medication,
 Maximum Strength Tablets
◆Sinutab Sinus Medication, Maximum
 Strength Without Drowsiness Formula
 Tablets & Caplets
◆Sinutab Sinus Medication, Regular
 Strength Without Drowsiness Formula
 Thera-Combex H-P Kapseals
 Tucks Cream
◆Tucks Premoistened Pads
 Tucks Take-Alongs

THE PARTHENON COMPANY,   638
 INC.
 3311 West 2400 South
 Salt Lake City, UT 84119
 Address inquiries to:
        (801) 972-5184
        FAX (801) 972-4734
 For Medical Emergency Contact:
 Nick G. Mihalopoulos   (801) 972-5184
 OTC Products Available
 Devrom Chewable Tablets

PFIZER CONSUMER   420, 638
 HEALTH CARE DIVISION
 Division of Pfizer Inc.
 100 Jefferson Road
 Parsippany, NJ 07054
 Address inquiries to:
 Research and Development Dept.
        (201) 887-2100
 OTC Products Available
 Ben-Gay External Analgesic Products
 Ben-Gay Ultra Strength Pain Relieving
 Rub
 Bonine Tablets
◆Desitin Ointment
 Rheaban Maximum Strength Tablets
 Rid Lice Control Spray
 Rid Lice Killing Shampoo
 Unisom Nighttime Sleep Aid
 Unisom with Pain Relief Nighttime
 Sleep Aid/Analgesic
◆Visine A.C. Eye Drops
◆Visine EXTRA Eye Drops
◆Visine Eye Drops
◆Visine L.R. Eye Drops
 Wart-Off Wart Remover

PLOUGH, INC.
 See SCHERING-PLOUGH HEALTHCARE
 PRODUCTS

PROCTER & GAMBLE   642
 P.O. Box 5516
 Cincinnati, OH 45201
 Also see Richardson-Vicks Inc.
 Address inquiries to:
 Arnold P. Austin   (800) 358-8707
 For Medical Emergencies Contact:
 J.B. Lucas, M.D.   (513) 626-3350
 After hours, call Collect
        (513) 751-5525

 For full descriptions of all the
 Metamucil products, see 1992
 Physicians' Desk Reference.
 OTC Products Available
 Denquel Sensitive Teeth Toothpaste
 Head & Shoulders Antidandruff
 Shampoo
 Head & Shoulders Antidandruff
 Shampoo 2-in-1 plus Conditioner
 Head & Shoulders Dry Scalp Shampoo
 Head & Shoulders Dry Scalp Shampoo
 2-in-1 plus Conditioner
 Head & Shoulders Intensive Treatment
 Dandruff Shampoo
 Head & Shoulders Intensive Treatment
 Dandruff Shampoo 2-in-1 plus
 Conditioner
 Metamucil Effervescent Sugar Free,
 Lemon-Lime Flavor
 Metamucil Effervescent Sugar Free,
 Orange Flavor
 Metamucil Powder, Orange Flavor
 Metamucil Powder, Regular Flavor

(◆ Shown in Product Identification Section)

Metamucil Powder, Strawberry Flavor
Metamucil Powder, Sugar Free, Orange
  Flavor
◆Metamucil Powder, Sugar Free, Regular
  Flavor
Pepto-Bismol Liquid & Tablets
Maximum Strength Pepto-Bismol Liquid

REED & CARNRICK   **420, 645**
Division of Block Drug Company, Inc.
257 Cornelison Avenue
Jersey City, NJ 07302-9988
    Address Inquiries to:
Professional Service Dept.
                    (201) 434-3000
    For Medical Emergencies Contact:
Medical Director   (201) 434-3000
    OTC Products Available
Alphosyl Lotion
◆Phazyme Drops
Phazyme Tablets
◆Phazyme-125 Softgels Maximum
  Strength
◆Phazyme-95 Tablets
proctoFoam/non-steroid
◆R&C Lice Treatment Kit
◆R&C Shampoo
◆R&C Spray
Trichotine Liquid, Vaginal Douche
Trichotine Powder, Vaginal Douche

THE REESE CHEMICAL   **420, 647**
COMPANY
10617 Frank Avenue
Cleveland, OH 44106
    Address inquiries to:
George W. Reese, III
                    (216) 231-6441
    OTC Products Available
Bi-Zet Throat Lozenges
Cold Control+ Intense Cold Medicine
Colicon Drops
Dentapaine Gel
Dermatox Skin Lotion
Keep Alert Caplets
Licide Lice Control Kit
Licide Lice Control Shampoo
Licide Lice Control Spray
Podactin Anti-Fungal Cream
Recort Plus (Hydrocortisone 1%)
Redacon DX
Red Hearts Vitamin Tonic Tablets
◆Reese's Pinworm Medicine
Sleep-ettes-D Tablets
Theracof Cough & Cold Liquid
Tri-Biozene Ointment

REQUA, INC.   **647**
Box 4008
1 Seneca Place
Greenwich, CT 06830
    Address inquiries to:
Geoffrey Geils   (203) 869-2445
                       (800) 321-1085
    OTC Products Available
Charcoaid
Charcoal Tablets
Charcocaps

RHONE-POULENC RORER   **420, 648**
PHARMACEUTICALS INC.
Consumer Pharmaceutical Products
500 Arcola Road
Collegeville, PA 19426-0107
    For Medical Emergencies/
    Product Information Contact:
Drug Product Safety and Product
Information Call   (215) 454-8870
    For Regulatory
    Questions Contact:
Margaret Masters
Assoc. Director, Regulatory Control
                       (215) 628-6085
    OTC Products Available
◆Ascriptin A/D Caplets
◆Regular Strength Ascriptin Tablets
◆Maalox HRF Heartburn Relief Formula
◆Maalox Plus Suspension/Tablets
◆Extra Strength Maalox Plus Suspension
◆Perdiem Fiber Granules
◆Perdiem Granules

RICHARDSON-VICKS, INC.   **652**
One Far Mill Crossings
Shelton, CT 06484
    Address inquiries to:
Vicks Research Center:
                    (203) 925-7888
    For Medical Emergencies Contact:
                    (301) 328-2425
    OTC Products Available
Children's Chloraseptic Lozenges
Children's Chloraseptic Spray
Chloraseptic Liquid, Cherry, Menthol
  and Cool Mint
Chloraseptic Liquid - Nitrogen Propelled
  Spray
Chloraseptic Lozenges, Cherry, Cool
  Mint and Menthol
Oil of Olay Daily UV Protectant SPF 15
  Beauty Fluid-Regular & Fragrance
  Free (Olay Co. Inc.)
Oil of Olay Daily UV Protectant SPF 15
  Moisture Replenishing Cream-Regular
  & Fragrance Free (Olay Co. Inc.)
Oil of Olay Foaming Face Wash (Olay
  Co. Inc.)
Percogesic Analgesic Tablets
Vicks Children's Cough Syrup
Vicks Children's NyQuil Nighttime
  Cold/Cough Medicine
Vicks Children's NyQuil Nighttime Head
  Cold/Allergy Medicine
Vicks Cough Drops
Extra Strength Vicks Cough Drops
Vicks Daycare Daytime Cold Medicine
  Caplets
Vicks Daycare Daytime Cold Medicine
  Liquid
Vicks Formula 44 Cough Control Discs
Vicks Formula 44 Cough Medicine
Vicks Formula 44D Cough and
  Decongestant Medicine
Vicks Formula 44E Cough &
  Expectorant Medicine
Vicks Formula 44M Multi-Symptom
  Cough & Cold Medicine
Vicks Inhaler
Vicks NyQuil LiquiCaps Adult Nighttime
  Cold/Flu Medicine
Vicks NyQuil Nighttime Cold/Flu
  Medicine-Regular & Cherry Flavor
Vicks Pediatric Formula 44 Cough
  Medicine
Vicks Pediatric Formula 44d Cough &
  Decongestant Medicine
Vicks Pediatric Formula 44e Cough &
  Expectorant Medicine
Vicks Pediatric Formula 44m
  Multi-Symptom Cough & Cold
  Medicine
Vicks Sinex Decongestant Nasal Spray
Vicks Sinex Decongestant Nasal Ultra
  Fine Mist
Vicks Sinex Long-Acting Decongestant
  Nasal Spray
Vicks Sinex Long-Acting Decongestant
  Nasal Ultra Fine Mist
Vicks Vaporub
Vicks Vaposteam
Vicks Vatronol Nose Drops

ROBERTS   **421, 663**
PHARMACEUTICAL
CORPORATION
6 Industrial Way West
Eatonton, NJ 07724
    Address inquiries to:
Customer Service Department
                    (800) 828-2088
    For Medical Emergencies Contact:
Medical Services Department
                    (908) 389-1705
                    (800) 992-9306
    OTC Products Available
Alkets Tablets
Calcium Lactate Tablets
Cheracol Cough Syrup
◆Cheracol-D Cough Formula
Cheracol Nasal Spray Pump
◆Cheracol Plus Head Cold/Cough
  Formula
Cheracol Sore Throat Spray
Cheracol Throat Discs
Citrocarbonate Antacid

Clocort Cream with Aloe
Clocream Skin Protectant Cream
Clomycin Antibiotic Ointment
Diostate D Tablets
◆Haltran Tablets
Kasof Capsules
Lipomul Oral Liquid
Orexin Tablets
Orthoxicol Cough Syrup
◆P-A-C Analgesic Tablets
Probec-T Tablets
◆Pyrroxate Capsules
◆Sigtab Tablets
Super D Perles
Zymacap Capsules

A. H. ROBINS CONSUMER   **421, 666**
PRODUCTS DIVISION
Subsidiary of American Home Products
  Corporation
1405 Cummings Drive
Richmond, VA 23220
    Address inquiries to:
The Medical Department
                    (804) 257-2000
    For Medical Emergencies Contact:
Medical Department   (804) 257-2000
(day or night)
If no answer, call answering service
                    (804) 257-7788
    OTC Products Available
Allbee with C Caplets
Allbee C-800 Plus Iron Tablets
Allbee C-800 Tablets
◆Chap Stick Lip Balm
◆Chap Stick Petroleum Jelly Plus
◆Chap Stick Petroleum Jelly Plus with
  Sunblock 15
◆Chap Stick Sunblock 15 Lip Balm
Dimacol Caplets
Dimetane Decongestant Caplets
Dimetane Decongestant Elixir
Dimetane Elixir
Dimetane Extentabs 8 mg
Dimetane Extentabs 12 mg
Dimetane Tablets
◆Dimetapp Cold & Flu Caplets
◆Dimetapp Elixir
◆Dimetapp DM Elixir
◆Dimetapp Extentabs
◆Dimetapp Tablets
◆Donnagel Liquid and Chewable Tablets
◆Robitussin
Robitussin Cough Calmers
◆Robitussin Cough Drops
◆Robitussin Maximum Strength Cough
  Suppressant
◆Robitussin Night Relief
◆Robitussin Pediatric Cough & Cold
  Formula
◆Robitussin Pediatric Cough
  Suppressant
◆Robitussin-CF
◆Robitussin-DM
◆Robitussin-PE
Z-BEC Tablets

ROSS LABORATORIES   **422, 677**
Division of Abbott Laboratories USA
P.O. Box 1317
Columbus, OH 43216-1317
    Address Inquiries to:
Medical Director   (614) 227-3333
    OTC Products Available
◆Clear Eyes ACR Astringent/Lubricating
  Eye Redness Reliever
◆Clear Eyes Lubricating Eye Redness
  Reliever
◆Ear Drops by Murine—(See Murine Ear
  Wax Removal System/Murine Ear
  Drops)
◆Murine Ear Drops
◆Murine Ear Wax Removal System
◆Murine Eye Lubricant
◆Murine Plus Lubricating Eye Redness
  Reliever
Pedialyte Oral Electrolyte Maintenance
  Solution
Rehydralyte Oral Electrolyte
  Rehydration Solution
Ross Pediatric Nutritional Products
  Alimentum Protein Hydrolysate
  Formula With Iron

(◆ Shown in Product Identification Section)

Isomil Soy Protein Formula With Iron
Isomil SF Sucrose-Free Soy Protein
Formula With Iron
PediaSure Liquid Nutrition for
Children
RCF Ross Carbohydrate Free
Low-Iron Soy Protein Formula Base
Similac Low-Iron Infant Formula
Similac PM 60/40 Low-Iron Infant
Formula
Similac Special Care With Iron 24
Premature Infant Formula
Similac With Iron Infant Formula
◆Selsun Blue Dandruff Shampoo
◆Selsun Blue Dandruff Shampoo-Extra
Medicated
◆Selsun Blue Extra Conditioning
Dandruff Shampoo
◆Tronolane Anesthetic Cream for
Hemorrhoids
◆Tronolane Hemorrhoidal Suppositories

RUSS PHARMACEUTICALS, INC.
See WHITBY PHARMACEUTICALS, INC.

RYDELLE LABORATORIES   423, 680
Division of S.C. Johnson & Son, Inc.
1525 Howe Street
Racine, WI 53403
Address inquiries to:
Thomas Conrarby
Consumer Resource Center Director
(414) 631-4000
For Medical Emergencies Contact:
Marvin G. Parker, M.D., F.A.C.P.
(414) 631-2111
OTC Products Available
◆Aveeno Anti-Itch Concentrated Lotion
◆Aveeno Anti-Itch Cream
◆Aveeno Bath Oilated
◆Aveeno Bath Regular
◆Aveeno Cleansing Bar for Acne
◆Aveeno Cleansing Bar for Combination
Skin
◆Aveeno Cleansing Bar for Dry Skin
◆Aveeno Moisturizing Cream
◆Aveeno Moisturizing Lotion
◆Aveeno Shower and Bath Oil
◆Rhulicream
◆Rhuligel
◆Rhulispray

SANDOZ   423, 682
PHARMACEUTICALS/
CONSUMER DIVISION
59 Route 10
East Hanover NJ 07936
Address Medical Inquiries To:
Medical Department
Sandoz Pharmaceuticals Corporation
East Hanover, NJ 07936
(201) 503-7500
Other Inquiries To:
(201) 503-7500
FAX (201) 503-8265
OTC Products Available
Acid Mantle Creme
◆BiCozene Creme
Cama Arthritis Pain Reliever
◆Dorcol Children's Cough Syrup
◆Dorcol Children's Decongestant Liquid
◆Dorcol Children's Liquid Cold Formula
◆Ex-Lax Chocolated Laxative Tablets
◆Extra Gentle Ex-Lax Laxative Pills
◆Maximum Relief Formula Ex-Lax
Laxative Pills
◆Regular Strength Ex-Lax Laxative Pills
◆Gas-X Tablets
◆Extra Strength Gas-X Tablets
◆Gentle Nature Natural Vegetable
Laxative Tablets
◆TheraFlu Flu and Cold Medicine
◆TheraFlu Flu, Cold and Cough Medicine
Triaminic Allergy Tablets
Triaminic Chewables
◆Triaminic Cold Tablets
◆Triaminic Expectorant
◆Triaminic Nite Light
◆Triaminic Syrup
◆Triaminic-12 Tablets
◆Triaminic-DM Syrup
◆Triaminicin Tablets
◆Triaminicol Multi-Symptom Cold Tablets

◆Triaminicol Multi-Symptom Relief
Ursinus Inlay-Tabs

SANOFI WINTHROP   689
PHARMACEUTICALS
Main Office
90 Park Avenue
New York, NY 10016
(212) 907-2000
Address Medical Inquiries to:
Product Information Services
(800) 446-6267
All Other Information:
Customer Relations/Orders
(800) 223-5511
OTC Products Available
Anti-Rust Tablets
Breonsin Capsules
Bronkolixir
Bronkotabs Tablets
Drisdol
pHisoderm (See Sterling Health)
Pontocaine Cream
Pontocaine Ointment
Zephiran Chloride Aqueous Solution
Zephiran Chloride Concentrate Solution
Zephiran Chloride Spray
Zephiran Chloride Tinted Tincture
Zephiran Towelettes

SCHERING CORPORATION
See SCHERING-PLOUGH HEALTHCARE
PRODUCTS

SCHERING-PLOUGH   424, 692
HEALTHCARE PRODUCTS
110 Allen Road
Liberty Corner, NJ 07938
Address product requests to:
Public Relations   (908) 604-1969
For Medical Emergencies Contact:
Clinical Department
(901) 320-2998
OTC Products Available
◆A and D Ointment
◆Afrin Cherry Scented Nasal Spray
0.05%
◆Afrin Children's Strength Nose Drops
0.025%
◆Afrin Menthol Nasal Spray, 0.05%
◆Afrin Nasal Spray 0.05% and Nasal
Spray Pump
◆Afrin Nose Drops 0.05%
◆Afrin Saline Mist
◆Afrin Tablets
◆Aftate for Athlete's Foot
◆Aftate for Jock Itch
Aspergum
◆Chlor-Trimeton Allergy Syrup, Tablets &
Long-Acting Repetabs Tablets
◆Chlor-Trimeton Antihistamine and
Decongestant Tablets
◆Chlor-Trimeton Long Acting
Antihistamine and Decongestant
Repetabs Tablets
◆Chlor-Trimeton Maximum Strength
Timed Release Allergy Tablets
◆Chlor-Trimeton Sinus Caplets
◆Chooz Antacid Gum
◆Complex 15 Hand & Body Moisturizing
Cream
◆Complex 15 Hand & Body Moisturizing
Lotion
◆Complex 15 Moisturizing Face Cream
◆Coricidin 'D' Decongestant Tablets
◆Coricidin Demilets Tablets for Children
◆Coricidin Tablets
◆Correctol Laxative Tablets
Cushion Grip Denture Adhesive
◆Di-Gel Antacid/Anti-Gas
Drixoral Antihistamine/Nasal
Decongestant Syrup
◆Drixoral Non-Drowsy Formula
◆Drixoral Plus Extended-Release Tablets
◆Drixoral Sinus
◆Drixoral Sustained-Action Tablets
◆DuoFilm Liquid
◆DuoPlant Gel
◆Duration 12 Hour Nasal Spray
◆Duration 12 Hour Nasal Spray Pump
◆Feen-A-Mint Gum
◆Feen-A-Mint Laxative Pills
◆Gyne-Lotrimin Vaginal Cream Antifungal

◆Gyne-Lotrimin Vaginal Inserts
◆Gyne-Moistrin Vaginal Gel
◆Lotrimin AF Antifungal Cream, Lotion
and Solution
Muskol Insect Repellent Aerosol Liquid
Muskol Insect Repellent Lotion
Muskol Insect Repellent Pump Spray
Muskol Insect Repellent Roll-on
◆OcuClear Eye Drops (See PDR For
Ophthalmology)
St. Joseph Adult Chewable Aspirin (81
mg.)
St. Joseph Aspirin-Free Fever Reducer
for Children Chewable Tablets
St. Joseph Cold Tablets for Children
St. Joseph Cough Suppressant for
Children
◆Tinactin Aerosol Liquid 1%
◆Tinactin Aerosol Powder 1%
◆Tinactin Antifungal Cream, Solution &
Powder 1%
Tinactin Deodorant Powder Aerosol 1%
◆Tinactin Jock Itch Cream 1%
◆Tinactin Jock Itch Spray Powder 1%

SMITHKLINE BEECHAM   426, 704
CONSUMER BRANDS
Unit of SmithKline Beecham, Inc.
P.O. Box 1467
Pittsburgh, PA 15230
Address inquiries to:
Professional Services Department
(800) BEECHAM
(412) 928-1050
OTC Products Available
◆A-200 Pediculicide Shampoo & Gel
◆Clear by Design Medicated Acne Gel
◆Contac Continuous Action
Decongestant/Antihistamine Capsules
◆Contac Cough and Chest Cold
◆Contac Cough & Sore Throat Formula
◆Contac Jr. Non-Drowsy Cold Liquid
◆Contac Maximum Strength Continuous
Action Decongestant/Antihistamine
Caplets
◆Contac Severe Cold and Flu Formula
Caplets
◆Contac Severe Cold & Flu Nighttime
◆Contac Sinus Caplets Maximum
Strength Non-Drowsy Formula
◆Contac Sinus Tablets Maximum
Strength Non-Drowsy Formula
◆Ecotrin Enteric Coated Aspirin
Maximum Strength Tablets and
Caplets
◆Ecotrin Enteric Coated Aspirin Regular
Strength Tablets and Caplets
◆Feosol Capsules
◆Feosol Elixir
◆Feosol Tablets
Geritol Complete Tablets
Geritol Extend Caplets
Geritol Liquid - High Potency Iron &
Vitamin Tonic
Massengill Baby Powder Soft Cloth
Towelette and Fragrance Free Soft
Cloth Towelette
◆Massengill Disposable Douches
Massengill Liquid Concentrate
◆Massengill Medicated Disposable
Douche
Massengill Medicated Liquid
Concentrate
Massengill Medicated Soft Cloth
Towelette
Massengill Powder
◆Nature's Remedy Enema, Mineral Oil
◆Nature's Remedy Enema, Regular
◆Nature's Remedy Natural Vegetable
Laxative Tablets
◆N'ICE Medicated Sugarless Sore Throat
and Cough Lozenges
◆N'ICE Sugarless Vitamin C Drops
◆Oxy Lathering Facial Scrub
◆Oxy Medicated Cleanser
◆Oxy Medicated Pads - Regular,
Sensitive Skin, and Maximum
Strength
◆Oxy Medicated Soap

(◆ Shown in Product Identification Section)

◆Oxy Night Watch Nighttime Acne Medication-Maximum Strength and Sensitive Skin Formulas
◆Oxy 10 Daily Face Wash Antibacterial Skin Wash
◆Oxy-5 and Oxy-10 Tinted and Vanishing Formulas with Sorboxyl
◆Sine-Off Maximum Strength Allergy/Sinus Formula Caplets
◆Sine-Off Maximum Strength No Drowsiness Formula Caplets
◆Sine-Off Sinus Medicine Tablets-Aspirin Formula
◆Sominex Caplets and Tablets
Sominex Liquid
◆Sominex Pain Relief Formula
◆Sucrets Original Mint
◆Sucrets Children's Cherry Flavored Sore Throat Lozenges
◆Sucrets Cold Formula
◆Sucrets Maximum Strength Wintergreen and Sucrets Wild Cherry (Regular Strength) Sore Throat Lozenges
◆Sucrets Maximum Strength Sprays
◆Teldrin Timed-Release Allergy Capsules, 12 mg.
◆Tums Antacid Tablets
◆Tums E-X Antacid Tablets
◆Tums Plus Antacid Anti-gas Tablets, Assorted Fruit or Peppermint
Vivarin Stimulant Tablets

SMITHKLINE CONSUMER PRODUCTS
See SMITHKLINE BEECHAM CONSUMER BRANDS.

E. R. SQUIBB & SONS, INC.   **722**
A Bristol-Myers Squibb Company
P.O. Box 4000
Princeton, NJ 08543-4000

Theragran line is now being distributed by Apothecon, page 505

STANDARD HOMEOPATHIC   **722**
COMPANY
210 West 131st Street
Box 61067
Los Angeles, CA 90061
      OTC Products Available
Hyland's Bed Wetting Tablets
Hyland's Calms Forté Tablets
Hyland's Colic Tablets
Hyland's Cough Syrup with Honey
Hyland's C-Plus Cold Tablets
Hyland's Teething Tablets
Hyland's Vitamin C for Children

STELLAR PHARMACAL   **428, 723**
CORPORATION
1990 N.W. 44th Street
Pompano Beach, FL 33064-8712
      Address inquiries to:
Scott L. Davidson   (305) 972-6060
Customer Service & Order Department
           (800) 845-7827
      OTC Products Available
◆Star-Optic Eye Wash
◆Star-Otic Ear Solution

STERLING HEALTH   **428, 724**
Division of Sterling Winthrop Inc.
90 Park Avenue
New York, NY 10016
      Address inquiries to:
Medical Director   (212) 907-2764
For Medical Emergencies Contact:
John T. Watters, MD, Medical Director
           (212) 907-2210
      OTC Products Available
◆Children's Bayer Chewable Aspirin
◆Genuine Bayer Aspirin Tablets & Caplets
◆Maximum Bayer Aspirin Tablets & Caplets
◆Bayer Plus Aspirin Tablets
◆Extra Strength Bayer Plus Aspirin Caplets
◆Therapy Bayer Enteric Aspirin Caplets
◆8 Hour Bayer Timed-Release Aspirin
◆Bronkaid Mist
Bronkaid Mist Suspension
◆Bronkaid Tablets
◆Campho-Phenique Cold Sore Gel
◆Campho-Phenique Liquid

◆Campho-Phenique Triple Antibiotic Ointment Plus Pain Reliever
◆Dairy Ease Caplets and Tablets
◆Dairy Ease Drops
Dairy Ease Real Milk
Fergon Elixir
◆Fergon Iron Supplement Tablets
◆Haley's M-O, Regular & Flavored
◆Midol IB Cramp Relief Formula
◆Maximum Strength Midol Multi-Symptom Menstrual Formula
◆Maximum Strength Midol Premenstrual Pain Formula
◆Regular Strength Midol Multi-Symptom Menstrual Formula
◆Teen Formula Midol
NTZ Long Acting Nasal Spray & Drops 0.05%
◆NāSal Moisturizing Nasal Spray
◆NāSal Moisturizing Nose Drops
Neo-Synephrine Maximum Strength 12 Hour Nasal Spray
◆Neo-Synephrine Maximum Strength 12 Hour Nasal Spray Pump
Neo-Synephrine Nasal Solutions, Pediatric, Mild, Regular & Extra Strength
◆Neo-Synephrine Nasal Sprays, Pediatric, Mild, Regular & Extra Strength
◆Neo-Synephrine Nose Drops
◆pHisoDerm Cleansing Bar
◆pHisoDerm For Baby
◆pHisoDerm Skin Cleanser and Conditioner - Regular and Oily
◆pHisoPUFF
◆Children's Panadol Chewable Tablets, Liquid, Infants' Drops
◆Junior Strength Panadol
◆Maximum Strength Panadol Tablets and Caplets
◆Phillips' LaxCaps
◆Concentrated Phillips' Milk of Magnesia
◆Phillips' Milk of Magnesia Liquid
◆Phillips' Milk of Magnesia Tablets
◆Stri-Dex Dual Textured Maximum Strength Pads
Stri-Dex Dual Textured Maximum Strength Big Pads
◆Stri-Dex Dual Textured Regular Strength Pads
Stri-Dex Dual Textured Regular Strength Big Pads
Stri-Dex Dual Textured Sensitive Skin Pads
Stri-Dex Super Scrub Pads
◆Vanquish Analgesic Caplets
WinGel Liquid

STUART   **431, 740**
PHARMACEUTICALS
a business unit of ICI Americas Inc.
Wilmington, DE 19897 USA
      Address inquiries to:
Yvonne A. Graham, Manager
Professional Services
           (302) 886-2231
      For Medical Emergencies:
After hours & on weekends
           (302) 886-3000
      OTC Products Available
◆HIBICLENS Antimicrobial Skin Ckeanser
HIBISTAT Germicidal Hand Rinse
HIBISTAT Towelette
◆STUART PRENATAL Tablets

SUBLINGUAL PRODUCTS   **431, 742**
INTERNATIONAL, INC.
1229 West Corporate Drive
Arlington, TX 76006
      Address inquiries to:
Elisa Miller, R.N.   (800) 338-4788
          FAX (817) 633-8146
      OTC Products Available
◆Sublingual B-Total
Sublingual C with Niacin
Sublingual Zinc

SYNTEX LABORATORIES, INC.   **743**
3401 Hillview Avenue
P.O. Box 10850
Palo Alto, CA 94304

Direct General/Sales/Order inquiries for U.S. Marketed products to:
Marketing Information Department
Specify product   (415) 855-5050
Direct Medical inquiries on U.S. marketed products to:
Medical Services Department
General Medical Inquiries
           (415) 855-5545
Adverse Reactions Inquiries
           (415) 852-1386
      OTC Products Available
Carmol 20 Cream
Carmol 10 Lotion

THOMPSON MEDICAL   **431, 743**
COMPANY, INC.
222 Lakeview Avenue
West Palm Beach, FL 33401
      Address inquiries to:
Consumer Services   (800) 352-8466
      OTC Products Available
Appedrine, Maximum Strength Tablets
Aqua-Ban, Maximum Strength Plus Tablets
Aqua-Ban Tablets
Arthritis Hot
Aspercreme Creme, Lotion Analgesic Rub
Breathe Free
Control Capsules
◆Cortizone-5 Creme and Ointment
Cortizone-5 Wipes
Cortizone-10 Creme and Ointment
Dexatrim Capsules, Caplets, Tablets
Dexatrim Maximum Strength Caffeine-Free Caplets
Dexatrim Maximum Strength Caffeine-Free Capsules
Dexatrim Maximum Strength Extended Duration Time Tablets
◆Dexatrim Maximum Strength Plus Vitamin C/Caffeine-free Caplets
◆Dexatrim Maximum Strength Plus Vitamin C/Caffeine-free Capsules
Diar Aid Tablets
Encare Vaginal Contraceptive Suppositories
End Lice
Ibuprin
◆Lactogest Softgel Capsules
◆NP-27 Cream, Solution, Spray Powder & Powder Antifungal
Prolamine Maximum Strength Capsules
Sleepinal Medicated Night Tea
◆Sleepinal Night-time Sleep Aid Capsules
Sportscreme Analgesic Rub
Tempo Antacid with Antigas Action
Tribiotic Plus

TRITON CONSUMER PRODUCTS,   **747**
INC.
561 West Golf Road
Arlington Heights, IL 60005
      Address inquiries to:
Karen Shrader   (800) 942-2009
      For Medical Emergencies Contact
           (800) 942-2009
      OTC Products Available
MG 217 Psoriasis Ointment and Lotion
MG 217 Psoriasis Shampoo and Conditioner
ProTech First-Aid Stik
Retro G Medicated Cold Sore Gel
Skeeter Stik Insect Bite Medication
Skeeter Stop 100 Insect Repellent
Tick Away Insect Repellent

UAS LABORATORIES   **747**
9201 Penn Avenue South #10
Minneapolis, MN 55431
      Address inquiries to:
Dr. S. K. Dash   (612) 881-1915
          (800) 422-3371
      OTC Products Available
DDS-Acidophilus

THE UPJOHN COMPANY   **431, 747**
7000 Portage Road
Kalamazoo, MI 49001
      For Medical and Pharmaceutical Information, Including Emergencies:
           (616) 329-8244
           (616) 323-6615

(◆ **Shown in Product Identification Section**)

Pharmaceutical Sales Areas and Distribution Centers

Atlanta (Chamblee)
GA 30341-2626   (404) 451-4822
Boston (Wellesley)
MA 02181   (617) 431-7970
Buffalo (Amherst)
NY 14221   (716) 632-5942
Chicago (Oak Brook Terrace)
IL 60181   (708) 574-3300
Cincinnati, OH 45202
(513) 723-1010
Dallas (Irving)
TX 75062   (214) 256-0022
Denver, CO 80216   (303) 399-3113
Hartford (Enfield)
CT 06082   (203) 741-3421
Honolulu, HI 96818   (808) 422-2777
Kalamazoo, MI 49001
(616) 323-4000
Kansas City (Overland Park)
KS 66210   (913) 469-8863
Los Angeles, CA 90038
(213) 463-8101
Memphis, TN 38119 (901) 685-8192
Minneapolis (Bloomington).
MN 55437   (612) 921-8484
New York (Uniondale)
NY 11553   (516) 745-6100
Orlando, FL 32809   (407) 859-4591
Philadelphia (Berwyn)
PA 19312   (215) 993-0100
Pittsburgh (Bridgeville)
PA 15017   (412) 257-0200
Portland, OR 97232 (503) 232-2133
St. Louis, MO 63141 (314) 872-8626
San Francisco (Foster City)
CA 94404   (415) 377-0203
Shreveport, LA 71129
(318) 688-3700
Washington, DC 20011
(202) 726-1517

OTC Products Available

◆Cortaid Cream with Aloe
◆Cortaid Lotion
◆Cortaid Ointment with Aloe
◆Cortaid Spray
◆Maximum Strength Cortaid Cream
◆Maximum Strength Cortaid Ointment
◆Maximum Strength Cortaid Spray
Cortef Feminine Itch Cream
◆Doxidan Liqui-Gels
◆Dramamine Chewable Tablets
◆Dramamine Liquid
◆Dramamine Tablets
◆Kaopectate Concentrated Anti-Diarrheal, Peppermint Flavor
◆Kaopectate Concentrated Anti-Diarrheal, Regular Flavor
◆Kaopectate Children's Chewable Tablets
◆Kaopectate Children's Liquid
◆Kaopectate Maximum Strength Caplets
◆Motrin IB Caplets and Tablets
◆Mycitracin Plus Pain Reliever
◆Maximum Strength Mycitracin Triple Antibiotic First Aid Ointment
Phenolax Wafers
Progaine Shampoo
◆Surfak Liqui-Gels
◆Unicap Softgel Capsules & Tablets
Unicap Jr. Chewable Tablets
◆Unicap M Tablets
Unicap Plus Iron Vitamin Formula Tablets
◆Unicap Sr. Tablets
◆Unicap T Tablets

WAKUNAGA OF AMERICA   432, 752 CO., LTD.
Subsidiary of Wakunaga Pharmaceutical Co., Ltd.
23501 Madero
Mission Viejo, CA 92691
Address inquires to:
(714) 855-2776
OTC Products Available
◆Kyolic
Kyo-Dophilus, Capsules: Acidophilus, Bifidus, S. Faecium

Kyo-Green, Powder: Barley & Wheat Grass, Chlorella, Brown Rice, Kelp
Kyolic Formula 106 Capsules: Aged Garlic Extract Powder (300 mg) & Vitamin E
Kyolic Super Formula 104 Capsules: Aged Garlic Extract Powder (300 mg)
Kyolic Super Formula 105 Capsules: Aged Garlic Extract Powder (200 mg)
Kyolic Super Formula 100 Capsules & Tablets: Aged Garlic Extract Powder (300 mg)
Kyolic Super Formula 100 Tablets: Aged Garlic Extract Powder (270 mg)
◆ Kyolic-Aged Garlic Extract Flavor & Odor Modified Enriched with Vitamins B_1 and B_{12}
Kyolic-Aged Garlic Extract Flavor & Odor Modified Plain
Kyolic-Aged Garlic Extract Liquid Enriched with Vitamin B & Vitamin B_{12}
Kyolic-Aged Garlic Extract Liquid Plain
◆ Kyolic-Formula 101 Capsules: Aged Garlic Extract (270 mg)
Kyolic-Formula 103 Capsules: Aged Garlic Extract Powder (220 mg)
Kyolic-Formula 101 Tablets: Aged Garlic Extract Powder (270 mg)
Kyolic-Super Formula 104 Capsules: Aged Garlic Extract Powder (300 mg) with Lecithin
Kyolic-Super Formula 103, Capsules: Aged Garlic Extract Powder (220 mg) with Vitamin C, Astragalus, Calcium
Kyolic-Super Formula 105, Capsules: Aged Garlic Extract Powder (250 mg) with Selenium, Vitamins A & E
Kyolic-Super Formula 106, Capsules: Aged Garlic Extract Powder (300 mg) with Vitamin E, Cayenne Pepper, Hawthorn Berry
◆ Kyolic-Super Formula 101 Garlic Plus Tablets & Capsules: Aged Garlic Extract Powder (270 mg) with Brewer's Yeast, Kelp & Algin
Kyolic-Super Formula 102, Tablets & Capsules: Aged Garlic Extract Powder (350 mg) with Enzyme Complex

WALKER, CORP & CO., INC.   432, 753
203 E. Hampton Place
Syracuse, NY 13206
Address inquiries to:
P.O. Box 1320
Syracuse, NY 13201 (315) 463-4511
For Medical Emergencies Contact:
George J. Eschenfelder
(315) 492-0947
OTC Products Available
◆Evac-U-Gen Mild Laxative

WALKER PHARMACAL COMPANY   753
4200 Laclede
St. Louis, MO 63108
Address Inquiries to:
Customer Service   (314) 533-9600
OTC Products Available
HIKE Antiseptic Ointment
PRID Salve

WALLACE LABORATORIES   432, 753
Half Acre Road
Cranbury, NJ 08512
Address inquiries to:
Wallace Laboratories
Div. of Carter-Wallace, Inc.
P.O. Box 1001
Cranbury, NJ 08512 (609) 655-6000
For Medical Emergencies:
(609) 799-1167
OTC Products Available
◆Maltsupex Liquid, Powder & Tablets
◆Ryna Liquid
◆Ryna-C Liquid

◆Ryna-CX Liquid
◆Syllact Powder

WARNER-LAMBERT   432, 755 COMPANY
Consumer Health Products Group
201 Tabor Road
Morris Plains, NJ 07950
See also Parke-Davis
Address Inquiries to:
Robert Kirpitch   (201) 540-3204
For Medical Emergencies Call:
(201) 540-2000
OTC Products Available
Bromo-Seltzer
Corn Husker's Lotion
Efferdent Extra Strength Denture Cleanser
◆Professional Strength Efferdent
◆Halls Mentho-Lyptus Cough Suppressant Tablets
◆Halls Plus Cough Suppressant Tablets
◆Halls Vitamin C Drops
Listerex Lotion
◆Listerine Antiseptic
◆Listermint with Fluoride
◆Lubriderm Bath Oil
◆Lubriderm Body Bar
◆Lubriderm Lotion
◆Replens
◆Rolaids
◆Rolaids (Calcium Rich/Sodium Free)
◆Extra Strength Rolaids
◆Soothers Throat Drops
Super Anahist Tablets

WATER-JEL TECHNOLOGIES, INC.   758
243 Veterans Boulevard
Carlstadt, NJ 07072
Address inquiries to:
Bob Daniels   (201) 507-8300
FAX (201) 507-8325
For Medical Emergencies Contact:
Bob Daniels   (201) 507-8300
FAX (201) 507-8325
OTC Products Available
Water-Jel Burn Wrap
Water-Jel Face Mask for Facial Burns
Water-Jel Fire Blanket Plus
Water-Jel Heat Shield
Water-Jel Sterile Burn Dressings

WESTWOOD-SQUIBB   433, 758 PHARMACEUTICALS INC.
100 Forest Avenue
Buffalo, NY 14213
(716) 887-3400
Address inquiries to:
Consumer Affairs Department
(716) 887-3773
OTC Products Available
Balnetar
Estar Gel
Fostril Lotion
Lowila Cake
◆Moisturel Cream
◆Moisturel Lotion
◆Moisturel Sensitive Skin Cleanser
Pernox Lotion
Pernox Medicated Scrub
Pernox Shampoo
Sebucare Lotion
◆Sebulex Antiseborrheic Treatment Shampoo
Sebulex Shampoo with Conditioners
Sebulon Dandruff Shampoo
◆Sebutone and Sebutone Cream Antiseborrheic Tar Shampoos

WHITBY   433, 759 PHARMACEUTICALS, INC.
1211 Sherwood Avenue
P.O. Box 85054
Richmond, VA 23261-5054
(804) 254-4400
Address inquiries to:
Susan Leake   (800) 477-7877
OTC Products Available
Amesec
◆Corticaine External Analgesic
◆Vicon Plus
◆Vicon-C Capsules
◆Vi-Zac

(◆ Shown in Product Identification Section)

WHITEHALL   **434, 761, 783**
LABORATORIES INC.
Division of American Home Products
  Corporation
685 Third Avenue
New York, NY 10017
  Address inquiries to:
Consumer Affairs
Professional Samples
                            (800) 343-0856
Other information
                            (800) 322-3129
  OTC Products Available
◆Advil Cold and Sinus (formerly CoAdvil)
◆Advil Ibuprofen Caplets and Tablets
◆Anacin Coated Analgesic Caplets
◆Anacin Coated Analgesic Tablets
  Anacin Maximum Strength Analgesic
    Coated Tablets
◆Aspirin Free Anacin Acetaminophen
    Film Coated Caplets
◆Aspirin Free Anacin Acetaminophen
    Film Coated Tablets
◆Anbesol Baby Teething Gel Anesthetic
◆Anbesol Gel
    Antiseptic-Anesthetic-Regular
    Strength
◆Anbesol Gel Antiseptic-Anesthetic -
    Maximum Strength
◆Anbesol Liquid Antiseptic-Anesthetic
◆Anbesol Liquid Antiseptic-Anesthetic -
    Maximum Strength
  Maximum Strength Arthritis Pain
    Formula by the Makers of Anacin
    Analgesic Tablets and Caplets
  Bronitin Asthma Tablets
  Bronitin Mist
◆Clearblue Easy
◆Clearplan Easy
  Clusivol Syrup
  CoAdvil (See Advil Cold and Sinus)
  Compound W Gel
  Compound W Liquid
  Denalan Denture Cleanser
◆Denorex Medicated Shampoo and
    Conditioner
◆Denorex Medicated Shampoo, Extra
    Strength
◆Denorex Medicated Shampoo, Extra
    Strength With Conditioners
◆Denorex Medicated Shampoo, Regular
    & Mountain Fresh Herbal Scent
  Dermoplast Anesthetic Pain Relief
    Lotion
  Dermoplast Anesthetic Pain Relief
    Spray
◆Dristan Allergy Nasal
    Decongestant/Antihistamine Caplets
◆Dristan Cold and Flu
◆Dristan Cold Nasal Decongestant/
    Antihistamine/Analgesic Coated
    Tablets
  Dristan Inhaler
◆Maximum Strength Dristan
    Cold Nasal Decongestant/
    Analgesic Coated Caplets
  Dristan Nasal Spray
  Dristan Menthol Nasal Spray
  Dristan Nasal Spray, Metered Dose
    Pump, Regular
  Dristan Room Vaporizer
◆Dristan Sinus Pain Reliever/Nasal
    Decongestant Caplets
  Dristan-AF
    Decongestant/Antihistamine/
    Analgesic Tablets
  Dristan 12-hour Nasal Spray, Regular
    and Menthol
  Dristan 12-hour Nasal Spray, Metered
    Dose Pump
  Enzactin Cream
  Fiber Guard
  Freezone Solution
  Heather Feminine Deodorant Spray
  Heet Analgesic Liniment
  Heet Analgesic Spray
  InfraRub Analgesic Cream
  Kerodex Cream 51 (for dry or oily
    work)
  Kerodex Cream 71 (for wet work)

Larylgan Throat Spray
Momentum Muscular Backache
  Formula
Outgro Solution
Oxipor VHC Lotion for Psoriasis
Posture 600 mg
Posture-D 600 mg
◆Preparation H Cleansing Tissues
◆Preparation H Hemorrhoidal Cream
◆Preparation H Hemorrhoidal Ointment
◆Preparation H Hemorrhoidal
    Suppositories
◆Primatene Mist
  Primatene Mist Suspension
◆Primatene Tablets-M Formula
◆Primatene Tablets-P Formula
◆Primatene Tablets-Regular Formula
  Quiet World Nighttime Pain Formula
  Riopan Antacid Suspension
  Riopan Antacid Swallow Tablets
  Riopan Plus Suspension
  Riopan Plus Chew Tablets
  Riopan Plus Chew Tablets in Rollpacks
◆Riopan Plus 2 Suspension-Mint and
    Cherry flavors
◆Riopan Plus 2 Chew Tablets-Mint and
    Cherry Vanilla flavors
  Semicid Vaginal Contraceptive Inserts
  Sleep-eze 3 Tablets
  Today Personal Lubricant
◆Today Vaginal Contraceptive Sponge
  Trendar Ibuprofen Tablets
  Viro-Med Tablets
  Youth Garde Moisturizer Plus PABA

WINTHROP CONSUMER PRODUCTS
Division of Sterling Winthrop Inc.
90 Park Avenue
New York, NY 10016
See STERLING HEALTH, page 724.

WINTHROP PHARMACEUTICALS
90 Park Avenue
New York, NY 10016
See SANOFI WINTHROP
PHARMACETUCALS, page 689.

WYETH-AYERST   **435, 773**
LABORATORIES
Division of American Home Products
Corporation
P.O. Box 8299
Philadelphia, PA 19101
  Address inquiries to:
Professional Service   (215) 688-4400
For EMERGENCY Medical Information
Day or night call   (215) 688-4400
  WYETH-AYERST DISTRIBUTION
  CENTERS
Atlanta, GA—P.O. Box 1773
  Paoli, PA 19301-1773
                            (800) 666-7248
  Freight address:
  221 Armour Drive NE
  Atlanta, GA 30324
  Mail DEA order forms to:
  P.O. Box 4365
  Atlanta, GA 30302
Boston MA—P.O. Box 1773
  Paoli, PA 19301-1773
                            (800) 666-7248
  Freight address:
  7 Connector Road
  Andover, MA 01810
  Mail DEA order forms to:
  P.O. Box 1776
  Andover, MA 01810

Chamblee, GA—P.O. Box 1773
  Paoli, PA 19301-1773
                            (800) 666-7248
  Freight address:
  3600 American Drive
  Chamblee, GA 30341
Chicago, IL—P.O. Box 1773
  Paoli, PA 19301-1773
                            (800) 666-7248
  Freight address:
  745 N. Gary Avenue
  Carol Stream, IL 60188
  Mail DEA order forms to:
  P.O. Box 140
  Wheaton, IL 60189-0140
Dallas, TX—P.O. Box 1773
  Paoli, PA 19301-1773
                            (800) 666-7248
  Freight address:
  11240 Petal Street
  Dallas, TX 75238
  Mail DEA order forms to:
  P.O. Box 650231
  Dallas, TX 75265-0231
Foster City, CA—P.O. Box 1773
  Paoli, PA 19301-1773
                            (800) 666-7248
  Freight address:
  1147 Chess Drive
  Foster City, CA 94404
Hawaii—P.O. Box 1773
  Paoli, PA 19301-1773
                            (800) 666-7248
  Mail DEA order forms to:
  96-1185 Waihona, Street, Unit C1
  Pearl City, HI 96782
Kansas City, MO—P.O. Box 1773
  Paoli, PA 19301-1773
                            (800) 666-7248
  Freight address:
  1340 Taney Street
  North Kansas City, MO 64116
  Mail DEA order forms to:
  P.O. Box 7588
  North Kansas City, MO 64116
Los Angeles, CA—P.O. Box 1773
  Paoli, PA 19301-1773
                            (800) 666-7248
  Freight address:
  6530 Altura Blvd.
  Buena Park, CA 90622
  Mail DEA order forms to:
  P.O. Box 5000
  Buena Park, CA 90622-5000
Philadelphia, PA—P.O. Box 1773
  Paoli, PA 19301-1773
                            (800) 666-7248
  Freight address:
  31 Morehall Road
  Frazer, PA 19355
  Mail DEA order forms to:
  P.O. Box 61
  Paoli, PA 19301
Seattle, WA—P.O. Box 1773
  Paoli, PA 19301-1773
                            (800) 666-7248
  Freight address:
  19255 80th Ave. South
  Kent, WA 98032
  Mail DEA order forms to:
  P.O. Box 5609
  Kent, WA 98064-5609
South Plainfield, NJ—P.O. Box 1773
  Paoli, PA 19301-1773
                            (800) 666-7248
  Freight address:
  4000 Hadley Road
  South Plainfield, NJ 07080
  OTC Products Available
◆Aludrox Oral Suspension
◆Amphojel Suspension
◆Amphojel Suspension without Flavor
◆Amphojel Tablets
◆Basaljel Capsules
◆Basaljel Suspension
◆Basaljel Tablets
◆Cerose-DM
◆Collyrium for Fresh Eyes

(◆ Shown in Product Identification Section)

◆Collyrium Fresh
◆Nursoy, Soy Protein Isolate Formula for Infants, Concentrated Liquid, Ready-to-Feed, and Powder
◆SMA Iron Fortified Infant Formula, Concentrated, Ready-to-Feed and Powder
◆SMA lo-iron Infant Formula, Concentrated, Ready-to-Feed, and Powder

◆Wyanoids Relief Factor Hemorrhoidal Suppositories

ZILA PHARMACEUTICALS, INC.   *435, 777*
5227 North 7th Street
Phoenix, AZ 85014

Address inquiries to:

Ed Pomerantz,
Vice President, Marketing
(602) 266-6700

OTC Products Available
◆Zilactin Medicated Gel
Zilactol Medicated Liquid
ZilaDent Oral Analgesic Gel

SECTION 2
Product Name Index

In this section only described products are listed in alphabetical sequence by brand name or generic name. They have page numbers to assist you in locating the descriptions. For additional information on other products, you may wish to contact the manufacturer directly. The symbol ◆ indicates the product is shown in the Product Identification Section.

A

◆ **A and D Ointment** (Schering-Plough HealthCare) p 424, 692

◆ **A-200 Pediculicide Shampoo & Gel** (SmithKline Beecham) p 426, 704

◆ **A.R.M. Allergy Relief Medicine Caplets** (Menley & James) p 415, 607

Acid Mantle Creme (Sandoz Consumer) p 682

◆ **Acnomel Cream** (Menley & James) p 415, 607

Actidose with Sorbitol (Paddock) p 628

Actidose-Aqua, Activated Charcoal (Paddock) p 628

◆ **Actifed Plus Caplets** (Burroughs Wellcome) p 406, 537

◆ **Actifed Plus Tablets** (Burroughs Wellcome) p 406, 538

◆ **Actifed Syrup** (Burroughs Wellcome) p 406, 537

◆ **Actifed Tablets** (Burroughs Wellcome) p 406, 537

◆ **Acutrim 16 Hour Steady Control Appetite Suppressant** (CIBA Consumer) p 407, 549

◆ **Acutrim Late Day Strength Appetite Suppressant** (CIBA Consumer) p 407, 549

◆ **Acutrim II Maximum Strength Appetite Suppressant** (CIBA Consumer) p 407, 549

◆ **Advance Pregnancy Test** (Ortho Pharmaceutical) p 418, 781

◆ **Advil Cold and Sinus (formerly CoAdvil)** (Whitehall) p 434, 761

◆ **Advil Ibuprofen Caplets and Tablets** (Whitehall) p 434, 761

◆ **Afrin Cherry Scented Nasal Spray 0.05 %** (Schering-Plough HealthCare) p 428, 692

◆ **Afrin Children's Strength Nose Drops 0.025 %** (Schering-Plough HealthCare) p 424, 692

◆ **Afrin Menthol Nasal Spray** (Schering-Plough HealthCare) p 424, 692

◆ **Afrin Nasal Spray 0.05 % and Nasal Spray Pump** (Schering-Plough HealthCare) p 424, 692

◆ **Afrin Nose Drops 0.05 %** (Schering-Plough HealthCare) p 424, 692

◆ **Afrin Saline Mist** (Schering-Plough HealthCare) p 424, 692

◆ **Afrin Tablets** (Schering-Plough HealthCare) p 424, 693

◆ **Aftate for Athlete's Foot** (Schering-Plough HealthCare) p 424, 693

◆ **Aftate for Jock Itch** (Schering-Plough HealthCare) p 424, 693

Agoral, Marshmallow Flavor (Parke-Davis) p 628

Agoral, Raspberry Flavor (Parke-Davis) p 628

◆ **Alka-Mints Chewable Antacid** (Miles Consumer) p 416, 612

◆ **Alka-Seltzer Effervescent Antacid** (Miles Consumer) p 416, 614

◆ **Alka-Seltzer Effervescent Antacid and Pain Reliever** (Miles Consumer) p 416, 612

◆ **Alka-Seltzer Extra Strength Effervescent Antacid and Pain Reliever** (Miles Consumer) p 416, 615

◆ **Alka-Seltzer (Flavored) Effervescent Antacid and Pain Reliever** (Miles Consumer) p 416, 613

◆ **Alka-Seltzer Plus Cold Medicine** (Miles Consumer) p 416, 615

◆ **Alka-Seltzer Plus Cold & Cough Medicine** (Miles Consumer) p 416, 616

◆ **Alka-Seltzer Plus Night-Time Cold Medicine** (Miles Consumer) p 416, 615

◆ **Alka Seltzer Plus Sinus Allergy Medicine** (Miles Consumer) p 416, 616

Allbee with C Caplets (Robins Consumer) p 667

Allbee C-800 Plus Iron Tablets (Robins Consumer) p 666

Allbee C-800 Tablets (Robins Consumer) p 666

Allerest Children's Chewable Tablets (Fisons Consumer Health) p 558

Allerest Headache Strength Tablets (Fisons Consumer Health) p 558

Allerest 12 Hour Caplets (Fisons Consumer Health) p 558

◆ **Allerest Maximum Strength Tablets** (Fisons Consumer Health) p 408, 558

◆ **Allerest No Drowsiness Tablets** (Fisons Consumer Health) p 408, 558

Allerest Sinus Pain Formula (Fisons Consumer Health) p 558

◆ **Allergy Drops** (Bausch & Lomb Personal) p 403, 513

◆ **Alpha Keri Moisture Rich Body Oil** (Bristol-Myers Products) p 405, 519

Alpha Keri Moisture Rich Cleansing Bar (Bristol-Myers Products) p 519

◆ **ALternaGEL Liquid** (J&J•Merck Consumer) p 409, 565

◆ **Aludrox Oral Suspension** (Wyeth-Ayerst) p 435, 773

◆ **Americaine Hemorrhoidal Ointment** (Fisons Consumer Health) p 409, 559

◆ **Americaine Topical Anesthetic First Aid Ointment** (Fisons Consumer Health) p 409, 559

◆ **Americaine Topical Anesthetic Spray** (Fisons Consumer Health) p 409, 559

Amesec (Whitby) p 759

◆ **Amphojel Suspension** (Wyeth-Ayerst) p 435, 773

◆ **Amphojel Suspension without Flavor** (Wyeth-Ayerst) p 435, 773

◆ **Amphojel Tablets** (Wyeth-Ayerst) p 435, 773

◆ **Anacin Coated Analgesic Caplets** (Whitehall) p 434, 762

◆ **Anacin Coated Analgesic Tablets** (Whitehall) p 434, 762

Anacin Maximum Strength Analgesic Coated Tablets (Whitehall) p 762

◆ **Aspirin Free Anacin Acetaminophen Film Coated Caplets** (Whitehall) p 434, 762

◆ **Aspirin Free Anacin Acetaminophen Film Coated Tablets** (Whitehall) p 434, 762

◆ **Anbesol Baby Teething Gel Anesthetic** (Whitehall) p 434, 763

(◆ **Shown in Product Identification Section**)

◆Anbesol Gel
   Antiseptic-Anesthetic-Regular
   Strength (Whitehall) p 434, 763
◆Anbesol Gel Antiseptic-Anesthetic -
   Maximum Strength (Whitehall) p 434,
   763
◆Anbesol Liquid Antiseptic-Anesthetic
   (Whitehall) p 434, 763
◆Anbesol Liquid Antiseptic-Anesthetic -
   Maximum Strength (Whitehall) p 434,
   763
◆Anticon (Neutrin) p 417, 622
◆Anusol Hemorrhoidal Suppositories
   (Parke-Davis) p 418, 629
◆Anusol Ointment (Parke-Davis) p 418, 629
◆Aqua Care Cream (Menley & James)
   p 415, 607
◆Aqua Care Lotion (Menley & James)
   p 415, 607
   Aqua Glycolic Lotion (Herald Pharmacal)
   p 564
   Aqua Glycolic Shampoo (Herald
   Pharmacal) p 564
   Aqua Glyde Cleanser (Herald Pharmacal)
   p 564
   Aqua-A Cream (Baker Cummins
   Pharmaceuticals) p 511
   Aquaderm Combination
   Treatment/Moisturizer (SPF 15
   Formula) (Baker Cummins
   Pharmaceuticals) p 511
   Aquaderm Cream (Baker Cummins
   Pharmaceuticals) p 511
   Aquaderm Lotion (Baker Cummins
   Pharmaceuticals) p 511
◆Aquaphor Antibiotic Ointment
   (Beiersdorf) p 404, 515
◆Aquaphor Healing Ointment, Original
   Formula (Beiersdorf) p 404, 514
◆Aquaphor Natural Healing Ointment
   (Beiersdorf) p 404, 515
   Aquaray 20 Sunscreen (Herald
   Pharmacal) p 564
   Arm & Hammer Pure Baking Soda
   (Church & Dwight) p 548
   Maximum Strength Arthritis Pain
   Formula by the Makers of Anacin
   Analgesic Tablets and Caplets
   (Whitehall) p 763
   Arthritis Strength BC Powder (Block)
   p 516
◆Ascriptin A/D Caplets (Rhone-Poulenc
   Rorer Consumer) p 420, 649
◆Regular Strength Ascriptin Tablets
   (Rhone-Poulenc Rorer Consumer) p 420,
   648
   Aspercreme Creme, Lotion Analgesic
   Rub (Thompson Medical) p 743
   AsthmaHaler Mist Epinephrine
   Bitartrate Bronchodilator (Menley &
   James) p 608
   AsthmaNefrin Solution "A"
   Bronchodilator (Menley & James) p 608
   Aurum Analgesic Lotion (Au
   Pharmaceuticals) p 510
◆Aveeno Anti-Itch Concentrated Lotion
   (Rydelle) p 423, 680
◆Aveeno Anti-Itch Cream (Rydelle) p 423,
   680
◆Aveeno Bath Oilated (Rydelle) p 423, 680
◆Aveeno Bath Regular (Rydelle) p 423, 680
◆Aveeno Cleansing Bar for Acne
   (Rydelle) p 423, 680
◆Aveeno Cleansing Bar for Combination
   Skin (Rydelle) p 423, 680
◆Aveeno Cleansing Bar for Dry Skin
   (Rydelle) p 423, 681
◆Aveeno Moisturizing Cream (Rydelle)
   p 423, 681
◆Aveeno Moisturizing Lotion (Rydelle)
   p 423, 681
◆Aveeno Shower and Bath Oil (Rydelle)
   p 423, 681
◆Ayr Saline Nasal Drops (Ascher) p 403,
   509
◆Ayr Saline Nasal Mist (Ascher) p 403,
   509

                        B

BC Powder (Block) p 517
BC Cold Powder Multi-Symptom
   Formula (Block) p 516

BC Cold Powder Multi-Symptom
   Non-Drowsy Formula (Block) p 516
◆Bactine Antiseptic/Anesthetic First Aid
   Liquid (Miles Consumer) p 416, 617
◆Bactine First Aid Antibiotic Plus
   Anesthetic Ointment (Miles Consumer)
   p 416, 617
◆Bactine Hydrocortisone Anti-Itch
   Cream (Miles Consumer) p 416, 617
   Balmex Baby Powder (Macsil) p 579
   Balmex Emollient Lotion (Macsil) p 579
   Balmex Ointment (Macsil) p 579
   Barri-Care Antimicrobial Barrier
   Ointment (Care-Tech) p 544
◆Basaljel Capsules (Wyeth-Ayerst) p 435,
   774
◆Basaljel Suspension (Wyeth-Ayerst)
   p 435, 774
◆Basaljel Tablets (Wyeth-Ayerst) p 435,
   774
◆Children's Bayer Chewable Aspirin
   (Sterling Health) p 429, 724
◆Genuine Bayer Aspirin Tablets &
   Caplets (Sterling Health) p 428, 724
◆Maximum Bayer Aspirin Tablets &
   Caplets (Sterling Health) p 429, 725
◆Bayer Plus Aspirin Tablets (Sterling
   Health) p 429, 726
◆Extra Strength Bayer Plus Aspirin
   Caplets (Sterling Health) p 429, 727
◆Therapy Bayer Enteric Aspirin Caplets
   (Sterling Health) p 429, 728
◆8 Hour Bayer Timed-Release Aspirin
   (Sterling Health) p 429, 726
   Beelith Tablets (Beach) p 514
◆Benadryl Anti-Itch Cream, Regular
   Strength 1% and Maximum Strength
   2% (Parke-Davis) p 418, 629
◆Benadryl Cold Tablets (Parke-Davis)
   p 418, 631
◆Benadryl Cold Nighttime Formula
   (Parke-Davis) p 419, 631
◆Benadryl Decongestant Elixir
   (Parke-Davis) p 419, 630
◆Benadryl Decongestant Kapseals
   (Parke-Davis) p 418, 630
◆Benadryl Decongestant Tablets
   (Parke-Davis) p 418, 630
◆Benadryl Elixir (Parke-Davis) p 419, 630
◆Benadryl Spray, Maximum Strength
   2% (Parke-Davis) p 418, 632
◆Benadryl Spray, Regular Strength 1%
   (Parke-Davis) p 418, 632
◆Benadryl 25 Kapseals (Parke-Davis)
   p 418, 631
◆Benadryl 25 Tablets (Parke-Davis) p 418,
   631
   Ben-Gay External Analgesic Products
   (Pfizer Consumer) p 638
   Ben-Gay Ultra Strength Pain Relieving
   Rub (Pfizer Consumer) p 638
◆Benylin Cough Syrup (Parke-Davis)
   p 419, 632
◆Benylin Decongestant (Parke-Davis)
   p 419, 633
◆Benylin DM Pediatric Cough Formula
   (Parke-Davis) p 419, 632
◆Benylin Expectorant (Parke-Davis) p 419,
   633
◆Benzedrex Inhaler (Menley & James)
   p 415, 608
◆BiCozene Creme (Sandoz Consumer)
   p 423, 682
   Bonine Tablets (Pfizer Consumer) p 638
   Borofax Ointment (Burroughs Wellcome)
   p 538
   Bromfed Syrup (Muro) p 621
◆Bronkaid Mist (Sterling Health) p 429,
   729
   Bronkaid Mist Suspension (Sterling
   Health) p 730
◆Bronkaid Tablets (Sterling Health) p 429,
   730
   Bronkolixir (Sanofi Winthrop
   Pharmaceuticals) p 689
   Bronkotabs Tablets (Sanofi Winthrop
   Pharmaceuticals) p 689
◆Arthritis Strength Bufferin Analgesic
   Caplets (Bristol-Myers Products) p 404,
   521
◆Extra Strength Bufferin Analgesic
   Tablets (Bristol-Myers Products) p 404,
   522

◆Bufferin Analgesic Tablets and Caplets
   (Bristol-Myers Products) p 404, 519
◆Bufferin A/F Nite Time
   Analgesic/Sleeping Aid Caplets
   (Bristol-Myers Products) p 404, 521
◆Bugs Bunny Children's Chewable
   Vitamins (Sugar Free) (Miles
   Consumer) p 416, 617
◆Bugs Bunny Complete Children's
   Chewable Vitamins + Minerals with
   Iron and Calcium (Sugar Free) (Miles
   Consumer) p 416, 618
◆Bugs Bunny With Extra C Children's
   Chewable Vitamins (Sugar Free)
   (Miles Consumer) p 416, 617
◆Bugs Bunny Plus Iron Children's
   Chewable Vitamins (Sugar Free)
   (Miles Consumer) p 416, 617

                        C

◆Caladryl Clear Lotion (Parke-Davis)
   p 419, 633
◆Caladryl Cream, Lotion, Spray
   (Parke-Davis) p 419, 633
◆Caldecort Anti-Itch Hydrocortisone
   Cream (Fisons Consumer Health) p 409,
   559
◆Caldecort Anti-Itch Hydrocortisone
   Spray (Fisons Consumer Health) p 409,
   559
◆Caldecort Light Cream (Fisons Consumer
   Health) p 409, 559
◆Caldesene Medicated Ointment (Fisons
   Consumer Health) p 409, 559
◆Caldesene Medicated Powder (Fisons
   Consumer Health) p 409, 559
◆Caltrate 600 (Lederle) p 410, 571
◆Caltrate 600 + Iron & Vitamin D
   (Lederle) p 410, 572
◆Caltrate 600 + Vitamin D (Lederle)
   p 410, 572
   Cam Lotion (Herald Pharmacal) p 564
   Cama Arthritis Pain Reliever (Sandoz
   Consumer) p 682
◆Campho-Phenique Cold Sore Gel
   (Sterling Health) p 429, 731
◆Campho-Phenique Liquid (Sterling
   Health) p 429, 731
◆Campho-Phenique Triple Antibiotic
   Ointment Plus Pain Reliever (Sterling
   Health) p 429, 731
   Care Creme (Care-Tech) p 544
   Carmol 20 Cream (Syntex) p 743
   Carmol 10 Lotion (Syntex) p 743
   Cellufresh Lubricant Ophthalmic
   Solution (Allergan Pharmaceuticals)
   p 504
   Celluvisc Lubricant Ophthalmic
   Solution (Allergan Pharmaceuticals)
   p 504
◆Centrum (Lederle) p 410, 572
◆Centrum, Jr. (Children's Chewable) +
   Extra C (Lederle) p 410, 573
◆Centrum, Jr. (Children's Chewable) +
   Extra Calcium (Lederle) p 411, 573
◆Centrum, Jr. (Children's Chewable) +
   Iron (Lederle) p 410, 573
◆Centrum Liquid (Lederle) p 411, 572
◆Centrum Silver (Lederle) p 411, 575
◆Cēpacol Anesthetic Lozenges (Troches)
   (Marion Merrell Dow) p 411, 580
◆Cēpacol/Cēpacol Mint
   Mouthwash/Gargle (Marion Merrell
   Dow) p 411, 579
◆Cēpacol Dry Throat Lozenges, Cherry
   Flavor (Marion Merrell Dow) p 411, 579
◆Cēpacol Dry Throat Lozenges,
   Honey-Lemon Flavor (Marion Merrell
   Dow) p 411, 579
◆Cēpacol Dry Throat Lozenges,
   Menthol-Eucalyptus Flavor (Marion
   Merrell Dow) p 411, 580
◆Cēpacol Dry Throat Lozenges, Original
   Flavor (Marion Merrell Dow) p 411, 580
◆Cēpastat Cherry Flavor Sore Throat
   Lozenges (Marion Merrell Dow) p 411,
   580
◆Cēpastat Extra Strength Sore Throat
   Lozenges (Marion Merrell Dow) p 411,
   580
◆Cerose-DM (Wyeth-Ayerst) p 435, 774
◆Chap Stick Lip Balm (Robins Consumer)
   p 421, 667

(◆ Shown in Product Identification Section)

◆Chap Stick Petroleum Jelly Plus (Robins Consumer) p 421, 668

◆Chap Stick Petroleum Jelly Plus with Sunblock 15 (Robins Consumer) p 421, 668

◆Chap Stick Sunblock 15 Lip Balm (Robins Consumer) p 421, 667

Charcoaid (Requa) p 647

Charcocaps (Requa) p 648

◆Cheracol-D Cough Formula (Roberts) p 421, 663

Cheracol Nasal Spray Pump (Roberts) p 663

◆Cheracol Plus Head Cold/Cough Formula (Roberts) p 421, 663

Cheracol Sore Throat Spray (Roberts) p 663

Children's Chloraseptic Lozenges (Richardson-Vicks) p 652

Children's Chloraseptic Spray (Richardson-Vicks) p 654

Chlor-3 Condiment (Fleming) p 563

Chloraseptic Liquid, Cherry, Menthol and Cool Mint (Richardson-Vicks) p 652

Chloraseptic Liquid - Nitrogen Propelled Spray (Richardson-Vicks) p 652

Chloraseptic Lozenges, Cherry, Cool Mint and Menthol (Richardson-Vicks) p 653

◆Chlor-Trimeton Allergy Syrup, Tablets & Long-Acting Repetabs Tablets (Schering-Plough HealthCare) p 424,425, 693

◆Chlor-Trimeton Antihistamine and Decongestant Tablets (Schering-Plough HealthCare) p 425, 694

◆Chlor-Trimeton Long Acting Antihistamine and Decongestant Repetabs Tablets (Schering-Plough HealthCare) p 425, 694

◆Chlor-Trimeton Maximum Strength Timed Release Allergy Tablets (Schering-Plough HealthCare) p 425

◆Chlor-Trimeton Sinus Caplets (Schering-Plough HealthCare) p 425

◆Chooz Antacid Gum (Schering-Plough HealthCare) p 425, 694

Citrocarbonate Antacid (Roberts) p 664

◆Citrucel Orange Flavor (Marion Merrell Dow) p 411, 581

◆Citrucel Sugar Free Orange Flavor (Marion Merrell Dow) p 411, 581

◆Clear by Design Medicated Acne Gel (SmithKline Beecham) p 426, 704

◆Clear Eyes ACR Astringent/Lubricating Eye Redness Reliever (Ross) p 422, 677

◆Clear Eyes Lubricating Eye Redness Reliever (Ross) p 422, 677

◆Clearblue Easy (Whitehall) p 434, 783

◆Clearplan Easy (Whitehall) p 434, 783

Clinical Care Dermal Wound Cleanser (Care-Tech) p 545

Clocream Skin Protectant Cream (Roberts) p 664

◆Colace (Mead Johnson Pharmaceuticals) p 415, 606

Cold Control+ Intense Cold Medicine (Reese Chemical) p 647

Colicon Drops (Reese Chemical) p 647

◆Collyrium for Fresh Eyes (Wyeth-Ayerst) p 435, 775

◆Collyrium Fresh (Wyeth-Ayerst) p 435, 775

◆Complex 15 Hand & Body Moisturizing Cream (Schering-Plough HealthCare) p 425, 694

◆Complex 15 Hand & Body Moisturizing Lotion (Schering-Plough HealthCare) p 425, 694

◆Complex 15 Moisturizing Face Cream (Schering-Plough HealthCare) p 425, 695

Compound W Gel (Whitehall) p 763

Compound W Liquid (Whitehall) p 763

◆Allergy-Sinus Comtrex Multi-Symptom Allergy-Sinus Formula Tablets & Caplets (Bristol-Myers Products) p 404, 523

◆Cough Formula Comtrex (Bristol-Myers Products) p 405, 524

◆Comtrex Multi-Symptom Cold Reliever Tablets/Caplets/Liqui-Gels/Liquid (Bristol-Myers Products) p 404, 522

◆Comtrex Multi-Symptom Day-Night Caplet-Tablet (Bristol-Myers Products) p 404, 525

◆Comtrex Multi-Symptom Non-Drowsy Caplets (Bristol-Myers Products) p 405, 526

Concept (Care-Tech) p 545

◆Conceptrol Contraceptive Gel • Single Use Contraceptive (Ortho Pharmaceutical) p 418, 625

◆Conceptrol Contraceptive Inserts (Ortho Pharmaceutical) p 418, 625

◆Congespirin For Children Aspirin Free Chewable Cold Tablets (Bristol-Myers Products) p 405, 527

◆Congestac Caplets (Menley & James) p 415, 609

◆Contac Continuous Action Decongestant/Antihistamine Capsules (SmithKline Beecham) p 426, 705

◆Contac Cough and Chest Cold (SmithKline Beecham) p 427, 706

◆Contac Cough & Sore Throat Formula (SmithKline Beecham) p 427, 707

◆Contac Jr. Non-Drowsy Cold Liquid (SmithKline Beecham) p 427, 707

◆Contac Maximum Strength Continuous Action Decongestant/Antihistamine Caplets (SmithKline Beecham) p 426, 704

◆Contac Severe Cold and Flu Formula Caplets (SmithKline Beecham) p 427, 706

◆Contac Severe Cold & Flu Nighttime (SmithKline Beecham) p 427, 708

◆Contac Sinus Caplets Maximum Strength Non-Drowsy Formula (SmithKline Beecham) p 427, 705

◆Contac Sinus Tablets Maximum Strength Non-Drowsy Formula (SmithKline Beecham) p 427, 705

◆Coricidin 'D' Decongestant Tablets (Schering-Plough HealthCare) p 425, 695

◆Coricidin Demilets Tablets for Children (Schering-Plough HealthCare) p 425, 696

◆Coricidin Tablets (Schering-Plough HealthCare) p 425, 695

◆Correctol Laxative Tablets (Schering-Plough HealthCare) p 425, 696

◆Cortaid Cream with Aloe (Upjohn) p 431, 747

◆Cortaid Lotion (Upjohn) p 431, 747

◆Cortaid Ointment with Aloe (Upjohn) p 431, 747

◆Cortaid Spray (Upjohn) p 431, 747

◆Maximum Strength Cortaid Cream (Upjohn) p 431, 748

◆Maximum Strength Cortaid Ointment (Upjohn) p 431, 748

◆Maximum Strength Cortaid Spray (Upjohn) p 431, 748

Cortef Feminine Itch Cream (Upjohn) p 748

◆Corticaine External Analgesic (Whitby) p 433, 760

◆Cortizone-5 Creme and Ointment (Thompson Medical) p 431, 743

Cortizone-5 Wipes (Thompson Medical) p 743

Cortizone-10 Creme and Ointment (Thompson Medical) p 744

◆Cramp End Tablets (Ohm Laboratories) p 418, 624

◆Cruex Antifungal Cream (Fisons Consumer Health) p 409, 560

◆Cruex Antifungal Powder (Fisons Consumer Health) p 409, 560

◆Cruex Antifungal Spray Powder (Fisons Consumer Health) p 409, 560

D

DDS-Acidophilus (UAS Laboratories) p 747

◆Dairy Ease Caplets and Tablets (Sterling Health) p 429, 731

◆Dairy Ease Drops (Sterling Health) p 429, 732

Dairy Ease Real Milk (Sterling Health) p 429, 732

◆Datril Extra-Strength Analgesic Tablets (Bristol-Myers Products) p 405, 527

Dayalets Filmtab (Abbott) p 502

Dayalets Plus Iron Filmtab (Abbott) p 502

◆Debrox Drops (Marion Merrell Dow) p 411, 581

◆Delfen Contraceptive Foam (Ortho Pharmaceutical) p 418, 625

Delsym Cough Formula (Fisons Corporation) p 562

◆Denorex Medicated Shampoo and Conditioner (Whitehall) p 434, 764

◆Denorex Medicated Shampoo, Extra Strength (Whitehall) p 434, 764

◆Denorex Medicated Shampoo, Extra Strength With Conditioners (Whitehall) p 434, 764

◆Denorex Medicated Shampoo, Regular & Mountain Fresh Herbal Scent (Whitehall) p 434, 764

Denquel Sensitive Teeth Toothpaste (Procter & Gamble) p 642

Dentapaine Gel (Reese Chemical) p 647

Dermoplast Anesthetic Pain Relief Lotion (Whitehall) p 764

Dermoplast Anesthetic Pain Relief Spray (Whitehall) p 764

Desenex Antifungal Cream (Fisons Consumer Health) p 560

Desenex Antifungal Foam (Fisons Consumer Health) p 560

◆Desenex Antifungal Ointment (Fisons Consumer Health) p 409, 560

◆Desenex Antifungal Powder (Fisons Consumer Health) p 409, 560

◆Desenex Antifungal Spray Powder (Fisons Consumer Health) p 409, 560

◆Desenex Foot & Sneaker Deodorant Spray Powder (Fisons Consumer Health) p 409, 560

◆Desitin Ointment (Pfizer Consumer) p 420, 638

Devrom Chewable Tablets (Parthenon) p 638

Dexatrim Capsules, Caplets, Tablets (Thompson Medical) p 744

Dexatrim Maximum Strength Caffeine-Free Caplets (Thompson Medical) p 744

Dexatrim Maximum Strength Caffeine-Free Capsules (Thompson Medical) p 744

Dexatrim Maximum Strength Extended Duration Time Tablets (Thompson Medical) p 744

◆Dexatrim Maximum Strength Plus Vitamin C/Caffeine-free Caplets (Thompson Medical) p 431, 744

◆Dexatrim Maximum Strength Plus Vitamin C/Caffeine-free Capsules (Thompson Medical) p 431, 744

◆Dialose Tablets (J&J•Merck Consumer) p 409, 565

◆Dialose Plus Tablets (J&J•Merck Consumer) p 409, 566

◆Diasorb Liquid (Columbia) p 408, 556

◆Diasorb Tablets (Columbia) p 408, 556

◆Di-Gel Antacid/Anti-Gas (Schering-Plough HealthCare) p 425, 696

Dimacol Caplets (Robins Consumer) p 668

Dimetane Decongestant Caplets (Robins Consumer) p 669

Dimetane Decongestant Elixir (Robins Consumer) p 669

Dimetane Elixir (Robins Consumer) p 668

Dimetane Extentabs 8 mg (Robins Consumer) p 668

Dimetane Extentabs 12 mg (Robins Consumer) p 668

Dimetane Tablets (Robins Consumer) p 668

◆Dimetapp Cold & Flu Caplets (Robins Consumer) p 421, 670

◆Dimetapp Elixir (Robins Consumer) p 421, 670

◆Dimetapp DM Elixir (Robins Consumer) p 421, 671

◆Dimetapp Extentabs (Robins Consumer) p 421, 671

◆Dimetapp Tablets (Robins Consumer) p 421, 672

◆Doan's - Extra-Strength Analgesic (CIBA Consumer) p 407, 549

(◆ Shown in Product Identification Section)

◆Extra Strength Doan's P.M. (CIBA Consumer) p 407, 549

◆Doan's - Regular Strength Analgesic (CIBA Consumer) p 407, 549

◆Domeboro Astringent Solution Effervescent Tablets (Miles Consumer) p 417, 619

◆Domeboro Astringent Solution Powder Packets (Miles Consumer) p 417, 618

◆Donnagel Liquid and Chewable Tablets (Robins Consumer) p 422, 672

◆Dorcol Children's Cough Syrup (Sandoz Consumer) p 423, 682

◆Dorcol Children's Decongestant Liquid (Sandoz Consumer) p 423, 683

◆Dorcol Children's Liquid Cold Formula (Sandoz Consumer) p 423, 683

Dove Bar (Lever Brothers) p 578

◆Doxidan Liqui-Gels (Upjohn) p 431, 748

◆Dramamine Chewable Tablets (Upjohn) p 431, 748

◆Dramamine Liquid (Upjohn) p 431, 748

◆Dramamine Tablets (Upjohn) p 431, 748

◆Dristan Allergy Nasal Decongestant/Antihistamine Caplets (Whitehall) p 434, 765

◆Dristan Cold and Flu (Whitehall) p 434, 766

Drisdol (Sanofi Winthrop Pharmaceuticals) p 689

◆Dristan Cold Nasal Decongestant/ Antihistamine/Analgesic Coated Tablets (Whitehall) p 434, 765

◆Maximum Strength Dristan Cold Nasal Decongestant/ Analgesic Coated Caplets (Whitehall) p 434, 765

Dristan Nasal Spray (Whitehall) p 764

Dristan Menthol Nasal Spray (Whitehall) p 764

Dristan Nasal Spray, Metered Dose Pump, Regular (Whitehall) p 764

◆Dristan Sinus Pain Reliever/Nasal Decongestant Caplets (Whitehall) p 434, 766

Dristan 12-hour Nasal Spray, Regular and Menthol (Whitehall) p 767

Dristan 12-hour Nasal Spray, Metered Dose Pump (Whitehall) p 767

Drixoral Antihistamine/Nasal Decongestant Syrup (Schering-Plough HealthCare) p 696

◆Drixoral Non-Drowsy Formula (Schering-Plough HealthCare) p 425, 697

◆Drixoral Plus Extended-Release Tablets (Schering-Plough HealthCare) p 425, 698

◆Drixoral Sinus (Schering-Plough HealthCare) p 426, 698

◆Drixoral Sustained-Action Tablets (Schering-Plough HealthCare) p 425, 697

◆Dry Eye Therapy Lubricating Eye Drops (Bausch & Lomb Personal) p 403, 513

◆Dulcolax Suppositories (CIBA Consumer) p 407, 550

◆Dulcolax Tablets (CIBA Consumer) p 407, 550

◆DuoFilm Liquid (Schering-Plough HealthCare) p 426, 698

◆Duolube Eye Ointment (Bausch & Lomb Personal) p 403, 514

◆DuoPlant Gel (Schering-Plough HealthCare) p 426, 699

◆Duration 12 Hour Nasal Spray (Schering-Plough HealthCare) p 426, 699

◆Duration 12 Hour Nasal Spray Pump (Schering-Plough HealthCare) p 426, 699

E

◆e.p.t. Early Pregnancy Test (Parke-Davis) p 419, 781

◆Ear Drops by Murine—(See Murine Ear Wax Removal System/Murine Ear Drops) (Ross) p 422, 677

◆Ecotrin Enteric Coated Aspirin Maximum Strength Tablets and Caplets (SmithKline Beecham) p 427, 708

◆Ecotrin Enteric Coated Aspirin Regular Strength Tablets and Caplets (SmithKline Beecham) p 427, 708

◆Professional Strength Efferdent (Warner-Lambert) p 432, 755

◆Effer-Syllium Natural Fiber Bulking Agent (J&J•Merck Consumer) p 409, 566

◆Emetrol (Adria) p 403, 503

◆Empirin Aspirin (Burroughs Wellcome) p 406, 538

Encare Vaginal Contraceptive Suppositories (Thompson Medical) p 745

◆Ener-B Vitamin B₁₂ Nasal Gel Dietary Supplement (Nature's Bounty) p 417, 622

Ester-C Tablets (Inter-Cal) p 564

◆Eucalyptamint 100% All Natural Ointment (CIBA Consumer) p 407, 551

◆Eucerin Cleansing Lotion Dry Skin Care (Beiersdorf) p 404, 515

◆Eucerin Dry Skin Care Daily Facial Lotion SPF 20 (Beiersdorf) p 404, 515

◆Eucerin Dry Skin Care Cleansing Bar (Beiersdorf) p 404, 515

◆Eucerin Dry Skin Care Creme (Beiersdorf) p 404, 515

◆Eucerin Lotion (Beiersdorf) p 404, 516

◆Eucerin Dry Skin Care Lotion (Fragrance-free) (Beiersdorf) p 404, 516

◆Evac-U-Gen Mild Laxative (Walker, Corp) p 432, 753

◆Aspirin Free Excedrin Analgesic Caplets (Bristol-Myers Products) p 405, 528

◆Excedrin Extra-Strength Analgesic Tablets & Caplets (Bristol-Myers Products) p 405, 529

◆Excedrin P.M. Analgesic/Sleeping Aid Tablets, Caplets and Liquid (Bristol-Myers Products) p 405, 530

◆Sinus Excedrin Analgesic, Decongestant Tablets & Caplets (Bristol-Myers Products) p 405, 531

◆Ex-Lax Chocolated Laxative Tablets (Sandoz Consumer) p 423, 683

◆Extra Gentle Ex-Lax Laxative Pills (Sandoz Consumer) p 423, 683

◆Maximum Relief Formula Ex-Lax Laxative Pills (Sandoz Consumer) p 423, 683

◆Regular Strength Ex-Lax Laxative Pills (Sandoz Consumer) p 423, 683

◆Eye Wash (Bausch & Lomb Personal) p 404, 514

F

◆4-Way Cold Tablets (Bristol-Myers Products) p 405, 531

◆4-Way Fast Acting Nasal Spray (regular & mentholated) & Metered Spray Pump (regular) (Bristol-Myers Products) p 405, 532

◆4-Way Long Lasting Nasal Spray & Metered Spray Pump (Bristol-Myers Products) p 405, 533

◆Fact Plus Pregnancy Test (Ortho Pharmaceutical) p 418, 781

◆Feen-A-Mint Gum (Schering-Plough HealthCare) p 426, 699

◆Feen-A-Mint Laxative Pills (Schering-Plough HealthCare) p 426, 699

Feminine Gold Analgesic Lotion (Au Pharmaceuticals) p 511

◆FemIron Multi Vitamins and Iron (Menley & James) p 415, 609

◆Feosol Capsules (SmithKline Beecham) p 427, 710

◆Feosol Elixir (SmithKline Beecham) p 427, 711

◆Feosol Tablets (SmithKline Beecham) p 427, 711

Ferancee Chewable Tablets (J&J•Merck Consumer) p 566

◆Ferancee-HP Tablets (J&J•Merck Consumer) p 409, 566

Fergon Elixir (Sterling Health) p 732

◆Fergon Iron Supplement Tablets (Sterling Health) p 429, 732

◆Ferro-Sequels (Lederle) p 411, 575

Fiberall Chewable Tablets, Lemon Creme Flavor (CIBA Consumer) p 551

◆Fiberall Fiber Wafers - Fruit & Nut (CIBA Consumer) p 407, 551

◆Fiberall Fiber Wafers - Oatmeal Raisin (CIBA Consumer) p 407, 551

◆Fiberall Powder Natural Flavor (CIBA Consumer) p 407, 551

◆Fiberall Powder Orange Flavor (CIBA Consumer) p 407, 551

◆FiberCon (Lederle) p 411, 575

Filibon Prenatal Vitamin Tablets (Lederle) p 575

◆Filteray Broad Spectrum Sunscreen Lotion (Burroughs Wellcome) p 406, 538

Flex-all 454 Pain Relieving Gel (Chattem) p 545

◆Flintstones Children's Chewable Vitamins (Miles Consumer) p 416, 617

◆Flintstones Children's Chewable Vitamins With Extra C (Miles Consumer) p 416, 618

◆Flintstones Children's Chewable Vitamins Plus Iron (Miles Consumer) p 416, 617

◆Flintstones Complete With Calcium, Iron & Minerals Children's Chewable Vitamins (Miles Consumer) p 416, 618

Formula Magic Antibacterial Powder (Care-Tech) p 545

Freezone Solution (Whitehall) p 767

G

◆Gas-X Tablets (Sandoz Consumer) p 423, 684

◆Extra Strength Gas-X Tablets (Sandoz Consumer) p 423, 684

◆Gaviscon Antacid Tablets (Marion Merrell Dow) p 412, 582

◆Gaviscon-2 Antacid Tablets (Marion Merrell Dow) p 412, 583

◆Gaviscon Extra Strength Relief Formula Liquid Antacid (Marion Merrell Dow) p 412, 582

◆Gaviscon Extra Strength Relief Formula Antacid Tablets (Marion Merrell Dow) p 412, 582

◆Gaviscon Liquid Antacid (Marion Merrell Dow) p 412, 583

◆Gelusil Liquid & Tablets (Parke-Davis) p 419, 634

◆Gentle Nature Natural Vegetable Laxative Tablets (Sandoz Consumer) p 423, 684

Geriplex-FS Kapseals (Parke-Davis) p 634

Geriplex-FS Liquid (Parke-Davis) p 634

Geritol Complete Tablets (SmithKline Beecham) p 711

Geritol Extend Caplets (SmithKline Beecham) p 712

Geritol Liquid - High Potency Iron & Vitamin Tonic (SmithKline Beecham) p 712

Gevrabon Liquid (Lederle) p 576

Gevral T Tablets (Lederle) p 576

Gevral Tablets (Lederle) p 576

Glutose (Paddock) p 628

◆Gly-Oxide Liquid (Marion Merrell Dow) p 412, 583

Guaifed Syrup (Muro) p 621

Guaitab Tablets (Muro) p 621

◆Gyne-Lotrimin Vaginal Cream Antifungal (Schering-Plough HealthCare) p 426, 699

◆Gyne-Lotrimin Vaginal Inserts (Schering-Plough HealthCare) p 426, 700

◆Gyne-Moistrin Vaginal Gel (Schering-Plough HealthCare) p 426, 700

◆Gynol II Extra Strength Contraceptive Jelly (Ortho Pharmaceutical) p 418, 626

◆Gynol II Original Formula Contraceptive Jelly (Ortho Pharmaceutical) p 418, 626

H

◆Haley's M-O, Regular & Flavored (Sterling Health) p 429, 732

◆Halfprin Low Strength Aspirin Tablets (Kramer) p 410, 570

◆Halls Mentho-Lyptus Cough Suppressant Tablets (Warner-Lambert) p 432, 755

◆Halls Plus Cough Suppressant Tablets (Warner-Lambert) p 432, 756

(◆ Shown in Product Identification Section)

◆Halls Vitamin C Drops (Warner-Lambert) p 433, 756

◆Haltran Tablets (Roberts) p 421, 664

Head & Shoulders Antidandruff Shampoo (Procter & Gamble) p 643

Head & Shoulders Antidandruff Shampoo 2-in-1 plus Conditioner (Procter & Gamble) p 643

Head & Shoulders Dry Scalp Shampoo (Procter & Gamble) p 643

Head & Shoulders Dry Scalp Shampoo 2-in-1 plus Conditioner (Procter & Gamble) p 643

Head & Shoulders Intensive Treatment Dandruff Shampoo (Procter & Gamble) p 643

Head & Shoulders Intensive Treatment Dandruff Shampoo 2-in-1 plus Conditioner (Procter & Gamble) p 643

Herpecin-L Cold Sore Lip Balm (Campbell) p 544

◆Hibiclens Antimicrobial Skin Cleanser (Stuart) p 431, 740

Hibistat Germicidal Hand Rinse (Stuart) p 741

Hibistat Towelette (Stuart) p 741

◆Hold Cough Suppressant Lozenge (Menley & James) p 415, 609

Hyland's Bed Wetting Tablets (Standard Homeopathic) p 722

Hyland's Calms Forté Tablets (Standard Homeopathic) p 722

Hyland's Colic Tablets (Standard Homeopathic) p 722

Hyland's Cough Syrup with Honey (Standard Homeopathic) p 722

Hyland's C-Plus Cold Tablets (Standard Homeopathic) p 722

Hyland's Teething Tablets (Standard Homeopathic) p 723

Hyland's Vitamin C for Children (Standard Homeopathic) p 723

I

◆Ibuprohm Ibuprofen Caplets (Ohm Laboratories) p 418, 625

◆Ibuprohm Ibuprofen Tablets (Ohm Laboratories) p 418, 625

Icy Hot Balm (Chattem) p 546

Icy Hot Cream (Chattem) p 546

Icy Hot Stick (Chattem) p 546

◆Imodium A-D Caplets and Liquid (McNeil Consumer Products) p 414, 587

Impregon Concentrate (Fleming) p 563

Incremin w/Iron Syrup (Lederle) p 576

◆Insta-Glucose (ICN Pharmaceuticals) p 409, 564

Ipecac Syrup, USP (Paddock) p 628

◆Isoclor Timesule Capsules (Fisons Consumer Health) p 409, 561

◆Itch-X Gel (Ascher) p 403, 509

K

◆Kaopectate Concentrated Anti-Diarrheal, Peppermint Flavor (Upjohn) p 431, 749

◆Kaopectate Concentrated Anti-Diarrheal, Regular Flavor (Upjohn) p 431, 749

◆Kaopectate Children's Chewable Tablets (Upjohn) p 431, 749

◆Kaopectate Children's Liquid (Upjohn) p 431, 749

◆Kaopectate Maximum Strength Caplets (Upjohn) p 431, 749

Kasof Capsules (Roberts) p 664

◆Keri Lotion - Original Formula (Bristol-Myers Products) p 405, 533

◆Keri Lotion - Silky Smooth Formula (Bristol-Myers Products) p 405, 533

◆Keri Lotion - Silky Smooth Fragrance Free Formula (Bristol-Myers Products) p 405, 533

◆Kyolic (Wakunaga) p 432, 752

◆ Kyolic-Aged Garlic Extract Flavor & Odor Modified Enriched with Vitamins B_1 and B_{12} (Wakunaga) p 432

◆ Kyolic-Formula 101 Capsules: Aged Garlic Extract (270 mg) (Wakunaga) p 432

◆ Kyolic-Super Formula 101 Garlic Plus Tablets & Capsules: Aged Garlic Extract Powder (270 mg) with Brewer's Yeast, Kelp & Algin (Wakunaga) p 432

L

Lacri-Lube NP Lubricant Ophthalmic Ointment (Allergan Pharmaceuticals) p 504

Lacri-Lube S.O.P. Sterile Ophthalmic Ointment (Allergan Pharmaceuticals) p 504

◆Lactaid Caplets (Now marketed by McNeil Consumer Products Co.) (Lactaid) p 414, 571

◆Lactaid Drops (Now marketed by McNeil Consumer Products Co.) (Lactaid) p 414, 571

◆Lactogest Softgel Capsules (Thompson Medical) p 431, 745

Lavoptik Eye Cup (Lavoptik) p 781

Lavoptik Eye Wash (Lavoptik) p 571

◆Legatrin Rub (Columbia) p 408, 556

◆Legatrin Tablets (Columbia) p 408, 556

Lever 2000 (Lever Brothers) p 578

◆Lice•Enz Foam (Copley) p 408, 556

◆Liquiprin Infants' Drops (Menley & James) p 415, 610

◆Listerine Antiseptic (Warner-Lambert) p 433, 756

◆Listermint with Fluoride (Warner-Lambert) p 433, 756

◆Lotrimin AF Antifungal Cream, Lotion and Solution (Schering-Plough HealthCare) p 426, 700

◆Lubriderm Bath Oil (Warner-Lambert) p 433, 757

◆Lubriderm Body Bar (Warner-Lambert) p 433, 756

◆Lubriderm Lotion (Warner-Lambert) p 433, 756

M

MG 217 Psoriasis Ointment and Lotion (Triton Consumer) p 747

MG 217 Psoriasis Shampoo and Conditioner (Triton Consumer) p 747

◆Maalox HRF Heartburn Relief Formula (Rhone-Poulenc Rorer Consumer) p 420, 649

◆Maalox Plus Suspension/Tablets (Rhone-Poulenc Rorer Consumer) p 421, 649

◆Extra Strength Maalox Plus Suspension (Rhone-Poulenc Rorer Consumer) p 420, 650

Magonate Tablets and Liquid (Fleming) p 563

Mag-Ox 400 (Blaine) p 516

MagTab SR Caplets (Niché Pharmaceuticals) p 624

◆Maltsupex Liquid, Powder & Tablets (Wallace) p 432, 753

Marblen Suspension Peach/Apricot (Fleming) p 563

Marblen Suspension Unflavored (Fleming) p 563

Marblen Tablets (Fleming) p 563

◆Marezine Tablets (Burroughs Wellcome) p 406, 539

Marlyn Formula 50 (Marlyn) p 586

Marlyn Formula 50 Mega Forte (Marlyn) p 587

Massengill Baby Powder Soft Cloth Towelette and Fragrance Free Soft Cloth Towelette (SmithKline Beecham) p 713

◆Massengill Disposable Douches (SmithKline Beecham) p 427, 712

Massengill Liquid Concentrate (SmithKline Beecham) p 712

◆Massengill Medicated Disposable Douche (SmithKline Beecham) p 427, 713

Massengill Medicated Liquid Concentrate (SmithKline Beecham) p 713

Massengill Medicated Soft Cloth Towelette (SmithKline Beecham) p 713

Massengill Powder (SmithKline Beecham) p 712

◆Medi-Flu Caplet, Liquid (Parke-Davis) p 419, 634

◆Medi-Flu Without Drowsiness Caplets (Parke-Davis) p 419, 635

◆Medipren ibuprofen Caplets and Tablets (McNeil Consumer Products) p 414, 587

◆Metamucil Powder, Sugar Free, Regular Flavor (Procter & Gamble)

◆Micatin Antifungal Cream (Ortho Pharmaceutical) p 418, 627

◆Micatin Antifungal Deodorant Spray Powder (Ortho Pharmaceutical) p 418, 627

◆Micatin Antifungal Powder (Ortho Pharmaceutical) p 418, 627

◆Micatin Antifungal Spray Liquid (Ortho Pharmaceutical) p 418, 627

◆Micatin Antifungal Spray Powder (Ortho Pharmaceutical) p 418, 627

Micatin Jock Itch Cream (Ortho Pharmaceutical) p 627

Micatin Jock Itch Spray Powder (Ortho Pharmaceutical) p 627

◆Midol IB Cramp Relief Formula (Sterling Health) p 430, 733

◆Maximum Strength Midol Multi-Symptom Menstrual Formula (Sterling Health) p 430, 733

◆Maximum Strength Midol Premenstrual Pain Formula (Sterling Health) p 430, 733

◆Regular Strength Midol Multi-Symptom Menstrual Formula (Sterling Health) p 430, 732

◆Teen Formula Midol (Sterling Health) p 430, 734

◆Miles Nervine Nighttime Sleep-Aid (Miles Consumer) p 417, 619

◆Mobigesic Analgesic Tablets (Ascher) p 403, 509

◆Mobisyl Analgesic Creme (Ascher) p 403, 510

◆Moisture Drops (Bausch & Lomb Personal) p 404, 514

◆Moisturel Cream (Westwood) p 433, 758

◆Moisturel Lotion (Westwood) p 433, 758

◆Moisturel Sensitive Skin Cleanser (Westwood) p 433, 759

Momentum Muscular Backache Formula (Whitehall) p 767

◆Monistat 7 Vaginal Cream (Ortho Pharmaceutical) p 418, 627

◆Monistat 7 Vaginal Suppositories (Ortho Pharmaceutical) p 418, 627

◆Motrin IB Caplets and Tablets (Upjohn) p 432, 750

◆Murine Ear Drops (Ross) p 422, 677

◆Murine Ear Wax Removal System (Ross) p 422, 677

◆Murine Eye Lubricant (Ross) p 422, 678

◆Murine Plus Lubricating Eye Redness Reliever (Ross) p 422, 678

◆Myadec (Parke-Davis) p 419, 635

◆Mycelex OTC Cream Antifungal (Miles Consumer) p 417, 619

◆Mycelex OTC Solution Antifungal (Miles Consumer) p 417, 619

◆Mycitracin Plus Pain Reliever (Upjohn) p 432, 750

◆Maximum Strength Mycitracin Triple Antibiotic First Aid Ointment (Upjohn) p 432, 750

◆Mylanta Gas Tablets-40 mg (J&J•Merck Consumer) p 410, 568

◆Mylanta Gas Tablets-80 mg (J&J•Merck Consumer) p 410, 569

◆Mylanta Liquid (J&J•Merck Consumer) p 410, 567

◆Mylanta Tablets (J&J•Merck Consumer) p 410, 567

◆Mylanta Double Strength Liquid (J&J•Merck Consumer) p 410, 567

◆Mylanta Double Strength Tablets (J&J•Merck Consumer) p 410, 567

◆Maximum Strength Mylanta Gas Tablets-125 mg (J&J•Merck Consumer) p 410, 569

◆Mylicon Drops (J&J•Merck Consumer) p 410, 568

(◆ Shown in Product Identification Section)

◆Myoflex Analgesic Creme (Fisons Consumer Health) p 409, 561

N

◆NP-27 (Thompson Medical) p 431, 746
NTZ Long Acting Nasal Spray & Drops 0.05% (Sterling Health) p 735
Naldecon CX Adult Liquid (Apothecon) p 505
Naldecon DX Adult Liquid (Apothecon) p 505
Naldecon DX Children's Syrup (Apothecon) p 506
Naldecon DX Pediatric Drops (Apothecon) p 506
Naldecon EX Children's Syrup (Apothecon) p 507
Naldecon EX Pediatric Drops (Apothecon) p 507
Naldecon Senior DX Cough/Cold Liquid (Apothecon) p 507
Naldecon Senior EX Cough/Cold Liquid (Apothecon) p 508
◆NāSal Moisturizing Nasal Spray (Sterling Health) p 430, 734
◆NāSal Moisturizing Nose Drops (Sterling Health) p 430, 734
Natabec Kapseals (Parke-Davis) p 636
◆Natural Best Vitamin E 1000 I.U. and 400 I.U. (Neutrin) p 417, 622
◆Nature's Remedy Enema, Mineral Oil (SmithKline Beecham) p 427, 714
◆Nature's Remedy Enema, Regular (SmithKline Beecham) p 427, 714
◆Nature's Remedy Natural Vegetable Laxative Tablets (SmithKline Beecham) p 427, 714
Neoloid (Lederle) p 577
◆Neosporin Cream (Burroughs Wellcome) p 406, 539
◆Neosporin Ointment (Burroughs Wellcome) p 406, 539
◆Neosporin Maximum Strength Ointment (Burroughs Wellcome) p 406, 539
Neo-Synephrine Maximum Strength 12 Hour Nasal Spray (Sterling Health) p 734
◆Neo-Synephrine Maximum Strength 12 Hour Nasal Spray Pump (Sterling Health) p 430, 734
Neo-Synephrine Nasal Solutions, Pediatric, Mild, Regular & Extra Strength (Sterling Health) p 734
◆Neo-Synephrine Nasal Sprays, Pediatric, Mild, Regular & Extra Strength (Sterling Health) p 430, 734
◆Neo-Synephrine Nose Drops (Sterling Health) p 430, 734
Nephrox Suspension (Fleming) p 563
◆Neutrogena Cleansing Wash (Neutrogena) p 417, 622
◆Neutrogena Moisture (Neutrogena) p 417, 622
◆Neutrogena Moisture SPF 15 Untinted (Neutrogena) p 417, 623
◆Neutrogena Moisture SPF 15 with Sheer Tint (Neutrogena) p 417, 623
◆Neutrogena Norwegian Formula Emulsion (Neutrogena) p 417, 623
◆Neutrogena Norwegian Formula Hand Cream (Neutrogena) p 417, 623
◆Neutrogena Sunblock (Neutrogena) p 417, 623
Neutrogena T/Derm Tar Emollient (Neutrogena) p 623
◆Neutrogena T/Gel Therapeutic Shampoo (Neutrogena) p 417, 623
◆Neutrogena T/Sal Therapeutic Shampoo (Neutrogena) p 417, 624
◆N'ICE Medicated Sugarless Sore Throat and Cough Lozenges (SmithKline Beecham) p 427, 714
◆N'ICE Sugarless Vitamin C Drops (SmithKline Beecham) p 427, 714
Nicotinex Elixir (Fleming) p 563
◆Nix Creme Rinse (Burroughs Wellcome) p 540, 407
◆No Doz Fast Acting Alertness Aid Tablets (Bristol-Myers Products) p 406, 533

◆No Doz Maximum Strength Caplets (Bristol-Myers Products) p 405, 533
Norwich Maximum Strength Aspirin (Chattem) p 546
Norwich Regular Strength Aspirin (Chattem) p 546
◆Nōstril Nasal Decongestant (CIBA Consumer) p 407, 552
◆Nōstrilla Long Acting Nasal Decongestant (CIBA Consumer) p 407, 552
◆Novahistine DMX (Marion Merrell Dow) p 412, 583
◆Novahistine Elixir (Marion Merrell Dow) p 412, 584
◆Nupercainal Hemorrhoidal and Anesthetic Ointment (CIBA Consumer) p 408, 552
◆Nupercainal Pain Relief Cream (CIBA Consumer) p 408, 553
◆Nupercainal Suppositories (CIBA Consumer) p 408, 553
◆Nuprin Ibuprofen/Analgesic Tablets & Caplets (Bristol-Myers Products) p 406, 534
◆Nursoy (Wyeth-Ayerst) p 435, 775
Nytol Tablets (Block) p 517

O

Ocean Mist (Fleming) p 563
◆OcuClear Eye Drops (See PDR For Ophthalmology) (Schering-Plough HealthCare) p 426
Oil of Olay Daily UV Protectant SPF 15 Beauty Fluid-Regular & Fragrance Free (Olay Co. Inc.) (Richardson-Vicks) p 653
Oil of Olay Daily UV Protectant SPF 15 Moisture Replenishing Cream-Regular & Fragrance Free (Olay Co. Inc.) (Richardson-Vicks) p 653
Oil of Olay Foaming Face Wash (Olay Co. Inc.) (Richardson-Vicks) p 654
◆One-A-Day Essential Vitamins (Miles Consumer) p 417, 620
◆One-A-Day Maximum Formula Vitamins and Minerals (Miles Consumer) p 417, 620
◆One-A-Day Plus Extra C Vitamins (Miles Consumer) p 417, 620
◆One-A-Day Stressgard Formula Vitamins (Miles Consumer) p 417, 620
◆One-A-Day Women's Formula Multivitamins with Calcium, Extra Iron, Zinc and Beta Carotene (Miles Consumer) p 417, 620
◆Optilets-500 Filmtab (Abbott) p 403, 502
◆Optilets-M-500 Filmtab (Abbott) p 403, 502
◆Baby Orajel (Del Pharmaceuticals) p 408, 557
◆Maximum Strength Orajel (Del Pharmaceuticals) p 408, 557
◆Orajel Mouth-Aid (Del Pharmaceuticals) p 408, 557
Orchid Fresh II Perineal/Ostomy Cleanser (Care-Tech) p 545
◆Ornex Caplets (Menley & James) p 415, 610
◆Maximum Strength Ornex Caplets (Menley & James) p 415, 610
◆Ortho-Gynol Contraceptive Jelly (Ortho Pharmaceutical) p 418, 626
Orthoxicol Cough Syrup (Roberts) p 665
◆Os-Cal 500 Chewable Tablets (Marion Merrell Dow) p 412, 585
◆Os-Cal 500 Tablets (Marion Merrell Dow) p 412, 585
◆Os-Cal 250+D Tablets (Marion Merrell Dow) p 412, 585
◆Os-Cal 500+D Tablets (Marion Merrell Dow) p 412, 585
◆Os-Cal Fortified Tablets (Marion Merrell Dow) p 412, 585
◆Os-Cal Plus Tablets (Marion Merrell Dow) p 412, 586
◆Oscillococcinum (Boiron) p 404, 519
◆Otrivin Nasal Drops (CIBA Consumer) p 408, 553
◆Otrivin Pediatric Nasal Drops (CIBA Consumer) p 408, 553
Outgro Solution (Whitehall) p 767

Oxipor VHC Lotion for Psoriasis (Whitehall) p 768
◆Oxy Lathering Facial Scrub (SmithKline Beecham) p 428, 715
◆Oxy Medicated Cleanser (SmithKline Beecham) p 428, 715
◆Oxy Medicated Pads - Regular, Sensitive Skin, and Maximum Strength (SmithKline Beecham) p 427, 716
◆Oxy Medicated Soap (SmithKline Beecham) p 428, 715
◆Oxy Night Watch Nighttime Acne Medication-Maximum Strength and Sensitive Skin Formulas (SmithKline Beecham) p 428, 716
◆Oxy 10 Daily Face Wash Antibacterial Skin Wash (SmithKline Beecham) p 427, 716
◆Oxy-5 and Oxy-10 Tinted and Vanishing Formulas with Sorboxyl (SmithKline Beecham) p 427, 715

P

◆P-A-C Analgesic Tablets (Roberts) p 421, 665
◆pHisoDerm Cleansing Bar (Sterling Health) p 430, 738
◆pHisoDerm For Baby (Sterling Health) p 430, 738
◆pHisoDerm Skin Cleanser and Conditioner - Regular and Oily (Sterling Health) p 430, 738
◆pHisoPUFF (Sterling Health) p 430, 738
PRID Salve (Walker Pharmacal) p 753
P & S Liquid (Baker Cummins Pharmaceuticals) p 511
P & S Plus Tar Gel (Baker Cummins Pharmaceuticals) p 512
P & S Shampoo (Baker Cummins Pharmaceuticals) p 512
Extra Strength Pamprin Multi-Symptom Formula Tablets and Caplets (Chattem) p 547
Maximum Strength Pamprin Cramp Relief Formula Caplets (Chattem) p 547
◆Children's Panadol Chewable Tablets, Liquid, Infants' Drops (Sterling Health) p 430, 735
◆Junior Strength Panadol (Sterling Health) p 430, 736
◆Maximum Strength Panadol Tablets and Caplets (Sterling Health) p 430, 736
◆Pazo Hemorrhoid Ointment & Suppositories (Bristol-Myers Products) p 406, 534
◆PediaCare Allergy Formula Liquid (McNeil Consumer Products) p 414, 588
◆PediaCare Cough-Cold Formula Liquid and Chewable Tablets (McNeil Consumer Products) p 414, 588
◆PediaCare Decongestant Drops (McNeil Consumer Products) p 414, 588
◆PediaCare Night Rest Cough-Cold Formula Liquid (McNeil Consumer Products) p 414, 588
◆PediaCare 6-12 Cough-Cold Formula Chewable Tablets (McNeil Consumer Products) p 414, 588
Pedialyte Oral Electrolyte Maintenance Solution (Ross) p 678
◆Pen•Kera Creme (Ascher) p 403, 510
Pepto-Bismol Liquid & Tablets (Procter & Gamble) p 644
Maximum Strength Pepto-Bismol Liquid (Procter & Gamble) p 644
Percogesic Analgesic Tablets (Richardson-Vicks) p 654
◆Perdiem Fiber Granules (Rhone-Poulenc Rorer Consumer) p 421, 652
◆Perdiem Granules (Rhone-Poulenc Rorer Consumer) p 421, 651
◆Peri-Colace (Mead Johnson Pharmaceuticals) p 415, 606
◆Phazyme Drops (Reed & Carnrick) p 420, 645
Phazyme Tablets (Reed & Carnrick) p 645
◆Phazyme-125 Softgels Maximum Strength (Reed & Carnrick) p 420, 645
◆Phazyme-95 Tablets (Reed & Carnrick) p 420, 645

(◆ Shown in Product Identification Section)

◆Phillips' LaxCaps (Sterling Health) p 430, 736
◆Concentrated Phillips' Milk of Magnesia (Sterling Health) p 430, 737
◆Phillips' Milk of Magnesia Liquid (Sterling Health) p 430, 737
◆Phillips' Milk of Magnesia Tablets (Sterling Health) p 430, 737
◆Polysporin Ointment (Burroughs Wellcome) p 407, 540
◆Polysporin Powder (Burroughs Wellcome) p 407, 540
◆Poly-Vi-Sol Vitamins, Chewable Tablets and Drops (without Iron) (Mead Johnson Nutritionals) p 414, 603
◆Poly-Vi-Sol Vitamins, Circus Shapes Chewable (without Iron) (Mead Johnson Nutritionals) p 414, 603
◆Poly-Vi-Sol Vitamins with Iron, Chewable Tablets and Circus Shapes Chewable (Mead Johnson Nutritionals) p 414, 604
◆Poly-Vi-Sol Vitamins with Iron, Drops (Mead Johnson Nutritionals) p 414, 604
Posture 600 mg (Whitehall) p 768
Posture-D 600 mg (Whitehall) p 768
Prēmsyn PMS (Chattem) p 547
◆Preparation H Cleansing Tissues (Whitehall) p 434, 769
◆Preparation H Hemorrhoidal Cream (Whitehall) p 434, 768
◆Preparation H Hemorrhoidal Ointment (Whitehall) p 434, 768
◆Preparation H Hemorrhoidal Suppositories (Whitehall) p 434, 768
PreSun Active 15 and 30 Clear Gel Sunscreens (Bristol-Myers Products) p 535
◆PreSun for Kids Lotion (Bristol-Myers Products) p 406, 535
◆PreSun 23 and For Kids, Spray Mist Sunscreens (Bristol-Myers Products) p 406, 535
PreSun 8 and 15 Moisturizing Sunscreens with KERI Moisturizers (Bristol-Myers Products) p 535
PreSun 25 Moisturizing Sunscreen with KERI Moisturizer (Bristol-Myers Products) p 535
◆PreSun 15 and 29 Sensitive Skin Sunscreens (Bristol-Myers Products) p 406, 536
PreSun 46 Moisturizing Sunscreen (Bristol-Myers Products) p 536
◆Primatene Mist (Whitehall) p 435, 769
Primatene Mist Suspension (Whitehall) p 770
◆Primatene Tablets-M Formula (Whitehall) p 435, 770
◆Primatene Tablets-P Formula (Whitehall) p 435, 770
◆Primatene Tablets-Regular Formula (Whitehall) p 435, 770
◆Privine Nasal Solution and Drops (CIBA Consumer) p 408, 554
◆Privine Nasal Spray (CIBA Consumer) p 408, 554
proctoFoam/non-steroid (Reed & Carnrick) p 645
Progaine Shampoo (Upjohn) p 750
Promise Toothpaste (Block) p 517
◆Pronto Lice Killing Shampoo Kit (Del Pharmaceuticals) p 408, 557
◆Pronto Lice Killing Spray (Del Pharmaceuticals) p 408
Purge Concentrate (Fleming) p 563
◆Pyrroxate Capsules (Roberts) p 421, 665

Q

◆Q-vel Muscle Relaxant Pain Reliever (CIBA Consumer) p 408, 554

R

◆R&C Lice Treatment Kit (Reed & Carnrick) p 420
◆R&C Shampoo (Reed & Carnrick) p 420, 646
◆R&C Spray (Reed & Carnrick) p 420, 646
◆Reese's Pinworm Medicine (Reese Chemical) p 420, 647

Refresh P.M. Lubricant Ophthalmic Ointment (Allergan Pharmaceuticals) p 505
Rehydralyte Oral Electrolyte Rehydration Solution (Ross) p 679
◆Replens (Warner-Lambert) p 433, 757
Rheaban Maximum Strength Tablets (Pfizer Consumer) p 639
◆Rhulicream (Rydelle) p 423, 681
◆Rhuligel (Rydelle) p 423, 681
◆Rhulispray (Rydelle) p 423, 681
◆Ricelyte, Rice-Based Oral Electrolyte Maintenance Solution (Mead Johnson Nutritionals) p 415, 604
Rid Lice Control Spray (Pfizer Consumer) p 639
Rid Lice Killing Shampoo (Pfizer Consumer) p 640
Riopan Antacid Suspension (Whitehall) p 770
Riopan Antacid Swallow Tablets (Whitehall) p 770
Riopan Plus Suspension (Whitehall) p 771
Riopan Plus Chew Tablets (Whitehall) p 771
Riopan Plus Chew Tablets in Rollpacks (Whitehall) p 771
◆Riopan Plus 2 Suspension-Mint and Cherry flavors (Whitehall) p 435, 771
◆Riopan Plus 2 Chew Tablets-Mint and Cherry Vanilla flavors (Whitehall) p 435, 771
◆Robitussin (Robins Consumer) p 422, 672
Robitussin Cough Calmers (Robins Consumer) p 674
◆Robitussin Cough Drops (Robins Consumer) p 422, 674
◆Robitussin Maximum Strength Cough Suppressant (Robins Consumer) p 422, 675
◆Robitussin Night Relief (Robins Consumer) p 422, 675
◆Robitussin Pediatric Cough & Cold Formula (Robins Consumer) p 422, 675
◆Robitussin Pediatric Cough Suppressant (Robins Consumer) p 422, 676
◆Robitussin-CF (Robins Consumer) p 422, 673
◆Robitussin-DM (Robins Consumer) p 422, 673
◆Robitussin-PE (Robins Consumer) p 422, 674
◆Rolaids (Warner-Lambert) p 433, 757
◆Rolaids (Calcium Rich/Sodium Free) (Warner-Lambert) p 433, 757
◆Extra Strength Rolaids (Warner-Lambert) p 433, 758
Ross Pediatric Nutritional Products (Ross) p 677
◆Ryna Liquid (Wallace) p 432, 754
◆Ryna-C Liquid (Wallace) p 432, 754
◆Ryna-CX Liquid (Wallace) p 432, 754

S

◆SMA Iron Fortified Infant Formula, Concentrated, Ready-to-Feed and Powder (Wyeth-Ayerst) p 435, 776
◆SMA lo-iron Infant Formula, Concentrated, Ready-to-Feed, and Powder (Wyeth-Ayerst) p 435, 776
S.T.37 Antiseptic Solution (Menley & James) p 611
Salinex Nasal Mist and Drops (Muro) p 621
Salivart Saliva Substitute (Gebauer) p 564
Satin Antimicrobial Skin Cleanser (Care-Tech) p 545
◆Sebulex Antiseborrheic Treatment Shampoo (Westwood) p 433, 759
◆Sebutone and Sebutone Cream Antiseborrheic Tar Shampoos (Westwood) p 433, 759
◆Selsun Blue Dandruff Shampoo (Ross) p 422, 679
◆Selsun Blue Dandruff Shampoo-Extra Medicated (Ross) p 422, 679
◆Selsun Blue Extra Conditioning Dandruff Shampoo (Ross) p 422, 679

Semicid Vaginal Contraceptive Inserts (Whitehall) p 772
Mint Gel Sensodyne (Block) p 518
Mint Sensodyne Toothpaste (Block) p 518
Original Sensodyne Toothpaste (Block) p 517
◆Serutan Toasted Granules (Menley & James) p 415, 611
◆Sigtab Tablets (Roberts) p 421, 666
Sinarest No Drowsiness Tablets (Fisons Consumer Health) p 561
Sinarest Tablets (Fisons Consumer Health) p 561
Sinarest Extra Strength Tablets (Fisons Consumer Health) p 561
◆Sine-Aid Maximum Strength Sinus Headache Gelcaps, Caplets and Tablets (McNeil Consumer Products) p 414, 589
◆Sine-Off Maximum Strength Allergy/Sinus Formula Caplets (SmithKline Beecham) p 428, 717
◆Sine-Off Maximum Strength No Drowsiness Formula Caplets (SmithKline Beecham) p 428, 717
◆Sine-Off Sinus Medicine Tablets-Aspirin Formula (SmithKline Beecham) p 428, 718
Singlet Tablets (Marion Merrell Dow) p 586
◆Sinutab Sinus Medication, Maximum Strength Caplets (Parke-Davis) p 419, 636
◆Sinutab Sinus Allergy Medication, Maximum Strength Tablets (Parke-Davis) p 419, 636
◆Sinutab Sinus Medication, Maximum Strength Without Drowsiness Formula Tablets & Caplets (Parke-Davis) p 419, 637
◆Sinutab Sinus Medication, Regular Strength Without Drowsiness Formula (Parke-Davis) p 419, 636
Sleep-ettes-D Tablets (Reese Chemical) p 647
Sleep-eze 3 Tablets (Whitehall) p 772
Sleepinal Medicated Night Tea (Thompson Medical) p 746
◆Sleepinal Night-time Sleep Aid Capsules (Thompson Medical) p 431, 746
◆Slow Fe Tablets (CIBA Consumer) p 408, 554
◆Sominex Caplets and Tablets (SmithKline Beecham) p 428, 718
◆Sominex Pain Relief Formula (SmithKline Beecham) p 428, 718
◆Soothers Throat Drops (Warner-Lambert) p 433, 758
St. Joseph Adult Chewable Aspirin (81 mg.) (Schering-Plough HealthCare) p 701
St. Joseph Aspirin-Free Fever Reducer for Children Chewable Tablets (Schering-Plough HealthCare) p 701
St. Joseph Cold Tablets for Children (Schering-Plough HealthCare) p 702
St. Joseph Cough Suppressant for Children (Schering-Plough HealthCare) p 702
◆Star-Optic Eye Wash (Stellar) p 428, 723
◆Star-Optic Ear Solution (Stellar) p 428, 723
◆Stresstabs (Lederle) p 411, 577
◆Stresstabs + Iron, Advanced Formula (Lederle) p 411, 577
◆Stresstabs + Zinc (Lederle) p 411, 577
◆Stri-Dex Dual Textured Maximum Strength Pads (Sterling Health) p 431, 739
Stri-Dex Dual Textured Maximum Strength Big Pads (Sterling Health) p 739
◆Stri-Dex Dual Textured Regular Strength Pads (Sterling Health) p 431, 739
Stri-Dex Dual Textured Regular Strength Big Pads (Sterling Health) p 739
Stri-Dex Dual Textured Sensitive Skin Pads (Sterling Health) p 739
Stri-Dex Super Scrub Pads (Sterling Health) p 739
◆Stuart Prenatal Tablets (Stuart) p 431, 742

(◆ Shown in Product Identification Section)

◆The Stuart Formula Tablets (J&J•Merck Consumer) p 410, 569
◆Stuartinic Tablets (J&J•Merck Consumer) p 410, 570
◆Sublingual B-Total (Sublingual Products) p 431, 742
Sublingual C with Niacin (Sublingual Products) p 743
Sublingual Zinc (Sublingual Products) p 743
◆Sucrets Original Mint (SmithKline Beecham) p 428, 719
◆Sucrets Children's Cherry Flavored Sore Throat Lozenges (SmithKline Beecham) p 428, 719
◆Sucrets Cold Formula (SmithKline Beecham) p 428, 719
◆Sucrets Maximum Strength Wintergreen and Sucrets Wild Cherry (Regular Strength) Sore Throat Lozenges (SmithKline Beecham) p 428, 719
◆Sucrets Maximum Strength Sprays (SmithKline Beecham) p 428, 720
◆Sudafed Children's Liquid (Burroughs Wellcome) p 407, 540
◆Sudafed Cough Syrup (Burroughs Wellcome) p 407, 541
◆Sudafed Plus Liquid (Burroughs Wellcome) p 407, 541
◆Sudafed Plus Tablets (Burroughs Wellcome) p 407, 542
◆Sudafed Severe Cold Formula Caplets (Burroughs Wellcome) p 407, 542
◆Sudafed Severe Cold Formula Tablets (Burroughs Wellcome) p 407, 542
◆Sudafed Sinus Caplets (Burroughs Wellcome) p 407, 543
◆Sudafed Sinus Tablets (Burroughs Wellcome) p 407, 543
◆Sudafed Tablets, 30 mg (Burroughs Wellcome) p 407, 541
◆Sudafed Tablets, Adult Strength, 60 mg (Burroughs Wellcome) p 407, 541
◆Sudafed 12 Hour Tablets (Burroughs Wellcome) p 407, 543
◆Sunkist Children's Chewable Multivitamins - Complete (CIBA Consumer) p 408, 555
◆Sunkist Children's Chewable Multivitamins - Plus Extra C (CIBA Consumer) p 408, 555
◆Sunkist Children's Chewable Multivitamins - Plus Iron (CIBA Consumer) p 408, 555
◆Sunkist Children's Chewable Multivitamins - Regular (CIBA Consumer) p 408, 554
◆Sunkist Vitamin C - Chewable (CIBA Consumer) p 408, 555
◆Sunkist Vitamin C - Easy to Swallow (CIBA Consumer) p 408, 555
Surbex (Abbott) p 502
Surbex with C (Abbott) p 502
◆Surbex-750 with Iron (Abbott) p 403, 503
◆Surbex-750 with Zinc (Abbott) p 403, 503
◆Surbex-T (Abbott) p 403, 502
Surelac Chewable Lactase Enzyme Tablets (Caraco) p 544
◆Surfak Liqui-Gels (Upjohn) p 432, 751
◆Syllact Powder (Wallace) p 432, 755

T

Tears Plus Lubricant Ophthalmic Solution (Allergan Pharmaceuticals) p 505
Techni-Care Surgical Scrub (Care-Tech) p 545
Tegrin Dandruff Shampoo (Block) p 518
Tegrin for Psoriasis Lotion, Skin Cream & Medicated Soap (Block) p 518
Tegrin-HC with Hydrocortisone Anti-Itch Ointment (Block) p 518
◆Teldrin Timed-Release Allergy Capsules, 12 mg. (SmithKline Beecham) p 428, 720
◆Tempra 1 Acetaminophen Infant Drops (Mead Johnson Nutritionals) p 415, 605
◆Tempra 2 Acetaminophen Toddlers Syrup (Mead Johnson Nutritionals) p 415, 605

◆Tempra 3 Chewable Tablets, Regular or Double-Strength (Mead Johnson Nutritionals) p 415, 605
Thera-Combex H-P (Parke-Davis) p 637
◆TheraFlu Flu and Cold Medicine (Sandoz Consumer) p 423, 684
◆TheraFlu Flu, Cold and Cough Medicine (Sandoz Consumer) p 423, 684
Theragold Analgesic Lotion (Au Pharmaceuticals) p 510
◆Theragran Liquid (Apothecon) p 403, 508
◆Theragran Stress Formula (Apothecon) p 403, 509
◆Theragran Tablets (Apothecon) p 403, 508
◆Theragran-M Tablets (Apothecon) p 403, 508
Therapeutic Gold Analgesic Lotion (Au Pharmaceuticals) p 510
◆Therapeutic Mineral Ice, Pain Relieving Gel (Bristol-Myers Products) p 406, 536
◆Therapeutic Mineral Ice Exercise Formula, Pain Relieving Gel (Bristol-Myers Products) p 406, 536
Thermotabs (Menley & James) p 611
◆Throat Discs Throat Lozenges (Marion Merrell Dow) p 412, 586
◆Tinactin Aerosol Liquid 1% (Schering-Plough HealthCare) p 426, 703
◆Tinactin Aerosol Powder 1% (Schering-Plough HealthCare) p 426, 703
◆Tinactin Antifungal Cream, Solution & Powder 1% (Schering-Plough HealthCare) p 426, 703
Tinactin Deodorant Powder Aerosol 1% (Schering-Plough HealthCare) p 703
◆Tinactin Jock Itch Cream 1% (Schering-Plough HealthCare) p 426, 703
◆Tinactin Jock Itch Spray Powder 1% (Schering-Plough HealthCare) p 426, 703
◆Ting Antifungal Cream (Fisons Consumer Health) p 409, 562
◆Ting Antifungal Powder (Fisons Consumer Health) p 409, 562
◆Ting Antifungal Spray Liquid (Fisons Consumer Health) p 409, 562
◆Ting Antifungal Spray Powder (Fisons Consumer Health) p 409, 562
◆Today Vaginal Contraceptive Sponge (Whitehall) p 435, 772
Triaminic Allergy Tablets (Sandoz Consumer) p 685
Triaminic Chewables (Sandoz Consumer) p 685
◆Triaminic Cold Tablets (Sandoz Consumer) p 424, 685
◆Triaminic Expectorant (Sandoz Consumer) p 424, 686
◆Triaminic Nite Light (Sandoz Consumer) p 424, 686
◆Triaminic Syrup (Sandoz Consumer) p 423, 686
◆Triaminic-12 Tablets (Sandoz Consumer) p 424, 687
◆Triaminic-DM Syrup (Sandoz Consumer) p 423, 687
◆Triaminicin Tablets (Sandoz Consumer) p 424, 687
◆Triaminicol Multi-Symptom Cold Tablets (Sandoz Consumer) p 424, 688
◆Triaminicol Multi-Symptom Relief (Sandoz Consumer) p 424, 688
◆Tri-Vi-Sol Vitamin Drops (Mead Johnson Nutritionals) p 415, 606
◆Tri-Vi-Sol Vitamin Drops with Iron (Mead Johnson Nutritionals) p 415, 606
◆Tronolane Anesthetic Cream for Hemorrhoids (Ross) p 422, 679
◆Tronolane Hemorrhoidal Suppositories (Ross) p 422, 680
Troph-Iron Liquid (Menley & James) p 611
Trophite Liquid (Menley & James) p 612
Tucks Cream (Parke-Davis) p 637
◆Tucks Premoistened Pads (Parke-Davis) p 420, 637
Tucks Take-Alongs (Parke-Davis) p 637
◆Tums Antacid Tablets (SmithKline Beecham) p 428, 720
◆Tums E-X Antacid Tablets (SmithKline Beecham) p 428, 720
◆Tums Plus Antacid Anti-gas Tablets, Assorted Fruit or Peppermint (SmithKline Beecham) p 428, 721

◆Tylenol acetaminophen Children's Chewable Tablets & Elixir (McNeil Consumer Products) p 413, 590
◆Tylenol Allergy Sinus Medication Maximum Strength Gelcaps and Caplets (McNeil Consumer Products) p 413, 600
◆Children's Tylenol Cold Multi Symptom Liquid Formula and Chewable Tablets (McNeil Consumer Products) p 413, 594
◆Tylenol Cold & Flu Hot Medication, Packets (McNeil Consumer Products) p 413, 595
◆Tylenol Cold & Flu No Drowsiness Hot Medication, Packets (McNeil Consumer Products) p 413, 598
◆Tylenol Cold Multi Symptom Medication Caplets and Tablets (McNeil Consumer Products) p 413, 596
◆Tylenol Cold Medication, Effervescent Tablets (McNeil Consumer Products) p 413, 595
◆Tylenol Cold Medication No Drowsiness Formula Caplets (McNeil Consumer Products) p 413, 597
◆Tylenol Cold Night Time Medication Liquid (McNeil Consumer Products) p 413, 599
◆Tylenol Cough Medication Maximum Strength Liquid (McNeil Consumer Products) p 414, 601
◆Tylenol Cough Medication Maximum Strength Liquid with Decongestant (McNeil Consumer Products) p 414, 601
Tylenol, Extra Strength, acetaminophen Adult Liquid Pain Reliever (McNeil Consumer Products) p 593
◆Tylenol, Extra Strength, acetaminophen Gelcaps, Caplets, Tablets (McNeil Consumer Products) p 412, 413, 592
◆Tylenol, Infants' Drops (McNeil Consumer Products) p 413, 590
◆Tylenol, Junior Strength, acetaminophen Coated Caplets, Grape and Fruit Chewable Tablets (McNeil Consumer Products) p 413, 414, 591
◆Tylenol, Maximum Strength, Sinus Medication Gelcaps, Caplets and Tablets (McNeil Consumer Products) p 413, 602
◆Tylenol, Regular Strength, acetaminophen Caplets and Tablets (McNeil Consumer Products) p 412, 591
◆Tylenol PM Extra Strength Pain Reliever/Sleep Aid Caplets and Tablets (McNeil Consumer Products) p 414, 593

U

Ultra Mide 25 (Baker Cummins Pharmaceuticals) p 512
◆Unicap Softgel Capsules & Tablets (Upjohn) p 432, 751
Unicap Jr. Chewable Tablets (Upjohn) p 751
◆Unicap M Tablets (Upjohn) p 432, 751
Unicap Plus Iron Vitamin Formula Tablets (Upjohn) p 751
◆Unicap Sr. Tablets (Upjohn) p 432, 752
◆Unicap T (Upjohn) p 432, 752
Unisom Nighttime Sleep Aid (Pfizer Consumer) p 640
Unisom with Pain Relief Nighttime Sleep Aid/Analgesic (Pfizer Consumer) p 640
Uro-Mag (Blaine) p 516
Ursinus Inlay-Tabs (Sandoz Consumer) p 688

V

◆Vanquish Analgesic Caplets (Sterling Health) p 431, 739
Vaseline Intensive Care Moisturizing Sunblock Lotion (Chese-Pond's) p 548
Vaseline Intensive Care U.V. Daily Defense Lotion for Hand and Body (Chese-Pond's) p 548
Extra Strength Vaseline Intensive Care Lotion (Chese-Pond's) p 548

(◆ Shown in Product Identification Section)

Vaseline Pure Petroleum Jelly Skin Protectant/Lip Therapy (Chese-Pond's) p 548

Vicks Children's Cough Syrup (Richardson-Vicks) p 654

Vicks Children's NyQuil Nighttime Cold/Cough Medicine (Richardson-Vicks) p 659

Vicks Children's NyQuil Nighttime Head Cold/Allergy Medicine (Richardson-Vicks) p 659

Vicks Cough Drops (Richardson-Vicks) p 655

Extra Strength Vicks Cough Drops (Richardson-Vicks) p 655

Vicks Daycare Daytime Cold Medicine Caplets (Richardson-Vicks) p 655

Vicks Daycare Daytime Cold Medicine Liquid (Richardson-Vicks) p 655

Vicks Formula 44 Cough Control Discs (Richardson-Vicks) p 656

Vicks Formula 44 Cough Medicine (Richardson-Vicks) p 656

Vicks Formula 44D Cough and Decongestant Medicine (Richardson-Vicks) p 656

Vicks Formula 44E Cough & Expectorant Medicine (Richardson-Vicks) p 657

Vicks Formula 44M Multi-Symptom Cough & Cold Medicine (Richardson-Vicks) p 657

Vicks Inhaler (Richardson-Vicks) p 659

Vicks NyQuil LiquiCaps Adult Nighttime Cold/Flu Medicine (Richardson-Vicks) p 661

Vicks NyQuil Nighttime Cold/Flu Medicine-Regular & Cherry Flavor (Richardson-Vicks) p 660

Vicks Pediatric Formula 44 Cough Medicine (Richardson-Vicks) p 657

Vicks Pediatric Formula 44d Cough & Decongestant Medicine (Richardson-Vicks) p 658

Vicks Pediatric Formula 44e Cough & Expectorant Medicine (Richardson-Vicks) p 659

Vicks Pediatric Formula 44m Multi-Symptom Cough & Cold Medicine (Richardson-Vicks) p 658

Vicks Sinex Decongestant Nasal Spray (Richardson-Vicks) p 661

Vicks Sinex Decongestant Nasal Ultra Fine Mist (Richardson-Vicks) p 661

Vicks Sinex Long-Acting Decongestant Nasal Spray (Richardson-Vicks) p 661

Vicks Sinex Long-Acting Decongestant Nasal Ultra Fine Mist (Richardson-Vicks) p 661

Vicks Vaporub (Richardson-Vicks) p 662

Vicks Vaposteam (Richardson-Vicks) p 662

Vicks Vatronol Nose Drops (Richardson-Vicks) p 662

◆Vicon Plus (Whitby) p 433, 760

◆Vicon-C Capsules (Whitby) p 433, 760

◆Visine A.C. Eye Drops (Pfizer Consumer) p 420, 641

◆Visine EXTRA Eye Drops (Pfizer Consumer) p 420, 642

◆Visine Eye Drops (Pfizer Consumer) p 420, 641

◆Visine L.R. Eye Drops (Pfizer Consumer) p 420, 642

Vitron-C Tablets (Fisons Consumer Health) p 562

Vivarin Stimulant Tablets (SmithKline Beecham) p 721

◆Vi-Zac (Whitby) p 433, 760

W

Wart-Off Wart Remover (Pfizer Consumer) p 642

Water-Jel Sterile Burn Dressings (Water-Jel Technologies) p 758

Wellcome Lanoline (Burroughs Wellcome) p 544

WinGel Liquid (Sterling Health) p 740

◆Wyanoids Relief Factor Hemorrhoidal Suppositories (Wyeth-Ayerst) p 435, 777

X

X-Seb Shampoo (Baker Cummins Pharmaceuticals) p 512

X-Seb Plus Conditioning Shampoo (Baker Cummins Pharmaceuticals) p 512

X-Seb T Shampoo (Baker Cummins Pharmaceuticals) p 513

X-Seb T Plus Conditioning Shampoo (Baker Cummins Pharmaceuticals) p 513

◆Xylocaine 2.5% Ointment (Astra) p 403, 510

Y

Yellolax (Luyties) p 578

Z

Z-BEC Tablets (Robins Consumer) p 676

Zephiran Chloride Aqueous Solution (Sanofi Winthrop Pharmaceuticals) p 689

Zephiran Chloride Spray (Sanofi Winthrop Pharmaceuticals) p 689

Zephiran Chloride Tinted Tincture (Sanofi Winthrop Pharmaceuticals) p 689

◆Zilactin Medicated Gel (Zila Pharmaceuticals) p 435, 777

Zilactol Medicated Liquid (Zila Pharmaceuticals) p 777

ZilaDent Oral Analgesic Gel (Zila Pharmaceuticals) p 777

◆Zincon Dandruff Shampoo (Lederle) p 411, 578

Zymacap Capsules (Roberts) p 666

(◆ Shown in Product Identification Section)

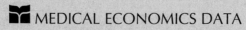

SECTION 3

Product Category Index

Products described in the Product Information (White) Section are listed according to their classifications. The headings and subheadings have been determined by the OTC Review process of the U.S. Food and Drug Administration. Classification of products have been determined by the Publisher with the cooperation of individual manufacturers. In cases where there were differences of opinion or where the manufacturer had no opinion, the Publisher made the final decision.

A

ACNE PRODUCTS
(see under DERMATOLOGICALS, ACNE PREPARATIONS)

ALLERGY RELIEF PRODUCTS
(see under COLD & COUGH PREPARATIONS, NASAL PREPARATIONS & ALLERGY RELIEF PRODUCTS, OPHTHALMIC)

ALLERGY RELIEF PRODUCTS, OPHTHALMIC
Allergy Drops (Bausch & Lomb Personal) p 403, 513
Clear Eyes ACR Astringent/Lubricating Eye Redness Reliever (Ross) p 422, 677
Visine A.C. Eye Drops (Pfizer Consumer) p 420, 641

AMEBICIDES & TRICHOMONACIDES
(see under ANTIPARASITICS)

AMINO ACID PREPARATIONS
Marlyn Formula 50 (Marlyn) p 586
Marlyn Formula 50 Mega Forte (Marlyn) p 587

ANALGESICS
ACETAMINOPHEN & COMBINATIONS
Actifed Plus Caplets (Burroughs Wellcome) p 406, 537
Actifed Plus Tablets (Burroughs Wellcome) p 406, 538
Aspirin Free Anacin Acetaminophen Film Coated Caplets (Whitehall) p 434, 762
Aspirin Free Anacin Acetaminophen Film Coated Tablets (Whitehall) p 434, 762
Bufferin A/F Nite Time Analgesic/Sleeping Aid Caplets (Bristol-Myers Products) p 404, 521
Datril Extra-Strength Analgesic Tablets (Bristol-Myers Products) p 405, 527
Aspirin Free Excedrin Analgesic Caplets (Bristol-Myers Products) p 405, 528

Excedrin Extra-Strength Analgesic Tablets & Caplets (Bristol-Myers Products) p 405, 529
Excedrin P.M. Analgesic/Sleeping Aid Tablets, Caplets and Liquid (Bristol-Myers Products) p 405, 530
Liquiprin Infants' Drops (Menley & James) p 415, 610
Maximum Strength Midol Multi-Symptom Menstrual Formula (Sterling Health) p 430, 733
Maximum Strength Midol Premenstrual Pain Formula (Sterling Health) p 430, 733
Regular Strength Midol Multi-Symptom Menstrual Formula (Sterling Health) p 430, 732
Teen Formula Midol (Sterling Health) p 430, 734
Extra Strength Pamprin Multi-Symptom Formula Tablets and Caplets (Chattem) p 547
Maximum Strength Pamprin Cramp Relief Formula Caplets (Chattem) p 547
Children's Panadol Chewable Tablets, Liquid, Infants' Drops (Sterling Health) p 430, 735
Junior Strength Panadol (Sterling Health) p 430, 736
Maximum Strength Panadol Tablets and Caplets (Sterling Health) p 430, 736
Percogesic Analgesic Tablets (Richardson-Vicks) p 654
Sominex Pain Relief Formula (SmithKline Beecham) p 428, 718
St. Joseph Aspirin-Free Fever Reducer for Children Chewable Tablets (Schering-Plough HealthCare) p 701
Tempra 1 Acetaminophen Infant Drops (Mead Johnson Nutritionals) p 415, 605
Tempra 2 Acetaminophen Toddlers Syrup (Mead Johnson Nutritionals) p 415, 605

Tempra 3 Chewable Tablets, Regular or Double-Strength (Mead Johnson Nutritionals) p 415, 605
Tylenol acetaminophen Children's Chewable Tablets & Elixir (McNeil Consumer Products) p 413, 590
Tylenol, Extra Strength, acetaminophen Adult Liquid Pain Reliever (McNeil Consumer Products) p 593
Tylenol, Extra Strength, acetaminophen Gelcaps, Caplets, Tablets (McNeil Consumer Products) p 412, 413, 592
Tylenol, Infants' Drops (McNeil Consumer Products) p 413, 590
Tylenol, Junior Strength, acetaminophen Coated Caplets, Grape and Fruit Chewable Tablets (McNeil Consumer Products) p 413, 414, 591
Tylenol, Regular Strength, acetaminophen Caplets and Tablets (McNeil Consumer Products) p 412, 591
Tylenol PM Extra Strength Pain Reliever/Sleep Aid Caplets and Tablets (McNeil Consumer Products) p 414, 593
Unisom with Pain Relief Nighttime Sleep Aid/Analgesic (Pfizer Consumer) p 640
Vanquish Analgesic Caplets (Sterling Health) p 431, 739

ASPIRIN
Children's Bayer Chewable Aspirin (Sterling Health) p 429, 724
Genuine Bayer Aspirin Tablets & Caplets (Sterling Health) p 428, 724
Maximum Bayer Aspirin Tablets & Caplets (Sterling Health) p 429, 725
Therapy Bayer Enteric Aspirin Caplets (Sterling Health) p 429, 728
8 Hour Bayer Timed-Release Aspirin (Sterling Health) p 429, 726
Empirin Aspirin (Burroughs Wellcome) p 406, 538
Halfprin Low Strength Aspirin Tablets (Kramer) p 410, 570

Norwich Maximum Strength Aspirin (Chattem) p 546
Norwich Regular Strength Aspirin (Chattem) p 546
St. Joseph Adult Chewable Aspirin (81 mg.) (Schering-Plough HealthCare) p 701

ASPIRIN COMBINATIONS
Alka-Seltzer Effervescent Antacid and Pain Reliever (Miles Consumer) p 416, 612
Alka-Seltzer Extra Strength Effervescent Antacid and Pain Reliever (Miles Consumer) p 416, 615
Alka-Seltzer (Flavored) Effervescent Antacid and Pain Reliever (Miles Consumer) p 416, 613
Anacin Coated Analgesic Caplets (Whitehall) p 434, 762
Anacin Coated Analgesic Tablets (Whitehall) p 434, 762
Anacin Maximum Strength Analgesic Coated Tablets (Whitehall) p 762
Arthritis Strength BC Powder (Block) p 516
Ascriptin A/D Caplets (Rhone-Poulenc Rorer Consumer) p 420, 649
Regular Strength Ascriptin Tablets (Rhone-Poulenc Rorer Consumer) p 420, 648
BC Powder (Block) p 517
BC Cold Powder Multi-Symptom Formula (Block) p 516
BC Cold Powder Multi-Symptom Non-Drowsy Formula (Block) p 516
Bayer Plus Aspirin Tablets (Sterling Health) p 429, 726
Extra Strength Bayer Plus Aspirin Caplets (Sterling Health) p 429, 727
Arthritis Strength Bufferin Analgesic Caplets (Bristol-Myers Products) p 404, 521
Extra Strength Bufferin Analgesic Tablets (Bristol-Myers Products) p 404, 522
Bufferin Analgesic Tablets and Caplets (Bristol-Myers Products) p 404, 519
Cama Arthritis Pain Reliever (Sandoz Consumer) p 682
Ecotrin Enteric Coated Aspirin Maximum Strength Tablets and Caplets (SmithKline Beecham) p 427, 708
Ecotrin Enteric Coated Aspirin Regular Strength Tablets and Caplets (SmithKline Beecham) p 427, 708
Excedrin Extra-Strength Analgesic Tablets & Caplets (Bristol-Myers Products) p 405, 529
Momentum Muscular Backache Formula (Whitehall) p 767
P-A-C Analgesic Tablets (Roberts) p 421, 665
Ursinus Inlay-Tabs (Sandoz Consumer) p 688
Vanquish Analgesic Caplets (Sterling Health) p 431, 739

ASPIRIN WITH ANTACIDS
Maximum Strength Arthritis Pain Formula by the Makers of Anacin Analgesic Tablets and Caplets (Whitehall) p 763

COLD GELS
Campho-Phenique Cold Sore Gel (Sterling Health) p 429, 731
Dentapaine Gel (Reese Chemical) p 647
Myoflex Analgesic Creme (Fisons Consumer Health) p 409, 561

IBUPROFEN
(see under ANALGESICS, NSAIDS)

NSAIDS
Advil Ibuprofen Caplets and Tablets (Whitehall) p 408, 761
Cramp End Tablets (Ohm Laboratories) p 418, 624
Haltran Tablets (Roberts) p 421, 664
Ibuprohm Ibuprofen Caplets (Ohm Laboratories) p 418, 625
Ibuprohm Ibuprofen Tablets (Ohm Laboratories) p 418, 625

Medipren ibuprofen Caplets and Tablets (McNeil Consumer Products) p 414, 587
Midol IB Cramp Relief Formula (Sterling Health) p 430, 733
Motrin IB Caplets and Tablets (Upjohn) p 432, 750
Nuprin Ibuprofen/Analgesic Tablets & Caplets (Bristol-Myers Products) p 406, 534

OTHER SALICYLATES & COMBINATIONS
Extra Strength Doan's P.M. (CIBA Consumer) p 407, 549
Myoflex Analgesic Creme (Fisons Consumer Health) p 409, 561

TOPICAL-ANALGESIC
Americaine Topical Anesthetic First Aid Ointment (Fisons Consumer Health) p 409, 559
Americaine Topical Anesthetic Spray (Fisons Consumer Health) p 409, 559
Anbesol Baby Teething Gel Anesthetic (Whitehall) p 434, 763
Anbesol Gel Antiseptic-Anesthetic-Regular Strength (Whitehall) p 434, 763
Anbesol Gel Antiseptic-Anesthetic - Maximum Strength (Whitehall) p 434, 763
Anbesol Liquid Antiseptic-Anesthetic (Whitehall) p 434, 763
Anbesol Liquid Antiseptic-Anesthetic - Maximum Strength (Whitehall) p 434, 763
Aveeno Anti-Itch Concentrated Lotion (Rydelle) p 423, 680
Aveeno Anti-Itch Cream (Rydelle) p 423, 680
Bactine Antiseptic/Anesthetic First Aid Liquid (Miles Consumer) p 416, 617
BiCozene Creme (Sandoz Consumer) p 423, 682
Campho-Phenique Cold Sore Gel (Sterling Health) p 429, 731
Campho-Phenique Liquid (Sterling Health) p 429, 731
Cepacol Anesthetic Lozenges (Troches) (Marion Merrell Dow) p 411, 580
Cepastat Cherry Flavor Sore Throat Lozenges (Marion Merrell Dow) p 411, 580
Cepastat Extra Strength Sore Throat Lozenges (Marion Merrell Dow) p 411, 580
Cheracol Sore Throat Spray (Roberts) p 663
Children's Chloraseptic Lozenges (Richardson-Vicks) p 652
Children's Chloraseptic Spray (Richardson-Vicks) p 654
Chloraseptic Liquid, Cherry, Menthol and Cool Mint (Richardson-Vicks) p 652
Chloraseptic Liquid - Nitrogen Propelled Spray (Richardson-Vicks) p 652
Corticaine External Analgesic (Whitby) p 433, 760
Dentapaine Gel (Reese Chemical) p 647
Dermoplast Anesthetic Pain Relief Lotion (Whitehall) p 764
Dermoplast Anesthetic Pain Relief Spray (Whitehall) p 764
Nupercainal Hemorrhoidal and Anesthetic Ointment (CIBA Consumer) p 408, 552
Nupercainal Pain Relief Cream (CIBA Consumer) p 408, 553
Baby Orajel (Del Pharmaceuticals) p 408, 557
Maximum Strength Orajel (Del Pharmaceuticals) p 408, 557
Rhulicream (Rydelle) p 423, 681
Rhuligel (Rydelle) p 423, 681
Rhulispray (Rydelle) p 423, 681
Sucrets Maximum Strength Sprays (SmithKline Beecham) p 428, 720
Tronolane Anesthetic Cream for Hemorrhoids (Ross) p 422, 679

Vicks Formula 44 Cough Control Discs (Richardson-Vicks) p 656
Xylocaine 2.5% Ointment (Astra) p 403, 510
Zilactin Medicated Gel (Zila Pharmaceuticals) p 435, 777
Zilactol Medicated Liquid (Zila Pharmaceuticals) p 777
ZilaDent Oral Analgesic Gel (Zila Pharmaceuticals) p 777

TOPICAL-COUNTERIRRITANT
Aurum Analgesic Lotion (Au Pharmaceuticals) p 510
Ben-Gay External Analgesic Products (Pfizer Consumer) p 638
Ben-Gay Ultra Strength Pain Relieving Rub (Pfizer Consumer) p 638
Eucalyptamint 100% All Natural Ointment (CIBA Consumer) p 407, 551
Feminine Gold Analgesic Lotion (Au Pharmaceuticals) p 511
Flex-all 454 Pain Relieving Gel (Chattem) p 545
Icy Hot Balm (Chattem) p 546
Icy Hot Cream (Chattem) p 546
Icy Hot Stick (Chattem) p 546
Legatrin Rub (Columbia) p 408, 556
Theragold Analgesic Lotion (Au Pharmaceuticals) p 510
Therapeutic Gold Analgesic Lotion (Au Pharmaceuticals) p 510
Therapeutic Mineral Ice, Pain Relieving Gel (Bristol-Myers Products) p 406, 536
Therapeutic Mineral Ice Exercise Formula, Pain Relieving Gel (Bristol-Myers Products) p 406, 536
Zilactin Medicated Gel (Zila Pharmaceuticals) p 435, 777
Zilactol Medicated Liquid (Zila Pharmaceuticals) p 777
ZilaDent Oral Analgesic Gel (Zila Pharmaceuticals) p 777

TOPICAL-SALICYLATES & COMBINATIONS
Aspercreme Creme, Lotion Analgesic Rub (Thompson Medical) p 743
Ben-Gay External Analgesic Products (Pfizer Consumer) p 638
Ben-Gay Ultra Strength Pain Relieving Rub (Pfizer Consumer) p 638
Icy Hot Balm (Chattem) p 546
Icy Hot Cream (Chattem) p 546
Icy Hot Stick (Chattem) p 546
Mobisyl Analgesic Creme (Ascher) p 403, 510

OTHER
Doan's - Extra-Strength Analgesic (CIBA Consumer) p 407, 549
Doan's - Regular Strength Analgesic (CIBA Consumer) p 407, 549
Hyland's Colic Tablets (Standard Homeopathic) p 722
Magonate Tablets and Liquid (Fleming) p 563
Mobigesic Analgesic Tablets (Ascher) p 403, 509
Momentum Muscular Backache Formula (Whitehall) p 767

ANEMIA PREPARATIONS
(see under HEMATINICS)

ANESTHETICS

TOPICAL
Anbesol Baby Teething Gel Anesthetic (Whitehall) p 434, 763
Anbesol Gel Antiseptic-Anesthetic-Regular Strength (Whitehall) p 434, 763
Anbesol Gel Antiseptic-Anesthetic - Maximum Strength (Whitehall) p 434, 763
Anbesol Liquid Antiseptic-Anesthetic (Whitehall) p 434, 763
Anbesol Liquid Antiseptic-Anesthetic - Maximum Strength (Whitehall) p 434, 763
Campho-Phenique Cold Sore Gel (Sterling Health) p 429, 731

Cheracol Sore Throat Spray (Roberts) p 663

Chloraseptic Lozenges, Cherry, Cool Mint and Menthol (Richardson-Vicks) p 653

Baby Orajel (Del Pharmaceuticals) p 408, 557

Maximum Strength Orajel (Del Pharmaceuticals) p 408, 557

Orajel Mouth-Aid (Del Pharmaceuticals) p 408, 557

proctoFoam/non-steroid (Reed & Carnrick) p 645

ZilaDent Oral Analgesic Gel (Zila Pharmaceuticals) p 777

ANORECTAL PRODUCTS

CREAMS, FOAMS, LOTIONS, OINTMENTS
Americaine Hemorrhoidal Ointment (Fisons Consumer Health) p 409, 559

Anusol Ointment (Parke-Davis) p 418, 629

BiCozene Creme (Sandoz Consumer) p 423, 682

Cortaid Cream with Aloe (Upjohn) p 431, 747

Cortaid Lotion (Upjohn) p 431, 747

Cortaid Ointment with Aloe (Upjohn) p 431, 747

Maximum Strength Cortaid Cream (Upjohn) p 431, 748

Maximum Strength Cortaid Ointment (Upjohn) p 431, 748

Maximum Strength Cortaid Spray (Upjohn) p 431, 748

Corticaine External Analgesic (Whitby) p 433, 760

Nupercainal Hemorrhoidal and Anesthetic Ointment (CIBA Consumer) p 408, 552

Pazo Hemorrhoid Ointment & Suppositories (Bristol-Myers Products) p 406, 534

Preparation H Hemorrhoidal Cream (Whitehall) p 434, 768

Preparation H Hemorrhoidal Ointment (Whitehall) p 434, 768

proctoFoam/non-steroid (Reed & Carnrick) p 645

Tronolane Anesthetic Cream for Hemorrhoids (Ross) p 422, 679

Tucks Cream (Parke-Davis) p 637

SUPPOSITORIES
Anusol Hemorrhoidal Suppositories (Parke-Davis) p 418, 629

Nupercainal Suppositories (CIBA Consumer) p 408, 553

Pazo Hemorrhoid Ointment & Suppositories (Bristol-Myers Products) p 406, 534

Preparation H Hemorrhoidal Suppositories (Whitehall) p 434, 768

Tronolane Hemorrhoidal Suppositories (Ross) p 422, 680

Wyanoids Relief Factor Hemorrhoidal Suppositories (Wyeth-Ayerst) p 435, 777

OTHER
Aveeno Bath Oilated (Rydelle) p 423, 680

Preparation H Cleansing Tissues (Whitehall) p 434, 769

Tucks Premoistened Pads (Parke-Davis) p 420, 637

Tucks Take-Alongs (Parke-Davis) p 637

ANOREXICS
(see under APPETITE SUPPRESSANTS)

ANTACIDS

ANTACID COMBINATIONS
Alka-Seltzer Effervescent Antacid (Miles Consumer) p 416, 614

Alka-Seltzer Extra Strength Effervescent Antacid and Pain Reliever (Miles Consumer) p 416, 615

Aludrox Oral Suspension (Wyeth-Ayerst) p 435, 773

Citrocarbonate Antacid (Roberts) p 664

Di-Gel Antacid/Anti-Gas (Schering-Plough HealthCare) p 425, 696

Gaviscon Antacid Tablets (Marion Merrell Dow) p 412, 582

Gaviscon-2 Antacid Tablets (Marion Merrell Dow) p 412, 583

Gaviscon Extra Strength Relief Formula Liquid Antacid (Marion Merrell Dow) p 412, 582

Gaviscon Extra Strength Relief Formula Antacid Tablets (Marion Merrell Dow) p 412, 582

Gaviscon Liquid Antacid (Marion Merrell Dow) p 412, 583

Gelusil Liquid & Tablets (Parke-Davis) p 419, 634

Marblen Suspension Peach/Apricot (Fleming) p 563

Marblen Suspension Unflavored (Fleming) p 563

Marblen Tablets (Fleming) p 563

Riopan Plus Suspension (Whitehall) p 771

Riopan Plus Chew Tablets (Whitehall) p 771

Riopan Plus Chew Tablets in Rollpacks (Whitehall) p 771

WinGel Liquid (Sterling Health) p 740

ANTACIDS
Alka-Mints Chewable Antacid (Miles Consumer) p 416, 612

Alka-Seltzer Effervescent Antacid and Pain Reliever (Miles Consumer) p 416, 612

Alka-Seltzer (Flavored) Effervescent Antacid and Pain Reliever (Miles Consumer) p 416, 613

ALternaGEL Liquid (J&J•Merck Consumer) p 409, 565

Amphojel Suspension (Wyeth-Ayerst) p 435, 773

Amphojel Suspension without Flavor (Wyeth-Ayerst) p 435, 773

Amphojel Tablets (Wyeth-Ayerst) p 435, 773

Arm & Hammer Pure Baking Soda (Church & Dwight) p 548

Basaljel Capsules (Wyeth-Ayerst) p 435, 774

Basaljel Suspension (Wyeth-Ayerst) p 435, 774

Basaljel Tablets (Wyeth-Ayerst) p 435, 774

Chooz Antacid Gum (Schering-Plough HealthCare) p 425, 694

Citrocarbonate Antacid (Roberts) p 664

Maalox HRF Heartburn Relief Formula (Rhone-Poulenc Rorer Consumer) p 420, 649

Mag-Ox 400 (Blaine) p 516

Nephrox Suspension (Fleming) p 563

Concentrated Phillips' Milk of Magnesia (Sterling Health) p 430, 737

Phillips' Milk of Magnesia Liquid (Sterling Health) p 430, 737

Phillips' Milk of Magnesia Tablets (Sterling Health) p 430, 737

Riopan Antacid Suspension (Whitehall) p 770

Riopan Antacid Swallow Tablets (Whitehall) p 770

Rolaids (Warner-Lambert) p 433, 757

Rolaids (Calcium Rich/Sodium Free) (Warner-Lambert) p 433, 757

Extra Strength Rolaids (Warner-Lambert) p 433, 758

Tums Antacid Tablets (SmithKline Beecham) p 428, 720

Tums E-X Antacid Tablets (SmithKline Beecham) p 428, 720

Uro-Mag (Blaine) p 516

WinGel Liquid (Sterling Health) p 740

ANTACIDS WITH ANTIFLATULENTS
Di-Gel Antacid/Anti-Gas (Schering-Plough HealthCare) p 425, 696

Gelusil Liquid & Tablets (Parke-Davis) p 419, 634

Maalox Plus Suspension/Tablets (Rhone-Poulenc Rorer Consumer) p 421, 649

Extra Strength Maalox Plus Suspension (Rhone-Poulenc Rorer Consumer) p 420, 650

Mylanta Liquid (J&J•Merck Consumer) p 410, 567

Mylanta Tablets (J&J•Merck Consumer) p 410, 567

Mylanta Double Strength Liquid (J&J•Merck Consumer) p 410, 567

Mylanta Double Strength Tablets (J&J•Merck Consumer) p 410, 567

Riopan Plus Suspension (Whitehall) p 771

Riopan Plus Chew Tablets (Whitehall) p 771

Riopan Plus Chew Tablets in Rollpacks (Whitehall) p 771

Riopan Plus 2 Suspension-Mint and Cherry flavors (Whitehall) p 435, 771

Riopan Plus 2 Chew Tablets-Mint and Cherry Vanilla flavors (Whitehall) p 435, 771

Tums Plus Antacid Anti-gas Tablets, Assorted Fruit or Peppermint (SmithKline Beecham) p 428, 721

ANTHELMINTICS
(see under ANTIPARASITICS)

ANTIARTHRITICS
(see under ARTHRITIS MEDICATIONS)

ANTIBACTERIALS
(see under ANTISEPTICS)

ANTIDOTES

ACUTE TOXIC INGESTION
Charcoaid (Requa) p 647

ANTIEMETICS
(see under NAUSEA MEDICATIONS)

ANTIHISTAMINES
Actifed Plus Caplets (Burroughs Wellcome) p 406, 537

Actifed Plus Tablets (Burroughs Wellcome) p 406, 538

Actifed Syrup (Burroughs Wellcome) p 406, 537

Actifed Tablets (Burroughs Wellcome) p 406, 537

Alka Seltzer Plus Sinus Allergy Medicine (Miles Consumer) p 416, 616

Allerest Children's Chewable Tablets (Fisons Consumer Health) p 558

Allerest Headache Strength Tablets (Fisons Consumer Health) p 558

Allerest Maximum Strength Tablets (Fisons Consumer Health) p 408, 558

Allerest Sinus Pain Formula (Fisons Consumer Health) p 558

BC Cold Powder Multi-Symptom Formula (Block) p 516

Comtrex Multi-Symptom Day-Night Caplet-Tablet (Bristol-Myers Products) p 404, 525

Dristan Allergy Nasal Decongestant/Antihistamine Caplets (Whitehall) p 434, 765

Dristan Cold Nasal Decongestant/Antihistamine/Analgesic Coated Tablets (Whitehall) p 434, 765

Isoclor Timesule Capsules (Fisons Consumer Health) p 409, 561

PediaCare Night Rest Cough-Cold Formula Liquid (McNeil Consumer Products) p 414, 588

Sinarest Tablets (Fisons Consumer Health) p 561

Sudafed Plus Liquid (Burroughs Wellcome) p 407, 541

Sudafed Plus Tablets (Burroughs Wellcome) p 407, 542

Tylenol PM Extra Strength Pain Reliever/Sleep Aid Caplets and Tablets (McNeil Consumer Products) p 414, 593

ANTI-INFLAMMATORY AGENTS

NON-STEROIDALS

Midol IB Cramp Relief Formula (Sterling Health) p 430, 733

SALICYLATES

Maximum Strength Arthritis Pain Formula by the Makers of Anacin Analgesic Tablets and Caplets (Whitehall) p 763

Children's Bayer Chewable Aspirin (Sterling Health) p 429, 724

Genuine Bayer Aspirin Tablets & Caplets (Sterling Health) p 428, 724

Maximum Bayer Aspirin Tablets & Caplets (Sterling Health) p 429, 725

Bayer Plus Aspirin Tablets (Sterling Health) p 429, 726

Extra Strength Bayer Plus Aspirin Caplets (Sterling Health) p 429, 727

8 Hour Bayer Timed-Release Aspirin (Sterling Health) p 429, 726

OTHER

Herpecin-L Cold Sore Lip Balm (Campbell) p 544

ANTIPARASITICS

ARTHROPODS

LICE

A-200 Pediculicide Shampoo & Gel (SmithKline Beecham) p 426, 704

Lice•Enz Foam (Copley) p 408, 556

Nix Creme Rinse (Burroughs Wellcome) p 540, 407

Pronto Lice Killing Shampoo Kit (Del Pharmaceuticals) p 408, 557

R&C Shampoo (Reed & Carnrick) p 420, 646

R&C Spray (Reed & Carnrick) p 420, 646

Rid Lice Control Spray (Pfizer Consumer) p 639

Rid Lice Killing Shampoo (Pfizer Consumer) p 640

HELMINTHS

ENTEROBIUS (PINWORM)

Reese's Pinworm Medicine (Reese Chemical) p 420, 647

ANTIPERSPIRANTS (see under DEODORANTS & DERMATOLOGICALS, ANTIPERSPIRANTS)

ANTIPYRETICS

Advil Ibuprofen Caplets and Tablets (Whitehall) p 434, 761

BC Cold Powder Multi-Symptom Formula (Block) p 516

BC Cold Powder Multi-Symptom Non-Drowsy Formula (Block) p 516

Children's Bayer Chewable Aspirin (Sterling Health) p 429, 724

Genuine Bayer Aspirin Tablets & Caplets (Sterling Health) p 428, 724

Bayer Plus Aspirin Tablets (Sterling Health) p 429, 726

Extra Strength Bayer Plus Aspirin Caplets (Sterling Health) p 429, 727

Empirin Aspirin (Burroughs Wellcome) p 406, 538

Ibuprofen Ibuprofen Caplets (Ohm Laboratories) p 418, 625

Ibuprofen Ibuprofen Tablets (Ohm Laboratories) p 418, 625

Tempra 1 Acetaminophen Infant Drops (Mead Johnson Nutritionals) p 415, 605

Tempra 2 Acetaminophen Toddlers Syrup (Mead Johnson Nutritionals) p 415, 605

Tempra 3 Chewable Tablets, Regular or Double-Strength (Mead Johnson Nutritionals) p 415, 605

Tylenol PM Extra Strength Pain Reliever/Sleep Aid Caplets and Tablets (McNeil Consumer Products) p 414, 593

Vanquish Analgesic Caplets (Sterling Health) p 431, 739

ANTISEPTICS

Anbesol Gel Antiseptic-Anesthetic-Regular Strength (Whitehall) p 434, 763

Anbesol Gel Antiseptic-Anesthetic - Maximum Strength (Whitehall) p 434, 763

Anbesol Liquid Antiseptic-Anesthetic (Whitehall) p 434, 763

Anbesol Liquid Antiseptic-Anesthetic - Maximum Strength (Whitehall) p 434, 763

Bactine Antiseptic/Anesthetic First Aid Liquid (Miles Consumer) p 416, 617

Children's Chloraseptic Spray (Richardson-Vicks) p 654

Hibiclens Antimicrobial Skin Cleanser (Stuart) p 431, 740

Hibistat Germicidal Hand Rinse (Stuart) p 741

Hibistat Towelette (Stuart) p 741

Impregon Concentrate (Fleming) p 563

Listerine Antiseptic (Warner-Lambert) p 433, 756

Orajel Mouth-Aid (Del Pharmaceuticals) p 408, 557

S.T.37 Antiseptic Solution (Menley & James) p 611

Sucrets Maximum Strength Sprays (SmithKline Beecham) p 428, 720

Techni-Care Surgical Scrub (Care-Tech) p 545

Zephiran Chloride Aqueous Solution (Sanofi Winthrop Pharmaceuticals) p 689

Zephiran Chloride Spray (Sanofi Winthrop Pharmaceuticals) p 689

Zephiran Chloride Tinted Tincture (Sanofi Winthrop Pharmaceuticals) p 689

ANTITUSSIVES (see under COLD & COUGH PREPARATIONS)

APPETITE SUPPRESSANTS

Acutrim 16 Hour Steady Control Appetite Suppressant (CIBA Consumer) p 407, 549

Acutrim Late Day Strength Appetite Suppressant (CIBA Consumer) p 407, 549

Acutrim II Maximum Strength Appetite Suppressant (CIBA Consumer) p 407, 549

Dexatrim Capsules, Caplets, Tablets (Thompson Medical) p 744

Dexatrim Maximum Strength Caffeine-Free Caplets (Thompson Medical) p 744

Dexatrim Maximum Strength Caffeine-Free Capsules (Thompson Medical) p 744

Dexatrim Maximum Strength Extended Duration Time Tablets (Thompson Medical) p 744

Dexatrim Maximum Strength Plus Vitamin C/Caffeine-free Caplets (Thompson Medical) p 431, 744

Dexatrim Maximum Strength Plus Vitamin C/Caffeine-free Capsules (Thompson Medical) p 431, 744

ARTHRITIS MEDICATIONS

NSAIDS

Maximum Strength Arthritis Pain Formula by the Makers of Anacin Analgesic Tablets and Caplets (Whitehall) p 763

Ibuprohm Ibuprofen Caplets (Ohm Laboratories) p 418, 625

Ibuprohm Ibuprofen Tablets (Ohm Laboratories) p 418, 625

SALICYLATES

Maximum Bayer Aspirin Tablets & Caplets (Sterling Health) p 429, 725

Bayer Plus Aspirin Tablets (Sterling Health) p 429, 726

Extra Strength Bayer Plus Aspirin Caplets (Sterling Health) p 429, 727

Therapy Bayer Enteric Aspirin Caplets (Sterling Health) p 429, 728

8 Hour Bayer Timed-Release Aspirin (Sterling Health) p 429, 726

Norwich Maximum Strength Aspirin (Chattem) p 546

Norwich Regular Strength Aspirin (Chattem) p 546

ARTIFICIAL TEARS PREPARATIONS

Celluvisc Lubricant Ophthalmic Solution (Allergan Pharmaceuticals) p 504

Tears Plus Lubricant Ophthalmic Solution (Allergan Pharmaceuticals) p 505

ASTHMA PREPARATIONS

Amesec (Whitby) p 759

AsthmaHaler Mist Epinephrine Bitartrate Bronchodilator (Menley & James) p 608

AsthmaNefrin Solution "A" Bronchodilator (Menley & James) p 608

Bronkaid Mist (Sterling Health) p 429, 729

Bronkaid Mist Suspension (Sterling Health) p 730

Bronkaid Tablets (Sterling Health) p 429, 730

Bronkolixir (Sanofi Winthrop Pharmaceuticals) p 689

Bronkotabs Tablets (Sanofi Winthrop Pharmaceuticals) p 689

Primatene Mist (Whitehall) p 435, 769

Primatene Mist Suspension (Whitehall) p 770

Primatene Tablets-M Formula (Whitehall) p 435, 770

Primatene Tablets-P Formula (Whitehall) p 435, 770

Primatene Tablets-Regular Formula (Whitehall) p 435, 770

ASTRINGENTS (see under DERMATOLOGICALS, ASTRINGENTS)

ATHLETE'S FOOT TREATMENT (see under DERMATOLOGICALS, FUNGICIDES)

B

BABY PRODUCTS

Anbesol Baby Teething Gel Anesthetic (Whitehall) p 434, 763

Caldesene Medicated Ointment (Fisons Consumer Health) p 409, 559

Caldesene Medicated Powder (Fisons Consumer Health) p 409, 559

Desitin Ointment (Pfizer Consumer) p 420, 638

Baby Orajel (Del Pharmaceuticals) p 408, 557

pHisoDerm For Baby (Sterling Health) p 430, 738

BACKACHE REMEDIES (see under ANALGESICS)

BAD BREATH PREPARATIONS (see under ORAL HYGIENE AID & MOUTHWASHES)

BEE STING RELIEF (see under INSECT BITE & STING PREPARATIONS)

BRONCHIAL DILATORS

SYMPATHOMIMETICS

Bronkaid Mist (Sterling Health) p 429, 729

Bronkaid Mist Suspension (Sterling Health) p 730

Primatene Mist (Whitehall) p 435, 769

Primatene Mist Suspension (Whitehall) p 770

Primatene Tablets-M Formula (Whitehall) p 435, 770

Primatene Tablets-P Formula (Whitehall) p 435, 770
Primatene Tablets-Regular Formula (Whitehall) p 435, 770

SYMPATHOMIMETICS & COMBINATIONS
Bronkaid Tablets (Sterling Health) p 429, 730
Bronkolixir (Sanofi Winthrop Pharmaceuticals) p 689
Bronkotabs Tablets (Sanofi Winthrop Pharmaceuticals) p 689

XANTHINE DERIVATIVES & COMBINATIONS
Bronkaid Tablets (Sterling Health) p 429, 730
Bronkolixir (Sanofi Winthrop Pharmaceuticals) p 689
Bronkotabs Tablets (Sanofi Winthrop Pharmaceuticals) p 689

BRONCHITIS PREPARATIONS
(see under COLD & COUGH PREPARATIONS)

BURN PREPARATIONS
(see under DERMATOLOGICALS, BURN RELIEF)

BURSITIS RELIEF
(see under ANALGESICS)

C

CALCIUM PREPARATIONS

CALCIUM SUPPLEMENTS
Alka-Mints Chewable Antacid (Miles Consumer) p 416, 612
Bugs Bunny Complete Children's Chewable Vitamins + Minerals with Iron and Calcium (Sugar Free) (Miles Consumer) p 416, 618
Caltrate 600 (Lederle) p 410, 571
Caltrate 600 + Iron & Vitamin D (Lederle) p 410, 572
Caltrate 600 + Vitamin D (Lederle) p 410, 572
Centrum, Jr. (Children's Chewable) + Extra Calcium (Lederle) p 411, 573
Flintstones Complete With Calcium, Iron & Minerals Children's Chewable Vitamins (Miles Consumer) p 416, 618
One-A-Day Women's Formula Multivitamins with Calcium, Extra Iron, Zinc and Beta Carotene (Miles Consumer) p 417, 620
Os-Cal 500 Chewable Tablets (Marion Merrell Dow) p 412, 585
Os-Cal 500 Tablets (Marion Merrell Dow) p 412, 585
Os-Cal 250+D Tablets (Marion Merrell Dow) p 412, 585
Os-Cal 500+D Tablets (Marion Merrell Dow) p 412, 585
Os-Cal Fortified Tablets (Marion Merrell Dow) p 412, 585
Os-Cal Plus Tablets (Marion Merrell Dow) p 412, 586
Posture 600 mg (Whitehall) p 768
Posture-D 600 mg (Whitehall) p 768
Rolaids (Calcium Rich/Sodium Free) (Warner-Lambert) p 433, 757

CANKER SORE PREPARATIONS
Gly-Oxide Liquid (Marion Merrell Dow) p 412, 583
Orajel Mouth-Aid (Del Pharmaceuticals) p 408, 557
Zilactin Medicated Gel (Zila Pharmaceuticals) p 435, 777

CENTRAL NERVOUS SYSTEM STIMULANTS
No Doz Maximum Strength Caplets (Bristol-Myers Products) p 405, 533

CERUMENOLYTICS
Debrox Drops (Marion Merrell Dow) p 411, 581
Ear Drops by Murine—(See Murine Ear Wax Removal System/Murine Ear Drops) (Ross) p 422, 677

Murine Ear Drops (Ross) p 422, 677
Murine Ear Wax Removal System (Ross) p 422, 677

COLD & COUGH PREPARATIONS

ANTIHISTAMINES & COMBINATIONS
A.R.M. Allergy Relief Medicine Caplets (Menley & James) p 415, 607
Actifed Plus Caplets (Burroughs Wellcome) p 406, 537
Actifed Plus Tablets (Burroughs Wellcome) p 406, 538
Actifed Syrup (Burroughs Wellcome) p 406, 537
Actifed Tablets (Burroughs Wellcome) p 406, 537
Alka-Seltzer Plus Cold Medicine (Miles Consumer) p 416, 615
Alka-Seltzer Plus Cold & Cough Medicine (Miles Consumer) p 416, 616
Alka-Seltzer Plus Night-Time Cold Medicine (Miles Consumer) p 416, 615
Alka Seltzer Plus Sinus Allergy Medicine (Miles Consumer) p 416, 616
Allerest Children's Chewable Tablets (Fisons Consumer Health) p 558
Allerest Headache Strength Tablets (Fisons Consumer Health) p 558
Allerest 12 Hour Caplets (Fisons Consumer Health) p 558
Allerest Maximum Strength Tablets (Fisons Consumer Health) p 408, 558
Allerest Sinus Pain Formula (Fisons Consumer Health) p 558
Benadryl Cold Tablets (Parke-Davis) p 418, 631
Benadryl Cold Nighttime Formula (Parke-Davis) p 419, 631
Benadryl Elixir (Parke-Davis) p 419, 630
Benadryl 25 Kapseals (Parke-Davis) p 418, 631
Benadryl 25 Tablets (Parke-Davis) p 418, 631
Bromfed Syrup (Muro) p 621
Cerose-DM (Wyeth-Ayerst) p 435, 774
Cheracol Plus Head Cold/Cough Formula (Roberts) p 421, 663
Chlor-Trimeton Allergy Syrup, Tablets & Long-Acting Repetabs Tablets (Schering-Plough HealthCare) p 424,425, 693
Chlor-Trimeton Antihistamine and Decongestant Tablets (Schering-Plough HealthCare) p 425, 694
Chlor-Trimeton Long Acting Antihistamine and Decongestant Repetabs Tablets (Schering-Plough HealthCare) p 425, 694
Cold Control+ Intense Cold Medicine (Reese Chemical) p 647
Allergy-Sinus Comtrex Multi-Symptom Allergy-Sinus Formula Tablets & Caplets (Bristol-Myers Products) p 404, 523
Comtrex Multi-Symptom Cold Reliever Tablets/Caplets/Liqui-Gels/Liquid (Bristol-Myers Products) p 404, 522
Comtrex Multi-Symptom Day-Night Caplet-Tablet (Bristol-Myers Products) p 404, 525
Contac Continuous Action Decongestant/Antihistamine Capsules (SmithKline Beecham) p 426, 705
Contac Maximum Strength Continuous Action Decongestant/Antihistamine Caplets (SmithKline Beecham) p 426, 704
Contac Severe Cold and Flu Formula Caplets (SmithKline Beecham) p 427, 706
Contac Severe Cold & Flu Nighttime (SmithKline Beecham) p 427, 708
Coricidin 'D' Decongestant Tablets (Schering-Plough HealthCare) p 425, 695

Coricidin Demilets Tablets for Children (Schering-Plough HealthCare) p 425, 696
Coricidin Tablets (Schering-Plough HealthCare) p 425, 695
Dimetane Decongestant Caplets (Robins Consumer) p 669
Dimetane Decongestant Elixir (Robins Consumer) p 669
Dimetane Elixir (Robins Consumer) p 668
Dimetane Extentabs 8 mg (Robins Consumer) p 668
Dimetane Extentabs 12 mg (Robins Consumer) p 668
Dimetane Tablets (Robins Consumer) p 668
Dimetapp Cold & Flu Caplets (Robins Consumer) p 421, 670
Dimetapp Elixir (Robins Consumer) p 421, 670
Dimetapp DM Elixir (Robins Consumer) p 421, 671
Dimetapp Extentabs (Robins Consumer) p 421, 671
Dimetapp Tablets (Robins Consumer) p 421, 672
Dorcol Children's Liquid Cold Formula (Sandoz Consumer) p 423, 683
Dristan Allergy Nasal Decongestant/Antihistamine Caplets (Whitehall) p 434, 765
Dristan Cold and Flu (Whitehall) p 434, 766
Dristan Cold Nasal Decongestant/ Antihistamine/Analgesic Coated Tablets (Whitehall) p 434, 765
Drixoral Antihistamine/Nasal Decongestant Syrup (Schering-Plough HealthCare) p 696
Drixoral Plus Extended-Release Tablets (Schering-Plough HealthCare) p 425, 698
Drixoral Sustained-Action Tablets (Schering-Plough HealthCare) p 425, 697
Isoclor Timesule Capsules (Fisons Consumer Health) p 409, 561
Medi-Flu Caplet, Liquid (Parke-Davis) p 419, 634
Novahistine Elixir (Marion Merrell Dow) p 412, 584
Orthoxicol Cough Syrup (Roberts) p 665
PediaCare Allergy Formula Liquid (McNeil Consumer Products) p 414, 588
PediaCare Cough-Cold Formula Liquid and Chewable Tablets (McNeil Consumer Products) p 414, 588
Pyrroxate Capsules (Roberts) p 421, 665
Robitussin Night Relief (Robins Consumer) p 422, 675
Ryna Liquid (Wallace) p 432, 754
Ryna-C Liquid (Wallace) p 432, 754
Sinarest Tablets (Fisons Consumer Health) p 561
Sinarest Extra Strength Tablets (Fisons Consumer Health) p 561
Sine-Off Sinus Medicine Tablets-Aspirin Formula (SmithKline Beecham) p 428, 718
Singlet Tablets (Marion Merrell Dow) p 586
Sinutab Sinus Medication, Maximum Strength Caplets (Parke-Davis) p 419, 636
Sinutab Sinus Allergy Medication, Maximum Strength Tablets (Parke-Davis) p 419, 636
Sudafed Plus Liquid (Burroughs Wellcome) p 407, 541
Sudafed Plus Tablets (Burroughs Wellcome) p 407, 542
Teldrin Timed-Release Allergy Capsules, 12 mg. (SmithKline Beecham) p 428, 720
Triaminic Allergy Tablets (Sandoz Consumer) p 685
Triaminic Chewables (Sandoz Consumer) p 685

Triaminic Cold Tablets (Sandoz Consumer) p 424, 685

Triaminic Syrup (Sandoz Consumer) p 423, 686

Triaminic-12 Tablets (Sandoz Consumer) p 424, 687

Triaminicin Tablets (Sandoz Consumer) p 424, 687

Triaminicol Multi-Symptom Cold Tablets (Sandoz Consumer) p 424, 688

Triaminicol Multi-Symptom Relief (Sandoz Consumer) p 424, 688

Tylenol Allergy Sinus Medication Maximum Strength Gelcaps and Caplets (McNeil Consumer Products) p 413, 600

Children's Tylenol Cold Multi Symptom Liquid Formula and Chewable Tablets (McNeil Consumer Products) p 413, 594

Tylenol Cold & Flu Hot Medication, Packets (McNeil Consumer Products) p 413, 595

Tylenol Cold Multi Symptom Medication Caplets and Tablets (McNeil Consumer Products) p 413, 596

Tylenol Cold Medication, Effervescent Tablets (McNeil Consumer Products) p 413, 595

Tylenol Cold Night Time Medication Liquid (McNeil Consumer Products) p 413, 599

Vicks Children's NyQuil Nighttime Cold/Cough Medicine (Richardson-Vicks) p 659

Vicks Formula 44M Multi-Symptom Cough & Cold Medicine (Richardson-Vicks) p 657

Vicks NyQuil LiquiCaps Adult Nighttime Cold/Flu Medicine (Richardson-Vicks) p 661

Vicks NyQuil Nighttime Cold/Flu Medicine-Regular & Cherry Flavor (Richardson-Vicks) p 660

Vicks Pediatric Formula 44m Multi-Symptom Cough & Cold Medicine (Richardson-Vicks) p 658

ANTITUSSIVES & COMBINATIONS

Alka-Seltzer Plus Cold & Cough Medicine (Miles Consumer) p 416, 616

Benylin Cough Syrup (Parke-Davis) p 419, 632

Benylin Decongestant (Parke-Davis) p 419, 633

Benylin DM Pediatric Cough Formula (Parke-Davis) p 419, 632

Cerose-DM (Wyeth-Ayerst) p 435, 774

Cheracol-D Cough Formula (Roberts) p 421, 663

Cheracol Plus Head Cold/Cough Formula (Roberts) p 421, 663

Comtrex Multi-Symptom Cold Reliever Tablets/Caplets/Liqui-Gels/Liquid (Bristol-Myers Products) p 404, 522

Comtrex Multi-Symptom Day-Night Caplet-Tablet (Bristol-Myers Products) p 404, 525

Comtrex Multi-Symptom Non-Drowsy Caplets (Bristol-Myers Products) p 405, 526

Contac Cough and Chest Cold (SmithKline Beecham) p 427, 706

Contac Cough & Sore Throat Formula (SmithKline Beecham) p 427, 707

Contac Jr. Non-Drowsy Cold Liquid (SmithKline Beecham) p 427, 707

Contac Severe Cold and Flu Formula Caplets (SmithKline Beecham) p 427, 706

Contac Severe Cold & Flu Nighttime (SmithKline Beecham) p 427, 708

Delsym Cough Formula (Fisons Corporation) p 562

Dimacol Caplets (Robins Consumer) p 668

Dimetapp DM Elixir (Robins Consumer) p 421, 671

Dorcol Children's Cough Syrup (Sandoz Consumer) p 423, 682

Dristan Cold and Flu (Whitehall) p 434, 766

Halls Mentho-Lyptus Cough Suppressant Tablets (Warner-Lambert) p 432, 755

Halls Plus Cough Suppressant Tablets (Warner-Lambert) p 432, 756

Hold Cough Suppressant Lozenge (Menley & James) p 415, 609

Hyland's Cough Syrup with Honey (Standard Homeopathic) p 722

Naldecon CX Adult Liquid (Apothecon) p 505

Naldecon DX Adult Liquid (Apothecon) p 505

Naldecon DX Children's Syrup (Apothecon) p 506

Naldecon DX Pediatric Drops (Apothecon) p 506

Naldecon Senior DX Cough/Cold Liquid (Apothecon) p 507

Novahistine DMX (Marion Merrell Dow) p 412, 583

PediaCare Cough-Cold Formula Liquid and Chewable Tablets (McNeil Consumer Products) p 414, 588

PediaCare Night Rest Cough-Cold Formula Liquid (McNeil Consumer Products) p 414, 588

PediaCare 6-12 Cough-Cold Formula Chewable Tablets (McNeil Consumer Products) p 414, 588

Robitussin Cough Calmers (Robins Consumer) p 674

Robitussin Cough Drops (Robins Consumer) p 422, 674

Robitussin Maximum Strength Cough Suppressant (Robins Consumer) p 422, 675

Robitussin Night Relief (Robins Consumer) p 422, 675

Robitussin Pediatric Cough & Cold Formula (Robins Consumer) p 422, 675

Robitussin Pediatric Cough Suppressant (Robins Consumer) p 422, 676

Robitussin-CF (Robins Consumer) p 422, 673

Robitussin-DM (Robins Consumer) p 422, 673

Ryna-C Liquid (Wallace) p 432, 754

Ryna-CX Liquid (Wallace) p 432, 754

St. Joseph Cough Suppressant for Children (Schering-Plough HealthCare) p 702

Sudafed Cough Syrup (Burroughs Wellcome) p 407, 541

Sudafed Severe Cold Formula Caplets (Burroughs Wellcome) p 407, 542

Sudafed Severe Cold Formula Tablets (Burroughs Wellcome) p 407, 542

TheraFlu Flu and Cold Medicine (Sandoz Consumer) p 423, 684

TheraFlu Flu, Cold and Cough Medicine (Sandoz Consumer) p 423, 684

Triaminic Nite Light (Sandoz Consumer) p 424, 686

Triaminic-DM Syrup (Sandoz Consumer) p 423, 687

Triaminicol Multi-Symptom Cold Tablets (Sandoz Consumer) p 424, 688

Triaminicol Multi-Symptom Relief (Sandoz Consumer) p 424, 688

Tylenol Cold & Flu No Drowsiness Hot Medication, Packets (McNeil Consumer Products) p 413, 598

Tylenol Cold Medication No Drowsiness Formula Caplets (McNeil Consumer Products) p 413, 597

Tylenol Cough Medication Maximum Strength Liquid (McNeil Consumer Products) p 414, 601

Tylenol Cough Medication Maximum Strength Liquid with Decongestant (McNeil Consumer Products) p 414, 601

Vicks Children's Cough Syrup (Richardson-Vicks) p 654

Vicks Children's NyQuil Nighttime Cold/Cough Medicine (Richardson-Vicks) p 659

Vicks Daycare Daytime Cold Medicine Caplets (Richardson-Vicks) p 655

Vicks Daycare Daytime Cold Medicine Liquid (Richardson-Vicks) p 655

Vicks Formula 44 Cough Control Discs (Richardson-Vicks) p 656

Vicks Formula 44 Cough Medicine (Richardson-Vicks) p 656

Vicks Formula 44D Cough and Decongestant Medicine (Richardson-Vicks) p 656

Vicks Formula 44E Cough & Expectorant Medicine (Richardson-Vicks) p 657

Vicks Formula 44M Multi-Symptom Cough & Cold Medicine (Richardson-Vicks) p 657

Vicks NyQuil LiquiCaps Adult Nighttime Cold/Flu Medicine (Richardson-Vicks) p 661

Vicks NyQuil Nighttime Cold/Flu Medicine-Regular & Cherry Flavor (Richardson-Vicks) p 660

Vicks Pediatric Formula 44 Cough Medicine (Richardson-Vicks) p 657

Vicks Pediatric Formula 44d Cough & Decongestant Medicine (Richardson-Vicks) p 658

Vicks Pediatric Formula 44e Cough & Expectorant Medicine (Richardson-Vicks) p 659

Vicks Pediatric Formula 44m Multi-Symptom Cough & Cold Medicine (Richardson-Vicks) p 658

Vicks Vaporub (Richardson-Vicks) p 662

Vicks Vaposteam (Richardson-Vicks) p 662

DECONGESTANTS

DECONGESTANTS, EXPECTORANTS & COMBINATIONS

Cheracol Plus Head Cold/Cough Formula (Roberts) p 421, 663

Cough Formula Comtrex (Bristol-Myers Products) p 405, 524

Guaifed Syrup (Muro) p 621

Guaitab Tablets (Muro) p 621

Sudafed Cough Syrup (Burroughs Wellcome) p 407, 541

ORAL & COMBINATIONS

Actifed Plus Caplets (Burroughs Wellcome) p 406, 537

Actifed Plus Tablets (Burroughs Wellcome) p 406, 538

Actifed Syrup (Burroughs Wellcome) p 406, 537

Actifed Tablets (Burroughs Wellcome) p 406, 537

Advil Cold and Sinus (formerly CoAdvil) (Whitehall) p 434, 761

Afrin Tablets (Schering-Plough HealthCare) p 424, 693

Alka-Seltzer Plus Cold Medicine (Miles Consumer) p 416, 615

Alka-Seltzer Plus Cold & Cough Medicine (Miles Consumer) p 416, 616

Alka-Seltzer Plus Night-Time Cold Medicine (Miles Consumer) p 416, 615

Alka Seltzer Plus Sinus Allergy Medicine (Miles Consumer) p 416, 616

Allerest Children's Chewable Tablets (Fisons Consumer Health) p 558

Allerest Headache Strength Tablets (Fisons Consumer Health) p 558

Allerest 12 Hour Caplets (Fisons Consumer Health) p 558

Allerest Maximum Strength Tablets (Fisons Consumer Health) p 408, 558

Allerest No Drowsiness Tablets (Fisons Consumer Health) p 408, 558

Allerest Sinus Pain Formula (Fisons Consumer Health) p 558

BC Cold Powder Multi-Symptom Formula (Block) p 516

BC Cold Powder Multi-Symptom Non-Drowsy Formula (Block) p 516

Benadryl Decongestant Elixir (Parke-Davis) p 419, 630

Benadryl Decongestant Kapseals (Parke-Davis) p 418, 630
Benadryl Decongestant Tablets (Parke-Davis) p 418, 630
Benylin Decongestant (Parke-Davis) p 419, 633
Benylin Expectorant (Parke-Davis) p 419, 633
Bromfed Syrup (Muro) p 621
Cerose-DM (Wyeth-Ayerst) p 435, 774
Cheracol Plus Head Cold/Cough Formula (Roberts) p 421, 663
Chlor-Trimeton Antihistamine and Decongestant Tablets (Schering-Plough HealthCare) p 425, 694
Chlor-Trimeton Long Acting Antihistamine and Decongestant Repetabs Tablets (Schering-Plough HealthCare) p 425, 694
Cold Control+ Intense Cold Medicine (Reese Chemical) p 647
Allergy-Sinus Comtrex Multi-Symptom Allergy-Sinus Formula Tablets & Caplets (Bristol-Myers Products) p 404, 523
Cough Formula Comtrex (Bristol-Myers Products) p 405, 524
Comtrex Multi-Symptom Cold Reliever Tablets/Caplets/Liqui-Gels/Liquid (Bristol-Myers Products) p 404, 522
Comtrex Multi-Symptom Day-Night Caplet-Tablet (Bristol-Myers Products) p 404, 525
Comtrex Multi-Symptom Non-Drowsy Caplets (Bristol-Myers Products) p 405, 526
Congespirin For Children Aspirin Free Chewable Cold Tablets (Bristol-Myers Products) p 405, 527
Congestac Caplets (Menley & James) p 415, 609
Contac Continuous Action Decongestant/Antihistamine Capsules (SmithKline Beecham) p 426, 705
Contac Jr. Non-Drowsy Cold Liquid (SmithKline Beecham) p 427, 707
Contac Maximum Strength Continuous Action Decongestant/Antihistamine Caplets (SmithKline Beecham) p 426, 704
Contac Severe Cold and Flu Formula Caplets (SmithKline Beecham) p 427, 706
Contac Severe Cold & Flu Nighttime (SmithKline Beecham) p 427, 708
Contac Sinus Caplets Maximum Strength Non-Drowsy Formula (SmithKline Beecham) p 427, 705
Contac Sinus Tablets Maximum Strength Non-Drowsy Formula (SmithKline Beecham) p 427, 705
Coricidin 'D' Decongestant Tablets (Schering-Plough HealthCare) p 425, 695
Coricidin Demilets Tablets for Children (Schering-Plough HealthCare) p 425, 696
Dimacol Caplets (Robins Consumer) p 668
Dimetane Decongestant Caplets (Robins Consumer) p 669
Dimetane Decongestant Elixir (Robins Consumer) p 669
Dimetapp Cold & Flu Caplets (Robins Consumer) p 421, 670
Dimetapp Elixir (Robins Consumer) p 421, 670
Dimetapp DM Elixir (Robins Consumer) p 421, 671
Dimetapp Extentabs (Robins Consumer) p 421, 671
Dimetapp Tablets (Robins Consumer) p 421, 672
Dorcol Children's Cough Syrup (Sandoz Consumer) p 423, 682
Dorcol Children's Decongestant Liquid (Sandoz Consumer) p 423, 683
Dorcol Children's Liquid Cold Formula (Sandoz Consumer) p 423, 683
Dristan Allergy Nasal Decongestant/Antihistamine Caplets (Whitehall) p 434, 765

Dristan Cold and Flu (Whitehall) p 434, 766
Dristan Cold Nasal Decongestant/ Antihistamine/Analgesic Coated Tablets (Whitehall) p 434, 765
Maximum Strength Dristan Cold Nasal Decongestant/ Analgesic Coated Caplets (Whitehall) p 434, 765
Dristan Sinus Pain Reliever/Nasal Decongestant Caplets (Whitehall) p 434, 766
Drixoral Antihistamine/Nasal Decongestant Syrup (Schering-Plough HealthCare) p 696
Drixoral Non-Drowsy Formula (Schering-Plough HealthCare) p 425, 697
Drixoral Plus Extended-Release Tablets (Schering-Plough HealthCare) p 425, 698
Drixoral Sinus (Schering-Plough HealthCare) p 426, 698
Drixoral Sustained-Action Tablets (Schering-Plough HealthCare) p 425, 697
Sinus Excedrin Analgesic, Decongestant Tablets & Caplets (Bristol-Myers Products) p 405, 531
4-Way Cold Tablets (Bristol-Myers Products) p 405, 531
Guaifed Syrup (Muro) p 621
Guaitab Tablets (Muro) p 621
Hyland's C-Plus Cold Tablets (Standard Homeopathic) p 722
Isoclor Timesule Capsules (Fisons Consumer Health) p 409, 561
Medi-Flu Caplet, Liquid (Parke-Davis) p 419, 634
Medi-Flu Without Drowsiness Caplets (Parke-Davis) p 419, 635
Naldecon CX Adult Liquid (Apothecon) p 505
Naldecon DX Adult Liquid (Apothecon) p 505
Naldecon DX Children's Syrup (Apothecon) p 506
Naldecon DX Pediatric Drops (Apothecon) p 506
Naldecon EX Children's Syrup (Apothecon) p 507
Naldecon EX Pediatric Drops (Apothecon) p 507
Novahistine DMX (Marion Merrell Dow) p 412, 583
Novahistine Elixir (Marion Merrell Dow) p 412, 584
Ornex Caplets (Menley & James) p 415, 610
Maximum Strength Ornex Caplets (Menley & James) p 415, 610
Orthoxicol Cough Syrup (Roberts) p 665
PediaCare Allergy Formula Liquid (McNeil Consumer Products) p 414, 588
PediaCare Cough-Cold Formula Liquid and Chewable Tablets (McNeil Consumer Products) p 414, 588
PediaCare Decongestant Drops (McNeil Consumer Products) p 414, 588
PediaCare Night Rest Cough-Cold Formula Liquid (McNeil Consumer Products) p 414, 588
Pyrroxate Capsules (Roberts) p 421, 665
Robitussin Night Relief (Robins Consumer) p 422, 675
Robitussin Pediatric Cough & Cold Formula (Robins Consumer) p 422, 675
Robitussin-CF (Robins Consumer) p 422, 673
Robitussin-PE (Robins Consumer) p 422, 674
Ryna Liquid (Wallace) p 432, 754
Ryna-C Liquid (Wallace) p 432, 754
Ryna-CX Liquid (Wallace) p 432, 754
Sinarest No Drowsiness Tablets (Fisons Consumer Health) p 561
Sinarest Tablets (Fisons Consumer Health) p 561

Sinarest Extra Strength Tablets (Fisons Consumer Health) p 561
Sine-Aid Maximum Strength Sinus Headache Gelcaps, Caplets and Tablets (McNeil Consumer Products) p 414, 589
Sine-Off Maximum Strength Allergy/Sinus Formula Caplets (SmithKline Beecham) p 428, 717
Sine-Off Maximum Strength No Drowsiness Formula Caplets (SmithKline Beecham) p 428, 717
Sine-Off Sinus Medicine Tablets-Aspirin Formula (SmithKline Beecham) p 428, 718
Singlet Tablets (Marion Merrell Dow) p 586
Sinutab Sinus Medication, Maximum Strength Caplets (Parke-Davis) p 419, 636
Sinutab Sinus Allergy Medication, Maximum Strength Tablets (Parke-Davis) p 419, 636
Sinutab Sinus Medication, Maximum Strength Without Drowsiness Formula Tablets & Caplets (Parke-Davis) p 419, 637
Sinutab Sinus Medication, Regular Strength Without Drowsiness Formula (Parke-Davis) p 419, 636
St. Joseph Cold Tablets for Children (Schering-Plough HealthCare) p 702
Sudafed Children's Liquid (Burroughs Wellcome) p 407, 540
Sudafed Cough Syrup (Burroughs Wellcome) p 407, 541
Sudafed Plus Liquid (Burroughs Wellcome) p 407, 541
Sudafed Plus Tablets (Burroughs Wellcome) p 407, 541
Sudafed Severe Cold Formula Caplets (Burroughs Wellcome) p 407, 542
Sudafed Severe Cold Formula Tablets (Burroughs Wellcome) p 407, 542
Sudafed Sinus Caplets (Burroughs Wellcome) p 407, 543
Sudafed Sinus Tablets (Burroughs Wellcome) p 407, 543
Sudafed Tablets, 30 mg (Burroughs Wellcome) p 407, 541
Sudafed Tablets, Adult Strength, 60 mg (Burroughs Wellcome) p 407, 541
Sudafed 12 Hour Tablets (Burroughs Wellcome) p 407, 543
TheraFlu Flu and Cold Medicine (Sandoz Consumer) p 423, 684
TheraFlu Flu, Cold and Cough Medicine (Sandoz Consumer) p 423, 684
Triaminic Chewables (Sandoz Consumer) p 685
Triaminic Cold Tablets (Sandoz Consumer) p 424, 685
Triaminic Expectorant (Sandoz Consumer) p 424, 686
Triaminic Nite Light (Sandoz Consumer) p 424, 686
Triaminic Syrup (Sandoz Consumer) p 423, 686
Triaminic-12 Tablets (Sandoz Consumer) p 424, 687
Triaminic-DM Syrup (Sandoz Consumer) p 423, 687
Triaminicin Tablets (Sandoz Consumer) p 424, 687
Triaminicol Multi-Symptom Cold Tablets (Sandoz Consumer) p 424, 688
Triaminicol Multi-Symptom Relief (Sandoz Consumer) p 424, 688
Tylenol Allergy Sinus Medication Maximum Strength Gelcaps and Caplets (McNeil Consumer Products) p 413, 600
Children's Tylenol Cold Multi Symptom Liquid Formula and Chewable Tablets (McNeil Consumer Products) p 413, 594
Tylenol Cold & Flu No Drowsiness Hot Medication, Packets (McNeil Consumer Products) p 413, 598
Tylenol Cold Multi Symptom Medication Caplets and Tablets (McNeil Consumer Products) p 413, 596

Tylenol Cold Medication No Drowsiness Formula Caplets (McNeil Consumer Products) p 413, 597

Tylenol Cold Night Time Medication Liquid (McNeil Consumer Products) p 413, 599

Tylenol Cough Medication Maximum Strength Liquid with Decongestant (McNeil Consumer Products) p 414, 601

Tylenol, Maximum Strength, Sinus Medication Gelcaps, Caplets and Tablets (McNeil Consumer Products) p 413, 602

Vicks Children's NyQuil Nighttime Cold/Cough Medicine (Richardson-Vicks) p 659

Vicks Children's NyQuil Nighttime Head Cold/Allergy Medicine (Richardson-Vicks) p 660

Vicks Daycare Daytime Cold Medicine Caplets (Richardson-Vicks) p 655

Vicks Daycare Daytime Cold Medicine Liquid (Richardson-Vicks) p 655

Vicks Formula 44D Cough and Decongestant Medicine (Richardson-Vicks) p 656

Vicks Formula 44M Multi-Symptom Cough & Cold Medicine (Richardson-Vicks) p 657

Vicks NyQuil LiquiCaps Adult Nighttime Cold/Flu Medicine (Richardson-Vicks) p 661

Vicks NyQuil Nighttime Cold/Flu Medicine-Regular & Cherry Flavor (Richardson-Vicks) p 660

Vicks Pediatric Formula 44d Cough & Decongestant Medicine (Richardson-Vicks) p 658

Vicks Pediatric Formula 44m Multi-Symptom Cough & Cold Medicine (Richardson-Vicks) p 658

TOPICAL

Afrin Cherry Scented Nasal Spray 0.05% (Schering-Plough HealthCare) p 428, 692

Afrin Children's Strength Nose Drops 0.025% (Schering-Plough HealthCare) p 424, 692

Afrin Menthol Nasal Spray (Schering-Plough HealthCare) p 424, 692

Afrin Nasal Spray 0.05% and Nasal Spray Pump (Schering-Plough HealthCare) p 424, 692

Afrin Nose Drops 0.05% (Schering-Plough HealthCare) p 424, 692

Ayr Saline Nasal Drops (Ascher) p 403, 509

Ayr Saline Nasal Mist (Ascher) p 403, 509

Benzedrex Inhaler (Menley & James) p 415, 608

Cheracol Nasal Spray Pump (Roberts) p 663

Dristan Nasal Spray (Whitehall) p 764

Dristan Menthol Nasal Spray (Whitehall) p 764

Dristan Nasal Spray, Metered Dose Pump, Regular (Whitehall) p 764

Dristan 12-hour Nasal Spray, Regular and Menthol (Whitehall) p 767

Dristan 12-hour Nasal Spray, Metered Dose Pump (Whitehall) p 767

Duration 12 Hour Nasal Spray (Schering-Plough HealthCare) p 426, 699

Duration 12 Hour Nasal Spray Pump (Schering-Plough HealthCare) p 426, 699

4-Way Fast Acting Nasal Spray (regular & mentholated) & Metered Spray Pump (regular) (Bristol-Myers Products) p 405, 532

4-Way Long Lasting Nasal Spray & Metered Spray Pump (Bristol-Myers Products) p 405, 533

NTZ Long Acting Nasal Spray & Drops 0.05% (Sterling Health) p 735

NāSal Moisturizing Nasal Spray (Sterling Health) p 430, 734

NāSal Moisturizing Nose Drops (Sterling Health) p 430, 734

Neo-Synephrine Maximum Strength 12 Hour Nasal Spray (Sterling Health) p 734

Neo-Synephrine Maximum Strength 12 Hour Nasal Spray Pump (Sterling Health) p 430, 734

Neo-Synephrine Nasal Solutions, Pediatric, Mild, Regular & Extra Strength (Sterling Health) p 734

Neo-Synephrine Nasal Sprays, Pediatric, Mild, Regular & Extra Strength (Sterling Health) p 430, 734

Neo-Synephrine Nose Drops (Sterling Health) p 430, 734

Nōstril Nasal Decongestant (CIBA Consumer) p 407, 552

Nōstrilla Long Acting Nasal Decongestant (CIBA Consumer) p 407, 552

Otrivin Nasal Drops (CIBA Consumer) p 408, 553

Otrivin Pediatric Nasal Drops (CIBA Consumer) p 408, 553

Privine Nasal Solution and Drops (CIBA Consumer) p 408, 554

Privine Nasal Spray (CIBA Consumer) p 408, 554

Vicks Inhaler (Richardson-Vicks) p 659

Vicks Sinex Decongestant Nasal Spray (Richardson-Vicks) p 661

Vicks Sinex Decongestant Nasal Ultra Fine Mist (Richardson-Vicks) p 661

Vicks Sinex Long-Acting Decongestant Nasal Spray (Richardson-Vicks) p 661

Vicks Sinex Long-Acting Decongestant Nasal Ultra Fine Mist (Richardson-Vicks) p 661

Vicks Vaporub (Richardson-Vicks) p 662

Vicks Vaposteam (Richardson-Vicks) p 662

Vicks Vatronol Nose Drops (Richardson-Vicks) p 662

EXPECTORANTS & COMBINATIONS

Benylin Expectorant (Parke-Davis) p 419, 633

Cheracol-D Cough Formula (Roberts) p 421, 663

Cough Formula Comtrex (Bristol-Myers Products) p 405, 524

Congestac Caplets (Menley & James) p 415, 609

Contac Cough and Chest Cold (SmithKline Beecham) p 427, 706

Contac Cough & Sore Throat Formula (SmithKline Beecham) p 427, 707

Dimacol Caplets (Robins Consumer) p 668

Dorcol Children's Cough Syrup (Sandoz Consumer) p 423, 682

Naldecon CX Adult Liquid (Apothecon) p 505

Naldecon DX Adult Liquid (Apothecon) p 505

Naldecon DX Children's Syrup (Apothecon) p 506

Naldecon DX Pediatric Drops (Apothecon) p 506

Naldecon EX Children's Syrup (Apothecon) p 507

Naldecon EX Pediatric Drops (Apothecon) p 507

Naldecon Senior DX Cough/Cold Liquid (Apothecon) p 507

Naldecon Senior EX Cough/Cold Liquid (Apothecon) p 508

Novahistine DMX (Marion Merrell Dow) p 412, 583

Robitussin (Robins Consumer) p 422, 672

Robitussin-CF (Robins Consumer) p 422, 673

Robitussin-DM (Robins Consumer) p 422, 673

Robitussin-PE (Robins Consumer) p 422, 674

Ryna-CX Liquid (Wallace) p 432, 754

Sudafed Cough Syrup (Burroughs Wellcome) p 407, 541

Triaminic Expectorant (Sandoz Consumer) p 424, 686

Vicks Children's Cough Syrup (Richardson-Vicks) p 654

Vicks Daycare Daytime Cold Medicine Caplets (Richardson-Vicks) p 655

Vicks Daycare Daytime Cold Medicine Liquid (Richardson-Vicks) p 655

Vicks Formula 44E Cough & Expectorant Medicine (Richardson-Vicks) p 657

Vicks Pediatric Formula 44e Cough & Expectorant Medicine (Richardson-Vicks) p 659

LOZENGES

Children's Chloraseptic Lozenges (Richardson-Vicks) p 652

Chloraseptic Lozenges, Cherry, Cool Mint and Menthol (Richardson-Vicks) p 653

Halls Plus Cough Suppressant Tablets (Warner-Lambert) p 432, 756

Hold Cough Suppressant Lozenge (Menley & James) p 415, 609

N'ICE Medicated Sugarless Sore Throat and Cough Lozenges (SmithKline Beecham) p 427, 714

Robitussin Cough Calmers (Robins Consumer) p 674

Robitussin Cough Drops (Robins Consumer) p 422, 674

Soothers Throat Drops (Warner-Lambert) p 433, 758

Sucrets Original Mint (SmithKline Beecham) p 428, 719

Sucrets Children's Cherry Flavored Sore Throat Lozenges (SmithKline Beecham) p 428, 719

Sucrets Cold Formula (SmithKline Beecham) p 428, 719

Sucrets Maximum Strength Wintergreen and Sucrets Wild Cherry (Regular Strength) Sore Throat Lozenges (SmithKline Beecham) p 428, 719

Vicks Cough Drops (Richardson-Vicks) p 655

Extra Strength Vicks Cough Drops (Richardson-Vicks) p 655

Vicks Formula 44 Cough Control Discs (Richardson-Vicks) p 656

OTHER

Cheracol Sore Throat Spray (Roberts) p 663

Children's Chloraseptic Spray (Richardson-Vicks) p 654

Chloraseptic Liquid, Cherry, Menthol and Cool Mint (Richardson-Vicks) p 652

Chloraseptic Liquid - Nitrogen Propelled Spray (Richardson-Vicks) p 652

NāSal Moisturizing Nasal Spray (Sterling Health) p 430, 734

NāSal Moisturizing Nose Drops (Sterling Health) p 430, 734

N'ICE Medicated Sugarless Sore Throat and Cough Lozenges (SmithKline Beecham) p 427, 714

Ocean Mist (Fleming) p 563

COLD SORE PREPARATIONS
(see under HERPES TREATMENT)

COLOSTOMY DEODORIZERS

Charcocaps (Requa) p 648

Devrom Chewable Tablets (Parthenon) p 638

CONSTIPATION AIDS
(see under LAXATIVES)

CONTRACEPTIVES

DEVICES

Today Vaginal Contraceptive Sponge (Whitehall) p 435, 772

TOPICAL

Conceptrol Contraceptive Gel • Single Use Contraceptive (Ortho Pharmaceutical) p 418, 625

Conceptrol Contraceptive Inserts (Ortho Pharmaceutical) p 418, 625

Delfen Contraceptive Foam (Ortho Pharmaceutical) p 418, 625

Encare Vaginal Contraceptive Suppositories (Thompson Medical) p 745

Gynol II Extra Strength Contraceptive Jelly (Ortho Pharmaceutical) p 418, 626

Gynol II Original Formula Contraceptive Jelly (Ortho Pharmaceutical) p 418, 626

Ortho-Gynol Contraceptive Jelly (Ortho Pharmaceutical) p 418, 626

Semicid Vaginal Contraceptive Inserts (Whitehall) p 772

CORN & CALLUS REMOVERS

Freezone Solution (Whitehall) p 767

COSMETICS

Herpecin-L Cold Sore Lip Balm (Campbell) p 544

COUGH PREPARATIONS (see under COLD & COUGH PREPARATIONS)

D

DANDRUFF & SEBORRHEA PREPARATIONS (see under DERMATOLOGICALS, DANDRUFF MEDICATIONS & SEBORRHEA TREATMENT)

DECONGESTANTS (see under COLD & COUGH PREPARATIONS)

DECONGESTANTS, OPHTHALMIC

DECONGESTANT COMBINATIONS

Visine EXTRA Eye Drops (Pfizer Consumer) p 420, 642

DECONGESTANT/ASTRINGENT COMBINATIONS

Clear Eyes ACR Astringent/Lubricating Eye Redness Reliever (Ross) p 422, 677

Visine A.C. Eye Drops (Pfizer Consumer) p 420, 641

DECONGESTANTS

Clear Eyes Lubricating Eye Redness Reliever (Ross) p 422, 677

Collyrium Fresh (Wyeth-Ayerst) p 435, 775

Murine Plus Lubricating Eye Redness Reliever (Ross) p 422, 678

Visine Eye Drops (Pfizer Consumer) p 420, 641

Visine L.R. Eye Drops (Pfizer Consumer) p 420, 642

VASOCONSTRICTORS

Visine L.R. Eye Drops (Pfizer Consumer) p 420, 642

DEMULCENT

Celluvisc Lubricant Ophthalmic Solution (Allergan Pharmaceuticals) p 504

Clear Eyes ACR Astringent/Lubricating Eye Redness Reliever (Ross) p 422, 677

Murine Eye Lubricant (Ross) p 422, 678

Murine Plus Lubricating Eye Redness Reliever (Ross) p 422, 678

Tears Plus Lubricant Ophthalmic Solution (Allergan Pharmaceuticals) p 505

Visine EXTRA Eye Drops (Pfizer Consumer) p 420, 642

DENTAL PREPARATIONS

CAVITY AGENTS

Listermint with Fluoride (Warner-Lambert) p 433, 756

DENTIFRICES

Denquel Sensitive Teeth Toothpaste (Procter & Gamble) p 642

Promise Toothpaste (Block) p 517

Mint Gel Sensodyne (Block) p 518

Mint Sensodyne Toothpaste (Block) p 518

Original Sensodyne Toothpaste (Block) p 517

RINSES

Chloraseptic Liquid, Cherry, Menthol and Cool Mint (Richardson-Vicks) p 652

Chloraseptic Liquid - Nitrogen Propelled Spray (Richardson-Vicks) p 652

Listerine Antiseptic (Warner-Lambert) p 433, 756

Listermint with Fluoride (Warner-Lambert) p 433, 756

OTHER

Anbesol Gel Antiseptic-Anesthetic-Regular Strength (Whitehall) p 434, 763

Anbesol Gel Antiseptic-Anesthetic - Maximum Strength (Whitehall) p 434, 763

Anbesol Liquid Antiseptic-Anesthetic (Whitehall) p 434, 763

Anbesol Liquid Antiseptic-Anesthetic - Maximum Strength (Whitehall) p 434, 763

Chloraseptic Lozenges, Cherry, Cool Mint and Menthol (Richardson-Vicks) p 653

Gly-Oxide Liquid (Marion Merrell Dow) p 412, 583

Maximum Strength Orajel (Del Pharmaceuticals) p 408, 557

Zilactin Medicated Gel (Zila Pharmaceuticals) p 435, 777

Zilactol Medicated Liquid (Zila Pharmaceuticals) p 777

ZilaDent Oral Analgesic Gel (Zila Pharmaceuticals) p 777

DENTURE PREPARATIONS

Professional Strength Efferdent (Warner-Lambert) p 432, 755

ZilaDent Oral Analgesic Gel (Zila Pharmaceuticals) p 777

DEODORANTS

TOPICAL

Orchid Fresh II Perineal/Ostomy Cleanser (Care-Tech) p 545

DERMATOLOGICALS

ABRADANT

Oxy Lathering Facial Scrub (SmithKline Beecham) p 428, 715

pHisoPUFF (Sterling Health) p 430, 738

ACNE PREPARATIONS

Acnomel Cream (Menley & James) p 415, 607

Aqua Glyde Cleanser (Herald Pharmacal) p 564

Aveeno Cleansing Bar for Acne (Rydelle) p 423, 680

Clear by Design Medicated Acne Gel (SmithKline Beecham) p 426, 704

DDS-Acidophilus (UAS Laboratories) p 747

Oxy Medicated Cleanser (SmithKline Beecham) p 428, 715

Oxy Medicated Pads - Regular, Sensitive Skin, and Maximum Strength (SmithKline Beecham) p 427, 716

Oxy Medicated Soap (SmithKline Beecham) p 428, 715

Oxy Night Watch Nighttime Acne Medication-Maximum Strength and Sensitive Skin Formulas (SmithKline Beecham) p 428, 716

Oxy 10 Daily Face Wash Antibacterial Skin Wash (SmithKline Beecham) p 427, 716

Oxy-5 and Oxy-10 Tinted and Vanishing Formulas with Sorboxyl (SmithKline Beecham) p 427, 715

Stri-Dex Dual Textured Maximum Strength Pads (Sterling Health) p 431, 739

Stri-Dex Dual Textured Maximum Strength Big Pads (Sterling Health) p 739

Stri-Dex Dual Textured Regular Strength Pads (Sterling Health) p 431, 739

Stri-Dex Dual Textured Regular Strength Big Pads (Sterling Health) p 739

Stri-Dex Dual Textured Sensitive Skin Pads (Sterling Health) p 739

Stri-Dex Super Scrub Pads (Sterling Health) p 739

ANALGESIC

Americaine Topical Anesthetic First Aid Ointment (Fisons Consumer Health) p 409, 559

Americaine Topical Anesthetic Spray (Fisons Consumer Health) p 409, 559

Aspercreme Creme, Lotion Analgesic Rub (Thompson Medical) p 743

Benadryl Anti-Itch Cream, Regular Strength 1% and Maximum Strength 2% (Parke-Davis) p 418, 629

Benadryl Spray, Maximum Strength 2% (Parke-Davis) p 418, 632

Benadryl Spray, Regular Strength 1% (Parke-Davis) p 418, 632

Corticaine External Analgesic (Whitby) p 433, 760

Icy Hot Balm (Chattem) p 546

Icy Hot Cream (Chattem) p 546

Icy Hot Stick (Chattem) p 546

Mycitracin Plus Pain Reliever (Upjohn) p 432, 750

Therapeutic Mineral Ice, Pain Relieving Gel (Bristol-Myers Products) p 406, 536

ANESTHETICS, TOPICAL

Americaine Topical Anesthetic First Aid Ointment (Fisons Consumer Health) p 409, 559

Americaine Topical Anesthetic Spray (Fisons Consumer Health) p 409, 559

Bactine Antiseptic/Anesthetic First Aid Liquid (Miles Consumer) p 416, 617

Campho-Phenique Triple Antibiotic Ointment Plus Pain Reliever (Sterling Health) p 429, 731

Dermoplast Anesthetic Pain Relief Lotion (Whitehall) p 764

Dermoplast Anesthetic Pain Relief Spray (Whitehall) p 764

Itch-X Gel (Ascher) p 403, 509

ZilaDent Oral Analgesic Gel (Zila Pharmaceuticals) p 777

ANTIBACTERIAL

Anbesol Gel Antiseptic-Anesthetic-Regular Strength (Whitehall) p 434, 763

Anbesol Gel Antiseptic-Anesthetic - Maximum Strength (Whitehall) p 434, 763

Anbesol Liquid Antiseptic-Anesthetic (Whitehall) p 434, 763

Anbesol Liquid Antiseptic-Anesthetic - Maximum Strength (Whitehall) p 434, 763

Aquaphor Antibiotic Ointment (Beiersdorf) p 404, 515

Bactine Antiseptic/Anesthetic First Aid Liquid (Miles Consumer) p 416, 617

Bactine First Aid Antibiotic Plus Anesthetic Ointment (Miles Consumer) p 416, 617

Barri-Care Antimicrobial Barrier Ointment (Care-Tech) p 544

Campho-Phenique Cold Sore Gel (Sterling Health) p 429, 731

Campho-Phenique Liquid (Sterling Health) p 429, 731

Campho-Phenique Triple Antibiotic Ointment Plus Pain Reliever (Sterling Health) p 429, 731

Care Creme (Care-Tech) p 544

Clinical Care Dermal Wound Cleanser (Care-Tech) p 545

Concept (Care-Tech) p 545

Formula Magic Antibacterial Powder (Care-Tech) p 545

Hibiclens Antimicrobial Skin Cleanser (Stuart) p 431, 740

Hibistat Germicidal Hand Rinse (Stuart) p 741

Hibistat Towelette (Stuart) p 741

Neosporin Cream (Burroughs
Wellcome) p 406, 539
Neosporin Ointment (Burroughs
Wellcome) p 406, 539
Neosporin Maximum Strength Ointment
(Burroughs Wellcome) p 406, 539
Orchid Fresh II Perineal/Ostomy
Cleanser (Care-Tech) p 545
Oxy Medicated Cleanser (SmithKline
Beecham) p 428, 715
Oxy Medicated Pads - Regular,
Sensitive Skin, and Maximum
Strength (SmithKline Beecham)
p 427, 716
Oxy Medicated Soap (SmithKline
Beecham) p 428, 715
Oxy 10 Daily Face Wash Antibacterial
Skin Wash (SmithKline Beecham)
p 427, 716
Oxy-5 and Oxy-10 Tinted and
Vanishing Formulas with Sorboxyl
(SmithKline Beecham) p 427, 715
PRID Salve (Walker Pharmacal) p 753
Polysporin Ointment (Burroughs
Wellcome) p 407, 540
Polysporin Powder (Burroughs
Wellcome) p 407, 540
Satin Antimicrobial Skin Cleanser
(Care-Tech) p 545
Stri-Dex Dual Textured Maximum
Strength Pads (Sterling Health)
p 431, 739
Stri-Dex Dual Textured Regular
Strength Pads (Sterling Health)
p 431, 739
Stri-Dex Dual Textured Sensitive Skin
Pads (Sterling Health) p 739
Stri-Dex Super Scrub Pads (Sterling
Health) p 739
Techni-Care Surgical Scrub (Care-Tech)
p 545

**ANTIBACTERIAL, ANTIFUNGAL &
COMBINATIONS**
Caldesene Medicated Powder (Fisons
Consumer Health) p 409, 559

ANTIBIOTIC
Aquaphor Antibiotic Ointment
(Beiersdorf) p 404, 515
Bactine First Aid Antibiotic Plus
Anesthetic Ointment (Miles
Consumer) p 416, 617
Campho-Phenique Triple Antibiotic
Ointment Plus Pain Reliever (Sterling
Health) p 429, 731
Mycitracin Plus Pain Reliever (Upjohn)
p 432, 750
Maximum Strength Mycitracin Triple
Antibiotic First Aid Ointment (Upjohn)
p 432, 750
Neosporin Cream (Burroughs
Wellcome) p 406, 539
Neosporin Ointment (Burroughs
Wellcome) p 406, 539
Neosporin Maximum Strength Ointment
(Burroughs Wellcome) p 406, 539
Polysporin Ointment (Burroughs
Wellcome) p 407, 540
Polysporin Powder (Burroughs
Wellcome) p 407, 540

ANTI-INFLAMMATORY AGENTS
Massengill Medicated Soft Cloth
Towelette (SmithKline Beecham)
p 713

ASTRINGENTS
Acid Mantle Creme (Sandoz Consumer)
p 682
Domeboro Astringent Solution
Effervescent Tablets (Miles
Consumer) p 417, 619
Domeboro Astringent Solution Powder
Packets (Miles Consumer) p 417,
618
Tucks Premoistened Pads (Parke-Davis)
p 420, 637
Tucks Take-Alongs (Parke-Davis) p 637

BARRIER
Barri-Care Antimicrobial Barrier
Ointment (Care-Tech) p 544

BATH OILS
Alpha Keri Moisture Rich Body Oil
(Bristol-Myers Products) p 405, 519

Aveeno Bath Oilated (Rydelle) p 423,
680
Aveeno Shower and Bath Oil (Rydelle)
p 423, 681

BURN RELIEF
A and D Ointment (Schering-Plough
HealthCare) p 424, 692
Americaine Topical Anesthetic First Aid
Ointment (Fisons Consumer Health)
p 409, 559
Americaine Topical Anesthetic Spray
(Fisons Consumer Health) p 409,
559
Aquaphor Natural Healing Ointment
(Beiersdorf) p 404, 515
Bactine Antiseptic/Anesthetic First Aid
Liquid (Miles Consumer) p 416, 617
Bactine First Aid Antibiotic Plus
Anesthetic Ointment (Miles
Consumer) p 416, 617
Balmex Ointment (Macsil) p 579
Barri-Care Antimicrobial Barrier
Ointment (Care-Tech) p 544
BiCozene Creme (Sandoz Consumer)
p 423, 682
Borofax Ointment (Burroughs
Wellcome) p 538
Campho-Phenique Triple Antibiotic
Ointment Plus Pain Reliever (Sterling
Health) p 429,.731
Care Creme (Care-Tech) p 544
Dermoplast Anesthetic Pain Relief
Lotion (Whitehall) p 764
Dermoplast Anesthetic Pain Relief
Spray (Whitehall) p 764
Desitin Ointment (Pfizer Consumer)
p 420, 638
Neosporin Cream (Burroughs
Wellcome) p 406, 539
Neosporin Ointment (Burroughs
Wellcome) p 406, 539
Neosporin Maximum Strength Ointment
(Burroughs Wellcome) p 406, 539
Nupercainal Pain Relief Cream (CIBA
Consumer) p 408, 553
Polysporin Ointment (Burroughs
Wellcome) p 407, 540
Polysporin Powder (Burroughs
Wellcome) p 407, 540
Water-Jel Sterile Burn Dressings
(Water-Jel Technologies) p 758

CLEANSING AGENTS
Aqua Glyde Cleanser (Herald
Pharmacal) p 564
Aveeno Bath Oilated (Rydelle) p 423,
680
Aveeno Bath Regular (Rydelle) p 423,
680
Aveeno Cleansing Bar for Acne
(Rydelle) p 423, 680
Aveeno Cleansing Bar for Combination
Skin (Rydelle) p 423, 680
Aveeno Cleansing Bar for Dry Skin
(Rydelle) p 423, 681
Aveeno Shower and Bath Oil (Rydelle)
p 423, 681
Cam Lotion (Herald Pharmacal) p 564
Concept (Care-Tech) p 545
Dove Bar (Lever Brothers) p 578
Eucerin Cleansing Lotion Dry Skin Care
(Beiersdorf) p 404, 515
Eucerin Dry Skin Care Cleansing Bar
(Beiersdorf) p 404, 515
Lubriderm Bath Oil (Warner-Lambert)
p 433, 757
Lubriderm Body Bar (Warner-Lambert)
p 433, 756
Massengill Baby Powder Soft Cloth
Towelette and Fragrance Free Soft
Cloth Towelette (SmithKline
Beecham) p 713
Moisturel Sensitive Skin Cleanser
(Westwood) p 433, 759
Neutrogena Cleansing Wash
(Neutrogena) p 417, 622
Oil of Olay Foaming Face Wash (Olay
Co. Inc.) (Richardson-Vicks) p 654
Orchid Fresh II Perineal/Ostomy
Cleanser (Care-Tech) p 545
Oxy Lathering Facial Scrub (SmithKline
Beecham) p 428, 715

Oxy Medicated Cleanser (SmithKline
Beecham) p 428, 715
Oxy Medicated Pads - Regular,
Sensitive Skin, and Maximum
Strength (SmithKline Beecham)
p 427, 716
Oxy Medicated Soap (SmithKline
Beecham) p 428, 715
Oxy Night Watch Nighttime Acne
Medication-Maximum Strength and
Sensitive Skin Formulas (SmithKline
Beecham) p 428, 716
Oxy 10 Daily Face Wash Antibacterial
Skin Wash (SmithKline Beecham)
p 427, 716
pHisoDerm Cleansing Bar (Sterling
Health) p 430, 738
pHisoDerm For Baby (Sterling Health)
p 430, 738
pHisoDerm Skin Cleanser and
Conditioner - Regular and Oily
(Sterling Health) p 430, 738
Satin Antimicrobial Skin Cleanser
(Care-Tech) p 545
Techni-Care Surgical Scrub (Care-Tech)
p 545

COAL TAR
Denorex Medicated Shampoo and
Conditioner (Whitehall) p 434, 764
Denorex Medicated Shampoo, Extra
Strength (Whitehall) p 434, 764
Denorex Medicated Shampoo, Extra
Strength With Conditioners
(Whitehall) p 434, 764
Denorex Medicated Shampoo, Regular
& Mountain Fresh Herbal Scent
(Whitehall) p 434, 764
Neutrogena T/Derm Tar Emollient
(Neutrogena) p 623
Neutrogena T/Gel Therapeutic
Shampoo (Neutrogena) p 417, 623
Neutrogena T/Sal Therapeutic
Shampoo (Neutrogena) p 417, 624
Oxipor VHC Lotion for Psoriasis
(Whitehall) p 768
P & S Plus Tar Gel (Baker Cummins
Pharmaceuticals) p 512
Tegrin Dandruff Shampoo (Block)
p 518
Tegrin for Psoriasis Lotion, Skin Cream
& Medicated Soap (Block) p 518
X-Seb T Shampoo (Baker Cummins
Pharmaceuticals) p 513
X-Seb T Plus Conditioning Shampoo
(Baker Cummins Pharmaceuticals)
p 513

COAL TAR & SULFUR
MG 217 Psoriasis Ointment and Lotion
(Triton Consumer) p 747
MG 217 Psoriasis Shampoo and
Conditioner (Triton Consumer) p 747

CONDITIONING RINSES
Denorex Medicated Shampoo and
Conditioner (Whitehall) p 434, 764
Denorex Medicated Shampoo, Extra
Strength With Conditioners
(Whitehall) p 434, 764

CONTACT DERMATITIS
Care Creme (Care-Tech) p 544
Maximum Strength Cortaid Cream
(Upjohn) p 431, 748
Maximum Strength Cortaid Ointment
(Upjohn) p 431, 748
Maximum Strength Cortaid Spray
(Upjohn) p 431, 748
Satin Antimicrobial Skin Cleanser
(Care-Tech) p 545

DANDRUFF MEDICATIONS
Denorex Medicated Shampoo and
Conditioner (Whitehall) p 434, 764
Denorex Medicated Shampoo, Extra
Strength (Whitehall) p 434, 764
Denorex Medicated Shampoo, Extra
Strength With Conditioners
(Whitehall) p 434, 764
Denorex Medicated Shampoo, Regular
& Mountain Fresh Herbal Scent
(Whitehall) p 434, 764
Head & Shoulders Antidandruff
Shampoo (Procter & Gamble) p 643

Head & Shoulders Antidandruff
Shampoo 2-in-1 plus Conditioner
(Procter & Gamble) p 643
Head & Shoulders Dry Scalp Shampoo
(Procter & Gamble) p 643
Head & Shoulders Dry Scalp Shampoo
2-in-1 plus Conditioner (Procter &
Gamble) p 643
Head & Shoulders Intensive Treatment
Dandruff Shampoo (Procter &
Gamble) p 643
Head & Shoulders Intensive Treatment
Dandruff Shampoo 2-in-1 plus
Conditioner (Procter & Gamble)
p 643
P & S Plus Tar Gel (Baker Cummins
Pharmaceuticals) p 512
P & S Shampoo (Baker Cummins
Pharmaceuticals) p 512
Sebulex Antiseborrheic Treatment
Shampoo (Westwood) p 433, 759
Sebutone and Sebutone Cream
Antiseborrheic Tar Shampoos
(Westwood) p 433, 759
Selsun Blue Dandruff Shampoo (Ross)
p 422, 679
Selsun Blue Dandruff Shampoo-Extra
Medicated (Ross) p 422, 679
Selsun Blue Extra Conditioning
Dandruff Shampoo (Ross) p 422,
679
Tegrin Dandruff Shampoo (Block)
p 518
X-Seb Shampoo (Baker Cummins
Pharmaceuticals) p 512
X-Seb Plus Conditioning Shampoo
(Baker Cummins Pharmaceuticals)
p 512
X-Seb T Shampoo (Baker Cummins
Pharmaceuticals) p 513
X-Seb T Plus Conditioning Shampoo
(Baker Cummins Pharmaceuticals)
p 513
Zincon Dandruff Shampoo (Lederle)
p 411, 578

DERMATITIS RELIEF
A and D Ointment (Schering-Plough
HealthCare) p 424, 692
Acid Mantle Creme (Sandoz Consumer)
p 682
Alpha Keri Moisture Rich Body Oil
(Bristol-Myers Products) p 405, 519
Aqua Care Cream (Menley & James)
p 415, 607
Aqua Care Lotion (Menley & James)
p 415, 607
Aveeno Bath Oilated (Rydelle) p 423,
680
Aveeno Bath Regular (Rydelle) p 423,
680
Aveeno Moisturizing Cream (Rydelle)
p 423, 681
Aveeno Moisturizing Lotion (Rydelle)
p 423, 681
Aveeno Shower and Bath Oil (Rydelle)
p 423, 681
Bactine Hydrocortisone Anti-Itch Cream
(Miles Consumer) p 416, 617
Balmex Baby Powder (Macsil) p 579
Balmex Emollient Lotion (Macsil) p 579
Balmex Ointment (Macsil) p 579
BiCozene Creme (Sandoz Consumer)
p 423, 682
Caladryl Clear Lotion (Parke-Davis)
p 419, 633
Caladryl Cream, Lotion, Spray
(Parke-Davis) p 419, 633
Caldecort Anti-Itch Hydrocortisone
Cream (Fisons Consumer Health)
p 409, 559
Caldecort Anti-Itch Hydrocortisone
Spray (Fisons Consumer Health)
p 409, 559
Caldecort Light Cream (Fisons
Consumer Health) p 409, 559
Caldesene Medicated Ointment (Fisons
Consumer Health) p 409, 559
Caldesene Medicated Powder (Fisons
Consumer Health) p 409, 559
Cam Lotion (Herald Pharmacal) p 564
Clocream Skin Protectant Cream
(Roberts) p 664
Concept (Care-Tech) p 545

Cortaid Cream with Aloe (Upjohn)
p 431, 747
Cortaid Lotion (Upjohn) p 431, 747
Cortaid Ointment with Aloe (Upjohn)
p 431, 747
Cortaid Spray (Upjohn) p 431, 747
Maximum Strength Cortaid Cream
(Upjohn) p 431, 748
Maximum Strength Cortaid Ointment
(Upjohn) p 431, 748
Maximum Strength Cortaid Spray
(Upjohn) p 431, 748
Cortef Feminine Itch Cream (Upjohn)
p 748
Corticaine External Analgesic (Whitby)
p 433, 760
Cortizone-5 Creme and Ointment
(Thompson Medical) p 431, 743
Cortizone-5 Wipes (Thompson Medical)
p 743
Cortizone-10 Creme and Ointment
(Thompson Medical) p 744
Desitin Ointment (Pfizer Consumer)
p 420, 638
Domeboro Astringent Solution
Effervescent Tablets (Miles
Consumer) p 417, 619
Domeboro Astringent Solution Powder
Packets (Miles Consumer) p 417,
618
Eucerin Dry Skin Care Daily Facial
Lotion SPF 20 (Beiersdorf) p 404,
515
Eucerin Lotion (Beiersdorf) p 404, 516
Massengill Medicated Soft Cloth
Towelette (SmithKline Beecham)
p 713
Moisturel Cream (Westwood) p 433,
758
Moisturel Lotion (Westwood) p 433,
758
P & S Liquid (Baker Cummins
Pharmaceuticals) p 511
P & S Plus Tar Gel (Baker Cummins
Pharmaceuticals) p 512
P & S Shampoo (Baker Cummins
Pharmaceuticals) p 512
Satin Antimicrobial Skin Cleanser
(Care-Tech) p 545
Tegrin-HC with Hydrocortisone Anti-Itch
Ointment (Block) p 518
X-Seb Plus Conditioning Shampoo
(Baker Cummins Pharmaceuticals)
p 512
X-Seb T Shampoo (Baker Cummins
Pharmaceuticals) p 513
X-Seb T Plus Conditioning Shampoo
(Baker Cummins Pharmaceuticals)
p 513

DETERGENTS
pHisoDerm For Baby (Sterling Health)
p 430, 738
pHisoDerm Skin Cleanser and
Conditioner - Regular and Oily
(Sterling Health) p 430, 738
Selsun Blue Dandruff Shampoo (Ross)
p 422, 679
Selsun Blue Dandruff Shampoo-Extra
Medicated (Ross) p 422, 679
Selsun Blue Extra Conditioning
Dandruff Shampoo (Ross) p 422,
679
X-Seb Shampoo (Baker Cummins
Pharmaceuticals) p 512
X-Seb Plus Conditioning Shampoo
(Baker Cummins Pharmaceuticals)
p 512
X-Seb T Shampoo (Baker Cummins
Pharmaceuticals) p 513
X-Seb T Plus Conditioning Shampoo
(Baker Cummins Pharmaceuticals)
p 513
Zincon Dandruff Shampoo (Lederle)
p 411, 578

DIAPER RASH RELIEF
Clocream Skin Protectant Cream
(Roberts) p 664
Vaseline Pure Petroleum Jelly Skin
Protectant/Lip Therapy
(Chese-Pond's) p 548

EMOLLIENTS
A and D Ointment (Schering-Plough
HealthCare) p 424, 692
Alpha Keri Moisture Rich Body Oil
(Bristol-Myers Products) p 405, 519
Alpha Keri Moisture Rich Cleansing Bar
(Bristol-Myers Products) p 519
Aqua Care Cream (Menley & James)
p 415, 607
Aqua Care Lotion (Menley & James)
p 415, 607
Aqua-A Cream (Baker Cummins
Pharmaceuticals) p 511
Aquaderm Combination
Treatment/Moisturizer (SPF 15
Formula) (Baker Cummins
Pharmaceuticals) p 511
Aquaderm Cream (Baker Cummins
Pharmaceuticals) p 511
Aquaderm Lotion (Baker Cummins
Pharmaceuticals) p 511
Aquaphor Healing Ointment, Original
Formula (Beiersdorf) p 404, 514
Aquaphor Natural Healing Ointment
(Beiersdorf) p 404, 514
Aveeno Bath Oilated (Rydelle) p 423,
680
Aveeno Bath Regular (Rydelle) p 423,
680
Aveeno Moisturizing Cream (Rydelle)
p 423, 681
Aveeno Moisturizing Lotion (Rydelle)
p 423, 681
Aveeno Shower and Bath Oil (Rydelle)
p 423, 681
Balmex Baby Powder (Macsil) p 579
Balmex Emollient Lotion (Macsil) p 579
Balmex Ointment (Macsil) p 579
Borofax Ointment (Burroughs
Wellcome) p 538
Care Creme (Care-Tech) p 544
Carmol 20 Cream (Syntex) p 743
Carmol 10 Lotion (Syntex) p 743
Chap Stick Lip Balm (Robins
Consumer) p 421, 667
Chap Stick Petroleum Jelly Plus
(Robins Consumer) p 421, 668
Chap Stick Petroleum Jelly Plus with
Sunblock 15 (Robins Consumer)
p 421, 668
Chap Stick Sunblock 15 Lip Balm
(Robins Consumer) p 421, 667
Clocream Skin Protectant Cream
(Roberts) p 664
Complex 15 Hand & Body Moisturizing
Cream (Schering-Plough HealthCare)
p 425, 694
Complex 15 Hand & Body Moisturizing
Lotion (Schering-Plough HealthCare)
p 425, 694
Complex 15 Moisturizing Face Cream
(Schering-Plough HealthCare) p 425,
695
Concept (Care-Tech) p 545
Desitin Ointment (Pfizer Consumer)
p 420, 638
Eucerin Dry Skin Care Daily Facial
Lotion SPF 20 (Beiersdorf) p 404,
515
Eucerin Dry Skin Care Creme
(Beiersdorf) p 404, 515
Eucerin Lotion (Beiersdorf) p 404, 516
Eucerin Dry Skin Care Lotion
(Fragrance-free) (Beiersdorf) p 404,
516
Herpecin-L Cold Sore Lip Balm
(Campbell) p 544
Keri Lotion - Original Formula
(Bristol-Myers Products) p 405, 533
Keri Lotion - Silky Smooth Formula
(Bristol-Myers Products) p 405, 533
Keri Lotion - Silky Smooth Fragrance
Free Formula (Bristol-Myers
Products) p 405, 533
Lubriderm Bath Oil (Warner-Lambert)
p 433, 757
Lubriderm Lotion (Warner-Lambert)
p 433, 756
Moisturel Cream (Westwood) p 433,
758
Moisturel Lotion (Westwood) p 433,
758

Moisturel Sensitive Skin Cleanser (Westwood) p 433, 759
Neutrogena Norwegian Formula Emulsion (Neutrogena) p 417, 623
Neutrogena Norwegian Formula Hand Cream (Neutrogena) p 417, 623
Oil of Olay Daily UV Protectant SPF 15 Beauty Fluid-Regular & Fragrance Free (Olay Co. Inc.) (Richardson-Vicks) p 653
Oil of Olay Daily UV Protectant SPF 15 Moisture Replenishing Cream-Regular & Fragrance Free (Olay Co. Inc.) (Richardson-Vicks) p 653
pHisoDerm Cleansing Bar (Sterling Health) p 430, 738
pHisoDerm For Baby (Sterling Health) p 430, 738
pHisoDerm Skin Cleanser and Conditioner - Regular and Oily (Sterling Health) p 430, 738
Pen•Kera Creme (Ascher) p 403, 510
Satin Antimicrobial Skin Cleanser (Care-Tech) p 545
Ultra Mide 25 (Baker Cummins Pharmaceuticals) p 512
Extra Strength Vaseline Intensive Care Lotion (Chese-Pond's) p 548
Vaseline Pure Petroleum Jelly Skin Protectant/Lip Therapy (Chese-Pond's) p 548
Wellcome Lanoline (Burroughs Wellcome) p 544

FOOT CARE
Desenex Foot & Sneaker Deodorant Spray Powder (Fisons Consumer Health) p 409, 560
Formula Magic Antibacterial Powder (Care-Tech) p 545
Freezone Solution (Whitehall) p 767
Lotrimin AF Antifungal Cream, Lotion and Solution (Schering-Plough HealthCare) p 426, 700
Outgro Solution (Whitehall) p 767

FUNGICIDES
Caldesene Medicated Powder (Fisons Consumer Health) p 409, 559
Cruex Antifungal Cream (Fisons Consumer Health) p 409, 560
Cruex Antifungal Powder (Fisons Consumer Health) p 409, 560
Cruex Antifungal Spray Powder (Fisons Consumer Health) p 409, 560
Desenex Antifungal Cream (Fisons Consumer Health) p 560
Desenex Antifungal Foam (Fisons Consumer Health) p 560
Desenex Antifungal Ointment (Fisons Consumer Health) p 409, 560
Desenex Antifungal Powder (Fisons Consumer Health) p 409, 560
Desenex Antifungal Spray Powder (Fisons Consumer Health) p 409, 560
Hibiclens Antimicrobial Skin Cleanser (Stuart) p 431, 740
Hibistat Germicidal Hand Rinse (Stuart) p 741
Hibistat Towelette (Stuart) p 741
Impregon Concentrate (Fleming) p 563
Lotrimin AF Antifungal Cream, Lotion and Solution (Schering-Plough HealthCare) p 426, 700
Massengill Medicated Disposable Douche (SmithKline Beecham) p 427, 713
Massengill Medicated Liquid Concentrate (SmithKline Beecham) p 713
Micatin Antifungal Cream (Ortho Pharmaceutical) p 418, 627
Micatin Antifungal Deodorant Spray Powder (Ortho Pharmaceutical) p 418, 627
Micatin Antifungal Powder (Ortho Pharmaceutical) p 418, 627
Micatin Antifungal Spray Liquid (Ortho Pharmaceutical) p 418, 627
Micatin Antifungal Spray Powder (Ortho Pharmaceutical) p 418, 627
Micatin Jock Itch Cream (Ortho Pharmaceutical) p 627

Micatin Jock Itch Spray Powder (Ortho Pharmaceutical) p 627
Mycelex OTC Cream Antifungal (Miles Consumer) p 417, 619
Mycelex OTC Solution Antifungal (Miles Consumer) p 417, 619
NP-27 (Thompson Medical) p 431, 746
Tinactin Aerosol Liquid 1% (Schering-Plough HealthCare) p 426, 703
Tinactin Aerosol Powder 1% (Schering-Plough HealthCare) p 426, 703
Tinactin Antifungal Cream, Solution & Powder 1% (Schering-Plough HealthCare) p 426, 703
Tinactin Deodorant Powder Aerosol 1% (Schering-Plough HealthCare) p 703
Tinactin Jock Itch Cream 1% (Schering-Plough HealthCare) p 426, 703
Tinactin Jock Itch Spray Powder 1% (Schering-Plough HealthCare) p 426, 703
Ting Antifungal Cream (Fisons Consumer Health) p 409, 562
Ting Antifungal Powder (Fisons Consumer Health) p 409, 562
Ting Antifungal Spray Liquid (Fisons Consumer Health) p 409, 562
Ting Antifungal Spray Powder (Fisons Consumer Health) p 409, 562

GENERAL
A and D Ointment (Schering-Plough HealthCare) p 424, 692
Acid Mantle Creme (Sandoz Consumer) p 682
Aveeno Bath Regular (Rydelle) p 423, 680
Aveeno Moisturizing Lotion (Rydelle) p 423, 681
Bactine First Aid Antibiotic Plus Anesthetic Ointment (Miles Consumer) p 416, 617
Bactine Hydrocortisone Anti-Itch Cream (Miles Consumer) p 416, 617
Balmex Ointment (Macsil) p 579
Caldesene Medicated Ointment (Fisons Consumer Health) p 409, 559
Cortaid Cream with Aloe (Upjohn) p 431, 747
Cortaid Lotion (Upjohn) p 431, 747
Cortaid Ointment with Aloe (Upjohn) p 431, 747
Cortaid Spray (Upjohn) p 431, 747
Maximum Strength Cortaid Cream (Upjohn) p 431, 748
Maximum Strength Cortaid Ointment (Upjohn) p 431, 748
Maximum Strength Cortaid Spray (Upjohn) p 431, 748
Corticaine External Analgesic (Whitby) p 433, 760
Cortizone-5 Creme and Ointment (Thompson Medical) p 431, 743
Cortizone-5 Wipes (Thompson Medical) p 743
Cortizone-10 Creme and Ointment (Thompson Medical) p 744
Desitin Ointment (Pfizer Consumer) p 420, 638
Lubriderm Lotion (Warner-Lambert) p 433, 756
Massengill Baby Powder Soft Cloth Towelette and Fragrance Free Soft Cloth Towelette (SmithKline Beecham) p 713

HERPES TREATMENT
Campho-Phenique Cold Sore Gel (Sterling Health) p 429, 731
Campho-Phenique Liquid (Sterling Health) p 429, 731
Herpecin-L Cold Sore Lip Balm (Campbell) p 544
Zilactin Medicated Gel (Zila Pharmaceuticals) p 435, 777
Zilactol Medicated Liquid (Zila Pharmaceuticals) p 777

INSECT BITES & STINGS
Benadryl Spray, Maximum Strength 2% (Parke-Davis) p 418, 632

Benadryl Spray, Regular Strength 1% (Parke-Davis) p 418, 632
Maximum Strength Cortaid Cream (Upjohn) p 431, 748
Maximum Strength Cortaid Ointment (Upjohn) p 431, 748
Maximum Strength Cortaid Spray (Upjohn) p 431, 748
Dermoplast Anesthetic Pain Relief Lotion (Whitehall) p 764
Dermoplast Anesthetic Pain Relief Spray (Whitehall) p 764
Domeboro Astringent Solution Effervescent Tablets (Miles Consumer) p 417, 619
Domeboro Astringent Solution Powder Packets (Miles Consumer) p 417, 618
Itch-X Gel (Ascher) p 403, 509
Massengill Medicated Soft Cloth Towelette (SmithKline Beecham) p 713

KERATOLYTICS
Carmol 20 Cream (Syntex) p 743
Carmol 10 Lotion (Syntex) p 743
Compound W Gel (Whitehall) p 763
Compound W Liquid (Whitehall) p 763
Freezone Solution (Whitehall) p 767
Neutrogena T/Sal Therapeutic Shampoo (Neutrogena) p 417, 624
Ultra Mide 25 (Baker Cummins Pharmaceuticals) p 512

MOISTURIZERS
Alpha Keri Moisture Rich Body Oil (Bristol-Myers Products) p 405, 519
Alpha Keri Moisture Rich Cleansing Bar (Bristol-Myers Products) p 519
Aqua Care Cream (Menley & James) p 415, 607
Aqua Care Lotion (Menley & James) p 415, 607
Aqua Glycolic Lotion (Herald Pharmacal) p 564
Aqua-A Cream (Baker Cummins Pharmaceuticals) p 511
Aquaderm Combination Treatment/Moisturizer (SPF 15 Formula) (Baker Cummins Pharmaceuticals) p 511
Aquaderm Cream (Baker Cummins Pharmaceuticals) p 511
Aquaderm Lotion (Baker Cummins Pharmaceuticals) p 511
Aquaphor Healing Ointment, Original Formula (Beiersdorf) p 404, 514
Aquaphor Natural Healing Ointment (Beiersdorf) p 404, 515
Aveeno Bath Oilated (Rydelle) p 423, 680
Aveeno Moisturizing Cream (Rydelle) p 423, 681
Aveeno Moisturizing Lotion (Rydelle) p 423, 681
Aveeno Shower and Bath Oil (Rydelle) p 423, 681
Balmex Emollient Lotion (Macsil) p 579
Carmol 20 Cream (Syntex) p 743
Carmol 10 Lotion (Syntex) p 743
Chap Stick Lip Balm (Robins Consumer) p 421, 667
Chap Stick Petroleum Jelly Plus (Robins Consumer) p 421, 668
Chap Stick Petroleum Jelly Plus with Sunblock 15 (Robins Consumer) p 421, 668
Chap Stick Sunblock 15 Lip Balm (Robins Consumer) p 421, 667
Clocream Skin Protectant Cream (Roberts) p 664
Complex 15 Hand & Body Moisturizing Cream (Schering-Plough HealthCare) p 425, 694
Complex 15 Hand & Body Moisturizing Lotion (Schering-Plough HealthCare) p 425, 694
Complex 15 Moisturizing Face Cream (Schering-Plough HealthCare) p 425, 695
Eucerin Dry Skin Care Daily Facial Lotion SPF 20 (Beiersdorf) p 404, 515

Eucerin Dry Skin Care Cleansing Bar (Beiersdorf) p 404, 515
Eucerin Dry Skin Care Creme (Beiersdorf) p 404, 515
Eucerin Lotion (Beiersdorf) p 404, 516
Eucerin Dry Skin Care Lotion (Fragrance-free) (Beiersdorf) p 404, 516
Keri Lotion - Original Formula (Bristol-Myers Products) p 405, 533
Keri Lotion - Silky Smooth Formula (Bristol-Myers Products) p 405, 533
Keri Lotion - Silky Smooth Fragrance Free Formula (Bristol-Myers Products) p 405, 533
Lubriderm Bath Oil (Warner-Lambert) p 433, 757
Lubriderm Lotion (Warner-Lambert) p 433, 756
Moisturel Cream (Westwood) p 433, 758
Moisturel Lotion (Westwood) p 433, 758
Moisturel Sensitive Skin Cleanser (Westwood) p 433, 759
Neutrogena Moisture (Neutrogena) p 417, 622
Neutrogena Moisture SPF 15 Untinted (Neutrogena) p 417, 623
Neutrogena Moisture SPF 15 with Sheer Tint (Neutrogena) p 417, 623
Neutrogena Norwegian Formula Emulsion (Neutrogena) p 417, 623
Neutrogena Norwegian Formula Hand Cream (Neutrogena) p 417, 623
Oil of Olay Daily UV Protectant SPF 15 Beauty Fluid-Regular & Fragrance Free (Olay Co. Inc.) (Richardson-Vicks) p 653
Oil of Olay Daily UV Protectant SPF 15 Moisture Replenishing Cream-Regular & Fragrance Free (Olay Co. Inc.) (Richardson-Vicks) p 653
Pen•Kera Creme (Ascher) p 403, 510
Ultra Mide 25 (Baker Cummins Pharmaceuticals) p 512
Vaseline Intensive Care Moisturizing Sunblock Lotion (Chese-Pond's) p 548
Vaseline Intensive Care U.V. Daily Defense Lotion for Hand and Body (Chese-Pond's) p 548
Extra Strength Vaseline Intensive Care Lotion (Chese-Pond's) p 548

POISON IVY, OAK OR SUMAC
Aveeno Anti-Itch Concentrated Lotion (Rydelle) p 423, 680
Aveeno Anti-Itch Cream (Rydelle) p 423, 680
Aveeno Bath Oilated (Rydelle) p 423, 680
Aveeno Bath Regular (Rydelle) p 423, 680
Benadryl Spray, Maximum Strength 2% (Parke-Davis) p 418, 632
Benadryl Spray, Regular Strength 1% (Parke-Davis) p 418, 632
Caladryl Clear Lotion (Parke-Davis) p 419, 633
Caladryl Cream, Lotion, Spray (Parke-Davis) p 419, 633
Cortizone-5 Creme and Ointment (Thompson Medical) p 431, 743
Cortizone-5 Wipes (Thompson Medical) p 743
Cortizone-10 Creme and Ointment (Thompson Medical) p 744
Domeboro Astringent Solution Effervescent Tablets (Miles Consumer) p 417, 619
Domeboro Astringent Solution Powder Packets (Miles Consumer) p 417, 618
Itch-X Gel (Ascher) p 403, 509
Rhulicream (Rydelle) p 423, 681
Rhuligel (Rydelle) p 423, 681
Rhulispray (Rydelle) p 423, 681

POWDERS
Balmex Baby Powder (Macsil) p 579
Caldesene Medicated Powder (Fisons Consumer Health) p 409, 559

Cruex Antifungal Powder (Fisons Consumer Health) p 409, 560
Cruex Antifungal Spray Powder (Fisons Consumer Health) p 409, 560
Desenex Antifungal Powder (Fisons Consumer Health) p 409, 560
Desenex Antifungal Spray Powder (Fisons Consumer Health) p 409, 560
Formula Magic Antibacterial Powder (Care-Tech) p 545
NP-27 (Thompson Medical) p 431, 746
Tinactin Aerosol Powder 1% (Schering-Plough HealthCare) p 426, 703
Tinactin Deodorant Powder Aerosol 1% (Schering-Plough HealthCare) p 703
Tinactin Jock Itch Spray Powder 1% (Schering-Plough HealthCare) p 426, 703
Ting Antifungal Powder (Fisons Consumer Health) p 409, 562
Ting Antifungal Spray Powder (Fisons Consumer Health) p 409, 562

PRURITUS MEDICATIONS
Alpha Keri Moisture Rich Body Oil (Bristol-Myers Products) p 405, 519
Americaine Topical Anesthetic First Aid Ointment (Fisons Consumer Health) p 409, 559
Americaine Topical Anesthetic Spray (Fisons Consumer Health) p 409, 559
Aveeno Anti-Itch Concentrated Lotion (Rydelle) p 423, 680
Aveeno Anti-Itch Cream (Rydelle) p 423, 680
Aveeno Bath Oilated (Rydelle) p 423, 680
Aveeno Bath Regular (Rydelle) p 423, 680
Aveeno Cleansing Bar for Acne (Rydelle) p 423, 680
Aveeno Cleansing Bar for Combination Skin (Rydelle) p 423, 680
Aveeno Cleansing Bar for Dry Skin (Rydelle) p 423, 681
Aveeno Moisturizing Cream (Rydelle) p 423, 681
Aveeno Moisturizing Lotion (Rydelle) p 423, 681
Aveeno Shower and Bath Oil (Rydelle) p 423, 681
Benadryl Anti-Itch Cream, Regular Strength 1% and Maximum Strength 2% (Parke-Davis) p 418, 629
Benadryl Spray, Maximum Strength 2% (Parke-Davis) p 418, 632
Benadryl Spray, Regular Strength 1% (Parke-Davis) p 418, 632
BiCozene Creme (Sandoz Consumer) p 423, 682
Caladryl Clear Lotion (Parke-Davis) p 419, 633
Caladryl Cream, Lotion, Spray (Parke-Davis) p 419, 633
Caldecort Anti-Itch Hydrocortisone Cream (Fisons Consumer Health) p 409, 559
Caldecort Anti-Itch Hydrocortisone Spray (Fisons Consumer Health) p 409, 559
Caldecort Light Cream (Fisons Consumer Health) p 409, 559
Campho-Phenique Cold Sore Gel (Sterling Health) p 429, 731
Campho-Phenique Liquid (Sterling Health) p 429, 731
Campho-Phenique Triple Antibiotic Ointment Plus Pain Reliever (Sterling Health) p 429, 731
Cortaid Cream with Aloe (Upjohn) p 431, 747
Cortaid Lotion (Upjohn) p 431, 747
Cortaid Ointment with Aloe (Upjohn) p 431, 747
Cortaid Spray (Upjohn) p 431, 747
Maximum Strength Cortaid Cream (Upjohn) p 431, 748
Maximum Strength Cortaid Ointment (Upjohn) p 431, 748

Maximum Strength Cortaid Spray (Upjohn) p 431, 748
Cortef Feminine Itch Cream (Upjohn) p 748
Corticaine External Analgesic (Whitby) p 433, 760
Cortizone-5 Creme and Ointment (Thompson Medical) p 431, 743
Cortizone-5 Wipes (Thompson Medical) p 743
Cortizone-10 Creme and Ointment (Thompson Medical) p 744
Denorex Medicated Shampoo and Conditioner (Whitehall) p 434, 764
Denorex Medicated Shampoo, Extra Strength (Whitehall) p 434, 764
Denorex Medicated Shampoo, Extra Strength With Conditioners (Whitehall) p 434, 764
Denorex Medicated Shampoo, Regular & Mountain Fresh Herbal Scent (Whitehall) p 434, 764
Dermoplast Anesthetic Pain Relief Lotion (Whitehall) p 764
Dermoplast Anesthetic Pain Relief Spray (Whitehall) p 764
Formula Magic Antibacterial Powder (Care-Tech) p 545
Itch-X Gel (Ascher) p 403, 509
Keri Lotion - Original Formula (Bristol-Myers Products) p 405, 533
Keri Lotion - Silky Smooth Formula (Bristol-Myers Products) p 405, 533
Keri Lotion - Silky Smooth Fragrance Free Formula (Bristol-Myers Products) p 405, 533
Massengill Medicated Soft Cloth Towelette (SmithKline Beecham) p 713
Moisturel Cream (Westwood) p 433, 758
Moisturel Lotion (Westwood) p 433, 758
Rhulicream (Rydelle) p 423, 681
Rhuligel (Rydelle) p 423, 681
Rhulispray (Rydelle) p 423, 681
Tegrin-HC with Hydrocortisone Anti-Itch Ointment (Block) p 518
Tucks Cream (Parke-Davis) p 637
Tucks Premoistened Pads (Parke-Davis) p 420, 637
Tucks Take-Alongs (Parke-Davis) p 637
Xylocaine 2.5% Ointment (Astra) p 403, 510

PSORIASIS AGENTS
Aveeno Bath Oilated (Rydelle) p 423, 680
Aveeno Bath Regular (Rydelle) p 423, 680
Care Creme (Care-Tech) p 544
Cortizone-5 Creme and Ointment (Thompson Medical) p 431, 743
Cortizone-5 Wipes (Thompson Medical) p 743
Cortizone-10 Creme and Ointment (Thompson Medical) p 744
Denorex Medicated Shampoo and Conditioner (Whitehall) p 434, 764
Denorex Medicated Shampoo, Extra Strength (Whitehall) p 434, 764
Denorex Medicated Shampoo, Extra Strength With Conditioners (Whitehall) p 434, 764
Denorex Medicated Shampoo, Regular & Mountain Fresh Herbal Scent (Whitehall) p 434, 764
MG 217 Psoriasis Ointment and Lotion (Triton Consumer) p 747
MG 217 Psoriasis Shampoo and Conditioner (Triton Consumer) p 747
Neutrogena T/Derm Tar Emollient (Neutrogena) p 623
Neutrogena T/Gel Therapeutic Shampoo (Neutrogena) p 417, 623
Neutrogena T/Sal Therapeutic Shampoo (Neutrogena) p 417, 624
Oxipor VHC Lotion for Psoriasis (Whitehall) p 768
P & S Liquid (Baker Cummins Pharmaceuticals) p 511
P & S Plus Tar Gel (Baker Cummins Pharmaceuticals) p 512

P & S Shampoo (Baker Cummins Pharmaceuticals) p 512

Satin Antimicrobial Skin Cleanser (Care-Tech) p 545

Sebutone and Sebutone Cream Antiseborrheic Tar Shampoos (Westwood) p 433, 759

Tegrin Dandruff Shampoo (Block) p 518

Tegrin for Psoriasis Lotion, Skin Cream & Medicated Soap (Block) p 518

Tegrin-HC with Hydrocortisone Anti-Itch Ointment (Block) p 518

Vaseline Pure Petroleum Jelly Skin Protectant/Lip Therapy (Chese-Pond's) p 548

X-Seb T Shampoo (Baker Cummins Pharmaceuticals) p 513

X-Seb T Plus Conditioning Shampoo (Baker Cummins Pharmaceuticals) p 513

SEBORRHEA TREATMENT

Denorex Medicated Shampoo and Conditioner (Whitehall) p 434, 764

Denorex Medicated Shampoo, Extra Strength (Whitehall) p 434, 764

Denorex Medicated Shampoo, Extra Strength With Conditioners (Whitehall) p 434, 764

Denorex Medicated Shampoo, Regular & Mountain Fresh Herbal Scent (Whitehall) p 434, 764

Head & Shoulders Antidandruff Shampoo (Procter & Gamble) p 643

Head & Shoulders Antidandruff Shampoo 2-in-1 plus Conditioner (Procter & Gamble) p 643

Head & Shoulders Dry Scalp Shampoo (Procter & Gamble) p 643

Head & Shoulders Dry Scalp Shampoo 2-in-1 plus Conditioner (Procter & Gamble) p 643

Head & Shoulders Intensive Treatment Dandruff Shampoo (Procter & Gamble) p 643

Head & Shoulders Intensive Treatment Dandruff Shampoo 2-in-1 plus Conditioner (Procter & Gamble) p 643

Neutrogena T/Derm Tar Emollient (Neutrogena) p 623

Neutrogena T/Gel Therapeutic Shampoo (Neutrogena) p 417, 623

Neutrogena T/Sal Therapeutic Shampoo (Neutrogena) p 417, 624

Sebulex Antiseborrheic Treatment Shampoo (Westwood) p 433, 759

Sebutone and Sebutone Cream Antiseborrheic Tar Shampoos (Westwood) p 433, 759

Tegrin Dandruff Shampoo (Block) p 518

Tegrin-HC with Hydrocortisone Anti-Itch Ointment (Block) p 518

Zincon Dandruff Shampoo (Lederle) p 411, 578

SHAMPOOS

Aqua Glycolic Shampoo (Herald Pharmacal) p 564

Concept (Care-Tech) p 545

Denorex Medicated Shampoo and Conditioner (Whitehall) p 434, 764

Denorex Medicated Shampoo, Extra Strength (Whitehall) p 434, 764

Denorex Medicated Shampoo, Extra Strength With Conditioners (Whitehall) p 434, 764

Denorex Medicated Shampoo, Regular & Mountain Fresh Herbal Scent (Whitehall) p 434, 764

Head & Shoulders Antidandruff Shampoo (Procter & Gamble) p 643

Head & Shoulders Antidandruff Shampoo 2-in-1 plus Conditioner (Procter & Gamble) p 643

Head & Shoulders Dry Scalp Shampoo (Procter & Gamble) p 643

Head & Shoulders Dry Scalp Shampoo 2-in-1 plus Conditioner (Procter & Gamble) p 643

Head & Shoulders Intensive Treatment Dandruff Shampoo (Procter & Gamble) p 643

Head & Shoulders Intensive Treatment Dandruff Shampoo 2-in-1 plus Conditioner (Procter & Gamble) p 643

MG 217 Psoriasis Shampoo and Conditioner (Triton Consumer) p 747

Neutrogena T/Gel Therapeutic Shampoo (Neutrogena) p 417, 623

Neutrogena T/Sal Therapeutic Shampoo (Neutrogena) p 417, 624

P & S Shampoo (Baker Cummins Pharmaceuticals) p 512

Progaine Shampoo (Upjohn) p 750

R&C Shampoo (Reed & Carnrick) p 420, 646

Sebulex Antiseborrheic Treatment Shampoo (Westwood) p 433, 759

Sebutone and Sebutone Cream Antiseborrheic Tar Shampoos (Westwood) p 433, 759

Selsun Blue Dandruff Shampoo (Ross) p 422, 679

Selsun Blue Dandruff Shampoo-Extra Medicated (Ross) p 422, 679

Selsun Blue Extra Conditioning Dandruff Shampoo (Ross) p 422, 679

Tegrin Dandruff Shampoo (Block) p 518

X-Seb Shampoo (Baker Cummins Pharmaceuticals) p 512

X-Seb Plus Conditioning Shampoo (Baker Cummins Pharmaceuticals) p 512

X-Seb T Shampoo (Baker Cummins Pharmaceuticals) p 513

X-Seb T Plus Conditioning Shampoo (Baker Cummins Pharmaceuticals) p 513

Zincon Dandruff Shampoo (Lederle) p 411, 578

SKIN PROTECTANT

Barri-Care Antimicrobial Barrier Ointment (Care-Tech) p 544

Caldesene Medicated Ointment (Fisons Consumer Health) p 409, 559

Caldesene Medicated Powder (Fisons Consumer Health) p 409, 559

Chap Stick Petroleum Jelly Plus (Robins Consumer) p 421, 668

Clocream Skin Protectant Cream (Roberts) p 664

Desitin Ointment (Pfizer Consumer) p 420, 638

Vaseline Pure Petroleum Jelly Skin Protectant/Lip Therapy (Chese-Pond's) p 548

Wellcome Lanoline (Burroughs Wellcome) p 544

SOAPS

Alpha Keri Moisture Rich Cleansing Bar (Bristol-Myers Products) p 519

Lever 2000 (Lever Brothers) p 578

Neutrogena Cleansing Wash (Neutrogena) p 417, 622

Oxy Medicated Soap (SmithKline Beecham) p 428, 715

STEROIDS & COMBINATIONS

Corticaine External Analgesic (Whitby) p 433, 760

SULFUR & SALICYLIC ACID

Sebulex Antiseborrheic Treatment Shampoo (Westwood) p 433, 759

Sebutone and Sebutone Cream Antiseborrheic Tar Shampoos (Westwood) p 433, 759

SUNBURN PREPARATIONS

Americaine Topical Anesthetic First Aid Ointment (Fisons Consumer Health) p 409, 559

Americaine Topical Anesthetic Spray (Fisons Consumer Health) p 409, 559

Aveeno Bath Oilated (Rydelle) p 423, 680

Aveeno Bath Regular (Rydelle) p 423, 680

Bactine Antiseptic/Anesthetic First Aid Liquid (Miles Consumer) p 416, 617

Balmex Ointment (Macsil) p 579

BiCozene Creme (Sandoz Consumer) p 423, 682

Dermoplast Anesthetic Pain Relief Lotion (Whitehall) p 764

Dermoplast Anesthetic Pain Relief Spray (Whitehall) p 764

Desitin Ointment (Pfizer Consumer) p 420, 638

Itch-X Gel (Ascher) p 403, 509

Keri Lotion - Original Formula (Bristol-Myers Products) p 405, 533

Keri Lotion - Silky Smooth Formula (Bristol-Myers Products) p 405, 533

Keri Lotion - Silky Smooth Fragrance Free Formula (Bristol-Myers Products) p 405, 533

Moisturel Cream (Westwood) p 433, 758

Moisturel Lotion (Westwood) p 433, 758

Nupercainal Pain Relief Cream (CIBA Consumer) p 408, 553

Rhuligel (Rydelle) p 423, 681

SUNSCREENS

Aquaderm Combination Treatment/Moisturizer (SPF 15 Formula) (Baker Cummins Pharmaceuticals) p 511

Aquaray 20 Sunscreen (Herald Pharmacal) p 564

Chap Stick Lip Balm (Robins Consumer) p 421, 667

Chap Stick Petroleum Jelly Plus with Sunblock 15 (Robins Consumer) p 421, 668

Chap Stick Sunblock 15 Lip Balm (Robins Consumer) p 421, 667

Desitin Ointment (Pfizer Consumer) p 420, 638

Eucerin Dry Skin Care Daily Facial Lotion SPF 20 (Beiersdorf) p 404, 515

Filteray Broad Spectrum Sunscreen Lotion (Burroughs Wellcome) p 406, 538

Herpecin-L Cold Sore Lip Balm (Campbell) p 544

Neutrogena Moisture (Neutrogena) p 417, 622

Neutrogena Moisture SPF 15 Untinted (Neutrogena) p 417, 623

Neutrogena Moisture SPF 15 with Sheer Tint (Neutrogena) p 417, 623

Neutrogena Sunblock (Neutrogena) p 417, 623

Oil of Olay Daily UV Protectant SPF 15 Beauty Fluid-Regular & Fragrance Free (Olay Co. Inc.) (Richardson-Vicks) p 653

Oil of Olay Daily UV Protectant SPF 15 Moisture Replenishing Cream-Regular & Fragrance Free (Olay Co. Inc.) (Richardson-Vicks) p 653

PreSun Active 15 and 30 Clear Gel Sunscreens (Bristol-Myers Products) p 535

PreSun for Kids Lotion (Bristol-Myers Products) p 406, 535

PreSun 23 and For Kids, Spray Mist Sunscreens (Bristol-Myers Products) p 406, 535

PreSun 8 and 15 Moisturizing Sunscreens with KERI Moisturizers (Bristol-Myers Products) p 535

PreSun 25 Moisturizing Sunscreen with KERI Moisturizer (Bristol-Myers Products) p 535

PreSun 15 and 29 Sensitive Skin Sunscreens (Bristol-Myers Products) p 406, 536

PreSun 46 Moisturizing Sunscreen (Bristol-Myers Products) p 536

Vaseline Intensive Care Moisturizing Sunblock Lotion (Chese-Pond's) p 548

Vaseline Intensive Care U.V. Daily Defense Lotion for Hand and Body (Chese-Pond's) p 548

WART REMOVERS

Compound W Gel (Whitehall) p 763

Compound W Liquid (Whitehall) p 763

DuoFilm Liquid (Schering-Plough HealthCare) p 426, 698
DuoPlant Gel (Schering-Plough HealthCare) p 426, 699
Wart-Off Wart Remover (Pfizer Consumer) p 642

WET DRESSINGS
Domeboro Astringent Solution Effervescent Tablets (Miles Consumer) p 417, 619
Domeboro Astringent Solution Powder Packets (Miles Consumer) p 417, 618
Tucks Premoistened Pads (Parke-Davis) p 420, 637
Tucks Take-Alongs (Parke-Davis) p 637

WOUND CLEANSER
Bactine Antiseptic/Anesthetic First Aid Liquid (Miles Consumer) p 416, 617
Clinical Care Dermal Wound Cleanser (Care-Tech) p 545
S.T.37 Antiseptic Solution (Menley & James) p 611
Techni-Care Surgical Scrub (Care-Tech) p 545

WOUND DRESSINGS
Aquaphor Antibiotic Ointment (Beiersdorf) p 404, 515
Bactine First Aid Antibiotic Plus Anesthetic Ointment (Miles Consumer) p 416, 617
Barri-Care Antimicrobial Barrier Ointment (Care-Tech) p 544
Care Creme (Care-Tech) p 544

OTHER
Bactine Hydrocortisone Anti-Itch Cream (Miles Consumer) p 416, 617
Borofax Ointment (Burroughs Wellcome) p 538
Cortaid Cream with Aloe (Upjohn) p 431, 747
Cortaid Lotion (Upjohn) p 431, 747
Cortaid Ointment with Aloe (Upjohn) p 431, 747
Cortaid Spray (Upjohn) p 431, 747
Maximum Strength Cortaid Cream (Upjohn) p 431, 748
Maximum Strength Cortaid Ointment (Upjohn) p 431, 748
Maximum Strength Cortaid Spray (Upjohn) p 431, 748
Cortef Feminine Itch Cream (Upjohn) p 748
PRID Salve (Walker Pharmacal) p 753

DEVICES, OPHTHALMOLOGICAL
Lavoptik Eye Cup (Lavoptik) p 781

DIAGNOSTICS
OVULATION PREDICTION TEST
Clearplan Easy (Whitehall) p 434, 783
PREGNANCY TESTS
Advance Pregnancy Test (Ortho Pharmaceutical) p 418, 781
Clearblue Easy (Whitehall) p 434, 783
e.p.t. Early Pregnancy Test (Parke-Davis) p 419, 781
Fact Plus Pregnancy Test (Ortho Pharmaceutical) p 418, 781

DIAPER RASH RELIEF
(see also under DERMATOLOGICALS, DERMATITIS RELIEF & DIAPER RASH RELIEF)
A and D Ointment (Schering-Plough HealthCare) p 424, 692
Aveeno Bath Oilated (Rydelle) p 423, 680
Aveeno Bath Regular (Rydelle) p 423, 680
Aveeno Moisturizing Lotion (Rydelle) p 423, 681
Balmex Baby Powder (Macsil) p 579
Balmex Emollient Lotion (Macsil) p 579
Balmex Ointment (Macsil) p 579
Borofax Ointment (Burroughs Wellcome) p 538
Desitin Ointment (Pfizer Consumer) p 420, 638
Impregon Concentrate (Fleming) p 563
Keri Lotion - Original Formula (Bristol-Myers Products) p 405, 533

Keri Lotion - Silky Smooth Formula (Bristol-Myers Products) p 405, 533
Keri Lotion - Silky Smooth Fragrance Free Formula (Bristol-Myers Products) p 405, 533
Moisturel Cream (Westwood) p 433, 758
Moisturel Lotion (Westwood) p 433, 758

DIARRHEA MEDICATIONS
Charcocaps (Requa) p 648
Diasorb Liquid (Columbia) p 408, 556
Diasorb Tablets (Columbia) p 408, 556
Donnagel Liquid and Chewable Tablets (Robins Consumer) p 422, 672
Imodium A-D Caplets and Liquid (McNeil Consumer Products) p 414, 587
Kaopectate Concentrated Anti-Diarrheal, Peppermint Flavor (Upjohn) p 431, 749
Kaopectate Concentrated Anti-Diarrheal, Regular Flavor (Upjohn) p 431, 749
Kaopectate Children's Chewable Tablets (Upjohn) p 431, 749
Kaopectate Children's Liquid (Upjohn) p 431, 749
Kaopectate Maximum Strength Caplets (Upjohn) p 431, 749
Pepto-Bismol Liquid & Tablets (Procter & Gamble) p 644
Maximum Strength Pepto-Bismol Liquid (Procter & Gamble) p 644
Rheaban Maximum Strength Tablets (Pfizer Consumer) p 639

DIET AIDS
(see under APPETITE SUPPRESSANTS OR FOODS)

DIETARY SUPPLEMENTS
Allbee with C Caplets (Robins Consumer) p 667
Allbee C-800 Plus Iron Tablets (Robins Consumer) p 666
Allbee C-800 Tablets (Robins Consumer) p 666
Beelith Tablets (Beach) p 514
Ester-C Tablets (Inter-Cal) p 564
FemIron Multi Vitamins and Iron (Menley & James) p 415, 609
Geritol Complete Tablets (SmithKline Beecham) p 711
Geritol Liquid - High Potency Iron & Vitamin Tonic (SmithKline Beecham) p 712
Incremin w/Iron Syrup (Lederle) p 576
Kyolic (Wakunaga) p 432, 752
Mag-Ox 400 (Blaine) p 516
MagTab SR Caplets (Niché Pharmaceuticals) p 624
Marlyn Formula 50 (Marlyn) p 586
Marlyn Formula 50 Mega Forte (Marlyn) p 587
Optilets-500 Filmtab (Abbott) p 403, 502
Poly-Vi-Sol Vitamins, Chewable Tablets and Drops (without Iron) (Mead Johnson Nutritionals) p 414, 603
Poly-Vi-Sol Vitamins, Circus Shapes Chewable (without Iron) (Mead Johnson Nutritionals) p 414, 603
Poly-Vi-Sol Vitamins with Iron, Chewable Tablets and Circus Shapes Chewable (Mead Johnson Nutritionals) p 414, 604
Poly-Vi-Sol Vitamins with Iron, Drops (Mead Johnson Nutritionals) p 414, 604
Sublingual B-Total (Sublingual Products) p 431, 742
Sublingual C with Niacin (Sublingual Products) p 743
Sublingual Zinc (Sublingual Products) p 743
Sunkist Children's Chewable Multivitamins - Complete (CIBA Consumer) p 408, 555
Sunkist Children's Chewable Multivitamins - Plus Extra C (CIBA Consumer) p 408, 555

Sunkist Children's Chewable Multivitamins - Plus Iron (CIBA Consumer) p 408, 555
Sunkist Children's Chewable Multivitamins - Regular (CIBA Consumer) p 408, 554
Tri-Vi-Sol Vitamin Drops (Mead Johnson Nutritionals) p 415, 606
Tri-Vi-Sol Vitamin Drops with Iron (Mead Johnson Nutritionals) p 415, 606
Uro-Mag (Blaine) p 516
Z-BEC Tablets (Robins Consumer) p 676

DIGESTIVE AIDS
Charcocaps (Requa) p 648
DDS-Acidophilus (UAS Laboratories) p 747
Pepto-Bismol Liquid & Tablets (Procter & Gamble) p 644
Maximum Strength Pepto-Bismol Liquid (Procter & Gamble) p 644

DISHPAN HANDS AIDS
(see under DERMATOLOGICALS, DERMATITIS RELIEF)

DRY SKIN PREPARATIONS
(see under DERMATOLOGICALS, EMOLLIENTS & MOISTURIZERS)

E

ECZEMA PREPARATIONS
(see under DERMATOLOGICALS, DERMATITIS RELIEF)

ELECTROLYTES
FLUID MAINTENANCE THERAPY
Mag-Ox 400 (Blaine) p 516
Pedialyte Oral Electrolyte Maintenance Solution (Ross) p 678
Ricelyte, Rice-Based Oral Electrolyte Maintenance Solution (Mead Johnson Nutritionals) p 415, 604
Uro-Mag (Blaine) p 516
FLUID REPLACEMENT THERAPY
Mag-Ox 400 (Blaine) p 516
Rehydralyte Oral Electrolyte Rehydration Solution (Ross) p 679
Uro-Mag (Blaine) p 516

EMETICS
Ipecac Syrup, USP (Paddock) p 628

EMOLLIENTS, OPHTHALMIC
Lacri-Lube NP Lubricant Ophthalmic Ointment (Allergan Pharmaceuticals) p 504
Lacri-Lube S.O.P. Sterile Ophthalmic Ointment (Allergan Pharmaceuticals) p 504
Refresh P.M. Lubricant Ophthalmic Ointment (Allergan Pharmaceuticals) p 505

ENURESIS
Hyland's Bed Wetting Tablets (Standard Homeopathic) p 722

ENZYMES & DIGESTANTS
DIGESTANTS
Dairy Ease Caplets and Tablets (Sterling Health) p 429, 731
Dairy Ease Drops (Sterling Health) p 429, 732
Lactaid Caplets (Now marketed by McNeil Consumer Products Co.) (Lactaid) p 414, 571
Lactaid Drops (Now marketed by McNeil Consumer Products Co.) (Lactaid) p 414, 571
Lactogest Softgel Capsules (Thompson Medical) p 431, 745
Surelac Chewable Lactase Enzyme Tablets (Caraco) p 544

EXPECTORANTS
(see under COLD & COUGH PREPARATIONS)

EYEWASHES

Collyrium for Fresh Eyes (Wyeth-Ayerst) p 435, 775

Eye Wash (Bausch & Lomb Personal) p 404, 514

Lavoptik Eye Wash (Lavoptik) p 571

Star-Optic Eye Wash (Stellar) p 428, 723

F

FEVER BLISTER AIDS
(see under HERPES TREATMENT)

FEVER PREPARATIONS
(see under ANALGESICS)

FLATULENCE RELIEF
(see also under ANTACIDS)

Charcocaps (Requa) p 648

Colicon Drops (Reese Chemical) p 647

Di-Gel Antacid/Anti-Gas (Schering-Plough HealthCare) p 425, 696

Gas-X Tablets (Sandoz Consumer) p 423, 684

Extra Strength Gas-X Tablets (Sandoz Consumer) p 423, 684

Maalox Plus Suspension/Tablets (Rhone-Poulenc Rorer Consumer) p 421, 649

Extra Strength Maalox Plus Suspension (Rhone-Poulenc Rorer Consumer) p 420, 650

Mylanta Gas Tablets-40 mg (J&J•Merck Consumer) p 410, 568

Mylanta Gas Tablets-80 mg (J&J•Merck Consumer) p 410, 569

Mylanta Liquid (J&J•Merck Consumer) p 410, 567

Mylanta Tablets (J&J•Merck Consumer) p 410, 567

Mylanta Double Strength Liquid (J&J•Merck Consumer) p 410, 567

Mylanta Double Strength Tablets (J&J•Merck Consumer) p 410, 567

Maximum Strength Mylanta Gas Tablets-125 mg (J&J•Merck Consumer) p 410, 569

Mylicon Drops (J&J•Merck Consumer) p 410, 568

Phazyme Drops (Reed & Carnrick) p 420, 645

Phazyme Tablets (Reed & Carnrick) p 645

Phazyme-125 Softgels Maximum Strength (Reed & Carnrick) p 420, 645

Phazyme-95 Tablets (Reed & Carnrick) p 420, 645

FOODS

ALLERGY DIET

Ross Pediatric Nutritional Products (Ross) p 677

COMPLETE THERAPEUTIC

Ross Pediatric Nutritional Products (Ross) p 677

INFANT
(see under INFANT FORMULAS)

FORMULAS
(see under INFANT FORMULAS)

FUNGAL MEDICATIONS

TOPICAL
(see under DERMATOLOGICALS, FUNGICIDES & VAGINAL PREPARATIONS

G

GASTRITIS AIDS
(see under ANTACIDS)

GERMICIDES/MICROBICIDES
(see under ANTIBIOTICS & ANTISEPTICS)

H

HALITOSIS PREPARATIONS
(see under ORAL HYGIENE AID & MOUTHWASHES)

HEAD LICE RELIEF
(see under ANTIPARASITICS)

HEADACHE RELIEF
(see under ANALGESICS)

HEARTBURN AIDS
(see under ANTACIDS)

HEMATINICS

Feosol Capsules (SmithKline Beecham) p 427, 710

Feosol Elixir (SmithKline Beecham) p 427, 711

Feosol Tablets (SmithKline Beecham) p 427, 711

Ferancee Chewable Tablets (J&J•Merck Consumer) p 566

Ferancee-HP Tablets (J&J•Merck Consumer) p 409, 566

Fergon Elixir (Sterling Health) p 732

Fergon Iron Supplement Tablets (Sterling Health) p 429, 732

Ferro-Sequels (Lederle) p 411, 575

Geritol Liquid - High Potency Iron & Vitamin Tonic (SmithKline Beecham) p 712

Incremin w/Iron Syrup (Lederle) p 576

Slow Fe Tablets (CIBA Consumer) p 408, 554

Stuartinic Tablets (J&J•Merck Consumer) p 410, 570

Troph-Iron Liquid (Menley & James) p 611

IRON & COMBINATIONS

Fergon Elixir (Sterling Health) p 732

Fergon Iron Supplement Tablets (Sterling Health) p 429, 732

Geritol Extend Caplets (SmithKline Beecham) p 712

Vitron-C Tablets (Fisons Consumer Health) p 562

HEMORRHOIDAL PREPARATIONS
(see under ANORECTAL PRODUCTS)

HERPES TREATMENT

Anbesol Gel Antiseptic-Anesthetic-Regular Strength (Whitehall) p 434, 763

Anbesol Gel Antiseptic-Anesthetic - Maximum Strength (Whitehall) p 434, 763

Anbesol Liquid Antiseptic-Anesthetic (Whitehall) p 434, 763

Anbesol Liquid Antiseptic-Anesthetic - Maximum Strength (Whitehall) p 434, 763

Herpecin-L Cold Sore Lip Balm (Campbell) p 544

Orajel Mouth-Aid (Del Pharmaceuticals) p 408, 557

Zilactin Medicated Gel (Zila Pharmaceuticals) p 435, 777

Zilactol Medicated Liquid (Zila Pharmaceuticals) p 777

HOMEOPATHIC MEDICATIONS

Hyland's Bed Wetting Tablets (Standard Homeopathic) p 722

Hyland's Calms Forté Tablets (Standard Homeopathic) p 722

Hyland's Colic Tablets (Standard Homeopathic) p 722

Hyland's Cough Syrup with Honey (Standard Homeopathic) p 722

Hyland's C-Plus Cold Tablets (Standard Homeopathic) p 722

Hyland's Teething Tablets (Standard Homeopathic) p 723

Oscillococcinum (Boiron) p 404, 519

Yellolax (Luyties) p 578

HOUSEWIVES' DERMATITIS AIDS
(see under DERMATOLOGICALS, DERMATITIS RELIEF)

HYPOGLYCEMIC AGENTS
(see also under DIABETES AGENTS)

Glutose (Paddock) p 628

Insta-Glucose (ICN Pharmaceuticals) p 409, 564

HYPOMAGNESEMIA

Magonate Tablets and Liquid (Fleming) p 563

I

INFANT FORMULAS, REGULAR

LIQUID CONCENTRATE

SMA Iron Fortified Infant Formula, Concentrated, Ready-to-Feed and Powder (Wyeth-Ayerst) p 435, 776

SMA lo-iron Infant Formula, Concentrated, Ready-to-Feed, and Powder (Wyeth-Ayerst) p 435, 776

LIQUID READY-TO-FEED

SMA Iron Fortified Infant Formula, Concentrated, Ready-to-Feed and Powder (Wyeth-Ayerst) p 435, 776

SMA lo-iron Infant Formula, Concentrated, Ready-to-Feed, and Powder (Wyeth-Ayerst) p 435, 776

POWDER

SMA Iron Fortified Infant Formula, Concentrated, Ready-to-Feed and Powder (Wyeth-Ayerst) p 435, 776

SMA lo-iron Infant Formula, Concentrated, Ready-to-Feed, and Powder (Wyeth-Ayerst) p 435, 776

INFANT FORMULAS, SPECIAL PURPOSE

CORN FREE

LIQUID CONCENTRATE
Nursoy (Wyeth-Ayerst) p 435, 775

LIQUID READY-TO-FEED
Nursoy (Wyeth-Ayerst) p 435, 775

IRON SUPPLEMENT

LIQUID CONCENTRATE
Nursoy (Wyeth-Ayerst) p 435, 775
SMA Iron Fortified Infant Formula, Concentrated, Ready-to-Feed and Powder (Wyeth-Ayerst) p 435, 776

LIQUID READY-TO-FEED
Nursoy (Wyeth-Ayerst) p 435, 775
Ross Pediatric Nutritional Products (Ross) p 677
SMA Iron Fortified Infant Formula, Concentrated, Ready-to-Feed and Powder (Wyeth-Ayerst) p 435, 776

POWDER
Nursoy (Wyeth-Ayerst) p 435, 775
SMA Iron Fortified Infant Formula, Concentrated, Ready-to-Feed and Powder (Wyeth-Ayerst) p 435, 776

LACTOSE FREE

LIQUID CONCENTRATE
Nursoy (Wyeth-Ayerst) p 435, 775

LIQUID READY-TO-FEED
Nursoy (Wyeth-Ayerst) p 435, 775

POWDER
Nursoy (Wyeth-Ayerst) p 435, 775

LOW IRON

LIQUID READY-TO-FEED
Ross Pediatric Nutritional Products (Ross) p 677

MILK FREE

LIQUID CONCENTRATE
Nursoy (Wyeth-Ayerst) p 435, 775

LIQUID READY-TO-FEED
Nursoy (Wyeth-Ayerst) p 435, 775

POWDER
Nursoy (Wyeth-Ayerst) p 435, 775

INGROWN TOENAIL PREPARATIONS
Outgro Solution (Whitehall) p 767

INSECT BITE & STING PREPARATIONS
Americaine Topical Anesthetic First Aid Ointment (Fisons Consumer Health) p 409, 559
Americaine Topical Anesthetic Spray (Fisons Consumer Health) p 409, 559
Aveeno Anti-Itch Concentrated Lotion (Rydelle) p 423, 680
Aveeno Anti-Itch Cream (Rydelle) p 423, 680
Aveeno Bath Oilated (Rydelle) p 423, 680
Bactine Antiseptic/Anesthetic First Aid Liquid (Miles Consumer) p 416, 617
Bactine Hydrocortisone Anti-Itch Cream (Miles Consumer) p 416, 617
BiCozene Creme (Sandoz Consumer) p 423, 682
Domeboro Astringent Solution Effervescent Tablets (Miles Consumer) p 417, 619
Domeboro Astringent Solution Powder Packets (Miles Consumer) p 417, 618
Nupercainal Hemorrhoidal and Anesthetic Ointment (CIBA Consumer) p 408, 552
Nupercainal Pain Relief Cream (CIBA Consumer) p 408, 553
Rhulicream (Rydelle) p 423, 681
Rhuligel (Rydelle) p 423, 681
Rhulispray (Rydelle) p 423, 681

IRON DEFICIENCY PREPARATIONS
(see under HEMATINICS)

IRRIGATING SOLUTION, OPHTHALMIC

FOR EXTERNAL USE
Collyrium for Fresh Eyes (Wyeth-Ayerst) p 435, 775
Lavoptik Eye Wash (Lavoptik) p 571

L

LAXATIVES

BULK
Citrucel Orange Flavor (Marion Merrell Dow) p 411, 581
Citrucel Sugar Free Orange Flavor (Marion Merrell Dow) p 411, 581
Effer-Syllium Natural Fiber Bulking Agent (J&J•Merck Consumer) p 409, 566
Fiberall Chewable Tablets, Lemon Creme Flavor (CIBA Consumer) p 551
Fiberall Fiber Wafers - Fruit & Nut (CIBA Consumer) p 407, 551
Fiberall Fiber Wafers - Oatmeal Raisin (CIBA Consumer) p 407, 551
Fiberall Powder Natural Flavor (CIBA Consumer) p 407, 551
Fiberall Powder Orange Flavor (CIBA Consumer) p 407, 551
FiberCon (Lederle) p 411, 575
Maltsupex Liquid, Powder & Tablets (Wallace) p 432, 753
Perdiem Fiber Granules (Rhone-Poulenc Rorer Consumer) p 421, 652
Perdiem Granules (Rhone-Poulenc Rorer Consumer) p 421, 651
Serutan Toasted Granules (Menley & James) p 415, 611
Syllact Powder (Wallace) p 432, 755

COMBINATIONS
Anticon (Neutrin) p 417, 622
Correctol Laxative Tablets (Schering-Plough HealthCare) p 425, 696
Dialose Plus Tablets (J&J•Merck Consumer) p 409, 566
Extra Gentle Ex-Lax Laxative Pills (Sandoz Consumer) p 423, 683
Feen-A-Mint Laxative Pills (Schering-Plough HealthCare) p 426, 699
Haley's M-O, Regular & Flavored (Sterling Health) p 429, 732
Nature's Remedy Natural Vegetable Laxative Tablets (SmithKline Beecham) p 427, 714
Perdiem Granules (Rhone-Poulenc Rorer Consumer) p 421, 651
Peri-Colace (Mead Johnson Pharmaceuticals) p 415, 606
Phillips' LaxCaps (Sterling Health) p 430, 736

ENEMAS
Nature's Remedy Enema, Mineral Oil (SmithKline Beecham) p 427, 714
Nature's Remedy Enema, Regular (SmithKline Beecham) p 427, 714

FECAL SOFTENERS
Colace (Mead Johnson Pharmaceuticals) p 415, 606
Correctol Laxative Tablets (Schering-Plough HealthCare) p 425, 696
Dialose Tablets (J&J•Merck Consumer) p 409, 565
Dialose Plus Tablets (J&J•Merck Consumer) p 409, 566
Doxidan Liqui-Gels (Upjohn) p 431, 748
Extra Gentle Ex-Lax Laxative Pills (Sandoz Consumer) p 423, 683
Feen-A-Mint Laxative Pills (Schering-Plough HealthCare) p 426, 699
Kasof Capsules (Roberts) p 664
Perdiem Fiber Granules (Rhone-Poulenc Rorer Consumer) p 421, 652
Perdiem Granules (Rhone-Poulenc Rorer Consumer) p 421, 651
Phillips' LaxCaps (Sterling Health) p 430, 736
Surfak Liqui-Gels (Upjohn) p 432, 751

MINERAL OIL
Haley's M-O, Regular & Flavored (Sterling Health) p 429, 732

SALINE
Haley's M-O, Regular & Flavored (Sterling Health) p 429, 732
Concentrated Phillips' Milk of Magnesia (Sterling Health) p 430, 737
Phillips' Milk of Magnesia Liquid (Sterling Health) p 430, 737
Phillips' Milk of Magnesia Tablets (Sterling Health) p 430, 737

STIMULANT
Agoral, Marshmallow Flavor (Parke-Davis) p 628
Agoral, Raspberry Flavor (Parke-Davis) p 628
Correctol Laxative Tablets (Schering-Plough HealthCare) p 425, 696
Dialose Plus Tablets (J&J•Merck Consumer) p 409, 566
Doxidan Liqui-Gels (Upjohn) p 431, 748
Dulcolax Suppositories (CIBA Consumer) p 407, 550
Dulcolax Tablets (CIBA Consumer) p 407, 550
Evac-U-Gen Mild Laxative (Walker, Corp) p 432, 753
Ex-Lax Chocolated Laxative Tablets (Sandoz Consumer) p 423, 683
Extra Gentle Ex-Lax Laxative Pills (Sandoz Consumer) p 423, 683
Maximum Relief Formula Ex-Lax Laxative Pills (Sandoz Consumer) p 423, 683
Regular Strength Ex-Lax Laxative Pills (Sandoz Consumer) p 423, 683

Feen-A-Mint Gum (Schering-Plough HealthCare) p 426, 699
Feen-A-Mint Laxative Pills (Schering-Plough HealthCare) p 426, 699
Gentle Nature Natural Vegetable Laxative Tablets (Sandoz Consumer) p 423, 684
Nature's Remedy Natural Vegetable Laxative Tablets (SmithKline Beecham) p 427, 714
Neoloid (Lederle) p 577
Perdiem Granules (Rhone-Poulenc Rorer Consumer) p 421, 651
Phillips' LaxCaps (Sterling Health) p 430, 736
Purge Concentrate (Fleming) p 563
Yellolax (Luyties) p 578

LEG MUSCLE CRAMP PREPARATIONS
(see under MUSCLE RELAXANTS, SKELETAL)

LICE TREATMENTS
(see under ANTIPARASITICS, ARTHROPODS)

LIP BALM
Campho-Phenique Cold Sore Gel (Sterling Health) p 429, 731
Campho-Phenique Liquid (Sterling Health) p 429, 731
Chap Stick Lip Balm (Robins Consumer) p 421, 667
Chap Stick Petroleum Jelly Plus (Robins Consumer) p 421, 668
Chap Stick Petroleum Jelly Plus with Sunblock 15 (Robins Consumer) p 421, 668
Chap Stick Sunblock 15 Lip Balm (Robins Consumer) p 421, 667
Herpecin-L Cold Sore Lip Balm (Campbell) p 544

LUBRICANTS, OPHTHALMIC
Cellufresh Lubricant Ophthalmic Solution (Allergan Pharmaceuticals) p 504
Celluvisc Lubricant Ophthalmic Solution (Allergan Pharmaceuticals) p 504
Clear Eyes ACR Astringent/Lubricating Eye Redness Reliever (Ross) p 422, 677
Clear Eyes Lubricating Eye Redness Reliever (Ross) p 422, 677
Collyrium Fresh (Wyeth-Ayerst) p 435, 775
Dry Eye Therapy Lubricating Eye Drops (Bausch & Lomb Personal) p 403, 513
Duolube Eye Ointment (Bausch & Lomb Personal) p 403, 514
Lacri-Lube NP Lubricant Ophthalmic Ointment (Allergan Pharmaceuticals) p 504
Lacri-Lube S.O.P. Sterile Ophthalmic Ointment (Allergan Pharmaceuticals) p 504
Moisture Drops (Bausch & Lomb Personal) p 404, 514
Murine Eye Lubricant (Ross) p 422, 678
Murine Plus Lubricating Eye Redness Reliever (Ross) p 422, 678
Refresh P.M. Lubricant Ophthalmic Ointment (Allergan Pharmaceuticals) p 505
Tears Plus Lubricant Ophthalmic Solution (Allergan Pharmaceuticals) p 505
Visine EXTRA Eye Drops (Pfizer Consumer) p 420, 642

M

MAGNESIUM PREPARATIONS
Magonate Tablets and Liquid (Fleming) p 563
Mag-Ox 400 (Blaine) p 516
MagTab SR Caplets (Niché Pharmaceuticals) p 624
Uro-Mag (Blaine) p 516

MENSTRUAL PREPARATIONS

Cramp End Tablets (Ohm Laboratories) p 418, 624

Feminine Gold Analgesic Lotion (Au Pharmaceuticals) p 511

Haltran Tablets (Roberts) p 421, 664

Ibuprohm Ibuprofen Caplets (Ohm Laboratories) p 418, 625

Ibuprohm Ibuprofen Tablets (Ohm Laboratories) p 418, 625

Midol IB Cramp Relief Formula (Sterling Health) p 430, 733

Maximum Strength Midol Multi-Symptom Menstrual Formula (Sterling Health) p 430, 733

Maximum Strength Midol Premenstrual Pain Formula (Sterling Health) p 430, 733

Regular Strength Midol Multi-Symptom Menstrual Formula (Sterling Health) p 430, 732

Teen Formula Midol (Sterling Health) p 430, 734

Motrin IB Caplets and Tablets (Upjohn) p 432, 750

Extra Strength Pamprin Multi-Symptom Formula Tablets and Caplets (Chattem) p 547

Maximum Strength Pamprin Cramp Relief Formula Caplets (Chattem) p 547

Maximum Strength Panadol Tablets and Caplets (Sterling Health) p 430, 736

Premsyn PMS (Chattem) p 547

MINERALS

Beelith Tablets (Beach) p 514

Magonate Tablets and Liquid (Fleming) p 563

Mag-Ox 400 (Blaine) p 516

MagTab SR Caplets (Niché Pharmaceuticals) p 624

One-A-Day Maximum Formula Vitamins and Minerals (Miles Consumer) p 417, 620

One-A-Day Stressgard Formula Vitamins (Miles Consumer) p 417, 620

Os-Cal 500 Chewable Tablets (Marion Merrell Dow) p 412, 585

Os-Cal 500 Tablets (Marion Merrell Dow) p 412, 585

Os-Cal 250+D Tablets (Marion Merrell Dow) p 412, 585

Os-Cal 500+D Tablets (Marion Merrell Dow) p 412, 585

Os-Cal Fortified Tablets (Marion Merrell Dow) p 412, 585

Os-Cal Plus Tablets (Marion Merrell Dow) p 412, 586

Sublingual Zinc (Sublingual Products) p 743

Uro-Mag (Blaine) p 516

MOISTURIZING AGENT, OPHTHALMIC

Dry Eye Therapy Lubricating Eye Drops (Bausch & Lomb Personal) p 403, 513

Moisture Drops (Bausch & Lomb Personal) p 404, 514

MOISTURIZING AGENT, VAGINAL

Replens (Warner-Lambert) p 433, 757

MOTION SICKNESS REMEDIES
(see also under NAUSEA MEDICATIONS)

Bonine Tablets (Pfizer Consumer) p 638

Dramamine Chewable Tablets (Upjohn) p 431, 748

Dramamine Liquid (Upjohn) p 431, 748

Dramamine Tablets (Upjohn) p 431, 748

Marezine Tablets (Burroughs Wellcome) p 406, 539

MOUTHWASHES

ANTIBACTERIAL

Cepacol/Cepacol Mint Mouthwash/Gargle (Marion Merrell Dow) p 411, 579

Chloraseptic Liquid, Cherry, Menthol and Cool Mint (Richardson-Vicks) p 652

Chloraseptic Liquid - Nitrogen Propelled Spray (Richardson-Vicks) p 652

S.T.37 Antiseptic Solution (Menley & James) p 611

DEODORANT

Cepacol/Cepacol Mint Mouthwash/Gargle (Marion Merrell Dow) p 411, 579

Chloraseptic Liquid, Cherry, Menthol and Cool Mint (Richardson-Vicks) p 652

Chloraseptic Liquid - Nitrogen Propelled Spray (Richardson-Vicks) p 652

MUSCLE ACHE RELIEF
(see under ANALGESICS)

MUSCLE RELAXANTS

SKELETAL MUSCLE RELAXANTS

Legatrin Tablets (Columbia) p 408, 556

Q-vel Muscle Relaxant Pain Reliever (CIBA Consumer) p 408, 554

N

NSAIDS
(see under ANALGESICS, ANTI-INFLAMMATORY AGENTS, NON-STEROIDAL & ARTHRITIS MEDICATIONS)

NASAL DECONGESTANTS
(see under COLD & COUGH PREPARATIONS)

NASAL PREPARATIONS
(see also under COLD & COUGH PREPARATIONS)

Afrin Cherry Scented Nasal Spray 0.05% (Schering-Plough HealthCare) p 428, 692

Afrin Children's Strength Nose Drops 0.025% (Schering-Plough HealthCare) p 424, 692

Afrin Menthol Nasal Spray (Schering-Plough HealthCare) p 424, 692

Afrin Nasal Spray 0.05% and Nasal Spray Pump (Schering-Plough HealthCare) p 424, 692

Afrin Nose Drops 0.05% (Schering-Plough HealthCare) p 424, 692

Afrin Saline Mist (Schering-Plough HealthCare) p 424, 692

Ayr Saline Nasal Drops (Ascher) p 403, 509

Ayr Saline Nasal Mist (Ascher) p 403, 509

Cheracol Nasal Spray Pump (Roberts) p 663

Dristan Nasal Spray (Whitehall) p 764

Dristan Menthol Nasal Spray (Whitehall) p 764

Dristan Nasal Spray, Metered Dose Pump, Regular (Whitehall) p 764

Dristan 12-hour Nasal Spray, Regular and Menthol (Whitehall) p 767

Dristan 12-hour Nasal Spray, Metered Dose Pump (Whitehall) p 767

Duration 12 Hour Nasal Spray (Schering-Plough HealthCare) p 426, 699

Duration 12 Hour Nasal Spray Pump (Schering-Plough HealthCare) p 426, 699

4-Way Fast Acting Nasal Spray (regular & mentholated) & Metered Spray Pump (regular) (Bristol-Myers Products) p 405, 532

4-Way Long Lasting Nasal Spray & Metered Spray Pump (Bristol-Myers Products) p 405, 533

NTZ Long Acting Nasal Spray & Drops 0.05% (Sterling Health) p 735

NaSal Moisturizing Nasal Spray (Sterling Health) p 430, 734

NaSal Moisturizing Nose Drops (Sterling Health) p 430, 734

Neo-Synephrine Maximum Strength 12 Hour Nasal Spray (Sterling Health) p 734

Neo-Synephrine Maximum Strength 12 Hour Nasal Spray Pump (Sterling Health) p 430, 734

Neo-Synephrine Nasal Sprays, Pediatric, Mild, Regular & Extra Strength (Sterling Health) p 430, 734

Neo-Synephrine Nose Drops (Sterling Health) p 430, 734

Nostril Nasal Decongestant (CIBA Consumer) p 407, 552

Nostrilla Long Acting Nasal Decongestant (CIBA Consumer) p 407, 552

Ocean Mist (Fleming) p 563

Otrivin Nasal Drops (CIBA Consumer) p 408, 553

Otrivin Pediatric Nasal Drops (CIBA Consumer) p 408, 553

Privine Nasal Solution and Drops (CIBA Consumer) p 408, 554

Privine Nasal Spray (CIBA Consumer) p 408, 554

Salinex Nasal Mist and Drops (Muro) p 621

Vicks Inhaler (Richardson-Vicks) p 659

Vicks Sinex Decongestant Nasal Spray (Richardson-Vicks) p 661

Vicks Sinex Decongestant Nasal Ultra Fine Mist (Richardson-Vicks) p 661

Vicks Sinex Long-Acting Decongestant Nasal Spray (Richardson-Vicks) p 661

Vicks Sinex Long-Acting Decongestant Nasal Ultra Fine Mist (Richardson-Vicks) p 661

Vicks Vatronol Nose Drops (Richardson-Vicks) p 662

NASAL SPRAYS

SALINE

Afrin Saline Mist (Schering-Plough HealthCare) p 424, 692

Ayr Saline Nasal Drops (Ascher) p 403, 509

Ayr Saline Nasal Mist (Ascher) p 403, 509

NaSal Moisturizing Nasal Spray (Sterling Health) p 430, 734

NaSal Moisturizing Nose Drops (Sterling Health) p 430, 734

Ocean Mist (Fleming) p 563

Salinex Nasal Mist and Drops (Muro) p 621

OTHER

Duration 12 Hour Nasal Spray (Schering-Plough HealthCare) p 426, 699

Duration 12 Hour Nasal Spray Pump (Schering-Plough HealthCare) p 426, 699

4-Way Fast Acting Nasal Spray (regular & mentholated) & Metered Spray Pump (regular) (Bristol-Myers Products) p 405, 532

4-Way Long Lasting Nasal Spray & Metered Spray Pump (Bristol-Myers Products) p 405, 533

NAUSEA MEDICATIONS

Dramamine Chewable Tablets (Upjohn) p 431, 748

Dramamine Liquid (Upjohn) p 431, 748

Dramamine Tablets (Upjohn) p 431, 748

Emetrol (Adria) p 403, 503

Marezine Tablets (Burroughs Wellcome) p 406, 539

Pepto-Bismol Liquid & Tablets (Procter & Gamble) p 644

Maximum Strength Pepto-Bismol Liquid (Procter & Gamble) p 644

O

OBESITY PREPARATIONS
(see under APPETITE
SUPPRESSANTS)

OPHTHALMOLOGICALS

DEVICES
(see under DEVICES,
OPHTHALMOLOGICAL)

EMOLLIENTS
(see under EMOLLIENTS,
OPHTHALMIC)

MOISTURIZERS
(see under MOISTURIZING AGENT,
OPHTHALMIC)

ORAL HYGIENE AID

Listerine Antiseptic (Warner-Lambert)
p 433, 756
S.T.37 Antiseptic Solution (Menley &
James) p 611

P

PAIN RELIEVERS
(see under ANALGESICS)

PEDICULICIDES
(see under ANTIPARASITICS)

PLATELET INHIBITORS

Children's Bayer Chewable Aspirin
(Sterling Health) p 429, 724
Genuine Bayer Aspirin Tablets &
Caplets (Sterling Health) p 428, 724
Bayer Plus Aspirin Tablets (Sterling
Health) p 429, 726
Therapy Bayer Enteric Aspirin Caplets
(Sterling Health) p 429, 728

POISON IVY & OAK PREPARATIONS

Aveeno Anti-Itch Concentrated Lotion
(Rydelle) p 423, 680
Aveeno Anti-Itch Cream (Rydelle)
p 423, 680
Aveeno Bath Oilated (Rydelle) p 423,
680
Aveeno Bath Regular (Rydelle) p 423,
680
Bactine Hydrocortisone Anti-Itch Cream
(Miles Consumer) p 416, 617
Caladryl Clear Lotion (Parke-Davis)
p 419, 633
Caladryl Cream, Lotion, Spray
(Parke-Davis) p 419, 633
Caldecort Anti-Itch Hydrocortisone
Cream (Fisons Consumer Health)
p 409, 559
Caldecort Anti-Itch Hydrocortisone
Spray (Fisons Consumer Health)
p 409, 559
Caldecort Light Cream (Fisons
Consumer Health) p 409, 559
Cortaid Cream with Aloe (Upjohn)
p 431, 747
Cortaid Lotion (Upjohn) p 431, 747
Cortaid Ointment with Aloe (Upjohn)
p 431, 747
Cortaid Spray (Upjohn) p 431, 747
Cortizone-5 Creme and Ointment
(Thompson Medical) p 431, 743
Cortizone-5 Wipes (Thompson Medical)
p 743
Cortizone-10 Creme and Ointment
(Thompson Medical) p 744
Domeboro Astringent Solution
Effervescent Tablets (Miles
Consumer) p 417, 619
Domeboro Astringent Solution Powder
Packets (Miles Consumer) p 417,
618
Rhulicream (Rydelle) p 423, 681
Rhuligel (Rydelle) p 423, 681
Rhulispray (Rydelle) p 423, 681

PREGNANCY TESTS
(see under DIAGNOSTICS,
PREGNANCY TESTS)

PREMENSTRUAL THERAPEUTICS
(see under MENSTRUAL
PREPARATIONS)

PRICKLY HEAT AIDS
(see under DERMATOLOGICALS,
DERMATITIS RELIEF & POWDERS)

PYRETICS
(see under ANTIPYRETICS)

S

SALIVA SUBSTITUTES

Salivart Saliva Substitute (Gebauer)
p 564

SALT SUBSTITUTES

Chlor-3 Condiment (Fleming) p 563

SALT TABLETS

Thermotabs (Menley & James) p 611

SCABICIDES
(see under ANTIPARASITICS)

SEDATIVES

NON-BARBITURATES
Bufferin A/F Nite Time
Analgesic/Sleeping Aid Caplets
(Bristol-Myers Products) p 404, 521
Extra Strength Doan's P.M. (CIBA
Consumer) p 407, 549
Excedrin P.M. Analgesic/Sleeping Aid
Tablets, Caplets and Liquid
(Bristol-Myers Products) p 405, 530
Hyland's Calms Forté Tablets (Standard
Homeopathic) p 722
Miles Nervine Nighttime Sleep-Aid
(Miles Consumer) p 417, 619
Nytol Tablets (Block) p 517
Sleep-ettes-D Tablets (Reese Chemical)
p 647
Sleep-eze 3 Tablets (Whitehall) p 772
Sleepinal Medicated Night Tea
(Thompson Medical) p 746
Sleepinal Night-time Sleep Aid Capsules
(Thompson Medical) p 431, 746
Sominex Caplets and Tablets
(SmithKline Beecham) p 428, 718
Sominex Pain Relief Formula
(SmithKline Beecham) p 428, 718
Unisom Nighttime Sleep Aid (Pfizer
Consumer) p 640
Unisom with Pain Relief Nighttime
Sleep Aid/Analgesic (Pfizer
Consumer) p 640

SHAMPOOS
(see under DERMATOLOGICALS,
SHAMPOOS)

SHINGLES RELIEF
(see under ANALGESICS)

SINUSITIS AIDS
(see under COLD & COUGH
PREPARATIONS)

SKIN BLEACHES
(see under DERMATOLOGICALS, SKIN
BLEACHES)

SKIN CARE PRODUCTS
(see under DERMATOLOGICALS)

SKIN PROTECTANTS

Borofax Ointment (Burroughs
Wellcome) p 538
Caldesene Medicated Ointment (Fisons
Consumer Health) p 409, 559
Caldesene Medicated Powder (Fisons
Consumer Health) p 409, 559
Chap Stick Lip Balm (Robins
Consumer) p 421, 667
Chap Stick Petroleum Jelly Plus
(Robins Consumer) p 421, 668
Chap Stick Petroleum Jelly Plus with
Sunblock 15 (Robins Consumer)
p 421, 668

Chap Stick Sunblock 15 Lip Balm
(Robins Consumer) p 421, 667
Impregon Concentrate (Fleming) p 563

SKIN WOUND PREPARATIONS

CLEANSERS
(see under DERMATOLOGICALS,
WOUND CLEANSER)
HEALING AGENTS
PRID Salve (Walker Pharmacal) p 753
PROTECTANTS
S.T.37 Antiseptic Solution (Menley &
James) p 611

SLEEP AIDS
(see under HYPNOTICS &
SEDATIVES)

SORE THROAT PREPARATIONS
(see under COLD & COUGH
PREPARATIONS, LOZENGES &
THROAT LOZENGES)

STIFF NECK RELIEF
(see under ANALGESICS)

STIMULANTS

No Doz Fast Acting Alertness Aid
Tablets (Bristol-Myers Products)
p 406, 533
Vivarin Stimulant Tablets (SmithKline
Beecham) p 721

SUNSCREENS
(see under DERMATOLOGICALS,
SUNSCREENS)

SUPPLEMENTS
(see under DIETARY SUPPLEMENTS)

SWIMMER'S EAR PREVENTION

Star-Otic Ear Solution (Stellar) p 428,
723

T

TEETHING REMEDIES

Anbesol Baby Teething Gel Anesthetic
(Whitehall) p 434, 763
Anbesol Gel
Antiseptic-Anesthetic-Regular
Strength (Whitehall) p 434, 763
Anbesol Gel Antiseptic-Anesthetic -
Maximum Strength (Whitehall) p 434,
763
Hyland's Teething Tablets (Standard
Homeopathic) p 723
Baby Orajel (Del Pharmaceuticals)
p 408, 557

TENNIS ELBOW RELIEF
(see under ANALGESICS)

THROAT LOZENGES

Cēpacol Anesthetic Lozenges (Troches)
(Marion Merrell Dow) p 411, 580
Cēpacol Dry Throat Lozenges, Cherry
Flavor (Marion Merrell Dow) p 411,
579
Cēpacol Dry Throat Lozenges,
Honey-Lemon Flavor (Marion Merrell
Dow) p 411, 579
Cēpacol Dry Throat Lozenges,
Menthol-Eucalyptus Flavor (Marion
Merrell Dow) p 411, 580
Cēpacol Dry Throat Lozenges, Original
Flavor (Marion Merrell Dow) p 411,
580
Cēpastat Cherry Flavor Sore Throat
Lozenges (Marion Merrell Dow)
p 411, 580
Cēpastat Extra Strength Sore Throat
Lozenges (Marion Merrell Dow)
p 411, 580
Children's Chloraseptic Lozenges
(Richardson-Vicks) p 652
Chloraseptic Lozenges, Cherry, Cool
Mint and Menthol (Richardson-Vicks)
p 653
Hold Cough Suppressant Lozenge
(Menley & James) p 415, 609
N'ICE Medicated Sugarless Sore Throat
and Cough Lozenges (SmithKline
Beecham) p 427, 714

Robitussin Cough Calmers (Robins Consumer) p 674
Robitussin Cough Drops (Robins Consumer) p 422, 674
Soothers Throat Drops (Warner-Lambert) p 433, 758
Sucrets Original Mint (SmithKline Beecham) p 428, 719
Sucrets Children's Cherry Flavored Sore Throat Lozenges (SmithKline Beecham) p 428, 719
Sucrets Cold Formula (SmithKline Beecham) p 428, 719
Sucrets Maximum Strength Wintergreen and Sucrets Wild Cherry (Regular Strength) Sore Throat Lozenges (SmithKline Beecham) p 428, 719
Throat Discs Throat Lozenges (Marion Merrell Dow) p 412, 586
Vicks Cough Drops (Richardson-Vicks) p 655
Extra Strength Vicks Cough Drops (Richardson-Vicks) p 655
Vicks Formula 44 Cough Control Discs (Richardson-Vicks) p 656

TOOTH DESENSITIZERS
Maximum Strength Orajel (Del Pharmaceuticals) p 408, 557
Promise Toothpaste (Block) p 517
Mint Gel Sensodyne (Block) p 518
Mint Sensodyne Toothpaste (Block) p 518
Original Sensodyne Toothpaste (Block) p 517

U

UNIT DOSE SYSTEMS
Allbee with C Caplets (Robins Consumer) p 667
Dimetapp Elixir (Robins Consumer) p 421, 670
Dimetapp Extentabs (Robins Consumer) p 421, 671
Peri-Colace (Mead Johnson Pharmaceuticals) p 415, 606
Z-BEC Tablets (Robins Consumer) p 676

V

VAGINAL PREPARATIONS
CLEANSERS, EXTERNAL
Massengill Baby Powder Soft Cloth Towelette and Fragrance Free Soft Cloth Towelette (SmithKline Beecham) p 713
CONTRACEPTIVES
(see under CONTRACEPTIVES)
CREAMS
Gyne-Lotrimin Vaginal Cream Antifungal (Schering-Plough HealthCare) p 426, 699
Massengill Medicated Soft Cloth Towelette (SmithKline Beecham) p 713
Monistat 7 Vaginal Cream (Ortho Pharmaceutical) p 418, 627
DOUCHES
Massengill Disposable Douches (SmithKline Beecham) p 427, 712
Massengill Liquid Concentrate (SmithKline Beecham) p 712
Massengill Medicated Disposable Douche (SmithKline Beecham) p 427, 713
Massengill Medicated Liquid Concentrate (SmithKline Beecham) p 713
Massengill Powder (SmithKline Beecham) p 712
INSERTS, SUPPOSITORIES
Encare Vaginal Contraceptive Suppositories (Thompson Medical) p 745
Gyne-Lotrimin Vaginal Inserts (Schering-Plough HealthCare) p 426, 700
Monistat 7 Vaginal Suppositories (Ortho Pharmaceutical) p 418, 627

Semicid Vaginal Contraceptive Inserts (Whitehall) p 772
JELLIES, OINTMENTS
Replens (Warner-Lambert) p 433, 757
LUBRICANTS
Replens (Warner-Lambert) p 433, 757
MOISTURIZERS
Gyne-Moistrin Vaginal Gel (Schering-Plough HealthCare) p 426, 700
Replens (Warner-Lambert) p 433, 757
OTHER
Cortef Feminine Itch Cream (Upjohn) p 748

VASOCONSTRICTOR
Clear Eyes ACR Astringent/Lubricating Eye Redness Reliever (Ross) p 422, 677
Murine Plus Lubricating Eye Redness Reliever (Ross) p 422, 678
Visine EXTRA Eye Drops (Pfizer Consumer) p 420, 642

VERTIGO AGENTS
Marezine Tablets (Burroughs Wellcome) p 406, 539
Nicotinex Elixir (Fleming) p 563

VIRAL AGENTS
Herpecin-L Cold Sore Lip Balm (Campbell) p 544

VITAMINS
GERIATRIC
Geritol Extend Caplets (SmithKline Beecham) p 712
INTRANASAL APPLICATION
Ener-B Vitamin B_{12} Nasal Gel Dietary Supplement (Nature's Bounty) p 417, 622
MULTIVITAMINS
Allbee with C Caplets (Robins Consumer) p 667
Allbee C-800 Tablets (Robins Consumer) p 666
Bugs Bunny Children's Chewable Vitamins (Sugar Free) (Miles Consumer) p 416, 617
Bugs Bunny With Extra C Children's Chewable Vitamins (Sugar Free) (Miles Consumer) p 416, 618
Centrum, Jr. (Children's Chewable) + Extra Calcium (Lederle) p 411, 573
Dayalets Filmtab (Abbott) p 502
Flintstones Children's Chewable Vitamins (Miles Consumer) p 416, 617
Flintstones Children's Chewable Vitamins With Extra C (Miles Consumer) p 416, 618
Geriplex-FS Kapseals (Parke-Davis) p 634
Geriplex-FS Liquid (Parke-Davis) p 634
One-A-Day Essential Vitamins (Miles Consumer) p 417, 620
One-A-Day Plus Extra C Vitamins (Miles Consumer) p 417, 620
One-A-Day Women's Formula Multivitamins with Calcium, Extra Iron, Zinc and Beta Carotene (Miles Consumer) p 417, 620
Optilets-500 Filmtab (Abbott) p 403, 502
Poly-Vi-Sol Vitamins, Chewable Tablets and Drops (without Iron) (Mead Johnson Nutritionals) p 414, 603
Poly-Vi-Sol Vitamins, Circus Shapes Chewable (without Iron) (Mead Johnson Nutritionals) p 414, 603
Sigtab Tablets (Roberts) p 421, 666
Stresstabs (Lederle) p 411, 577
Sublingual B-Total (Sublingual Products) p 431, 742
Sublingual C with Niacin (Sublingual Products) p 743
Surbex (Abbott) p 502
Surbex with C (Abbott) p 502
Surbex-750 with Iron (Abbott) p 403, 503
Surbex-T (Abbott) p 403, 502

Thera-Combex H-P (Parke-Davis) p 637
Theragran Liquid (Apothecon) p 403, 508
Theragran Tablets (Apothecon) p 403, 508
Tri-Vi-Sol Vitamin Drops (Mead Johnson Nutritionals) p 415, 606
Trophite Liquid (Menley & James) p 612
Unicap Softgel Capsules & Tablets (Upjohn) p 432, 751
Unicap Jr. Chewable Tablets (Upjohn) p 751
Zymacap Capsules (Roberts) p 666
MULTIVITAMINS WITH MINERALS
Allbee C-800 Plus Iron Tablets (Robins Consumer) p 666
Bugs Bunny Complete Children's Chewable Vitamins + Minerals with Iron and Calcium (Sugar Free) (Miles Consumer) p 416, 618
Bugs Bunny Plus Iron Children's Chewable Vitamins (Sugar Free) (Miles Consumer) p 416, 617
Centrum (Lederle) p 410, 572
Centrum, Jr. (Children's Chewable) + Extra C (Lederle) p 410, 573
Centrum, Jr. (Children's Chewable) + Extra Calcium (Lederle) p 411, 573
Centrum, Jr. (Children's Chewable) + Iron (Lederle) p 410, 573
Centrum Liquid (Lederle) p 411, 572
Centrum Silver (Lederle) p 411, 575
Dayalets Plus Iron Filmtab (Abbott) p 502
FemIron Multi Vitamins and Iron (Menley & James) p 415, 609
Flintstones Children's Chewable Vitamins Plus Iron (Miles Consumer) p 416, 617
Flintstones Complete With Calcium, Iron & Minerals Children's Chewable Vitamins (Miles Consumer) p 416, 618
Geriplex-FS Kapseals (Parke-Davis) p 634
Geriplex-FS Liquid (Parke-Davis) p 634
Geritol Complete Tablets (SmithKline Beecham) p 711
Geritol Extend Caplets (SmithKline Beecham) p 712
Geritol Liquid - High Potency Iron & Vitamin Tonic (SmithKline Beecham) p 712
Gevrabon Liquid (Lederle) p 576
Gevral T Tablets (Lederle) p 576
Gevral Tablets (Lederle) p 576
Myadec (Parke-Davis) p 419, 635
Natabec Kapseals (Parke-Davis) p 636
One-A-Day Maximum Formula Vitamins and Minerals (Miles Consumer) p 417, 620
One-A-Day Stressgard Formula Vitamins (Miles Consumer) p 417, 620
One-A-Day Women's Formula Multivitamins with Calcium, Extra Iron, Zinc and Beta Carotene (Miles Consumer) p 417, 620
Optilets-M-500 Filmtab (Abbott) p 403, 502
Os-Cal Fortified Tablets (Marion Merrell Dow) p 412, 585
Os-Cal Plus Tablets (Marion Merrell Dow) p 412, 586
Poly-Vi-Sol Vitamins with Iron, Chewable Tablets and Circus Shapes Chewable (Mead Johnson Nutritionals) p 414, 604
Poly-Vi-Sol Vitamins with Iron, Drops (Mead Johnson Nutritionals) p 414, 604
Stresstabs + Iron, Advanced Formula (Lederle) p 411, 577
Stresstabs + Zinc (Lederle) p 411, 577
Stuart Prenatal Tablets (Stuart) p 431, 742
The Stuart Formula Tablets (J&J•Merck Consumer) p 410, 569
Sunkist Children's Chewable Multivitamins - Complete (CIBA Consumer) p 408, 555

Sunkist Children's Chewable Multivitamins - Plus Extra C (CIBA Consumer) p 408, 555
Sunkist Children's Chewable Multivitamins - Plus Iron (CIBA Consumer) p 408, 555
Sunkist Children's Chewable Multivitamins - Regular (CIBA Consumer) p 408, 554
Surbex-750 with Zinc (Abbott) p 403, 503
Theragran Stress Formula (Apothecon) p 403, 509
Theragran-M Tablets (Apothecon) p 403, 508
Tri-Vi-Sol Vitamin Drops with Iron (Mead Johnson Nutritionals) p 415, 606
Troph-Iron Liquid (Menley & James) p 611
Unicap M Tablets (Upjohn) p 432, 751
Unicap Plus Iron Vitamin Formula Tablets (Upjohn) p 751
Unicap Sr. Tablets (Upjohn) p 432, 752
Unicap T Tablets (Upjohn) p 432, 752
Vicon Plus (Whitby) p 433, 760
Vicon-C Capsules (Whitby) p 433, 760
Vi-Zac (Whitby) p 433, 760
Z-BEC Tablets (Robins Consumer) p 676

PEDIATRIC
Bugs Bunny Children's Chewable Vitamins (Sugar Free) (Miles Consumer) p 416, 617
Bugs Bunny Complete Children's Chewable Vitamins + Minerals with Iron and Calcium (Sugar Free) (Miles Consumer) p 416, 618
Bugs Bunny With Extra C Children's Chewable Vitamins (Sugar Free) (Miles Consumer) p 416, 618
Centrum, Jr. (Children's Chewable) + Extra C (Lederle) p 410, 573
Centrum, Jr. (Children's Chewable) + Extra Calcium (Lederle) p 411, 573
Centrum, Jr. (Children's Chewable) + Iron (Lederle) p 410, 573
Flintstones Children's Chewable Vitamins (Miles Consumer) p 416, 617

Flintstones Children's Chewable Vitamins With Extra C (Miles Consumer) p 416, 618
Flintstones Complete With Calcium, Iron & Minerals Children's Chewable Vitamins (Miles Consumer) p 416, 618
Hyland's Vitamin C for Children (Standard Homeopathic) p 723
Poly-Vi-Sol Vitamins, Chewable Tablets and Drops (without Iron) (Mead Johnson Nutritionals) p 414, 603
Poly-Vi-Sol Vitamins, Circus Shapes Chewable (without Iron) (Mead Johnson Nutritionals) p 414, 603
Poly-Vi-Sol Vitamins with Iron, Chewable Tablets and Circus Shapes Chewable (Mead Johnson Nutritionals) p 414, 604
Poly-Vi-Sol Vitamins with Iron, Drops (Mead Johnson Nutritionals) p 414, 604
Sunkist Children's Chewable Multivitamins - Complete (CIBA Consumer) p 408, 555
Sunkist Children's Chewable Multivitamins - Plus Extra C (CIBA Consumer) p 408, 555
Sunkist Children's Chewable Multivitamins - Plus Iron (CIBA Consumer) p 408, 555
Sunkist Children's Chewable Multivitamins - Regular (CIBA Consumer) p 408, 554
Tri-Vi-Sol Vitamin Drops (Mead Johnson Nutritionals) p 415, 606
Tri-Vi-Sol Vitamin Drops with Iron (Mead Johnson Nutritionals) p 415, 606
Unicap Jr. Chewable Tablets (Upjohn) p 751

PRENATAL
Filibon Prenatal Vitamin Tablets (Lederle) p 575
Natabec Kapseals (Parke-Davis) p 636
Stuart Prenatal Tablets (Stuart) p 431, 742

SUBLINGUAL
Sublingual B-Total (Sublingual Products) p 431, 742
Sublingual C with Niacin (Sublingual Products) p 743

THERAPEUTIC
Centrum, Jr. (Children's Chewable) + Extra C (Lederle) p 410, 573
Centrum, Jr. (Children's Chewable) + Extra Calcium (Lederle) p 411, 573
Centrum, Jr. (Children's Chewable) + Iron (Lederle) p 410, 573
Gevral T Tablets (Lederle) p 576
N'ICE Sugarless Vitamin C Drops (SmithKline Beecham) p 427, 714
Sigtab Tablets (Roberts) p 421, 666
Stresstabs (Lederle) p 411, 577
Stresstabs + Iron, Advanced Formula (Lederle) p 411, 577
Stresstabs + Zinc (Lederle) p 411, 577
Vicon Plus (Whitby) p 433, 760
Vicon-C Capsules (Whitby) p 433, 760
Vi-Zac (Whitby) p 433, 760
Zymacap Capsules (Roberts) p 666

VITAMINS
Drisdol (Sanofi Winthrop Pharmaceuticals) p 689
Ester-C Tablets (Inter-Cal) p 564
Natural Best Vitamin E 1000 I.U. and 400 I.U. (Neutrin) p 417, 622

OTHER
Beelith Tablets (Beach) p 514
Halls Vitamin C Drops (Warner-Lambert) p 433, 756
Nicotinex Elixir (Fleming) p 563
Posture-D 600 mg (Whitehall) p 768
Sunkist Vitamin C - Chewable (CIBA Consumer) p 408, 555
Sunkist Vitamin C - Easy to Swallow (CIBA Consumer) p 408, 555

W

WART REMOVERS
(see under DERMATOLOGICALS, WART REMOVERS)

WEIGHT CONTROL PREPARATIONS
(see under APPETITE SUPPRESSANTS OR FOODS)

WET DRESSINGS
(see under DERMATOLOGICALS, WET DRESSINGS)

SECTION 4

Active Ingredients Index

In this section the products described in the Product Information (White) Section are listed under their chemical (generic) name according to their principal ingredient(s). Products have been included under specific headings by the Publisher with the cooperation of individual manufacturers.

A

ACETAMINOPHEN

Actifed Plus Caplets (Burroughs Wellcome) p 406, 537
Actifed Plus Tablets (Burroughs Wellcome) p 406, 538
Allerest Headache Strength Tablets (Fisons Consumer Health) p 558
Allerest No Drowsiness Tablets (Fisons Consumer Health) p 408, 558
Allerest Sinus Pain Formula (Fisons Consumer Health) p 558
Aspirin Free Anacin Acetaminophen Film Coated Caplets (Whitehall) p 434, 762
Aspirin Free Anacin Acetaminophen Film Coated Tablets (Whitehall) p 434, 762
Benadryl Cold Tablets (Parke-Davis) p 418, 631
Benadryl Cold Nighttime Formula (Parke-Davis) p 419, 631
Bufferin A/F Nite Time Analgesic/Sleeping Aid Caplets (Bristol-Myers Products) p 404, 521
Cold Control+ Intense Cold Medicine (Reese Chemical) p 647
Allergy-Sinus Comtrex Multi-Symptom Allergy-Sinus Formula Tablets & Caplets (Bristol-Myers Products) p 404, 523
Cough Formula Comtrex (Bristol-Myers Products) p 405, 524
Comtrex Multi-Symptom Cold Reliever Tablets/Caplets/Liqui-Gels/Liquid (Bristol-Myers Products) p 404, 522
Comtrex Multi-Symptom Day-Night Caplet-Tablet (Bristol-Myers Products) p 404, 525
Comtrex Multi-Symptom Non-Drowsy Caplets (Bristol-Myers Products) p 405, 526
Congespirin For Children Aspirin Free Chewable Cold Tablets (Bristol-Myers Products) p 405, 527
Contac Cough and Chest Cold (SmithKline Beecham) p 427, 706

Contac Cough & Sore Throat Formula (SmithKline Beecham) p 427, 707
Contac Jr. Non-Drowsy Cold Liquid (SmithKline Beecham) p 427, 707
Contac Severe Cold and Flu Formula Caplets (SmithKline Beecham) p 427, 706
Contac Severe Cold & Flu Nighttime (SmithKline Beecham) p 427, 708
Contac Sinus Caplets Maximum Strength Non-Drowsy Formula (SmithKline Beecham) p 427, 705
Contac Sinus Tablets Maximum Strength Non-Drowsy Formula (SmithKline Beecham) p 427, 705
Coricidin 'D' Decongestant Tablets (Schering-Plough HealthCare) p 425, 695
Coricidin Demilets Tablets for Children (Schering-Plough HealthCare) p 425, 696
Coricidin Tablets (Schering-Plough HealthCare) p 425, 695
Datril Extra-Strength Analgesic Tablets (Bristol-Myers Products) p 405, 527
Dimetapp Cold & Flu Caplets (Robins Consumer) p 421, 670
Dristan Cold and Flu (Whitehall) p 434, 766
Dristan Cold Nasal Decongestant/ Antihistamine/Analgesic Coated Tablets (Whitehall) p 434, 765
Maximum Strength Dristan Cold Nasal Decongestant/ Analgesic Coated Caplets (Whitehall) p 434, 765
Drixoral Plus Extended-Release Tablets (Schering-Plough HealthCare) p 425, 698
Drixoral Sinus (Schering-Plough HealthCare) p 426, 698
Aspirin Free Excedrin Analgesic Caplets (Bristol-Myers Products) p 405, 528
Excedrin Extra-Strength Analgesic Tablets & Caplets (Bristol-Myers Products) p 405, 529

Excedrin P.M. Analgesic/Sleeping Aid Tablets, Caplets and Liquid (Bristol-Myers Products) p 405, 530
Sinus Excedrin Analgesic, Decongestant Tablets & Caplets (Bristol-Myers Products) p 405, 531
Liquiprin Infants' Drops (Menley & James) p 415, 610
Medi-Flu Caplet, Liquid (Parke-Davis) p 419, 634
Medi-Flu Without Drowsiness Caplets (Parke-Davis) p 419, 635
Maximum Strength Midol Multi-Symptom Menstrual Formula (Sterling Health) p 430, 733
Maximum Strength Midol Premenstrual Pain Formula (Sterling Health) p 430, 733
Regular Strength Midol Multi-Symptom Menstrual Formula (Sterling Health) p 430, 732
Teen Formula Midol (Sterling Health) p 430, 734
Ornex Caplets (Menley & James) p 415, 610
Maximum Strength Ornex Caplets (Menley & James) p 415, 610
Extra Strength Pamprin Multi-Symptom Formula Tablets and Caplets (Chattem) p 547
Maximum Strength Pamprin Cramp Relief Formula Caplets (Chattem) p 547
Children's Panadol Chewable Tablets, Liquid, Infants' Drops (Sterling Health) p 430, 735
Junior Strength Panadol (Sterling Health) p 430, 736
Maximum Strength Panadol Tablets and Caplets (Sterling Health) p 430, 736
Percogesic Analgesic Tablets (Richardson-Vicks) p 654
Premsyn PMS (Chattem) p 547
Pyrroxate Capsules (Roberts) p 421, 665
Robitussin Night Relief (Robins Consumer) p 422, 675

Sinarest No Drowsiness Tablets (Fisons Consumer Health) p 561
Sinarest Tablets (Fisons Consumer Health) p 561
Sinarest Extra Strength Tablets (Fisons Consumer Health) p 561
Sine-Aid Maximum Strength Sinus Headache Gelcaps, Caplets and Tablets (McNeil Consumer Products) p 414, 589
Sine-Off Maximum Strength Allergy/Sinus Formula Caplets (SmithKline Beecham) p 428, 717
Sine-Off Maximum Strength No Drowsiness Formula Caplets (SmithKline Beecham) p 428, 717
Singlet Tablets (Marion Merrell Dow) p 586
Sinutab Sinus Medication, Maximum Strength Caplets (Parke-Davis) p 419, 636
Sinutab Sinus Allergy Medication, Maximum Strength Tablets (Parke-Davis) p 419, 636
Sinutab Sinus Medication, Maximum Strength Without Drowsiness Formula Tablets & Caplets (Parke-Davis) p 419, 637
Sinutab Sinus Medication, Regular Strength Without Drowsiness Formula (Parke-Davis) p 419, 636
Sominex Pain Relief Formula (SmithKline Beecham) p 428, 718
St. Joseph Aspirin-Free Fever Reducer for Children Chewable Tablets (Schering-Plough HealthCare) p 701
St. Joseph Cold Tablets for Children (Schering-Plough HealthCare) p 702
Sudafed Severe Cold Formula Caplets (Burroughs Wellcome) p 407, 542
Sudafed Severe Cold Formula Tablets (Burroughs Wellcome) p 407, 542
Sudafed Sinus Caplets (Burroughs Wellcome) p 407, 543
Sudafed Sinus Tablets (Burroughs Wellcome) p 407, 543
Tempra 1 Acetaminophen Infant Drops (Mead Johnson Nutritionals) p 415, 605
Tempra 2 Acetaminophen Toddlers Syrup (Mead Johnson Nutritionals) p 415, 605
Tempra 3 Chewable Tablets, Regular or Double-Strength (Mead Johnson Nutritionals) p 415, 605
TheraFlu Flu and Cold Medicine (Sandoz Consumer) p 423, 684
TheraFlu Flu, Cold and Cough Medicine (Sandoz Consumer) p 423, 684
Triaminicin Tablets (Sandoz Consumer) p 424, 687
Tylenol acetaminophen Children's Chewable Tablets & Elixir (McNeil Consumer Products) p 413, 590
Tylenol Allergy Sinus Medication Maximum Strength Gelcaps and Caplets (McNeil Consumer Products) p 413, 600
Children's Tylenol Cold Multi Symptom Liquid Formula and Chewable Tablets (McNeil Consumer Products) p 413, 594
Tylenol Cold & Flu Hot Medication, Packets (McNeil Consumer Products) p 413, 595
Tylenol Cold & Flu No Drowsiness Hot Medication, Packets (McNeil Consumer Products) p 413, 598
Tylenol Cold Multi Symptom Medication Caplets and Tablets (McNeil Consumer Products) p 413, 596
Tylenol Cold Medication, Effervescent Tablets (McNeil Consumer Products) p 413, 595
Tylenol Cold Medication No Drowsiness Formula Caplets (McNeil Consumer Products) p 413, 597
Tylenol Cold Night Time Medication Liquid (McNeil Consumer Products) p 413, 599
Tylenol Cough Medication Maximum Strength Liquid (McNeil Consumer Products) p 414, 601

Tylenol Cough Medication Maximum Strength Liquid with Decongestant (McNeil Consumer Products) p 414, 601
Tylenol, Extra Strength, acetaminophen Adult Liquid Pain Reliever (McNeil Consumer Products) p 593
Tylenol, Extra Strength, acetaminophen Gelcaps, Caplets, Tablets (McNeil Consumer Products) p 412, 413, 592
Tylenol, Infants' Drops (McNeil Consumer Products) p 413, 590
Tylenol, Junior Strength, acetaminophen Coated Caplets, Grape and Fruit Chewable Tablets (McNeil Consumer Products) p 413, 414, 591
Tylenol, Maximum Strength, Sinus Medication Gelcaps, Caplets and Tablets (McNeil Consumer Products) p 413, 602
Tylenol, Regular Strength, acetaminophen Caplets and Tablets (McNeil Consumer Products) p 412, 591
Tylenol PM Extra Strength Pain Reliever/Sleep Aid Caplets and Tablets (McNeil Consumer Products) p 414, 593
Unisom with Pain Relief Nighttime Sleep Aid/Analgesic (Pfizer Consumer) p 640
Vanquish Analgesic Caplets (Sterling Health) p 431, 739
Vicks Daycare Daytime Cold Medicine Caplets (Richardson-Vicks) p 655
Vicks Daycare Daytime Cold Medicine Liquid (Richardson-Vicks) p 655
Vicks Formula 44M Multi-Symptom Cough & Cold Medicine (Richardson-Vicks) p 657
Vicks NyQuil LiquiCaps Adult Nighttime Cold/Flu Medicine (Richardson-Vicks) p 661
Vicks NyQuil Nighttime Cold/Flu Medicine-Regular & Cherry Flavor (Richardson-Vicks) p 660

ACETIC ACID

Star-Otic Ear Solution (Stellar) p 428, 723

ACETYLSALICYLIC ACID
(see under ASPIRIN)

ACONITE

Hyland's Cough Syrup with Honey (Standard Homeopathic) p 722

ALLANTOIN

Herpecin-L Cold Sore Lip Balm (Campbell) p 544

ALOE

Cortaid Cream with Aloe (Upjohn) p 431, 747
Cortaid Ointment with Aloe (Upjohn) p 431, 747
Nature's Remedy Natural Vegetable Laxative Tablets (SmithKline Beecham) p 427, 714

ALPHA TOCOPHERAL ACETATE
(see under VITAMIN E)

ALUMINUM ACETATE

Acid Mantle Creme (Sandoz Consumer) p 682
Domeboro Astringent Solution Effervescent Tablets (Miles Consumer) p 417, 619
Domeboro Astringent Solution Powder Packets (Miles Consumer) p 417, 618

ALUMINUM CARBONATE

Basaljel Capsules (Wyeth-Ayerst) p 435, 774
Basaljel Suspension (Wyeth-Ayerst) p 435, 774
Basaljel Tablets (Wyeth-Ayerst) p 435, 774

ALUMINUM CHLOROHYDRATE

Desenex Foot & Sneaker Deodorant Spray Powder (Fisons Consumer Health) p 409, 560

ALUMINUM HYDROXIDE

Cama Arthritis Pain Reliever (Sandoz Consumer) p 682
Gaviscon Extra Strength Relief Formula Liquid Antacid (Marion Merrell Dow) p 412, 582
Gaviscon Extra Strength Relief Formula Antacid Tablets (Marion Merrell Dow) p 412, 582
Gaviscon Liquid Antacid (Marion Merrell Dow) p 412, 583
Gelusil Liquid & Tablets (Parke-Davis) p 419, 634
Maalox HRF Heartburn Relief Formula (Rhone-Poulenc Rorer Consumer) p 420, 649
Maalox Plus Suspension/Tablets (Rhone-Poulenc Rorer Consumer) p 421, 649
Extra Strength Maalox Plus Suspension (Rhone-Poulenc Rorer Consumer) p 420, 650
Nephrox Suspension (Fleming) p 563
WinGel Liquid (Sterling Health) p 740

ALUMINUM HYDROXIDE GEL

ALternaGEL Liquid (J&J•Merck Consumer) p 409, 565
Aludrox Oral Suspension (Wyeth-Ayerst) p 435, 773
Amphojel Suspension (Wyeth-Ayerst) p 435, 773
Amphojel Suspension without Flavor (Wyeth-Ayerst) p 435, 773
Mylanta Liquid (J&J•Merck Consumer) p 410, 567
Mylanta Double Strength Liquid (J&J•Merck Consumer) p 410, 567

ALUMINUM HYDROXIDE GEL, DRIED

Amphojel Tablets (Wyeth-Ayerst) p 435, 773
Ascriptin A/D Caplets (Rhone-Poulenc Rorer Consumer) p 420, 649
Regular Strength Ascriptin Tablets (Rhone-Poulenc Rorer Consumer) p 420, 648
Gaviscon Antacid Tablets (Marion Merrell Dow) p 412, 582
Gaviscon-2 Antacid Tablets (Marion Merrell Dow) p 412, 582
Mylanta Tablets (J&J•Merck Consumer) p 410, 567
Mylanta Double Strength Tablets (J&J•Merck Consumer) p 410, 567

AMINO ACID PREPARATIONS

Marlyn Formula 50 (Marlyn) p 586
Marlyn Formula 50 Mega Forte (Marlyn) p 587

AMINOPHYLLINE

Amesec (Whitby) p 759

AMMONIUM ALUM

Massengill Powder (SmithKline Beecham) p 712

ASCORBIC ACID
(see under VITAMIN C)

ASPIRIN

Alka-Seltzer Effervescent Antacid and Pain Reliever (Miles Consumer) p 416, 612
Alka-Seltzer Extra Strength Effervescent Antacid and Pain Reliever (Miles Consumer) p 416, 615
Alka-Seltzer (Flavored) Effervescent Antacid and Pain Reliever (Miles Consumer) p 416, 613
Alka-Seltzer Plus Cold Medicine (Miles Consumer) p 416, 615
Alka-Seltzer Plus Cold & Cough Medicine (Miles Consumer) p 416, 616

Alka-Seltzer Plus Night-Time Cold Medicine (Miles Consumer) p 416, 615

Alka Seltzer Plus Sinus Allergy Medicine (Miles Consumer) p 416, 616

Anacin Coated Analgesic Caplets (Whitehall) p 434, 762

Anacin Coated Analgesic Tablets (Whitehall) p 434, 762

Anacin Maximum Strength Analgesic Coated Tablets (Whitehall) p 762

Maximum Strength Arthritis Pain Formula by the Makers of Anacin Analgesic Tablets and Caplets (Whitehall) p 763

Arthritis Strength BC Powder (Block) p 516

Ascriptin A/D Caplets (Rhone-Poulenc Rorer Consumer) p 420, 649

Regular Strength Ascriptin Tablets (Rhone-Poulenc Rorer Consumer) p 420, 648

BC Powder (Block) p 517

BC Cold Powder Multi-Symptom Formula (Block) p 516

BC Cold Powder Multi-Symptom Non-Drowsy Formula (Block) p 516

Children's Bayer Chewable Aspirin (Sterling Health) p 429, 724

Genuine Bayer Aspirin Tablets & Caplets (Sterling Health) p 428, 724

Maximum Bayer Aspirin Tablets & Caplets (Sterling Health) p 429, 725

Bayer Plus Aspirin Tablets (Sterling Health) p 429, 726

Extra Strength Bayer Plus Aspirin Caplets (Sterling Health) p 429, 727

Therapy Bayer Enteric Aspirin Caplets (Sterling Health) p 429, 728

8 Hour Bayer Timed-Release Aspirin (Sterling Health) p 429, 726

Arthritis Strength Bufferin Analgesic Caplets (Bristol-Myers Products) p 404, 521

Extra Strength Bufferin Analgesic Tablets (Bristol-Myers Products) p 404, 522

Bufferin Analgesic Tablets and Caplets (Bristol-Myers Products) p 404, 519

Cama Arthritis Pain Reliever (Sandoz Consumer) p 682

Ecotrin Enteric Coated Aspirin Maximum Strength Tablets and Caplets (SmithKline Beecham) p 427, 708

Ecotrin Enteric Coated Aspirin Regular Strength Tablets and Caplets (SmithKline Beecham) p 427, 708

Empirin Aspirin (Burroughs Wellcome) p 406, 538

Excedrin Extra-Strength Analgesic Tablets & Caplets (Bristol-Myers Products) p 405, 529

4-Way Cold Tablets (Bristol-Myers Products) p 405, 531

Halfprin Low Strength Aspirin Tablets (Kramer) p 410, 570

Momentum Muscular Backache Formula (Whitehall) p 767

Norwich Maximum Strength Aspirin (Chattem) p 546

Norwich Regular Strength Aspirin (Chattem) p 546

P-A-C Analgesic Tablets (Roberts) p 421, 665

Sine-Off Sinus Medicine Tablets-Aspirin Formula (SmithKline Beecham) p 428, 718

St. Joseph Adult Chewable Aspirin (81 mg.) (Schering-Plough HealthCare) p 701

Ursinus Inlay-Tabs (Sandoz Consumer) p 688

Vanquish Analgesic Caplets (Sterling Health) p 431, 739

ASPIRIN BUFFERED

Maximum Strength Arthritis Pain Formula by the Makers of Anacin Analgesic Tablets and Caplets (Whitehall) p 763

Ascriptin A/D Caplets (Rhone-Poulenc Rorer Consumer) p 420, 649

Regular Strength Ascriptin Tablets (Rhone-Poulenc Rorer Consumer) p 420, 648

Extra Strength Bayer Plus Aspirin Caplets (Sterling Health) p 429, 727

Arthritis Strength Bufferin Analgesic Caplets (Bristol-Myers Products) p 404, 521

Extra Strength Bufferin Analgesic Tablets (Bristol-Myers Products) p 404, 522

Bufferin Analgesic Tablets and Caplets (Bristol-Myers Products) p 404, 519

ASPIRIN, ENTERIC COATED

Therapy Bayer Enteric Aspirin Caplets (Sterling Health) p 429, 728

Halfprin Low Strength Aspirin Tablets (Kramer) p 410, 570

ATTAPULGITE

Diasorb Liquid (Columbia) p 408, 556

Diasorb Tablets (Columbia) p 408, 556

Donnagel Liquid and Chewable Tablets (Robins Consumer) p 422, 672

Kaopectate Concentrated Anti-Diarrheal, Peppermint Flavor (Upjohn) p 431, 749

Kaopectate Concentrated Anti-Diarrheal, Regular Flavor (Upjohn) p 431, 749

Kaopectate Children's Chewable Tablets (Upjohn) p 431, 749

Kaopectate Children's Liquid (Upjohn) p 431, 749

Kaopectate Maximum Strength Caplets (Upjohn) p 431, 749

ATTAPULGITE, ACTIVATED

Rheaban Maximum Strength Tablets (Pfizer Consumer) p 639

ATTAPULGITE, NONFIBROUS ACTIVATED

Diasorb Liquid (Columbia) p 408, 556

Diasorb Tablets (Columbia) p 408, 556

AVOBENZONE

Filteray Broad Spectrum Sunscreen Lotion (Burroughs Wellcome) p 406, 538

B

BACITRACIN

Bactine First Aid Antibiotic Plus Anesthetic Ointment (Miles Consumer) p 416, 617

Campho-Phenique Triple Antibiotic Ointment Plus Pain Reliever (Sterling Health) p 429, 731

Mycitracin Plus Pain Reliever (Upjohn) p 432, 750

Maximum Strength Mycitracin Triple Antibiotic First Aid Ointment (Upjohn) p 432, 750

BACITRACIN ZINC

Aquaphor Antibiotic Ointment (Beiersdorf) p 404, 515

Neosporin Ointment (Burroughs Wellcome) p 406, 539

Neosporin Maximum Strength Ointment (Burroughs Wellcome) p 406, 539

Polysporin Ointment (Burroughs Wellcome) p 407, 540

Polysporin Powder (Burroughs Wellcome) p 407, 540

BALSAM PERU, SPECIAL FRACTION OF

Balmex Baby Powder (Macsil) p 579

Balmex Ointment (Macsil) p 579

BELLADONNA ALKALOIDS

Hyland's Bed Wetting Tablets (Standard Homeopathic) p 722

Hyland's Teething Tablets (Standard Homeopathic) p 723

BENZALKONIUM CHLORIDE

Bactine Antiseptic/Anesthetic First Aid Liquid (Miles Consumer) p 416, 617

Orajel Mouth-Aid (Del Pharmaceuticals) p 408, 557

Zephiran Chloride Aqueous Solution (Sanofi Winthrop Pharmaceuticals) p 689

Zephiran Chloride Spray (Sanofi Winthrop Pharmaceuticals) p 689

Zephiran Chloride Tinted Tincture (Sanofi Winthrop Pharmaceuticals) p 689

BENZETHONIUM CHLORIDE

Clinical Care Dermal Wound Cleanser (Care-Tech) p 545

Formula Magic Antibacterial Powder (Care-Tech) p 545

Orchid Fresh II Perineal/Ostomy Cleanser (Care-Tech) p 545

BENZOCAINE

Americaine Hemorrhoidal Ointment (Fisons Consumer Health) p 409, 559

Americaine Topical Anesthetic First Aid Ointment (Fisons Consumer Health) p 409, 559

Americaine Topical Anesthetic Spray (Fisons Consumer Health) p 409, 559

Anbesol Baby Teething Gel Anesthetic (Whitehall) p 434, 763

Anbesol Gel Antiseptic-Anesthetic-Regular Strength (Whitehall) p 434, 763

Anbesol Gel Antiseptic-Anesthetic - Maximum Strength (Whitehall) p 434, 763

Anbesol Liquid Antiseptic-Anesthetic (Whitehall) p 434, 763

Anbesol Liquid Antiseptic-Anesthetic - Maximum Strength (Whitehall) p 434, 763

BiCozene Creme (Sandoz Consumer) p 423, 682

Cēpacol Anesthetic Lozenges (Troches) (Marion Merrell Dow) p 411, 580

Children's Chloraseptic Lozenges (Richardson-Vicks) p 652

Chloraseptic Lozenges, Cherry, Cool Mint and Menthol (Richardson-Vicks) p 653

Dentapaine Gel (Reese Chemical) p 647

Dermoplast Anesthetic Pain Relief Lotion (Whitehall) p 764

Dermoplast Anesthetic Pain Relief Spray (Whitehall) p 764

Legatrin Rub (Columbia) p 408, 556

Baby Orajel (Del Pharmaceuticals) p 408, 557

Maximum Strength Orajel (Del Pharmaceuticals) p 408, 557

Orajel Mouth-Aid (Del Pharmaceuticals) p 408, 557

Oxipor VHC Lotion for Psoriasis (Whitehall) p 768

Rhulispray (Rydelle) p 423, 681

Vicks Formula 44 Cough Control Discs (Richardson-Vicks) p 656

ZilaDent Oral Analgesic Gel (Zila Pharmaceuticals) p 777

BENZOPHENONE-3

Neutrogena Moisture SPF 15 Untinted (Neutrogena) p 417, 623

Neutrogena Moisture SPF 15 with Sheer Tint (Neutrogena) p 417, 623

BENZOYL PEROXIDE

Clear by Design Medicated Acne Gel (SmithKline Beecham) p 426, 704

Oxy 10 Daily Face Wash Antibacterial Skin Wash (SmithKline Beecham) p 427, 716

Oxy-5 and Oxy-10 Tinted and Vanishing Formulas with Sorboxyl (SmithKline Beecham) p 427, 715

BENZYL ALCOHOL

Cēpacol Dry Throat Lozenges, Original Flavor (Marion Merrell Dow) p 411, 580

Itch-X Gel (Ascher) p 403, 509

Rhuligel (Rydelle) p 423, 681

BETA CAROTENE
Bugs Bunny Children's Chewable Vitamins (Sugar Free) (Miles Consumer) p 416, 617
Bugs Bunny Complete Children's Chewable Vitamins + Minerals with Iron and Calcium (Sugar Free) (Miles Consumer) p 416, 618
Bugs Bunny With Extra C Children's Chewable Vitamins (Sugar Free) (Miles Consumer) p 416, 618
Bugs Bunny Plus Iron Children's Chewable Vitamins (Sugar Free) (Miles Consumer) p 416, 617
Flintstones Children's Chewable Vitamins (Miles Consumer) p 416, 617
Flintstones Children's Chewable Vitamins With Extra C (Miles Consumer) p 416, 618
Flintstones Children's Chewable Vitamins Plus Iron (Miles Consumer) p 416, 617
Flintstones Complete With Calcium, Iron & Minerals Children's Chewable Vitamins (Miles Consumer) p 416, 618
One-A-Day Women's Formula Multivitamins with Calcium, Extra Iron, Zinc and Beta Carotene (Miles Consumer) p 417, 620
Theragran-M Tablets (Apothecon) p 403, 508

BISACODYL
Dulcolax Suppositories (CIBA Consumer) p 407, 550
Dulcolax Tablets (CIBA Consumer) p 407, 550

BISMUTH SUBGALLATE
Devrom Chewable Tablets (Parthenon) p 638

BISMUTH SUBNITRATE
Balmex Ointment (Macsil) p 579

BISMUTH SUBSALICYLATE
Pepto-Bismol Liquid & Tablets (Procter & Gamble) p 644
Maximum Strength Pepto-Bismol Liquid (Procter & Gamble) p 644

BONESET
Hyland's C-Plus Cold Tablets (Standard Homeopathic) p 722

BORIC ACID
Borofax Ointment (Burroughs Wellcome) p 538
Collyrium for Fresh Eyes (Wyeth-Ayerst) p 435, 775
Collyrium Fresh (Wyeth-Ayerst) p 435, 775
Eye Wash (Bausch & Lomb Personal) p 404, 514
Star-Otic Ear Solution (Stellar) p 428, 723

BROMPHENIRAMINE MALEATE
Alka Seltzer Plus Sinus Allergy Medicine (Miles Consumer) p 416, 616
Bromfed Syrup (Muro) p 621
Dimetane Decongestant Caplets (Robins Consumer) p 669
Dimetane Decongestant Elixir (Robins Consumer) p 669
Dimetane Elixir (Robins Consumer) p 668
Dimetane Extentabs 8 mg (Robins Consumer) p 668
Dimetane Extentabs 12 mg (Robins Consumer) p 668
Dimetane Tablets (Robins Consumer) p 668
Dimetapp Cold & Flu Caplets (Robins Consumer) p 421, 670
Dimetapp Elixir (Robins Consumer) p 421, 670

Dimetapp DM Elixir (Robins Consumer) p 421, 671
Dimetapp Extentabs (Robins Consumer) p 421, 671
Dimetapp Tablets (Robins Consumer) p 421, 672
Dristan Allergy Nasal Decongestant/Antihistamine Caplets (Whitehall) p 434, 765
Drixoral Antihistamine/Nasal Decongestant Syrup (Schering-Plough HealthCare) p 696

BUROW'S SOLUTION
Star-Otic Ear Solution (Stellar) p 428, 723

C

CAFFEINE
Anacin Coated Analgesic Caplets (Whitehall) p 434, 762
Anacin Coated Analgesic Tablets (Whitehall) p 434, 762
Anacin Maximum Strength Analgesic Coated Tablets (Whitehall) p 762
Aspirin Free Excedrin Analgesic Caplets (Bristol-Myers Products) p 405, 528
Excedrin Extra-Strength Analgesic Tablets & Caplets (Bristol-Myers Products) p 405, 529
Maximum Strength Midol Multi-Symptom Menstrual Formula (Sterling Health) p 430, 733
No Doz Fast Acting Alertness Aid Tablets (Bristol-Myers Products) p 406, 533
No Doz Maximum Strength Caplets (Bristol-Myers Products) p 405, 533
P-A-C Analgesic Tablets (Roberts) p 421, 665
Vanquish Analgesic Caplets (Sterling Health) p 431, 739
Vivarin Stimulant Tablets (SmithKline Beecham) p 721

CALAMINE
Aveeno Anti-Itch Concentrated Lotion (Rydelle) p 423, 680
Aveeno Anti-Itch Cream (Rydelle) p 423, 680
Caladryl Cream, Lotion, Spray (Parke-Davis) p 419, 633
Rhulicream (Rydelle) p 423, 681
Rhulispray (Rydelle) p 423, 681

CALCIUM
Bugs Bunny Complete Children's Chewable Vitamins + Minerals with Iron and Calcium (Sugar Free) (Miles Consumer) p 416, 618
Flintstones Complete With Calcium, Iron & Minerals Children's Chewable Vitamins (Miles Consumer) p 416, 618
One-A-Day Maximum Formula Vitamins and Minerals (Miles Consumer) p 417, 620
One-A-Day Women's Formula Multivitamins with Calcium, Extra Iron, Zinc and Beta Carotene (Miles Consumer) p 417, 620
Os-Cal Fortified Tablets (Marion Merrell Dow) p 412, 585
Os-Cal Plus Tablets (Marion Merrell Dow) p 412, 586

CALCIUM ASCORBATE
Ester-C Tablets (Inter-Cal) p 564

CALCIUM CARBONATE
Alka-Mints Chewable Antacid (Miles Consumer) p 416, 612
Ascriptin A/D Caplets (Rhone-Poulenc Rorer Consumer) p 420, 649
Regular Strength Ascriptin Tablets (Rhone-Poulenc Rorer Consumer) p 420, 648
Balmex Baby Powder (Macsil) p 579
Extra Strength Bayer Plus Aspirin Caplets (Sterling Health) p 429, 727
Bufferin Analgesic Tablets and Caplets (Bristol-Myers Products) p 404, 519

Caltrate 600 (Lederle) p 410, 571
Caltrate 600 + Iron & Vitamin D (Lederle) p 410, 572
Caltrate 600 + Vitamin D (Lederle) p 410, 572
Centrum, Jr. (Children's Chewable) + Extra Calcium (Lederle) p 411, 573
Chooz Antacid Gum (Schering-Plough HealthCare) p 425, 694
Di-Gel Antacid/Anti-Gas (Schering-Plough HealthCare) p 425, 696
Marblen Suspension Peach/Apricot (Fleming) p 563
Marblen Suspension Unflavored (Fleming) p 563
Marblen Tablets (Fleming) p 563
Os-Cal 500 Chewable Tablets (Marion Merrell Dow) p 412, 585
Os-Cal 500 Tablets (Marion Merrell Dow) p 412, 585
Os-Cal 250+D Tablets (Marion Merrell Dow) p 412, 585
Os-Cal 500+D Tablets (Marion Merrell Dow) p 412, 585
Rolaids (Calcium Rich/Sodium Free) (Warner-Lambert) p 433, 757
Extra Strength Rolaids (Warner-Lambert) p 433, 758
Tums Plus Antacid Anti-gas Tablets, Assorted Fruit or Peppermint (SmithKline Beecham) p 428, 721

CALCIUM CARBONATE, PRECIPITATED
Tums Antacid Tablets (SmithKline Beecham) p 428, 720
Tums E-X Antacid Tablets (SmithKline Beecham) p 428, 720

CALCIUM PANTOTHENATE
(see also under PANTOTHENIC ACID)
Vicon Plus (Whitby) p 433, 760
Vicon-C Capsules (Whitby) p 433, 760

CALCIUM PHOSPHATE
Hyland's Teething Tablets (Standard Homeopathic) p 723

CALCIUM PHOSPHATE, DIBASIC
Centrum, Jr. (Children's Chewable) + Extra Calcium (Lederle) p 411, 573

CALCIUM PHOSPHATE, TRIBASIC
Posture 600 mg (Whitehall) p 768
Posture-D 600 mg (Whitehall) p 768

CALCIUM POLYCARBOPHIL
Fiberall Chewable Tablets, Lemon Creme Flavor (CIBA Consumer) p 551
FiberCon (Lederle) p 411, 575

CALCIUM UNDECYLENATE
Caldesene Medicated Powder (Fisons Consumer Health) p 409, 559
Cruex Antifungal Powder (Fisons Consumer Health) p 409, 560

CAMPHOR
Aurum Analgesic Lotion (Au Pharmaceuticals) p 510
Aveeno Anti-Itch Concentrated Lotion (Rydelle) p 423, 680
Aveeno Anti-Itch Cream (Rydelle) p 423, 680
Ben-Gay Ultra Strength Pain Relieving Rub (Pfizer Consumer) p 638
Caladryl Cream, Lotion, Spray (Parke-Davis) p 419, 633
Campho-Phenique Cold Sore Gel (Sterling Health) p 429, 731
Campho-Phenique Liquid (Sterling Health) p 429, 731
Feminine Gold Analgesic Lotion (Au Pharmaceuticals) p 511
Pazo Hemorrhoid Ointment & Suppositories (Bristol-Myers Products) p 406, 534
Rhulicream (Rydelle) p 423, 681
Rhuligel (Rydelle) p 423, 681
Rhulispray (Rydelle) p 423, 681
Theragold Analgesic Lotion (Au Pharmaceuticals) p 510

Therapeutic Gold Analgesic Lotion (Au Pharmaceuticals) p 510
Vicks Vaporub (Richardson-Vicks) p 662
Vicks Vaposteam (Richardson-Vicks) p 662

CARBAMIDE PEROXIDE

Debrox Drops (Marion Merrell Dow) p 411, 581
Ear Drops by Murine—(See Murine Ear Wax Removal System/Murine Ear Drops) (Ross) p 422, 677
Gly-Oxide Liquid (Marion Merrell Dow) p 412, 583
Murine Ear Drops (Ross) p 422, 677
Murine Ear Wax Removal System (Ross) p 422, 677

CARBOLIC ACID
(see under PHENOL)

CARBOXYMETHYLCELLULOSE SODIUM

Cellufresh Lubricant Ophthalmic Solution (Allergan Pharmaceuticals) p 504
Celluvisc Lubricant Ophthalmic Solution (Allergan Pharmaceuticals) p 504

CASANTHRANOL

Anticon (Neutrin) p 417, 622
Peri-Colace (Mead Johnson Pharmaceuticals) p 415, 606

CASCARA SAGRADA

Nature's Remedy Natural Vegetable Laxative Tablets (SmithKline Beecham) p 427, 714
Peri-Colace (Mead Johnson Pharmaceuticals) p 415, 606

CASTOR OIL

Neoloid (Lederle) p 577
Purge Concentrate (Fleming) p 563

CETYLPYRIDINIUM CHLORIDE

Cēpacol Anesthetic Lozenges (Troches) (Marion Merrell Dow) p 411, 580
Cēpacol/Cēpacol Mint Mouthwash/Gargle (Marion Merrell Dow) p 411, 579
Cēpacol Dry Throat Lozenges, Original Flavor (Marion Merrell Dow) p 411, 580

CHAMOMILE

Hyland's Calms Forté Tablets (Standard Homeopathic) p 722
Hyland's Colic Tablets (Standard Homeopathic) p 722
Hyland's Teething Tablets (Standard Homeopathic) p 723

CHARCOAL, ACTIVATED

Actidose with Sorbitol (Paddock) p 628
Actidose-Aqua, Activated Charcoal (Paddock) p 628
Charcoaid (Requa) p 647
Charcocaps (Requa) p 648

CHLORHEXIDINE GLUCONATE

Hibiclens Antimicrobial Skin Cleanser (Stuart) p 431, 740
Hibistat Germicidal Hand Rinse (Stuart) p 741
Hibistat Towelette (Stuart) p 741

CHLORIDE

One-A-Day Maximum Formula Vitamins and Minerals (Miles Consumer) p 417, 620

CHLOROBUTANOL

Outgro Solution (Whitehall) p 767

CHLOROXYLENOL

Barri-Care Antimicrobial Barrier Ointment (Care-Tech) p 544
Care Creme (Care-Tech) p 544
Concept (Care-Tech) p 545
Satin Antimicrobial Skin Cleanser (Care-Tech) p 545

Techni-Care Surgical Scrub (Care-Tech) p 545

CHLORPHENIRAMINE MALEATE

A.R.M. Allergy Relief Medicine Caplets (Menley & James) p 415, 607
Alka-Seltzer Plus Cold Medicine (Miles Consumer) p 416, 615
Alka-Seltzer Plus Cold & Cough Medicine (Miles Consumer) p 416, 616
Allerest Children's Chewable Tablets (Fisons Consumer Health) p 558
Allerest Headache Strength Tablets (Fisons Consumer Health) p 558
Allerest 12 Hour Caplets (Fisons Consumer Health) p 558
Allerest Maximum Strength Tablets (Fisons Consumer Health) p 408, 558
Allerest Sinus Pain Formula (Fisons Consumer Health) p 558
BC Cold Powder Multi-Symptom Formula (Block) p 516
Cerose-DM (Wyeth-Ayerst) p 435, 774
Cheracol Plus Head Cold/Cough Formula (Roberts) p 421, 663
Chlor-Trimeton Allergy Syrup, Tablets & Long-Acting Repetabs Tablets (Schering-Plough HealthCare) p 424,425, 693
Chlor-Trimeton Antihistamine and Decongestant Tablets (Schering-Plough HealthCare) p 425, 694
Chlor-Trimeton Long Acting Antihistamine and Decongestant Repetabs Tablets (Schering-Plough HealthCare) p 425, 694
Allergy-Sinus Comtrex Multi-Symptom Allergy-Sinus Formula Tablets & Caplets (Bristol-Myers Products) p 404, 523
Comtrex Multi-Symptom Cold Reliever Tablets/Caplets/Liqui-Gels/Liquid (Bristol-Myers Products) p 404, 522
Comtrex Multi-Symptom Day-Night Caplet-Tablet (Bristol-Myers Products) p 404, 525
Contac Continuous Action Decongestant/Antihistamine Capsules (SmithKline Beecham) p 426, 705
Contac Maximum Strength Continuous Action Decongestant/Antihistamine Caplets (SmithKline Beecham) p 426, 704
Contac Severe Cold and Flu Formula Caplets (SmithKline Beecham) p 427, 706
Contac Severe Cold & Flu Nighttime (SmithKline Beecham) p 427, 708
Coricidin 'D' Decongestant Tablets (Schering-Plough HealthCare) p 425, 695
Coricidin Demilets Tablets for Children (Schering-Plough HealthCare) p 425, 696
Coricidin Tablets (Schering-Plough HealthCare) p 425, 695
Dorcol Children's Liquid Cold Formula (Sandoz Consumer) p 423, 683
Dristan Cold and Flu (Whitehall) p 434, 766
Dristan Cold Nasal Decongestant/ Antihistamine/Analgesic Coated Tablets (Whitehall) p 434, 765
4-Way Cold Tablets (Bristol-Myers Products) p 405, 531
Isoclor Timesule Capsules (Fisons Consumer Health) p 409, 561
Medi-Flu Caplet, Liquid (Parke-Davis) p 419, 634
Novahistine Elixir (Marion Merrell Dow) p 412, 584
Orthoxicol Cough Syrup (Roberts) p 665
PediaCare Allergy Formula Liquid (McNeil Consumer Products) p 414, 588
PediaCare Cough-Cold Formula Liquid and Chewable Tablets (McNeil Consumer Products) p 414, 588

PediaCare Night Rest Cough-Cold Formula Liquid (McNeil Consumer Products) p 414, 588
PediaCare 6-12 Cough-Cold Formula Chewable Tablets (McNeil Consumer Products) p 414, 588
Pyrroxate Capsules (Roberts) p 421, 665
Ryna Liquid (Wallace) p 432, 754
Ryna-C Liquid (Wallace) p 432, 754
Sinarest Tablets (Fisons Consumer Health) p 561
Sinarest Extra Strength Tablets (Fisons Consumer Health) p 561
Sine-Off Maximum Strength Allergy/Sinus Formula Caplets (SmithKline Beecham) p 428, 717
Sine-Off Sinus Medicine Tablets-Aspirin Formula (SmithKline Beecham) p 428, 718
Singlet Tablets (Marion Merrell Dow) p 586
Sinutab Sinus Medication, Maximum Strength Caplets (Parke-Davis) p 419, 636
Sinutab Sinus Allergy Medication, Maximum Strength Tablets (Parke-Davis) p 419, 636
Sudafed Plus Liquid (Burroughs Wellcome) p 407, 541
Sudafed Plus Tablets (Burroughs Wellcome) p 407, 542
Teldrin Timed-Release Allergy Capsules, 12 mg. (SmithKline Beecham) p 428, 720
TheraFlu Flu and Cold Medicine (Sandoz Consumer) p 423, 684
TheraFlu Flu, Cold and Cough Medicine (Sandoz Consumer) p 423, 684
Triaminic Allergy Tablets (Sandoz Consumer) p 685
Triaminic Chewables (Sandoz Consumer) p 685
Triaminic Cold Tablets (Sandoz Consumer) p 424, 685
Triaminic Nite Light (Sandoz Consumer) p 424, 686
Triaminic Syrup (Sandoz Consumer) p 423, 686
Triaminic-12 Tablets (Sandoz Consumer) p 424, 687
Triaminicin Tablets (Sandoz Consumer) p 424, 687
Triaminicol Multi-Symptom Cold Tablets (Sandoz Consumer) p 424, 688
Triaminicol Multi-Symptom Relief (Sandoz Consumer) p 424, 688
Tylenol Allergy Sinus Medication Maximum Strength Gelcaps and Caplets (McNeil Consumer Products) p 413, 600
Children's Tylenol Cold Multi Symptom Liquid Formula and Chewable Tablets (McNeil Consumer Products) p 413, 594
Tylenol Cold & Flu Hot Medication, Packets (McNeil Consumer Products) p 413, 595
Tylenol Cold Multi Symptom Medication Caplets and Tablets (McNeil Consumer Products) p 413, 596
Tylenol Cold Medication, Effervescent Tablets (McNeil Consumer Products) p 413, 595
Vicks Children's NyQuil Nighttime Cold/Cough Medicine (Richardson-Vicks) p 659
Vicks Children's NyQuil Nighttime Head Cold/Allergy Medicine (Richardson-Vicks) p 660
Vicks Formula 44M Multi-Symptom Cough & Cold Medicine (Richardson-Vicks) p 657
Vicks Pediatric Formula 44m Multi-Symptom Cough & Cold Medicine (Richardson-Vicks) p 658

CHOLINE BITARTRATE

Geritol Liquid - High Potency Iron & Vitamin Tonic (SmithKline Beecham) p 712

CITRIC ACID

Alka-Seltzer Effervescent Antacid (Miles Consumer) p 416, 614
Alka-Seltzer Effervescent Antacid and Pain Reliever (Miles Consumer) p 416, 612
Alka-Seltzer Extra Strength Effervescent Antacid and Pain Reliever (Miles Consumer) p 416, 615
Alka-Seltzer (Flavored) Effervescent Antacid and Pain Reliever (Miles Consumer) p 416, 613
Ricelyte, Rice-Based Oral Electrolyte Maintenance Solution (Mead Johnson Nutritionals) p 415, 604

CLOTRIMAZOLE

Gyne-Lotrimin Vaginal Cream Antifungal (Schering-Plough HealthCare) p 426, 699
Gyne-Lotrimin Vaginal Inserts (Schering-Plough HealthCare) p 426, 700
Lotrimin AF Antifungal Cream, Lotion and Solution (Schering-Plough HealthCare) p 426, 700
Mycelex OTC Cream Antifungal (Miles Consumer) p 417, 619
Mycelex OTC Solution Antifungal (Miles Consumer) p 417, 619

COAL TAR

Denorex Medicated Shampoo and Conditioner (Whitehall) p 434, 764
Denorex Medicated Shampoo, Extra Strength (Whitehall) p 434, 764
Denorex Medicated Shampoo, Extra Strength With Conditioners (Whitehall) p 434, 764
Denorex Medicated Shampoo, Regular & Mountain Fresh Herbal Scent (Whitehall) p 434, 764
MG 217 Psoriasis Ointment and Lotion (Triton Consumer) p 747
MG 217 Psoriasis Shampoo and Conditioner (Triton Consumer) p 747
Neutrogena T/Derm Tar Emollient (Neutrogena) p 623
Neutrogena T/Gel Therapeutic Shampoo (Neutrogena) p 417, 623
Neutrogena T/Sal Therapeutic Shampoo (Neutrogena) p 417, 624
Oxipor VHC Lotion for Psoriasis (Whitehall) p 768
P & S Plus Tar Gel (Baker Cummins Pharmaceuticals) p 512
Sebutone and Sebutone Cream Antiseborrheic Tar Shampoos (Westwood) p 433, 759
Tegrin Dandruff Shampoo (Block) p 518
Tegrin for Psoriasis Lotion, Skin Cream & Medicated Soap (Block) p 518
X-Seb T Shampoo (Baker Cummins Pharmaceuticals) p 513
X-Seb T Plus Conditioning Shampoo (Baker Cummins Pharmaceuticals) p 513

COCOA BUTTER

Nupercainal Suppositories (CIBA Consumer) p 408, 553
Preparation H Hemorrhoidal Suppositories (Whitehall) p 434, 768
Wyanoids Relief Factor Hemorrhoidal Suppositories (Wyeth-Ayerst) p 435, 777

COCONUT OIL

pHisoDerm Cleansing Bar (Sterling Health) p 430, 738

COD LIVER OIL

Desitin Ointment (Pfizer Consumer) p 420, 638

CODEINE PHOSPHATE

Naldecon CX Adult Liquid (Apothecon) p 505
Ryna-C Liquid (Wallace) p 432, 754
Ryna-CX Liquid (Wallace) p 432, 754

COLLOIDAL OATMEAL

Aveeno Bath Oilated (Rydelle) p 423, 680
Aveeno Bath Regular (Rydelle) p 423, 680
Aveeno Cleansing Bar for Acne (Rydelle) p 423, 680
Aveeno Cleansing Bar for Combination Skin (Rydelle) p 423, 680
Aveeno Cleansing Bar for Dry Skin (Rydelle) p 423, 681
Aveeno Moisturizing Cream (Rydelle) p 423, 681
Aveeno Moisturizing Lotion (Rydelle) p 423, 681
Aveeno Shower and Bath Oil (Rydelle) p 423, 681

COPPER

One-A-Day Maximum Formula Vitamins and Minerals (Miles Consumer) p 417, 620
One-A-Day Stressgard Formula Vitamins (Miles Consumer) p 417, 620

CYANOCOBALAMIN

Bugs Bunny Children's Chewable Vitamins (Sugar Free) (Miles Consumer) p 416, 617
Bugs Bunny With Extra C Children's Chewable Vitamins (Sugar Free) (Miles Consumer) p 416, 618
Bugs Bunny Plus Iron Children's Chewable Vitamins (Sugar Free) (Miles Consumer) p 416, 617
Flintstones Children's Chewable Vitamins (Miles Consumer) p 416, 617
Flintstones Children's Chewable Vitamins With Extra C (Miles Consumer) p 416, 618
Flintstones Children's Chewable Vitamins Plus Iron (Miles Consumer) p 416, 617
Geritol Liquid - High Potency Iron & Vitamin Tonic (SmithKline Beecham) p 712
One-A-Day Essential Vitamins (Miles Consumer) p 417, 620
One-A-Day Maximum Formula Vitamins and Minerals (Miles Consumer) p 417, 620
One-A-Day Plus Extra C Vitamins (Miles Consumer) p 417, 620

CYCLIZINE HYDROCHLORIDE

Marezine Tablets (Burroughs Wellcome) p 406, 539

D

DESOXYEPHEDRINE

Vicks Inhaler (Richardson-Vicks) p 659

DEXBROMPHENIRAMINE MALEATE

Drixoral Plus Extended-Release Tablets (Schering-Plough HealthCare) p 425, 698
Drixoral Sinus (Schering-Plough HealthCare) p 426, 698
Drixoral Sustained-Action Tablets (Schering-Plough HealthCare) p 425, 697

DEXTRAN 70

Moisture Drops (Bausch & Lomb Personal) p 404, 514

DEXTROMETHORPHAN HYDROBROMIDE

Alka-Seltzer Plus Cold & Cough Medicine (Miles Consumer) p 416, 616
Benylin DM Pediatric Cough Formula (Parke-Davis) p 419, 632
Benylin Expectorant (Parke-Davis) p 419, 633
Cerose-DM (Wyeth-Ayerst) p 435, 774
Cheracol-D Cough Formula (Roberts) p 421, 663
Cheracol Plus Head Cold/Cough Formula (Roberts) p 421, 663

Cough Formula Comtrex (Bristol-Myers Products) p 405, 524
Comtrex Multi-Symptom Cold Reliever Tablets/Caplets/Liqui-Gels/Liquid (Bristol-Myers Products) p 404, 522
Comtrex Multi-Symptom Day-Night Caplet-Tablet (Bristol-Myers Products) p 404, 525
Comtrex Multi-Symptom Non-Drowsy Caplets (Bristol-Myers Products) p 405, 526
Contac Cough and Chest Cold (SmithKline Beecham) p 427, 706
Contac Cough & Sore Throat Formula (SmithKline Beecham) p 427, 707
Contac Jr. Non-Drowsy Cold Liquid (SmithKline Beecham) p 427, 707
Contac Severe Cold and Flu Formula Caplets (SmithKline Beecham) p 427, 706
Contac Severe Cold & Flu Nighttime (SmithKline Beecham) p 427, 708
Dimacol Caplets (Robins Consumer) p 668
Dimetapp DM Elixir (Robins Consumer) p 421, 671
Dorcol Children's Cough Syrup (Sandoz Consumer) p 423, 682
Dristan Cold and Flu (Whitehall) p 434, 766
Hold Cough Suppressant Lozenge (Menley & James) p 415, 609
Medi-Flu Caplet, Liquid (Parke-Davis) p 419, 634
Medi-Flu Without Drowsiness Caplets (Parke-Davis) p 419, 635
Naldecon DX Adult Liquid (Apothecon) p 505
Naldecon DX Children's Syrup (Apothecon) p 506
Naldecon DX Pediatric Drops (Apothecon) p 506
Naldecon Senior DX Cough/Cold Liquid (Apothecon) p 507
Novahistine DMX (Marion Merrell Dow) p 412, 583
Orthoxicol Cough Syrup (Roberts) p 665
PediaCare Cough-Cold Formula Liquid and Chewable Tablets (McNeil Consumer Products) p 414, 588
PediaCare Night Rest Cough-Cold Formula Liquid (McNeil Consumer Products) p 414, 588
PediaCare 6-12 Cough-Cold Formula Chewable Tablets (McNeil Consumer Products) p 414, 588
Robitussin Cough Calmers (Robins Consumer) p 674
Robitussin Maximum Strength Cough Suppressant (Robins Consumer) p 422, 675
Robitussin Night Relief (Robins Consumer) p 422, 675
Robitussin Pediatric Cough & Cold Formula (Robins Consumer) p 422, 675
Robitussin Pediatric Cough Suppressant (Robins Consumer) p 422, 676
Robitussin-CF (Robins Consumer) p 422, 673
Robitussin-DM (Robins Consumer) p 422, 673
St. Joseph Cough Suppressant for Children (Schering-Plough HealthCare) p 702
Sudafed Cough Syrup (Burroughs Wellcome) p 407, 541
Sudafed Severe Cold Formula Caplets (Burroughs Wellcome) p 407, 542
Sudafed Severe Cold Formula Tablets (Burroughs Wellcome) p 407, 542
TheraFlu Flu, Cold and Cough Medicine (Sandoz Consumer) p 423, 684
Triaminic Nite Light (Sandoz Consumer) p 424, 686
Triaminic-DM Syrup (Sandoz Consumer) p 423, 687
Triaminicol Multi-Symptom Cold Tablets (Sandoz Consumer) p 424, 688
Triaminicol Multi-Symptom Relief (Sandoz Consumer) p 424, 688

Tylenol Cold & Flu Hot Medication, Packets (McNeil Consumer Products) p 413, 595
Tylenol Cold & Flu No Drowsiness Hot Medication, Packets (McNeil Consumer Products) p 413, 598
Tylenol Cold Multi Symptom Medication Caplets and Tablets (McNeil Consumer Products) p 413, 596
Tylenol Cold Medication No Drowsiness Formula Caplets (McNeil Consumer Products) p 413, 597
Tylenol Cold Night Time Medication Liquid (McNeil Consumer Products) p 413, 599
Tylenol Cough Medication Maximum Strength Liquid (McNeil Consumer Products) p 414, 601
Tylenol Cough Medication Maximum Strength Liquid with Decongestant (McNeil Consumer Products) p 414, 601
Vicks Children's Cough Syrup (Richardson-Vicks) p 654
Vicks Children's NyQuil Nighttime Cold/Cough Medicine (Richardson-Vicks) p 659
Vicks Daycare Daytime Cold Medicine Caplets (Richardson-Vicks) p 655
Vicks Daycare Daytime Cold Medicine Liquid (Richardson-Vicks) p 655
Vicks Formula 44 Cough Control Discs (Richardson-Vicks) p 656
Vicks Formula 44 Cough Medicine (Richardson-Vicks) p 656
Vicks Formula 44D Cough and Decongestant Medicine (Richardson-Vicks) p 656
Vicks Formula 44E Cough & Expectorant Medicine (Richardson-Vicks) p 657
Vicks Formula 44M Multi-Symptom Cough & Cold Medicine (Richardson-Vicks) p 657
Vicks NyQuil LiquiCaps Adult Nighttime Cold/Flu Medicine (Richardson-Vicks) p 661
Vicks NyQuil Nighttime Cold/Flu Medicine-Regular & Cherry Flavor (Richardson-Vicks) p 660
Vicks Pediatric Formula 44 Cough Medicine (Richardson-Vicks) p 657
Vicks Pediatric Formula 44d Cough & Decongestant Medicine (Richardson-Vicks) p 658
Vicks Pediatric Formula 44e Cough & Expectorant Medicine (Richardson-Vicks) p 659
Vicks Pediatric Formula 44m Multi-Symptom Cough & Cold Medicine (Richardson-Vicks) p 658

DEXTROMETHORPHAN POLISTIREX
Delsym Cough Formula (Fisons Corporation) p 562

DEXTROSE
Emetrol (Adria) p 403, 503
Glutose (Paddock) p 628

DIBUCAINE
Nupercainal Hemorrhoidal and Anesthetic Ointment (CIBA Consumer) p 408, 552
Nupercainal Pain Relief Cream (CIBA Consumer) p 408, 553

DIHYDROXYALUMINUM SODIUM CARBONATE
Rolaids (Warner-Lambert) p 433, 757

DIMENHYDRINATE
Dramamine Chewable Tablets (Upjohn) p 431, 748
Dramamine Liquid (Upjohn) p 431, 748
Dramamine Tablets (Upjohn) p 431, 748

DIMETHICONE
Moisturel Cream (Westwood) p 433, 758

Moisturel Lotion (Westwood) p 433, 758

DIOCTYL SODIUM SULFOSUCCINATE (see under DOCUSATE SODIUM)

DIPERODON HYDROCHLORIDE
Bactine First Aid Antibiotic Plus Anesthetic Ointment (Miles Consumer) p 416, 617
Campho-Phenique Triple Antibiotic Ointment Plus Pain Reliever (Sterling Health) p 429, 731

DIPHENHYDRAMINE CITRATE
Alka-Seltzer Plus Night-Time Cold Medicine (Miles Consumer) p 416, 615
Bufferin A/F Nite Time Analgesic/Sleeping Aid Caplets (Bristol-Myers Products) p 404, 521
Excedrin P.M. Analgesic/Sleeping Aid Tablets, Caplets and Liquid (Bristol-Myers Products) p 405, 530

DIPHENHYDRAMINE HYDROCHLORIDE
Benadryl Anti-Itch Cream, Regular Strength 1% and Maximum Strength 2% (Parke-Davis) p 418, 629
Benadryl Cold Tablets (Parke-Davis) p 418, 631
Benadryl Cold Nighttime Formula (Parke-Davis) p 419, 631
Benadryl Decongestant Elixir (Parke-Davis) p 419, 630
Benadryl Decongestant Kapseals (Parke-Davis) p 418, 630
Benadryl Decongestant Tablets (Parke-Davis) p 418, 630
Benadryl Elixir (Parke-Davis) p 419, 630
Benadryl Spray, Maximum Strength 2% (Parke-Davis) p 418, 632
Benadryl Spray, Regular Strength 1% (Parke-Davis) p 418, 632
Benadryl 25 Kapseals (Parke-Davis) p 418, 631
Benadryl 25 Tablets (Parke-Davis) p 418, 631
Benylin Cough Syrup (Parke-Davis) p 419, 632
Benylin Decongestant (Parke-Davis) p 419, 633
Caladryl Clear Lotion (Parke-Davis) p 419, 633
Caladryl Cream, Lotion, Spray (Parke-Davis) p 419, 633
Cold Control+ Intense Cold Medicine (Reese Chemical) p 647
Extra Strength Doan's P.M. (CIBA Consumer) p 407, 549
Miles Nervine Nighttime Sleep-Aid (Miles Consumer) p 417, 619
Nytol Tablets (Block) p 517
Sleep-ettes-D Tablets (Reese Chemical) p 647
Sleep-eze 3 Tablets (Whitehall) p 772
Sleepinal Medicated Night Tea (Thompson Medical) p 746
Sleepinal Night-time Sleep Aid Capsules (Thompson Medical) p 431, 746
Sominex Caplets and Tablets (SmithKline Beecham) p 428, 718
Sominex Pain Relief Formula (SmithKline Beecham) p 428, 718
Tylenol Cold Night Time Medication Liquid (McNeil Consumer Products) p 413, 599
Tylenol PM Extra Strength Pain Reliever/Sleep Aid Caplets and Tablets (McNeil Consumer Products) p 414, 593
Unisom with Pain Relief Nighttime Sleep Aid/Analgesic (Pfizer Consumer) p 640
Vicks NyQuil LiquiCaps Adult Nighttime Cold/Flu Medicine (Richardson-Vicks) p 661

DISOCOREA
Hyland's Colic Tablets (Standard Homeopathic) p 722

DISODIUM PHOSPHATE
Afrin Saline Mist (Schering-Plough HealthCare) p 424, 692

DOCUSATE CALCIUM
Doxidan Liqui-Gels (Upjohn) p 431, 748
Surfak Liqui-Gels (Upjohn) p 432, 751

DOCUSATE POTASSIUM
Kasof Capsules (Roberts) p 664

DOCUSATE SODIUM
Anticon (Neutrin) p 417, 622
Colace (Mead Johnson Pharmaceuticals) p 415, 606
Correctol Laxative Tablets (Schering-Plough HealthCare) p 425, 696
Dialose Tablets (J&J•Merck Consumer) p 409, 565
Dialose Plus Tablets (J&J•Merck Consumer) p 409, 566
Extra Gentle Ex-Lax Laxative Pills (Sandoz Consumer) p 423, 683
Feen-A-Mint Laxative Pills (Schering-Plough HealthCare) p 426, 699
Ferro-Sequels (Lederle) p 411, 575
Geriplex-FS Kapseals (Parke-Davis) p 634
Geriplex-FS Liquid (Parke-Davis) p 634
Peri-Colace (Mead Johnson Pharmaceuticals) p 415, 606
Phillips' LaxCaps (Sterling Health) p 430, 736

DOXYLAMINE SUCCINATE
Unisom Nighttime Sleep Aid (Pfizer Consumer) p 640
Vicks NyQuil Nighttime Cold/Flu Medicine-Regular & Cherry Flavor (Richardson-Vicks) p 660

DYCLONINE HYDROCHLORIDE
Sucrets Children's Cherry Flavored Sore Throat Lozenges (SmithKline Beecham) p 428, 719
Sucrets Maximum Strength Wintergreen and Sucrets Wild Cherry (Regular Strength) Sore Throat Lozenges (SmithKline Beecham) p 428, 719
Sucrets Maximum Strength Sprays (SmithKline Beecham) p 428, 720

E

ELECTROLYTE SUPPLEMENT
Pedialyte Oral Electrolyte Maintenance Solution (Ross) p 678
Rehydralyte Oral Electrolyte Rehydration Solution (Ross) p 679

EPHEDRINE HYDROCHLORIDE
Amesec (Whitby) p 759
Primatene Tablets-M Formula (Whitehall) p 435, 770
Primatene Tablets-P Formula (Whitehall) p 435, 770
Primatene Tablets-Regular Formula (Whitehall) p 435, 770

EPHEDRINE SULFATE
Bronkaid Tablets (Sterling Health) p 429, 730
Bronkolixir (Sanofi Winthrop Pharmaceuticals) p 689
Bronkotabs Tablets (Sanofi Winthrop Pharmaceuticals) p 689
Pazo Hemorrhoid Ointment & Suppositories (Bristol-Myers Products) p 406, 534
Vicks Vatronol Nose Drops (Richardson-Vicks) p 662

EPINEPHRINE
Bronkaid Mist (Sterling Health) p 429, 729
Primatene Mist (Whitehall) p 435, 769

EPINEPHRINE BITARTRATE

AsthmaHaler Mist Epinephrine Bitartrate Bronchodilator (Menley & James) p 608

Bronkaid Mist Suspension (Sterling Health) p 730

Primatene Mist Suspension (Whitehall) p 770

EQUISETUM HYEMALE

Hyland's Bed Wetting Tablets (Standard Homeopathic) p 722

ETHYL ALCOHOL

Anbesol Gel Antiseptic-Anesthetic-Regular Strength (Whitehall) p 434, 763

Anbesol Gel Antiseptic-Anesthetic - Maximum Strength (Whitehall) p 434, 763

Anbesol Liquid Antiseptic-Anesthetic (Whitehall) p 434, 763

Anbesol Liquid Antiseptic-Anesthetic - Maximum Strength (Whitehall) p 434, 763

P & S Plus Tar Gel (Baker Cummins Pharmaceuticals) p 512

X-Seb T Shampoo (Baker Cummins Pharmaceuticals) p 513

X-Seb T Plus Conditioning Shampoo (Baker Cummins Pharmaceuticals) p 513

ETHYL AMINOBENZOATE (see under BENZOCAINE)

ETHYLHEXYL P-METHOXYCINNAMATE

Eucerin Dry Skin Care Daily Facial Lotion SPF 20 (Beiersdorf) p 404, 515

Oil of Olay Daily UV Protectant SPF 15 Beauty Fluid-Regular & Fragrance Free (Olay Co. Inc.) (Richardson-Vicks) p 653

Oil of Olay Daily UV Protectant SPF 15 Moisture Replenishing Cream-Regular & Fragrance Free (Olay Co. Inc.) (Richardson-Vicks) p 653

Vaseline Intensive Care Moisturizing Sunblock Lotion (Chese-Pond's) p 548

Vaseline Intensive Care U.V. Daily Defense Lotion for Hand and Body (Chese-Pond's) p 548

2-ETHYLHEXYL SALICYLATE

Eucerin Dry Skin Care Daily Facial Lotion SPF 20 (Beiersdorf) p 404, 515

Vaseline Intensive Care Moisturizing Sunblock Lotion (Chese-Pond's) p 548

EUCALYPTUS, OIL OF

Halls Mentho-Lyptus Cough Suppressant Tablets (Warner-Lambert) p 432, 755

Halls Plus Cough Suppressant Tablets (Warner-Lambert) p 432, 756

Listerine Antiseptic (Warner-Lambert) p 433, 756

Vicks Vaporub (Richardson-Vicks) p 662

Vicks Vaposteam (Richardson-Vicks) p 662

EUCERITE

Eucerin Dry Skin Care Cleansing Bar (Beiersdorf) p 404, 515

F

FAT, HARD

Anusol Hemorrhoidal Suppositories (Parke-Davis) p 418, 629

Tronolane Hemorrhoidal Suppositories (Ross) p 422, 680

FERRIC PYROPHOSPHATE

Troph-Iron Liquid (Menley & James) p 611

FERROUS FUMARATE

Bugs Bunny Plus Iron Children's Chewable Vitamins (Sugar Free) (Miles Consumer) p 416, 617

Caltrate 600 + Iron & Vitamin D (Lederle) p 410, 572

Centrum, Jr. (Children's Chewable) + Iron (Lederle) p 410, 573

FemIron Multi Vitamins and Iron (Menley & James) p 415, 609

Ferancee Chewable Tablets (J&J•Merck Consumer) p 566

Ferancee-HP Tablets (J&J•Merck Consumer) p 409, 566

Ferro-Sequels (Lederle) p 411, 575

Flintstones Children's Chewable Vitamins Plus Iron (Miles Consumer) p 416, 617

One-A-Day Maximum Formula Vitamins and Minerals (Miles Consumer) p 417, 620

One-A-Day Stressgard Formula Vitamins (Miles Consumer) p 417, 620

One-A-Day Women's Formula Multivitamins with Calcium, Extra Iron, Zinc and Beta Carotene (Miles Consumer) p 417, 620

Poly-Vi-Sol Vitamins with Iron, Chewable Tablets and Circus Shapes Chewable (Mead Johnson Nutritionals) p 414, 604

Stresstabs + Iron, Advanced Formula (Lederle) p 411, 577

Stuartinic Tablets (J&J•Merck Consumer) p 410, 570

Theragran-M Tablets (Apothecon) p 403, 508

Vitron-C Tablets (Fisons Consumer Health) p 562

FERROUS GLUCONATE

Fergon Elixir (Sterling Health) p 732

Fergon Iron Supplement Tablets (Sterling Health) p 429, 732

FERROUS SULFATE

Dayalets Plus Iron Filmtab (Abbott) p 502

Feosol Capsules (SmithKline Beecham) p 427, 710

Feosol Elixir (SmithKline Beecham) p 427, 711

Feosol Tablets (SmithKline Beecham) p 427, 711

Poly-Vi-Sol Vitamins with Iron, Drops (Mead Johnson Nutritionals) p 414, 604

Slow Fe Tablets (CIBA Consumer) p 408, 554

Tri-Vi-Sol Vitamin Drops with Iron (Mead Johnson Nutritionals) p 415, 606

FOLIC ACID

Allbee C-800 Plus Iron Tablets (Robins Consumer) p 666

Bugs Bunny Children's Chewable Vitamins (Sugar Free) (Miles Consumer) p 416, 617

Bugs Bunny With Extra C Children's Chewable Vitamins (Sugar Free) (Miles Consumer) p 416, 618

Bugs Bunny Plus Iron Children's Chewable Vitamins (Sugar Free) (Miles Consumer) p 416, 617

Flintstones Children's Chewable Vitamins (Miles Consumer) p 416, 617

Flintstones Children's Chewable Vitamins With Extra C (Miles Consumer) p 416, 618

Flintstones Children's Chewable Vitamins Plus Iron (Miles Consumer) p 416, 617

One-A-Day Essential Vitamins (Miles Consumer) p 417, 620

One-A-Day Maximum Formula Vitamins and Minerals (Miles Consumer) p 417, 620

One-A-Day Plus Extra C Vitamins (Miles Consumer) p 417, 620

One-A-Day Stressgard Formula Vitamins (Miles Consumer) p 417, 620

One-A-Day Women's Formula Multivitamins with Calcium, Extra Iron, Zinc and Beta Carotene (Miles Consumer) p 417, 620

Sigtab Tablets (Roberts) p 421, 666

Stuart Prenatal Tablets (Stuart) p 431, 742

The Stuart Formula Tablets (J&J•Merck Consumer) p 410, 569

Theragran Stress Formula (Apothecon) p 403, 509

Zymacap Capsules (Roberts) p 666

G

GARLIC EXTRACT

Kyolic (Wakunaga) p 432, 752

GLUCOSE, LIQUID

Glutose (Paddock) p 628

Insta-Glucose (ICN Pharmaceuticals) p 409, 564

GLYCERIN

Aqua Care Cream (Menley & James) p 415, 607

Campho-Phenique Cold Sore Gel (Sterling Health) p 429, 731

Clear Eyes ACR Astringent/Lubricating Eye Redness Reliever (Ross) p 422, 677

Clear Eyes Lubricating Eye Redness Reliever (Ross) p 422, 677

Collyrium Fresh (Wyeth-Ayerst) p 435, 775

Dry Eye Therapy Lubricating Eye Drops (Bausch & Lomb Personal) p 403, 513

Moisture Drops (Bausch & Lomb Personal) p 404, 514

Neutrogena Cleansing Wash (Neutrogena) p 417, 622

Neutrogena Norwegian Formula Emulsion (Neutrogena) p 417, 623

Neutrogena Norwegian Formula Hand Cream (Neutrogena) p 417, 623

pHisoDerm Cleansing Bar (Sterling Health) p 430, 738

Pen•Kera Creme (Ascher) p 403, 510

Replens (Warner-Lambert) p 433, 757

Rhulicream (Rydelle) p 423, 681

S.T.37 Antiseptic Solution (Menley & James) p 611

Extra Strength Vaseline Intensive Care Lotion (Chese-Pond's) p 548

Water-Jel Sterile Burn Dressings (Water-Jel Technologies) p 758

GLYCERYL GUAIACOLATE (see under GUAIFENESIN)

GLYCOLIC ACID

Aqua Glycolic Lotion (Herald Pharmacal) p 564

Aqua Glycolic Shampoo (Herald Pharmacal) p 564

Aqua Glyde Cleanser (Herald Pharmacal) p 564

GLYCYRRHIZA EXTRACT

Throat Discs Throat Lozenges (Marion Merrell Dow) p 412, 586

GUAIFENESIN

Benylin Expectorant (Parke-Davis) p 419, 633

Bronkaid Tablets (Sterling Health) p 429, 730

Bronkolixir (Sanofi Winthrop Pharmaceuticals) p 689

Bronkotabs Tablets (Sanofi Winthrop Pharmaceuticals) p 689

Cheracol-D Cough Formula (Roberts) p 421, 663

Cough Formula Comtrex (Bristol-Myers Products) p 405, 524

Congestac Caplets (Menley & James) p 415, 609

Contac Cough and Chest Cold (SmithKline Beecham) p 427, 706

Dimacol Caplets (Robins Consumer)
p 668
Dorcol Children's Cough Syrup (Sandoz
Consumer) p 423, 682
Guaifed Syrup (Muro) p 621
Guaitab Tablets (Muro) p 621
Naldecon CX Adult Liquid (Apothecon)
p 505
Naldecon DX Adult Liquid (Apothecon)
p 505
Naldecon DX Children's Syrup
(Apothecon) p 506
Naldecon DX Pediatric Drops
(Apothecon) p 506
Naldecon EX Children's Syrup
(Apothecon) p 507
Naldecon EX Pediatric Drops
(Apothecon) p 507
Naldecon Senior DX Cough/Cold Liquid
(Apothecon) p 507
Naldecon Senior EX Cough/Cold Liquid
(Apothecon) p 508
Novahistine DMX (Marion Merrell Dow)
p 412, 583
Robitussin (Robins Consumer) p 422,
672
Robitussin-CF (Robins Consumer)
p 422, 673
Robitussin-DM (Robins Consumer)
p 422, 673
Robitussin-PE (Robins Consumer)
p 422, 674
Ryna-CX Liquid (Wallace) p 432, 754
Sudafed Cough Syrup (Burroughs
Wellcome) p 407, 541
Triaminic Expectorant (Sandoz
Consumer) p 424, 686
Vicks Children's Cough Syrup
(Richardson-Vicks) p 654
Vicks Daycare Daytime Cold Medicine
Caplets (Richardson-Vicks) p 655
Vicks Daycare Daytime Cold Medicine
Liquid (Richardson-Vicks) p 655
Vicks Formula 44E Cough &
Expectorant Medicine
(Richardson-Vicks) p 657
Vicks Pediatric Formula 44e Cough &
Expectorant Medicine
(Richardson-Vicks) p 659

H

HCG MONOCLONAL ANTIBODY

Advance Pregnancy Test (Ortho
Pharmaceutical) p 418, 781
e.p.t. Early Pregnancy Test
(Parke-Davis) p 419, 781

HEXYLRESORCINOL

S.T.37 Antiseptic Solution (Menley &
James) p 611
Sucrets Original Mint (SmithKline
Beecham) p 428, 719
Sucrets Cold Formula (SmithKline
Beecham) p 428, 719

HOMEOPATHIC MEDICATIONS

Oscillococcinum (Boiron) p 404, 519
Yellolax (Luyties) p 578

HUMAN CHORIONIC GONADOTROPIN
(HCG)

Advance Pregnancy Test (Ortho
Pharmaceutical) p 418, 781
Fact Plus Pregnancy Test (Ortho
Pharmaceutical) p 418, 781

HYDROCORTISONE

Bactine Hydrocortisone Anti-Itch Cream
(Miles Consumer) p 416, 617
Caldecort Anti-Itch Hydrocortisone
Spray (Fisons Consumer Health)
p 409, 559
Cortaid Spray (Upjohn) p 431, 747
Maximum Strength Cortaid Spray
(Upjohn) p 431, 748
Cortizone-5 Creme and Ointment
(Thompson Medical) p 431, 743
Cortizone-5 Wipes (Thompson Medical)
p 743
Cortizone-10 Creme and Ointment
(Thompson Medical) p 744

Massengill Medicated Soft Cloth
Towelette (SmithKline Beecham)
p 713
Tegrin-HC with Hydrocortisone Anti-Itch
Ointment (Block) p 518

HYDROCORTISONE ACETATE

Caldecort Anti-Itch Hydrocortisone
Cream (Fisons Consumer Health)
p 409, 559
Caldecort Light Cream (Fisons
Consumer Health) p 409, 559
Cortaid Cream with Aloe (Upjohn)
p 431, 747
Cortaid Lotion (Upjohn) p 431, 747
Cortaid Ointment with Aloe (Upjohn)
p 431, 747
Maximum Strength Cortaid Cream
(Upjohn) p 431, 748
Maximum Strength Cortaid Ointment
(Upjohn) p 431, 748
Cortef Feminine Itch Cream (Upjohn)
p 748
Corticaine External Analgesic (Whitby)
p 433, 760

HYDROXYPROPYL METHYLCELLULOSE

Moisture Drops (Bausch & Lomb
Personal) p 404, 514

I

IBUPROFEN

Advil Cold and Sinus (formerly CoAdvil)
(Whitehall) p 434, 761
Advil Ibuprofen Caplets and Tablets
(Whitehall) p 434, 761
Cramp End Tablets (Ohm Laboratories)
p 418, 624
Dristan Sinus Pain Reliever/Nasal
Decongestant Caplets (Whitehall)
p 434, 766
Haltran Tablets (Roberts) p 421, 664
Ibuprohm Ibuprofen Caplets (Ohm
Laboratories) p 418, 625
Ibuprohm Ibuprofen Tablets (Ohm
Laboratories) p 418, 625
Medipren ibuprofen Caplets and
Tablets (McNeil Consumer Products)
p 414, 587
Midol IB Cramp Relief Formula (Sterling
Health) p 430, 733
Motrin IB Caplets and Tablets (Upjohn)
p 432, 750
Nuprin Ibuprofen/Analgesic Tablets &
Caplets (Bristol-Myers Products)
p 406, 534

ICHTHAMMOL

PRID Salve (Walker Pharmacal) p 753

IODINE

One-A-Day Maximum Formula Vitamins
and Minerals (Miles Consumer)
p 417, 620
Stuart Prenatal Tablets (Stuart) p 431,
742
The Stuart Formula Tablets
(J&J•Merck Consumer) p 410, 569

IPECAC

Hyland's Cough Syrup with Honey
(Standard Homeopathic) p 722
Ipecac Syrup, USP (Paddock) p 628

IRON POLYSACCHARIDE COMPLEX
(see under POLYSACCHARIDE-IRON
COMPLEX)

IRON PREPARATIONS

Allbee C-800 Plus Iron Tablets (Robins
Consumer) p 666
Bugs Bunny Complete Children's
Chewable Vitamins + Minerals with
Iron and Calcium (Sugar Free) (Miles
Consumer) p 416, 618
Bugs Bunny Plus Iron Children's
Chewable Vitamins (Sugar Free)
(Miles Consumer) p 416, 617

FemIron Multi Vitamins and Iron
(Menley & James) p 415, 609
Ferancee Chewable Tablets (J&J•Merck
Consumer) p 566
Ferancee-HP Tablets (J&J•Merck
Consumer) p 409, 566
Fergon Elixir (Sterling Health) p 732
Fergon Iron Supplement Tablets
(Sterling Health) p 429, 732
Ferro-Sequels (Lederle) p 411, 575
Flintstones Children's Chewable
Vitamins Plus Iron (Miles Consumer)
p 416, 617
Flintstones Complete With Calcium, Iron
& Minerals Children's Chewable
Vitamins (Miles Consumer) p 416,
618
Geritol Extend Caplets (SmithKline
Beecham) p 712
Geritol Liquid - High Potency Iron &
Vitamin Tonic (SmithKline Beecham)
p 712
Incremin w/Iron Syrup (Lederle) p 576
One-A-Day Maximum Formula Vitamins
and Minerals (Miles Consumer)
p 417, 620
Poly-Vi-Sol Vitamins with Iron,
Chewable Tablets and Circus Shapes
Chewable (Mead Johnson
Nutritionals) p 414, 604
Poly-Vi-Sol Vitamins with Iron, Drops
(Mead Johnson Nutritionals) p 414,
604
SMA Iron Fortified Infant Formula,
Concentrated, Ready-to-Feed and
Powder (Wyeth-Ayerst) p 435, 776
Slow Fe Tablets (CIBA Consumer)
p 408, 554
The Stuart Formula Tablets
(J&J•Merck Consumer) p 410, 569
Stuartinic Tablets (J&J•Merck
Consumer) p 410, 570
Surbex-750 with Iron (Abbott) p 403,
503
Unicap Plus Iron Vitamin Formula
Tablets (Upjohn) p 751

ISOPROPYL MYRISTATE

Eucerin Lotion (Beiersdorf) p 404, 516

L

LACTASE (BETA-D-GALACTOSIDASE)

Dairy Ease Caplets and Tablets
(Sterling Health) p 429, 731
Dairy Ease Drops (Sterling Health)
p 429, 732
Lactaid Caplets (Now marketed by
McNeil Consumer Products Co.)
(Lactaid) p 414, 571
Lactaid Drops (Now marketed by
McNeil Consumer Products Co.)
(Lactaid) p 414, 571
Lactogest Softgel Capsules (Thompson
Medical) p 431, 745
Surelac Chewable Lactase Enzyme
Tablets (Caraco) p 544

LACTIC ACID

Massengill Baby Powder Soft Cloth
Towelette and Fragrance Free Soft
Cloth Towelette (SmithKline
Beecham) p 713
Massengill Liquid Concentrate
(SmithKline Beecham) p 712

LACTOBACILLUS ACIDOPHILUS

DDS-Acidophilus (UAS Laboratories)
p 747

LANOLIN

A and D Ointment (Schering-Plough
HealthCare) p 424, 692
Borofax Ointment (Burroughs
Wellcome) p 538
Desitin Ointment (Pfizer Consumer)
p 420, 638
Eucerin Dry Skin Care Lotion
(Fragrance-free) (Beiersdorf) p 404,
516
Wellcome Lanoline (Burroughs
Wellcome) p 544

LANOLIN OIL

Alpha Keri Moisture Rich Body Oil
(Bristol-Myers Products) p 405, 519
Balmex Emollient Lotion (Macsil) p 579

LEVULOSE

Emetrol (Adria) p 403, 503

LIDOCAINE

Mycitracin Plus Pain Reliever (Upjohn)
p 432, 750
Xylocaine 2.5% Ointment (Astra)
p 403, 510

LIDOCAINE HYDROCHLORIDE

Bactine Antiseptic/Anesthetic First Aid
Liquid (Miles Consumer) p 416, 617

LIVE YEAST CELL DERIVATIVE

Preparation H Hemorrhoidal Cream
(Whitehall) p 434, 768
Preparation H Hemorrhoidal Ointment
(Whitehall) p 434, 768
Preparation H Hemorrhoidal
Suppositories (Whitehall) p 434, 768
Wyanoids Relief Factor Hemorrhoidal
Suppositories (Wyeth-Ayerst) p 435,
777

LOPERAMIDE HYDROCHLORIDE

Imodium A-D Caplets and Liquid
(McNeil Consumer Products) p 414,
587

M

MAGALDRATE

Riopan Antacid Suspension (Whitehall)
p 770
Riopan Antacid Swallow Tablets
(Whitehall) p 770
Riopan Plus Suspension (Whitehall)
p 771
Riopan Plus Chew Tablets (Whitehall)
p 771
Riopan Plus Chew Tablets in Rollpacks
(Whitehall) p 771
Riopan Plus 2 Suspension-Mint and
Cherry flavors (Whitehall) p 435,
771
Riopan Plus 2 Chew Tablets-Mint and
Cherry Vanilla flavors (Whitehall)
p 435, 771

MAGNESIUM

Beelith Tablets (Beach) p 514
Mag-Ox 400 (Blaine) p 516
MagTab SR Caplets (Niché
Pharmaceuticals) p 624
One-A-Day Maximum Formula Vitamins
and Minerals (Miles Consumer)
p 417, 620
Uro-Mag (Blaine) p 516

MAGNESIUM CARBONATE

Gaviscon Extra Strength Relief Formula
Liquid Antacid (Marion Merrell Dow)
p 412, 582
Gaviscon Extra Strength Relief Formula
Antacid Tablets (Marion Merrell Dow)
p 412, 582
Gaviscon Liquid Antacid (Marion
Merrell Dow) p 412, 583
Maalox HRF Heartburn Relief Formula
(Rhone-Poulenc Rorer Consumer)
p 420, 649
Marblen Suspension Peach/Apricot
(Fleming) p 563
Marblen Suspension Unflavored
(Fleming) p 563
Marblen Tablets (Fleming) p 563

MAGNESIUM CHLORIDE

Chlor-3 Condiment (Fleming) p 563

MAGNESIUM GLUCONATE

Magonate Tablets and Liquid (Fleming)
p 563

MAGNESIUM HYDROXIDE

Aludrox Oral Suspension
(Wyeth-Ayerst) p 435, 773
Ascriptin A/D Caplets (Rhone-Poulenc
Rorer Consumer) p 420, 649
Regular Strength Ascriptin Tablets
(Rhone-Poulenc Rorer Consumer)
p 420, 648
Di-Gel Antacid/Anti-Gas
(Schering-Plough HealthCare) p 425,
696
Gelusil Liquid & Tablets (Parke-Davis)
p 419, 634
Haley's M-O, Regular & Flavored
(Sterling Health) p 429, 732
Maalox Plus Suspension/Tablets
(Rhone-Poulenc Rorer Consumer)
p 421, 649
Extra Strength Maalox Plus Suspension
(Rhone-Poulenc Rorer Consumer)
p 420, 650
Mylanta Liquid (J&J•Merck Consumer)
p 410, 567
Mylanta Tablets (J&J•Merck
Consumer) p 410, 567
Mylanta Double Strength Liquid
(J&J•Merck Consumer) p 410, 567
Mylanta Double Strength Tablets
(J&J•Merck Consumer) p 410, 567
Concentrated Phillips' Milk of Magnesia
(Sterling Health) p 430, 737
Phillips' Milk of Magnesia Liquid
(Sterling Health) p 430, 737
Phillips' Milk of Magnesia Tablets
(Sterling Health) p 430, 737
WinGel Liquid (Sterling Health) p 740

MAGNESIUM LACTATE

MagTab SR Caplets (Niché
Pharmaceuticals) p 624

MAGNESIUM OXIDE

Beelith Tablets (Beach) p 514
Bufferin Analgesic Tablets and Caplets
(Bristol-Myers Products) p 404, 519
Cama Arthritis Pain Reliever (Sandoz
Consumer) p 682
Mag-Ox 400 (Blaine) p 516
Uro-Mag (Blaine) p 516

MAGNESIUM SALICYLATE

Doan's - Extra-Strength Analgesic (CIBA
Consumer) p 407, 549
Extra Strength Doan's P.M. (CIBA
Consumer) p 407, 549
Doan's - Regular Strength Analgesic
(CIBA Consumer) p 407, 549
Mobigesic Analgesic Tablets (Ascher)
p 403, 509

MAGNESIUM SULFATE

Vicon Plus (Whitby) p 433, 760
Vicon-C Capsules (Whitby) p 433, 760

MAGNESIUM TRISILICATE

Gaviscon Antacid Tablets (Marion
Merrell Dow) p 412, 582
Gaviscon-2 Antacid Tablets (Marion
Merrell Dow) p 412, 583

MALT SOUP EXTRACT

Maltsupex Liquid, Powder & Tablets
(Wallace) p 432, 753

MECLIZINE HYDROCHLORIDE

Bonine Tablets (Pfizer Consumer)
p 638

MENTHOL

Aurum Analgesic Lotion (Au
Pharmaceuticals) p 510
Ben-Gay External Analgesic Products
(Pfizer Consumer) p 638
Ben-Gay Ultra Strength Pain Relieving
Rub (Pfizer Consumer) p 638
Cēpacol Dry Throat Lozenges, Cherry
Flavor (Marion Merrell Dow) p 411,
579
Cēpacol Dry Throat Lozenges,
Honey-Lemon Flavor (Marion Merrell
Dow) p 411, 579

Cēpacol Dry Throat Lozenges,
Menthol-Eucalyptus Flavor (Marion
Merrell Dow) p 411, 580
Chloraseptic Lozenges, Cherry, Cool
Mint and Menthol (Richardson-Vicks)
p 653
Denorex Medicated Shampoo and
Conditioner (Whitehall) p 434, 764
Denorex Medicated Shampoo, Extra
Strength (Whitehall) p 434, 764
Denorex Medicated Shampoo, Extra
Strength With Conditioners
(Whitehall) p 434, 764
Denorex Medicated Shampoo, Regular
& Mountain Fresh Herbal Scent
(Whitehall) p 434, 764
Dermoplast Anesthetic Pain Relief
Lotion (Whitehall) p 764
Dermoplast Anesthetic Pain Relief
Spray (Whitehall) p 764
Desenex Foot & Sneaker Deodorant
Spray Powder (Fisons Consumer
Health) p 409, 560
Eucalyptamint 100% All Natural
Ointment (CIBA Consumer) p 407,
551
Feminine Gold Analgesic Lotion (Au
Pharmaceuticals) p 511
Flex-all 454 Pain Relieving Gel
(Chattem) p 545
Halls Mentho-Lyptus Cough
Suppressant Tablets
(Warner-Lambert) p 432, 755
Halls Plus Cough Suppressant Tablets
(Warner-Lambert) p 432, 756
Icy Hot Balm (Chattem) p 546
Icy Hot Cream (Chattem) p 546
Icy Hot Stick (Chattem) p 546
Legatrin Rub (Columbia) p 408, 556
Listerine Antiseptic (Warner-Lambert)
p 433, 756
N'ICE Medicated Sugarless Sore Throat
and Cough Lozenges (SmithKline
Beecham) p 427, 714
Rhuligel (Rydelle) p 423, 681
Robitussin Cough Drops (Robins
Consumer) p 422, 674
Selsun Blue Dandruff Shampoo-Extra
Medicated (Ross) p 422, 679
Soothers Throat Drops
(Warner-Lambert) p 433, 758
Sucrets Cold Formula (SmithKline
Beecham) p 428, 719
Theragold Analgesic Lotion (Au
Pharmaceuticals) p 510
Therapeutic Gold Analgesic Lotion (Au
Pharmaceuticals) p 510
Therapeutic Mineral Ice, Pain Relieving
Gel (Bristol-Myers Products) p 406,
536
Therapeutic Mineral Ice Exercise
Formula, Pain Relieving Gel
(Bristol-Myers Products) p 406, 536
Vicks Cough Drops (Richardson-Vicks)
p 655
Extra Strength Vicks Cough Drops
(Richardson-Vicks) p 655
Vicks Formula 44 Cough Control Discs
(Richardson-Vicks) p 656
Vicks Vaporub (Richardson-Vicks)
p 662
Vicks Vaposteam (Richardson-Vicks)
p 662

MENTHYL ANTHRANILATE

Neutrogena Sunblock (Neutrogena)
p 417, 623

METHIONINE

Geritol Liquid - High Potency Iron &
Vitamin Tonic (SmithKline Beecham)
p 712

METHYL SALICYLATE

Aurum Analgesic Lotion (Au
Pharmaceuticals) p 510
Ben-Gay External Analgesic Products
(Pfizer Consumer) p 638
Ben-Gay Ultra Strength Pain Relieving
Rub (Pfizer Consumer) p 638
Icy Hot Balm (Chattem) p 546
Icy Hot Cream (Chattem) p 546
Icy Hot Stick (Chattem) p 546

Listerine Antiseptic (Warner-Lambert)
p 433, 756
Theragold Analgesic Lotion (Au
Pharmaceuticals) p 510
Therapeutic Gold Analgesic Lotion (Au
Pharmaceuticals) p 510

METHYLCELLULOSE

Citrucel Orange Flavor (Marion Merrell
Dow) p 411, 581
Citrucel Sugar Free Orange Flavor
(Marion Merrell Dow) p 411, 581

MICONAZOLE NITRATE

Micatin Antifungal Cream (Ortho
Pharmaceutical) p 418, 627
Micatin Antifungal Deodorant Spray
Powder (Ortho Pharmaceutical)
p 418, 627
Micatin Antifungal Powder (Ortho
Pharmaceutical) p 418, 627
Micatin Antifungal Spray Liquid (Ortho
Pharmaceutical) p 418, 627
Micatin Antifungal Spray Powder (Ortho
Pharmaceutical) p 418, 627
Micatin Jock Itch Cream (Ortho
Pharmaceutical) p 627
Micatin Jock Itch Spray Powder (Ortho
Pharmaceutical) p 627
Monistat 7 Vaginal Cream (Ortho
Pharmaceutical) p 418, 627
Monistat 7 Vaginal Suppositories
(Ortho Pharmaceutical) p 418, 627

MILK, LACTASE REDUCED

Dairy Ease Real Milk (Sterling Health)
p 429, 732

MILK OF MAGNESIA

Concentrated Phillips' Milk of Magnesia
(Sterling Health) p 430, 737
Phillips' Milk of Magnesia Liquid
(Sterling Health) p 430, 737
Phillips' Milk of Magnesia Tablets
(Sterling Health) p 430, 737

MINERAL OIL

Agoral, Marshmallow Flavor
(Parke-Davis) p 628
Agoral, Raspberry Flavor (Parke-Davis)
p 628
Anusol Ointment (Parke-Davis) p 418,
629
Aqua Care Cream (Menley & James)
p 415, 607
Aqua Care Lotion (Menley & James)
p 415, 607
Aquaphor Healing Ointment, Original
Formula (Beiersdorf) p 404, 514
Aquaphor Natural Healing Ointment
(Beiersdorf) p 404, 515
Duolube Eye Ointment (Bausch & Lomb
Personal) p 403, 514
Eucerin Lotion (Beiersdorf) p 404, 516
Eucerin Dry Skin Care Lotion
(Fragrance-free) (Beiersdorf) p 404,
516
Haley's M-O, Regular & Flavored
(Sterling Health) p 429, 732
Keri Lotion - Original Formula
(Bristol-Myers Products) p 405, 533
Lacri-Lube NP Lubricant Ophthalmic
Ointment (Allergan Pharmaceuticals)
p 504
Lacri-Lube S.O.P. Sterile Ophthalmic
Ointment (Allergan Pharmaceuticals)
p 504
Nature's Remedy Enema, Mineral Oil
(SmithKline Beecham) p 427, 714
Nephrox Suspension (Fleming) p 563
pHisoDerm For Baby (Sterling Health)
p 430, 738
pHisoDerm Skin Cleanser and
Conditioner - Regular and Oily
(Sterling Health) p 430, 738
Refresh P.M. Lubricant Ophthalmic
Ointment (Allergan Pharmaceuticals)
p 505
Replens (Warner-Lambert) p 433, 757
Ultra Mide 25 (Baker Cummins
Pharmaceuticals) p 512

MINERAL WAX

Aquaphor Healing Ointment, Original
Formula (Beiersdorf) p 404, 514
Aquaphor Natural Healing Ointment
(Beiersdorf) p 404, 515

MULTIVITAMINS

Dayalets Filmtab (Abbott) p 502
Poly-Vi-Sol Vitamins, Circus Shapes
Chewable (without Iron) (Mead
Johnson Nutritionals) p 414, 603
Tri-Vi-Sol Vitamin Drops (Mead Johnson
Nutritionals) p 415, 606

MULTIVITAMINS WITH MINERALS

Centrum, Jr. (Children's Chewable) +
Extra C (Lederle) p 410, 573
Centrum Liquid (Lederle) p 411, 572
Centrum Silver (Lederle) p 411, 575
Dayalets Plus Iron Filmtab (Abbott)
p 502
Optilets-500 Filmtab (Abbott) p 403,
502
Optilets-M-500 Filmtab (Abbott) p 403,
502
Poly-Vi-Sol Vitamins, Chewable Tablets
and Drops (without Iron) (Mead
Johnson Nutritionals) p 414, 603
Poly-Vi-Sol Vitamins with Iron,
Chewable Tablets and Circus Shapes
Chewable (Mead Johnson
Nutritionals) p 414, 604
Poly-Vi-Sol Vitamins with Iron, Drops
(Mead Johnson Nutritionals) p 414,
604
Sunkist Children's Chewable
Multivitamins - Complete (CIBA
Consumer) p 408, 555
Sunkist Children's Chewable
Multivitamins - Plus Extra C (CIBA
Consumer) p 408, 555
Sunkist Children's Chewable
Multivitamins - Plus Iron (CIBA
Consumer) p 408, 555
Sunkist Children's Chewable
Multivitamins - Regular (CIBA
Consumer) p 408, 554
Surbex-750 with Iron (Abbott) p 403,
503
Surbex-750 with Zinc (Abbott) p 403,
503
Theragran-M Tablets (Apothecon)
p 403, 508

N

NAPHAZOLINE HYDROCHLORIDE

Allergy Drops (Bausch & Lomb
Personal) p 403, 513
Clear Eyes ACR Astringent/Lubricating
Eye Redness Reliever (Ross) p 422,
677
Clear Eyes Lubricating Eye Redness
Reliever (Ross) p 422, 677
4-Way Fast Acting Nasal Spray (regular
& mentholated) & Metered Spray
Pump (regular) (Bristol-Myers
Products) p 405, 532
Privine Nasal Solution and Drops (CIBA
Consumer) p 408, 554
Privine Nasal Spray (CIBA Consumer)
p 408, 554

NEOMYCIN SULFATE

Bactine First Aid Antibiotic Plus
Anesthetic Ointment (Miles
Consumer) p 416, 617
Campho-Phenique Triple Antibiotic
Ointment Plus Pain Reliever (Sterling
Health) p 429, 731
Mycitracin Plus Pain Reliever (Upjohn)
p 432, 750
Maximum Strength Mycitracin Triple
Antibiotic First Aid Ointment (Upjohn)
p 432, 750
Neosporin Cream (Burroughs
Wellcome) p 406, 539
Neosporin Ointment (Burroughs
Wellcome) p 406, 539
Neosporin Maximum Strength Ointment
(Burroughs Wellcome) p 406, 539

NIACIN

Allbee with C Caplets (Robins
Consumer) p 667
Allbee C-800 Plus Iron Tablets (Robins
Consumer) p 666
Allbee C-800 Tablets (Robins
Consumer) p 666
Bugs Bunny Children's Chewable
Vitamins (Sugar Free) (Miles
Consumer) p 416, 617
Bugs Bunny With Extra C Children's
Chewable Vitamins (Sugar Free)
(Miles Consumer) p 416, 618
Bugs Bunny Plus Iron Children's
Chewable Vitamins (Sugar Free)
(Miles Consumer) p 416, 617
Flintstones Children's Chewable
Vitamins (Miles Consumer) p 416,
617
Flintstones Children's Chewable
Vitamins With Extra C (Miles
Consumer) p 416, 618
Flintstones Children's Chewable
Vitamins Plus Iron (Miles Consumer)
p 416, 617
One-A-Day Essential Vitamins (Miles
Consumer) p 417, 620
One-A-Day Maximum Formula Vitamins
and Minerals (Miles Consumer)
p 417, 620
One-A-Day Plus Extra C Vitamins (Miles
Consumer) p 417, 620
One-A-Day Stressgard Formula
Vitamins (Miles Consumer) p 417,
620
One-A-Day Women's Formula
Multivitamins with Calcium, Extra
Iron, Zinc and Beta Carotene (Miles
Consumer) p 417, 620
Sigtab Tablets (Roberts) p 421, 666
Stuart Prenatal Tablets (Stuart) p 431,
742
The Stuart Formula Tablets
(J&J•Merck Consumer) p 410, 569
Stuartinic Tablets (J&J•Merck
Consumer) p 410, 570
Sublingual C with Niacin (Sublingual
Products) p 743
Theragran Liquid (Apothecon) p 403,
508
Z-BEC Tablets (Robins Consumer)
p 676
Zymacap Capsules (Roberts) p 666

NIACINAMIDE

Geritol Liquid - High Potency Iron &
Vitamin Tonic (SmithKline Beecham)
p 712
Vicon Plus (Whitby) p 433, 760
Vicon-C Capsules (Whitby) p 433, 760

NICOTINIC ACID
(see also under NIACIN)

Nicotinex Elixir (Fleming) p 563

NONOXYNOL-9

Conceptrol Contraceptive Gel • Single
Use Contraceptive (Ortho
Pharmaceutical) p 418, 625
Conceptrol Contraceptive Inserts (Ortho
Pharmaceutical) p 418, 625
Delfen Contraceptive Foam (Ortho
Pharmaceutical) p 418, 625
Encare Vaginal Contraceptive
Suppositories (Thompson Medical)
p 745
Gynol II Extra Strength Contraceptive
Jelly (Ortho Pharmaceutical) p 418,
626
Gynol II Original Formula Contraceptive
Jelly (Ortho Pharmaceutical) p 418,
626
Semicid Vaginal Contraceptive Inserts
(Whitehall) p 772
Today Vaginal Contraceptive Sponge
(Whitehall) p 435, 772

O

OCTOXYNOL-3

pHisoDerm For Baby (Sterling Health)
p 430, 738

pHisoDerm Skin Cleanser and Conditioner - Regular and Oily (Sterling Health) p 430, 738

OCTOXYNOL-9

Massengill Liquid Concentrate (SmithKline Beecham) p 712
Ortho-Gynol Contraceptive Jelly (Ortho Pharmaceutical) p 418, 626
Water-Jel Sterile Burn Dressings (Water-Jel Technologies) p 758

OCTYL DIMETHYL PABA

Herpecin-L Cold Sore Lip Balm (Campbell) p 544
PreSun 8 and 15 Moisturizing Sunscreens with KERI Moisturizers (Bristol-Myers Products) p 535
PreSun 46 Moisturizing Sunscreen (Bristol-Myers Products) p 536

OCTYL METHOXYCINNAMATE

Aquaderm Combination Treatment/Moisturizer (SPF 15 Formula) (Baker Cummins Pharmaceuticals) p 511
Neutrogena Moisture (Neutrogena) p 417, 622
Neutrogena Moisture SPF 15 Untinted (Neutrogena) p 417, 623
Neutrogena Moisture SPF 15 with Sheer Tint (Neutrogena) p 417, 623
Neutrogena Sunblock (Neutrogena) p 417, 623
PreSun Active 15 and 30 Clear Gel Sunscreens (Bristol-Myers Products) p 535
PreSun for Kids Lotion (Bristol-Myers Products) p 406, 535
PreSun 23 and For Kids, Spray Mist Sunscreens (Bristol-Myers Products) p 406, 535
PreSun 25 Moisturizing Sunscreen with KERI Moisturizer (Bristol-Myers Products) p 535
PreSun 15 and 29 Sensitive Skin Sunscreens (Bristol-Myers Products) p 406, 536

OCTYL SALICYLATE

Neutrogena Sunblock (Neutrogena) p 417, 623
PreSun Active 15 and 30 Clear Gel Sunscreens (Bristol-Myers Products) p 535
PreSun for Kids Lotion (Bristol-Myers Products) p 406, 535
PreSun 23 and For Kids, Spray Mist Sunscreens (Bristol-Myers Products) p 406, 535
PreSun 25 Moisturizing Sunscreen with KERI Moisturizer (Bristol-Myers Products) p 535
PreSun 15 and 29 Sensitive Skin Sunscreens (Bristol-Myers Products) p 406, 536

OIL OF MELALEUCA ALTERNIFOLIA

Water-Jel Sterile Burn Dressings (Water-Jel Technologies) p 758

OXYBENZONE

Aquaderm Combination Treatment/Moisturizer (SPF 15 Formula) (Baker Cummins Pharmaceuticals) p 511
Chap Stick Petroleum Jelly Plus with Sunblock 15 (Robins Consumer) p 421, 668
Chap Stick Sunblock 15 Lip Balm (Robins Consumer) p 421, 667
PreSun Active 15 and 30 Clear Gel Sunscreens (Bristol-Myers Products) p 535
PreSun for Kids Lotion (Bristol-Myers Products) p 406, 535
PreSun 23 and For Kids, Spray Mist Sunscreens (Bristol-Myers Products) p 406, 535
PreSun 8 and 15 Moisturizing Sunscreens with KERI Moisturizers (Bristol-Myers Products) p 535

PreSun 25 Moisturizing Sunscreen with KERI Moisturizer (Bristol-Myers Products) p 535
PreSun 15 and 29 Sensitive Skin Sunscreens (Bristol-Myers Products) p 406, 536
PreSun 46 Moisturizing Sunscreen (Bristol-Myers Products) p 536
Vaseline Intensive Care Moisturizing Sunblock Lotion (Chese-Pond's) p 548
Vaseline Intensive Care U.V. Daily Defense Lotion for Hand and Body (Chese-Pond's) p 548

OXYMETAZOLINE HYDROCHLORIDE

Afrin Cherry Scented Nasal Spray 0.05% (Schering-Plough HealthCare) p 428, 692
Afrin Children's Strength Nose Drops 0.025% (Schering-Plough HealthCare) p 424, 692
Afrin Menthol Nasal Spray (Schering-Plough HealthCare) p 424, 692
Afrin Nasal Spray 0.05% and Nasal Spray Pump (Schering-Plough HealthCare) p 424, 692
Afrin Nose Drops 0.05% (Schering-Plough HealthCare) p 424, 692
Cheracol Nasal Spray Pump (Roberts) p 663
Dristan 12-hour Nasal Spray, Regular and Menthol (Whitehall) p 767
Dristan 12-hour Nasal Spray, Metered Dose Pump (Whitehall) p 767
Duration 12 Hour Nasal Spray (Schering-Plough HealthCare) p 426, 699
Duration 12 Hour Nasal Spray Pump (Schering-Plough HealthCare) p 426, 699
4-Way Long Lasting Nasal Spray & Metered Spray Pump (Bristol-Myers Products) p 405, 533
NTZ Long Acting Nasal Spray & Drops 0.05% (Sterling Health) p 735
Neo-Synephrine Maximum Strength 12 Hour Nasal Spray (Sterling Health) p 734
Neo-Synephrine Maximum Strength 12 Hour Nasal Spray Pump (Sterling Health) p 430, 734
Nōstrilla Long Acting Nasal Decongestant (CIBA Consumer) p 407, 552
Vicks Sinex Long-Acting Decongestant Nasal Spray (Richardson-Vicks) p 661
Vicks Sinex Long-Acting Decongestant Nasal Ultra Fine Mist (Richardson-Vicks) p 661
Visine L.R. Eye Drops (Pfizer Consumer) p 420, 642

P

PADIMATE O (OCTYL DIMETHYL PABA)

Chap Stick Lip Balm (Robins Consumer) p 421, 667
Chap Stick Petroleum Jelly Plus with Sunblock 15 (Robins Consumer) p 421, 668
Chap Stick Sunblock 15 Lip Balm (Robins Consumer) p 421, 667
Filteray Broad Spectrum Sunscreen Lotion (Burroughs Wellcome) p 406, 538

PAMABROM

Maximum Strength Midol Premenstrual Pain Formula (Sterling Health) p 430, 733
Teen Formula Midol (Sterling Health) p 430, 734
Extra Strength Pamprin Multi-Symptom Formula Tablets and Caplets (Chattem) p 547
Maximum Strength Pamprin Cramp Relief Formula Caplets (Chattem) p 547
Prēmsyn PMS (Chattem) p 547

PANTHENOL

Geritol Liquid - High Potency Iron & Vitamin Tonic (SmithKline Beecham) p 712

PANTOTHENATE, CALCIUM (see under CALCIUM PANTOTHENATE)

PANTOTHENIC ACID

Allbee with C Caplets (Robins Consumer) p 667
Allbee C-800 Plus Iron Tablets (Robins Consumer) p 666
Allbee C-800 Tablets (Robins Consumer) p 666
One-A-Day Essential Vitamins (Miles Consumer) p 417, 620
One-A-Day Maximum Formula Vitamins and Minerals (Miles Consumer) p 417, 620
One-A-Day Plus Extra C Vitamins (Miles Consumer) p 417, 620
One-A-Day Stressgard Formula Vitamins (Miles Consumer) p 417, 620
One-A-Day Women's Formula Multivitamins with Calcium, Extra Iron, Zinc and Beta Carotene (Miles Consumer) p 417, 620
Sigtab Tablets (Roberts) p 421, 666
Stuartinic Tablets (J&J•Merck Consumer) p 410, 570
Z-BEC Tablets (Robins Consumer) p 676
Zymacap Capsules (Roberts) p 666

PASSIFLORA

Hyland's Calms Forté Tablets (Standard Homeopathic) p 722

PERMETHRIN

Nix Creme Rinse (Burroughs Wellcome) p 540, 407

PETROLATUM

A and D Ointment (Schering-Plough HealthCare) p 424, 692
Aqua Care Cream (Menley & James) p 415, 607
Aqua Care Lotion (Menley & James) p 415, 607
Aquaphor Healing Ointment, Original Formula (Beiersdorf) p 404, 514
Aquaphor Natural Healing Ointment (Beiersdorf) p 404, 515
Chap Stick Lip Balm (Robins Consumer) p 421, 667
Chap Stick Sunblock 15 Lip Balm (Robins Consumer) p 421, 667
Desitin Ointment (Pfizer Consumer) p 420, 638
Eucerin Dry Skin Care Creme (Beiersdorf) p 404, 515
Keri Lotion - Silky Smooth Fragrance Free Formula (Bristol-Myers Products) p 405, 533
Moisturel Cream (Westwood) p 433, 758
pHisoDerm For Baby (Sterling Health) p 430, 738
pHisoDerm Skin Cleanser and Conditioner - Regular and Oily (Sterling Health) p 430, 738
Preparation H Hemorrhoidal Cream (Whitehall) p 434, 768
Preparation H Hemorrhoidal Ointment (Whitehall) p 434, 768
Extra Strength Vaseline Intensive Care Lotion (Chese-Pond's) p 548

PETROLATUM, WHITE

Vaseline Pure Petroleum Jelly Skin Protectant/Lip Therapy (Chese-Pond's) p 548

PHENIRAMINE MALEATE

Dristan Nasal Spray (Whitehall) p 764
Dristan Menthol Nasal Spray (Whitehall) p 764
Dristan Nasal Spray, Metered Dose Pump, Regular (Whitehall) p 764

PHENOBARBITAL

Bronkolixir (Sanofi Winthrop Pharmaceuticals) p 689
Bronkotabs Tablets (Sanofi Winthrop Pharmaceuticals) p 689
Primatene Tablets-P Formula (Whitehall) p 435, 770

PHENOL

Anbesol Gel Antiseptic-Anesthetic-Regular Strength (Whitehall) p 434, 763
Anbesol Liquid Antiseptic-Anesthetic (Whitehall) p 434, 763
Campho-Phenique Cold Sore Gel (Sterling Health) p 429, 731
Campho-Phenique Liquid (Sterling Health) p 429, 731
Cēpastat Cherry Flavor Sore Throat Lozenges (Marion Merrell Dow) p 411, 580
Cēpastat Extra Strength Sore Throat Lozenges (Marion Merrell Dow) p 411, 580
Cheracol Sore Throat Spray (Roberts) p 663
Children's Chloraseptic Spray (Richardson-Vicks) p 654
Chloraseptic Liquid, Cherry, Menthol and Cool Mint (Richardson-Vicks) p 652
Chloraseptic Liquid - Nitrogen Propelled Spray (Richardson-Vicks) p 652
PRID Salve (Walker Pharmacal) p 753

PHENOLPHTHALEIN

Agoral, Marshmallow Flavor (Parke-Davis) p 628
Agoral, Raspberry Flavor (Parke-Davis) p 628
Phillips' LaxCaps (Sterling Health) p 430, 736

PHENOLPHTHALEIN, YELLOW

Correctol Laxative Tablets (Schering-Plough HealthCare) p 425, 696
Dialose Plus Tablets (J&J•Merck Consumer) p 409, 566
Doxidan Liqui-Gels (Upjohn) p 431, 748
Evac-U-Gen Mild Laxative (Walker, Corp) p 432, 753
Ex-Lax Chocolated Laxative Tablets (Sandoz Consumer) p 423, 683
Extra Gentle Ex-Lax Laxative Pills (Sandoz Consumer) p 423, 683
Maximum Relief Formula Ex-Lax Laxative Pills (Sandoz Consumer) p 423, 683
Regular Strength Ex-Lax Laxative Pills (Sandoz Consumer) p 423, 683
Feen-A-Mint Gum (Schering-Plough HealthCare) p 426, 699
Feen-A-Mint Laxative Pills (Schering-Plough HealthCare) p 426, 699
Yellolax (Luyties) p 578

PHENOXYETHANOL

Preparation H Cleansing Tissues (Whitehall) p 434, 769

2-PHENYL-BENZIMIDAZOLE-5-SULFONIC ACID

Eucerin Dry Skin Care Daily Facial Lotion SPF 20 (Beiersdorf) p 404, 515
Oil of Olay Daily UV Protectant SPF 15 Beauty Fluid-Regular & Fragrance Free (Olay Co. Inc.) (Richardson-Vicks) p 653
Oil of Olay Daily UV Protectant SPF 15 Moisture Replenishing Cream-Regular & Fragrance Free (Olay Co. Inc.) (Richardson-Vicks) p 653

PHENYLEPHRINE HYDROCHLORIDE

Anusol Hemorrhoidal Suppositories (Parke-Davis) p 418, 629
Cerose-DM (Wyeth-Ayerst) p 435, 774

Congespirin For Children Aspirin Free Chewable Cold Tablets (Bristol-Myers Products) p 405, 527
Dimetane Decongestant Caplets (Robins Consumer) p 669
Dimetane Decongestant Elixir (Robins Consumer) p 669
Dristan Cold Nasal Decongestant/ Antihistamine/Analgesic Coated Tablets (Whitehall) p 434, 765
Dristan Nasal Spray (Whitehall) p 764
Dristan Menthol Nasal Spray (Whitehall) p 764
Dristan Nasal Spray, Metered Dose Pump, Regular (Whitehall) p 764
4-Way Fast Acting Nasal Spray (regular & mentholated) & Metered Spray Pump (regular) (Bristol-Myers Products) p 405, 532
Neo-Synephrine Nasal Solutions, Pediatric, Mild, Regular & Extra Strength (Sterling Health) p 734
Neo-Synephrine Nasal Sprays, Pediatric, Mild, Regular & Extra Strength (Sterling Health) p 430, 734
Neo-Synephrine Nose Drops (Sterling Health) p 430, 734
Nōstril Nasal Decongestant (CIBA Consumer) p 407, 552
Novahistine Elixir (Marion Merrell Dow) p 412, 584
Robitussin Night Relief (Robins Consumer) p 422, 675
Vicks Sinex Decongestant Nasal Spray (Richardson-Vicks) p 661
Vicks Sinex Decongestant Nasal Ultra Fine Mist (Richardson-Vicks) p 661

PHENYLPROPANOLAMINE BITARTRATE

Alka-Seltzer Plus Cold Medicine (Miles Consumer) p 416, 615
Alka-Seltzer Plus Cold & Cough Medicine (Miles Consumer) p 416, 616
Alka-Seltzer Plus Night-Time Cold Medicine (Miles Consumer) p 416, 615
Alka Seltzer Plus Sinus Allergy Medicine (Miles Consumer) p 416, 616

PHENYLPROPANOLAMINE HYDROCHLORIDE

A.R.M. Allergy Relief Medicine Caplets (Menley & James) p 415, 607
Acutrim 16 Hour Steady Control Appetite Suppressant (CIBA Consumer) p 407, 549
Acutrim Late Day Strength Appetite Suppressant (CIBA Consumer) p 407, 549
Acutrim II Maximum Strength Appetite Suppressant (CIBA Consumer) p 407, 549
Allerest Children's Chewable Tablets (Fisons Consumer Health) p 558
Allerest 12 Hour Caplets (Fisons Consumer Health) p 558
BC Cold Powder Multi-Symptom Formula (Block) p 516
BC Cold Powder Multi-Symptom Non-Drowsy Formula (Block) p 516
Cheracol Plus Head Cold/Cough Formula (Roberts) p 421, 663
Contac Continuous Action Decongestant/Antihistamine Capsules (SmithKline Beecham) p 426, 705
Contac Maximum Strength Continuous Action Decongestant/Antihistamine Caplets (SmithKline Beecham) p 426, 704
Contac Severe Cold and Flu Formula Caplets (SmithKline Beecham) p 427, 706
Coricidin 'D' Decongestant Tablets (Schering-Plough HealthCare) p 425, 695
Coricidin Demilets Tablets for Children (Schering-Plough HealthCare) p 425, 696
Dexatrim Capsules, Caplets, Tablets (Thompson Medical) p 744

Dexatrim Maximum Strength Caffeine-Free Caplets (Thompson Medical) p 744
Dexatrim Maximum Strength Caffeine-Free Capsules (Thompson Medical) p 744
Dexatrim Maximum Strength Extended Duration Time Tablets (Thompson Medical) p 744
Dexatrim Maximum Strength Plus Vitamin C/Caffeine-free Caplets (Thompson Medical) p 431, 744
Dexatrim Maximum Strength Plus Vitamin C/Caffeine-free Capsules (Thompson Medical) p 431, 744
Dimetapp Cold & Flu Caplets (Robins Consumer) p 421, 670
Dimetapp Elixir (Robins Consumer) p 421, 670
Dimetapp DM Elixir (Robins Consumer) p 421, 671
Dimetapp Extentabs (Robins Consumer) p 421, 671
Dimetapp Tablets (Robins Consumer) p 421, 672
4-Way Cold Tablets (Bristol-Myers Products) p 405, 531
Naldecon CX Adult Liquid (Apothecon) p 505
Naldecon DX Adult Liquid (Apothecon) p 505
Naldecon DX Children's Syrup (Apothecon) p 506
Naldecon DX Pediatric Drops (Apothecon) p 506
Naldecon EX Children's Syrup (Apothecon) p 507
Naldecon EX Pediatric Drops (Apothecon) p 507
Orthoxicol Cough Syrup (Roberts) p 665
Pyrroxate Capsules (Roberts) p 421, 665
Robitussin-CF (Robins Consumer) p 422, 673
Sine-Off Sinus Medicine Tablets-Aspirin Formula (SmithKline Beecham) p 428, 718
St. Joseph Cold Tablets for Children (Schering-Plough HealthCare) p 702
Triaminic Allergy Tablets (Sandoz Consumer) p 685
Triaminic Chewables (Sandoz Consumer) p 685
Triaminic Cold Tablets (Sandoz Consumer) p 424, 685
Triaminic Expectorant (Sandoz Consumer) p 424, 686
Triaminic Syrup (Sandoz Consumer) p 423, 686
Triaminic-12 Tablets (Sandoz Consumer) p 424, 687
Triaminic-DM Syrup (Sandoz Consumer) p 423, 687
Triaminicin Tablets (Sandoz Consumer) p 424, 687
Triaminicol Multi-Symptom Cold Tablets (Sandoz Consumer) p 424, 688
Triaminicol Multi-Symptom Relief (Sandoz Consumer) p 424, 688
Tylenol Cold Medication, Effervescent Tablets (McNeil Consumer Products) p 413, 595

PHENYLTOLOXAMINE CITRATE

Mobigesic Analgesic Tablets (Ascher) p 403, 509
Momentum Muscular Backache Formula (Whitehall) p 767
Percogesic Analgesic Tablets (Richardson-Vicks) p 654

PHOSPHORATED CARBOHYDRATE SOLUTION

Emetrol (Adria) p 403, 503

PHOSPHORUS

One-A-Day Maximum Formula Vitamins and Minerals (Miles Consumer) p 417, 620

PIPERONYL BUTOXIDE
A-200 Pediculicide Shampoo & Gel (SmithKline Beecham) p 426, 704
Lice•Enz Foam (Copley) p 408, 556
Pronto Lice Killing Shampoo Kit (Del Pharmaceuticals) p 408, 557
R&C Shampoo (Reed & Carnrick) p 420, 646
Rid Lice Killing Shampoo (Pfizer Consumer) p 640

POLYAMINO SUGAR CONDENSATE
Pen•Kera Creme (Ascher) p 403, 510

POLYCARBOPHIL
Replens (Warner-Lambert) p 433, 757

POLYETHYLENE GLYCOL
Allergy Drops (Bausch & Lomb Personal) p 403, 513
Visine EXTRA Eye Drops (Pfizer Consumer) p 420, 642

POLYGLYCERYLMETHACRYLATE
Gyne-Moistrin Vaginal Gel (Schering-Plough HealthCare) p 426, 700

POLYMYXIN B SULFATE
Aquaphor Antibiotic Ointment (Beiersdorf) p 404, 515
Bactine First Aid Antibiotic Plus Anesthetic Ointment (Miles Consumer) p 416, 617
Campho-Phenique Triple Antibiotic Ointment Plus Pain Reliever (Sterling Health) p 429, 731
Mycitracin Plus Pain Reliever (Upjohn) p 432, 750
Maximum Strength Mycitracin Triple Antibiotic First Aid Ointment (Upjohn) p 432, 750
Neosporin Cream (Burroughs Wellcome) p 406, 539
Neosporin Ointment (Burroughs Wellcome) p 406, 539
Neosporin Maximum Strength Ointment (Burroughs Wellcome) p 406, 539
Polysporin Ointment (Burroughs Wellcome) p 407, 540
Polysporin Powder (Burroughs Wellcome) p 407, 540

POLYSACCHARIDE-IRON COMPLEX
Sunkist Children's Chewable Multivitamins - Plus Iron (CIBA Consumer) p 408, 555

POLYVINYL ALCOHOL
Murine Eye Lubricant (Ross) p 422, 678
Murine Plus Lubricating Eye Redness Reliever (Ross) p 422, 678
Tears Plus Lubricant Ophthalmic Solution (Allergan Pharmaceuticals) p 505

POLYVINYLPYRROLIDONE
(see under POVIDONE)

POTASSIUM BICARBONATE
Alka-Seltzer Effervescent Antacid (Miles Consumer) p 416, 614

POTASSIUM CHLORIDE
Chlor-3 Condiment (Fleming) p 563
Salivart Saliva Substitute (Gebauer) p 564
Thermotabs (Menley & James) p 611

POTASSIUM CITRATE
Ricelyte, Rice-Based Oral Electrolyte Maintenance Solution (Mead Johnson Nutritionals) p 415, 604

POTASSIUM IODIDE
Hyland's C-Plus Cold Tablets (Standard Homeopathic) p 722

POTASSIUM MONOPERSULFATE
Professional Strength Efferdent (Warner-Lambert) p 432, 755

POTASSIUM NITRATE
Denquel Sensitive Teeth Toothpaste (Procter & Gamble) p 642
Promise Toothpaste (Block) p 517
Mint Gel Sensodyne (Block) p 518
Mint Sensodyne Toothpaste (Block) p 518

POTASSIUM SORBATE
Massengill Baby Powder Soft Cloth Towelette and Fragrance Free Soft Cloth Towelette (SmithKline Beecham) p 713

POVIDONE
Murine Eye Lubricant (Ross) p 422, 678
Murine Plus Lubricating Eye Redness Reliever (Ross) p 422, 678
Tears Plus Lubricant Ophthalmic Solution (Allergan Pharmaceuticals) p 505

POVIDONE IODINE
Massengill Medicated Disposable Douche (SmithKline Beecham) p 427, 713
Massengill Medicated Liquid Concentrate (SmithKline Beecham) p 713

PRAMOXINE HYDROCHLORIDE
Anusol Ointment (Parke-Davis) p 418, 629
Aveeno Anti-Itch Concentrated Lotion (Rydelle) p 423, 680
Aveeno Anti-Itch Cream (Rydelle) p 423, 680
Itch-X Gel (Ascher) p 403, 509
proctoFoam/non-steroid (Reed & Carnrick) p 645
Rhulicream (Rydelle) p 423, 681
Tronolane Anesthetic Cream for Hemorrhoids (Ross) p 422, 679

PROPYLENE GLYCOL
Eucerin Dry Skin Care Lotion (Fragrance-free) (Beiersdorf) p 404, 516
Preparation H Cleansing Tissues (Whitehall) p 434, 769

PROPYLHEXEDRINE
Benzedrex Inhaler (Menley & James) p 415, 608

PSEUDOEPHEDRINE HYDROCHLORIDE
Actifed Plus Caplets (Burroughs Wellcome) p 406, 537
Actifed Plus Tablets (Burroughs Wellcome) p 406, 538
Actifed Syrup (Burroughs Wellcome) p 406, 537
Actifed Tablets (Burroughs Wellcome) p 406, 537
Advil Cold and Sinus (formerly CoAdvil) (Whitehall) p 434, 761
Allerest Headache Strength Tablets (Fisons Consumer Health) p 558
Allerest Maximum Strength Tablets (Fisons Consumer Health) p 408, 558
Allerest No Drowsiness Tablets (Fisons Consumer Health) p 408, 558
Allerest Sinus Pain Formula (Fisons Consumer Health) p 558
Benadryl Cold Tablets (Parke-Davis) p 418, 631
Benadryl Cold Nighttime Formula (Parke-Davis) p 419, 631
Benadryl Decongestant Elixir (Parke-Davis) p 419, 630
Benadryl Decongestant Kapseals (Parke-Davis) p 418, 630
Benadryl Decongestant Tablets (Parke-Davis) p 418, 630
Benylin Decongestant (Parke-Davis) p 419, 633
Bromfed Syrup (Muro) p 621
Cold Control+ Intense Cold Medicine (Reese Chemical) p 647

Allergy-Sinus Comtrex Multi-Symptom Allergy-Sinus Formula Tablets & Caplets (Bristol-Myers Products) p 404, 523
Cough Formula Comtrex (Bristol-Myers Products) p 405, 524
Comtrex Multi-Symptom Cold Reliever Tablets/Caplets/Liqui-Gels/Liquid (Bristol-Myers Products) p 404, 522
Comtrex Multi-Symptom Day-Night Caplet-Tablet (Bristol-Myers Products) p 404, 525
Comtrex Multi-Symptom Non-Drowsy Caplets (Bristol-Myers Products) p 405, 526
Congestac Caplets (Menley & James) p 415, 609
Contac Cough and Chest Cold (SmithKline Beecham) p 427, 706
Contac Jr. Non-Drowsy Cold Liquid (SmithKline Beecham) p 427, 707
Contac Severe Cold & Flu Nighttime (SmithKline Beecham) p 427, 708
Contac Sinus Caplets Maximum Strength Non-Drowsy Formula (SmithKline Beecham) p 427, 705
Contac Sinus Tablets Maximum Strength Non-Drowsy Formula (SmithKline Beecham) p 427, 705
Dimacol Caplets (Robins Consumer) p 668
Dorcol Children's Cough Syrup (Sandoz Consumer) p 423, 682
Dorcol Children's Decongestant Liquid (Sandoz Consumer) p 423, 683
Dorcol Children's Liquid Cold Formula (Sandoz Consumer) p 423, 683
Dristan Allergy Nasal Decongestant/Antihistamine Caplets (Whitehall) p 434, 765
Dristan Cold and Flu (Whitehall) p 434, 766
Maximum Strength Dristan Cold Nasal Decongestant/ Analgesic Coated Caplets (Whitehall) p 434, 765
Dristan Sinus Pain Reliever/Nasal Decongestant Caplets (Whitehall) p 434, 766
Sinus Excedrin Analgesic, Decongestant Tablets & Caplets (Bristol-Myers Products) p 405, 531
Guaifed Syrup (Muro) p 621
Guaitab Tablets (Muro) p 621
Isoclor Timesule Capsules (Fisons Consumer Health) p 409, 561
Medi-Flu Caplet, Liquid (Parke-Davis) p 419, 634
Medi-Flu Without Drowsiness Caplets (Parke-Davis) p 419, 635
Novahistine DMX (Marion Merrell Dow) p 412, 583
Ornex Caplets (Menley & James) p 415, 610
Maximum Strength Ornex Caplets (Menley & James) p 415, 610
PediaCare Allergy Formula Liquid (McNeil Consumer Products) p 414, 588
PediaCare Cough-Cold Formula Liquid and Chewable Tablets (McNeil Consumer Products) p 414, 588
PediaCare Decongestant Drops (McNeil Consumer Products) p 414, 588
PediaCare Night Rest Cough-Cold Formula Liquid (McNeil Consumer Products) p 414, 588
PediaCare 6-12 Cough-Cold Formula Chewable Tablets (McNeil Consumer Products) p 414, 588
Robitussin Pediatric Cough & Cold Formula (Robins Consumer) p 422, 675
Robitussin-PE (Robins Consumer) p 422, 674
Ryna Liquid (Wallace) p 432, 754
Ryna-C Liquid (Wallace) p 432, 754
Ryna-CX Liquid (Wallace) p 432, 754
Sinarest No Drowsiness Tablets (Fisons Consumer Health) p 561
Sinarest Tablets (Fisons Consumer Health) p 561

Sinarest Extra Strength Tablets (Fisons Consumer Health) p 561
Sine-Aid Maximum Strength Sinus Headache Gelcaps, Caplets and Tablets (McNeil Consumer Products) p 414, 589
Sine-Off Maximum Strength Allergy/Sinus Formula Caplets (SmithKline Beecham) p 428, 717
Sine-Off Maximum Strength No Drowsiness Formula Caplets (SmithKline Beecham) p 428, 717
Singlet Tablets (Marion Merrell Dow) p 586
Sinutab Sinus Medication, Maximum Strength Caplets (Parke-Davis) p 419, 636
Sinutab Sinus Allergy Medication, Maximum Strength Tablets (Parke-Davis) p 419, 636
Sinutab Sinus Medication, Maximum Strength Without Drowsiness Formula Tablets & Caplets (Parke-Davis) p 419, 637
Sinutab Sinus Medication, Regular Strength Without Drowsiness Formula (Parke-Davis) p 419, 636
Sudafed Children's Liquid (Burroughs Wellcome) p 407, 540
Sudafed Cough Syrup (Burroughs Wellcome) p 407, 541
Sudafed Plus Liquid (Burroughs Wellcome) p 407, 541
Sudafed Plus Tablets (Burroughs Wellcome) p 407, 542
Sudafed Severe Cold Formula Caplets (Burroughs Wellcome) p 407, 542
Sudafed Severe Cold Formula Tablets (Burroughs Wellcome) p 407, 542
Sudafed Sinus Caplets (Burroughs Wellcome) p 407, 543
Sudafed Sinus Tablets (Burroughs Wellcome) p 407, 543
Sudafed Tablets, 30 mg (Burroughs Wellcome) p 407, 541
Sudafed Tablets, Adult Strength, 60 mg (Burroughs Wellcome) p 407, 541
TheraFlu Flu and Cold Medicine (Sandoz Consumer) p 423, 684
TheraFlu Flu, Cold and Cough Medicine (Sandoz Consumer) p 423, 684
Triaminic Nite Light (Sandoz Consumer) p 424, 686
Tylenol Allergy Sinus Medication Maximum Strength Gelcaps and Caplets (McNeil Consumer Products) p 413, 600
Children's Tylenol Cold Multi Symptom Liquid Formula and Chewable Tablets (McNeil Consumer Products) p 413, 594
Tylenol Cold & Flu Hot Medication, Packets (McNeil Consumer Products) p 413, 595
Tylenol Cold & Flu No Drowsiness Hot Medication, Packets (McNeil Consumer Products) p 413, 598
Tylenol Cold Multi Symptom Medication Caplets and Tablets (McNeil Consumer Products) p 413, 596
Tylenol Cold Medication No Drowsiness Formula Caplets (McNeil Consumer Products) p 413, 597
Tylenol Cold Night Time Medication Liquid (McNeil Consumer Products) p 413, 599
Tylenol Cough Medication Maximum Strength Liquid with Decongestant (McNeil Consumer Products) p 414, 601
Tylenol, Maximum Strength, Sinus Medication Gelcaps, Caplets and Tablets (McNeil Consumer Products) p 413, 602
Ursinus Inlay-Tabs (Sandoz Consumer) p 688
Vicks Children's NyQuil Nighttime Cold/Cough Medicine (Richardson-Vicks) p 659
Vicks Children's NyQuil Nighttime Head Cold/Allergy Medicine (Richardson-Vicks) p 660

Vicks Daycare Daytime Cold Medicine Caplets (Richardson-Vicks) p 655
Vicks Daycare Daytime Cold Medicine Liquid (Richardson-Vicks) p 655
Vicks Formula 44D Cough and Decongestant Medicine (Richardson-Vicks) p 656
Vicks Formula 44M Multi-Symptom Cough & Cold Medicine (Richardson-Vicks) p 657
Vicks NyQuil LiquiCaps Adult Nighttime Cold/Flu Medicine (Richardson-Vicks) p 661
Vicks NyQuil Nighttime Cold/Flu Medicine-Regular & Cherry Flavor (Richardson-Vicks) p 660
Vicks Pediatric Formula 44d Cough & Decongestant Medicine (Richardson-Vicks) p 658
Vicks Pediatric Formula 44m Multi-Symptom Cough & Cold Medicine (Richardson-Vicks) p 658

PSEUDOEPHEDRINE SULFATE
Afrin Tablets (Schering-Plough HealthCare) p 424, 693
Chlor-Trimeton Antihistamine and Decongestant Tablets (Schering-Plough HealthCare) p 425, 694
Chlor-Trimeton Long Acting Antihistamine and Decongestant Repetabs Tablets (Schering-Plough HealthCare) p 425, 694
Drixoral Antihistamine/Nasal Decongestant Syrup (Schering-Plough HealthCare) p 696
Drixoral Non-Drowsy Formula (Schering-Plough HealthCare) p 425, 697
Drixoral Plus Extended-Release Tablets (Schering-Plough HealthCare) p 425, 698
Drixoral Sinus (Schering-Plough HealthCare) p 426, 698
Drixoral Sustained-Action Tablets (Schering-Plough HealthCare) p 425, 697
Sudafed 12 Hour Tablets (Burroughs Wellcome) p 407, 543

PSYLLIUM PREPARATIONS
Effer-Syllium Natural Fiber Bulking Agent (J&J•Merck Consumer) p 409, 566
Fiberall Fiber Wafers - Fruit & Nut (CIBA Consumer) p 407, 551
Fiberall Fiber Wafers - Oatmeal Raisin (CIBA Consumer) p 407, 551
Fiberall Powder Natural Flavor (CIBA Consumer) p 407, 551
Fiberall Powder Orange Flavor (CIBA Consumer) p 407, 551
Perdiem Fiber Granules (Rhone-Poulenc Rorer Consumer) p 421, 652
Perdiem Granules (Rhone-Poulenc Rorer Consumer) p 421, 651
Serutan Toasted Granules (Menley & James) p 415, 611
Syllact Powder (Wallace) p 432, 755

PYRANTEL PAMOATE
Reese's Pinworm Medicine (Reese Chemical) p 420, 647

PYRETHRINS
A-200 Pediculicide Shampoo & Gel (SmithKline Beecham) p 426, 704
Lice•Enz Foam (Copley) p 408, 556
Pronto Lice Killing Shampoo Kit (Del Pharmaceuticals) p 408, 557
R&C Shampoo (Reed & Carnrick) p 420, 646
Rid Lice Killing Shampoo (Pfizer Consumer) p 640

PYRETHROIDS
R&C Spray (Reed & Carnrick) p 420, 646
Rid Lice Control Spray (Pfizer Consumer) p 639

PYRIDOXINE HYDROCHLORIDE
(see under VITAMIN B₆)

PYRILAMINE MALEATE
4-Way Fast Acting Nasal Spray (regular & mentholated) & Metered Spray Pump (regular) (Bristol-Myers Products) p 405, 532
Maximum Strength Midol Multi-Symptom Menstrual Formula (Sterling Health) p 430, 733
Maximum Strength Midol Premenstrual Pain Formula (Sterling Health) p 430, 733
Regular Strength Midol Multi-Symptom Menstrual Formula (Sterling Health) p 430, 732
Extra Strength Pamprin Multi-Symptom Formula Tablets and Caplets (Chattem) p 547
Maximum Strength Pamprin Cramp Relief Formula Caplets (Chattem) p 547
Premsyn PMS (Chattem) p 547
Primatene Tablets-M Formula (Whitehall) p 435, 770
Robitussin Night Relief (Robins Consumer) p 422, 675

PYRITHIONE ZINC
Head & Shoulders Antidandruff Shampoo (Procter & Gamble) p 643
Head & Shoulders Antidandruff Shampoo 2-in-1 plus Conditioner (Procter & Gamble) p 643
Head & Shoulders Dry Scalp Shampoo (Procter & Gamble) p 643
Head & Shoulders Dry Scalp Shampoo 2-in-1 plus Conditioner (Procter & Gamble) p 643
X-Seb Shampoo (Baker Cummins Pharmaceuticals) p 512
X-Seb Plus Conditioning Shampoo (Baker Cummins Pharmaceuticals) p 512
Zincon Dandruff Shampoo (Lederle) p 411, 578

Q

QUININE SULFATE
Legatrin Tablets (Columbia) p 408, 556
Q-vel Muscle Relaxant Pain Reliever (CIBA Consumer) p 408, 554

R

RACEPINEPHRINE HYDROCHLORIDE
AsthmaNefrin Solution "A" Bronchodilator (Menley & James) p 608

RESORCINOL
Acnomel Cream (Menley & James) p 415, 607
BiCozene Creme (Sandoz Consumer) p 423, 682

RHUS AROMATICA
Hyland's Bed Wetting Tablets (Standard Homeopathic) p 722

RIBOFLAVIN
(see under VITAMIN B₂)

RICE SYRUP SOLIDS
Ricelyte, Rice-Based Oral Electrolyte Maintenance Solution (Mead Johnson Nutritionals) p 415, 604

S

SD ALCOHOL
Oxy Medicated Pads - Regular, Sensitive Skin, and Maximum Strength (SmithKline Beecham) p 427, 716
Stri-Dex Dual Textured Maximum Strength Pads (Sterling Health) p 431, 739

Stri-Dex Dual Textured Maximum Strength Big Pads (Sterling Health) p 739

Stri-Dex Dual Textured Regular Strength Pads (Sterling Health) p 431, 739

Stri-Dex Dual Textured Regular Strength Big Pads (Sterling Health) p 739

Stri-Dex Dual Textured Sensitive Skin Pads (Sterling Health) p 739

Stri-Dex Super Scrub Pads (Sterling Health) p 739

SALICYLIC ACID

Aveeno Cleansing Bar for Acne (Rydelle) p 423, 680

Compound W Gel (Whitehall) p 763

Compound W Liquid (Whitehall) p 763

DuoFilm Liquid (Schering-Plough HealthCare) p 426, 698

DuoPlant Gel (Schering-Plough HealthCare) p 426, 699

Freezone Solution (Whitehall) p 767

MG 217 Psoriasis Ointment and Lotion (Triton Consumer) p 747

MG 217 Psoriasis Shampoo and Conditioner (Triton Consumer) p 747

Oxipor VHC Lotion for Psoriasis (Whitehall) p 768

Oxy Medicated Cleanser (SmithKline Beecham) p 428, 715

Oxy Medicated Pads - Regular, Sensitive Skin, and Maximum Strength (SmithKline Beecham) p 427, 716

Oxy Night Watch Nighttime Acne Medication-Maximum Strength and Sensitive Skin Formulas (SmithKline Beecham) p 428, 716

P & S Plus Tar Gel (Baker Cummins Pharmaceuticals) p 512

P & S Shampoo (Baker Cummins Pharmaceuticals) p 512

Sebulex Antiseborrheic Treatment Shampoo (Westwood) p 433, 759

Sebutone and Sebutone Cream Antiseborrheic Tar Shampoos (Westwood) p 433, 759

Stri-Dex Dual Textured Maximum Strength Pads (Sterling Health) p 431, 739

Stri-Dex Dual Textured Maximum Strength Big Pads (Sterling Health) p 739

Stri-Dex Dual Textured Regular Strength Pads (Sterling Health) p 431, 739

Stri-Dex Dual Textured Regular Strength Big Pads (Sterling Health) p 739

Stri-Dex Dual Textured Sensitive Skin Pads (Sterling Health) p 739

Stri-Dex Super Scrub Pads (Sterling Health) p 739

Wart-Off Wart Remover (Pfizer Consumer) p 642

SELENIUM SULFIDE

Head & Shoulders Intensive Treatment Dandruff Shampoo (Procter & Gamble) p 643

Head & Shoulders Intensive Treatment Dandruff Shampoo 2-in-1 plus Conditioner (Procter & Gamble) p 643

Selsun Blue Dandruff Shampoo (Ross) p 422, 679

Selsun Blue Dandruff Shampoo-Extra Medicated (Ross) p 422, 679

Selsun Blue Extra Conditioning Dandruff Shampoo (Ross) p 422, 679

SENNA CONCENTRATES

Gentle Nature Natural Vegetable Laxative Tablets (Sandoz Consumer) p 423, 684

Perdiem Granules (Rhone-Poulenc Rorer Consumer) p 421, 651

SHARK LIVER OIL

Preparation H Hemorrhoidal Cream (Whitehall) p 434, 768

Preparation H Hemorrhoidal Ointment (Whitehall) p 434, 768

Preparation H Hemorrhoidal Suppositories (Whitehall) p 434, 768

Wyanoids Relief Factor Hemorrhoidal Suppositories (Wyeth-Ayerst) p 435, 777

SIMETHICONE

Colicon Drops (Reese Chemical) p 647

Di-Gel Antacid/Anti-Gas (Schering-Plough HealthCare) p 425, 696

Gas-X Tablets (Sandoz Consumer) p 423, 684

Extra Strength Gas-X Tablets (Sandoz Consumer) p 423, 684

Gelusil Liquid & Tablets (Parke-Davis) p 419, 634

Maalox Plus Suspension/Tablets (Rhone-Poulenc Rorer Consumer) p 421, 649

Extra Strength Maalox Plus Suspension (Rhone-Poulenc Rorer Consumer) p 420, 650

Mylanta Gas Tablets-40 mg (J&J•Merck Consumer) p 410, 568

Mylanta Gas Tablets-80 mg (J&J•Merck Consumer) p 410, 569

Mylanta Liquid (J&J•Merck Consumer) p 410, 567

Mylanta Tablets (J&J•Merck Consumer) p 410, 567

Mylanta Double Strength Liquid (J&J•Merck Consumer) p 410, 567

Mylanta Double Strength Tablets (J&J•Merck Consumer) p 410, 567

Maximum Strength Mylanta Gas Tablets-125 mg (J&J•Merck Consumer) p 410, 569

Mylicon Drops (J&J•Merck Consumer) p 410, 568

Phazyme Drops (Reed & Carnrick) p 420, 645

Phazyme Tablets (Reed & Carnrick) p 645

Phazyme-125 Softgels Maximum Strength (Reed & Carnrick) p 420, 645

Phazyme-95 Tablets (Reed & Carnrick) p 420, 645

Riopan Plus Suspension (Whitehall) p 771

Riopan Plus Chew Tablets (Whitehall) p 771

Riopan Plus Chew Tablets in Rollpacks (Whitehall) p 771

Riopan Plus 2 Suspension-Mint and Cherry flavors (Whitehall) p 435, 771

Riopan Plus 2 Chew Tablets-Mint and Cherry Vanilla flavors (Whitehall) p 435, 771

Tums Plus Antacid Anti-gas Tablets, Assorted Fruit or Peppermint (SmithKline Beecham) p 428, 721

SODIUM ASCORBATE

Hyland's Vitamin C for Children (Standard Homeopathic) p 723

SODIUM BICARBONATE

Alka-Seltzer Effervescent Antacid (Miles Consumer) p 416, 614

Alka-Seltzer Effervescent Antacid and Pain Reliever (Miles Consumer) p 416, 612

Alka-Seltzer Extra Strength Effervescent Antacid and Pain Reliever (Miles Consumer) p 416, 615

Alka-Seltzer (Flavored) Effervescent Antacid and Pain Reliever (Miles Consumer) p 416, 613

Arm & Hammer Pure Baking Soda (Church & Dwight) p 548

Citrocarbonate Antacid (Roberts) p 664

Massengill Liquid Concentrate (SmithKline Beecham) p 712

SODIUM BIPHOSPHATE

Nature's Remedy Enema, Regular (SmithKline Beecham) p 427, 714

SODIUM BORATE

Collyrium for Fresh Eyes (Wyeth-Ayerst) p 435, 775

Collyrium Fresh (Wyeth-Ayerst) p 435, 775

Eye Wash (Bausch & Lomb Personal) p 404, 514

SODIUM CARBOXYMETHYLCELLULOSE

Salivart Saliva Substitute (Gebauer) p 564

SODIUM CHLORIDE

Afrin Saline Mist (Schering-Plough HealthCare) p 424, 692

Ayr Saline Nasal Drops (Ascher) p 403, 509

Ayr Saline Nasal Mist (Ascher) p 403, 509

Chlor-3 Condiment (Fleming) p 563

NäSal Moisturizing Nasal Spray (Sterling Health) p 430, 734

NäSal Moisturizing Nose Drops (Sterling Health) p 430, 734

Ocean Mist (Fleming) p 563

Ricelyte, Rice-Based Oral Electrolyte Maintenance Solution (Mead Johnson Nutritionals) p 415, 604

Salinex Nasal Mist and Drops (Muro) p 621

Star-Optic Eye Wash (Stellar) p 428, 723

Thermotabs (Menley & James) p 611

SODIUM CITRATE

Citrocarbonate Antacid (Roberts) p 664

Ricelyte, Rice-Based Oral Electrolyte Maintenance Solution (Mead Johnson Nutritionals) p 415, 604

SODIUM COCOATE

Lever 2000 (Lever Brothers) p 578

SODIUM COCOYL ISETHIONATE

Dove Bar (Lever Brothers) p 578

Lubriderm Body Bar (Warner-Lambert) p 433, 756

SODIUM FLUORIDE

Listermint with Fluoride (Warner-Lambert) p 433, 756

SODIUM LACTATE

Massengill Baby Powder Soft Cloth Towelette and Fragrance Free Soft Cloth Towelette (SmithKline Beecham) p 713

SODIUM LAURYL SULFATE

Eucerin Cleansing Lotion Dry Skin Care (Beiersdorf) p 404, 515

Moisturel Sensitive Skin Cleanser (Westwood) p 433, 759

SODIUM OCTOXYNOL-2 ETHANE SULFONATE

pHisoDerm For Baby (Sterling Health) p 430, 738

pHisoDerm Skin Cleanser and Conditioner - Regular and Oily (Sterling Health) p 430, 738

SODIUM PERBORATE

Professional Strength Efferdent (Warner-Lambert) p 432, 755

SODIUM PHENOLATE

Chloraseptic Liquid - Nitrogen Propelled Spray (Richardson-Vicks) p 652

SODIUM PHOSPHATE

Nature's Remedy Enema, Regular (SmithKline Beecham) p 427, 714

SODIUM PHOSPHATE DIBASIC

Star-Optic Eye Wash (Stellar) p 428, 723

SODIUM PHOSPHATE MONOBASIC

Star-Optic Eye Wash (Stellar) p 428, 723

SODIUM TALLOWATE

Alpha Keri Moisture Rich Cleansing Bar (Bristol-Myers Products) p 519
Dove Bar (Lever Brothers) p 578
Lever 2000 (Lever Brothers) p 578
pHisoDerm Cleansing Bar (Sterling Health) p 430, 738

SORBITOL

Actidose with Sorbitol (Paddock) p 628
Salivart Saliva Substitute (Gebauer) p 564

STARCH

Balmex Baby Powder (Macsil) p 579

STRONTIUM CHLORIDE HEXAHYDRATE

Original Sensodyne Toothpaste (Block) p 517

SULFUR

Acnomel Cream (Menley & James) p 415, 607
Sebulex Antiseborrheic Treatment Shampoo (Westwood) p 433, 759
Sebutone and Sebutone Cream Antiseborrheic Tar Shampoos (Westwood) p 433, 759

SULFUR (COLLOIDAL)

MG 217 Psoriasis Ointment and Lotion (Triton Consumer) p 747
MG 217 Psoriasis Shampoo and Conditioner (Triton Consumer) p 747

T

TANNIC ACID

Outgro Solution (Whitehall) p 767
Zilactin Medicated Gel (Zila Pharmaceuticals) p 435, 777
Zilactol Medicated Liquid (Zila Pharmaceuticals) p 777

TETRACHLOROSALICYLANILIDE

Impregon Concentrate (Fleming) p 563

TETRAHYDROZOLINE HYDROCHLORIDE

Collyrium Fresh (Wyeth-Ayerst) p 435, 775
Murine Plus Lubricating Eye Redness Reliever (Ross) p 422, 678
Visine A.C. Eye Drops (Pfizer Consumer) p 420, 641
Visine EXTRA Eye Drops (Pfizer Consumer) p 420, 642
Visine Eye Drops (Pfizer Consumer) p 420, 641

THEOPHYLLINE

Bronkaid Tablets (Sterling Health) p 429, 730
Bronkolixir (Sanofi Winthrop Pharmaceuticals) p 689
Bronkotabs Tablets (Sanofi Winthrop Pharmaceuticals) p 689

THEOPHYLLINE ANHYDROUS

Primatene Tablets-M Formula (Whitehall) p 435, 770
Primatene Tablets-Regular Formula (Whitehall) p 435, 770

THEOPHYLLINE HYDROUS

Primatene Tablets-P Formula (Whitehall) p 435, 770

THIAMINE

Bugs Bunny Children's Chewable Vitamins (Sugar Free) (Miles Consumer) p 416, 617
Bugs Bunny With Extra C Children's Chewable Vitamins (Sugar Free) (Miles Consumer) p 416, 618
Bugs Bunny Plus Iron Children's Chewable Vitamins (Sugar Free) (Miles Consumer) p 416, 617

Flintstones Children's Chewable Vitamins (Miles Consumer) p 416, 617
Flintstones Children's Chewable Vitamins With Extra C (Miles Consumer) p 416, 618
Flintstones Children's Chewable Vitamins Plus Iron (Miles Consumer) p 416, 617
Geritol Liquid - High Potency Iron & Vitamin Tonic (SmithKline Beecham) p 712
One-A-Day Essential Vitamins (Miles Consumer) p 417, 620
One-A-Day Maximum Formula Vitamins and Minerals (Miles Consumer) p 417, 620
One-A-Day Plus Extra C Vitamins (Miles Consumer) p 417, 620
Sigtab Tablets (Roberts) p 421, 666
The Stuart Formula Tablets (J&J•Merck Consumer) p 410, 569
Stuartinic Tablets (J&J•Merck Consumer) p 410, 570
Vicon-C Capsules (Whitby) p 433, 760
Zymacap Capsules (Roberts) p 666

THIAMINE MONONITRATE

Allbee with C Caplets (Robins Consumer) p 667
Allbee C-800 Plus Iron Tablets (Robins Consumer) p 666
Allbee C-800 Tablets (Robins Consumer) p 666
Stuart Prenatal Tablets (Stuart) p 431, 742
Vicon Plus (Whitby) p 433, 760
Z-BEC Tablets (Robins Consumer) p 676

THYMOL

Listerine Antiseptic (Warner-Lambert) p 433, 756

TITANIUM DIOXIDE

Aquaderm Combination Treatment/Moisturizer (SPF 15 Formula) (Baker Cummins Pharmaceuticals) p 511
Eucerin Dry Skin Care Daily Facial Lotion SPF 20 (Beiersdorf) p 404, 515

TOLNAFTATE

Aftate for Athlete's Foot (Schering-Plough HealthCare) p 424, 693
Aftate for Jock Itch (Schering-Plough HealthCare) p 424, 693
NP-27 (Thompson Medical) p 431, 746
Tinactin Aerosol Liquid 1% (Schering-Plough HealthCare) p 426, 703
Tinactin Aerosol Powder 1% (Schering-Plough HealthCare) p 426, 703
Tinactin Antifungal Cream, Solution & Powder 1% (Schering-Plough HealthCare) p 426, 703
Tinactin Deodorant Powder Aerosol 1% (Schering-Plough HealthCare) p 703
Tinactin Jock Itch Cream 1% (Schering-Plough HealthCare) p 426, 703
Tinactin Jock Itch Spray Powder 1% (Schering-Plough HealthCare) p 426, 703
Ting Antifungal Cream (Fisons Consumer Health) p 409, 562
Ting Antifungal Powder (Fisons Consumer Health) p 409, 562
Ting Antifungal Spray Liquid (Fisons Consumer Health) p 409, 562
Ting Antifungal Spray Powder (Fisons Consumer Health) p 409, 562

TRICLOSAN

Oxy Medicated Soap (SmithKline Beecham) p 428, 715

TRIPROLIDINE HYDROCHLORIDE

Actifed Plus Caplets (Burroughs Wellcome) p 406, 537
Actifed Plus Tablets (Burroughs Wellcome) p 406, 538
Actifed Syrup (Burroughs Wellcome) p 406, 537
Actifed Tablets (Burroughs Wellcome) p 406, 537

TROLAMINE SALICYLATE

Aspercreme Creme, Lotion Analgesic Rub (Thompson Medical) p 743
Mobisyl Analgesic Creme (Ascher) p 403, 510
Myoflex Analgesic Creme (Fisons Consumer Health) p 409, 561

U

UNDECYLENIC ACID

Cruex Antifungal Cream (Fisons Consumer Health) p 409, 560
Cruex Antifungal Spray Powder (Fisons Consumer Health) p 409, 560
Desenex Antifungal Cream (Fisons Consumer Health) p 560
Desenex Antifungal Foam (Fisons Consumer Health) p 560
Desenex Antifungal Ointment (Fisons Consumer Health) p 409, 560
Desenex Antifungal Powder (Fisons Consumer Health) p 409, 560
Desenex Antifungal Spray Powder (Fisons Consumer Health) p 409, 560

UREA

Aqua Care Cream (Menley & James) p 415, 607
Aqua Care Lotion (Menley & James) p 415, 607
Carmol 20 Cream (Syntex) p 743
Carmol 10 Lotion (Syntex) p 743
Pen•Kera Creme (Ascher) p 403, 510
Ultra Mide 25 (Baker Cummins Pharmaceuticals) p 512

V

VINEGAR

Massengill Disposable Douches (SmithKline Beecham) p 427, 712

VITAMIN A

Bugs Bunny Children's Chewable Vitamins (Sugar Free) (Miles Consumer) p 416, 617
Bugs Bunny With Extra C Children's Chewable Vitamins (Sugar Free) (Miles Consumer) p 416, 618
Bugs Bunny Plus Iron Children's Chewable Vitamins (Sugar Free) (Miles Consumer) p 416, 617
Centrum Silver (Lederle) p 411, 575
Flintstones Children's Chewable Vitamins (Miles Consumer) p 416, 617
Flintstones Children's Chewable Vitamins With Extra C (Miles Consumer) p 416, 618
Flintstones Children's Chewable Vitamins Plus Iron (Miles Consumer) p 416, 617
Myadec (Parke-Davis) p 419, 635
One-A-Day Essential Vitamins (Miles Consumer) p 417, 620
One-A-Day Maximum Formula Vitamins and Minerals (Miles Consumer) p 417, 620
One-A-Day Plus Extra C Vitamins (Miles Consumer) p 417, 620
One-A-Day Stressgard Formula Vitamins (Miles Consumer) p 417, 620
One-A-Day Women's Formula Multivitamins with Calcium, Extra Iron, Zinc and Beta Carotene (Miles Consumer) p 417, 620
Os-Cal Fortified Tablets (Marion Merrell Dow) p 412, 585

Os-Cal Plus Tablets (Marion Merrell Dow) p 412, 586
Tri-Vi-Sol Vitamin Drops (Mead Johnson Nutritionals) p 415, 606
Tri-Vi-Sol Vitamin Drops with Iron (Mead Johnson Nutritionals) p 415, 606
Unicap T Tablets (Upjohn) p 432, 752
Vicon Plus (Whitby) p 433, 760
Vi-Zac (Whitby) p 433, 760
Zymacap Capsules (Roberts) p 666

VITAMIN A & VITAMIN D

Clocream Skin Protectant Cream (Roberts) p 664
Dairy Ease Real Milk (Sterling Health) p 429, 732
Sigtab Tablets (Roberts) p 421, 666
Stuart Prenatal Tablets (Stuart) p 431, 742
The Stuart Formula Tablets (J&J•Merck Consumer) p 410, 569

VITAMIN B COMPLEX

Stuart Prenatal Tablets (Stuart) p 431, 742
The Stuart Formula Tablets (J&J•Merck Consumer) p 410, 569
Surbex (Abbott) p 502
Unicap T Tablets (Upjohn) p 432, 752

VITAMIN B COMPLEX WITH VITAMIN C

Os-Cal Fortified Tablets (Marion Merrell Dow) p 412, 585
Os-Cal Plus Tablets (Marion Merrell Dow) p 412, 586
Sigtab Tablets (Roberts) p 421, 666
Stresstabs (Lederle) p 411, 577
Stresstabs + Iron, Advanced Formula (Lederle) p 411, 577
Stresstabs + Zinc (Lederle) p 411, 577
Sublingual B-Total (Sublingual Products) p 431, 742
Sunkist Children's Chewable Multivitamins - Regular (CIBA Consumer) p 408, 554
Surbex with C (Abbott) p 502
Surbex-T (Abbott) p 403, 502
Thera-Combex H-P (Parke-Davis) p 637
Theragran Stress Formula (Apothecon) p 403, 509
Theragran Tablets (Apothecon) p 403, 508
Theragran-M Tablets (Apothecon) p 403, 508
Vicon Plus (Whitby) p 433, 760
Vicon-C Capsules (Whitby) p 433, 760
Zymacap Capsules (Roberts) p 666

VITAMIN B$_1$

Allbee with C Caplets (Robins Consumer) p 667
Allbee C-800 Plus Iron Tablets (Robins Consumer) p 666
Allbee C-800 Tablets (Robins Consumer) p 666
Bugs Bunny Children's Chewable Vitamins (Sugar Free) (Miles Consumer) p 416, 617
Bugs Bunny With Extra C Children's Chewable Vitamins (Sugar Free) (Miles Consumer) p 416, 618
Bugs Bunny Plus Iron Children's Chewable Vitamins (Sugar Free) (Miles Consumer) p 416, 617
Flintstones Children's Chewable Vitamins (Miles Consumer) p 416, 617
Flintstones Children's Chewable Vitamins With Extra C (Miles Consumer) p 416, 618
Flintstones Children's Chewable Vitamins Plus Iron (Miles Consumer) p 416, 617
One-A-Day Essential Vitamins (Miles Consumer) p 417, 620
One-A-Day Maximum Formula Vitamins and Minerals (Miles Consumer) p 417, 620
One-A-Day Plus Extra C Vitamins (Miles Consumer) p 417, 620

One-A-Day Stressgard Formula Vitamins (Miles Consumer) p 417, 620
One-A-Day Women's Formula Multivitamins with Calcium, Extra Iron, Zinc and Beta Carotene (Miles Consumer) p 417, 620
Troph-Iron Liquid (Menley & James) p 611
Trophite Liquid (Menley & James) p 612
Z-BEC Tablets (Robins Consumer) p 676

VITAMIN B$_2$

Allbee with C Caplets (Robins Consumer) p 667
Allbee C-800 Plus Iron Tablets (Robins Consumer) p 666
Allbee C-800 Tablets (Robins Consumer) p 666
Bugs Bunny Children's Chewable Vitamins (Sugar Free) (Miles Consumer) p 416, 617
Bugs Bunny With Extra C Children's Chewable Vitamins (Sugar Free) (Miles Consumer) p 416, 618
Bugs Bunny Plus Iron Children's Chewable Vitamins (Sugar Free) (Miles Consumer) p 416, 617
Flintstones Children's Chewable Vitamins (Miles Consumer) p 416, 617
Flintstones Children's Chewable Vitamins With Extra C (Miles Consumer) p 416, 618
Flintstones Children's Chewable Vitamins Plus Iron (Miles Consumer) p 416, 617
Geritol Liquid - High Potency Iron & Vitamin Tonic (SmithKline Beecham) p 712
One-A-Day Essential Vitamins (Miles Consumer) p 417, 620
One-A-Day Maximum Formula Vitamins and Minerals (Miles Consumer) p 417, 620
One-A-Day Plus Extra C Vitamins (Miles Consumer) p 417, 620
One-A-Day Stressgard Formula Vitamins (Miles Consumer) p 417, 620
One-A-Day Women's Formula Multivitamins with Calcium, Extra Iron, Zinc and Beta Carotene (Miles Consumer) p 417, 620
Stuart Prenatal Tablets (Stuart) p 431, 742
The Stuart Formula Tablets (J&J•Merck Consumer) p 410, 569
Stuartinic Tablets (J&J•Merck Consumer) p 410, 570
Vicon-C Capsules (Whitby) p 433, 760
Z-BEC Tablets (Robins Consumer) p 676

**VITAMIN B$_3$
(see under NIACIN)**

VITAMIN B$_6$

Allbee with C Caplets (Robins Consumer) p 667
Allbee C-800 Plus Iron Tablets (Robins Consumer) p 666
Allbee C-800 Tablets (Robins Consumer) p 666
Beelith Tablets (Beach) p 514
Bugs Bunny Children's Chewable Vitamins (Sugar Free) (Miles Consumer) p 416, 617
Bugs Bunny With Extra C Children's Chewable Vitamins (Sugar Free) (Miles Consumer) p 416, 618
Bugs Bunny Plus Iron Children's Chewable Vitamins (Sugar Free) (Miles Consumer) p 416, 617
Flintstones Children's Chewable Vitamins (Miles Consumer) p 416, 617
Flintstones Children's Chewable Vitamins With Extra C (Miles Consumer) p 416, 618

Flintstones Children's Chewable Vitamins Plus Iron (Miles Consumer) p 416, 617
Geritol Liquid - High Potency Iron & Vitamin Tonic (SmithKline Beecham) p 712
Marlyn Formula 50 (Marlyn) p 586
Marlyn Formula 50 Mega Forte (Marlyn) p 587
One-A-Day Essential Vitamins (Miles Consumer) p 417, 620
One-A-Day Maximum Formula Vitamins and Minerals (Miles Consumer) p 417, 620
One-A-Day Plus Extra C Vitamins (Miles Consumer) p 417, 620
One-A-Day Stressgard Formula Vitamins (Miles Consumer) p 417, 620
One-A-Day Women's Formula Multivitamins with Calcium, Extra Iron, Zinc and Beta Carotene (Miles Consumer) p 417, 620
Stuart Prenatal Tablets (Stuart) p 431, 742
The Stuart Formula Tablets (J&J•Merck Consumer) p 410, 569
Sunkist Children's Chewable Multivitamins - Complete (CIBA Consumer) p 408, 555
Z-BEC Tablets (Robins Consumer) p 676

VITAMIN B$_{12}$

Allbee C-800 Plus Iron Tablets (Robins Consumer) p 666
Allbee C-800 Tablets (Robins Consumer) p 666
Bugs Bunny Children's Chewable Vitamins (Sugar Free) (Miles Consumer) p 416, 617
Bugs Bunny With Extra C Children's Chewable Vitamins (Sugar Free) (Miles Consumer) p 416, 618
Bugs Bunny Plus Iron Children's Chewable Vitamins (Sugar Free) (Miles Consumer) p 416, 617
Centrum Silver (Lederle) p 411, 575
Ener-B Vitamin B$_{12}$ Nasal Gel Dietary Supplement (Nature's Bounty) p 417, 622
Flintstones Children's Chewable Vitamins (Miles Consumer) p 416, 617
Flintstones Children's Chewable Vitamins With Extra C (Miles Consumer) p 416, 618
Flintstones Children's Chewable Vitamins Plus Iron (Miles Consumer) p 416, 617
Geritol Liquid - High Potency Iron & Vitamin Tonic (SmithKline Beecham) p 712
One-A-Day Essential Vitamins (Miles Consumer) p 417, 620
One-A-Day Maximum Formula Vitamins and Minerals (Miles Consumer) p 417, 620
One-A-Day Plus Extra C Vitamins (Miles Consumer) p 417, 620
One-A-Day Stressgard Formula Vitamins (Miles Consumer) p 417, 620
One-A-Day Women's Formula Multivitamins with Calcium, Extra Iron, Zinc and Beta Carotene (Miles Consumer) p 417, 620
Stuart Prenatal Tablets (Stuart) p 431, 742
The Stuart Formula Tablets (J&J•Merck Consumer) p 410, 569
Stuartinic Tablets (J&J•Merck Consumer) p 410, 570
Troph-Iron Liquid (Menley & James) p 611
Trophite Liquid (Menley & James) p 612
Z-BEC Tablets (Robins Consumer) p 676

VITAMIN B₁₂, NASAL DELIVERY

Ener-B Vitamin B₁₂ Nasal Gel Dietary Supplement (Nature's Bounty) p 417, 622

VITAMIN C

Allbee with C Caplets (Robins Consumer) p 667
Allbee C-800 Plus Iron Tablets (Robins Consumer) p 666
Allbee C-800 Tablets (Robins Consumer) p 666
Bugs Bunny Children's Chewable Vitamins (Sugar Free) (Miles Consumer) p 416, 617
Bugs Bunny With Extra C Children's Chewable Vitamins (Sugar Free) (Miles Consumer) p 416, 618
Bugs Bunny Plus Iron Children's Chewable Vitamins (Sugar Free) (Miles Consumer) p 416, 617
Centrum, Jr. (Children's Chewable) + Extra C (Lederle) p 410, 573
Ester-C Tablets (Inter-Cal) p 564
Ferancee Chewable Tablets (J&J•Merck Consumer) p 566
Ferancee-HP Tablets (J&J•Merck Consumer) p 409, 566
Flintstones Children's Chewable Vitamins (Miles Consumer) p 416, 617
Flintstones Children's Chewable Vitamins With Extra C (Miles Consumer) p 416, 618
Flintstones Children's Chewable Vitamins Plus Iron (Miles Consumer) p 416, 617
Halls Vitamin C Drops (Warner-Lambert) p 433, 756
Hyland's Vitamin C for Children (Standard Homeopathic) p 723
N'ICE Sugarless Vitamin C Drops (SmithKline Beecham) p 427, 714
One-A-Day Essential Vitamins (Miles Consumer) p 417, 620
One-A-Day Maximum Formula Vitamins and Minerals (Miles Consumer) p 417, 620
One-A-Day Plus Extra C Vitamins (Miles Consumer) p 417, 620
One-A-Day Stressgard Formula Vitamins (Miles Consumer) p 417, 620
One-A-Day Women's Formula Multivitamins with Calcium, Extra Iron, Zinc and Beta Carotene (Miles Consumer) p 417, 620
Stuart Prenatal Tablets (Stuart) p 431, 742
The Stuart Formula Tablets (J&J•Merck Consumer) p 410, 569
Stuartinic Tablets (J&J•Merck Consumer) p 410, 570
Sublingual C with Niacin (Sublingual Products) p 743
Sunkist Children's Chewable Multivitamins - Plus Extra C (CIBA Consumer) p 408, 555
Sunkist Vitamin C - Chewable (CIBA Consumer) p 408, 555
Sunkist Vitamin C - Easy to Swallow (CIBA Consumer) p 408, 555
Surbex with C (Abbott) p 502
Theragran Liquid (Apothecon) p 403, 508
Tri-Vi-Sol Vitamin Drops (Mead Johnson Nutritionals) p 415, 606
Tri-Vi-Sol Vitamin Drops with Iron (Mead Johnson Nutritionals) p 415, 606
Vi-Zac (Whitby) p 433, 760
Z-BEC Tablets (Robins Consumer) p 676

VITAMIN D

Bugs Bunny Children's Chewable Vitamins (Sugar Free) (Miles Consumer) p 416, 617
Bugs Bunny With Extra C Children's Chewable Vitamins (Sugar Free) (Miles Consumer) p 416, 618

Bugs Bunny Plus Iron Children's Chewable Vitamins (Sugar Free) (Miles Consumer) p 416, 617
Caltrate 600 + Iron & Vitamin D (Lederle) p 410, 572
Caltrate 600 + Vitamin D (Lederle) p 410, 572
Flintstones Children's Chewable Vitamins (Miles Consumer) p 416, 617
Flintstones Children's Chewable Vitamins With Extra C (Miles Consumer) p 416, 618
Flintstones Children's Chewable Vitamins Plus Iron (Miles Consumer) p 416, 617
One-A-Day Essential Vitamins (Miles Consumer) p 417, 620
One-A-Day Maximum Formula Vitamins and Minerals (Miles Consumer) p 417, 620
One-A-Day Plus Extra C Vitamins (Miles Consumer) p 417, 620
One-A-Day Stressgard Formula Vitamins (Miles Consumer) p 417, 620
One-A-Day Women's Formula Multivitamins with Calcium, Extra Iron, Zinc and Beta Carotene (Miles Consumer) p 417, 620
Os-Cal 250+D Tablets (Marion Merrell Dow) p 412, 585
Os-Cal 500+D Tablets (Marion Merrell Dow) p 412, 585
Os-Cal Fortified Tablets (Marion Merrell Dow) p 412, 585
Os-Cal Plus Tablets (Marion Merrell Dow) p 412, 586
Posture-D 600 mg (Whitehall) p 768
Tri-Vi-Sol Vitamin Drops (Mead Johnson Nutritionals) p 415, 606
Tri-Vi-Sol Vitamin Drops with Iron (Mead Johnson Nutritionals) p 415, 606
Zymacap Capsules (Roberts) p 666

VITAMIN D₂

Drisdol (Sanofi Winthrop Pharmaceuticals) p 689

VITAMIN E

Allbee C-800 Plus Iron Tablets (Robins Consumer) p 666
Allbee C-800 Tablets (Robins Consumer) p 666
Bugs Bunny Children's Chewable Vitamins (Sugar Free) (Miles Consumer) p 416, 617
Bugs Bunny With Extra C Children's Chewable Vitamins (Sugar Free) (Miles Consumer) p 416, 618
Bugs Bunny Plus Iron Children's Chewable Vitamins (Sugar Free) (Miles Consumer) p 416, 617
Flintstones Children's Chewable Vitamins (Miles Consumer) p 416, 617
Flintstones Children's Chewable Vitamins With Extra C (Miles Consumer) p 416, 618
Flintstones Children's Chewable Vitamins Plus Iron (Miles Consumer) p 416, 617
Natural Best Vitamin E 1000 I.U. and 400 I.U. (Neutrin) p 417, 622
One-A-Day Essential Vitamins (Miles Consumer) p 417, 620
One-A-Day Maximum Formula Vitamins and Minerals (Miles Consumer) p 417, 620
One-A-Day Plus Extra C Vitamins (Miles Consumer) p 417, 620
One-A-Day Stressgard Formula Vitamins (Miles Consumer) p 417, 620
One-A-Day Women's Formula Multivitamins with Calcium, Extra Iron, Zinc and Beta Carotene (Miles Consumer) p 417, 620
Q-vel Muscle Relaxant Pain Reliever (CIBA Consumer) p 408, 554
Stuart Prenatal Tablets (Stuart) p 431, 742

The Stuart Formula Tablets (J&J•Merck Consumer) p 410, 569
Vicon Plus (Whitby) p 433, 760
Vi-Zac (Whitby) p 433, 760
Z-BEC Tablets (Robins Consumer) p 676

VITAMIN K

One-A-Day Maximum Formula Vitamins and Minerals (Miles Consumer) p 417, 620

VITAMINS WITH IRON

Geritol Extend Caplets (SmithKline Beecham) p 712

VITAMINS WITH MINERALS

Bugs Bunny Complete Children's Chewable Vitamins + Minerals with Iron and Calcium (Sugar Free) (Miles Consumer) p 416, 618
Centrum (Lederle) p 410, 572
Centrum, Jr. (Children's Chewable) + Extra C (Lederle) p 410, 573
Centrum, Jr. (Children's Chewable) + Extra Calcium (Lederle) p 411, 573
Centrum, Jr. (Children's Chewable) + Iron (Lederle) p 410, 573
Centrum Liquid (Lederle) p 411, 572
Centrum Silver (Lederle) p 411, 575
Femiron Multi Vitamins and Iron (Menley & James) p 415, 609
Filibon Prenatal Vitamin Tablets (Lederle) p 575
Flintstones Complete With Calcium, Iron & Minerals Children's Chewable Vitamins (Miles Consumer) p 416, 618
Geritol Complete Tablets (SmithKline Beecham) p 711
Geritol Extend Caplets (SmithKline Beecham) p 712
Gevrabon Liquid (Lederle) p 576
Gevral T Tablets (Lederle) p 576
Gevral Tablets (Lederle) p 576
Myadec (Parke-Davis) p 419, 635
Natabec Kapseals (Parke-Davis) p 636
One-A-Day Maximum Formula Vitamins and Minerals (Miles Consumer) p 417, 620
Optilets-M-500 Filmtab (Abbott) p 403, 502
Stuart Prenatal Tablets (Stuart) p 431, 742
The Stuart Formula Tablets (J&J•Merck Consumer) p 410, 569
Stuartinic Tablets (J&J•Merck Consumer) p 410, 570
Sunkist Children's Chewable Multivitamins - Complete (CIBA Consumer) p 408, 555
Sunkist Children's Chewable Multivitamins - Plus Extra C (CIBA Consumer) p 408, 555
Sunkist Children's Chewable Multivitamins - Plus Iron (CIBA Consumer) p 408, 555
Sunkist Children's Chewable Multivitamins - Regular (CIBA Consumer) p 408, 554
Theragran Stress Formula (Apothecon) p 403, 509
Theragran-M Tablets (Apothecon) p 403, 508
Unicap M Tablets (Upjohn) p 432, 751
Unicap Plus Iron Vitamin Formula Tablets (Upjohn) p 751
Unicap T Tablets (Upjohn) p 432, 752
Vicon Plus (Whitby) p 433, 760
Vicon-C Capsules (Whitby) p 433, 760
Vi-Zac (Whitby) p 433, 760

VITAMINS, MULTIPLE

Centrum, Jr. (Children's Chewable) + Extra C (Lederle) p 410, 573
Optilets-500 Filmtab (Abbott) p 403, 502
Unicap Softgel Capsules & Tablets (Upjohn) p 432, 751
Unicap Jr. Chewable Tablets (Upjohn) p 751
Unicap Sr. Tablets (Upjohn) p 432, 752

VITAMINS, SUPPLEMENT

Natabec Kapseals (Parke-Davis) p 636
Sigtab Tablets (Roberts) p 421, 666
Theragran Liquid (Apothecon) p 403, 508
Theragran Tablets (Apothecon) p 403, 508

W

WHITE PETROLATUM

Caldesene Medicated Ointment (Fisons Consumer Health) p 409, 559
Chap Stick Petroleum Jelly Plus (Robins Consumer) p 421, 668
Chap Stick Petroleum Jelly Plus with Sunblock 15 (Robins Consumer) p 421, 668
Duolube Eye Ointment (Bausch & Lomb Personal) p 403, 514
Lacri-Lube NP Lubricant Ophthalmic Ointment (Allergan Pharmaceuticals) p 504
Lacri-Lube S.O.P. Sterile Ophthalmic Ointment (Allergan Pharmaceuticals) p 504
Refresh P.M. Lubricant Ophthalmic Ointment (Allergan Pharmaceuticals) p 505

WITCH HAZEL

Tucks Cream (Parke-Davis) p 637
Tucks Premoistened Pads (Parke-Davis) p 420, 637
Tucks Take-Alongs (Parke-Davis) p 637

WOOL WAX ALCOHOL

Eucerin Dry Skin Care Creme (Beiersdorf) p 404, 515

X

XYLOMETAZOLINE HYDROCHLORIDE

Otrivin Nasal Drops (CIBA Consumer) p 408, 553
Otrivin Pediatric Nasal Drops (CIBA Consumer) p 408, 553

Z

ZINC

One-A-Day Maximum Formula Vitamins and Minerals (Miles Consumer) p 417, 620
One-A-Day Stressgard Formula Vitamins (Miles Consumer) p 417, 620
One-A-Day Women's Formula Multivitamins with Calcium, Extra Iron, Zinc and Beta Carotene (Miles Consumer) p 417, 620
Stuart Prenatal Tablets (Stuart) p 431, 742
Sublingual Zinc (Sublingual Products) p 743
Vicon Plus (Whitby) p 433, 760
Vicon-C Capsules (Whitby) p 433, 760
Vi-Zac (Whitby) p 433, 760
Z-BEC Tablets (Robins Consumer) p 676

ZINC CHLORIDE

Orajel Mouth-Aid (Del Pharmaceuticals) p 408, 557

ZINC OXIDE

Anusol Ointment (Parke-Davis) p 418, 629
Balmex Baby Powder (Macsil) p 579
Balmex Ointment (Macsil) p 579

Caladryl Clear Lotion (Parke-Davis) p 419, 633
Caldesene Medicated Ointment (Fisons Consumer Health) p 409, 559
Desitin Ointment (Pfizer Consumer) p 420, 638
Nupercainal Suppositories (CIBA Consumer) p 408, 553
Pazo Hemorrhoid Ointment & Suppositories (Bristol-Myers Products) p 406, 534
Tronolane Hemorrhoidal Suppositories (Ross) p 422, 680
Extra Strength Vaseline Intensive Care Lotion (Chese-Pond's) p 548

ZINC PYRITHIONE
(see under PYRITHIONE ZINC)

ZINC SULFATE

Clear Eyes ACR Astringent/Lubricating Eye Redness Reliever (Ross) p 422, 677
Surbex-750 with Zinc (Abbott) p 403, 503
Visine A.C. Eye Drops (Pfizer Consumer) p 420, 641

ZINC UNDECYLENATE

Cruex Antifungal Cream (Fisons Consumer Health) p 409, 560
Cruex Antifungal Spray Powder (Fisons Consumer Health) p 409, 560
Desenex Antifungal Cream (Fisons Consumer Health) p 560
Desenex Antifungal Ointment (Fisons Consumer Health) p 409, 560
Desenex Antifungal Powder (Fisons Consumer Health) p 409, 560
Desenex Antifungal Spray Powder (Fisons Consumer Health) p 409, 560

DRUG INFORMATION CENTERS

Centers in each state are listed alphabetically by city.

ALABAMA

Drug Information Service
University of Alabama Hospital
Birmingham
Mon-Fri 8 AM-5 PM
(205) 934-2162

Samford Global Drug Information Center
Samford University
Birmingham
Mon-Fri 8 AM-4:30 PM
(205) 870-2891

Huntsville Hospital Drug Information Center
Huntsville
Mon-Fri 8 AM-5 PM
(205) 533-8284

ARIZONA

Arizona Poison and Drug Information Center
Arizona Health Science Center
Tucson
7 days/week, 24 hours
(602) 626-6016; (800) 362-0101

ARKANSAS

Arkansas Poison and Drug Information Center
University of Arkansas for Medical Sciences
Little Rock
Mon-Fri 8 AM-9 PM
(501) 666-5532

CALIFORNIA

Alta Bates-Herrick Hospital
Drug Information Service
Berkeley
Mon-Fri 8 AM-4:30 PM
(415) 540-1503

Drug Information Analysis Center
Valley Medical Center
Fresno
Mon-Fri 8 AM-4:30 PM
(209) 453-4596

Los Angeles County-University of Southern California
Drug Information Center
Los Angeles
Mon-Fri 7:45 AM-4:15 PM
(213) 226-7741

Drug Information Analysis Service
Veterans Administration Medical Center
San Diego
Mon-Fri 8 AM-4:30 PM
(619) 453-7500, ext 3026

Drug Information Center
US Naval Hospital
San Diego
Mon-Fri, 24-hour service
(619) 532-8414

UCSD Drug Information Service
San Diego
Mon-Fri 9 AM-5 PM
(619) 294-6085

Drug Information Analysis Service
University of California
San Francisco
Mon-Fri 8 AM-6 PM
(415) 476-4346

Drug Information Services
St. Johns Hospital and Health Center
Santa Monica
Mon-Fri 8 AM-5 PM
(213) 829-8243;
after hours (213) 829-8250

Drug Information Center
Stanford University Hospital
Stanford
Mon-Fri 9 AM-5 PM
(415) 723-6422

COLORADO

Rocky Mountain Drug Consultation Center
Denver
Mon-Fri 8:30 AM-3:30 PM
(303) 893-3784

Drug Information Center
University of Colorado Health Science Center
Denver
Mon-Fri 8 AM-4:30 PM
(303) 270-8489

CONNECTICUT

Drug Information Service
University of Connecticut Health Center
Farmington
Mon-Fri 8 AM-4:30 PM
(203) 679-2783

Drug Information Center
Hartford Hospital
Hartford
Mon-Fri 8:30 AM-5 PM
(203) 524-2221;
after hours (203) 524-2961

Drug Information Center
Yale-New Haven Hospital
New Haven
Mon-Fri 8:15 AM-4:45 PM
(203) 785-2248

DISTRICT OF COLUMBIA

Drug Information Center
Children's National Medical Center
Washington
Mon-Fri 8 AM-4:30 PM
(202) 745-2055; (202) 745-3171;
(202) 745-3172

Drug Information Center
Washington Hospital Center
Washington
Mon-Fri 7:30 AM-4 PM
(202) 877-6646

Drug Information Service
Howard University Hospital
Washington
Mon-Fri 8:30 AM-5 PM
(202) 865-1325

FLORIDA

Drug Information & Pharmacy Center
Shands Hospital at University of Florida
Gainesville
Mon-Fri 9 AM-5 PM
(904) 395-0408

Drug Information Service
University Medical Center
Jacksonville
Mon - Fri 8 AM-5 PM
(904) 549-4095

Drug Information Center
University of Miami/Jackson Memorial Center
Miami
Mon-Fri 9 AM-5 PM
(305) 585-6898

Drug Information Center
VA Medical Center
Miami
Mon-Fri 7:30 AM-4 PM
(305) 324-4455, ext 3237

Drug Information Service
Southeastern University of the Health Sciences
North Miami Beach
Mon-Fri 9 AM-5 PM
(305) 948-8255

GEORGIA

Drug Information Center
Emory University Hospital
Atlanta
Mon-Fri 8:30 AM-5 PM
(404) 727-4644

Drug Information Service
Northside Hospital
Atlanta
Mon-Fri 8 AM-5 PM
(404) 851-8676

Drug Information Center
University of Georgia
Medical College of Georgia
Augusta
Mon-Fri 8:30 AM-5 PM
(404) 721-2887

Drug Information Center
Mercer University School of Pharmacy
Atlanta
Mon-Fri 8 AM-4 PM
(404) 223-7725

IDAHO

Idaho Drug Information Service
Pocatello Regional Medical Center
Pocatello
Mon-Fri 8 AM-4:30 PM
(208) 234-0777

ILLINOIS

Drug Information Center
Northwestern Memorial Hospital
Chicago
Mon-Fri 8:30 AM-5 PM
(312) 908-7573

Drug Information Center
University of Illinois at Chicago
Chicago
Mon-Fri 8 AM-5 PM
(312) 996-3681

Drug Information Service
Saint Joseph Hospital and Health Care Center
Chicago
7 days/week, 24 hours
(312) 975-3199

Drug Information Services
University of Chicago
Chicago
Mon-Fri 8 AM-5 PM
(312) 702-1388

Drug Information Center
Ingalls Memorial Hospital
Harvey
Mon-Fri 8 AM-4:30 PM
(708) 333-2300, ext 4430

Edgar M. Stevenson Drug Information
Resource Center
Brokaw Hospital
Normal
Mon-Fri 8 AM-4:30 PM
(309) 454-1400

Drug Information Center
Lutheran General Hospital
Park Ridge
Mon-Fri 8 AM-5 PM
(708) 696-8128

Drug Information Center
Swedish-American Hospital
Rockford
7 days/week, 24 hours
(815) 968-4400, ext 4577

INDIANA

Drug Information Center
St. Vincent Hospital
Indianapolis
Mon-Fri 8 AM-4 PM
(317) 871-3200

Drug Information Services
Indiana University Medical Center
Indianapolis
Mon-Fri 8 AM-4:30 PM
(317) 274-3581

IOWA

Drug Information Center
Mercy Hospital Medical Center
Des Moines
7 days/week, 24 hours
(515) 247-3286

Variety Club Drug and Poison
Information Center
Iowa Methodist Medical Center
Des Moines
7 days/week, 24 hours
(515) 283-6254;
(800) 362-2327 (Iowa only)

Drug Information Center
University of Iowa Hospital and Clinics
Iowa City
Open 24 hours, 7 days
(319) 356-2600

KANSAS

Drug Information Center
Kansas University Medical Center
Kansas City
Mon-Fri 8 AM-4 PM
(913) 588-2328

KENTUCKY

Drug Information Center
Chandler Medical Center
College of Pharmacy
University of Kentucky
Lexington
Mon-Fri 8 AM-5 PM
(606) 233-5320

LOUISIANA

Drug Information Center- Poison Control Center
St. Francis Medical Center
Monroe
7 days/week, 24 hours
(318) 325-6454

Xavier University
Drug Information Center at
Tulane Medical Center Hospital and Clinic
New Orleans
Mon-Fri 9 AM-5 PM
(504) 588-5670

MARYLAND

Drug Information Services
The Anne Arundel Medical Center
Annapolis
7 days, 24 hours
(301) 267-1130; (301) 267-1000

Drug Information Center
Franklin Square Hospital Center
Baltimore
Mon-Fri 8 AM-5 PM
(301) 682-7700;
after hours (301) 682-7374

Drug Information Center
University of Maryland Medical System
Baltimore
Mon-Fri 8:30 AM-5 PM
(301) 328-5668

Drug Information Service
Baltimore
Mon-Fri 8 AM-5 PM
(301) 955-6348

Drug Information Service
Clinical Pharmacy Department
National Institutes of Health
Bethesda
Mon-Fri 8:30 AM-5 PM
(301) 496-2407

Drug Information Services
Malcolm Grow USAF Medical Center
Camp Springs
Mon-Fri 7:30 AM-6 PM
(301) 981-4209

Drug Information Center
Memorial Hospital
Easton
7 days/week, 24 hours
(301) 822-1000, ext 5645

MASSACHUSETTS

Drug Information Service
Brigham and Women's Hospital
Boston
5 days, 7 AM-5 PM
(617) 732-7166

Drug Information Service
New England Medical Center
Boston
Mon-Fri 8 AM-4:30 PM
(617) 956-5377

Drug Information Center
UMMC Hospital
Worcester
Mon-Fri 8:30 AM-5 PM
(508) 856-3456;
after hours (508) 856-2775

MICHIGAN

Drug Information Service
University of Michigan Medical Center
Ann Arbor
Mon-Fri 8 AM-5 PM
(313) 936-8200;
after hours (313) 936-8251

Drug Information Center
Henry Ford Hospital
Detroit
Mon-Fri 8 AM-5 PM
(313) 876-1229

Drug Information Service
Sinai Hospital
Detroit
Mon-Fri 8 AM-4:30 PM
(313) 493-5692

Drug Information Services
Harper Hospital
Detroit
Mon-Fri 8 AM-5 PM
(313) 745-2006;
after hours (313) 745-8638

Bronson Drug & Poison Information Center
Bronson Methodist Hospital
Kalamazoo
7 days/week, 24 hours
(616) 341-6409

Drug Information Center
Sparrow Hospital
Lansing
Mon-Fri 8 AM-4:30 PM
(517) 483-2444

Drug Information Center
St. Joseph Mercy Hospital
Pontiac
Mon-Fri 8 AM-4:30 PM
(313) 858-3055

Drug Information Services
William Beaumont Hospital
Royal Oak
Mon-Fri 8 AM-4:30 PM
(313) 551-4077

Drug Information Center
Saginaw General Hospital
Saginaw
7 days/week, 24 hours
(517) 755-1111

Drug Information Service
Providence Hospital
Southfield
Mon-Fri 8 AM-4:30 PM
(313) 424-3125

MINNESOTA

Drug Information Center
St. Mary's Hospital
Rochester
Mon-Fri 8 AM-4:30 PM
(507) 255-5062;
after hours (507) 255-5732

Drug Information Center
United Hospital and Children's Hospital of St. Paul
St. Paul
Mon-Fri 9 AM-5 PM
(612) 220-8566

MISSISSIPPI

Drug Information Center
University of Mississippi Medical Center
Jackson
Mon-Fri 8 AM-5 PM; on call 24 hours
(601) 984-2060

MISSOURI

Drug Information Center
St. John's Regional Health Center
Springfield
Mon-Fri 7:30 AM-4:30 PM
(417) 885-3488

Drug Information Service
Heartland Hospital West
St. Joseph
7 days/week, 24 hours
(816) 271-7582

St. Louis Drug Information Center
St. Louis
7 days/week, 24 hours
(314) 454-8399

NEBRASKA

Drug Information Service
School of Pharmacy
Creighton University
Omaha
Mon-Fri 8:30 AM-4:30 PM
(402) 280-5101
FAX: (402) 280-5147

Drug Information and Education Services
University of Nebraska Medical Center
Omaha
Mon-Fri 8 AM-4:30 PM
(402) 559-4114

NEW HAMPSHIRE

Drug Information Center
Dartmouth-Hitchcock Medical Center
Lebanon
Mon-Fri 7:30 AM-4 PM
(603) 650-5590

NEW MEXICO

New Mexico Poison & Drug Information Center
University of New Mexico
Albuquerque
7 days/week, 24 hours
(505) 843-2551;
(800) 432-6866 (NM only)

NEW YORK

Drug Information Service
Bellevue Hospital Center
New York
Mon-Fri 9 AM-5 PM
(212) 561-6504

Drug Information Center
Memorial Sloan-Kettering Cancer Center
New York
Mon-Fri 9 AM-5 PM
(212) 639-7552

Drug Information Center
Bronx Municipal Hospital Center
Bronx
Mon-Fri 9 AM-5 PM
(212) 918-4556; (212) 918-1574

International Drug Information Center
Long Island University
Arnold & Marie Schwartz College of Pharmacy
Brooklyn
Mon-Fri 9 AM-5 PM
(718) 403-1064;
(718) 834-6000, ext 3728

Drug Information Center
Erie County Medical Center
Buffalo
Mon-Fri 8 AM-5 PM
(716) 898-3000, ext 5061

Drug Information Center
The Mary Imogene Bassett Hospital
Cooperstown
Mon-Fri 8:30 AM-5 PM
(607) 547-3686

Drug Information Center
St. John's University at Long Island
Jewish Medical Center
New Hyde Park
Mon-Fri 9 AM-3 PM
(718) 470-DRUG

Drug Information Center
Lenox Hill Hospital
New York
Mon-Fri 9 AM-5 PM
(212) 439-3190

Drug Information Center
Mount Sinai Medical Center
New York
Mon-Fri 9 AM-5 PM
(212) 241-6619

Drug Information Service
The New York Hospital
New York
Mon-Fri 9 AM-5 PM
(212) 746-0741

Drug Information Service
University of Rochester/Strong Memorial Hospital
Rochester
Mon-Fri 8 AM-5 PM
(716) 275-3718;
after hours (716) 275-2681

Suffolk Drug Information Center
University Hospital
SUNY-Stony Brook
Stony Brook
Mon-Fri 8 AM-4:30 PM
(516) 444-2672;
after hours (516) 444-2680

NORTH CAROLINA

Drug Information Center
University of North Carolina Hospitals
University of North Carolina
Chapel Hill
Mon-Fri 8 AM-5 PM
(919) 966-2373;
after hours (919) 966-4131, pager 3866

Triad Poison and Drug Information Center
Moses H. Cone Memorial Hospital
Greensboro
7 days/week, 24 hours
(919) 379-4105

Eastern Carolina Drug Information Center
Pitt County Memorial Hospital
Greenville
Mon-Fri 8 AM-4:30 PM
(919) 551-4257

Drug Information Service Center
North Carolina Baptist Hospital/Bowman-Gray
Medical Center
Winston-Salem
Mon-Fri 8 AM-5 PM
(919) 748-2037

OHIO

Drug Information Center
Ohio Northern University
Ada
Mon-Fri 9 AM-3 PM
(419) 772-2307

Cleveland Clinic Foundation Drug Information Center
Cleveland
Mon-Fri 8 AM-4:30 PM
(216) 444-6456

Drug Information Center
Ohio State University Hospital
Columbus
Mon-Fri 8 AM-4 PM
(614) 293-8679

Drug Information Center
Riverside Methodist Hospitals
Columbus
Mon-Fri 8 AM-5 PM
(614) 566-5425

Western Ohio Poison & Drug Information Center
The Children's Medical Center
Dayton
7 days/week, 24 hours
(513) 222-2227;
(1-800) 762-0727 (Ohio only)

Drug Information Service
The Toledo Hospital
Toledo
Mon-Fri 8 AM-4:30 PM
(419) 471-2171;
after hours (419) 471-5637

Drug Information/Poison Center
Bethesda Hospital
Zanesville
7 days/week, 24 hours
(614) 454-4221; (614) 454-4300;
(800) 686-4221

OKLAHOMA

Drug Information Center
Presbyterian Hospital
Oklahoma City
Mon-Fri 7 AM-3:30 PM
(405) 271-6226

Drug Information Service
University of Oklahoma
Health Sciences Center
Oklahoma City
Mon-Fri 8 AM-5 PM
(405) 271-8080

Drug Information Service
St. Francis Hospital
Tulsa
Mon-Fri 9 AM-5:30 PM
(918) 494-6339
FAX: (918) 494-1893

OREGON

University Drug Consultation Service
The Oregon Health Sciences University
Portland
Mon-Fri 8:30 AM-5 PM
(503) 494-7530

PENNSYLVANIA

Drug Information and Pharmacoepidemiology Center
University of Pittsburgh Medical Center
Pittsburgh
8 AM-6 PM
(412) 624-3784

Pharmacy and Drug Information Services
Hamot Medical Center
Erie
7 days/week, 24 hours
(814) 870-6022

Drug Information Center
Temple University Hospital
Philadelphia
Mon-Fri 8 AM-4:30 PM
(215) 221-4644

Drug Information Center
Thomas Jefferson University Hospital
Philadelphia
Mon-Fri 8 AM-5 PM;
on call after hours (215) 955-8877

Drug Information Center
Medical College of Pennsylvania
Philadelphia
7 days/week, 24 hours
(215) 842-6550

Center for Drug Information
Mercy Hospital of Pittsburgh
Pittsburgh, PA
Mon-Fri 7:30 AM-8 PM
(412) 232-7903; (412) 232-7907

Drug Information Center
Allegheny General Hospital
Pittsburgh
Mon-Fri 8 AM-4:30 PM
(412) 359-3192

Drug Information Center
Crozer-Chester Medical Center
Upland
Mon-Fri 8 AM-4:30 PM
(215) 447-2843;
after hours (215) 447-2862

Drug Information Center
Williamsport Hospital and Medical Center
Williamsport
Mon-Fri 8 AM-4:30 PM;
on call 7 days/week, 24 hours
(717) 321-3289

PUERTO RICO

Centro de Informacion de Medicamentos
Colegio de Farmacia RCM
San Juan
Mon-Fri 8 AM-4 PM
(809) 758-2525, ext 1516;
(809) 763-0196

RHODE ISLAND

Drug Information Service
Rhode Island Hospital
Providence
Mon-Fri 8:30 AM-5 PM
(401) 277-5547

University of Rhode Island
Drug Information Center
Roger Williams Hospital
Providence
Mon-Fri 8 AM-4 PM
(401) 456-2260

SOUTH CAROLINA

Drug Information Service
Medical University of South Carolina
Charleston
Mon-Fri 8 AM-4 PM
(803) 792-3896;
(800) 922-5250 (SC only)

Drug Information Center
Spartanburg Regional Medical Center
Spartanburg
Mon-Fri 8 AM-5 PM
(803) 591-6910;
after hours (803) 591-6779

SOUTH DAKOTA

South Dakota Drug Information Center
Brookings
7 days/week, 8 AM-4:30 PM
(800) 456-1004

Drug Information Center
McKennan Hospital
Sioux Falls
7 days/week, 24 hours
(605) 336-3894;
(800) 952-0123 (Iowa only);
(800) 843-0505 (out of state)

TENNESSEE

Drug Information Center
University of Tennessee Medical Center
Knoxville
Mon-Fri 8 AM-4:30 PM
(615) 544-9125

Drug Information Center
University of Tennessee
Memphis
Mon-Fri 8 AM-5 PM
(901) 528-5555

South East Regional Drug Information Center
Memphis
Mon-Fri 7:30 AM-4 PM
(901) 523-8990, ext 5191

TEXAS

Drug Information Center
University of Texas Medical Branch
Galveston
Mon-Fri 8 AM-5 PM
(409) 772-2734

Drug Information Center
M.D. Anderson Cancer Center
Houston
Mon-Fri 8 AM-4:30 PM
(713) 792-2858;
after hours (713) 792-2875

Drug Information Center
Methodist Hospital
Houston
Mon-Fri 8 AM-5 PM
(713) 790-4190

Drug Information Center
St. Luke's Episcopal Hospital/Texas Heart Institute
Houston
7 days/week, 24 hours
(713) 791-3098

Hermann Drug Information Center
Hermann Hospital
Houston
Mon-Fri 8 AM-4:30 PM
(713) 797-2073

Drug Information Center
Wilford Hall USAF Medical Center
Lackland AFB
Mon-Fri 7:30 AM-5 PM
(512) 670-6291

Methodist Hospital Drug Information &
Consultation Service
Lubbock
Mon-Fri 8 AM-5 PM
(806) 793-4012

Drug Information Center
Scott and White Memorial Hospital
Temple
Mon-Fri 8 AM-5 PM
(817) 774-4636

Drug Information Center
Ben Taub General Hospital
Texas Southern University College of Pharmacy
and Health Sciences
Houston
8 AM-4 PM
(713) 793-2915

UTAH

Drug Information Center
University of Utah Hospital
Salt Lake City
Mon-Fri 8:30 AM-4:30 PM
(801) 581-2073

VIRGINIA

Drug Information Center
Santara Hampton General Hospital
Hampton
Mon-Fri 7:30 AM-4 PM
(804) 727-7185

Drug Information Center
St. Mary's Hospital
Richmond
Mon-Fri 7:30 AM-12 midnight
(804) 281-8058

WASHINGTON

Drug Information Center
Washington State University
College of Pharmacy
Spokane
Mon-Fri 8 AM-4:30 PM
(509) 456-4409

WEST VIRGINIA

West Virginia Drug Information Center
School of Pharmacy
Morgantown
Mon-Fri 9 AM-5 PM
(304) 293-5101;
(800) 352-2501 (WV only)

WISCONSIN

Drug Information Center
University of Wisconsin Hospital
Madison
7 days/week, 24 hours
(608) 262-1315

WYOMING

Drug Information Center
University of Wyoming
Laramie
Mon-Fri 8 AM-5 PM
(307) 766-6128

SECTION 5
Product Identification Section

This section is designed to help you identify products and their packaging.

Participating manufacturers have included selected products in full color. Where capsules and tablets are included they are shown in actual size. Packages generally are reduced in size.

For more information on products included, refer to the description in the PRODUCT INFORMATION SECTION or check directly with the manufacturer.

While every effort has been made to reproduce products faithfully, this section should be considered only as a quick-reference identification aid.

INDEX BY MANUFACTURER

Abbott Laboratories 403
Adria Laboratories... 403
Apothecon 403
B.F. Ascher & Company, Inc............................... 403
Astra Pharmaceutical Products, Inc. 403

Bausch & Lomb 403
Beiersdorf Inc. 404
Boiron 404
Bristol-Myers Products 404
Burroughs Wellcome Company 406

CIBA Consumer Pharmaceuticals 407
Columbia Laboratories, Inc. 408
Copley Pharmaceutical 408

Fisons Consumer Health Division 408

ICN Pharmaceuticals, Inc. 409

Johnson & Johnson - Merck 409

Kramer Laboratories 410

Lederle Laboratories 410

Marion Merrell Dow, Inc. 411
McNeil Consumer Products Co. 412
Mead Johnson Nutritionals 414
Mead Johnson Pharmaceuticals 415
Menley & James Laboratories 415
Miles Inc. Consumer Healthcare Division 416

Nature's Bounty, Inc. 417
Neutrin Drug, Inc. 417
Neutrogena Dermatologics 417

Ohm Laboratories, Inc. 418
Ortho Advanced Care Products 418

Parke-Davis 418
Pfizer Consumer Health Care 420

Reed & Carnrick 420
Reese Chemical Co. 420
Rhône-Poulenc Rorer Pharmaceuticals Inc. ... 420
Roberts Pharmaceutical Corporation 421
A.H. Robins Company, Inc. 421
Ross Laboratories 422
Rydelle Laboratories, Inc. 423

Sandoz Pharmaceuticals/Consumer Div. 423
Schering-Plough Health Care Products 424
SmithKline Beecham Consumer Brands 426
Stellar Pharmacal Corporation 428
Sterling Health 428
Stuart Pharmaceuticals 431
Sublingual Products International 431

Thompson Medical Company, Inc. 431

The Upjohn Company 431

Wakunaga of America Co., Ltd. 432
Walker, Corp & Company, Inc. 432
Wallace Laboratories 432
Warner-Lambert Company 432
Westwood-Squibb Pharmaceuticals 433
Whitby Pharmaceuticals, Inc. 433
Whitehall Laboratories 434
Wyeth-Ayerst Laboratories 435

Zila Pharmaceuticals, Inc. 435

ABBOTT

Optilets®-500
(high potency thera-
peutic vitamin
formulation)

Optilets-M-500®
(high potency thera-
peutic vitamin formu-
lation with minerals)

Abbott

Surbex-T® Filmtab®
(high-potency B-complex
with 500 mg vitamin C)

Surbex®-750 With Iron Filmtab®
(high-potency B-complex with iron,
vitamin E and 750 mg of vitamin C)

Surbex®-750 With Zinc Filmtab®
(high-potency B-complex vitamins with zinc,
vitamin E and 750 mg of vitamin C)

ADRIA

Original
Flavor

Cherry
Flavor

EMETROL®
(phosphorated carbohydrate solution)

APOTHECON

**COMPLETE FORMULA
THERAGRAN-M®**
High Potency Multivitamin
Formula with Minerals

Apothecon

**COMPLETE FORMULA
THERAGRAN®**
High Potency Multivitamin
Formula

Apothecon

THERAGRAN® STRESS FORMULA
High Potency Multivitamin Formula
with Iron and Biotin

Apothecon

**THERAGRAN®
LIQUID**
High Potency Liquid
Vitamin Supplement

ASCHER

AYR® SALINE NASAL MIST

AYR® SALINE NASAL DROPS

B. F. Ascher & Co., Inc.

Available in 1.25 oz tube
ITCH-X® GEL
(benzyl alcohol 10% &
pramoxine hydrochloride 1%)

B. F. Ascher & Co., Inc.

Available: 18's, 50's & 100's
**MOBIGESIC®
ANALGESIC TABLETS**

B. F. Ascher & Co., Inc.

Also Available: 1.25 oz
**MOBISYL®
ANALGESIC CREME**

B. F. Ascher & Co., Inc.

Available in 8 oz bottle
PEN•KERA®

**Therapeutic Creme
for Chronic Dry Skin**

ASTRA

Available in 35g Tube

XYLOCAINE® 2.5% OINTMENT
(lidocaine)

BAUSCH & LOMB

0.5 fl. oz.

ALLERGY DROPS
Lubricant/Redness Reliever
Eye Drops

Bausch & Lomb

Preservative Free Artificial Tears
32 Sterile Single-Use Containers
0.01 fl. oz. Each
**DRY EYE THERAPY™
Lubricating Eye Drops**

Bausch & Lomb

⅛ oz.

DUOLUBE®
Lubricant Eye Ointment
Nighttime Relief for Dry Eyes

Bausch & Lomb

4 fl. oz.

EYE WASH

Cleanses, Refreshes and Soothes
Irritated Eyes

Beiersdorf

Cleansing Bar

Cleansing
Lotion

**EUCERIN®
Fragrance-Free Dry
Skin Care**

Bristol-Myers Products

Bottles of 30,
50 and 100
coated caplets

BUFFERIN® CAPLET
(buffered aspirin)

Bristol-Myers Products

Caplets: Blister packs of 24 and
bottles of 50. Tablets: Blister packs
of 24, bottles of 50, vials of 10.

**COMTREX®
CAPLETS AND TABLETS**

Bausch & Lomb

0.5 and 1.0 fl. oz. sizes
**MOISTURE DROPS®
ARTIFICIAL TEARS**

Lubricant Eye Drops
Soothing Relief for Dry Eyes

BOIRON

OSCILLOCOCCINUM®

Homeopathic remedy for the natural
relief of flu-like symptoms.
Now also available in new family
value pak. (6 doses)

Bristol-Myers Products

Bottles of 30,
50 and 100
coated tablets

**EXTRA STRENGTH
BUFFERIN® TABLET**
(buffered aspirin)

Bristol-Myers Products

Blister packs of 24 and 50

**COMTREX®
LIQUI-GELS**

BEIERSDORF

**AQUAPHOR®
Healing Ointment**
For dry skin, minor cuts and burns

Bristol-Myers Products

Bottles of 40
and 100
coated caplets

**ARTHRITIS STRENGTH
BUFFERIN® CAPLET**
(buffered aspirin)

Bristol-Myers Products

Bottles of
24 and 50
caplets

BUFFERIN® A/F NITE TIME
Analgesic/Sleeping Aid Caplets
(acetaminophen and diphenhydramine citrate)

Bristol-Myers Products

Available in blister packs of 24 and
bottles of 50
**COMTREX® A/S MULTI-SYMPTOM
CAPLETS AND TABLETS
ALLERGY-SINUS FORMULA**
(acetaminophen, pseudoephedrine,
chlorpheniramine)

Beiersdorf

Creme

Moisturizing

Daily
Facial
Cleanser

**EUCERIN®
Fragrance-Free Dry
Skin Care**

Bristol-Myers Products

Bottles of 12, 30, 50,
100, 200 and 1000,
and vials of 10

Hospital/Institutional
packs of 150 x 2
tablets in foil packets

BUFFERIN® TABLET
(buffered aspirin)

Bristol-Myers Products

Bottles of
6 oz.

COMTREX® LIQUID

Bristol-Myers Products

Muti-
Symptom
Cold
Reliever

Day   Night

Blister packs of 24
DAY-NIGHT COMTREX®
Caplets: (acetaminophen, pseudoephedrine HCl, dextromethorphan HBr)
Tablets: (acetaminophen, pseudoephedrine HCl, dextromethorphan HBr,
chlorpheniramine maleate)

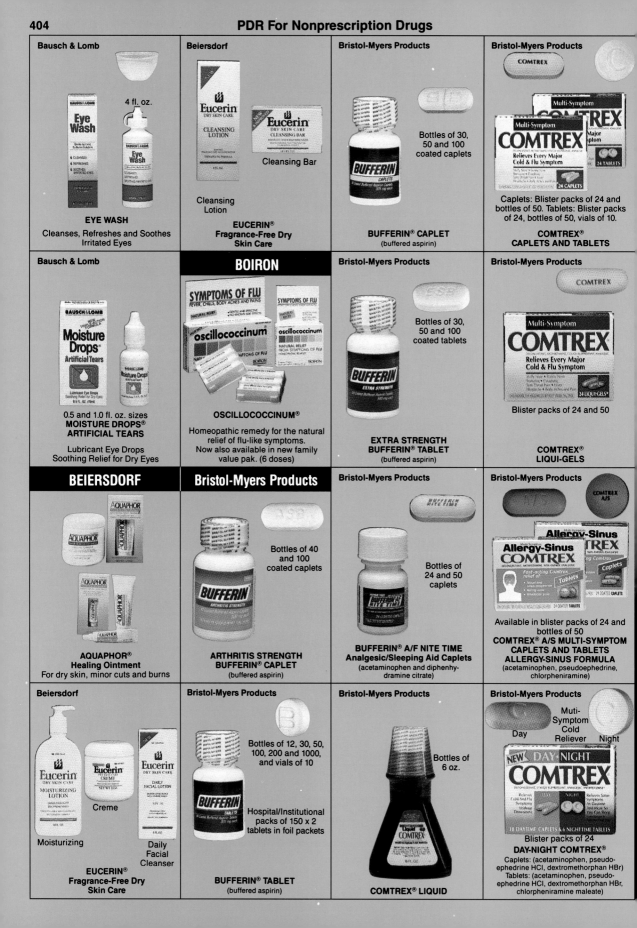

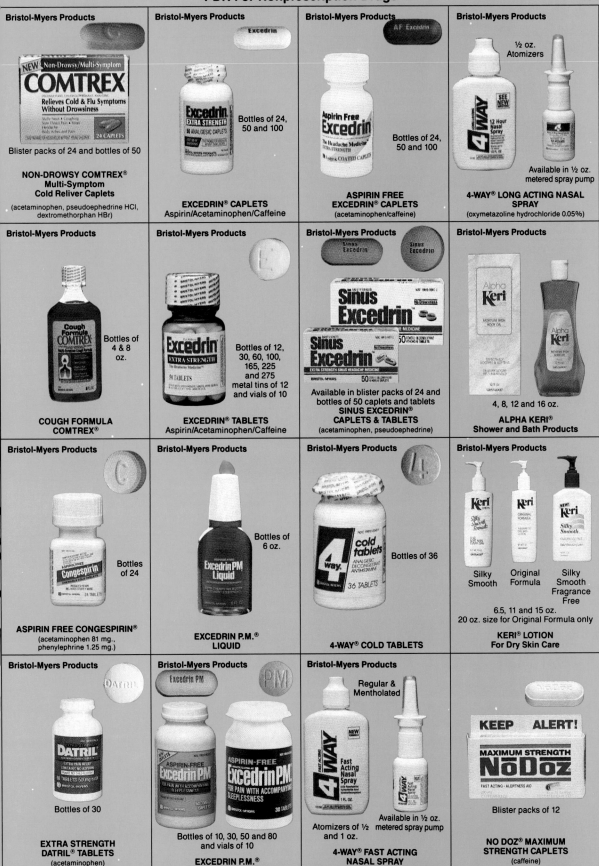

Bristol-Myers Products

NEW Non-Drowsy/Multi-Symptom
COMTREX
Relieves Cold & Flu Symptoms
Without Drowsiness

Blister packs of 24 and bottles of 50

NON-DROWSY COMTREX®
Multi-Symptom
Cold Reliver Caplets
(acetaminophen, pseudoephedrine HCl,
dextromethorphan HBr)

Bristol-Myers Products

Excedrin

Bottles of 24,
50 and 100

EXCEDRIN® CAPLETS
Aspirin/Acetaminophen/Caffeine

Bristol-Myers Products

AF Excedrin

Aspirin Free
Excedrin
The Headache Medicine
EXTRA STRENGTH

Bottles of 24,
50 and 100

ASPIRIN FREE
EXCEDRIN® CAPLETS
(acetaminophen/caffeine)

Bristol-Myers Products

½ oz.
Atomizers

4-WAY
12 Hour
Nasal
Spray

Available in ½ oz.
metered spray pump

4-WAY® LONG ACTING NASAL
SPRAY
(oxymetazoline hydrochloride 0.05%)

Bristol-Myers Products

Cough
Formula
COMTREX

Bottles of
4 & 8
oz.

COUGH FORMULA
COMTREX®

Bristol-Myers Products

Excedrin
EXTRA STRENGTH
50 TABLETS

Bottles of 12,
30, 60, 100,
165, 225
and 275
metal tins of 12
and vials of 10

EXCEDRIN® TABLETS
Aspirin/Acetaminophen/Caffeine

Bristol-Myers Products

Sinus
Excedrin

Sinus
Excedrin

Sinus
Excedrin

Sinus
Excedrin
EXTRA STRENGTH SINUS HEADACHE MEDICINE

Available in blister packs of 24 and
bottles of 50 caplets and tablets
SINUS EXCEDRIN®
CAPLETS & TABLETS
(acetaminophen, pseudoephedrine)

Bristol-Myers Products

Alpha
Keri

Alpha
Keri

4, 8, 12 and 16 oz.

ALPHA KERI®
Shower and Bath Products

Bristol-Myers Products

Congespirin

Bottles
of 24

ASPIRIN FREE CONGESPIRIN®
(acetaminophen 81 mg.,
phenylephrine 1.25 mg.)

Bristol-Myers Products

Excedrin PM
Liquid

Bottles of
6 oz.

EXCEDRIN P.M.®
LIQUID

Bristol-Myers Products

4
way.
cold
tablets
ANALGESIC
DECONGESTANT
ANTIHISTAMINE
36 TABLETS

Bottles of 36

4-WAY® COLD TABLETS

Bristol-Myers Products

Keri
Silky
Smooth
Formula

Keri
ORIGINAL
FORMULA

NEW!
Keri
Silky
Smooth

Silky
Smooth

Original
Formula

Silky
Smooth
Fragrance
Free

6.5, 11 and 15 oz.
20 oz. size for Original Formula only

KERI® LOTION
For Dry Skin Care

Bristol-Myers Products

DATRIL
DATRIL
EXTRA STRENGTH

Bottles of 30

EXTRA STRENGTH
DATRIL® TABLETS
(acetaminophen)

Bristol-Myers Products

Excedrin PM
PM

ASPIRIN-FREE
Excedrin PM
FOR PAIN WITH ACCOMPANYING
SLEEPLESSNESS

ASPIRIN-FREE
Excedrin P.M.
FOR PAIN WITH ACCOMPANYING
SLEEPLESSNESS
30 TABLETS

Bottles of 10, 30, 50 and 80
and vials of 10

EXCEDRIN P.M.®

Bristol-Myers Products

Regular &
Mentholated

NEW
4 WAY
Fast
Acting
Nasal
Spray

4 WAY
Fast
Acting
Nasal
Spray

Available in ½ oz.
Atomizers of ½ metered spray pump
and 1 oz.

4-WAY® FAST ACTING
NASAL SPRAY

Bristol-Myers Products

NODOZ

KEEP   ALERT!
MAXIMUM STRENGTH
NoDoz
FAST ACTING · ALERTNESS AID

Blister packs of 12

NO DOZ® MAXIMUM
STRENGTH CAPLETS
(caffeine)

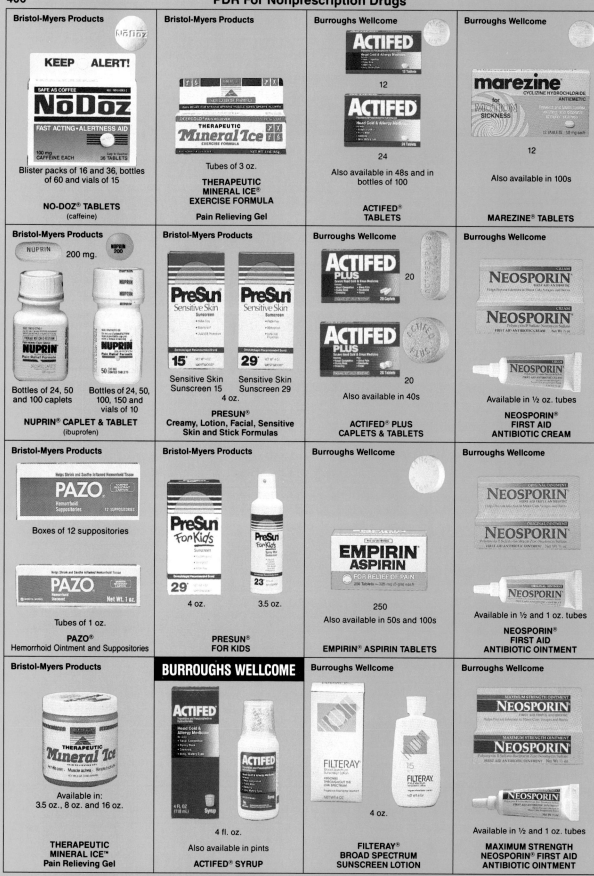

Bristol-Myers Products

KEEP ALERT!

SAFE AS COFFEE

NoDoz

FAST ACTING • ALERTNESS AID

100 mg CAFFEINE EACH   36 TABLETS

Blister packs of 16 and 36, bottles of 60 and vials of 15

NO-DOZ® TABLETS
(caffeine)

Bristol-Myers Products

NEW EXERCISE FORMULA

THERAPEUTIC
Mineral Ice
EXERCISE FORMULA

Tubes of 3 oz.

THERAPEUTIC MINERAL ICE® EXERCISE FORMULA

Pain Relieving Gel

Burroughs Wellcome

ACTIFED
Head Cold & Allergy Medicine
12 Tablets

12

ACTIFED
Head Cold & Allergy Medicine
24 Tablets

24

Also available in 48s and in bottles of 100

ACTIFED® TABLETS

Burroughs Wellcome

marezine
CYCLIZINE HYDROCHLORIDE
ANTIEMETIC
for MOTION SICKNESS

12 TABLETS   50 mg each

12

Also available in 100s

MAREZINE® TABLETS

Bristol-Myers Products

NUPRIN   200 mg.   NUPRIN 200

NUPRIN
Pain Relief Formula

NUPRIN
Pain Relief Formula

Bottles of 24, 50 and 100 caplets

Bottles of 24, 50, 100, 150 and vials of 10

NUPRIN® CAPLET & TABLET
(ibuprofen)

Bristol-Myers Products

PreSun
Sensitive Skin
Sunscreen

15

PreSun
Sensitive Skin
Sunscreen

29

Sensitive Skin Sunscreen 15

Sensitive Skin Sunscreen 29

4 oz.

PRESUN®
Creamy, Lotion, Facial, Sensitive Skin and Stick Formulas

Burroughs Wellcome

ACTIFED
PLUS
Severe Head Cold & Sinus Medicine
20 Caplets

20

ACTIFED
PLUS
Severe Head Cold & Sinus Medicine
20 Tablets

20

Also available in 40s

ACTIFED® PLUS CAPLETS & TABLETS

Burroughs Wellcome

NEOSPORIN
CREAM
FIRST AID ANTIBIOTIC

NEOSPORIN
CREAM
FIRST AID ANTIBIOTIC CREAM

NEOSPORIN

Available in ½ oz. tubes

NEOSPORIN® FIRST AID ANTIBIOTIC CREAM

Bristol-Myers Products

Helps Shrink and Soothe Inflamed Hemorrhoid Tissue

PAZO
Hemorrhoid Suppositories   12 SUPPOSITORIES

Boxes of 12 suppositories

Helps Shrink and Soothe Inflamed Hemorrhoid Tissue

PAZO
Hemorrhoid Ointment   Net Wt. 1 oz.

Tubes of 1 oz.

PAZO®
Hemorrhoid Ointment and Suppositories

Bristol-Myers Products

PreSun
For Kids
Sunscreen

29

PreSun
For Kids
Spray Mist Sunscreen

23

4 oz.   3.5 oz.

PRESUN® FOR KIDS

Burroughs Wellcome

EMPIRIN
ASPIRIN
FOR RELIEF OF PAIN
250 Tablets — 325 mg (5 gms) each

250

Also available in 50s and 100s

EMPIRIN® ASPIRIN TABLETS

Burroughs Wellcome

NEOSPORIN
ORIGINAL OINTMENT
FIRST AID TRIPLE ANTIBIOTIC

NEOSPORIN
ORIGINAL OINTMENT
FIRST AID ANTIBIOTIC OINTMENT

NEOSPORIN
ORIGINAL OINTMENT

Available in ½ and 1 oz. tubes

NEOSPORIN® FIRST AID ANTIBIOTIC OINTMENT

Bristol-Myers Products

THERAPEUTIC
Mineral Ice
Arthritis pain • Muscle aches • Simple backache

Available in:
3.5 oz., 8 oz. and 16 oz.

THERAPEUTIC MINERAL ICE™
Pain Relieving Gel

BURROUGHS WELLCOME

ACTIFED
Head Cold & Allergy Medicine

ACTIFED
Head Cold & Allergy Medicine
Syrup

4 FL OZ (118 mL)   Syrup

4 fl. oz.

Also available in pints

ACTIFED® SYRUP

Burroughs Wellcome

FILTERAY
Broad Spectrum Sunscreen Lotion

FILTERAY
15

4 oz.

FILTERAY® BROAD SPECTRUM SUNSCREEN LOTION

Burroughs Wellcome

NEOSPORIN
MAXIMUM STRENGTH OINTMENT
FIRST AID TRIPLE ANTIBIOTIC

NEOSPORIN
MAXIMUM STRENGTH OINTMENT
FIRST AID ANTIBIOTIC OINTMENT

NEOSPORIN

Available in ½ and 1 oz. tubes

MAXIMUM STRENGTH NEOSPORIN® FIRST AID ANTIBIOTIC OINTMENT

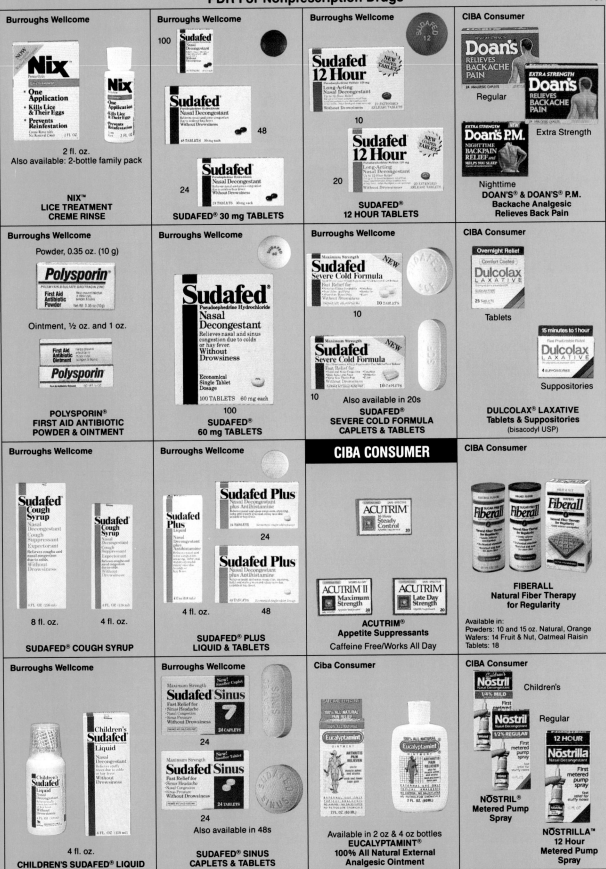

Burroughs Wellcome

2 fl. oz.
Also available: 2-bottle family pack

**NIX™
LICE TREATMENT
CREME RINSE**

Burroughs Wellcome

100

48

24

SUDAFED® 30 mg TABLETS

Burroughs Wellcome

10

20

**SUDAFED®
12 HOUR TABLETS**

CIBA Consumer

Regular

Extra Strength

Nighttime

**DOAN'S® & DOAN'S® P.M.
Backache Analgesic
Relieves Back Pain**

Burroughs Wellcome

Powder, 0.35 oz. (10 g)

Ointment, ½ oz. and 1 oz.

**POLYSPORIN®
FIRST AID ANTIBIOTIC
POWDER & OINTMENT**

Burroughs Wellcome

Sudafed®
Pseudoephedrine Hydrochloride
Nasal Decongestant
Relieves nasal and sinus congestion due to colds or hay fever. Without Drowsiness
Economical Single Tablet Dosage
100 TABLETS   60 mg each

100

**SUDAFED®
60 mg TABLETS**

Burroughs Wellcome

10

10

10

Also available in 20s

**SUDAFED®
SEVERE COLD FORMULA
CAPLETS & TABLETS**

CIBA Consumer

Tablets

Suppositories

**DULCOLAX® LAXATIVE
Tablets & Suppositories**
(bisacodyl USP)

Burroughs Wellcome

8 fl. oz.   4 fl. oz.

SUDAFED® COUGH SYRUP

Burroughs Wellcome

24

4 fl. oz.   48

**SUDAFED® PLUS
LIQUID & TABLETS**

CIBA CONSUMER

20

20   20

**ACUTRIM®
Appetite Suppressants**

Caffeine Free/Works All Day

CIBA Consumer

**FIBERALL
Natural Fiber Therapy
for Regularity**

Available in:
Powders: 10 and 15 oz. Natural, Orange
Wafers: 14 Fruit & Nut, Oatmeal Raisin
Tablets: 18

Burroughs Wellcome

4 fl. oz.

CHILDREN'S SUDAFED® LIQUID

Burroughs Wellcome

24

24

Also available in 48s

**SUDAFED® SINUS
CAPLETS & TABLETS**

Ciba Consumer

Available in 2 oz & 4 oz bottles
**EUCALYPTAMINT®
100% All Natural External
Analgesic Ointment**

CIBA Consumer

Children's

Regular

**NŌSTRIL®
Metered Pump
Spray**

**NŌSTRILLA™
12 Hour
Metered Pump
Spray**

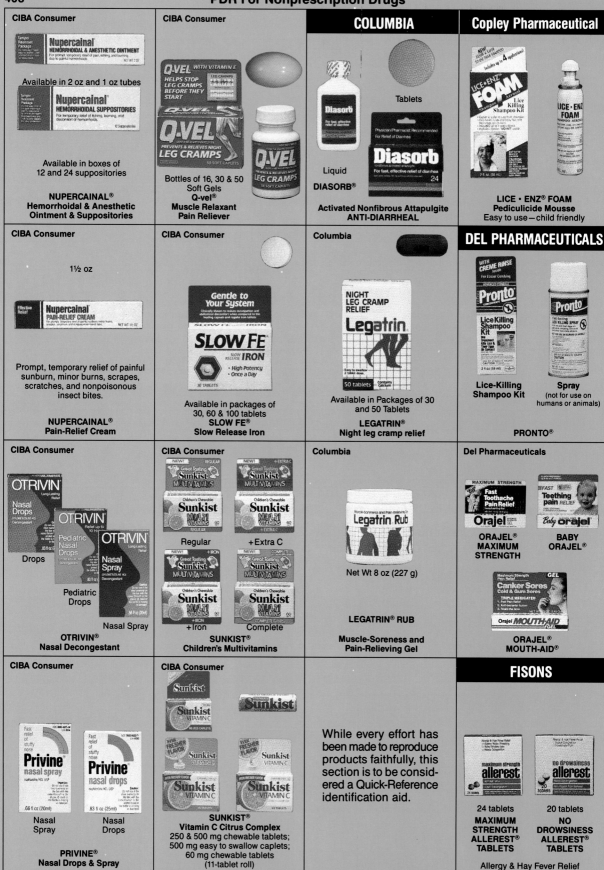

CIBA Consumer

Available in 2 oz and 1 oz tubes

Available in boxes of
12 and 24 suppositories

NUPERCAINAL®
Hemorrhoidal & Anesthetic
Ointment & Suppositories

CIBA Consumer

Bottles of 16, 30 & 50
Soft Gels
Q-vel®
Muscle Relaxant
Pain Reliever

COLUMBIA

Tablets

Liquid

DIASORB®

Activated Nonfibrous Attapulgite
ANTI-DIARRHEAL

Copley Pharmaceutical

LICE • ENZ® FOAM
Pediculicide Mousse
Easy to use — child friendly

CIBA Consumer

1½ oz

Prompt, temporary relief of painful
sunburn, minor burns, scrapes,
scratches, and nonpoisonous
insect bites.

NUPERCAINAL®
Pain-Relief Cream

CIBA Consumer

SLOW FE®
IRON
· High Potency
· Once a Day

Available in packages of
30, 60 & 100 tablets
SLOW FE®
Slow Release Iron

Columbia

NIGHT
LEG CRAMP
RELIEF

Legatrin

50 tablets

Available in Packages of 30
and 50 Tablets

LEGATRIN®
Night leg cramp relief

DEL PHARMACEUTICALS

Pronto
Lice Killing
Shampoo
Kit

Pronto

Lice-Killing
Shampoo Kit

Spray
(not for use on
humans or animals)

PRONTO®

CIBA Consumer

OTRIVIN
Nasal Drops

OTRIVIN
Pediatric
Nasal
Drops

OTRIVIN
Nasal
Spray

Drops

Pediatric
Drops

Nasal Spray

OTRIVIN®
Nasal Decongestant

CIBA Consumer

Sunkist
MULTIVITAMINS

Sunkist
MULTIVITAMINS

Regular   +Extra C

Sunkist
MULTIVITAMINS

Sunkist
MULTIVITAMINS

+Iron   Complete

SUNKIST®
Children's Multivitamins

Columbia

Legatrin Rub

Net Wt 8 oz (227 g)

LEGATRIN® RUB

Muscle-Soreness and
Pain-Relieving Gel

Del Pharmaceuticals

Orajel
Fast
Toothache
Pain Relief

Baby orajel
Teething
pain RELIEF

ORAJEL®
MAXIMUM
STRENGTH

BABY
ORAJEL®

Canker Sores
Cold & Gum Sores

Orajel MOUTH-AID

ORAJEL®
MOUTH-AID®

CIBA Consumer

Privine®
nasal spray

Privine®
nasal drops

Nasal
Spray

Nasal
Drops

PRIVINE®
Nasal Drops & Spray

CIBA Consumer

Sunkist

Sunkist
VITAMIN C

Sunkist

Sunkist
VITAMIN C

Sunkist
VITAMIN C

Sunkist
VITAMIN C

SUNKIST®
Vitamin C Citrus Complex
250 & 500 mg chewable tablets;
500 mg easy to swallow caplets;
60 mg chewable tablets
(11-tablet roll)

While every effort has
been made to reproduce
products faithfully, this
section is to be consid-
ered a Quick-Reference
identification aid.

FISONS

maximum strength
allerest

no drowsiness
allerest

24 tablets

20 tablets

MAXIMUM
STRENGTH
ALLEREST®
TABLETS

NO
DROWSINESS
ALLEREST®
TABLETS

Allergy & Hay Fever Relief

Fisons

Ointment
¾ oz.

Spray
2 oz.

Hemorrhoidal Ointment
1 oz.

AMERICAINE®
(benzocaine)

Fisons

½ oz.

2.7 oz.

DESENEX®
Spray Powder, Powder, Cream &
Ointment
Relieves Symptoms of Athlete's Foot

Fisons

Cream 0.5 oz.

3 oz.

Powder

Spray
Liquid

Spray
Powder

TING®
For Athlete's Foot &
Jock Itch

---

12 oz

5 oz

ALternaGEL®
High Potency Aluminum Hydroxide
Antacid

Fisons

½ oz.

CALDECORT Light® – ½% Cream

½ oz.

1 oz.

CALDECORT® – 1% Cream
(hydrocortisone acetate)

Fisons

3 oz.

DESENEX®
FOOT & SNEAKER
DEODORANT
Soothes, Cools, Comforts
& Absorbs Moisture

An
Ounce
of
Prevention

Insta-Glucose

INSTA-GLUCOSE
For treatment of insulin
reaction/hypoglycemia

J&J-Merck

Bottles of 36 & 100 tablets

DIALOSE®
(docusate sodium,
100 mg)

DIALOSE® PLUS
(docusate sodium,
100 mg
yellow phenolph-
thalein, 65 mg)

Fisons

2 oz.

4 oz.

1.25 oz.

CALDESENE®
MEDICATED POWDER and OINTMENT

Fisons

94-44 94-44

ISOCLOR

10's

ISOCLOR

20's

ISOCLOR® TIMESULE® CAPSULES
Nasal Decongestant/Antihistamine

While every effort has
been made to reproduce
products faithfully, this
section is to be consid-
ered a Quick-Reference
identification aid.

J&J-Merck

Available in
9 oz and 16 oz
bottles

EFFER-
SYLLIUM

Packets in
cartons of
12s & 24s

EFFER-SYLLIUM®
Natural Fiber Bulking Agent

Fisons

Spray Powder

Cruex
spray powder
kills
jock itch
fungus

Cruex
antifungal
cream
relieves itching,
chafing, rash
kills
jock itch
fungus

Cruex
antifungal cream

Cream

CRUEX®
Antifungal Spray Powder & Cream
Relieves Itching, Chafing, Rash

Fisons

Works
where it hurts
to relieve
pain at the source

MYOFLEX
ANALGESIC CREME

MYOFLEX
ANALGESIC CREME

Available in 2 oz. and 4 oz. tubes,
8 oz. and 16 oz. jars

MYOFLEX®
Analgesic Cream
(trolamine salicylate)

For more detailed in-
formation on products
illustrated in this sec-
tion, consult the Prod-
uct Information Section
or manufacturers may
be contacted directly.

J&J-Merck

FERANCEE-HP
HIGH POTENCY
HEMATINIC

Bottles
of
60 tablets

FERANCEE®-HP
High Potency Hematinic

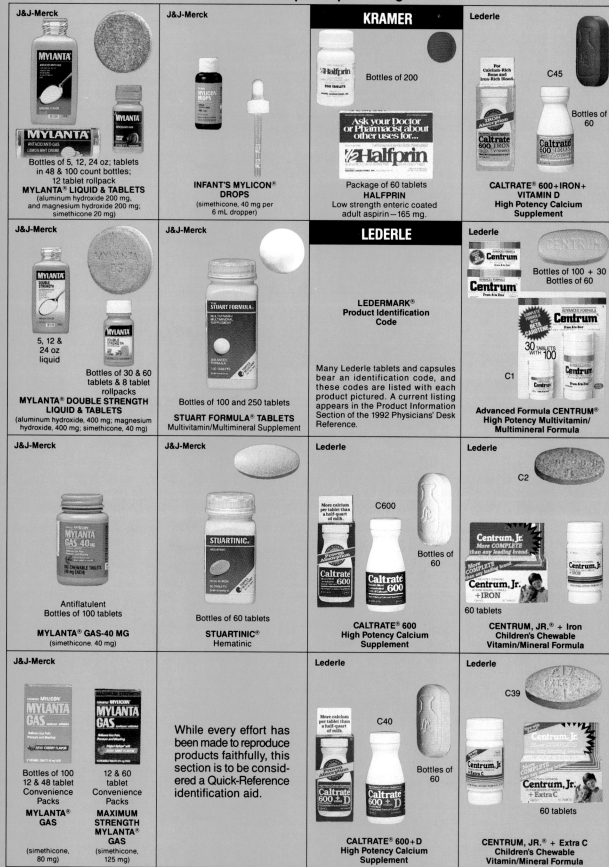

J&J-Merck

Bottles of 5, 12, 24 oz; tablets
in 48 & 100 count bottles;
12 tablet rollpack
MYLANTA® LIQUID & TABLETS
(aluminum hydroxide 200 mg,
and magnesium hydroxide 200 mg;
simethicone 20 mg)

J&J-Merck

**INFANT'S MYLICON®
DROPS**
(simethicone, 40 mg per
6 mL dropper)

KRAMER

Bottles of 200

Package of 60 tablets
HALFPRIN
Low strength enteric coated
adult aspirin—165 mg.

Ask your Doctor
or Pharmacist about
other uses for...
½ Halfprin

Lederle

C45

Bottles of
60

**CALTRATE® 600+IRON+
VITAMIN D
High Potency Calcium
Supplement**

J&J-Merck

5, 12 &
24 oz
liquid

Bottles of 30 & 60
tablets & 8 tablet
rollpacks
**MYLANTA® DOUBLE STRENGTH
LIQUID & TABLETS**
(aluminum hydroxide, 400 mg; magnesium
hydroxide, 400 mg; simethicone, 40 mg)

J&J-Merck

Bottles of 100 and 250 tablets
STUART FORMULA® TABLETS
Multivitamin/Multimineral Supplement

LEDERLE

**LEDERMARK®
Product Identification
Code**

Many Lederle tablets and capsules
bear an identification code, and
these codes are listed with each
product pictured. A current listing
appears in the Product Information
Section of the 1992 Physicians' Desk
Reference.

Lederle

Bottles of 100 + 30
Bottles of 60

C1

**Advanced Formula CENTRUM®
High Potency Multivitamin/
Multimineral Formula**

J&J-Merck

Antiflatulent
Bottles of 100 tablets

MYLANTA® GAS-40 MG
(simethicone, 40 mg)

J&J-Merck

Bottles of 60 tablets
STUARTINIC®
Hematinic

Lederle

C600

Bottles of
60

**CALTRATE® 600
High Potency Calcium
Supplement**

Lederle

C2

60 tablets

**CENTRUM, JR.® + Iron
Children's Chewable
Vitamin/Mineral Formula**

J&J-Merck

Bottles of 100
12 & 48 tablet
Convenience
Packs

**MYLANTA®
GAS**

(simethicone,
80 mg)

12 & 60
tablet
Convenience
Packs

**MAXIMUM
STRENGTH
MYLANTA®
GAS**

(simethicone,
125 mg)

While every effort has
been made to reproduce
products faithfully, this
section is to be consid-
ered a Quick-Reference
identification aid.

Lederle

C40

Bottles of
60

**CALTRATE® 600+D
High Potency Calcium
Supplement**

Lederle

C39

60 tablets

**CENTRUM, JR.® + Extra C
Children's Chewable
Vitamin/Mineral Formula**

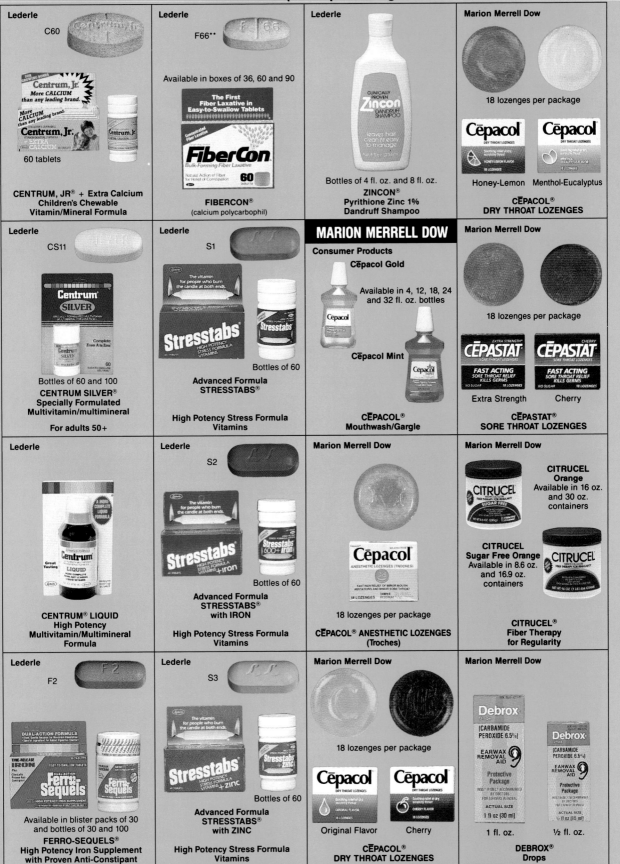

Lederle

C60

60 tablets

CENTRUM, JR® + Extra Calcium
Children's Chewable
Vitamin/Mineral Formula

Lederle

F66**

Available in boxes of 36, 60 and 90

FIBERCON®
(calcium polycarbophil)

Lederle

Bottles of 4 fl. oz. and 8 fl. oz.
ZINCON®
Pyrithione Zinc 1%
Dandruff Shampoo

Marion Merrell Dow

18 lozenges per package

Honey-Lemon   Menthol-Eucalyptus
CĒPACOL®
DRY THROAT LOZENGES

Lederle

CS11

Bottles of 60 and 100
CENTRUM SILVER®
Specially Formulated
Multivitamin/multimineral

For adults 50+

Lederle

S1

Bottles of 60
Advanced Formula
STRESSTABS®

High Potency Stress Formula
Vitamins

MARION MERRELL DOW

Consumer Products
Cēpacol Gold

Available in 4, 12, 18, 24
and 32 fl. oz. bottles

Cēpacol Mint

CĒPACOL®
Mouthwash/Gargle

Marion Merrell Dow

18 lozenges per package

Extra Strength   Cherry
CĒPASTAT®
SORE THROAT LOZENGES

Lederle

CENTRUM® LIQUID
High Potency
Multivitamin/Multimineral
Formula

Lederle

S2

Bottles of 60
Advanced Formula
STRESSTABS®
with IRON

High Potency Stress Formula
Vitamins

Marion Merrell Dow

18 lozenges per package

CĒPACOL® ANESTHETIC LOZENGES
(Troches)

Marion Merrell Dow

CITRUCEL
Orange
Available in 16 oz.
and 30 oz.
containers

CITRUCEL
Sugar Free Orange
Available in 8.6 oz.
and 16.9 oz.
containers

CITRUCEL®
Fiber Therapy
for Regularity

Lederle

F2

Available in blister packs of 30
and bottles of 30 and 100
FERRO-SEQUELS®
High Potency Iron Supplement
with Proven Anti-Constipant

Lederle

S3

Bottles of 60
Advanced Formula
STRESSTABS®
with ZINC

High Potency Stress Formula
Vitamins

Marion Merrell Dow

18 lozenges per package

Original Flavor   Cherry
CĒPACOL®
DRY THROAT LOZENGES

Marion Merrell Dow

1 fl. oz.   ½ fl. oz.
DEBROX®
Drops

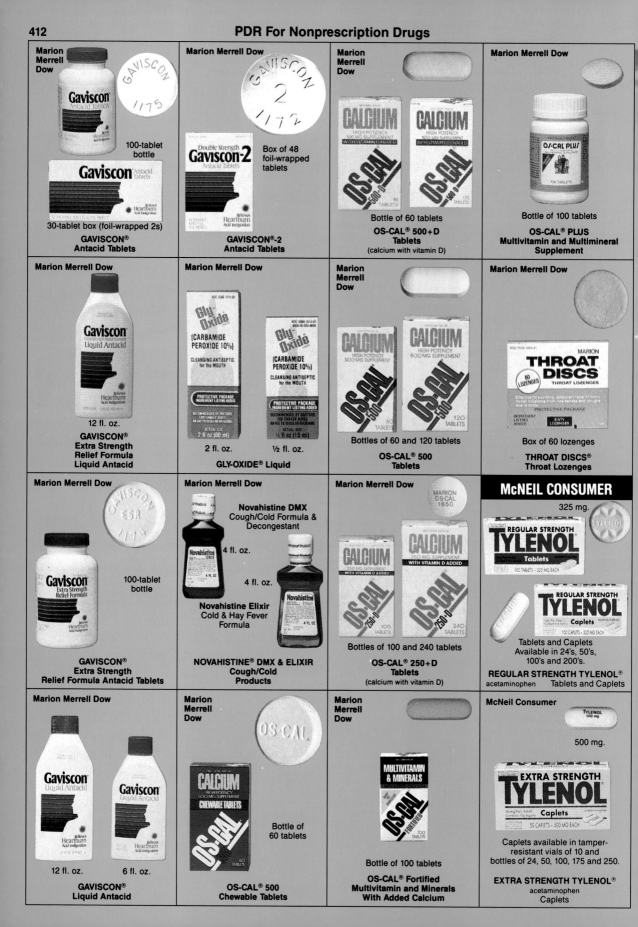

Marion Merrell Dow

100-tablet bottle

30-tablet box (foil-wrapped 2s)

GAVISCON®
Antacid Tablets

Marion Merrell Dow

Double Strength
Gaviscon-2
Antacid Tablets

Box of 48 foil-wrapped tablets

GAVISCON®-2
Antacid Tablets

Marion Merrell Dow

Bottle of 60 tablets

OS-CAL® 500+D
Tablets
(calcium with vitamin D)

Marion Merrell Dow

OS-CAL PLUS

Bottle of 100 tablets

OS-CAL® PLUS
Multivitamin and Multimineral
Supplement

Marion Merrell Dow

Gaviscon
Liquid Antacid

12 fl. oz.

GAVISCON®
Extra Strength
Relief Formula
Liquid Antacid

Marion Merrell Dow

Gly-Oxide
(CARBAMIDE PEROXIDE 10%)
CLEANSING ANTISEPTIC for the MOUTH

2 fl. oz.

Gly-Oxide
(CARBAMIDE PEROXIDE 10%)
CLEANSING ANTISEPTIC for the MOUTH

½ fl. oz.

GLY-OXIDE® Liquid

Marion Merrell Dow

Bottles of 60 and 120 tablets

OS-CAL® 500
Tablets

Marion Merrell Dow

MARION
THROAT DISCS
THROAT LOZENGES

Box of 60 lozenges

THROAT DISCS®
Throat Lozenges

Marion Merrell Dow

Gaviscon
Extra Strength
Relief Formula

100-tablet bottle

GAVISCON®
Extra Strength
Relief Formula Antacid Tablets

Marion Merrell Dow

Novahistine DMX
Cough/Cold Formula & Decongestant

4 fl. oz.

4 fl. oz.

Novahistine Elixir
Cold & Hay Fever Formula

NOVAHISTINE® DMX & ELIXIR
Cough/Cold
Products

Marion Merrell Dow

MARION
OS-CAL
650

Bottles of 100 and 240 tablets

OS-CAL® 250+D
Tablets
(calcium with vitamin D)

---

325 mg.

TYLENOL

REGULAR STRENGTH
TYLENOL
Tablets
100 TABLETS · 325 MG EACH

REGULAR STRENGTH
TYLENOL
Caplets
100 CAPLETS · 325 MG EACH

Tablets and Caplets
Available in 24's, 50's,
100's and 200's.

REGULAR STRENGTH TYLENOL®
acetaminophen   Tablets and Caplets

Marion Merrell Dow

Gaviscon
Liquid Antacid

Gaviscon
Liquid Antacid

12 fl. oz.   6 fl. oz.

GAVISCON®
Liquid Antacid

Marion Merrell Dow

OS-CAL

CALCIUM
HIGH POTENCY
500 MG SUPPLEMENT
CHEWABLE TABLETS
OS-CAL
500

Bottle of 60 tablets

OS-CAL® 500
Chewable Tablets

Marion Merrell Dow

MULTIVITAMIN
& MINERALS
OS-CAL
FORTIFIED

Bottle of 100 tablets

OS-CAL® Fortified
Multivitamin and Minerals
With Added Calcium

McNeil Consumer

TYLENOL
500 mg.

500 mg.

EXTRA STRENGTH
TYLENOL
Caplets
50 CAPLETS · 500 MG EACH

Caplets available in tamper-
resistant vials of 10 and
bottles of 24, 50, 100, 175 and 250.

EXTRA STRENGTH TYLENOL®
acetaminophen
Caplets

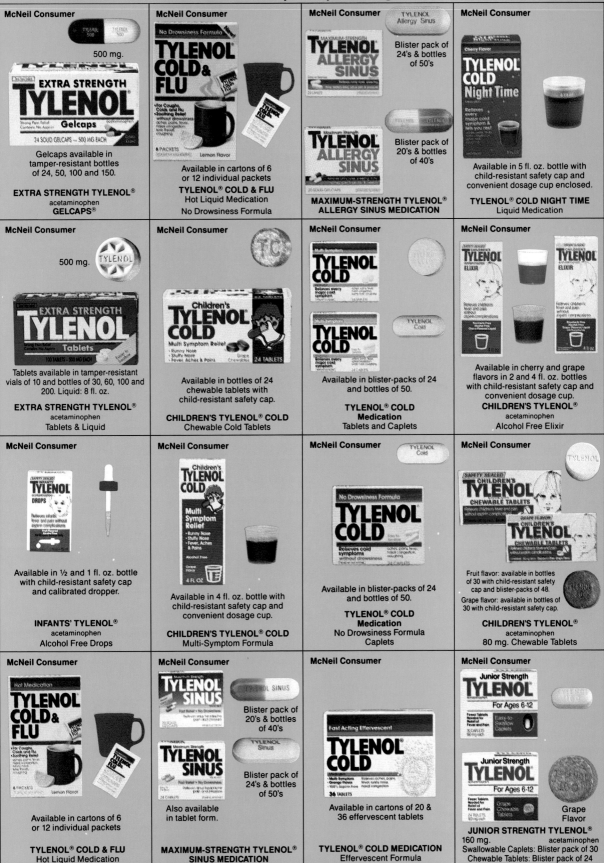

McNeil Consumer

500 mg.

Gelcaps available in tamper-resistant bottles of 24, 50, 100 and 150.

EXTRA STRENGTH TYLENOL®
acetaminophen
GELCAPS®

McNeil Consumer

Available in cartons of 6 or 12 individual packets

TYLENOL® COLD & FLU
Hot Liquid Medication
No Drowsiness Formula

McNeil Consumer

Blister pack of 24's & bottles of 50's

Blister pack of 20's & bottles of 40's

MAXIMUM-STRENGTH TYLENOL®
ALLERGY SINUS MEDICATION

McNeil Consumer

Available in 5 fl. oz. bottle with child-resistant safety cap and convenient dosage cup enclosed.

TYLENOL® COLD NIGHT TIME
Liquid Medication

McNeil Consumer

500 mg.

Tablets available in tamper-resistant vials of 10 and bottles of 30, 60, 100 and 200. Liquid: 8 fl. oz.

EXTRA STRENGTH TYLENOL®
acetaminophen
Tablets & Liquid

McNeil Consumer

Available in bottles of 24 chewable tablets with child-resistant safety cap.

CHILDREN'S TYLENOL® COLD
Chewable Cold Tablets

McNeil Consumer

Available in blister-packs of 24 and bottles of 50.

TYLENOL® COLD
Medication
Tablets and Caplets

McNeil Consumer

Available in cherry and grape flavors in 2 and 4 fl. oz. bottles with child-resistant safety cap and convenient dosage cup.

CHILDREN'S TYLENOL®
acetaminophen
Alcohol Free Elixir

McNeil Consumer

Available in ½ and 1 fl. oz. bottle with child-resistant safety cap and calibrated dropper.

INFANTS' TYLENOL®
acetaminophen
Alcohol Free Drops

McNeil Consumer

Available in 4 fl. oz. bottle with child-resistant safety cap and convenient dosage cup.

CHILDREN'S TYLENOL® COLD
Multi-Symptom Formula

McNeil Consumer

Available in blister-packs of 24 and bottles of 50.

TYLENOL® COLD
Medication
No Drowsiness Formula
Caplets

McNeil Consumer

Fruit flavor: available in bottles of 30 with child-resistant safety cap and blister-packs of 48.
Grape flavor: available in bottles of 30 with child-resistant safety cap.

CHILDREN'S TYLENOL®
acetaminophen
80 mg. Chewable Tablets

McNeil Consumer

Available in cartons of 6 or 12 individual packets

TYLENOL® COLD & FLU
Hot Liquid Medication

McNeil Consumer

Blister pack of 20's & bottles of 40's

Blister pack of 24's & bottles of 50's

Also available in tablet form.

MAXIMUM-STRENGTH TYLENOL®
SINUS MEDICATION

McNeil Consumer

Available in cartons of 20 & 36 effervescent tablets

TYLENOL® COLD MEDICATION
Effervescent Formula

McNeil Consumer

Grape Flavor

JUNIOR STRENGTH TYLENOL®
160 mg.   acetaminophen
Swallowable Caplets: Blister pack of 30
Chewable Tablets: Blister pack of 24

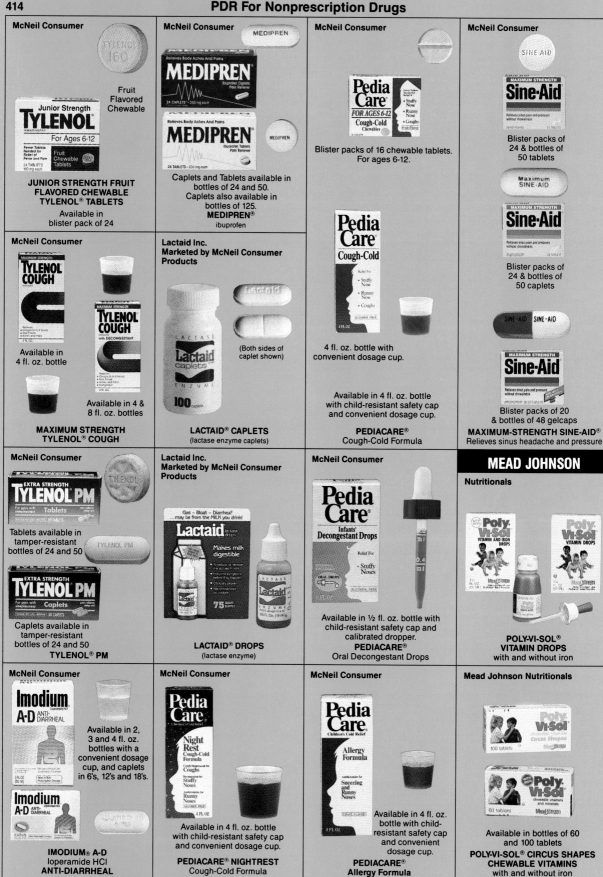

McNeil Consumer

Fruit Flavored Chewable

JUNIOR STRENGTH FRUIT FLAVORED CHEWABLE TYLENOL® TABLETS

Available in blister pack of 24

McNeil Consumer

Caplets and Tablets available in bottles of 24 and 50.
Caplets also available in bottles of 125.

MEDIPREN®
ibuprofen

McNeil Consumer

Blister packs of 16 chewable tablets. For ages 6-12.

McNeil Consumer

Blister packs of 24 & bottles of 50 tablets

Blister packs of 24 & bottles of 50 caplets

Blister packs of 20 & bottles of 48 gelcaps

MAXIMUM-STRENGTH SINE-AID®
Relieves sinus headache and pressure

McNeil Consumer

Available in 4 fl. oz. bottle

Available in 4 & 8 fl. oz. bottles

MAXIMUM STRENGTH TYLENOL® COUGH

**Lactaid Inc.
Marketed by McNeil Consumer Products**

(Both sides of caplet shown)

LACTAID® CAPLETS
(lactase enzyme caplets)

4 fl. oz. bottle with convenient dosage cup.

Available in 4 fl. oz. bottle with child-resistant safety cap and convenient dosage cup.

PEDIACARE®
Cough-Cold Formula

McNeil Consumer

Tablets available in tamper-resistant bottles of 24 and 50

Caplets available in tamper-resistant bottles of 24 and 50

TYLENOL® PM

**Lactaid Inc.
Marketed by McNeil Consumer Products**

Gas – Bloat – Diarrhea?
...may be from the MILK you drink!

Makes milk digestible

LACTAID® DROPS
(lactase enzyme)

McNeil Consumer

Available in ½ fl. oz. bottle with child-resistant safety cap and calibrated dropper.

PEDIACARE®
Oral Decongestant Drops

MEAD JOHNSON

Nutritionals

POLY-VI-SOL®
VITAMIN DROPS
with and without iron

McNeil Consumer

Available in 2, 3 and 4 fl. oz. bottles with a convenient dosage cup, and caplets in 6's, 12's and 18's.

IMODIUM® A-D
loperamide HCl
ANTI-DIARRHEAL

McNeil Consumer

Available in 4 fl. oz. bottle with child-resistant safety cap and convenient dosage cup.

PEDIACARE® NIGHTREST
Cough-Cold Formula

McNeil Consumer

Available in 4 fl. oz. bottle with child-resistant safety cap and convenient dosage cup.

PEDIACARE®
Allergy Formula

Mead Johnson Nutritionals

Available in bottles of 60 and 100 tablets

POLY-VI-SOL® CIRCUS SHAPES CHEWABLE VITAMINS
with and without iron

Mead Johnson Nutritionals

RICELYTE™
Rice-Based Oral
Electrolyte Maintenance
Solution

Mead Johnson Pharmaceuticals

NDC 0087-0718-02
CAPSULES
PERI-COLACE®
CASANTHRANOL AND DOCUSATE SODIUM
LAXATIVE PLUS
STOOL SOFTENER
A GENTLE,
PREDICTABLE
LAXATIVE
60 CAPSULES
Mead Johnson

Bottles of 30, 60, 250 and 1000
Laxative and Stool Softener

†PERI-COLACE®
(casanthranol and docusate sodium)

Menley & James

SAFETY SEALED
BENZEDREX·
INHALER
for
stuffed-up
noses
EDREX
ALER

1 inhaler per package

BENZEDREX® INHALER
(propylhexedrine)

Menley & James

Liquiprin
INFANTS'
DROPS
NO ASPIRIN
NO ALCOHOL

1.16 fl. oz.
Fruit Flavored Drops

Alcohol Free
Child Resistant Safety Cap

LIQUIPRIN®
Acetaminophen

Mead Johnson Nutritionals

Tempra 2
Tempra 1
Tempra 2
Tempra 3
Tempra 3

Alcohol-free
Aspirin-free
TEMPRA®
Acetaminophen for children

MENLEY & JAMES

ACNOMEL acne cream
NET WT. 1 OZ
(28 GRAMS)
The treatment for pimples and blemishes due to acne.

1 oz. tube

ACNOMEL® ACNE CREAM
(resorcinol, sulfur)

Menley & James

Congestac
CONGESTION
RELIEF MEDICINE
RELIEVES NASAL, SINUS
AND CHEST CONGESTION
HELPS YOU
BREATHE EASIER
NO ANTIHISTAMINE
DROWSINESS
12
CAPLETS

Packages of 12 and 24 caplets

CONGESTAC®
Congestion Relief Medicine
Decongestant/Expectorant

Menley & James

ORNEX

ORNEX
DECONGESTANT ANALGESIC
COLDS
SINUSITIS & FLU
24

MAXIMUM STRENGTH
ORNEX
DECONGESTANT/ANALGESIC
COLDS
SINUSITIS & FLU
24

Regular
Strength

Maximum
Strength

Packages of 24 and
48 caplets

ORNEX® CAPLETS
Decongestant/Analgesic

Mead Johnson Nutritionals

Tri·Vi·Sol
VITAMINS A, D, C AND IRON
DROPS

Tri·Vi·Sol
VITAMINS A, D, C AND
DROPS

Mead Johnson

TRI-VI-SOL®
VITAMIN DROPS
with and without iron

Menley & James

A.R.M.
MAXIMUM STRENGTH CAPLETS
ALLERGY
RELIEF
MEDICINE
FAST RELIEF OF HAY FEVER, ALLERGIES
AND SINUS CONGESTION
20
CAPLETS

Packages of 20 and 40 caplets
A.R.M.® ALLERGY RELIEF
MEDICINE
(chlorpheniramine maleate,
phenylpropanolamine HCl)

Menley & James

FILLS
YOUR
DAILY IRON
NEEDS
Femiron
DAILY IRON SUPPLEMENT
40 TABLETS

FEMIRON® REGULAR
Bottles of 40 and 120

IRON
PLUS
ALL-DAILY
VITAMIN
NEEDS
Femiron
MULTI-VITAMINS AND IRON
THE DAILY MULTI-VITAMIN AND IRON SUPPLEMENT
35 TABLETS

FEMIRON® WITH VITAMINS
Bottles of 35, 60 and 90

Menley & James   Toasted
Granules

Serutan

Serutan

6 oz.

18 oz.

SERUTAN®
Natural Fiber
Therapy For Regularity (psyllium)

Available in:
Toasted Granules—6 and 18 oz.
Regular Powder—7, 14 and 21 oz.
Fruit Flavored Powder—6, 12, and 18 oz.

MEAD JOHNSON PHARM.

NDC 0087-0713-02
CAPSULES
COLACE®
DOCUSATE SODIUM
STOOL
SOFTENER
Store below 86°F/30°C.
Protect from freezing.
60 CAPSULES
Mead Johnson

MJ
50 mg

100 mg

Bottles of 30, 60, 250 and 1000
Stool Softener

†COLACE®
(docusate sodium)

Menley & James

THERAPLASTIC
Aqua
Care
WITH 10% UREA
EFFECTIVE
MEDICATION
FOR DRY SKIN
RELIEF
CREAM
NET WT. 2.5 OZ

Aqua
Care
WITH 10% UREA
EFFECTIVE
MEDICATION
FOR DRY SKIN
RELIEF
LOTION
NET WT. 8 OZ.

2.5 oz. tube   8 oz. bottle

AQUA CARE® CREAM
AND LOTION
with 10% Urea

Menley & James

Original Flavor   Cherry

HOLD
DM

HOLD
DM

Each
contain
10
lozenges

HOLD®
Cough Suppressant
Lozenges with Dextromethorphan

For more detailed information on products illustrated in this section, consult the Product Information Section or manufacturers may be contacted directly.

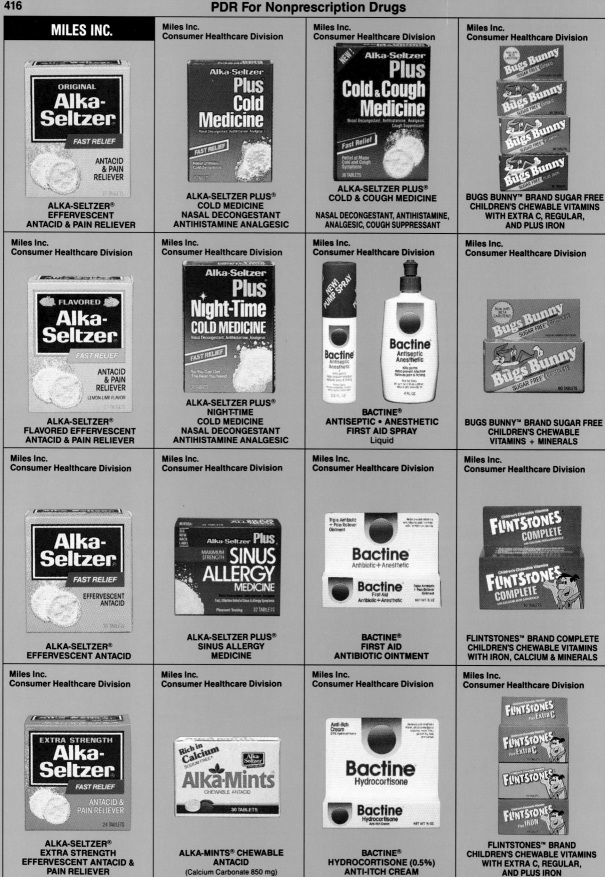

MILES INC.

Miles Inc.
Consumer Healthcare Division

ALKA-SELTZER®
EFFERVESCENT
ANTACID & PAIN RELIEVER

Miles Inc.
Consumer Healthcare Division

ALKA-SELTZER PLUS®
COLD MEDICINE
NASAL DECONGESTANT
ANTIHISTAMINE ANALGESIC

Miles Inc.
Consumer Healthcare Division

ALKA-SELTZER PLUS®
COLD & COUGH MEDICINE

NASAL DECONGESTANT, ANTIHISTAMINE,
ANALGESIC, COUGH SUPPRESSANT

Miles Inc.
Consumer Healthcare Division

BUGS BUNNY™ BRAND SUGAR FREE
CHILDREN'S CHEWABLE VITAMINS
WITH EXTRA C, REGULAR,
AND PLUS IRON

Miles Inc.
Consumer Healthcare Division

ALKA-SELTZER®
FLAVORED EFFERVESCENT
ANTACID & PAIN RELIEVER

Miles Inc.
Consumer Healthcare Division

ALKA-SELTZER PLUS®
NIGHT-TIME
COLD MEDICINE
NASAL DECONGESTANT
ANTIHISTAMINE ANALGESIC

Miles Inc.
Consumer Healthcare Division

BACTINE®
ANTISEPTIC • ANESTHETIC
FIRST AID SPRAY
Liquid

Miles Inc.
Consumer Healthcare Division

BUGS BUNNY™ BRAND SUGAR FREE
CHILDREN'S CHEWABLE
VITAMINS + MINERALS

Miles Inc.
Consumer Healthcare Division

ALKA-SELTZER®
EFFERVESCENT ANTACID

Miles Inc.
Consumer Healthcare Division

ALKA-SELTZER PLUS®
SINUS ALLERGY
MEDICINE

Miles Inc.
Consumer Healthcare Division

BACTINE®
FIRST AID
ANTIBIOTIC OINTMENT

Miles Inc.
Consumer Healthcare Division

FLINTSTONES™ BRAND COMPLETE
CHILDREN'S CHEWABLE VITAMINS
WITH IRON, CALCIUM & MINERALS

Miles Inc.
Consumer Healthcare Division

ALKA-SELTZER®
EXTRA STRENGTH
EFFERVESCENT ANTACID &
PAIN RELIEVER

Miles Inc.
Consumer Healthcare Division

ALKA-MINTS® CHEWABLE
ANTACID
(Calcium Carbonate 850 mg)

Miles Inc.
Consumer Healthcare Division

BACTINE®
HYDROCORTISONE (0.5%)
ANTI-ITCH CREAM

Miles Inc.
Consumer Healthcare Division

FLINTSTONES™ BRAND
CHILDREN'S CHEWABLE VITAMINS
WITH EXTRA C, REGULAR,
AND PLUS IRON

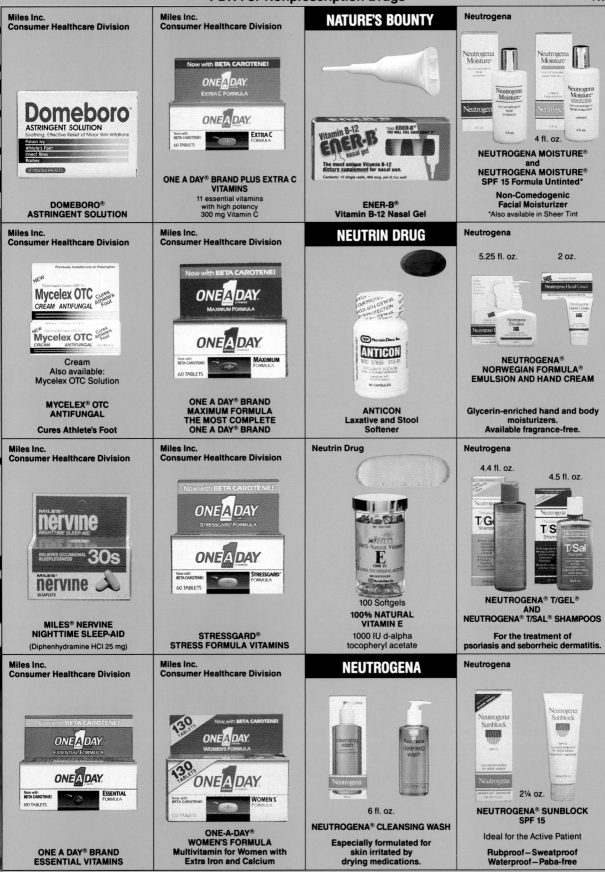

Miles Inc.
Consumer Healthcare Division

DOMEBORO®
ASTRINGENT SOLUTION

Miles Inc.
Consumer Healthcare Division

ONE A DAY® BRAND PLUS EXTRA C
VITAMINS
11 essential vitamins
with high potency
300 mg Vitamin C

NATURE'S BOUNTY

ENER-B®
Vitamin B-12 Nasal Gel

Neutrogena

4 fl. oz.

NEUTROGENA MOISTURE®
and
NEUTROGENA MOISTURE®
SPF 15 Formula Untinted*

Non-Comedogenic
Facial Moisturizer

*Also available in Sheer Tint

Miles Inc.
Consumer Healthcare Division

Cream
Also available:
Mycelex OTC Solution

MYCELEX® OTC
ANTIFUNGAL

Cures Athlete's Foot

Miles Inc.
Consumer Healthcare Division

ONE A DAY® BRAND
MAXIMUM FORMULA
THE MOST COMPLETE
ONE A DAY® BRAND

NEUTRIN DRUG

ANTICON
Laxative and Stool
Softener

Neutrogena

5.25 fl. oz.   2 oz.

NEUTROGENA®
NORWEGIAN FORMULA®
EMULSION AND HAND CREAM

Glycerin-enriched hand and body
moisturizers.
Available fragrance-free.

Miles Inc.
Consumer Healthcare Division

MILES® NERVINE
NIGHTTIME SLEEP-AID
(Diphenhydramine HCl 25 mg)

Miles Inc.
Consumer Healthcare Division

STRESSGARD®
STRESS FORMULA VITAMINS

Neutrin Drug

100 Softgels
100% NATURAL
VITAMIN E
1000 IU d-alpha
tocopheryl acetate

Neutrogena

4.4 fl. oz.   4.5 fl. oz.

NEUTROGENA® T/GEL®
AND
NEUTROGENA® T/SAL® SHAMPOOS

For the treatment of
psoriasis and seborrheic dermatitis.

Miles Inc.
Consumer Healthcare Division

ONE A DAY® BRAND
ESSENTIAL VITAMINS

Miles Inc.
Consumer Healthcare Division

ONE-A-DAY®
WOMEN'S FORMULA
Multivitamin for Women with
Extra Iron and Calcium

NEUTROGENA

6 fl. oz.

NEUTROGENA® CLEANSING WASH

Especially formulated for
skin irritated by
drying medications.

Neutrogena

2¼ oz.

NEUTROGENA® SUNBLOCK
SPF 15

Ideal for the Active Patient

Rubproof—Sweatproof
Waterproof—Paba-free

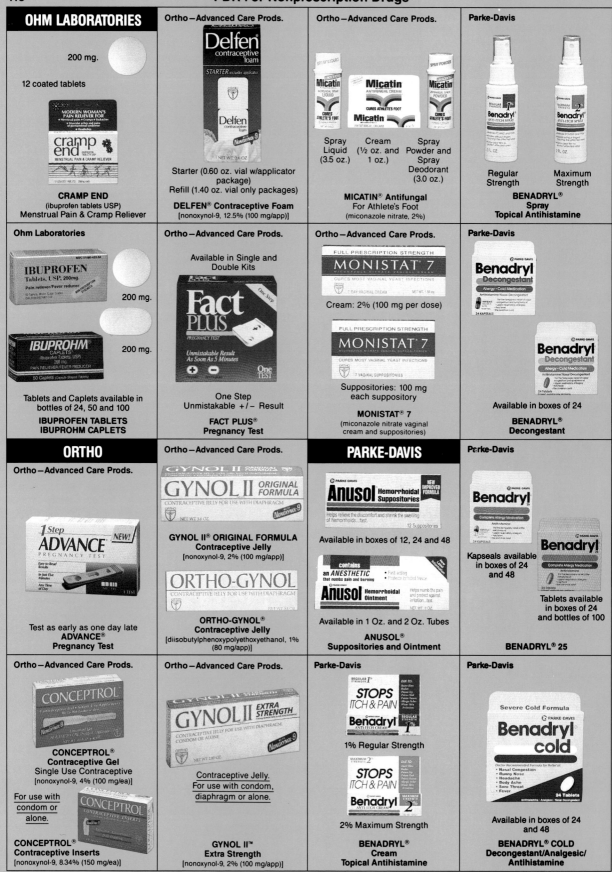

OHM LABORATORIES

200 mg.

12 coated tablets

CRAMP END
(ibuprofen tablets USP)
Menstrual Pain & Cramp Reliever

Ohm Laboratories

IBUPROFEN
Tablets, USP, 200mg.

200 mg.

IBUPROHM
CAPLETS

200 mg.

Tablets and Caplets available in
bottles of 24, 50 and 100
IBUPROFEN TABLETS
IBUPROHM CAPLETS

ORTHO

Ortho—Advanced Care Prods.

1 Step
ADVANCE
PREGNANCY TEST   NEW!

Test as early as one day late
ADVANCE®
Pregnancy Test

Ortho—Advanced Care Prods.

CONCEPTROL

CONCEPTROL®
Contraceptive Gel
Single Use Contraceptive
[nonoxynol-9, 4% (100 mg/ea)]

For use with
condom or
alone.

CONCEPTROL
INSERTS

CONCEPTROL®
Contraceptive Inserts
[nonoxynol-9, 8.34% (150 mg/ea)]

Ortho—Advanced Care Prods.

Delfen®
contraceptive
foam
STARTER includes applicator

Delfen
contraceptive
foam

NET WT 0.6 OZ

Starter (0.60 oz. vial w/applicator
package)
Refill (1.40 oz. vial only packages)
DELFEN® Contraceptive Foam
[nonoxynol-9, 12.5% (100 mg/app)]

Ortho—Advanced Care Prods.

Available in Single and
Double Kits

Fact
PLUS
One Step

Unmistakable Result
As Soon As 5 Minutes

One
TEST

One Step
Unmistakable +/– Result
FACT PLUS®
Pregnancy Test

Ortho—Advanced Care Prods.

GYNOL II   ORIGINAL
FORMULA
CONTRACEPTIVE JELLY FOR USE WITH DIAPHRAGM
NET WT 3.8 OZ

GYNOL II® ORIGINAL FORMULA
Contraceptive Jelly
[nonoxynol-9, 2% (100 mg/app)]

ORTHO-GYNOL
CONTRACEPTIVE JELLY FOR USE WITH DIAPHRAGM

ORTHO-GYNOL®
Contraceptive Jelly
[diisobutylphenoxypolyethoxyethanol, 1%
(80 mg/app)]

Ortho—Advanced Care Prods.

GYNOL II   EXTRA
STRENGTH
CONTRACEPTIVE JELLY FOR USE WITH DIAPHRAGM.
CONDOM OR ALONE
NET WT 2.85 OZ.

Contraceptive Jelly.
For use with condom,
diaphragm or alone.
GYNOL II™
Extra Strength
[nonoxynol-9, 2% (100 mg/app)]

Ortho—Advanced Care Prods.

Micatin
TOPICAL SPRAY
LIQUID
CURES
ATHLETE'S FOOT

Micatin
ANTIFUNGAL CREAM
CURES ATHLETE'S FOOT

Micatin
ANTIFUNGAL SPRAY POWDER
CURES
ATHLETE'S FOOT

Spray   Cream   Spray
Liquid   (½ oz. and   Powder and
(3.5 oz.)   1 oz.)   Spray
               Deodorant
               (3.0 oz.)

MICATIN® Antifungal
For Athlete's Foot
(miconazole nitrate, 2%)

Ortho—Advanced Care Prods.

FULL PRESCRIPTION STRENGTH
MONISTAT 7
MICONAZOLE NITRATE VAGINAL CREAM
NET WT. 1.59 OZ.

Cream: 2% (100 mg per dose)

FULL PRESCRIPTION STRENGTH
MONISTAT 7
MICONAZOLE NITRATE VAGINAL SUPPOSITORIES
7 VAGINAL SUPPOSITORIES

Suppositories: 100 mg
each suppository
MONISTAT® 7
(miconazole nitrate vaginal
cream and suppositories)

PARKE-DAVIS

PARKE-DAVIS
Anusol   Hemorrhoidal
Suppositories   NEW IMPROVED FORMULA
Helps relieve the discomfort and shrink the
swelling of hemorrhoids...fast.
12 Suppositories

Available in boxes of 12, 24 and 48

contains
an ANESTHETIC
that numbs pain and burning
Anusol   Hemorrhoidal
Ointment
NET WT. 2 OZ.

Available in 1 Oz. and 2 Oz. Tubes
ANUSOL®
Suppositories and Ointment

Parke-Davis

REGULAR STRENGTH 1%
STOPS
ITCH & PAIN
Benadryl
ANTI-ITCH CREAM   1

1% Regular Strength

MAXIMUM STRENGTH 2
STOPS
ITCH & PAIN
Benadryl
ANTI-ITCH CREAM   2

2% Maximum Strength

BENADRYL®
Cream
Topical Antihistamine

Parke-Davis

REGULAR STRENGTH 1%
Benadryl
ANTI-ITCH SPRAY

MAXIMUM STRENGTH 2
Benadryl
ANTI-ITCH SPRAY

Regular   Maximum
Strength   Strength

BENADRYL®
Spray
Topical Antihistamine

Parke-Davis

Benadryl
Decongestant
Allergy · Cold Medication

Benadryl
Decongestant
Allergy · Cold Medication

Available in boxes of 24
BENADRYL®
Decongestant

Parke-Davis

Benadryl
Complete Allergy Medication
Antihistamine

Kapseals available
in boxes of 24
and 48

Benadryl 25
Complete Allergy Medication

Tablets available
in boxes of 24
and bottles of 100
BENADRYL® 25

Parke-Davis

Severe Cold Formula
Benadryl
cold
Doctor Recommended Formula for Relief of:
• Nasal Congestion
• Runny Nose
• Headache
• Body Ache
• Sore Throat
• Fever
24 Tablets

Available in boxes of 24
and 48
BENADRYL® COLD
Decongestant/Analgesic/
Antihistamine

Parke-Davis

Honey-Lemon Flavor

Available in 6 Fl. Oz. Bottles

BENADRYL® COLD NIGHTTIME FORMULA

Parke-Davis

Available in 4 Oz. Bottles

BENYLIN® Decongestant Cough Formula

Parke-Davis

1 test kit

2 test kits

e·p·t® Simple to do. Easy to read. Accurate results.

e·p·t® STICK TEST Early Pregnancy Test

Parke-Davis

Available in bottles of 130 Tablets

MYADEC® Multivitamin-Multimineral Supplement

Parke-Davis

Available in 4 Oz. and 8 Oz. Bottles

BENADRYL® Elixir

Parke-Davis

Available in 4 Oz. Bottles

BENYLIN DM® Pediatric Cough Formula

Parke-Davis

100 tablets

12 Fl. Oz.

GELUSIL® Antacid-Anti-gas Sodium Free

Parke-Davis

SINUTAB® SINUS MEDICATION

Regular Strength Without Drowsiness Formula

Parke-Davis

Available in 4 Oz. Bottles

BENADRYL® Decongestant Elixir

Parke-Davis

Available in 4 Oz. and 8 Oz. Bottles

BENYLIN® EXPECTORANT

Parke-Davis

16 Caplets

6 Fl. Oz.

FLU STRENGTH RELIEF™ MEDI-FLU®

Parke-Davis

SINUTAB® SINUS ALLERGY MEDICATION

Maximum Strength Formula

Available in Caplets or Tablets

Parke-Davis

Available in 4 Oz. and 8 Oz. Bottles

BENYLIN® Cough Syrup

Parke-Davis

Spray

Lotion

Lotion

Cream

For relief from itching due to: Poison Ivy, Insect Bites, Poison Oak, Skin Irritation

CALADRYL® Topical Antihistamine/Skin Protectant

Parke-Davis

16 Caplets

MEDI-FLU®

Flu Strength Relief Without Drowsiness

Parke-Davis

SINUTAB® SINUS MEDICATION

Maximum Strength Without Drowsiness Formula

Available in Caplets or Tablets

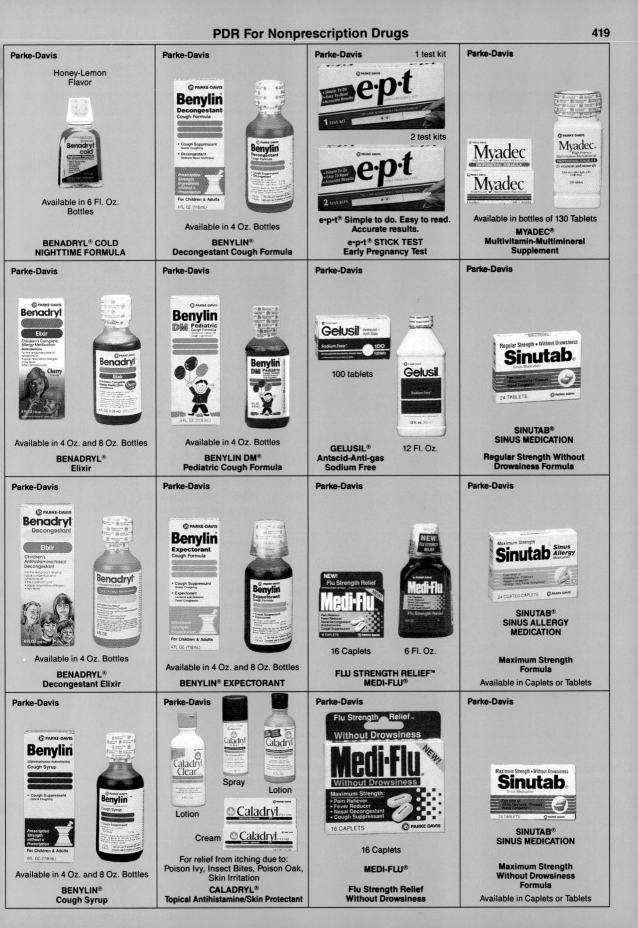

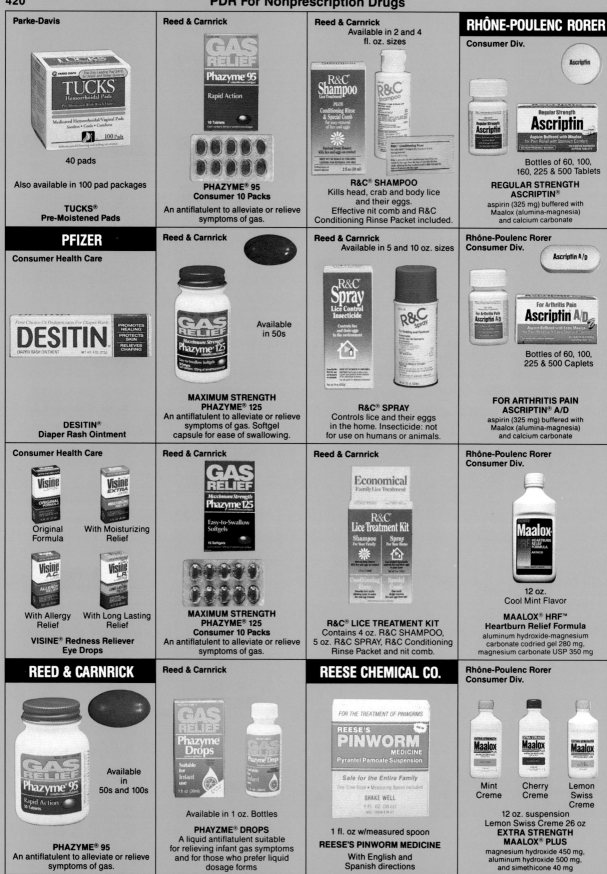

Parke-Davis

40 pads

Also available in 100 pad packages

**TUCKS®
Pre-Moistened Pads**

PFIZER

Consumer Health Care

**DESITIN®
Diaper Rash Ointment**

Consumer Health Care

Original
Formula

With Moisturizing
Relief

With Allergy
Relief

With Long Lasting
Relief

**VISINE® Redness Reliever
Eye Drops**

REED & CARNRICK

Available
in
50s and 100s

PHAZYME® 95

An antiflatulent to alleviate or relieve
symptoms of gas.

Reed & Carnrick

**PHAZYME® 95
Consumer 10 Packs**

An antiflatulent to alleviate or relieve
symptoms of gas.

Reed & Carnrick

Available
in 50s

**MAXIMUM STRENGTH
PHAZYME® 125**

An antiflatulent to alleviate or relieve
symptoms of gas. Softgel
capsule for ease of swallowing.

Reed & Carnrick

**MAXIMUM STRENGTH
PHAZYME® 125
Consumer 10 Packs**

An antiflatulent to alleviate or relieve
symptoms of gas.

Reed & Carnrick

Available
in
50s and 100s

Available in 1 oz. Bottles

PHAYZME® DROPS

A liquid antiflatulent suitable
for relieving infant gas symptoms
and for those who prefer liquid
dosage forms

Reed & Carnrick
Available in 2 and 4
fl. oz. sizes

R&C® SHAMPOO

Kills head, crab and body lice
and their eggs.

Effective nit comb and R&C
Conditioning Rinse Packet included.

Reed & Carnrick
Available in 5 and 10 oz. sizes

R&C® SPRAY

Controls lice and their eggs
in the home. Insecticide: not
for use on humans or animals.

Reed & Carnrick

R&C® LICE TREATMENT KIT

Contains 4 oz. R&C SHAMPOO,
5 oz. R&C SPRAY, R&C Conditioning
Rinse Packet and nit comb.

REESE CHEMICAL CO.

1 fl. oz w/measured spoon

REESE'S PINWORM MEDICINE

With English and
Spanish directions

RHÔNE-POULENC RORER

Consumer Div.

Bottles of 60, 100,
160, 225 & 500 Tablets

**REGULAR STRENGTH
ASCRIPTIN®**

aspirin (325 mg) buffered with
Maalox (alumina-magnesia)
and calcium carbonate

**Rhône-Poulenc Rorer
Consumer Div.**

Bottles of 60, 100,
225 & 500 Caplets

**FOR ARTHRITIS PAIN
ASCRIPTIN® A/D**

aspirin (325 mg) buffered with
Maalox (alumina-magnesia)
and calcium carbonate

**Rhône-Poulenc Rorer
Consumer Div.**

12 oz.
Cool Mint Flavor

**MAALOX® HRF™
Heartburn Relief Formula**

aluminum hydroxide-magnesium
carbonate codried gel 280 mg,
magnesium carbonate USP 350 mg

**Rhône-Poulenc Rorer
Consumer Div.**

Mint
Creme

Cherry
Creme

Lemon
Swiss
Creme

12 oz. suspension
Lemon Swiss Creme 26 oz

**EXTRA STRENGTH
MAALOX® PLUS**

magnesium hydroxide 450 mg,
aluminum hydroxide 500 mg,
and simethicone 40 mg

Rhône-Poulenc Rorer Consumer Div.

Mint Creme Tablets
EXTRA STRENGTH MAALOX® PLUS TABLETS
magnesium hydroxide 350 mg, dried aluminum hydroxide gel 350 mg and simethicone 30 mg

38's, 75's

Cheracol D COUGH FORMULA
Maximum Strength Cough Relief

Cheracol PLUS
Head Cold/Cough Formula

2 oz, 4 oz, 6 oz
CHERACOL D® Cough Formula

4 oz, 6 oz
CHERACOL PLUS® Head Cold/Cough Formula

Roberts Pharmaceutical

Sigtab Tablets
A high potency vitamin supplement
90 Tablets

Bottles of 90 and 500 tablets

SIGTAB® Tablets
High potency vitamin supplement

A. H. Robins

Dimetapp DM Cold & Cough Elixir
Relieves Cold Symptoms — Suppresses Coughs
Red Grape Taste
4 Fl. Oz.

Available in bottles of 4 Fl. Oz. and 8 Fl. Oz.

DIMETAPP® DM COLD & COUGH ELIXIR
(Brompheniramine Maleate, Phenylpropanolamine HCl, Dextromethorphan Hydrobromide)

Rhône-Poulenc Rorer Consumer Div.

Maalox PLUS — 50 TABLETS

Lemon Swiss Creme & Cherry Creme Tablets
50's, 100's

Lemon and Cherry 3 roll pack

Lemon Swiss Creme Cherry Creme

Maalox Plus

MAALOX® PLUS
magnesium hydroxide 200 mg, dried aluminum hydroxide gel 200 mg, and simethicone 25 mg

Roberts Pharmaceutical

HALTRAN
Relieves Cramps Right From The Start

HALTRAN
MENSTRUAL PAIN AND CRAMP RELIEVER
50 TABLETS - 200 mg EACH

200 mg

Bottles of 30

HALTRAN® Tablets
(ibuprofen tablets, USP)

ChapStick (×5)

Sunblock 15

CHAP STICK®   Lip Balm

A. H. Robins

Maximum Strength Dimetapp
NASAL DECONGESTANT, ANTIHISTAMINE
12-Hour Extentabs®
For Relief of Cold and Allergy Symptoms
Relieves nasal congestion, sneezing, runny nose, and itchy, watery eyes
24 TABLETS

Available in consumer cartons of 12, 24 and 48 and bottles of 100 and 500

DIMETAPP EXTENTABS®

Rhône-Poulenc Rorer Consumer Div.

Perdiem
RELIEF OF CONSTIPATION
100% NATURAL VEGETABLE LAXATIVE
NET WT. 8.8 OUNCE (250 g)

Granules
100 gm and 250 gm
PERDIEM®
100% Natural Vegetable Laxative
82 percent psyllium (Plantago Hydrocolloid)
18 percent senna (Cassia Pod Concentrate)

Roberts Pharmaceutical

P-A-C Analgesic Tablets
For the temporary relief of occasional minor aches, pains, headache, and the reduction of fever.
1000 Tablets

P-A-C Analgesic Tablets

1,000 tablets   100 tablets

P-A-C®
Analgesic Tablets

A. H. Robins

Petroleum Jelly Plus (×3)
for Dry, Chapped Lips

Cherry Flavored

for Dry, Chapped Lips   for Dry, Chapped Lips with SUNBLOCK 15

CHAP STICK® Petroleum Jelly Plus

A. H. Robins

Dimetapp
NASAL DECONGESTANT, ANTIHISTAMINE
4-Hour Tablets
For Relief of Cold and Allergy Symptoms
Relieves nasal congestion, sneezing, runny nose, and itchy, watery eyes
24 TABLETS

Available in consumer cartons of 24

DIMETAPP® TABLETS

Rhône-Poulenc Rorer Consumer Div.

Perdiem Fiber
AID TO REGULARITY
100% NATURAL DAILY FIBER SOURCE
33% MORE
NO SODIUM
NET WT. 8.8 OZ (250 grams)

Granules
100 gm and 250 gm
PERDIEM® FIBER
100% Natural Daily Fiber Source
100% Psyllium (Plantago Hydrocolloid)

Roberts Pharmaceutical

Pyrroxate
Just one capsule relieves Colds, Allergies & Sinus Congestion
Extra Strength
Colds, Allergies & Sinus Congestion 24

Pyrroxate
Colds, Allergies & Sinus Congestion 24

Pyrroxate
Colds, Allergies & Sinus Congestion

Bottles of 24 and 500 tablets

PYRROXATE® Capsules
Nasal Decongestant/Antihistamine/Analgesic

A. H. Robins

Dimetapp Elixir
Relieves Cold and Allergy Symptoms
Great Grape Taste
Relieves: nasal congestion, runny nose, itchy, watery eyes, sneezing
4 FL. OZ.

Dimetapp Elixir

Available in bottles of 4 Fl. Oz., 8 Fl. Oz., 16 Fl. Oz. and 128 Fl. Oz.

DIMETAPP® ELIXIR

A. H. Robins

Dimetapp Cold & Flu
NASAL DECONGESTANT, ANTIHISTAMINE, ANALGESIC
Cold & Flu Formula with Non-Aspirin Pain Reliever
for relief of Nasal Congestion, Sneezing, Runny Nose, Itchy, Watery Eyes, and Fever, Aches, and Pains
24 CAPLETS

Available in consumer cartons of 24 and bottles of 48

DIMETAPP® COLD AND FLU CAPLETS

A. H. Robins

Available in bottles of 4 Fl. Oz.,
8 Fl. Oz. and 16 Fl. Oz. and
chewable tablets in cartons of 18

DONNAGEL®

A. H. Robins

Available in bottles of 4 Fl. Oz.,
8 Fl. Oz. and 16 Fl. Oz.

ROBITUSSIN®-PE SYRUP

A. H. Robins

Available in bottles of 4 Fl. Oz.
and 8 Fl. Oz.

**ROBITUSSIN® MAXIMUM
STRENGTH COUGH**

(Dextromethorphan Hydrobromide)

Ross

0.5 Fl. Oz.   0.5 Fl. Oz.

**MURINE® EAR
WAX REMOVAL
SYSTEM**

**MURINE®
EAR DROPS**

A. H. Robins

Available in bottles of 4 Fl. Oz.,
8 Fl. Oz., 16 Fl. Oz. and 128 Fl. Oz.

ROBITUSSIN® SYRUP

(Guaifenesin Syrup, USP)

A. H. Robins

Available in bottles of
4 Fl. Oz. and 8 Fl. Oz.

**ROBITUSSIN® PEDIATRIC
COUGH SUPPRESSANT**

(Dextromethorphan Hydrobromide)

A. H. Robins

Available in packages of 25
and sticks of 9

**ROBITUSSIN®
Cough Drops**

Ross   4 Fl. Oz.

For Oily   For Dry   For Regular   For All
Hair   Hair   Hair   Hair Types

**SELSUN BLUE®
Dandruff Shampoo**

Also available in 7
and 11 Fl. Oz.

Extra Medicated
For All Hair Types

A. H. Robins

Available in bottles of 8 Fl. Oz.,
12 Fl. Oz. and 16 Fl. Oz.

ROBITUSSIN®-CF SYRUP

A. H. Robins

Available in bottles of 4 Fl. Oz.
and 8 Fl. Oz.

**ROBITUSSIN® PEDIATRIC
COUGH & COLD**

ROSS

**CLEAR EYES®
Lubricating Eye
Redness Reliever**

**CLEAR EYES® ACR
Astringent/Lubricat-
ing Eye Redness
Reliver Drops**

Ross

Cream
1 Oz. and 2 Oz. Tubes

Suppositories
10's and 20's

**TRONOLANE®
Anesthetic Cream and
Suppositories for Hemorrhoids**

A. H. Robins

Available in bottles of 4 Fl. Oz.,
8 Fl. Oz., 16 Fl. Oz. and 128 Fl. Oz.

ROBITUSSIN®-DM SYRUP

A. H. Robins

Available in bottles of 4 Fl. Oz. and
8 Fl. Oz. with convenient dosage cup.

ROBITUSSIN NIGHT RELIEF®

**MURINE® EYE
LUBRICANT
More Closely
Matches Natural
Tears**

**MURINE® PLUS
Lubricating Eye
Redness Reliever**

Available in:
0.5 and 1.0 Fl. Oz.

While every effort has
been made to reproduce
products faithfully, this
section is to be consid-
ered a Quick-Reference
identification aid.

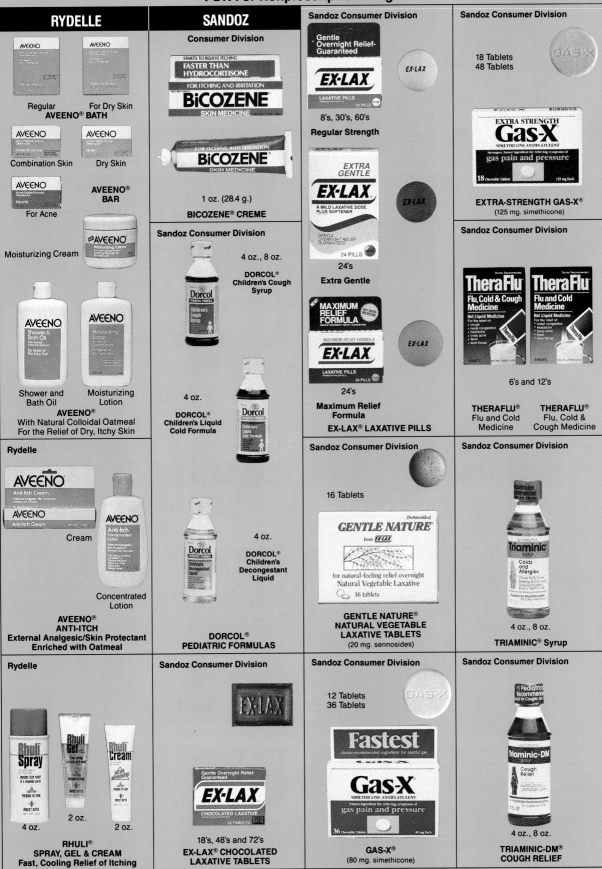

RYDELLE

Regular — **For Dry Skin**
AVEENO® BATH

Combination Skin — **Dry Skin**

For Acne
AVEENO® BAR

Moisturizing Cream

Shower and Bath Oil — **Moisturizing Lotion**
AVEENO®
With Natural Colloidal Oatmeal
For the Relief of Dry, Itchy Skin

Rydelle

Cream

Concentrated Lotion

AVEENO®
ANTI-ITCH
External Analgesic/Skin Protectant
Enriched with Oatmeal

Rydelle

4 oz. — 2 oz. — 2 oz.

RHULI®
SPRAY, GEL & CREAM
Fast, Cooling Relief of Itching

SANDOZ

Consumer Division

STARTS TO RELIEVE ITCHING
FASTER THAN HYDROCORTISONE
FOR ITCHING AND IRRITATION
BiCOZENE
SKIN MEDICINE

FOR ITCHING AND IRRITATION
BiCOZENE
SKIN MEDICINE

1 oz. (28.4 g.)

BICOZENE® CREME

Sandoz Consumer Division

4 oz., 8 oz.

DORCOL®
Children's Cough Syrup

4 oz.
DORCOL®
Children's Liquid Cold Formula

4 oz.
DORCOL®
Children's Decongestant Liquid

DORCOL®
PEDIATRIC FORMULAS

Sandoz Consumer Division

Gentle Overnight Relief- Guaranteed
EX-LAX
LAXATIVE PILLS

EX-LAX CHOCOLATED LAXATIVE TABLETS

18's, 48's and 72's

EX-LAX® CHOCOLATED LAXATIVE TABLETS

Sandoz Consumer Division

Gentle Overnight Relief- Guaranteed
EX-LAX
LAXATIVE PILLS
8's, 30's, 60's

Regular Strength

EXTRA GENTLE
EX-LAX
A MILD LAXATIVE DOSE PLUS SOFTENER
GENTLE OVERNIGHT RELIEF- GUARANTEED
24 PILLS
24's

Extra Gentle

NEW!
MAXIMUM RELIEF FORMULA
EX-LAX
LAXATIVE PILLS
24 PILLS
24's

Maximum Relief Formula
EX-LAX® LAXATIVE PILLS

Sandoz Consumer Division

16 Tablets

GENTLE NATURE®
(Sennosides)
from **EX-LAX**
for natural-feeling relief overnight
Natural Vegetable Laxative
16 tablets

GENTLE NATURE®
NATURAL VEGETABLE LAXATIVE TABLETS
(20 mg. sennosides)

Sandoz Consumer Division

12 Tablets
36 Tablets

Fastest
doctor-recommended ingredient for painful gas
Gas-X
SIMETHICONE ANTIFLATULENT
Fastest ingredient for relieving symptoms of
gas pain and pressure
36 Chewable Tablets

GAS-X®
(80 mg. simethicone)

Sandoz Consumer Division

18 Tablets
48 Tablets

GAS-X

EXTRA STRENGTH
Gas-X
SIMETHICONE ANTIFLATULENT
Strongest ingredient for relieving symptoms of
gas pain and pressure
18 Chewable Tablets
125 mg Each

EXTRA-STRENGTH GAS-X®
(125 mg. simethicone)

Sandoz Consumer Division

TheraFlu
Flu, Cold & Cough Medicine
Hot Liquid Medicine

TheraFlu
Flu and Cold Medicine
Hot Liquid Medicine

6's and 12's

THERAFLU®
Flu and Cold Medicine

THERAFLU®
Flu, Cold & Cough Medicine

Sandoz Consumer Division

Triaminic
SYRUP
Colds and Allergies

4 oz., 8 oz.

TRIAMINIC® Syrup

Sandoz Consumer Division

Triaminic-DM
SYRUP
Cough Relief

4 oz., 8 oz.

TRIAMINIC-DM®
COUGH RELIEF

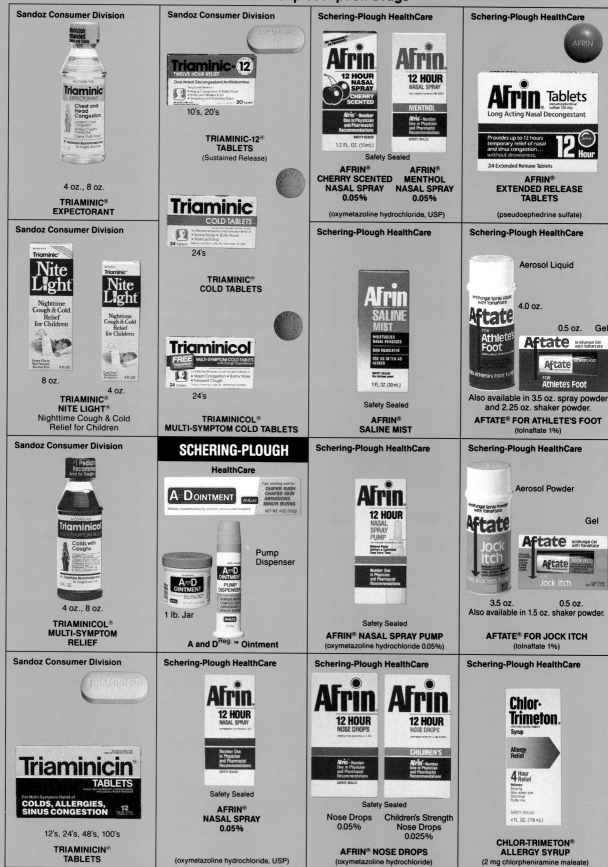

Sandoz Consumer Division

4 oz., 8 oz.

**TRIAMINIC®
EXPECTORANT**

Sandoz Consumer Division

8 oz.   4 oz.

**TRIAMINIC®
NITE LIGHT®**
Nighttime Cough & Cold
Relief for Children

Sandoz Consumer Division

4 oz., 8 oz.

**TRIAMINICOL®
MULTI-SYMPTOM
RELIEF**

Sandoz Consumer Division

12's, 24's, 48's, 100's

**TRIAMINICIN®
TABLETS**

Sandoz Consumer Division

10's, 20's

**TRIAMINIC-12®
TABLETS**
(Sustained Release)

24's

**TRIAMINIC®
COLD TABLETS**

24's

**TRIAMINICOL®
MULTI-SYMPTOM COLD TABLETS**

SCHERING-PLOUGH
HealthCare

Pump
Dispenser

1 lb. Jar

A and D Reg. ™ **Ointment**

Schering-Plough HealthCare

Safety Sealed

**AFRIN®
NASAL SPRAY
0.05%**

(oxymetazoline hydrochloride, USP)

Schering-Plough HealthCare

1/2 FL. OZ. (15mL)

Safety Sealed

**AFRIN®
CHERRY SCENTED
NASAL SPRAY
0.05%**

**AFRIN®
MENTHOL
NASAL SPRAY
0.05%**

(oxymetazoline hydrochloride, USP)

Schering-Plough HealthCare

1 FL. OZ. (30 mL)

Safety Sealed

**AFRIN®
SALINE MIST**

Schering-Plough HealthCare

Safety Sealed

AFRIN® NASAL SPRAY PUMP
(oxymetazoline hydrochloride 0.05%)

Schering-Plough HealthCare

Safety Sealed

Nose Drops
0.05%

Children's Strength
Nose Drops
0.025%

AFRIN® NOSE DROPS
(oxymetazoline hydrochloride)

Schering-Plough HealthCare

24 Extended Release Tablets

**AFRIN®
EXTENDED RELEASE
TABLETS**

(pseudoephedrine sulfate)

Schering-Plough HealthCare

Aerosol Liquid

4.0 oz.

0.5 oz.   Gel

Also available in 3.5 oz. spray powder
and 2.25 oz. shaker powder.

AFTATE® FOR ATHLETE'S FOOT
(tolnaftate 1%)

Schering-Plough HealthCare

Aerosol Powder

Gel

3.5 oz.   0.5 oz.
Also available in 1.5 oz. shaker powder.

AFTATE® FOR JOCK ITCH
(tolnaftate 1%)

Schering-Plough HealthCare

**CHLOR-TRIMETON®
ALLERGY SYRUP**
(2 mg chlorpheniramine maleate)

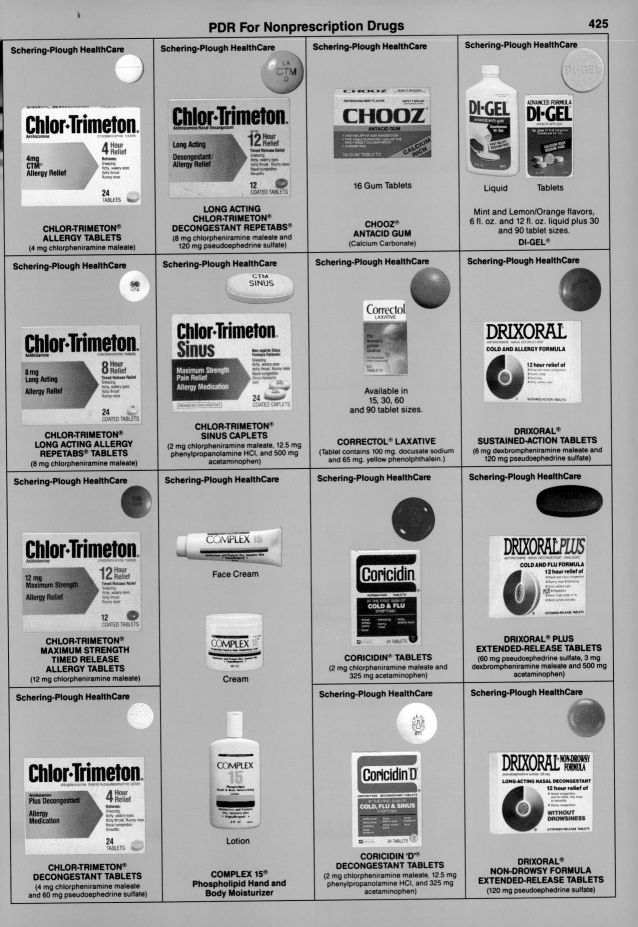

Schering-Plough HealthCare

**CHLOR-TRIMETON®
ALLERGY TABLETS**

(4 mg chlorpheniramine maleate)

Schering-Plough HealthCare

**LONG ACTING
CHLOR-TRIMETON®
DECONGESTANT REPETABS®**

(8 mg chlorpheniramine maleate and
120 mg pseudoephedrine sulfate)

Schering-Plough HealthCare

16 Gum Tablets

**CHOOZ®
ANTACID GUM**

(Calcium Carbonate)

Schering-Plough HealthCare

Liquid   Tablets

Mint and Lemon/Orange flavors,
6 fl. oz. and 12 fl. oz. liquid plus 30
and 90 tablet sizes.
DI-GEL®

Schering-Plough HealthCare

**CHLOR-TRIMETON®
LONG ACTING ALLERGY
REPETABS® TABLETS**

(8 mg chlorpheniramine maleate)

Schering-Plough HealthCare

**CHLOR-TRIMETON®
SINUS CAPLETS**

(2 mg chlorpheniramine maleate, 12.5 mg
phenylpropanolamine HCl, and 500 mg
acetaminophen)

Schering-Plough HealthCare

Available in
15, 30, 60
and 90 tablet sizes.

CORRECTOL® LAXATIVE

(Tablet contains 100 mg. docusate sodium
and 65 mg. yellow phenolphthalein.)

Schering-Plough HealthCare

**DRIXORAL®
SUSTAINED-ACTION TABLETS**

(6 mg dexbrompheniramine maleate and
120 mg pseudoephedrine sulfate)

Schering-Plough HealthCare

**CHLOR-TRIMETON®
MAXIMUM STRENGTH
TIMED RELEASE
ALLERGY TABLETS**

(12 mg chlorpheniramine maleate)

Schering-Plough HealthCare

Face Cream

Cream

**COMPLEX 15®
Phospholipid Hand and
Body Moisturizer**

Schering-Plough HealthCare

CORICIDIN® TABLETS

(2 mg chlorpheniramine maleate and
325 mg acetaminophen)

Schering-Plough HealthCare

**DRIXORAL® PLUS
EXTENDED-RELEASE TABLETS**

(60 mg pseudoephedrine sulfate, 3 mg
dexbrompheniramine maleate and 500 mg
acetaminophen)

Schering-Plough HealthCare

**CHLOR-TRIMETON®
DECONGESTANT TABLETS**

(4 mg chlorpheniramine maleate
and 60 mg pseudoephedrine sulfate)

Schering-Plough HealthCare

Lotion

**COMPLEX 15®
Phospholipid Hand and
Body Moisturizer**

Schering-Plough HealthCare

**CORICIDIN 'D'®
DECONGESTANT TABLETS**

(2 mg chlorpheniramine maleate, 12.5 mg
phenylpropanolamine HCl, and 325 mg
acetaminophen)

Schering-Plough HealthCare

**DRIXORAL®
NON-DROWSY FORMULA
EXTENDED-RELEASE TABLETS**

(120 mg pseudoephedrine sulfate)

Schering-Plough HealthCare

DRIXORAL® SINUS
(60 mg pseudoephedrine sulfate,
3 mg dexbrompheniramine maleate,
500 mg acetaminophen)

Schering-Plough HealthCare

Cream

Inserts

GYNE-LOTRIMIN®
Clotrimazole Vaginal
Antifungal

Schering-Plough HealthCare

TINACTIN®
CREAM AND SOLUTION
(tolnaftate 1%)

For more detailed information on products illustrated in this section, consult the Product Information Section or manufacturers may be contacted directly.

Schering-Plough HealthCare

DuoFilm Wart Remover

DuoPlant Plantar Wart
Remover for Feet

DUOFILM®/DUOPLANT®

Schering-Plough HealthCare

Available in 1.5 and 2.5 oz. sizes

GYNE-MOISTRIN™
Vaginal Moisturizing Gel
Relieves vaginal dryness

Schering-Plough HealthCare

TINACTIN® JOCK ITCH
CREAM AND SPRAY POWDER
(tolnaftate 1%)

SMITHKLINE BEECHAM

Consumer Brands

4 fl. oz.

A-200® PEDICULICIDE SHAMPOO
Also available:
A-200® Pediculicide Shampoo, 2 fl. oz.
A-200® Pediculicide Gel, 1 oz.

Schering-Plough HealthCare

Available in ½ oz., 1 oz. and ½ oz.
measured dosage pump spray.
(oxymetazoline HCl)

DURATION®
NASAL SPRAY

Schering-Plough HealthCare

LOTRIMIN® AF
(1% clotrimazole)

Schering-Plough HealthCare

TINACTIN® POWDER AEROSOL
AND POWDER
(tolnaftate 1%)

SmithKline Beecham Consumer Brands

1.5 oz. tube
CLEAR BY DESIGN®
Medicated Acne Gel
(benzoyl peroxide 2.5%)

Schering-Plough HealthCare

Laxative Gum

Laxative plus
Softener

FEEN-A-MINT® LAXATIVE
Gum contains:
97.2 mg. phenolphthalein.
Pills contain: 100 mg. docusate
sodium and 65 mg. phenolphthalein.

Schering-Plough HealthCare

Safety Sealed
OCUCLEAR®
EYE DROPS

(oxymetazoline HCl 0.025%)

Schering-Plough HealthCare

TINACTIN®
LIQUID AEROSOL
(tolnaftate 1%)

SmithKline Beecham Consumer Brands

Packages of 10, 20 and 40
capsules and caplets

CONTAC®
CONTINUOUS ACTION NASAL
DECONGESTANT ANTIHISTAMINE
CAPLETS & CAPSULES

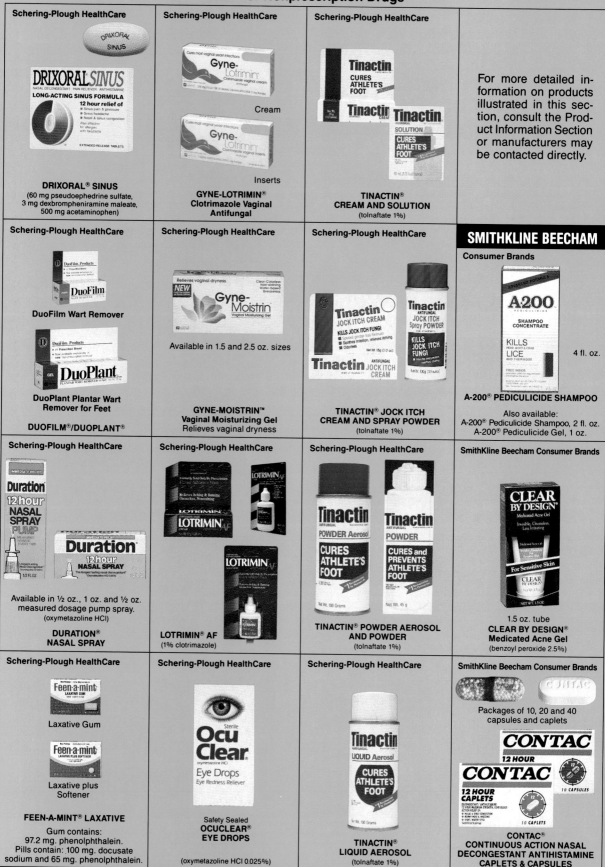

SmithKline Beecham Consumer Brands

CONTAC
SEVERE COLD & FLU
DECONGESTANT/ANTIHISTAMINE
ANALGESIC/COUGH SUPPRESSANT

RELIEVES YOUR SEVERE COLD & FLU SYMPTOMS:
● NASAL CONGESTION
● ACHES & PAINS, FEVER
● RUNNY NOSE, SNEEZING
● SORE THROAT
● COUGHING

10 CAPLETS

Packages of 10, 20 and 40 caplets
CONTAC®
SEVERE COLD FORMULA

SmithKline Beecham Consumer Brands

Regular Strength
Ecotrin
SAFETY-COATED ASPIRIN
for Arthritis Pain 100

Tablets in bottles of
100, 250 and 1000

Regular Strength
Ecotrin
SAFETY-COATED ASPIRIN
for Arthritis Pain 100

Caplets in bottles of 100
**REGULAR STRENGTH
ECOTRIN® TABLETS AND CAPLETS**
Enteric coated 5 gr. aspirin

SmithKline Beecham Consumer Brands

Feosol
TABLETS
Iron
Therapy

100 TABLETS

In 100 and 1000 tablet bottles
FEOSOL® TABLETS
(ferrous sulfate USP)

SmithKline Beecham Consumer Brands

N'ICE
RELIEVES SORE THROATS AND COUGHS
CHERRY

N'ICE
RELIEVES SORE THROATS AND COUGHS
CITRUS

Available in Cherry, Citrus,
Menthol Eucalyptus, Menthol
Mint, Children's Berry
N'ICE®
Sore Throat Lozenges

SmithKline Beecham Consumer Brands

CONTAC
CONTAC
SINUS
DECONGESTANT/ANALGESIC
NON-DROWSY FORMULA

24 TABLETS

24 TABLETS

Packages of 24
**CONTAC®
MAXIMUM STRENGTH
SINUS TABLETS AND CAPLETS
NON-DROWSY FORMULA**

SmithKline Beecham Consumer Brands

Maximum Strength
Ecotrin
SAFETY-COATED ASPIRIN
for Arthritis Pain 60

Tablets in bottles of
60 and 150

Maximum Strength
Ecotrin
SAFETY-COATED ASPIRIN
for Arthritis Pain 60

Caplets in bottles of 60
**MAXIMUM STRENGTH
ECOTRIN® TABLETS AND CAPLETS**
Enteric coated 7.7 gr. aspirin

SmithKline Beecham Consumer Brands

TRUST
Massengill
DISPOSABLE DOUCHE

MEDICATED

Available in single or twin packs

MASSENGILL® Medicated
Disposable Douche
With Povidone-iodine

SmithKline Beecham Consumer Brands

N'ICE
N'ICE
N'ICE
VITAMIN C DROPS

Available in Orange,
Lemon, Children's Grape
in 16 count packages
N'ICE®
Vitamin C Drops

SmithKline Beecham Consumer Brands

CONTAC Jr.
Non-Drowsy
Cold Liquid
Gentle Relief for Children:

BERRY FLAVOR

4 FL. OZ.

Includes dose-
by-weight cup

CONTAC JR.®
COLD MEDICINE FOR CHILDREN

SmithKline Beecham Consumer Brands

**FEOSOL
ELIXIR**
For iron

FL. OZ. (355 ML.)

16 oz. bottle
FEOSOL® ELIXIR
(ferrous sulfate USP)

SmithKline Beecham Consumer Brands

NEW!
**Nature's
Remedy**
ENEMA

Regular

NEW!
**Nature's
Remedy**

Mineral
Oil

**NATURE'S REMEDY®
ENEMAS**

SmithKline Beecham Consumer Brands

VANISHING
Sensitive
Skin
OXY5

VANISHING
Maximum
Strength
OXY10

OXY-5®

OXY-10®

Maximum
Strength
OXY10
DAILY
FACE WASH

OXY-10® DAILY FACE WASH

SmithKline Beecham Consumer Brands

Measured
dose cup

CONTAC
COUGH &
CHEST COLD

CONTAC
COUGH &
SORE THROAT

4 FL. OZ.

4 FL. OZ.

**CONTAC® COUGH AND
COUGH & SORE THROAT FORMULA**

SmithKline Beecham Consumer Brands

Feosol
CAPSULES
Iron
Therapy

30 CAPSULES

Packages of 30 and
60 capsules
FEOSOL® CAPSULES
(ferrous sulfate USP)

SmithKline Beecham Consumer Brands

SAFETY SEALED See back for instructions.
**Nature's
Remedy**
FAST ACTING LAXATIVE
for Gentle Overnight
Relief of Constipation
60 TABLETS

60 tablets
**NATURE'S REMEDY®
LAXATIVE TABLETS**
Also available:
Box 12s and 30s

SmithKline Beecham Consumer Brands

Regular
Strength
OXY
50 Medicated Pads

Maximum
Strength
OXY
50 Medicated Pads

Regular
Strength

Maximum
Strength

Sensitive
Skin

Sensitive
Skin
OXY
50 Medicated Pads

50 pads
Also available: 90 pads
**OXY CLEAN®
MEDICATED PADS**

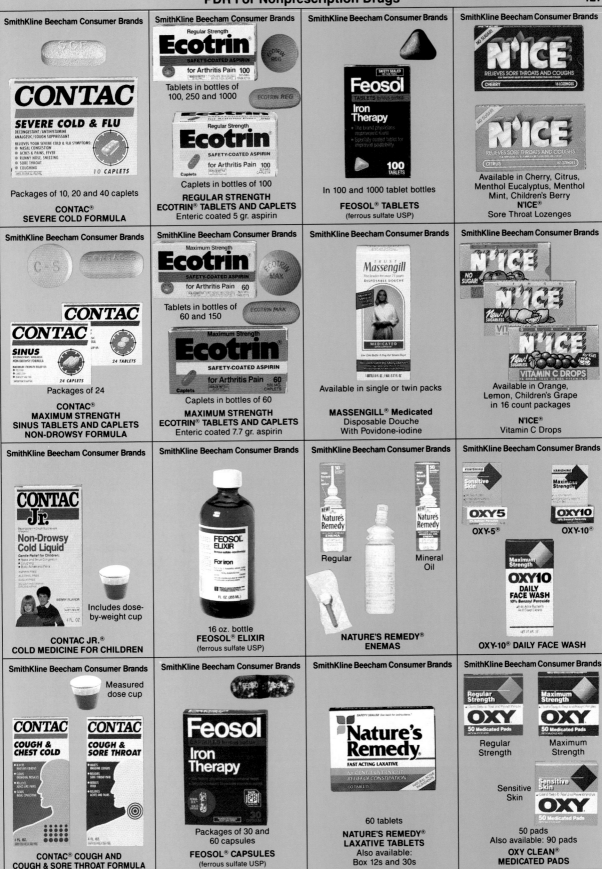

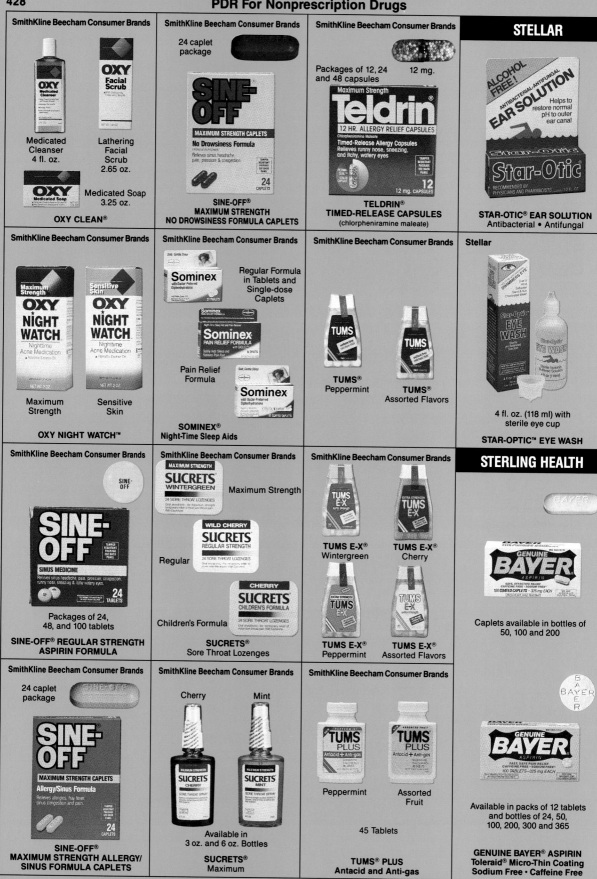

SmithKline Beecham Consumer Brands

Medicated
Cleanser
4 fl. oz.

Lathering
Facial
Scrub
2.65 oz.

Medicated Soap
3.25 oz.

OXY CLEAN®

SmithKline Beecham Consumer Brands

24 caplet
package

**SINE-OFF®
MAXIMUM STRENGTH
NO DROWSINESS FORMULA CAPLETS**

SmithKline Beecham Consumer Brands

Packages of 12, 24
and 48 capsules

12 mg.

**TELDRIN®
TIMED-RELEASE CAPSULES**
(chlorpheniramine maleate)

STELLAR

STAR-OTIC® EAR SOLUTION
Antibacterial • Antifungal

SmithKline Beecham Consumer Brands

Maximum
Strength

Sensitive
Skin

OXY NIGHT WATCH™

SmithKline Beecham Consumer Brands

Regular Formula
in Tablets and
Single-dose
Caplets

Pain Relief
Formula

**SOMINEX®
Night-Time Sleep Aids**

SmithKline Beecham Consumer Brands

TUMS®
Peppermint

TUMS®
Assorted Flavors

Stellar

4 fl. oz. (118 ml) with
sterile eye cup

STAR-OPTIC™ EYE WASH

SmithKline Beecham Consumer Brands

Packages of 24,
48, and 100 tablets

**SINE-OFF® REGULAR STRENGTH
ASPIRIN FORMULA**

SmithKline Beecham Consumer Brands

Maximum Strength

Regular

Children's Formula

SUCRETS®
Sore Throat Lozenges

SmithKline Beecham Consumer Brands

TUMS E-X®
Wintergreen

TUMS E-X®
Cherry

TUMS E-X®
Peppermint

TUMS E-X®
Assorted Flavors

STERLING HEALTH

Caplets available in bottles of
50, 100 and 200

SmithKline Beecham Consumer Brands

24 caplet
package

**SINE-OFF®
MAXIMUM STRENGTH ALLERGY/
SINUS FORMULA CAPLETS**

SmithKline Beecham Consumer Brands

Cherry   Mint

Available in
3 oz. and 6 oz. Bottles

SUCRETS®
Maximum

SmithKline Beecham Consumer Brands

Peppermint

Assorted
Fruit

45 Tablets

**TUMS® PLUS
Antacid and Anti-gas**

Available in packs of 12 tablets
and bottles of 24, 50,
100, 200, 300 and 365

GENUINE BAYER® ASPIRIN
Toleraid® Micro-Thin Coating
Sodium Free • Caffeine Free

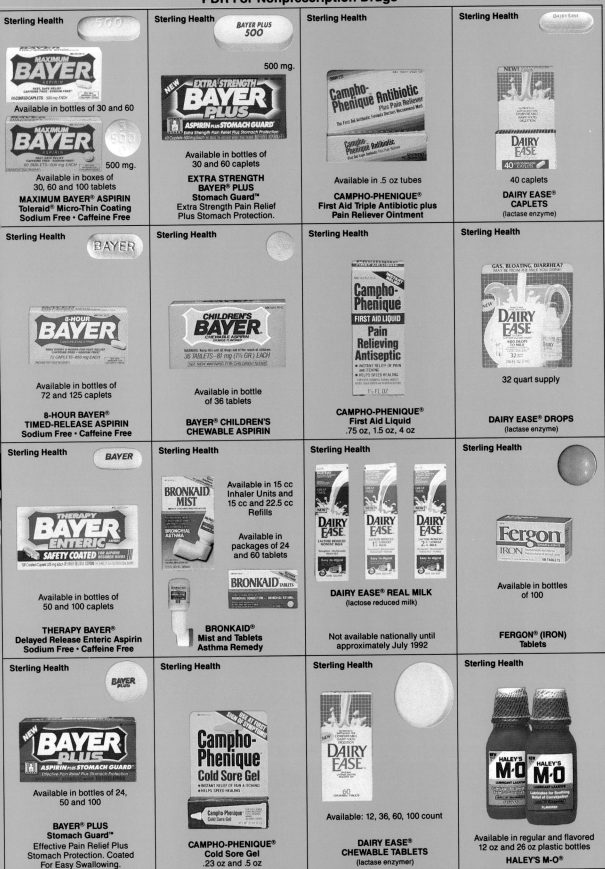

Sterling Health

500

Available in bottles of 30 and 60

500 mg.

Available in boxes of
30, 60 and 100 tablets

MAXIMUM BAYER® ASPIRIN
Toleraid® Micro-Thin Coating
Sodium Free • Caffeine Free

Sterling Health

BAYER PLUS
500

500 mg.

NEW
EXTRA STRENGTH
BAYER PLUS
ASPIRIN PLUS STOMACH GUARD®
Extra Strength Pain Relief Plus Stomach Protection

Available in bottles of
30 and 60 caplets

EXTRA STRENGTH
BAYER® PLUS
Stomach Guard™
Extra Strength Pain Relief
Plus Stomach Protection.

Sterling Health

Campho-
Phenique Antibiotic
Plus Pain Reliever

Campho-
Phenique Antibiotic

Available in .5 oz tubes

CAMPHO-PHENIQUE®
First Aid Triple Antibiotic plus
Pain Reliever Ointment

Sterling Health

DAIRY EASE

NEW

DAIRY
EASE

40 caplets

DAIRY EASE®
CAPLETS
(lactase enzyme)

Sterling Health

BAYER

8-HOUR
BAYER

Available in bottles of
72 and 125 caplets

8-HOUR BAYER®
TIMED-RELEASE ASPIRIN
Sodium Free • Caffeine Free

Sterling Health

BAYER

CHILDREN'S
BAYER
CHEWABLE ASPIRIN
ORANGE FLAVORED

Available in bottle
of 36 tablets

BAYER® CHILDREN'S
CHEWABLE ASPIRIN

Sterling Health

Campho-
Phenique
FIRST AID LIQUID
Pain
Relieving
Antiseptic

1½ FL OZ

CAMPHO-PHENIQUE®
First Aid Liquid
.75 oz, 1.5 oz, 4 oz

Sterling Health

GAS, BLOATING, DIARRHEA?
MAY BE FROM THE MILK YOU DRINK!

NEW

DAIRY
EASE
ADD DROPS
TO MILK
32

32 quart supply

DAIRY EASE® DROPS
(lactase enzyme)

Sterling Health

BAYER

THERAPY
BAYER
ENTERIC
SAFETY COATED

Available in bottles of
50 and 100 caplets

THERAPY BAYER®
Delayed Release Enteric Aspirin
Sodium Free • Caffeine Free

Sterling Health

BRONKAID
MIST
BRONCHIAL
ASTHMA

Available in 15 cc
Inhaler Units and
15 cc and 22.5 cc
Refills

Available in
packages of 24
and 60 tablets

BRONKAID TABLETS

BRONKAID®
Mist and Tablets
Asthma Remedy

Sterling Health

DAIRY
EASE
LACTOSE REDUCED
NONFAT MILK

DAIRY
EASE
LACTOSE REDUCED
1% LOWFAT MILK

DAIRY
EASE
LACTOSE REDUCED
2% LOWFAT MILK

DAIRY EASE® REAL MILK
(lactose reduced milk)

Not available nationally until
approximately July 1992

Sterling Health

Fergon
IRON

Available in bottles
of 100

FERGON® (IRON)
Tablets

Sterling Health

BAYER
PLUS

NEW
BAYER PLUS
ASPIRIN PLUS STOMACH GUARD®
Effective Pain Relief Plus Stomach Protection

Available in bottles of 24,
50 and 100

BAYER® PLUS
Stomach Guard™
Effective Pain Relief Plus
Stomach Protection. Coated
For Easy Swallowing.

Sterling Health

USE AT FIRST
SIGN OF SYMPTOMS

Campho-
Phenique
Cold Sore Gel
• INSTANT RELIEF OF PAIN & ITCHING
• HELPS SPEED HEALING

Campho-Phenique
Cold Sore Gel
NET WT .23 oz

CAMPHO-PHENIQUE®
Cold Sore Gel
.23 oz and .5 oz

Sterling Health

NEW

DAIRY
EASE
60
CHEWABLE TABLETS

Available: 12, 36, 60, 100 count

DAIRY EASE®
CHEWABLE TABLETS
(lactase enzymer)

Sterling Health

NEW
HALEY'S M·O
LUBRICANT LAXATIVE

NEW
HALEY'S M·O
LUBRICANT LAXATIVE

Available in regular and flavored
12 oz and 26 oz plastic bottles

HALEY'S M·O®

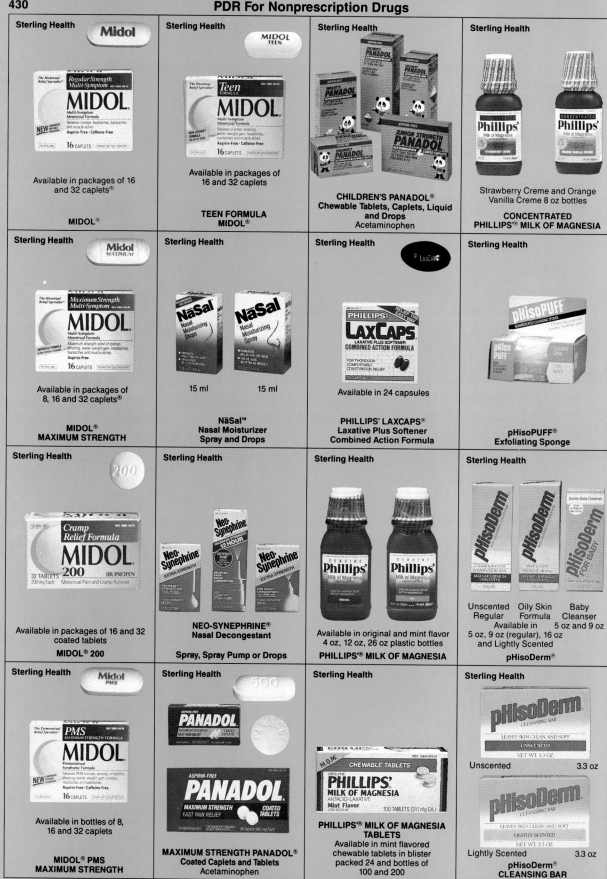

Sterling Health

MIDOL

The Menstrual Relief Specialist

Regular Strength Multi-Symptom

MIDOL.
Multi-Symptom Menstrual Formula

Relieves cramps, headaches, backaches and muscle aches

Aspirin-Free · Caffeine-Free

NEW

16 CAPLETS

Available in packages of 16 and 32 caplets®

MIDOL®

Sterling Health

MIDOL TEEN

The Menstrual Relief Specialist

Teen FORMULA

MIDOL.
Multi-Symptom Menstrual Formula

Relieves cramps, bloating, water-weight gain, headaches, backaches and muscle aches

Non-Drowsy

Aspirin-Free · Caffeine-Free

16 CAPLETS

Available in packages of 16 and 32 caplets

TEEN FORMULA MIDOL®

Sterling Health

PANADOL

JUNIOR STRENGTH PANADOL

CHILDREN'S PANADOL

CHILDREN'S PANADOL®
Chewable Tablets, Caplets, Liquid and Drops
Acetaminophen

Sterling Health

Phillips' Milk of Magnesia

STRAWBERRY CREME

Phillips' Milk of Magnesia

ORANGE VANILLA CREME

Strawberry Creme and Orange Vanilla Creme 8 oz bottles

CONCENTRATED PHILLIPS'® MILK OF MAGNESIA

Sterling Health

Midol MAXIMUM

The Menstrual Relief Specialist

Maximum Strength Multi-Symptom

MIDOL.
Multi-Symptom Menstrual Formula

Maximum strength relief of cramps, bloating, water-weight gain, headaches, backaches and muscle aches

Aspirin-Free

IMPROVED FORMULA

16 CAPLETS

Available in packages of 8, 16 and 32 caplets®

MIDOL® MAXIMUM STRENGTH

Sterling Health

NaSal
Nasal Moisturizing Drops

NaSal
Nasal Moisturizing Spray

15 ml   15 ml

**NāSal™
Nasal Moisturizer
Spray and Drops**

Sterling Health

LaxCaps

PHILLIPS'
LaxCaps
LAXATIVE PLUS SOFTENER
COMBINED ACTION FORMULA

FOR THOROUGH COMFORTABLE CONSTIPATION RELIEF

24 CAPSULES

Available in 24 capsules

**PHILLIPS' LAXCAPS®
Laxative Plus Softener
Combined Action Formula**

Sterling Health

pHisoPUFF

pHiso PUFF

CLEANS SKIN

TWO WAYS

**pHisoPUFF®
Exfoliating Sponge**

Sterling Health

200

Cramp Relief Formula

MIDOL. 200
IBUPROFEN

32 TABLETS   200 mg Each   Menstrual Pain and Cramp Reliever

Available in packages of 16 and 32 coated tablets

MIDOL® 200

Sterling Health

Neo-Synephrine
EXTRA STRENGTH

Neo-Synephrine
12 HOUR

Neo-Synephrine
EXTRA STRENGTH

**NEO-SYNEPHRINE®
Nasal Decongestant**

Spray, Spray Pump or Drops

Sterling Health

GENUINE
Phillips'
Milk of Magnesia

GENUINE
Phillips'
Milk of Magnesia

Available in original and mint flavor 4 oz, 12 oz, 26 oz plastic bottles

PHILLIPS'® MILK OF MAGNESIA

Sterling Health

pHisoDerm

pHisoDerm

Gentle Baby Cleanser
pHisoDerm FOR BABY

Unscented Regular   Oily Skin Formula   Baby Cleanser   5 oz and 9 oz

Available in 5 oz, 9 oz (regular), 16 oz and Lightly Scented

pHisoDerm®

Sterling Health

Midol PMS

The Premenstrual Relief Specialist

PMS
MAXIMUM STRENGTH FORMULA

MIDOL.
Premenstrual Syndrome Formula

Relieves PMS tension, anxiety, irritability, bloating, water-weight gain, cramps, headaches and backaches

Aspirin-Free · Caffeine-Free

NEW

16 CAPLETS

Available in bottles of 8, 16 and 32 caplets

**MIDOL® PMS
MAXIMUM STRENGTH**

Sterling Health

ASPIRIN-FREE
PANADOL
MAXIMUM STRENGTH   COATED CAPLETS
FAST PAIN RELIEF

ASPIRIN-FREE
PANADOL
MAXIMUM STRENGTH   COATED TABLETS
FAST PAIN RELIEF

Acetaminophen

**MAXIMUM STRENGTH PANADOL®
Coated Caplets and Tablets
Acetaminophen**

Sterling Health

M.O.M.

CHEWABLE TABLETS

GENUINE
**PHILLIPS'
MILK OF MAGNESIA**
ANTACID-LAXATIVE
Mint Flavor
LOW SODIUM

100 TABLETS (311 mg EA.)

PHILLIPS'® MILK OF MAGNESIA TABLETS
Available in mint flavored chewable tablets in blister packed 24 and bottles of 100 and 200

Sterling Health

pHisoDerm
CLEANSING BAR
LEAVES SKIN CLEAN AND SOFT
UNSCENTED
NET WT. 3.3 OZ.

Unscented   3.3 oz

pHisoDerm
CLEANSING BAR
LEAVES SKIN CLEAN AND SOFT
LIGHTLY SCENTED
NET WT. 3.3 OZ.

Lightly Scented   3.3 oz

**pHisoDerm®
CLEANSING BAR**

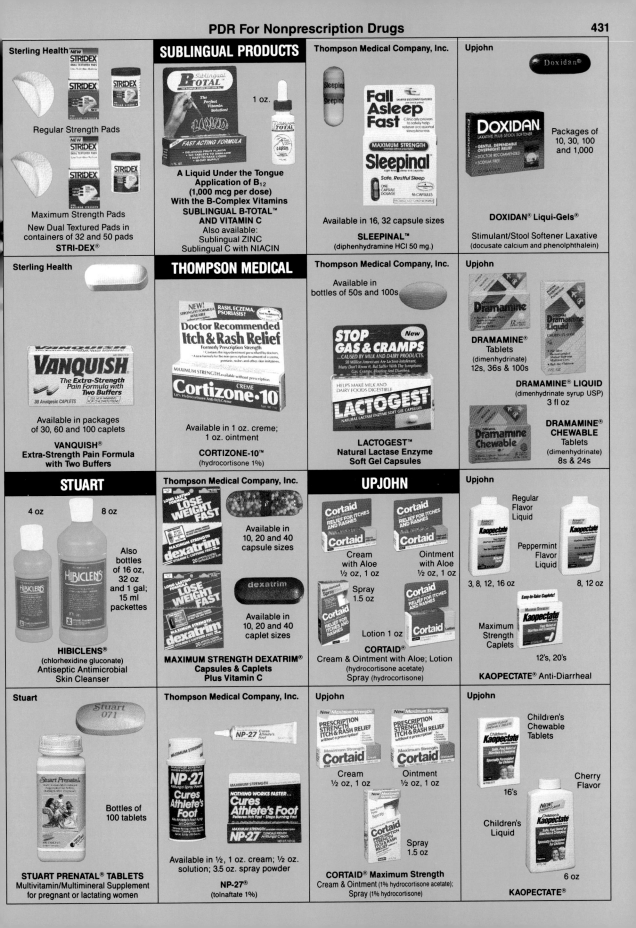

Sterling Health

STRIDEX

Regular Strength Pads

Maximum Strength Pads

New Dual Textured Pads in containers of 32 and 50 pads

STRI-DEX®

SUBLINGUAL PRODUCTS

Sublingual B-TOTAL

1 oz.

A Liquid Under the Tongue Application of B$_{12}$ (1,000 mcg per dose) With the B-Complex Vitamins SUBLINGUAL B-TOTAL™ AND VITAMIN C

Also available:
Sublingual ZINC
Sublingual C with NIACIN

Thompson Medical Company, Inc.

Fall Asleep Fast

MAXIMUM STRENGTH

Sleepinal

Safe, Restful Sleep

Available in 16, 32 capsule sizes

SLEEPINAL™
(diphenhydramine HCl 50 mg.)

Upjohn

Doxidan®

DOXIDAN
LAXATIVE PLUS STOOL SOFTENER

Packages of 10, 30, 100 and 1,000

DOXIDAN® Liqui-Gels®

Stimulant/Stool Softener Laxative
(docusate calcium and phenolphthalein)

Sterling Health

VANQUISH
The Extra-Strength Pain Formula with Two Buffers
30 Analgesic CAPLETS

Available in packages of 30, 60 and 100 caplets

VANQUISH®
Extra-Strength Pain Formula with Two Buffers

THOMPSON MEDICAL

NEW! STRONGEST FORMULA AVAILABLE
RASH, ECZEMA, PSORIASIS†

Doctor Recommended Itch & Rash Relief
Formerly Prescription Strength

MAXIMUM STRENGTH available without prescription

Cortizone·10
CREME
1.0% Hydrocortisone Anti-Itch Creme

Available in 1 oz. creme;
1 oz. ointment

CORTIZONE-10™
(hydrocortisone 1%)

Thompson Medical Company, Inc.

Available in bottles of 50s and 100s

STOP GAS & CRAMPS
New
...CAUSED BY MILK AND DAIRY PRODUCTS.

HELPS MAKE MILK AND DAIRY FOODS DIGESTIBLE

LACTOGEST
NATURAL LACTASE ENZYME SOFT GEL CAPSULES

LACTOGEST™
Natural Lactase Enzyme Soft Gel Capsules

Upjohn

Dramamine

DRAMAMINE®
Tablets
(dimenhydrinate)
12s, 36s & 100s

Dramamine Liquid

DRAMAMINE® LIQUID
(dimenhydrinate syrup USP)
3 fl oz

Dramamine Chewable

DRAMAMINE® CHEWABLE
Tablets
(dimenhydrinate)
8s & 24s

STUART

4 oz   8 oz

Also bottles of 16 oz, 32 oz and 1 gal; 15 ml packettes

HIBICLENS

HIBICLENS®
(chlorhexidine gluconate)
Antiseptic Antimicrobial Skin Cleanser

Thompson Medical Company, Inc.

LONG LASTING FORMULA
LOSE WEIGHT FAST
MAXIMUM STRENGTH
dexatrim

Available in 10, 20 and 40 capsule sizes

LONG LASTING FORMULA
LOSE WEIGHT FAST
MAXIMUM STRENGTH
dexatrim

dexatrim

Available in 10, 20 and 40 caplet sizes

MAXIMUM STRENGTH DEXATRIM®
Capsules & Caplets
Plus Vitamin C

UPJOHN

Cortaid
RELIEF FOR ITCHES AND RASHES

Cortaid
RELIEF FOR ITCHES AND RASHES

Cream with Aloe
½ oz, 1 oz

Ointment with Aloe
½ oz, 1 oz

Cortaid
Spray
1.5 oz

Cortaid
RELIEF FOR ITCHES AND RASHES

Cortaid
Lotion 1 oz

CORTAID®
Cream & Ointment with Aloe; Lotion
(hydrocortisone acetate)
Spray (hydrocortisone)

Upjohn

Regular Flavor Liquid

Kaopectate

Peppermint Flavor Liquid

Kaopectate

3, 8, 12, 16 oz   8, 12 oz

Easy-to-Take Caplets!

Kaopectate

Maximum Strength Caplets

12's, 20's

KAOPECTATE® Anti-Diarrheal

Stuart

Stuart 071

Stuart Prenatal

Bottles of 100 tablets

STUART PRENATAL® TABLETS
Multivitamin/Multimineral Supplement for pregnant or lactating women

---

Thompson Medical Company, Inc.

MAXIMUM STRENGTH
NP-27
Cures Athlete's Foot

MAXIMUM STRENGTH
Cures Athlete's Foot

NOTHING WORKS FASTER...
Cures Athlete's Foot
Relieves Itch Fast • Stops Burning Fast

MAXIMUM STRENGTH
NP-27

Available in ½, 1 oz. cream; ½ oz. solution; 3.5 oz. spray powder

NP-27®
(tolnaftate 1%)

Upjohn

New Maximum Strength!
PRESCRIPTION STRENGTH
ITCH & RASH RELIEF
without a prescription!

Cortaid
Maximum Strength

Cream
½ oz, 1 oz

New Maximum Strength!
PRESCRIPTION STRENGTH
ITCH & RASH RELIEF
without a prescription!

Cortaid
Maximum Strength

Ointment
½ oz, 1 oz

Cortaid
Spray
1.5 oz

CORTAID® Maximum Strength
Cream & Ointment (1% hydrocortisone acetate);
Spray (1% hydrocortisone)

Upjohn

Children's Chewable Tablets

Kaopectate
Children's

16's

Cherry Flavor

Children's Liquid

Kaopectate
Children's

6 oz

KAOPECTATE®

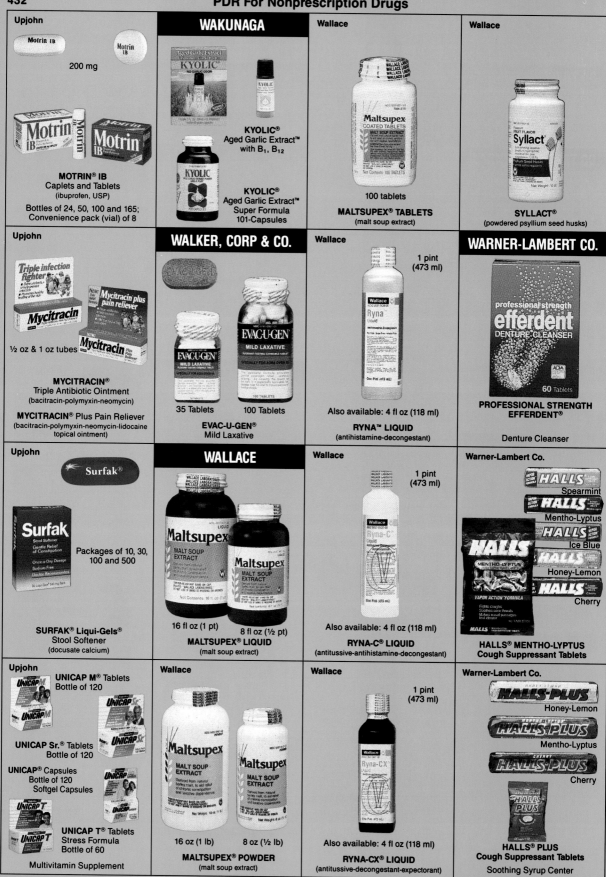

Upjohn

200 mg

MOTRIN® IB
Caplets and Tablets
(ibuprofen, USP)

Bottles of 24, 50, 100 and 165;
Convenience pack (vial) of 8

Upjohn

½ oz & 1 oz tubes

MYCITRACIN®
Triple Antibiotic Ointment
(bacitracin-polymyxin-neomycin)

MYCITRACIN® Plus Pain Reliever
(bacitracin-polymyxin-neomycin-lidocaine
topical ointment)

Upjohn

Surfak®

Packages of 10, 30,
100 and 500

SURFAK® Liqui-Gels®
Stool Softener
(docusate calcium)

Upjohn

UNICAP M® Tablets
Bottle of 120

UNICAP Sr.® Tablets
Bottle of 120

UNICAP® Capsules
Bottle of 120
Softgel Capsules

UNICAP T® Tablets
Stress Formula
Bottle of 60

Multivitamin Supplement

WAKUNAGA

KYOLIC®
Aged Garlic Extract™
with B₁, B₁₂

KYOLIC®
Aged Garlic Extract™
Super Formula
101-Capsules

WALKER, CORP & CO.

35 Tablets   100 Tablets

EVAC-U-GEN®
Mild Laxative

WALLACE

16 fl oz (1 pt)   8 fl oz (½ pt)

MALTSUPEX® LIQUID
(malt soup extract)

Wallace

16 oz (1 lb)   8 oz (½ lb)

MALTSUPEX® POWDER
(malt soup extract)

Wallace

100 tablets

MALTSUPEX® TABLETS
(malt soup extract)

Wallace

1 pint
(473 ml)

Also available: 4 fl oz (118 ml)

RYNA™ LIQUID
(antihistamine-decongestant)

Wallace

1 pint
(473 ml)

Also available: 4 fl oz (118 ml)

RYNA-C® LIQUID
(antitussive-antihistamine-decongestant)

Wallace

1 pint
(473 ml)

Also available: 4 fl oz (118 ml)

RYNA-CX® LIQUID
(antitussive-decongestant-expectorant)

Wallace

SYLLACT®
(powdered psyllium seed husks)

WARNER-LAMBERT CO.

professional strength
efferdent
DENTURE CLEANSER

60 Tablets

**PROFESSIONAL STRENGTH
EFFERDENT®**

Denture Cleanser

Warner-Lambert Co.

HALLS Spearmint
HALLS Mentho-Lyptus
HALLS Ice Blue
HALLS Honey-Lemon
HALLS Cherry

HALLS® MENTHO-LYPTUS
Cough Suppressant Tablets

Warner-Lambert Co.

HALLS-PLUS Honey-Lemon
HALLS-PLUS Mentho-Lyptus
HALLS-PLUS Cherry

HALLS® PLUS
Cough Suppressant Tablets
Soothing Syrup Center

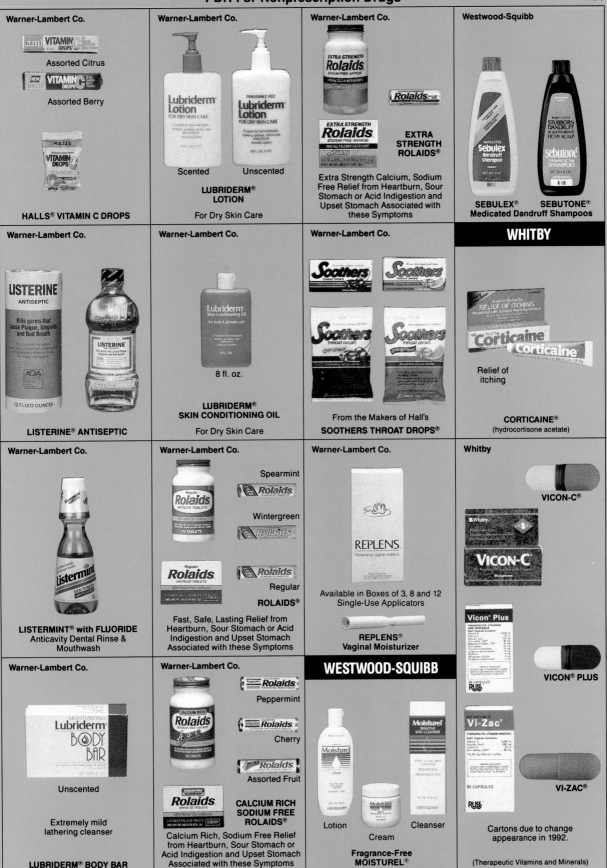

Warner-Lambert Co.

Assorted Citrus

Assorted Berry

HALLS® VITAMIN C DROPS

Warner-Lambert Co.

Scented   Unscented

**LUBRIDERM®
LOTION**

For Dry Skin Care

Warner-Lambert Co.

EXTRA STRENGTH ROLAIDS®

Extra Strength Calcium, Sodium Free Relief from Heartburn, Sour Stomach or Acid Indigestion and Upset Stomach Associated with these Symptoms

Westwood-Squibb

SEBULEX®   **SEBUTONE®**
Medicated Dandruff Shampoos

Warner-Lambert Co.

LISTERINE® ANTISEPTIC

Warner-Lambert Co.

8 fl. oz.

**LUBRIDERM®
SKIN CONDITIONING OIL**

For Dry Skin Care

Warner-Lambert Co.

From the Makers of Hall's
SOOTHERS THROAT DROPS®

WHITBY

Relief of itching

CORTICAINE®
(hydrocortisone acetate)

Warner-Lambert Co.

LISTERMINT® with FLUORIDE
Anticavity Dental Rinse & Mouthwash

Warner-Lambert Co.

Spearmint

Wintergreen

Regular

ROLAIDS®

Fast, Safe, Lasting Relief from Heartburn, Sour Stomach or Acid Indigestion and Upset Stomach Associated with these Symptoms

Warner-Lambert Co.

REPLENS.

Available in Boxes of 3, 8 and 12 Single-Use Applicators

**REPLENS®
Vaginal Moisturizer**

Whitby

VICON-C®

VICON-C

Vicon® Plus

VICON® PLUS

Warner-Lambert Co.

Unscented

Extremely mild lathering cleanser

LUBRIDERM® BODY BAR

Warner-Lambert Co.

Peppermint

Cherry

Assorted Fruit

**CALCIUM RICH
SODIUM FREE
ROLAIDS®**

Calcium Rich, Sodium Free Relief from Heartburn, Sour Stomach or Acid Indigestion and Upset Stomach Associated with these Symptoms

WESTWOOD-SQUIBB

Lotion   Cleanser
     Cream

**Fragrance-Free
MOISTUREL®**

Vi-Zac®

VI-ZAC®

Cartons due to change appearance in 1992.

(Therapeutic Vitamins and Minerals)

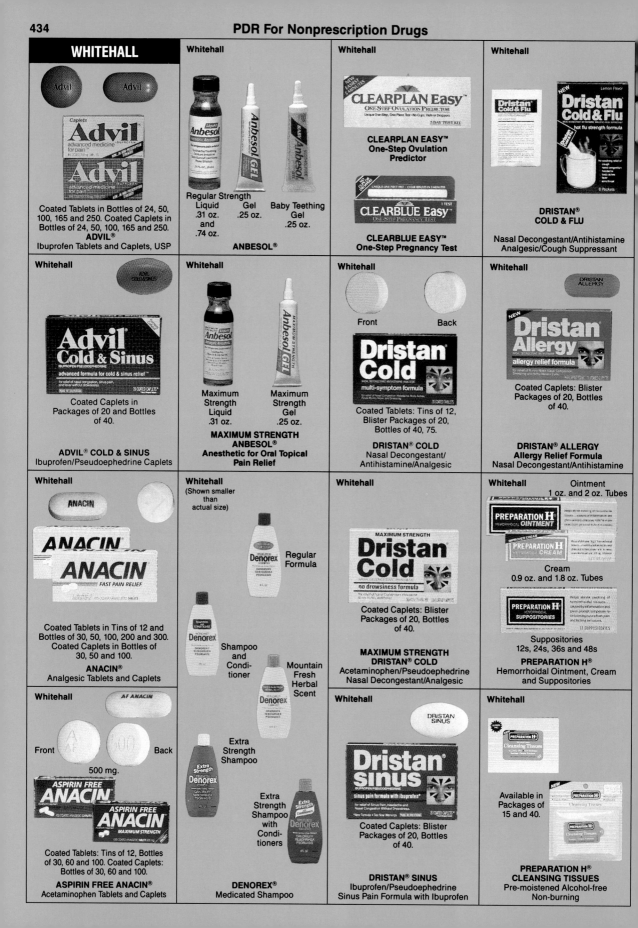

WHITEHALL

Coated Tablets in Bottles of 24, 50, 100, 165 and 250. Coated Caplets in Bottles of 24, 50, 100, 165 and 250.
ADVIL®
Ibuprofen Tablets and Caplets, USP

Whitehall

Regular Strength Liquid .31 oz. and .74 oz.

Gel .25 oz.

Baby Teething Gel .25 oz.

ANBESOL®

Whitehall

CLEARPLAN EASY™
One-Step Ovulation Predictor

CLEARBLUE EASY™
One-Step Pregnancy Test

Whitehall

DRISTAN®
COLD & FLU

Nasal Decongestant/Antihistamine Analgesic/Cough Suppressant

Whitehall

Coated Caplets in Packages of 20 and Bottles of 40.

ADVIL® COLD & SINUS
Ibuprofen/Pseudoephedrine Caplets

Whitehall

Maximum Strength Liquid .31 oz.

Maximum Strength Gel .25 oz.

MAXIMUM STRENGTH ANBESOL®
Anesthetic for Oral Topical Pain Relief

Whitehall

Front   Back

Coated Tablets: Tins of 12, Blister Packages of 20, Bottles of 40, 75.

DRISTAN® COLD
Nasal Decongestant/ Antihistamine/Analgesic

Whitehall

Coated Caplets: Blister Packages of 20, Bottles of 40.

DRISTAN® ALLERGY
Allergy Relief Formula
Nasal Decongestant/Antihistamine

Whitehall

Coated Tablets in Tins of 12 and Bottles of 30, 50, 100, 200 and 300. Coated Caplets in Bottles of 30, 50 and 100.
ANACIN®
Analgesic Tablets and Caplets

Whitehall
(Shown smaller than actual size)

Regular Formula

Shampoo and Conditioner

Mountain Fresh Herbal Scent

Extra Strength Shampoo

Extra Strength Shampoo with Conditioners

DENOREX®
Medicated Shampoo

Whitehall

MAXIMUM STRENGTH
Dristan Cold
no drowsiness formula

Coated Caplets: Blister Packages of 20, Bottles of 40.

MAXIMUM STRENGTH DRISTAN® COLD
Acetaminophen/Pseudoephedrine Nasal Decongestant/Analgesic

Whitehall

Ointment 1 oz. and 2 oz. Tubes

Cream 0.9 oz. and 1.8 oz. Tubes

Suppositories 12s, 24s, 36s and 48s

PREPARATION H®
Hemorrhoidal Ointment, Cream and Suppositories

Whitehall

Front   Back

500 mg.

Coated Tablets: Tins of 12, Bottles of 30, 60 and 100. Coated Caplets: Bottles of 30, 60 and 100.

ASPIRIN FREE ANACIN®
Acetaminophen Tablets and Caplets

Whitehall

Coated Caplets: Blister Packages of 20, Bottles of 40.

DRISTAN® SINUS
Ibuprofen/Pseudoephedrine Sinus Pain Formula with Ibuprofen

Whitehall

Available in Packages of 15 and 40.

PREPARATION H®
CLEANSING TISSUES
Pre-moistened Alcohol-free Non-burning

Whitehall

Available in 15 mL Inhaler Unit, 10 mL Suspension, 15 mL and 22.5 mL Refills.

PRIMATENE® MIST

Asthma Remedy

WYETH-AYERST

Tamper-Resistant/Evident Packaging

Statements alerting consumers to the specific type of Tamper-Resistant/Evident Packaging appear on the bottle labels and cartons of all over-the-counter products of Wyeth-Ayerst. This includes plastic cap seals on bottles, individually wrapped tablets or suppositories, and sealed cartons. This packaging has been developed to better protect the consumer.

Wyeth-Ayerst

12 Fl. Oz.

**BASALJEL®
SUSPENSION**

Antacid

Wyeth-Ayerst

Also available in Ready-to-Feed Liquid and Powder

13 Fl. Oz.

Iron Fortified

**NURSOY®
SOY PROTEIN ISOLATE FORMULA
Concentrated Liquid**

Whitehall

Regular

Front   Back

P Formula

Front   Back

M Formula

Front   Back

PRIMATENE® TABLETS

Asthma Remedy

Wyeth-Ayerst

Aludrox

12 Fl. Oz.

ALUDROX® SUSPENSION

Antacid

Wyeth-Ayerst

Cerose® DM
Cough & Cold Formula

- Cough Suppressant Quiets Coughing
- Decongestant Relieves Nasal Congestion
- Antihistamine Dries Runny Nose

SUGAR FREE

4 FL. OZ. (118 ml)

Cerose® DM
COUGH & COLD FORMULA

4 Fl. Oz.

CEROSE-DM®

Cough/Cold Formula with Dextromethorphan

Also available in 1-pint bottles

Wyeth-Ayerst

Also available in Ready-to-Feed Liquid and Powder

S·M·A   S·M·A

Lo-Iron   Iron Fortified

13 Fl. Oz.

**S • M • A® INFANT FORMULA
Concentrated Liquid**

Whitehall

Available in 12 fl. oz. Suspension and Chew Tablets (60s).

Available in Mint and Cherry Flavors.

Riopan Plus 2

RIOPAN PLUS® 2

High-Potency Antacid plus Anti-Gas
(magaldrate and simethicone)

Wyeth-Ayerst

Amphojel
ANTACID

100 tablets

Amphojel

0.6 gram (10 gr.)

**AMPHOJEL® TABLETS
and
SUSPENSION
Antacid**

12 Fl. Oz.
Also available in 0.3 gram (5 gr.) tablets

Wyeth-Ayerst

EYE WASH

Collyrium
for FRESH EYES
EYE WASH
PHARMACIST RECOMMENDED

Collyrium
for FRESH EYES
EYE WASH

Eye Wash 4 Fl. Oz. (118 ml) with separate eyecup bottle cap.

**COLLYRIUM for FRESH EYES
Eye Wash**

Wyeth-Ayerst

12 Suppositories

Wyanoids® 12 hemorrhoidal suppositories
Relief Factor
Wyeth
Prompt, temporary relief from pain and itching. Helps shrink swelling of hemorrhoidal tissues.

Also available in boxes of 24

**WYANOIDS®
RELIEF FACTOR**
Hemorrhoidal Suppositories

Whitehall

Today sponge

Available in Packages of 3, 6 and 12.

Contraceptive Sponge

TODAY®
Vaginal Contraceptive Sponge

Wyeth-Ayerst

472

Basaljel
ANTACID

Bottles of 100, 500

Basaljel
ANTACID

Bottles of 100

473

**BASALJEL®
TABLETS and CAPSULES**

Antacid

Wyeth-Ayerst

EYE DROPS

COLLYRIUM
FRESH
LUBRICANT
REDNESS RELIEVER
REMOVES REDNESS
MOISTURIZES
PHARMACIST RECOMMENDED
0.5 FL. OZ. (15 ml)

COLLYRIUM
FRESH

½ Fl. Oz. (15 ml)

COLLYRIUM FRESH™

Eye drops with tetrahydrozoline HCl plus glycerin

ZILA

FAST RELIEF
From the pain, itching or burning of
**CANKER SORES
FEVER BLISTERS
COLD SORES!**

Zilactin

ZILACTIN®
Fast relief from canker sores, fever blisters & cold sores.
Also from Zila:
ZilaDent™ treats brace & denture sores
Zilactol™ treats cold sores & fever blisters before they break out

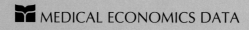
MEDICAL ECONOMICS DATA

SECTION 6
Product Information Section

This section is made possible through the courtesy of the manufacturers whose products appear on the following pages. The information concerning each product has been prepared, edited and approved by the manufacturer.

Products described in this edition comply with labeling regulations. Copy may include all the essential information necessary for informed usage such as active ingredients, indications, actions, warnings, drug interactions, precautions, symptoms and treatment of oral overdosage, dosage and administration, professional labeling, and how supplied. In some cases additional information has been supplied to complement the foregoing. The Publisher has emphasized to manufacturers the necessity of describing products comprehensively so that all information essential for intelligent and informed use is available. In organizing and presenting the material in this edition the Publisher is providing all the information made available by manufacturers.

In presenting the following material to the medical profession, the Publisher is not necessarily advocating the use of any product.

Abbott Laboratories
Pharmaceutical Products Division
NORTH CHICAGO, IL 60064

DAYALETS® Filmtab®
[dāy'a-lets]
Multivitamin Supplement for adults and children 4 or more years of age

DAYALETS® PLUS IRON Filmtab®
Multivitamin Supplement with Iron for adults and children 4 or more years of age

Description: Dayalets provide 100% of the recommended daily allowances of essential vitamins. Dayalets Plus Iron provides 100% of the recommended daily allowances of essential vitamins plus the mineral iron.
Daily dosage (one Dayalets tablet) provides:

VITAMINS			% U.S. RDA
Vitamin A.. (1.5 mg)..	5000	IU	100%
Vitamin D.. (10 mcg).	400	IU	100%
Vitamin E	30	IU	100%
Vitamin C	60	mg	100%
Folic Acid	0.4	mg	100%
Thiamine (Vitamin B₁)	1.5	mg	100%
Riboflavin (Vitamin B₂)	1.7	mg	100%
Niacin	20	mg	100%
Vitamin B₆..................	2	mg	100%
Vitamin B₁₂	6	mcg	100%

Ingredients: Ascorbic acid, cellulose, dl-alpha tocopheryl acetate, niacinamide, povidone, pyridoxine hydrochloride, riboflavin, thiamine hydrochloride, vitamin A acetate, vitamin A palmitate, folic acid, FD&C Yellow No. 6, cholecalciferol, and cyanocobalamin in a film-coated tablet with vanillin flavoring and artificial coloring added.
Each Dayalets Plus Iron Filmtab® represents all the vitamins in the Dayalets formula in the same concentrations, plus the mineral iron 18 mg (100% U.S. R.D.A.), as ferrous sulfate. Dayalets Plus Iron contain the same ingredients as Dayalets.
These products contain no sugar and essentially no calories.

Indications: Dietary supplement and supplement with iron for adults and children 4 or more years of age.

Administration and Dosage: One Filmtab tablet daily.

How Supplied: Dayalets® Filmtab® in bottles of 100 tablets (NDC 0074-3925-01).
Dayalets® Plus Iron Filmtab in bottles of 100 tablets (NDC 0074-6667-01).
® Filmtab—Film-sealed tablets, Abbott.
Abbott Laboratories
North Chicago, IL 60064
Ref. 02-6903-8/R9, Ref. 07-8057-7/R8

OPTILETS®–500
[op'te-lets]
High potency multivitamin for use in treatment of multivitamin deficiency.

OPTILETS-M-500®
High potency multivitamin for use in treatment of multivitamin deficiency. Mineral supplementation added.

Description: A therapeutic formula of ten important vitamins, with and without minerals, in a small tablet with the Abbott Filmtab® coating. Each Optilets-500 tablet provides:
Vitamin C
  (as sodium ascorbate) ....500 mg
Niacinamide ....100 mg
Calcium Pantothenate ....20 mg
Vitamin B₁
  (thiamine mononitrate) ....15 mg
Vitamin B₂ (riboflavin) ....10 mg
Vitamin B₆
  (pyridoxine hydrochloride) ....5 mg
Vitamin A (as palmitate
  1.5 mg, as acetate 1.5 mg—
  total 3 mg) ....10,000 IU
Vitamin B₁₂
  (cyanocobalamin) ....12 mcg
Vitamin D
  (cholecalciferol) ....(10 mcg) 400 IU
Vitamin E (as dl-alpha
  tocopheryl acetate) ....30 IU

Inactive Ingredients: Cellulosic polymers, corn starch, D&C Yellow No. 10, FD&C Yellow No. 6, iron oxide, polyethylene glycol, povidone, stearic acid, talc, titanium dioxide and vanillin.
Each Optilets-M-500 Filmtab contains all the vitamins (vitamin C—ascorbic acid) in the same quantities provided in Optilets-500, plus the following minerals and inactive ingredients:
Magnesium (as oxide) ....80 mg
Iron (as dried ferrous sulfate) ......20 mg
Copper (as sulfate) ....2 mg
Zinc (as sulfate) ....1.5 mg
Manganese (as sulfate) ....1 mg
Iodine (as calcium iodate) ....0.15 mg

Inactive Ingredients: Cellulosic polymers, colloidal silicon dioxide, corn starch, D&C Red No. 7, FD&C Blue No. 1, iron oxide, magnesium stearate, microcrystalline cellulose, polyethylene glycol, povidone, propylene glycol, sorbic acid and titanium dioxide.

Dosage and Administration: Usual adult dosage is one Filmtab tablet daily, or as directed by physician.

How Supplied: Optilets-500 tablets are supplied in bottles of 120 (**NDC** 0074-4287-22). Optilets-M-500 tablets are supplied in bottles of 120 (**NDC** 0074-4286-22).
®Filmtab—Film-sealed Tablets, Abbott.
Abbott Laboratories
North Chicago, IL 60064
Ref. 02-7063-7/R1, Ref. 02-7133-8/R2
Shown in Product Identification Section, page 403

SURBEX®
[sir'bex]
Vitamin B-complex
SURBEX® with C
Vitamin B-complex with vitamin C

Description: Each Surbex Filmtab tablet provides:
Niacinamide ....30 mg
Calcium Pantothenate ....10 mg
Vitamin B₁
  (thiamine mononitrate) ....6 mg
Vitamin B₂ (riboflavin) ....6 mg
Vitamin B₆
  (pyridoxine hydrochloride)........2.5 mg
Vitamin B₁₂ (cyanocobalamin) .....5 mcg
Each Surbex with C Filmtab tablet provides the same ingredients as Surbex, plus 250 mg Vitamin C (as sodium ascorbate).

Inactive Ingredients
Surbex tablets: Cellulosic polymers, corn starch, D&C Yellow No. 10, dibasic calcium phosphate, FD&C Yellow No. 6, magnesium stearate, polyethylene glycol, povidone, propylene glycol, stearic acid, titanium dioxide, and vanillin.
Surbex with C Tablets: Cellulosic polymers, corn starch, D&C Yellow No. 10, FD&C Yellow No. 6, lactose, magnesium stearate, microcrystalline cellulose, polyethylene glycol, povidone, propylene glycol, titanium dioxide, and vanillin.

Indications: Surbex is indicated for treatment of Vitamin B-Complex deficiency.
Surbex with C is indicated for use in treatment of Vitamin B-Complex with Vitamin C deficiency.

Dosage and Administration: Usual adult dosage is one tablet twice daily or as directed by physician.

How Supplied: Surbex is supplied as bright orange-colored tablets in bottles of 100 (NDC 0074-4876-13).
Surbex with C is supplied as yellow-colored tablets in bottles of 100 (NDC 0074-4877-13).
Abbott Laboratories
North Chicago, IL 60064
Ref. 03-1763-5/R12, 03-1616-5/R12

SURBEX-T®
High-potency vitamin B-complex with 500 mg of vitamin C

Description: Each Filmtab® tablet provides:
Vitamin C (ascorbic acid) ....500 mg
Niacinamide ....100 mg
Calcium Pantothenate ....20 mg
Vitamin B₁ (thiamine
  mononitrate) ....15 mg
Vitamin B₂ (riboflavin) ....10 mg
Vitamin B₆ (pyridoxine
  hydrochloride) ....5 mg
Vitamin B₁₂ (cyanocobalamin) ...10 mcg

Inactive Ingredients: Cellulosic polymers, colloidal silicon dioxide, corn starch, D&C Yellow No. 10, FD&C Yellow No. 6, magnesium stearate, microcrystalline cellulose, polyethylene glycol, povidone, propylene glycol, titanium dioxide, and vanillin.

Indications: For use in treatment of Vitamin B-Complex with Vitamin C deficiency.

Dosage and Administration: Usual adult dosage is one Filmtab tablet daily, or as directed by physician.

How Supplied: Orange-colored tablets in bottles of 100 (**NDC** 0074-4878-13). Also supplied in Abbo-Pac® unit dose packages of 100 tablets in strips of 10 tablets per strip (**NDC** 0074-4878-11). ®Filmtab—Film-sealed Tablets, Abbott. Abbott Laboratories
North Chicago, IL 60064
Ref. 03-1765-7/R13
Shown in Product Identification
Section, page 403

SURBEX®-750 with IRON
High-potency B-complex with iron, vitamin E and 750 mg vitamin C

Description: Each Filmtab® tablet provides:
VITAMINS
Vitamin C (as sodium ascorbate) 750 mg
Niacinamide .... 100 mg
Vitamin B6 (pyridoxine
  hydrochloride) .... 25 mg
Calcium Pantothenate .... 20 mg
Vitamin B1 (thiamine
  mononitrate) .... 15 mg
Vitamin B2 (riboflavin) .... 15 mg
Vitamin B12 (cyanocobalamin) 12 mcg
Folic Acid .... 400 mcg
Vitamin E (as dl-alpha tocopheryl
  acetate) .... 30 IU
MINERAL
Elemental Iron (as dried
  ferrous sulfate) .... 27 mg
  equivalent to 135 mg ferrous sulfate

Inactive Ingredients: Cellulosic polymers, colloidal silicon dioxide, FD&C Red No. 3, corn starch, iron oxide, magnesium stearate, microcrystalline cellulose, polyethylene glycol, povidone, and vanillin.

Indications: For the treatment of vitamin C and B-complex deficiencies and to supplement the daily intake of iron and vitamin E.

Dosage and Administration: Usual adult dosage is one tablet daily or as directed by physician.

How Supplied: Bottles of 50 tablets (**NDC** 0074-8029-50). Abbott Laboratories
North Chicago, IL 60064
Ref. 03-1800-4/R9
Shown in Product Identification
Section, page 403

SURBEX®-750 with ZINC
High-potency B-complex with zinc, vitamin E and 750 mg of vitamin C. For persons 12 years of age or older

Description: Daily dose (one Filmtab® tablet) provides:
[See table next column]

Ingredients: Ascorbic acid, niacinamide, cellulose, dl-alpha tocopheryl ace-

		%U.S. R.D.A.*
VITAMINS		
Vitamin E	30 IU	100%
Vitamin C	750 mg	1250%
Folic Acid	0.4 mg	100%
Thiamine (B1)	15 mg	1000%
Riboflavin (B2)	15 mg	882%
Niacin	100 mg	500%
Vitamin B6	20 mg	1000%
Vitamin B12	12 mcg	200%
Pantothenic Acid	20 mg	200%
MINERAL		
Zinc**	22.5 mg	150%

* % U.S. Recommended Daily Allowance for Adults.
** Equivalent to 100 mg of zinc sulfate.

tate, zinc sulfate, povidone, pyridoxine hydrochloride, calcium pantothenate, riboflavin, thiamine mononitrate, cyanocobalamin, magnesium stearate, colloidal silicon dioxide, folic acid, in a film-coated tablet with vanillin flavoring and artificial coloring added.

Usual Adult Dose: One tablet daily.

How Supplied: Bottles of 50 tablets (**NDC** 0074-8152-50).
Abbott Laboratories
North Chicago, IL 60064
Ref. 03-1767-4/R10
Shown in Product Identification
Section, page 403

If desired, additional information on any Abbott Product will be provided upon request to Abbott Laboratories.

Adria Laboratories
Division of Erbamont Inc.
7001 POST ROAD
DUBLIN, OH 43017

Professional Labeling
EMETROL®
(Phosphorated Carbohydrate Solution)
For the relief of nausea associated with upset stomach

Description: EMETROL is an oral solution containing balanced amounts of dextrose (glucose) and levulose (fructose) and phosphoric acid with controlled hydrogen ion concentration. Available in original lemon-mint or cherry flavor.

Ingredients: Each 5 mL teaspoonful contains dextrose (glucose), 1.87 g; levulose (fructose), 1.87 g; phosphoric acid, 21.5 mg; and the following inactive ingredients: glycerin, methylparaben, purified water; D&C yellow No. 10 and natural lemon-mint flavor in lemon-mint Emetrol; FD&C red No. 40 and artificial cherry flavor in cherry Emetrol.

Action: EMETROL quickly relieves nausea by local action on the wall of the hyperactive G.I. tract. It reduces smooth-muscle contraction in proportion to the amount used. Unlike systemic antinauseants, EMETROL works almost immediately to control nausea.

Indications: For the relief of nausea associated with upset stomach. For other

conditions, take only as directed by your physician.

Advantages:
1. **Fast Action**—works almost immediately by local action on contact with the hyperactive G.I. tract.
2. **Effectiveness**—reduces smooth-muscle contractions in proportion to the amount used—stops nausea.
3. **Safety**—non-toxic—won't mask symptoms of organic pathology.
4. **Convenience**—no ℞ required.
5. **Patient Acceptance**—a low cost that patients appreciate—pleasant lemon-mint or cherry flavor.

Usual Adult Dose: One or two tablespoonfuls. Repeat every 15 minutes until distress subsides.

Usual Children's Dose: One or two teaspoonfuls. Repeat dose every 15 minutes until distress subsides.

Important: Never dilute EMETROL or drink fluids of any kind immediately before or after taking a dose.

Caution: Not to be taken for more than one hour (5 doses) without consulting a physician. If upset stomach continues or recurs frequently, consult a physician promptly as it may be a sign of a serious condition.
WARNING: KEEP THIS AND ALL MEDICATIONS OUT OF THE REACH OF CHILDREN. As with any drug, if you are pregnant or nursing a baby, seek the advice of a health professional before using this product.
This product contains fructose and should not be taken by persons with hereditary fructose intolerance (HFI).

> **This product contains sugar and should not be taken by diabetics except under the advice and supervision of a physician.**

In case of accidental overdose, contact a poison control center, emergency medical facility, or physician immediately for advice.

How Supplied: Each 5 mL teaspoonful of EMETROL contains dextrose (glucose), 1.87 g; levulose (fructose), 1.87 g; and phosphoric acid, 21.5 mg in a yellow, lemon-mint or red, cherry-flavored syrup.
Yellow, Lemon-Mint
NDC 0013-2113-45—Bottle of 4 fluid ounces (118 mL)
NDC 0013-2113-65—Bottle of 8 fluid ounces (236 mL)
NDC 0013-2113-51—Bottle of 1 pint (473 mL)
Red, Cherry
NDC 0013-2114-45—Bottle of 4 fluid ounces (118 mL)
NDC 0013-2114-65—Bottle of 8 fluid ounces (236 mL)
NDC 0013-2114-51—Bottle of 1 pint (473 mL)

Continued on next page

Adria—Cont.

Store at room temperature.
NOTICE: Each bottle is protected by a printed band around the cap. Do not use if band is damaged or missing.

Shown in Product Identification Section, page 403

Allergan Pharmaceuticals
A Division of Allergan, Inc.
2525 DUPONT DRIVE
P.O. BOX 19534
IRVINE, CA 92713-9534

CELLUFRESH™
(carboxymethylcellulose sodium)
0.5%
Lubricant Ophthalmic Solution

Description: Cellufresh™ solution is a preservative-free ophthalmic lubricant formulated for the patient who may need relief from dryness or minor irritation of the eye that may be caused by exposure to wind, sun, or heat.
The special lubricating formula was designed to supplement the natural balance of essential ions found in your own tears.
The active ingredient combines with your own tears to provide comforting relief from the burning and irritation associated with a dry eye through proper lubrication.
Preservative-free to avoid the risk of preservative-induced irritation.

Contains: Active: Carboxymethylcellulose sodium 0.5%. **Inactive:** calcium chloride, magnesium chloride, potassium chloride, purified water, sodium chloride, and sodium lactate. May also contain hydrochloric acid or sodium hydroxide to adjust pH.

FDA APPROVED USES

Indications: FOR USE AS A LUBRICANT TO PREVENT FURTHER IRRITATION OR TO RELIEVE DRYNESS OF THE EYE.

Warnings: To avoid contamination, do not touch tip of container to any surface. Do not reuse. Once opened, discard. If you experience eye pain, changes in vision, continued redness or irritation of the eye, or if the condition worsens or persists for more than 72 hours, discontinue use and consult a doctor. If solution changes color or becomes cloudy, do not use. Keep this and all drugs out of the reach of children. In case of accidental ingestion, seek professional assistance or contact a Poison Control Center immediately.

Directions: Instill 1 or 2 drops in the affected eye(s) as needed.

Note: Do not touch unit-dose tip to eye.

How Supplied: Solution is supplied in sterile, preservative-free, disposable, single-use containers of 0.01 fluid ounce each in the following size:
30 SINGLE-USE CONTAINERS—
 NDC 0023-5487-30.

CELLUVISC®
(carboxymethylcellulose sodium) 1%
Lubricant Ophthalmic Solution

Celluvisc® Ophthalmic Solution is a preservative-free ophthalmic lubricant formulated specifically for the patient who needs frequent relief from dryness of the eye:
● Special lubricating formula helps maintain the natural electrolyte balance of your tears.
● Preservative-free for no preservative-induced irritation.
● Single, unit-dose containers for greater convenience.

Contains: Active: Carboxymethylcellulose sodium 1%. Inactives: calcium chloride, potassium chloride, purified water, sodium chloride, and sodium lactate.

FDA APPROVED USES

Indications: FOR USE AS A LUBRICANT TO PREVENT FURTHER IRRITATION OR TO RELIEVE DRYNESS OF THE EYE.

Warnings: To avoid contamination, do not touch tip of container to any surface. Do not reuse. Once opened, discard. If you experience eye pain, changes in vision, continued redness or irritation of the eye, or if the condition worsens or persists for more than 72 hours, discontinue use and consult a doctor. If solution changes color or becomes cloudy, do not use. Keep this and all drugs out of the reach of children. In case of accidental ingestion, seek professional assistance or contact a poison control center immediately.

Directions: Instill 1 or 2 drops in the affected eye(s) as needed.
NOTE: Do not touch unit-dose tip to eye. Celluvisc may cause temporary blurring due to its viscosity.

How Supplied: Celluvisc® (carboxymethylcellulose sodium) 1% Lubricant Ophthalmic Solution is supplied in sterile, preservative-free, disposable, single-use containers of 0.01 fluid ounce each, in the following size:
30 SINGLE-USE CONTAINERS—
 NDC 0023-4554-30

LACRI-LUBE® S.O.P.®
(white petrolatum 56.8%, mineral oil 42.5%)
Lubricant Ophthalmic Ointment

Contains: Actives: white petrolatum 56.8%, mineral oil 42.5%. Inactives: chlorobutanol (chloral deriv.) 0.5% and lanolin alcohols.

FDA APPROVED USES

Indications: FOR USE AS A LUBRICANT TO PREVENT FURTHER IRRITATION OR TO RELIEVE DRYNESS OF THE EYE.

Warnings: To avoid contamination, do not touch tip of container to any surface. Replace cap after using either the 3.5g or 7.0g tube. If you are using the unit-dose product, do not reuse it after it has been opened. Once the product is opened, it should be discarded. If you experience eye pain, changes in vision, continued redness or irritation of the eye, or if the condition worsens or persists for more than 72 hours, discontinue use and consult a doctor. Keep this and all drugs out of the reach of children. In case of accidental ingestion, seek professional assistance or contact a poison control center immediately.

Directions: Pull down the lower lid of the affected eye and apply a small amount (one-fourth inch) of ointment to the inside of the eyelid.

How Supplied: Lacri-Lube® S.O.P.® (white petrolatum 56.8%, mineral oil 42.5%) Lubricant Ophthalmic Ointment is supplied in sterile, disposable, unit-dose containers of 0.7 g each and sterile, ophthalmic ointment tubes as follows:
 24 UNIT-DOSE CONTAINERS—
 NDC 0023-0312-01
 3.5 g TUBE—NDC 0023-0312-04
 7.0 g TUBE—NDC 0023-0312-07

LACRI-LUBE® NP
(white petrolatum 57.3%, mineral oil 42.5%)
Lubricant Ophthalmic Ointment

Contains:
Actives:
white petrolatum 57.3%
mineral oil 42.5%
Inactive: lanolin alcohols.

FDA APPROVED USES

Indications: FOR USE AS A LUBRICANT TO PREVENT FURTHER IRRITATION OR TO RELIEVE DRYNESS OF THE EYE.

Warnings: To avoid contamination, do not touch tip of container to any surface. Do not reuse. Once the product is opened, discard. If you experience eye pain, changes in vision, continued redness or irritation of the eye, or if the condition worsens or persists for more than 72 hours, discontinue use and consult a doctor. Keep this and all drugs out of the reach of children. In case of accidental ingestion, seek professional assistance or contact a poison control center immediately.

Directions: Pull down the lower lid of the affected eye and apply a small amount (one-fourth inch) of ointment to the inside of the eyelid.

Note: Do not touch unit-dose tip to eye.

How Supplied: Lacri-Lube® NP (white petrolatum 57.3%, mineral oil 42.5%) Lubricant Ophthalmic Ointment is supplied in sterile, preservative-free, disposable, single-use containers of 0.025 oz (0.7 g) each, in the following size:
   SINGLE-USE CONTAINERS—
   NDC 0023-0240-01

REFRESH® P.M.
(white petrolatum 56.8%, mineral oil 41.5%)
Lubricant Ophthalmic Ointment

Contains: Actives: white petrolatum 56.8%, mineral oil 41.5%. Inactives: lanolin alcohols, purified water and sodium chloride.

FDA APPROVED USES

Indications: FOR USE AS A LUBRICANT TO PREVENT FURTHER IRRITATION OR TO RELIEVE DRYNESS OF THE EYE.

Warnings: To avoid contamination, do not touch tip of container to any surface. Replace cap after using. If you experience eye pain, changes in vision, continued redness or irritation of the eye, or if the condition worsens or persists for more than 72 hours, discontinue use and consult a doctor. Keep this and all drugs out of the reach of children. In case of accidental ingestion, seek professional assistance or contact a poison control center immediately.

Directions: Pull down the lower lid of the affected eye and apply a small amount (one-fourth inch) of ointment to the inside of the eyelid.

Note: Store away from heat. Protect from freezing.

How Supplied: Refresh® P.M. (white petrolatum 56.8%, mineral oil 41.5%) Lubricant Ophthalmic Ointment is supplied in sterile, preservative-free, ophthalmic ointment tubes in the following size:
   3.5 g—NDC 0023-0667-04

TEARS PLUS®
(polyvinyl alcohol 1.4%, povidone 0.6%)
Lubricant Ophthalmic Solution

Contains: Actives: Polyvinyl alcohol 1.4% and povidone 0.6%. Inactives: chlorobutanol (chloral deriv.) 0.5%, purified water and sodium chloride. May also contain hydrochloric acid or sodium hydroxide to adjust pH.

FDA APPROVED USES

Indications: FOR USE AS A LUBRICANT TO PREVENT FURTHER IRRITATION OR TO RELIEVE DRYNESS OF THE EYE.

Warnings: To avoid contamination, do not touch tip of container to any surface. Replace cap after using. If you experience eye pain, changes in vision, continued redness or irritation of the eye, or if the condition worsens or persists for more than 72 hours, discontinue use and consult a doctor. If solution changes color or becomes cloudy, do not use. Keep this and all drugs out of the reach of children. In case of accidental ingestion, seek professional assistance or contact a poison control center immediately.

Directions: Instill 1 or 2 drops in the affected eye(s) as needed.

Note: Not for use while wearing soft contact lenses.

How Supplied: Tears Plus® (polyvinyl alcohol 1.4%, povidone 0.6%) Lubricant Ophthalmic Solution is supplied in sterile, plastic dropper bottles in the following sizes:
   ½ fl oz—NDC 11980-165-15
   1 fl oz—NDC 11980-165-30

Apothecon
A Bristol-Myers Squibb Company
P.O. BOX 4000
PRINCETON, NJ 08540

NALDECON CX® ADULT LIQUID ©
[nal'dě-côn CX]
For dry, hacking coughs
Nasal Decongestant/
Expectorant/Cough Suppressant
                                    ⓤ

Description: Each teaspoonful (5 mL) of Naldecon CX Adult Liquid contains:
Phenylpropanolamine
   hydrochloride .... 12.5 mg
Guaifenesin (glyceryl
   guaiacolate) .... 200 mg
Codeine phosphate .... 10 mg
   (Warning: May be Habit-Forming)
This combination product is alcohol-free, and sugar-free.

Inactive Ingredients: Citric acid, FD&C Blue No. 1, FD&C Red No. 40, hydrogenated glucose syrup, natural and artificial flavor, polyethylene glycol, saccharin sodium, sodium benzoate, sodium citrate, and purified water.

Indications: For the temporary relief of nasal congestion due to the common cold (cold), hay fever or other respiratory allergies (allergic rhinitis), or associated with sinusitis. Helps loosen phlegm (sputum) and thin bronchial secretions to rid the bronchial passageways of bothersome mucus. Temporarily quiets cough due to minor throat and bronchial irritation as may occur with a cold or inhaled irritants.

Contraindications: Do not take if hypersensitive to guaifenesin, codeine, or sympathomimetic amines.

Warnings: As with any drug, if you are pregnant or nursing a baby, seek the advice of a health professional before using this product. Do not give this product to children under 12 years of age unless di-

rected by a physician. Do not exceed recommended dosage because at higher doses nervousness, dizziness, or sleeplessness may occur. Do not take this product for more than 7 days. If symptoms do not improve or are accompanied by fever, consult a physician. Do not take this product if you have heart disease, high blood pressure, thyroid disease, diabetes, or difficulty in urination due to enlargement of the prostate gland unless directed by a physician.

Drug Interaction Precaution: Do not take this product if you are presently taking a prescription drug for high blood pressure or depression, without first consulting your physician. A persistent cough may be a sign of a serious condition. If cough persists for more than 1 week, tends to recur, or is accompanied by fever, rash, or persistent headache, consult a physician. Do not take this product for persistent or chronic cough such as occurs with smoking, asthma, chronic bronchitis, or emphysema, or if cough is accompanied by excessive phlegm (sputum) unless directed by a physician. Do not take this product if you have a chronic pulmonary disease or shortness of breath unless directed by a physician. May cause or aggravate constipation. Keep this and all drugs out of the reach of children. In case of accidental overdose, seek professional assistance or contact a Poison Control Center immediately.

Directions: Adults and children 12 years of age and over: Oral dosage is 2 teaspoonfuls every 4 hours, not to exceed 6 doses in 24 hours, or as directed by a physician.

How Supplied: NALDECON CX Adult Liquid—4 ounce and pint bottles.
Store at room temperature. Avoid excessive heat.

NALDECON DX® ADULT LIQUID
[nal'dě-côn DX]
For dry, hacking coughs
Nasal Decongestant/
Expectorant/Cough Suppressant
                                    ⓤ

Description: Each teaspoonful (5 mL) of Naldecon DX Adult Liquid contains:
Phenylpropanolamine
   hydrochloride .... 12.5 mg
Guaifenesin (glyceryl
   guaiacolate) .... 200 mg
Dextromethorphan
   hydrobromide .... 10 mg
This combination product is sugar-free.

Inactive Ingredients: Alcohol (0.06% V/V), citric acid, FD&C Yellow No. 6, natural and artificial flavor, polyethylene glycol, saccharin sodium, sodium benzoate, sodium citrate, sorbitol solution, and purified water.

Indications: For the temporary relief of nasal congestion due to the common cold (cold), hay fever, or other respiratory allergies (allergic rhinitis), or associated

Continued on next page

Apothecon—Cont.

with sinusitis. Helps loosen phlegm (sputum) and thin bronchial secretions to rid the bronchial passageways of bothersome mucus. Temporarily quiets cough due to minor throat and bronchial irritation as may occur with a cold or inhaled irritants.

Contraindications: Do not take if hypersensitive to guaifenesin, dextromethorphan, or sympathomimetic amines.

Warnings: As with any drug, if you are pregnant or nursing a baby, seek the advice of a health professional before using this product. Do not give this product to children under 12 years of age unless directed by a physician. Do not exceed recommended dosage because at higher doses nervousness, dizziness or sleeplessness may occur. Do not take this product for more than 7 days. If symptoms do not improve or are accompanied by fever, consult a physician. Do not take this product if you have heart disease, high blood pressure, thyroid disease, diabetes, or difficulty in urination due to enlargement of the prostate gland unless directed by a physician.

Drug Interaction Precaution: Do not take this product if you are presently taking a prescription drug for high blood pressure or depression, without first consulting your physician. A persistent cough may be a sign of a serious condition. If cough persists for more than 1 week, tends to recur, or is accompanied by fever, rash, or persistent headache, consult a physician. Do not take this product for persistent or chronic cough such as occurs with smoking, asthma, chronic bronchitis, or emphysema, or if cough is accompanied by excessive phlegm (sputum) unless directed by a physician. Keep this and all drugs out of the reach of children. In case of accidental overdose, seek professional assistance or contact a poison control center immediately.

Directions: Adults and children 12 years of age and over: Oral dosage is 2 teaspoonfuls every 4 hours, not to exceed 6 doses in 24 hours, or as directed by a physician.

How Supplied: NALDECON DX Adult Liquid—4 ounce and pint bottles. Store at room temperature. Avoid excessive heat.

NALDECON DX®
[nal'dĕ-côn DX]
CHILDREN'S SYRUP
For dry, hacking coughs
Nasal Decongestant/
Expectorant/Cough Suppressant

℗

Description: Each teaspoonful (5 mL) of Naldecon DX Children's Syrup contains:
Phenylpropanolamine
hydrochloride .... 6.25 mg
Guaifenesin (glyceryl
guaiacolate) .... 100 mg

Dextromethorphan
hydrobromide .... 5 mg

Inactive Ingredients: Alcohol (5% V/V), FD&C Yellow No. 6, fructose, glycerin, natural and artificial flavors, sodium benzoate, sucrose, tartaric acid, and purified water.

Indications: For the temporary relief of nasal congestion due to the common cold (cold), hay fever, or other respiratory allergies (allergic rhinitis), or associated with sinusitis. Helps loosen phlegm (sputum) and thin bronchial secretions to rid the bronchial passageways of bothersome mucus. Temporarily quiets cough due to minor throat and bronchial irritation as may occur with a cold or inhaled irritants.

Contraindications: Do not take if hypersensitive to guaifenesin, dextromethorphan, or sympathomimetic amines.

Warnings: Do not exceed recommended dosage because at higher doses nervousness, dizziness, or sleeplessness may occur. Do not give this product to children for more than 7 days. If symptoms do not improve or are accompanied by fever, consult a physician. Do not give this product to children who have heart disease, high blood pressure, thyroid disease, or diabetes, unless directed by a physician.

Drug Interaction Precaution: Do not give this product to a child who is taking a prescription drug for high blood pressure or depression, without first consulting the child's physician. A persistent cough may be a sign of a serious condition. If cough persists for more than 1 week, tends to recur, or is accompanied by fever, rash, or persistent headache, consult a physician. Do not give this product for persistent or chronic cough such as occurs with smoking, asthma, chronic bronchitis, or emphysema, or if cough is accompanied by excessive phlegm (sputum) unless directed by a physician. Keep this and all drugs out of the reach of children. In case of accidental overdose, seek professional assistance or contact a poison control center immediately. Your physician or pharmacist is the best source of information on this medication.

Directions: Children 6 to under 12 years of age: Oral dosage is 2 teaspoonfuls every 4 hours, not to exceed 6 doses in 24 hours, or as directed by a physician. Children 2 to under 6 years of age: Oral dosage is 1 teaspoonful every 4 hours, not to exceed 6 doses in 24 hours, or as directed by a physician. Children under 2 years of age: consult a physician.

How Supplied: NALDECON DX Children's Syrup—4 ounce and pint bottles. Store at room temprature. Protect from excessive heat and freezing.

NALDECON DX® PEDIATRIC DROPS
For dry, hacking coughs
[nal'dĕ-côn DX]
Nasal Decongestant/
Expectorant/Cough Suppressant

℗

Description: Each 1 mL of Naldecon DX Pediatric Drops contains:
Phenylpropanolamine
hydrochloride .... 6.25 mg
Guaifenesin (glyceryl
guaiacolate) .... 50 mg
Dextromethorphan
hydrobromide .... 5 mg
This combination product is sugar-free.

Inactive Ingredients: Citric acid, FD&C Yellow No. 6, natural and artificial flavors, polyethylene glycol 1450, propylene glycol, saccharin sodium, sodium benzoate, sorbitol solution, and purified water.

Indications: For the temporary relief of nasal congestion due to the common cold (cold), hay fever or other respiratory allergies (allergic rhinitis), or associated with sinusitis. Helps loosen phlegm (sputum) and thin bronchial secretions to rid the bronchial passageways of bothersome mucus. Temporarily quiets cough due to minor throat and bronchial irritation as may occur with a cold or inhaled irritants.

Contraindications: Do not take if hypersensitive to guaifenesin, dextromethorphan, or sympathomimetic amines.

Warnings: Take by mouth only. Do not exceed recommended dosage because at higher doses nervousness, dizziness, or sleeplessness may occur. Do not give this product to children for more than 7 days. If symptoms do not improve or are accompanied by fever, consult a physician. Do not give this product to children who have heart disease, high blood pressure, thyroid disease, or diabetes, unless directed by a physician.

Drug Interaction Precaution: Do not give this product to a child who is taking a prescription drug for high blood pressure or depression, without first consulting the child's physician. A persistent cough may be a sign of a serious condition. If cough persists for more than 1 week, tends to recur, or is accompanied by fever, rash, or persistent headache, consult a physician. Do not give this product for persistent or chronic cough such as occurs with smoking, asthma, chronic bronchitis, or emphysema, or if cough is accompanied by excessive phlegm (sputum) unless directed by a physician. Keep this and all drugs out of the reach of children. In case of accidental overdose, seek professional assistance or contact a poison control center immediately. Your physician or pharmacist is the best source of information on this product.

Directions: Children 2 to under 6 years of age: Oral dosage is 1 mL every 4 hours, not to exceed 6 doses in 24 hours, or as directed by a physician. Children under 2 years of age: consult a physician.

Professional Labeling—Children under 2 years of age: Dosage should be adjusted to age or weight and be administered every 4 hours as shown in the dosage table, not to exceed 6 doses in 24 hours.

Age	Weight	Dosage
1–3 months	8–12 lb	¼ mL
4–6 months	13–17 lb	½ mL
7–9 months	18–20 lb	¾ mL
10–24 months	21+ lb	1.0 mL

Bottle label reads as follows: Children under 2 years of age: Consult a physician.

How Supplied: NALDECON DX Pediatric Drops—30 mL bottle with calibrated dropper.
Store at room temperature.

NALDECON EX® CHILDREN'S SYRUP
For loose, productive coughs
[nal 'dĕ-cón EX]
Nasal Decongestant/Expectorant
Ⓤ

Description: Each teaspoonful (5 mL) of Naldecon EX Children's Syrup contains:
Phenylpropanolamine
  hydrochloride .... 6.25 mg
Guaifenesin (glyceryl
  guaiacolate) .... 100 mg
This combination product is sugar-free.

Inactive Ingredients: Alcohol (5% V/V), D&C Yellow No. 10, glycerin, natural and artificial flavors, propylene glycol, saccharin sodium, sodium benzoate, sorbitol solution, tartaric acid, and purified water.

Indications: For the temporary relief of nasal congestion due to the common cold (cold), hay fever, or other respiratory allergies (allergic rhinitis), or associated with sinusitis. Helps loosen phlegm (sputum) and thin bronchial secretions to rid the bronchial passageways of bothersome mucus.

Contraindications: Do not take if hypersensitive to guaifenesin or sympathomimetic amines.

Warnings: Do not exceed recommended dosage because at higher doses nervousness, dizziness, or sleeplessness may occur. Do not give this product to children for more than 7 days. If symptoms do not improve or are accompanied by fever, consult a physician. Do not give this product to children who have heart disease, high blood pressure, thyroid disease, or diabetes, unless directed by a physician.

Drug Interaction Precaution: Do not give this product to a child who is taking a prescription drug for high blood pressure or depression, without first consulting the child's physician. A persistent cough may be a sign of a serious condition. If cough persists for more than 1 week, tends to recur, or is accompanied by fever, rash, or persistent headache, consult a physician. Do not give this product for persistent or chronic cough such as occurs with smoking, asthma, chronic bronchitis, or emphysema, or if cough is accompanied by excessive phlegm (sputum) unless directed by a physician. Keep this and all drugs out of the reach of children. In case of accidental overdose, seek professional assistance or contact a poison control center immediately. Your physician or pharmacist is the best source of information on this medication.

Directions: Children 6 to under 12 years of age: Oral dosage is 2 teaspoonfuls every 4 hours, not to exceed 6 doses in 24 hours, or as directed by a physician. Children 2 to under 6 years of age: Oral dosage is 1 teaspoonful every 4 hours, not to exceed 6 doses in 24 hours, or as directed by a physician. Children under 2 years of age: consult a physician.

How Supplied: NALDECON EX Children's Syrup—4 ounce and pint bottles.
Store at room temperature.

NALDECON EX® PEDIATRIC DROPS
For loose, productive coughs
[nal 'dĕ-cón EX]
Nasal Decongestant/Expectorant
Ⓤ

Description: Each 1 mL of Naldecon EX Pediatric Drops contains:
Phenylpropanolamine
  hydrochloride ....6.25 mg
Guaifenesin (glyceryl
  guaiacolate) ....50 mg
This combination product is sugar-free.

Inactive Ingredients: Citric acid, D&C Yellow No. 10, natural and artificial flavors, polyethylene glycol 1450, propylene glycol, saccharin sodium, sodium benzoate, sorbitol solution, and purified water.

Indications: For the temporary relief of nasal congestion due to the common cold (cold), hay fever or other respiratory allergies (allergic rhinitis), or associated with sinusitis. Helps loosen phlegm (sputum) and thin bronchial secretions to rid the bronchial passageways of bothersome mucus.

Contraindications: Do not take if hypersensitive to guaifenesin or sympathomimetic amines.

Warnings: Take by mouth only. Do not exceed recommended dosage because at higher doses nervousness, dizziness, or sleeplessness may occur. Do not give this product to children for more than 7 days. If symptoms do not improve or are accompanied by fever, consult a physician. Do not give this product to children who have heart disease, high blood pressure, thyroid disease, or diabetes, unless directed by a physician.

Drug Interaction Precaution: Do not give this product to a child who is taking a prescription drug for high blood pressure or depression, without first consulting the child's physician. A persistent cough may be a sign of a serious condition. If cough persists for more than 1 week, tends to recur, or is accompanied by fever, rash, or persistent headache, consult a physician. Do not give this product for persistent or chronic cough such as occurs with smoking, asthma, chronic bronchitis, or emphysema, or if cough is accompanied by excessive phlegm (sputum) unless directed by a physician. Keep this and all drugs out of the reach of children. In case of accidental overdose, seek professional assistance or contact a poison control center immediately. Your physician or pharmacist is the best source of information on this medication.

Directions: Children 2 to under 6 years of age: Oral dosage is 1 mL every 4 hours, not to exceed 6 doses in 24 hours, or as directed by a physician. Children under 2 years of age: consult a physician.

Professional Labeling—Children under 2 years of age: Dosage should be adjusted to age or weight and be administered every 4 hours as shown in the dosage table, not to exceed 6 doses in 24 hours.

Age	Weight	Dosage
1–3 months	8–12 lb	¼ mL
4–6 months	13–17 lb	½ mL
7–9 months	18–20 lb	¾ mL
10–24 months	21+ lb	1.0 mL

Bottle label reads as follows: Children under 2 years of age: Use only as directed by a physician.

How Supplied: NALDECON EX Pediatric Drops—30 mL bottle with calibrated dropper.
Store at room temperature.

NALDECON SENIOR DX®
For dry, hacking coughs
Expectorant/Cough Suppressant
Cough/Cold Liquid
Ⓤ

Description: Each teaspoonful (5 mL) of Naldecon Senior DX Cough/Cold Liquid contains:
Guaifenesin .... 200 mg
Dextromethorphan
  hydrobromide .... 15 mg
This combination product is alcohol-free and sugar-free.

Inactive Ingredients: Citric acid, FD&C Blue No. 1, FD&C Red No. 40, natural and artificial flavor, polyethylene glycol, saccharin sodium, sodium benzoate, sodium citrate, sorbitol solution, and purified water.

Indications: Temporarily quiets coughs due to minor throat and bronchial irritation as may occur with a cold or inhaled irritants. Helps loosen phlegm (sputum) and thin bronchial secretions to rid the bronchial passageways of bothersome mucus.

Contraindications: Do not take if hypersensitive to guaifenesin or dextromethorphan.

Continued on next page

Apothecon—Cont.

Warnings: A persistent cough may be a sign of a serious condition. If cough persists for more than 1 week, tends to recur, or is accompanied by fever, rash, or persistent headache, consult a physician. Do not take this product for persistent or chronic cough such as occurs with smoking, asthma, chronic bronchitis, or emphysema, or if cough is accompanied by excessive phlegm (sputum) unless directed by a physician. Do not exceed recommended dose or give this product to children under 12 years of age unless directed by a physician. As with any drug, if you are pregnant or nursing a baby, seek the advice of a health professional before using this product. Keep this and all drugs out of the reach of children. In case of accidental overdose, seek professional assistance or contact a Poison Control Center immediately.

Directions: Adults and children 12 years of age and over: Oral dosage is 2 teaspoonfuls every 4 hours, not to exceed 6 doses in 24 hours, or as directed by a physician. Children under 12 years of age: consult a physician.

How Supplied: Naldecon Senior DX Cough/Cold Liquid—4 ounce and pint bottles.
Store at room temperature and protect from temperatures above 104°F (40°C).

NALDECON SENIOR EX®
For loose, productive coughs (guaifenesin)
Expectorant
Cough/Cold Liquid

Ⓤ

Description: Each teaspoonful (5 mL) of Naldecon Senior EX Cough/Cold Liquid contains:
Guaifenesin .... 200 mg
Contains no sugar or alcohol.

Inactive Ingredients: Citric acid, FD&C Blue No. 1, FD&C Red No. 40, natural and artificial flavor, polyethylene glycol, saccharin sodium, sodium benzoate, sodium citrate, sorbitol solution, and purified water.

Indications: Helps loosen phlegm (sputum) and thin bronchial secretions to rid the bronchial passageways of bothersome mucus.

Contraindications: Do not take if hypersensitive to guaifenesin.

Warnings: A persistent cough may be a sign of a serious condition. If cough persists for more than 1 week, tends to recur, or is accompanied by fever, rash, or persistent headache, consult a physician. Do not take this product for persistent or chronic cough such as occurs with smoking, asthma, chronic bronchitis, or emphysema, or where cough is accompanied by excessive phlegm (sputum) unless directed by a physician. Do not exceed recommended dose or give this product to children under 12 years of age unless di-

rected by a physician. As with any drug, if you are pregnant or nursing a baby, seek the advice of a health professional before using this product. Keep this and all drugs out of the reach of children. In case of accidental overdose, seek professional assistance or contact a Poison Control Center immediately.

Directions: Adults and children 12 years and over: Oral dosage is 2 teaspoonfuls every 4 hours, not to exceed 6 doses in 24 hours, or as directed by a physician. Children under 12 years of age: consult a physician.

How Supplied: Naldecon Senior EX Cough/Cold Liquid—4 ounce and pint bottles.
Store at room temperature.

THERAGRAN® LIQUID with Niacin & Vitamin C
High Potency Vitamin Supplement

Each 5 ml. teaspoonful contains:

		Percent US RDA*
Vitamin A	5,000 IU	100
Vitamin D	400 IU	100
Vitamin C	200 mg	333
Thiamine	10 mg	667
Riboflavin	10 mg	588
Niacin	100 mg	500
Vitamin B_6	4.1 mg	205
Vitamin B_{12}	5 mcg	83
Pantothenic Acid	21.4 mg	214

*US Recommended Daily Allowance

Ingredients: purified water, sucrose, glycerine, propylene glycol, sodium ascorbate, niacinamide, polysorbate 80, ascorbic acid, thiamine hydrochloride, d-panthenol, carboxymethylcellulose sodium, riboflavin-5-phosphate sodium, artificial and natural flavors, (sodium benzoate and methylparaben as preservatives), pyridoxine hydrochloride, vitamin A palmitate, cholecalciferol, ferric ammonium citrate, cyanocobalamin
Take 1 teaspoonful daily or as directed by physician.

How Supplied: In bottles of 4 fl. oz.
NO REFRIGERATION REQUIRED

Storage: Store at room temperature; avoid excessive heat.
(P9163-00)
Shown in Product Identification Section, page 403

ADVANCED FORMULA THERAGRAN® TABLETS
(High Potency Multivitamin Formula)

FOR ADULTS—PERCENTAGE OF U.S. RECOMMENDED DAILY ALLOWANCE

Vitamins	Quantity	US RDA
Vitamin A	5000 IU	100%
(as Acetate and Beta Carotene)		
Vitamin B_1	3 mg	200%
Vitamin B_2	3.4 mg	200%
Vitamin B_6	3 mg	150%
Vitamin B_{12}	9 mcg	150%
Vitamin C	90 mg	150%
Vitamin D	400 I.U.	100%
Vitamin E	30 I.U.	100%

Vitamins	Quantity	US RDA
Niacin	20 mg	100%
Folic Acid	400 mcg	100%
Pantothenic Acid	10.0 mg	100%
Biotin	30 mcg	10%

Ingredients: Lactose, ascorbic acid, microcrystalline cellulose, gelatin, dl-alpha-tocopheryl acetate, niacinamide, starch, calcium pantothenate, sodium caseinate, hydroxypropyl methylcellulose, sucrose, povidone, pyridoxine hydrochloride, riboflavin, silicon dioxide, magnesium stearate, thiamine mononitrate, vitamin A acetate, polyethylene glycol, triacetin, stearic acid, titanium dioxide, annatto, beta carotene, FD&C Red 40, folic acid, biotin, ergocalciferol, cyanocobalamin.

Warning: KEEP OUT OF REACH OF CHILDREN.

Recommended Adult Intake—1 tablet daily or as directed by physician.

How Supplied: Packs of 130; and Unimatic® cartons of 100.

Storage: Store at room temperature; avoid excessive heat; keep tightly closed. UNIMATIC® is a trademark of E.R. Squibb & Sons, Inc.
Shown in Product Identification Section, page 403

COMPLETE FORMULA with Beta Carotene
THERAGRAN-M® TABLETS
(High Potency Multivitamin Formula with Minerals)

TABLET CONTENTS:
FOR ADULTS—PERCENTAGE OF U.S. RECOMMENDED DAILY ALLOWANCE

Vitamins	Quantity	US RDA
Vitamin A	5000 IU	100%
(as Acetate and Beta Carotene)		
Vitamin B_1	3 mg	200%
Vitamin B_2	3.4 mg	200%
Vitamin B_6	3 mg	150%
Vitamin B_{12}	9 mcg	150%
Vitamin C	90 mg	150%
Vitamin D	400 IU	100%
Vitamin E	30 IU	100%
Niacin	20 mg	100%
Folic Acid	400 mcg	100%
Pantothenic Acid	10.0 mg	100%
Biotin	30 mcg	10%
Minerals		
Iron	27 mg	150%
Copper	2 mg	100%
Iodine	150 mcg	100%
Zinc	15 mg	100%
Magnesium	100 mg	25%
Calcium	40 mg	4%
Phosphorus	31 mg	3%
Chromium	15 mcg	*
Molybdenum	15 mcg	*
Selenium	10 mcg	*
Manganese	5 mg	*
ELECTROLYTES		
Chloride	7.5 mg	*
Potassium	7.5 mg	*

*US RDA not established.

Ingredients: Magnesium oxide, dibasic calcium phosphate, lactose, ascorbic acid, ferrous fumarate, gelatin, dl-alpha tocopheryl, acetate, crospovidone, niacinamide, hydroxypropyl methylcellulose, zinc oxide, povidone, manganese sulfate, potassium chloride, starch, calcium pantothenate, sodium caseinate, pyridoxine hydrochloride, cupric sulfate, magnesium stearate, sucrose, silicon dioxide, riboflavin, thiamine mononitrate, stearic acid, polyethylene glycol, triacetin, Vitamin A acetate, FD&C Red 40, potassium citrate, beta carotene, titanium dioxide, folic acid, potassium iodide, FD&C Blue No. 2, chromic chloride, sodium molybdate, biotin, sodium selenate, ergocalciferol, cyanocobalamin

Warning: KEEP OUT OF REACH OF CHILDREN.

Usage: For adults—1 tablet daily

How Supplied: Packs of 90, 130 and 240; and Unimatic® cartons of 100.

Storage: Store at room temperature; avoid excessive heat; keep tightly closed. UNIMATIC® is a trademark of E.R. Squibb & Sons, Inc.
Shown in Product Identification Section, page 403

THERAGRAN® STRESS FORMULA
High Potency Multivitamin Stress Formula with Iron and Vitamin C

TABLET CONTENTS: For Adults—Percentage of US Recommended Daily Allowance

Ingredients	Quantity	US RDA
Vitamin B$_1$	15 mg	1000%
Vitamin B$_2$	15 mg	882%
Vitamin B$_6$	25 mg	1250%
Vitamin B$_{12}$	12 mcg	200%
Vitamin C	600 mg	1000%
Vitamin E	30 IU	100%
Niacin	100 mg	500%
Pantothenic Acid	20 mg	200%
Iron	27 mg	150%
Folic Acid	400 mcg	100%
Biotin	45 mcg	15%

Ingredients: Ascorbic acid, niacinamide, ferrous fumarate, starch, lactose, pyridoxine hydrochloride, crospovidone, dl-alpha tocopheryl acetate, gelatin, riboflavin, povidone, thiamine mononitrate, hydroxypropyl methylcellulose, sodium caseinate, magnesium stearate, silicon dioxide, stearic acid, polyethylene glycol, triacetin, titanium dioxide, FD&C Red No. 40, FD&C Yellow No. 6, folic acid, biotin, cyanocobalamin

Warning: KEEP OUT OF REACH OF CHILDREN.

Recommended Adult Intake—1 tablet daily or as directed by physician.

How Supplied: Bottles of 75.

Storage: Store at room temperature; avoid excessive heat.
(P893-01)
Shown in Product Identification Section, page 403

B.F. Ascher & Company, Inc.
15501 WEST 109th STREET
LENEXA, KS 66219
Mailing address:
P.O. BOX 717
SHAWNEE MISSION, KS 66201-0717

AYR® Saline Nasal Mist and Drops
[ār]

AYR Mist or Drops restores vital moisture to provide prompt relief for dry, crusted and inflamed nasal membranes due to chronic sinusitis, colds, low humidity, overuse of nasal decongestant drops and sprays, allergies, minor nose bleeds and other minor nasal irritations. AYR provides a soothing way to thin thick secretions and aid their removal from the nose and sinuses. AYR can be used as often as needed without the side effects associated with overuse of decongestant nose drops and sprays.
SAFE AND GENTLE ENOUGH FOR CHILDREN AND INFANTS
AYR Drops are particularly convenient for easy application with infants and children. AYR is formulated to prevent stinging, burning and irritation of delicate nasal tissue, even that of babies.

Directions For Use: SPRAY—Squeeze twice in each nostril as often as needed. Hold bottle upright. To spray, give the bottle short, firm squeezes. Take care not to aspirate nasal contents back into bottle. DROPS—Two to four drops in each nostril every two hours as needed, or as directed by your physician.
AYR is a specially formulated, buffered, isotonic saline solution containing sodium chloride 0.65% adjusted to the proper tonicity and pH with monobasic potassium phosphate/sodium hydroxide buffer to prevent nasal irritation. AYR also contains the non-irritating antibacterial and antifungal preservatives thimerosal and benzalkonium chloride and is formulated with deionized water.

How Supplied: AYR Mist in 50 ml spray bottles, AYR Drops in 50 ml dropper bottles.
Shown in Product Identification Section, page 403

ITCH-X GEL®

Active Ingredients: Benzyl alcohol 10% and pramoxine HCl 1%.
Also contains: Aloe vera gel, carbomer 934, diazolidinyl urea, FD&C blue #1, methylparaben, propylene glycol, propylparaben, SD alcohol 40, styrene/acrylate copolymer, triethanolamine, and water.

Indications: For the temporary relief of pain and itching associated with minor skin irritations, allergic itches, rashes, hives, minor burns, insect bites, sunburns, poison ivy, poison oak, and poison sumac.

Warnings: For external use only. Avoid contact with the eyes. If condition worsens, or if symptoms persist for more than 7 days or clear up and occur again within a few days, discontinue use of this product and consult a physician. KEEP THIS AND ALL DRUGS OUT OF THE REACH OF CHILDREN. In case of accidental ingestion, seek professional assistance or contact a Poison Control Center immediately.

Directions: Adults and children 2 years of age and older: Apply to affected area not more than 3 to 4 times daily. Children under 2 years of age: consult a physician.

How Supplied: 1.25 oz tube
Shown in Product Identification Section, page 403

MOBIGESIC® Analgesic Tablets
[mō'bĭ-jē'zĭk]

Active Ingredients: Each tablet contains 325 mg of magnesium salicylate with 30 mg of phenyltoloxamine citrate.

Also Contains: Microcrystalline cellulose, magnesium stearate and colloidal silicon dioxide which aid in the formulation of the tablet and its dissolution in the gastrointestinal tract.

Indications: MOBIGESIC acts fast to provide relief from the pain and discomfort of simple headaches and colds; for temporary relief of the pain and tension accompanying muscle soreness and fatigue, neuralgia, minor menstrual cramps, T.M.J. and pain of tooth extraction. The unique formula provides relief of pain due to sinusitis and in the fever and inflammation of colds.

Caution: When used for the temporary symptomatic relief of colds, if relief does not occur within 7 days (3 days for fever), discontinue use and consult physician. This preparation may cause drowsiness. Do not drive or operate machinery while taking this medication. Do not administer to children under 6 years of age or exceed recommended dosage unless directed by physician.

Warnings: Keep this and all drugs out of the reach of children. In case of accidental overdose, call your doctor or poison control center immediately. As with any drug, if you are pregnant or nursing a baby, seek the advice of a health professional before using this product.

Usual Dosage: Adults—1 or 2 tablets every four hours, up to 10 tablets daily. Children (6 to 12 years)—1 tablet every 4 hours, up to 5 tablets daily. Do not use more than 10 days unless directed by physician.
Store at room temperature (59°–86°F).

How Supplied: Packages of 18's, 50's and 100's.
Shown in Product Identification Section, page 403

Continued on next page

Ascher—Cont.

MOBISYL® Analgesic Creme
[mō′bĭ-sĭl]

Active Ingredient: Trolamine salicylate 10%. Also Contains: Glycerin, methylparaben, mineral oil, polysorbate 60, propylparaben, sorbitan stearate, sorbitol, stearic acid, and water.

Description: MOBISYL is a greaseless, odorless, penetrating, non-burning, non-irritating analgesic creme.

Indications: For adults and children, 12 years of age and older, MOBISYL is indicated for the temporary relief of minor aches and pains of muscles and joints, such as simple backache, lumbago, arthritis, neuralgia, strains, bruises and sprains.

Actions: MOBISYL penetrates fast into sore, tender joints and muscles where pain originates. It works to reduce inflammation. Helps soothe stiff joints and muscles and gets you going again.

Warnings: For external use only. Avoid contact with the eyes. Discontinue use if condition worsens or if symptoms persist for more than 7 days, and consult a physician. Do not use on children under 12 years of age except under the advice and supervision of a physician. In case of accidental ingestion, seek professional assistance or contact a Poison Control Center immediately. Close cap tightly. Keep this and all drugs out of the reach of children. Store at room temperature.

Dosage and Administration: Place a liberal amount of MOBISYL Creme in your palm and massage into the area of pain and soreness three or four times a day, especially before retiring. MOBISYL may be worn under clothing or bandages.

How Supplied: MOBISYL is available in 1.25 oz tubes, 3.5 oz tubes, 8 oz jars.
Shown in Product Identification Section, page 403

PEN•KERA® Creme with Keratin Binding Factor
A Therapeutic Creme for Chronic Dry Skin

Ingredients: Water, octyl palmitate, glycerin, mineral oil, polysorbate 60, sorbitan stearate, polyamino sugar condensate, urea, wheat germ glycerides, carbomer 940, triethanolamine, DMDMH, iodo propynyl butyl carbamate, diazolidinyl urea, and dehydroacetic acid.

Indications: PEN•KERA Therapeutic Creme for Chronic Dry Skin contains Keratin Binding Factor, a polyamino sugar condensate and urea, which is synthesized to match the same biological components as those found in skin. The Keratin Binding Factor in PEN•KERA Creme replaces the missing elements of dehydrated skin which absorb and retain moisture. The Keratin Binding Factor actually simulates the natural moisturizing mechanism of the skin, relieving itching, flaking, sensitive, dry skin symptoms.
PEN•KERA is fragrance-free, dye-free, paraben-free, lanolin-free, non-comedogenic and non-greasy for smooth, fast absorption.

Dosage and Administration: Apply in a thin layer. Because it penetrates quickly and is non-greasy, PEN•KERA may be used under make-up or sun screens. Regular use will reduce the frequency of application and quantity required to achieve moisturized skin.

Precautions: FOR EXTERNAL USE ONLY

How Supplied: PEN•KERA Therapeutic Creme is available in 8 oz. bottles.
Shown in Product Identification Section, page 403

Astra Pharmaceutical Products, Inc.
50 OTIS ST.
WESTBORO, MA 01581-4500

XYLOCAINE® (lidocaine) 2.5%
[zī′lo-caine]
OINTMENT

For temporary relief of pain and itching due to minor burns, sunburn, minor cuts, abrasions, insect bites and minor skin irritations.

Composition: Diethylaminoacet-2,6-xylidide 2.5% in a water miscible ointment vehicle consisting of polyethylene glycols and propylene glycol.

Action and Uses: A topical anesthetic ointment for fast, temporary relief of pain and itching due to minor burns, sunburn, minor cuts, abrasions, insect bites and minor skin irritations. The ointment can be easily removed with water. It is ineffective when applied to intact skin.

Administration and Dosage: Apply topically in liberal amounts for adequate control of symptoms. When the anesthetic effect wears off additional ointment may be applied as needed.

Important Warning: *In persistent, severe or extensive skin disorders, advise patient to use only as directed. In case of accidental ingestion advise patient to seek professional assistance or to contact a poison control center immediately. Keep out of the reach of children.*

Caution: *Do not use in the eyes. Not for prolonged use. If the condition for which this preparation is used persists or if a rash or irritation develops, advise patient to discontinue use and consult a physician.*

How Supplied: Available in tube of 35 grams (approximately 1.25 ounces).
Shown in Product Identification Section, page 403

Au Pharmaceuticals, Inc.
P. O. BOX 476
GRAND SALINE, TX 75140

AURUM–Analgesic Lotion
Topical Analgesic
THERAGOLD–Analgesic Lotion
Topical Analgesic
THERAPEUTIC GOLD–Analgesic Lotion
Topical Analgesic

Active Ingredients: The active ingredients are methyl salicylate 10%; menthol 3%; camphor 2.5%. These are combined in a rich, nonpetroleum base for easy and effective topical application.

Other Selected Ingredients: Special inactive ingredients include Deionized Water, C12–15 Alcohols, Propylene Glycol, Eucalyptus Oil, Stearic Acid, DEA Cetyl Phosphate, PEG 8-Distearate, Carboxy Polymethylene, Methyl Hydroxybenzoate, Ginseng, Imidazolidinyl Urea, Triethanolamine, Disodium EDTA, Urea, Jojoba Oil, Vitamins A & D_3, Vitamin E, FD&C Yellow No. 5, 24 Karat Gold, Aloe.

Indications: These lotions give fast, deep-penetrating, effective temporary relief from stiff, sore, aching muscles and joints associated with arthritis, bursitis, tendinitis and muscle disorders.

Actions: Methyl salicylate, menthol and camphor are classified as counter-irritants which combine to provide both heat and cold stimulation to the pain receptors over and around the affected area. The lotions replace the perception of pain with the feeling of heat and/or cold to provide temporary relief of minor aches and pains.

Directions: Apply a liberal amount of lotion to painful area and allow to remain on skin for 30 seconds before rubbing lotion into the affected area. Apply product 3 or 4 times a day or as needed until pain is relieved, then reduce the frequency as needed.

Warnings: Use only as directed. For external use only. Avoid contact with eyes, mucous membranes, broken or irritated skin. Should contact occur, flush area with water. Do not use a heating pad with this lotion until one hour after application. Do not use on children under 12 years of age without advice of a physician. If condition worsens or persists for more than 7 days without relief, discontinue use of this product and consult a physician. Some individuals may experience sensitivity to some ingredients. If so, discontinue use immediately.

Caution: contains 10% Methyl Salicylate and 24K GOLD. Persons who are allergic or hypersensitive to these ingredients should consult their physician before using this product.

How Supplied: These products are available in 128 ounce, 8 ounce and 2 ounce bottles.
National Drug Code Registration #058796

FEMININE GOLD—
Analgesic Lotion
Topical Analgesic

Active Ingredients: The active ingredients are menthol 3%, camphor 2.5%. These are combined in a rich, non-petroleum base for easy and effective topical application.

Other Selected Ingredients: Special inactive ingredients include Deionized Water, C12–15 Alcohols, Propylene Glycol, Eucalyptus Oil, Stearic Acid, DEA Cetyl Phosphate, PEG 8-Distearate, Carboxy Polymethylene, Methyl Hydroxybenzoate, Ginseng, Imidazolidinyl Urea, Triethanolamine, Disodium EDTA, Urea, Jojoba Oil, Vitamin A & D_3, Vitamin E, FD&C Yellow No. 5, 24 Karat Gold, Aloe.

Indications: This lotion gives fast, deep-penetrating, effective temporary relief from pain and discomfort of cramps and backache suffered during the menstrual cycle.

Actions: Menthol and camphor are classified as counterirritants which combine to provide both heat and cold stimulation to the pain receptors over and around the affected area. The lotion replaces the perception of pain with the feeling of heat and/or cold to provide temporary relief of minor aches and pains.

Directions: Apply a liberal amount of lotion to painful area and allow to remain on skin for 30 seconds before rubbing lotion into the affected area. Apply product 3 or 4 times a day or as needed until pain is relieved, then reduce the frequency to as needed.

Warnings: Use only as directed. For external use only. Avoid contact with eyes, mucous membranes, broken or irritated skin. Should contact occur, flush area with water. Do not use a heating pad with this lotion untl one hour after application. Do not use on children under 12 years of age without advice of a physician. If condition worsens or persists for more than 7 days without relief, discontinue use of this product and consult a physician. Some individuals may experience sensitivity to some ingredients. If so discontinue use immediately.

Caution: contains 24K GOLD. Persons who are allergic or hypersensitive to these ingredients should consult their physician before using this product.

How Supplied: These products are available in 8 ounce and 2 ounce bottles. National Drug Code Registration #058796

Products are indexed by
generic and chemical names
in the
YELLOW SECTION.

Ayerst Laboratories
Division of American Home Products Corporation
685 THIRD AVE.
NEW YORK, NY 10017-4071

For information for Ayerst's consumer products, see product listings under Whitehall Laboratories.
Please turn to Whitehall Laboratories, page 761.

Baker Cummins Pharmaceuticals, Inc.
8800 NORTHWEST 36TH STREET
MIAMI, FL 33178

AQUA-A® Cream

Description: Contains the vitamin A derivative, retinyl palmitate. Moisture-enriched smoothing concentrate. Clinically proven for all skin types.

Ingredients: Water, Caprylic/Capric Triglyceride, Methyl Gluceth-10, Glyceryl Stearate, Squalane, Mineral Oil, PPG-20 Methyl Glucose Ether Distearate, Dimethicone, Stearic Acid, PEG-50 Stearate, Retinyl Palmitate, Sodium Hyaluronate, Lecithin, Sodium Polyglutamate, Ascorbyl Palmitate, Carbomer 934, Dichlorobenzyl Alcohol, Cetyl Alcohol, BHT, Diazolidinyl Urea, Xanthan Gum, Menthol, Sodium Hydroxide, Tetrasodium EDTA.

Directions for Use: Use morning or night or both.

How Supplied: 2 oz. jars

AQUADERM® Combination Treatment/Moisturizer

Description: Aquaderm® Combination Treatment/Moisturizer developed by leading dermatologists to deliver maximum moisturization. Regular daily use of Aquaderm's dual action moisturizer and sunscreen protects and preserves your youthful appearance. This specially developed formula contains sunscreens (SPF 15) that shield your skin from UVA and UVB rays, to protect it from wrinkles and reduce skin damage and possible skin cancer. Aquaderm® Combination Treatment/Moisturizer is safe and effective, hypo-allergenic, non-comedogenic, Paraben-free, and will not leave an artificial-feeling film. Aquaderm® Combination Treatment/Moisturizer is especially suited for patients undergoing Retin-A® therapy, who require maximum moisturization and sun protection. Retin-A® is a registered trademark of Johnson & Johnson.

Ingredients: Octyl Methoxycinnamate, 7.5%, Oybenzone, 6%, Titanium Dioxide, 2%, in a moisturizing cream base.

Indications: Protects against harmful skin-aging rays of the sun.

Warnings: FOR EXTERNAL USE ONLY. Avoid contact with eyes. If irritation develops, discontinue use. Keep this and all drugs out of the reach of children. In case of accidental ingestion, seek professional assistance or contact a Poison Control Center immediately.

Directions for Use: Apply to face and neck as needed. Effective and compatible for daily use under make-up.

How Supplied: 3.5 oz. tube

AQUADERM® Cream

Description: Ultrarich moisturizing cream concentrate. Softens, smooths, protects, absorbs quickly.

Ingredients: Water, Caprylic/Capric Triglyceride, Methyl Gluceth-10, Glyceryl Stearate, Mineral Oil, Squalane, Dimethicone, Stearic Acid, PEG-50 Stearate, Sodium Hyaluronate, Lecithin, Sodium Polyglutamate, Magnesium Aluminum Silicate, Carbomer 934, Dichlorobenzyl Alcohol, Cetyl Alcohol, BHT, Diazolidinyl Urea, Xanthan Gum, Menthol, Sodium Hydroxide, Tetrasodium EDTA.

Directions for Use: Apply to face or other dry areas morning or night or both.

How Supplied: 4 oz. jar (0575-2002-04)

AQUADERM® Lotion

Description: Ultrarich moisturizing lotion concentrate. Smooths, softens, protects, absorbs quickly.

Ingredients: Water, Caprylic/Capric Triglyceride, Methyl Gluceth-10, Glyceryl Stearate, Dimethicone, Petrolatum, Mineral Oil, Squalane, PEG-50 Stearate, Stearic Acid, Sodium Hyaluronate, Lecithin, Sodium Polyglutamate, Magnesium Aluminum Silicate, Carbomer 934, Dichlorobenzyl Alcohol, Cetyl Alcohol, BHT, Diazolidinyl Urea, Xanthan Gum, Menthol, Tetrasodium EDTA, Sodium Hydroxide.

Directions for Use: Apply to hands and body morning or night or both.

How Supplied: 7.5 fl. oz. bottle (0575-2001-75)

P&S® Liquid

Ingredients: Mineral Oil, Water, Fragrance, Glycerin, Phenol, Sodium Chloride, D&C Yellow #11, D&C Red #17, D&C Green #6.

Indications: P&S® Liquid, used regularly, helps loosen and remove crusts and scales on the scalp.

Caution: FOR EXTERNAL USE ONLY. Do not apply to large portions of body surfaces. Discontinue use if excessive skin irritation develops. Avoid contact with eyes or mucous membranes.

Continued on next page

Baker Pharm.—Cont.

Keep out of the reach of children. In case of accidental ingestion, seek professional assistance or contact a Poison Control Center immediately.

Directions for Use: Apply liberally to scalp lesions each night before retiring. Massage gently to loosen scales and crusts. Leave on overnight and shampoo the next morning. Use daily as needed.

How Supplied: 8 fl. oz. bottle (0575-4001-04); 4 fl. oz. bottle (0575-4001-08)

P&S® PLUS Tar Gel

Active Ingredients: 8% Coal Tar Solution (equivalent to 1.6% Crude Coal Tar), 6.4% Ethyl Alcohol, 2% Salicylic Acid.

Indications: For psoriasis and other scaling conditions. P&S® PLUS relieves the itching, irritation and skin flaking associated with seborrheic dermatitis, psoriasis and dandruff.

Warnings: FOR EXTERNAL USE ONLY. Avoid contact with the eyes; flush with water if product gets into eyes. If irritation develops, discontinue use. If condition worsens or does not improve after regular use of this product as directed, consult a physician. Do not use on children under 2 years of age except as directed by a physician. Use caution in exposing skin to sunlight after applying this product; it may increase your tendency to sunburn for up to 24 hours after application. Do not use this product with other forms of psoriasis therapy such as ultraviolet radiation or prescription drugs unless directed to do so by a doctor. If condition covers a large area of the body, consult your doctor before using this product.

Caution: Keep this and all drugs out of reach of children. In case of accidental ingestion, seek professional assistance or contact a Poison Control Center immediately.

Directions for Use: Apply to affected areas of skin and scalp daily or as directed by physician.

How Supplied: 3.5 oz. tube (NDC 0575-4009-35)

P&S® Shampoo

Active Ingredient: 2% Salicylic Acid.

Indications: P&S® Shampoo relieves the itching, irritation and skin flaking associated with seborrheic dermatitis of the scalp. It also relieves the itching, redness, and scaling associated with psoriasis of the scalp. P&S® Shampoo may be used alone as well as following treatment with P&S® Liquid. Its rich conditioning formula improves hair's manageability and helps prevent tangles.

Warnings: FOR EXTERNAL USE ONLY. Avoid contact with eyes or mu-

cous membranes. If this occurs, rinse thoroughly with water. If condition worsens or does not improve after regular use of this product as directed, consult a physician. Do not use on children under 2 years of age except as directed by a physician. If condition covers a large area of the body, consult your doctor before using this product.

Caution: Keep this and all drugs out of reach of children. In case of accidental ingestion, seek professional assistance or contact a Poison Control Center immediately.

Directions for Use: For best results use twice weekly or as directed by a physician. Wet hair, apply to scalp and massage vigorously. Rinse and repeat.

How Supplied: 4 fl. oz. bottle (NDC 0575-4007-04); 8 fl. oz. bottle (NDC 0575-4007-08)

ULTRA MIDE 25® Extra Strength Moisturizer

Ingredients: Water, Urea, Mineral Oil, Glycerin, Propylene Glycol, PEG-50 Stearate, Butyrolactone, Hydrogenated Lanolin, Sorbitan Laurate, Glyceryl Stearate, Magnesium Aluminum Silicate, Propylene Glycol Stearate SE, Cetyl Alcohol, Fragrance, Diazolidinyl Urea, Tetrasodium EDTA.

Indications: Intensive moisturizer for extra dry, scaly or calloused skin. Contains ingredients to soften and moisturize areas of very dry, rough, cracked or calloused skin. This unique keratolytic formula contains a stabilized form of urea (25%) to help prevent the stinging and irritation often associated with moisturizers containing urea. ULTRA MIDE 25® Lotion contains no parabens.

Warnings: FOR EXTERNAL USE ONLY. Keep out of reach of children. Discontinue use if irritation occurs. Caution should be taken when used near the eyes. In case of accidental ingestion, seek professional assistance or contact a Poison Control Center immediately.

Directions for Use: Apply four times daily, or as directed by a physician. Each application should be rubbed in completely.

How Supplied: 8 fl. oz. bottle (0575-4200-08)

X–SEB® Shampoo

Active Ingredient: 1% Zinc Pyrithione.

Inactive Ingredients: Purified Water, Ammonium Lauryl Sulfate, Ammonium Laureth Sulfate, Ethylene Glycol Distearate, Lauramide DEA, Salicylic Acid, PEG 75 Lanolin, Ammonium Xylene Sulfate, Triethanolamine, Menthol, Methylchloroisothiazolinone and Methylisothiazolinone, Fragrance, FD&C Blue #1.

Indications: X-SEB® Shampoo provides effective relief of the itching and

scalp flaking associated with dandruff. This unique formulation is gentle enough for daily use leaving hair healthy looking and manageable.

Warnings: FOR EXTERNAL USE ONLY. Avoid contact with the eyes. If this happens, rinse thoroughly with water. If condition worsens or does not improve after regular use of this product as directed, consult a physician. Do not use on children under 2 years of age except as directed by a physician.

Caution: Keep this and all drugs out of the reach of children. In case of accidental ingestion, seek professional assistance or contact a Poison Control Center immediately.

Directions for Use: For best results, use X-SEB® Shampoo twice a week or as directed by a physician. Wet hair, apply to scalp and massage vigorously. Rinse and repeat.

How Supplied: 4 fl. oz. bottle (NDC 0575-1006-04); 8 fl. oz. bottle (NDC 0575-1006-08)

X–SEB® PLUS Conditioning Shampoo

Active Ingredients: 1% Zinc Pyrithione.

Inactive Ingredients: Purified Water, Ammonium Lauryl Sulfate, Ammonium Laureth Sulfate, Ethylene Glycol Distearate, Lauramide DEA, Salicylic Acid, PEG 75 Lanolin, Polyquaternium-7, Ammonium Xylene Sulfate, Triethanolamine, Menthol, Methylchloroisothiazolinone and Methylisothiazolinone, Fragrance, FD&C Blue #1.

Indications: X-SEB® PLUS conditioning shampoo provides effective relief of the itching and scalp flaking associated with dandruff. Ideal for dry, brittle hair. This unique formulation is gentle enough for daily use giving hair extra body, a healthy look and ease of manageability.

Warnings: FOR EXTERNAL USE ONLY. Avoid contact with the eyes; if this happens, rinse thoroughly with water. If condition worsens or does not improve after regular use of this product as directed, consult a physician. Do not use on children under 2 years of age except as directed by a physician.

Caution: Keep this and all drugs out of the reach of children. In case of accidental ingestion, seek professional assistance or contact a Poison Control Center immediately.

Directions for Use: For best results, use X-SEB® PLUS conditioning shampoo twice a week or as directed by a physician. Wet hair, apply to scalp and massage vigorously. Rinse and repeat.

How Supplied: 4 fl. oz. bottle (NDC 0575-1016-04); 8 fl. oz. bottle (NDC 0575-1016-08)

X–SEB T® Shampoo

Active Ingredients: 10% Coal Tar Solution (2% Crude Coal Tar, 8% Ethyl Alcohol).

Inactive Ingredients: Purified water, Sodium Lauryl Sulfate, Laureth-23, Propylene Glycol, Salicylic Acid, Tetrasodium EDTA.

Indications: X–SEB T® Shampoo relieves the itching, irritation and skin flaking associated with dandruff, seborrheic dermatitis, and psoriasis.This formulation is designed to effectively treat scaly conditions in a mild, gentle cleansing base leaving hair healthy looking and manageable.

Warnings: FOR EXTERNAL USE ONLY. Avoid contact with the eyes; if this happens, rinse thoroughly with water. If irritation develops, discontinue use. If condition worsens or does not improve after regular use of this product as directed, consult a physician. Do not use on children under 2 years of age except as directed by a physician. Use caution in exposing skin to sunlight after applying this product; it may increase your tendency to sunburn for up to 24 hours after application. Do not use for prolonged periods without consulting a physician. Do not use this product with other forms of psoriasis therapy such as ultraviolet radiation or prescription drugs unless directed to do so by a physician. If condition covers a large area of the body, consult your physician before using this product.

Caution: Keep this and all drugs out of the reach of children. In case of accidental ingestion, seek professional assistance or contact a Poison Control Center immediately.

Directions for Use: For best results, use X–SEB T® shampoo at least twice a week or as directed by physician. Wet hair, apply to scalp and massage vigorously. Rinse and repeat or as directed by a physician.

How Supplied: 4 fl. oz. bottle (NDC 0575-1005-04); 8 fl. oz. bottle (NDC 0575-1005-08)

X–SEB T® PLUS Conditioning Shampoo

Active Ingredients: 10% Coal Tar Solution (equivalent to 2% Crude Coal Tar, 8% Ethyl Alcohol).

Inactive Ingredients: Purified water, TEA Lauryl Sulfate, Lauramide DEA, Ethylene Glycol Distearate, PEG-75 Lanolin, Salicylic Acid, Polyquaternium-7, Menthol, Hydroxypropyl Methylcellulose, Chloroxylenol, Disodium EDTA, Fragrance, FD&C BLUE #1.

Indications: X–SEB T® PLUS conditioning shampoo relieves the itching, irritation and skin flaking associated with dandruff, seborrheic dermatitis, and psoriasis. This formulation is designed to effectively treat scaly conditions in a mild, gentle cleansing base leaving hair healthy looking and manageable. X–SEB T® PLUS will not discolor or damage hair that has been color treated or permed.

Warnings: FOR EXTERNAL USE ONLY. Avoid contact with the eyes; if this happens, rinse thoroughly with water. If irritation develops, discontinue use. If condition worsens or does not improve after regular use of this product as directed, consult a physician. Do not use on children under 2 years of age except as directed by a physician. Use caution in exposing skin to sunlight after applying this product; it may increase your tendency to sunburn for up to 24 hours after application. Do not use for prolonged periods without consulting a physician. Do not use this product with other forms of psoriasis therapy such as ultraviolet radiation or prescription drugs unless directed to do so by a physician. If condition covers a large area of the body, consult your physician before using this product.

Caution: Keep this and all drugs out of the reach of children. In case of accidental ingestion, seek professional assistance or contact a Poison Control Center immediately.

Directions for Use: For best results, use X–SEB T® PLUS at least twice a week or as directed by physician. Wet hair, apply to scalp and massage vigorously. Rinse and repeat or as directed by physician.

How Supplied: 4 fl. oz. bottle (NDC 0575-1015-04); 8 fl. oz. bottle (NDC 0575-1015-08)

Bausch & Lomb
Personal Products
Division
**1400 N GOODMAN ST.
ROCHESTER, NY 14692-0450**

ALLERGY DROPS
Lubricant/Redness Reliever Eye Drops

Description: BAUSCH & LOMB Allergy Drops is a sterile lubricating eye drop that relieves minor irritation caused by allergens—pollen, dust, animal hair, air pollutants, and other common eye irritants. It relieves redness and keeps on working to protect eyes against further irritation.
Unlike other eye drops, BAUSCH & LOMB Allergy Drops contains a special ingredient that provides longer lasting relief from itching, burning, dry, irritated eyes.

Ingredients: Polyethylene glycol 300 (0.2%), naphazoline hydrochloride (0.012%). Also contains: boric acid, disodium edetate, sodium borate, sodium chloride; preserved with benzalkonium chloride (0.01%).

Indications: Relieves redness of the eye due to minor eye irritations. For the temporary relief of burning and irrita-

tion due to dryness of the eye and for use as a protectant against further irritation, or to relieve dryness of the eye.

Warnings: To avoid contamination, do not touch tip of container to any surface. Replace cap after using. If solution changes color or becomes cloudy, do not use. If you experience eye pain, changes in vision, continued redness or irritation of the eye, or if the condition worsens or persists for more than 72 hours, discontinue use and consult a doctor. If you have glaucoma, do not use this product except under the advice and supervision of a doctor. Overuse of this product may produce increased redness of the eye. Keep this and all medication out of the reach of children.
REMOVE CONTACT LENSES BEFORE USING.

Directions: Instill 1 or 2 drops in the affected eye(s) up to four times daily. Store at room temperature.

How Supplied: In plastic bottles of 0.5 fl oz.

Shown in Product Identification Section, page 403

DRY EYE THERAPY™
Lubricating Eye Drops
Preservative Free

Ingredients: Glycerin 0.3%, with: calcium chloride, magnesium chloride, purified water, potassium chloride, sodium chloride, sodium citrate, sodium phosphate, and zinc chloride.

Indications: For the temporary relief of burning and irritation due to dryness of the eye and for use as a lubricant to prevent further irritation. For the temporary relief of discomfort due to minor irritations of the eye or to exposure to wind or sun.

Description: Bausch & Lomb Dry Eye Therapy, like natural tears, contains a lubricant and four essential nutrients: calcium, zinc, potassium, and magnesium. It provides soothing relief for dry eyes.

Warnings: To avoid contamination, do not touch tip of container to any surface. Do not re-use. Once opened, discard. If you experience eye pain, changes in vision, continued redness or irritation of the eye, or if the condition worsens or persists for more than 72 hours, discontinue use and consult a doctor. If solution changes color or becomes cloudy, do not use.
Use only if single-use container is intact. Keep this and all drugs out of the reach of children.
Store at room temperature.

Directions:
- Make sure single-use container is intact before use.
- Separate one container from the strip of four.
- Open the single-use container by completely twisting off the top tab.

Continued on next page

Bausch & Lomb—Cont.

- Place thumb and forefinger on the marks on the center of the bubble.
- Gently squeeze 1 to 2 drops in the affected eye(s).
- After placing the drops in eye(s), throw away the container. Do not re-use.

Dry Eye Therapy may be used as often as needed.

How Supplied: 32 sterile, single-use containers, each 0.01 fl. oz.

Shown in Product Identification Section, page 403

DUOLUBE
Sterile Lubricant Eye Ointment

Description: White petrolatum 80% and mineral oil 20%. Contains no preservatives.

Indications: For use as a lubricant to prevent further irritation or to relieve dryness of the eye.

Directions: Pull down the lower lid of the affected eye and apply a small amount (one-fourth inch) of Duolube ointment to the inside of the eyelid.

Warnings: To avoid contamination, do not touch tip of container to any surface. Replace cap after using. If you experience eye pain, changes in vision, continued redness, irritation of the eye, or if the condition worsens or persists for more than 72 hours, discontinue use and consult a doctor. KEEP OUT OF REACH OF CHILDREN. NOT FOR USE WITH CONTACT LENSES.
DO NOT USE IF BOTTOM RIDGE OF CAP IS EXPOSED PRIOR TO INITIAL USE.
Store at room temperature.

How Supplied: In 1/8-oz (NDC 10119-020-13) tube.

Shown in Product Identification Section, page 403

EYE WASH
Sterile Isotonic Buffered Solution

Description: A sterile, isotonic solution that contains boric acid, purified water, sodium borate and sodium chloride; preserved with disodium edetate 0.025% and sorbic acid 0.1%. CONTAINS NO THIMEROSAL (MERCURY).

Indications: For cleansing the eye to help relieve irritation, burning, stinging and itching by removing loose, foreign material, air pollutants (smog or pollen) or chlorinated water.

Warnings: To avoid contamination, do not touch tip of container to any surface. Replace cap after using. If you experience eye pain, changes in vision, continued redness or irritation of the eye, or if the condition worsens or persists, consult a doctor. Obtain immediate medical treatment for all open wounds in or near the eyes. If solution changes color or becomes cloudy, do not use.

Use only as directed. If you experience any chemical burns, consult a doctor immediately. KEEP OUT OF REACH OF CHILDREN.

Directions: With Eye Cup—Rinse cup with BAUSCH & LOMB® Eye Wash immediately before and after each use. Avoid contamination of rim and inside surfaces of cup. Fill cup one-half full with BAUSCH & LOMB Eye Wash. Apply cup tightly to the affected eye to prevent spillage and tilt head backward. Open eyelids wide and rotate eyeball to thoroughly wash the eye.
NOTE: Enclosed eye cup is sterile if packaging intact.

Directions: Without Eye Cup—Flush the affected eye as needed, controlling the rate of flow of solution by pressure on the bottle.

How Supplied: In plastic dropper bottles of 4 fl oz, packaged with sterile eye cup.

Shown in Product Identification Section, page 404

MOISTURE DROPS®
Artificial Tears

Description: BAUSCH & LOMB MOISTURE DROPS Artificial Tears quickly provides soothing relief to dry, itchy, burning, irritated eyes. Its unique triple-action formula keeps on working, so your eyes stay moist, healthy, protected against further irritation. And unlike some eye drops, MOISTURE DROPS can be used as often as needed.

Ingredients: Hydroxypropyl methylcellulose (0.5%), dextran 70 (0.1%) and glycerin (0.2%). Also contains: boric acid, disodium edetate, potassium chloride, sodium borate, sodium chloride; preserved with benzalkonium chloride (0.01%).

Indications: For the temporary relief of burning and irritation due to dryness of the eye and for use as a protectant against further irritation, or to relieve dryness of the eye.

Warnings: To avoid contamination, do not touch tip of container to any surface. Replace cap after using. If you experience eye pain, changes in vision, continued redness or irritation of the eye, or if the condition worsens or persists for more than 72 hours, discontinue use and consult a doctor. If solution changes color or becomes cloudy, do not use.
Keep this and all medication out of the reach of children.
REMOVE CONTACT LENSES BEFORE USING.

Directions: Instill 1 or 2 drops in the affected eye(s) as needed.
Store at room temperature.

How Supplied: In plastic bottles of 0.5 and 1.0 fl oz.

Shown in Product Identification Section, page 404

Beach Pharmaceuticals
Division of Beach Products, Inc.
5220 SOUTH MANHATTAN AVE.
TAMPA, FL 33611

BEELITH Tablets
MAGNESIUM SUPPLEMENT
With PYRIDOXINE HCl
Each tablet supplies 362 mg of magnesium (31.83 mEq).

Directions: As a dietary supplement, take one tablet daily or as directed by a physician. Each tablet yields 362 mg of magnesium and supplies 90% of the Adult U.S. Recommended Daily Allowance (RDA) for magnesium and 1000% of the Adult RDA for vitamin B_6.
Each tablet contains magnesium oxide 600 mg and pyridoxine hydrochloride (Vitamin B_6) 25 mg equivalent to B_6 20 mg. *Also, castor oil, hydroxypropyl methylcellulose, magnesium stearate, microcrystalline cellulose, pharmaceutical glaze, povidone, sodium starch glycolate, D&C Yellow #10, FD&C Yellow #6 (Sunset Yellow), and titanium dioxide.*

Drug Interaction Precautions: Do not take this product if you are presently taking a prescription antibiotic drug containing any form of tetracycline.

Warnings: If you have kidney disease, take only under the supervision of a physician. Excessive dosage may cause laxation. **KEEP OUT OF THE REACH OF CHILDREN.** Do not use if protective printed band around cap is broken or missing.

How Supplied: Golden yellow, film coated tablet with the name **BEACH** and the number **1132** printed on each tablet. Packaged in bottles of 100 (NDC 0486-1132-01) tablets.

Storage: Keep tightly closed. Store at 15°–30°C (59°–86°F). Protect from light.
R4/90

Shown on page 405 in the 1992 PHYSICIANS' DESK REFERENCE

Beiersdorf Inc.
P.O. BOX 5529
NORWALK, CT 06856-5529

AQUAPHOR®—Original Formula
Ointment
NDC Numbers– 10356-020-01
10356-020-02

Composition: Petrolatum, mineral oil, mineral wax and wool wax alcohol.

Actions and Uses: Aquaphor is a stable, neutral, odorless, anhydrous ointment base. Miscible with water or aqueous solutions, Aquaphor will absorb several times its own weight, forming smooth, creamy water-in-oil emulsions. In its pure form, Aquaphor is recommended for use as a topical preparation to help heal severely dry skin. Aquaphor contains no preservatives, fragrances or known irritants.

Administration and Dosages: Use Aquaphor alone or in compounding virtually any ointment using aqueous solutions or in combination with other oil-based substances and all common topical medications. Apply Aquaphor liberally to affected area.

Precautions: For external use only. Avoid contact with eyes. Not to be applied over third degree burns, deep or puncture wounds, infections or lacerations. If condition worsens or does not improve within 7 days, patient should consult a doctor.

How Supplied: 16 oz. jar—List No. 45585; 5 lb. jar—List. No. 45586
Shown in Product Identification Section, page 404

AQUAPHOR® Antibiotic Ointment
NDC Number–10356-022-01

Composition: Polymyxin-B Sulfate/Bacitracin Zinc, Petrolatum, Mineral Wax, Mineral Oil, Wool Wax Alcohol.

Actions and Uses: Aquaphor Antibiotic Formula is formulated to help reduce wound healing time and the risk of infection.[1] Recommended for prevention of infection in minor first-aid wounds and for use as a post-operative dressing. Aquaphor Antibiotic Formula is preservative-free, fragrance-free and hypoallergenic. It is recommended for patients with sensitive skin.

Administration and Dosage: Use Aquaphor Antibiotic Formula whenever a topical antibiotic ointment is needed to help prevent infection in minor cuts, scrapes and burns. Apply Aquaphor Antibiotic Formula liberally to affected area two to three times a day as needed.

Precautions: For external use only. Avoid contact with eyes, Not to be applied over third degree burns, deep or puncture wounds, infections or lacerations. If condition worsens or does not improve within seven days, patient should consult a physician.

How Supplied: .5 oz. tube.
1. Data on file, BDF Inc
Shown in Product Identification Section, page 404

AQUAPHOR® Natural Healing Ointment
NDC Number–10356-021-01

Composition: Petrolatum, Mineral Oil, Mineral Wax, Wool Wax Alcohol, Panthenol, Bisabolol, Glycerin.

Actions and Uses: Aquaphor Natural Healing Formula is specially formulated for faster healing of severely dry skin, cracked skin and minor burns. It is recommended for patients suffering from severe skin chapping and from skin disorders that result in severely dry, damaged skin. This formula is also indicated as a follow-up skin treatment for patients undergoing radiation therapy or other drying/burning medical therapies. It is preservative-free, fragrance-free and hypoallergenic, and is clinically proven to reduce wound healing time.[1]

Administration and Dosage: Use Aquaphor Natural Healing Formula whenever a mild healing agent is needed. Apply liberally to affected areas two to three times a day. In the case of wounds, clean area prior to application.

Precautions: For external use only. Avoid contact with the eyes. Not to be applied over third degree burns, deep or puncture wounds, infections or lacerations. If condition worsens or does not improve within seven days, patient should consult a physician.

How Supplied: 1.75 oz. tube
1. Data on file, BDF Inc
Shown in Product Identification Section, page 404

EUCERIN®
[ū 'sir-in]
Dry Skin Care Cleansing Bar

Actions and Uses: Eucerin® Cleansing Bar has been specially formulated for use on sensitive skin. The formulation contains Eucerite®, a special blend of ingredients that closely resemble the natural oils of the skin, thus providing excellent moisturizing properties. This formulation is fragrance-free and non-comedogenic. Additionally, the pH value of Eucerin Cleansing Bar is neutral so as not to affect the skin's normal acid mantle.

Directions: Use during shower, bath, or regular cleansing, or as directed by physician.

How Supplied:
3 ounce bar
List Number 3852
Shown in Product Identification Section, page 404

EUCERIN® Cleansing Lotion
Dry Skin Care

Composition: Water, Sodium Laureth Sulfate, Cocoamphodiacetate, Cocamidopropyl Betaine, PEG-7 Glyceryl Cocoate, Glycol Distearate, PEG-5 Lanolate, Citric Acid, Imidazolidinyl Urea, Cocamide MEA, Lanolin Alcohol.

Actions and Uses: Eucerin Cleansing Lotion is formulated for the care of dry, sensitive or irritated skin. Its soap-free formula combines gentle cleansing with unique moisturizing ingredients to both clean skin and protect it against dryness. It contains no fragrances, is non-comedogenic, and leaves no soapy residue. It is ideal for atopic dermatitis and psoriasis.

Administration and Dosage: Wash with water; rinse thoroughly.

Precautions: For external use only.

How Supplied:
8 Fluid oz.—List Number 3962
1 Fluid oz.—List Number 3960
Shown in Product Identification Section, page 404

EUCERIN® Creme
[ū 'sir-in]
Dry Skin Care
NDC Numbers— 10356.090.01
10356.090.05
10356.090.04
10356.090.07

Composition: Water, petrolatum, mineral oil, wool wax alcohol, methylchloroisothiazolinone, methylisothiazolinone.

Actions and Uses: A gentle, non-comedogenic, fragrance-free water-in-oil emulsion. Eucerin can be used as a treatment for dry skin associated with eczema, psoriasis, chapped or chafed skin, sunburn, windburn and itching associated with dryness.

Administration and Dosages: Apply freely to affected areas of the skin as often as necessary or as directed by physician.

Precautions: For external use only.

How Supplied:
16 oz. jar—List Number 0090
8 oz. jar—List Number 3774
4 oz. jar—List Number 3797
2 oz. tube—List Number 3868
Shown in Product Identification Section, page 404

EUCERIN® DAILY FACIAL LOTION
NDC Number–10356-972-01

Composition: Active Ingredients: Ethylhexyl p-methoxycinnamate, micronized Titanium Dioxide, 2-Phenylbenzimidazole-5-Sulfonic Acid, 2-Ethylhexyl Salicylate. Other Ingredients: Triple Purified water, Caprylic/capric Triglyceride, Mineral Oil, Octyl Stearate, Cetearyl Alcohol, Glyceryl Stearate, sodium Hydroxide PEG-40, Castor Oil, Acrylamide/Sodium Acrylate Copolymer, Sodium Cetearyl Sulfate, Wool Wax Alcohol, EDTA, Methylchloroisothiazolinone, Methylisothiazolinone.

Actions and Uses: Eucerin Daily Facial Lotion is fragrance-free, non-comedogenic and non-acnegenic, with an SPF 20 non-sensitive sunscreen to protect skin from UVA and UVB rays. It is specially formulated for dry, sensitive skin or for those undergoing therapies which irritate delicate facial skin such as Retin-A® therapy, chemical peels and treatment with drying medications. This light, oil-in-water formula is non-greasy and is easily absorbed into the skin.

Administration and Dosage: Apply Eucerin Daily Facial Lotion twice a day (especially in the morning), or as directed by a physician, to nourish and moisture skin and protect it from harmful UVA and UVB rays.

Precautions: For external use only. Avoid contact with eyes.

Continued on next page

Beiersdorf—Cont.

How Supplied:
4-oz. bottle.

*Shown in Product Identification
Section, page 404*

EUCERIN® Lotion
[*ū 'sir-in*]
Dry Skin Care Lotion
NDC Numbers— 10356-793-01
                 10356-793-04
                 10356-793-06

Composition: Water, Mineral Oil, Isopropyl Myristate, PEG-40 Sorbitan Peroleate, Lanolin Acid Glycerin Ester, Sorbitol, Propylene Glycol, Cetyl Palmitate, Magnesium Sulfate, Aluminum Stearate, Wool Wax Alcohol, BHT, Methylchloroisothiazolinone, Methylisothiazolinone.

Actions and Uses: Eucerin Lotion is a non-comedogenic, fragrance-free, unique water-in-oil formulation that will help to alleviate and soothe excessively dry skin, and provide long-lasting moisturization.

Administration and Dosage: Use daily as preventative care for skin exposed to sun, water, wind, cold or other drying elements.

Precautions: For external use only.

How Supplied:
4 fluid oz. plastic bottle—
    List Number 3771
8 fluid oz. plastic bottle—
    List Number 3793
16 fluid oz. plastic bottle—
    List number 3794
*Shown in Product Identification
Section, page 404*

Blaine Company, Inc.
**2700 DIXIE HWY.
FT. MITCHELL, KY 41017**

MAG-OX 400

Description: Each tablet contains Magnesium Oxide 400 mg. U.S.P. (Heavy), or 241.3 mg. Elemental Magnesium (19.86 mEq.)

Indications and Usage: Hypomagnesemia, magnesium deficiencies and/or magnesium depletion resulting from malnutrition, restricted diet, alcoholism or magnesium depleting drugs. An antacid. For increasing urinary magnesium excretion. For magnesium supplementation during pregnancy.

Warnings: Do not use this product except under the advice and supervision of a physician if you have a kidney disease. May have laxative effect.

Dosage: Adult dose 1 or 2 tablets daily or as directed by a physician.

Professional Labeling: Mag-Ox 400 Tablets for recurring calcium oxalate urinary calculi; for maintenance of tocolysis; for PMS therapy.

How Supplied: Bottles of 100 and 1000.

URO-MAG

Description: Each capsule contains Magnesium Oxide 140 mg. U.S.P. (Heavy), or 84.5 mg. Elemental Magnesium (6.93 mEq.)

Indications and Usage: Hypomagnesemia, magnesium deficiencies and/or magnesium depletion resulting from malnutrition, restricted diet, alcoholism or magnesium depleting drugs. An antacid. For increasing urinary magnesium excretion. For magnesium supplementation during pregnancy.

Warnings: Do not use this product except under the advice and supervision of a physician if you have a kidney disease. May have laxative effect.

Dosage: Adult dose 3–4 capsules daily or as directed by a physician.

Professional Labeling: URO-MAG Capsules for recurring calcium oxalate urinary calculi; for maintenance of tocolysis; for PMS therapy.

How Supplied: Bottles of 100 and 1000.

EDUCATIONAL MATERIAL

Samples and literature available to physicians upon request.

Block Drug Company, Inc.
**257 CORNELISON AVENUE
JERSEY CITY, NJ 07302**

ARTHRITIS STRENGTH BC® POWDER

Active Ingredients: Aspirin 742 mg in combination with 222 mg Salicylamide and 36 mg Caffeine per powder.

Indications: Arthritis Strength BC Powder is specially formulated with more of the pain relieving ingredients to provide fast temporary relief of minor arthritis pain and inflammation, neuralgia, neuritis and sciatica; relief of muscular aches, discomfort and fever of colds; and pain of tooth extraction.

Warning: Children and teenagers should not use this medicine for chicken pox or flu symptoms before a doctor is consulted about Reye Syndrome, a rare but serious illness reported to be associated with aspirin. Do not exceed recommended dosage or administer to children, including teenagers, with chicken pox or flu, unless directed by a physician. Do not take this product if you are allergic to aspirin, have asthma, gastric ulcer, or are taking a medication that affects the clotting of blood, except under the advice and supervision of a physician. If pain persists for more than 10 days or redness is present, discontinue use of this product and consult a physician immediately. Keep this and all medication out of children's reach. As with any drug, if you are pregnant or nursing a baby, consult your physician before using this product. IT IS ESPECIALLY IMPORTANT NOT TO USE ASPIRIN DURING THE LAST 3 MONTHS OF PREGNANCY UNLESS SPECIFICALLY DIRECTED TO DO SO BY A DOCTOR BECAUSE IT MAY CAUSE PROBLEMS IN THE UNBORN CHILD OR COMPLICATIONS DURING DELIVERY. Discontinue use if ringing in the ears occurs.
In case of accidental overdosage, contact a physician or poison control center immediately.

Dosage and Administration: Place one powder on tongue and follow with liquid. If you prefer, stir powder into glass of water or other liquid. May be used every three to four hours, up to 4 powders each 24 hours. For children under 12, consult a physician.

How Supplied: Available in tamper resistant cellophane wrapped envelopes of 6 powders, and tamper resistant cellophane wrapped boxes of 24 and 50 powders.

BC COLD POWDER
**BC Cold Powder Multi-Symptom Formula
BC Cold Powder Multi-Symptom Non-Drowsy Formula**

Active Ingredients: *Multi-Symptom Formula*—Aspirin 650 mg, Phenylpropanolamine Hydrochloride 25 mg, and Chlorpheniramine Maleate 4 mg per powder. *Non-Drowsy Formula*—Aspirin 650 mg and Phenylpropanolamine Hydrochloride 25 mg per powder.

Indications: *BC Cold Powder Multi-Symptom Formula* is for relief of cold symptoms such as body aches, fever, nasal congestion, sneezing, running nose, and watery itchy eyes. *BC Cold Powder Multi-Symptom Non-Drowsy Formula* is for relief of such symptoms as body aches, fever, and nasal congestions.

Warnings: CHILDREN AND TEENAGERS SHOULD NOT USE THIS MEDICINE FOR CHICKEN POX OR FLU SYMPTOMS BEFORE A DOCTOR IS CONSULTED ABOUT REYE SYNDROME, A RARE BUT SERIOUS ILLNESS REPORTED TO BE ASSOCIATED WITH ASPIRIN. KEEP THIS AND ALL MEDICINES OUT OF CHILDREN'S REACH. IN CASE OF ACCIDENTAL OVERDOSE, CONTACT A PHYSICIAN IMMEDIATELY. As with any drug, if you are pregnant or nursing a baby, seek the advice of a health professional before using this product. IT IS ESPECIALLY IMPORTANT NOT TO USE ASPIRIN DURING THE LAST 3 MONTHS OF PREGNANCY UNLESS SPECIFICALLY DIRECTED TO DO SO

BY A DOCTOR BECAUSE IT MAY CAUSE PROBLEMS IN THE UNBORN CHILD OR COMPLICATIONS DURING DELIVERY. Do not exceed recommended dosage. If symptoms do not improve within 7 days, or are accompanied by high fever, consult a physician before continuing use. Do not take this product if you have high blood pressure, heart disease, diabetes, or thyroid disease except under the advice and supervision of a physician. Do not take this product if you are presently taking a prescription antihypertensive or antidepressant drug containing a monoamine oxidase inhibitor except under the advice and supervision of a physician. This product contains aspirin and should not be taken by individuals who are sensitive to aspirin. BC Cold Powder Multi-Symptom with antihistamine may cause drowsiness. Avoid alcoholic beverages while taking this product. Use caution when driving a motor vehicle or operating machinery.

Dosage and Administration: *Adults* —Stir one powder into a glass of water or other liquid, or place powder on tongue and follow with liquid. May be used every 4 hours up to 4 times a day. *For children under 12*—consult a physician.

How Supplied: Available in tamper-resistant cellophane-wrapped envelopes of 6 powders, as well as tamper-resistant boxes of 24 powders.

BC® POWDER
[*bee-see*]

Active Ingredients: Aspirin 650 mg per powder, Salicylamide 195 mg per powder and Caffeine 32 mg per powder.

Indications: BC Powder is for relief of simple headache; for temporary relief of minor arthritic pain, neuralgia, neuritis and sciatica; for relief of muscular aches, discomfort and fever of colds; and for relief of normal menstrual pain and pain of tooth extraction.

Warning: Children and teenagers should not use this medicine for chicken pox or flu symptoms before a doctor is consulted about Reye Syndrome, a rare but serious illness reported to be associated with aspirin. Do not exceed recommended dosage or administer to children, including teenagers, with chicken pox or flu, unless directed by a physician. Do not take this product if you are allergic to aspirin, have asthma, gastric ulcer, or are taking a medication that affects the clotting of blood, except under the advice and supervision of a physician. If pain persists for more than 10 days or redness is present, discontinue use of this product and consult a physician immediately. Keep this and all medication out of children's reach. As with any drug, if you are pregnant or nursing a baby, consult your physician before using this product. IT IS ESPECIALLY IMPORTANT NOT TO USE ASPIRIN DURING THE LAST 3 MONTHS OF PREGNANCY UNLESS SPECIFICALLY DIRECTED TO DO SO BY A DOCTOR BECAUSE IT MAY

CAUSE PROBLEMS IN THE UNBORN CHILD OR COMPLICATIONS DURING DELIVERY. Discontinue use if ringing in the ears occurs.

In case of accidental overdosage, contact a physician or poison control center immediately.

Dosage and Administration: Stir one powder into a glass of water or other liquid, or, place powder on tongue and follow with liquid. May be used every 3 or 4 hours up to 4 times a day. For children under 12 consult a physician.

How Supplied: Available in tamper-resistant cellophane wrapped envelopes of 2 or 6 powders, as well as tamper resistant boxes of 24 and 50 powders.

NYTOL® TABLETS

Active Ingredient: Diphenhydramine Hydrochloride, 25 mg per tablet (NYTOL with DPH) and 50 mg per tablet (Maximum Strength NYTOL).

Indications: Diphenhydramine Hydrochloride is an antihistamine with anticholinergic and sedative effects which induces drowsiness and helps in falling asleep.

Warnings: Do not give children under 12 years of age. If sleeplessness persists continuously for more than 2 weeks, consult your physician. Insomnia may be a symptom of serious underlying medical illness. If pregnant or nursing, consult your physician before taking this or any medicine. Do not take this product if you have asthma, glaucoma, emphysema, chronic pulmonary disorders, shortness of breath, difficulty in breathing or difficulty in urination due to enlargement of the prostate gland unless directed by a physician. Do not take this product if you are taking tranquilizers or sedatives, without first consulting a physician. Avoid alcoholic beverages while taking this product. Keep this and all drugs out of the reach of children. In case of accidental overdose, contact a physician immediately.

Drug Interaction: Alcohol and other drugs which cause CNS depression will heighten the depressant effect of this product. Monoamine oxidase (MAO) inhibitors will prolong and intensify the anticholinergic effects of antihistamines.

Symptoms and Treatment of Oral Overdosage: In adults overdose may cause CNS depression resulting in hypnosis and coma. In children CNS hyperexcitability may follow sedation; the stimulant phase may bring tremor, delirium and convulsions. Gastrointestinal reactions may include dry mouth, appetite loss, nausea and vomiting. Respiratory distress and cardiovascular complications (hypotension) may be evident. Treatment includes inducing emesis, and controlling symptoms.

Dosage and Administration: Take 2 NYTOL with DPH or 1 Maximum Strength NYTOL tablet 20 minutes before bed or as directed by a physician.

How Supplied: Available in tamper resistant packages of 16, 32, and 72 tablets NYTOL with DPH; of 8 and 16 tablets Maximum Strength NYTOL.

PROMISE® SENSITIVE TEETH TOOTHPASTE
Desensitizing Dentifrice

Active Ingredients: 5% Potassium Nitrate in a pleasantly mint-flavored dentifrice.

Promise contains Potassium Nitrate for relief of dentinal hypersensitivity resulting from the exposure of tooth dentin due to periodontal surgery, cervical (gumline) erosion, abrasion or recession which causes pain on contact with hot, cold, or tactile stimuli. The Council on Dental Therapeutics of the ADA has given Promise the ADA Seal of Acceptance as an effective desensitizing dentifrice for otherwise normal teeth sensitive to hot, cold, or pressure (tactile).

Actions: Promise significantly reduces tooth hypersensitivity, with response to therapy evident after two weeks of use. Controlled double-blind clinical studies provide substantial evidence of the safety and effectiveness of Promise. The current theory on mechanism of action is that the potassium nitrate in Promise has an effect on neural transmission, interrupting the signal which would result in the sensation of pain.

Warning: When you start with Promise, it is important to remember that you have to brush for at least two weeks before relief begins to occur. Greater improvement should occur as regular use continues. If you see no improvement after a month of regular use, consult your dentist.

Dosage and Administration: Use twice a day in place of regular toothpaste or as directed by a dental professional.

How Supplied: Promise Toothpaste is supplied in 1.6 oz. and 3.0 oz. tubes.

ORIGINAL SENSODYNE® TOOTHPASTE
Desensitizing Dentifrice

Description: Each tube contains strontium chloride hexahydrate (10%) in a pleasantly flavored cleansing/polishing dentifrice.

Actions/Indications: Tooth hypersensitivity is a condition in which individuals experience pain from exposure to hot, cold stimuli, from chewing fibrous foods, or from tactile stimuli (e.g. toothbrushing.) Hypersensitivity usually occurs when the protective enamel covering on teeth wears away (which happens most often at the gum line) or if gum tissue recedes and exposes the dentin underneath.

Running through the dentin are microscopic small "tubules" which, according

Continued on next page

Block—Cont.

to many authorities, carry the pain impulses to the nerve of the tooth.

Sensodyne provides a unique ingredient—strontium chloride which is believed to be deposited in the tubules where it blocks the pain. The longer Sensodyne is used, the more of a barrier it helps build against pain.

The effect of Sensodyne may not be manifested immediately and may require a few weeks or longer of use for relief to be obtained. A number of clinical studies in the U.S. and other countries have provided substantial evidence of Sensodyne's performance attributes. Complete relief of hypersensitivity has been reported in approximately 65% of users and measurable relief or reduction in hypersensitivity in approximately 90%. Sensodyne has been commercially available for over 25 years. The ADA Council on Dental Therapeutics has given Sensodyne the Seal of Acceptance as an effective desensitizing dentifrice in otherwise normal teeth sensitive to hot, cold, or pressure (tactile).

Contraindications: Subjects with severe dental erosion should brush properly and lightly with any dentifrice to avoid further removal of tooth structure.

Dosage: Use regularly in place of ordinary toothpaste or as recommended by dental professional.
NOTE: Individuals should be instructed to use SENSODYNE frequently since relief from pain tends to be cumulative. If relief does not occur after 3 months, a dentist should be consulted.

How Supplied: SENSODYNE Toothpaste is supplied in 2.1 oz. and 4.0 oz. tubes and in 4.0 oz. pumps.
(U.S. Patent No. 3,122,483)

MINT SENSODYNE®
MINT GEL SENSODYNE®
TOOTHPASTES
Desensitizing Dentifrice

Active Ingredients: 5% Potassium Nitrate in a pleasantly mint-flavored dentifrice.
Mint Sensodyne and Mint Gel Sensodyne contain Potassium Nitrate for relief of dentinal hypersensitivity resulting from the exposure of tooth dentin due to periodontal surgery, cervical (gum line) erosion, abrasion or recession which causes pain on contact with hot, cold, or tactile stimuli. Mint Sensodyne has been given the Seal of Acceptance by the ADA Council on Dental Therapeutics as an effective desensitizing dentifrice for otherwise normal teeth sensitive to hot, cold, or pressure (tactile).

Actions: Mint Sensodyne and Mint Gel Sensodyne significantly reduce tooth hypersensitivity, with response to therapy evident after two weeks of use. Controlled double-blind clinical studies provide substantial evidence of the safety and effectiveness of Mint Sensodyne and Mint Gel Sensodyne. The current theory

on mechanism of action is that the potassium nitrate has an effect on neural transmission, interrupting the signal which would result in the sensation of pain.

Warning: When used as directed, it is important to remember that you have to brush for at least two weeks before relief begins to occur. If no improvement is seen after one month of use, consult your dentist.

Dosage and Administration: Use twice a day in place of regular toothpaste or as directed by a dental professional.

How Supplied: Mint Sensodyne and Mint Gel Sensodyne Toothpastes are supplied in 2.1 and 4.0 oz. tubes and in 4 oz. pumps.
(U.S. Patent No. 3,863,006)

TEGRIN® DANDRUFF SHAMPOO
[tĕg´rĭn]

Description: Tegrin® Dandruff Shampoo contains 7% coal tar solution in a pleasantly scented, high-foaming, cleansing shampoo base with emollients, conditioners and other formula components.

Actions/Indications: Coal Tar is obtained in the destructive distillation of bituminous coal and is a highly effective agent for controlling the flaking and itching associated with dandruff, seborrheic dermatitis and psoriasis. The action of coal tar is believed to be keratolytic, antiseptic, antipruritic and astringent. The coal tar solution used in Tegrin Dandruff Shampoo is prepared in such a way as to reduce the pitch and other irritant components found in crude coal tar without reduction in therapeutic potency.
Coal tar solution has been used clinically for many years as a remedy for dandruff and for scaling associated with scalp disorders such as eczema, seborrhea, and psoriasis. Its mechanism of action has not been fully established, but it is believed to retard the rate of turnover of epidermal cells with regular use. A number of clinical studies have demonstrated the performance attributes of Tegrin Dandruff Shampoo against dandruff and seborrheic dermatitis. In addition to relieving the above symptoms, Tegrin shampoo, used regularly, maintains scalp and hair cleanliness and leaves the hair lustrous and manageable.

Contraindications: For External Use Only—Avoid contact with eyes—if this happens, rinse thoroughly with water. Should irritation develop, discontinue use. Keep out of reach of children.

Dosage: Use regularly as a shampoo. Wet hair thoroughly. Rub Tegrin liberally into hair and scalp. Rinse thoroughly. Briskly massage a second application of the shampoo into a rich lather. Rinse thoroughly.

How Supplied: Tegrin Dandruff Shampoo is supplied in 7 fl. oz. plastic bottles.

TEGRIN® for Psoriasis Lotion, Skin Cream and Medicated Soap
[tĕg´rĭn]

Description: Each tube of cream or bottle of lotion contains special coal tar solution (5%) in a greaseless, stainless vehicle; both also contain alcohol (4.6%). Tegrin Medicated Soap contains 2.0% coal tar solution.

Actions/Indications: Coal tar is obtained in the destructive distillation of bituminous coal and is a highly effective agent that helps to relieve the itching, redness and scaling associated with psoriasis. The action of coal tar is believed to be keratolytic, antiseptic, antipruritic and astringent. The coal tar solution used in the Tegrin products is prepared in such a way as to reduce the pitch and other irritant components found in crude coal tar.

Caution: For external use only. Avoid contact with eyes and mucous membranes. Should irritation develop, discontinue use. Keep out of reach of children.

Directions: Apply lotion or cream 2 to 4 times daily as needed, massaging thoroughly into affected areas. Lather with Tegrin Soap in a hot bath before application to help soften heavy scales. Once condition is under control, maintenance therapy should be individually adjusted. Occlusive dressings are not required.

How Supplied: Tegrin Lotion 6 fl. oz. bottle, Tegrin Cream 2 oz. and 4.4 oz. tubes, Tegrin Soap 4.5 oz. bars.

TEGRIN®-HC WITH HYDROCORTISONE ANTI-ITCH OINTMENT

Description: Tegrin-HC is a special fragrance-free ointment which contains 1.0% hydrocortisone, an effective anti-itch ingredient in the maximum strength available without a prescription.

Indications: Tegrin-HC is for the temporary relief of itching associated with minor skin irritations, inflammation, rashes due to psoriasis, eczema and seborrheic dermatitis; other uses of this product should be only under the advice and supervision of a doctor.

Warning: For external use only. Avoid contact with the eyes. If condition worsens, or if symptoms persist for more than 7 days, or clear up again within a few days, stop use of this product and do not use any other hydrocortisone products unless you have consulted a doctor. Do not use for the treatment of diaper rash; consult a doctor. In case of accidental ingestion, get professional assistance or contact a poison control center immediately. **KEEP OUT OF THE REACH OF CHILDREN.**

Directions: Adults and children 2 years of age and older: apply to affected area not more than 3 to 4 times daily. Children under 2 years of age: Do not use, consult a doctor.

Boiron
1208 AMOSLAND ROAD
NORWOOD, PA 19074

OSCILLOCOCCINUM®
[ah-sill 'o-cox-see 'num ']

Active Ingredient: Anas Barbariae Hepatis et Cordis Extractum HPUS 200CK

Indications: For the relief of flu-like symptoms such as fever, chills, body aches and pains.

Actions: Like most Homeopathic remedies, Oscillococcinum® acts gently by stimulating the patient's natural defense mechanisms.

Warnings: If symptoms persist for more than three days or worsen, consult your physician. Keep all medication out of reach of children. As with any drug if you are pregnant or nursing a baby, seek professional advice before using this product.

Dosage and Administration: (Adults and Children over 2 years)
At the onset of symptoms, place the entire contents of one tube in your mouth and allow to dissolve under your tongue. Repeat every 6 hours as necessary. For maximum results, Oscillococcinum® should be taken early, at the onset of symptoms, and at least 15 minutes before or 1 hour after meals.

How Supplied: boxes of 3 unit doses or 6 unit doses of 0.04 oz. (1 gram) each (NDC #51979-9756-43 and NDC #51979-9985-43) Tamper resistant package.
Manufactured by Boiron, France.
Distributor: Boiron, Norwood, PA
Shown in Product Identification Section, page 404

EDUCATIONAL MATERIAL

Boiron Product Catalogue
General description of the most popular Boiron remedies and lines.
Oscillococcinum ® Brochure
Brochure on Oscillococcinum® describing clinical research on the product and its general use.
"What's Homeopathy?"
Booklet free to physicians and pharmacists.
"An Introduction to Homeopathy for the Practicing Pharmacist"
A free continuing education booklet for pharmacists.

Products are
indexed alphabetically
in the
PINK SECTION.

Bristol Laboratories
A Bristol-Myers Squibb Company
2400 W. LLOYD EXPRESSWAY
EVANSVILLE, IN 47721

Naldecon DX®, EX®, and CX® are distributed by Apothecon. For the Naldecon listing, please see the Apothecon section.

Bristol-Myers Products
(A Bristol-Myers Squibb Company)
345 PARK AVENUE
NEW YORK, NY 10154

ALPHA KERI®
Moisture Rich Body Oil

Composition: Contains mineral oil, Hydroloc™ brand of Westwood's PEG-4 dilaurate, lanolin oil, fragrance, benzophenone-3, D&C green 6.

Indications: ALPHA KERI is a water-dispersible oil for the care of dry skin. ALPHA KERI effectively deposits a thin, uniform, emulsified film of oil over the skin. This film lubricates and softens the skin. ALPHA KERI Moisture Rich Body Oil is an all-over skin moisturizer. Only Alpha Keri contains Hydroloc™—the unique emulsifier that provides a more uniform distribution of the therapeutic oils to moisturize dry skin. ALPHA KERI is valuable as an aid for dry skin and mild skin irritations.

Directions for Use: ALPHA KERI *should always be used with water, either added to water or rubbed on to wet skin.* Because of its inherent cleansing properties it is not necessary to use soap when ALPHA KERI is being used.
For external use only.
Label directions should be followed for use in shower, bath and cleansing.

Precaution: The patient should be warned to guard against slipping in tub or shower.

How Supplied: 4 fl. oz., 8 fl. oz., 12 fl. oz., and 16 fl. oz., plastic bottles. Also available in non-aerosol pump spray, 3.5 oz.
Shown in Product Identification Section, page 405

ALPHA KERI®
Moisture Rich Cleansing Bar
Non-detergent Soap

Composition: Sodium tallowate, sodium cocoate, water, mineral oil, fragrance, PEG-75, glycerin, titanium dioxide, lanolin oil, sodium chloride. May contain: BHT, and/or Trisodium HEDTA, D&C Green 5, D&C Yellow 10.

Indications: ALPHA KERI Moisture Rich Cleansing Bar, rich in emollient oils, thoroughly cleanses as it soothes and softens the skin.

Indications: Adjunctive use in dry skin care.

Directions for Use: To be used as any other soap.

How Supplied: 4 oz. bar.

BUFFERIN®
[bŭf'fĕr-ĭn]
Analgesic

Composition:
Active Ingredient: Each coated tablet or caplet contains Aspirin 325 mg in a formulation buffered with Calcium Carbonate, Magnesium Oxide and Magnesium Carbonate.
Other Ingredients: Benzoic Acid, Citric Acid, Corn Starch, FD&C Blue No. 1, Hydroxypropyl Methylcellulose, Magnesium Stearate, Mineral Oil, Polysorbate 20, Povidone, Propylene Glycol, Simethicone Emulsion, Sodium Phosphate, Sorbitan Monolaurate, Titanium Dioxide. May also contain: Carnauba Wax, Zinc Stearate.

Indications: For temporary relief of headaches, pain and fever of colds, muscle aches, minor arthritis pain and inflammation, menstrual pain and toothaches.

Directions: Adults: 2 tablets or caplets with water every 4 hours while symptoms persist, not to exceed 12 tablets or caplets in 24 hours, or as directed by a doctor. Children 6 to under 12 years of age: One tablet or caplet with water every 4 hours, not to exceed 5 tablets or caplets in 24 hours or as directed by a doctor. Children under 6: Consult a doctor.

Warnings: Children and teenagers should not use this medicine for chicken pox or flu symptoms before a doctor is consulted about Reye syndrome, a rare but serious illness reported to be associated with aspirin. KEEP THIS AND ALL OTHER MEDICATIONS OUT OF THE REACH OF CHILDREN. IN CASE OF ACCIDENTAL OVERDOSE, SEEK PROFESSIONAL ASSISTANCE OR CONTACT A POISON CONTROL CENTER IMMEDIATELY. As with any drug, if you are pregnant or nursing a baby, seek the advice of a health professional before using this product. IT IS ESPECIALLY IMPORTANT NOT TO USE ASPIRIN DURING THE LAST 3 MONTHS OF PREGNANCY UNLESS SPECIFICALLY DIRECTED TO DO SO BY A DOCTOR BECAUSE IT MAY CAUSE PROBLEMS IN THE UNBORN CHILD OR COMPLICATIONS DURING DELIVERY. Do not take this product for pain for more than 10 days (for adults) or 5 days (for children) or for fever for more than 3 days unless directed by a doctor. If pain or fever persists or gets worse, if new symptoms occur, or if redness or swelling is present, consult a doctor because these could be signs of a serious condition. Consult a dentist promptly for toothache. Do not give this product to children for the pain of arthritis unless directed by a doctor. Do not take this product if you are allergic to aspirin,

Continued on next page

Bristol-Myers—Cont.

have asthma, have stomach problems (such as heartburn, upset stomach or stomach pain) that persist or recur, or if you have ulcers or bleeding problems, unless directed by a doctor. If ringing in the ears or loss of hearing occurs, consult a doctor before taking or giving any more of this product.

Drug Interaction Precaution: This product should not be taken by any adult or child who is taking a prescription drug for anticoagulation (thinning of blood), diabetes, gout or arthritis unless directed by a doctor.

How Supplied: BUFFERIN is supplied as:
Coated circular white tablet with letter "B" debossed on one surface.
NDC 19810-0073-2 Bottle of 12's
NDC 19810-0093-3 Bottle of 30's
NDC 19810-0093-4 Bottle of 50's
NDC 19810-0073-5 Bottle of 100's
NDC 19810-0073-6 Bottle of 200's
NDC 19810-0073-7 Bottle of 1000's for hospital and clinical use.
NDC 19810-0073-9 Boxed 150 × 2 tablet foil pack for hospital and clinical use.
NDC 19810-0073-0 Vials of 10
Coated scored white caplet with letter "B" debossed on each side of scoring.
NDC 19810-0072-7 Bottle of 30's
NDC 19810-0072-8 Bottle of 50's
NDC 19810-0072-3 Bottle of 100's
All consumer sizes have child resistant closures except 100's for tablets and 50's for caplets which are sizes recommended for households without young children. Store at room temperature.
Also described in *PDR* for prescription drugs.

Professional Labeling

1. BUFFERIN® FOR RECURRENT TRANSIENT ISCHEMIC ATTACKS

Indication: For reducing the risk of recurrent transient ischemic attacks (TIA's) or stroke in men who have had transient ischemia of the brain due to fibrin platelet emboli. There is inadequate evidence that aspirin or buffered aspirin is effective in reducing TIA's in women at the recommended dosage. There is no evidence that aspirin or buffered aspirin is of benefit in the treatment of completed strokes in men or women.

Clinical Trials: The indication is supported by the results of a Canadian study (1) in which 585 patients with threatened stroke were followed in a randomized clinical trial for an average of 26 months to determine whether aspirin or sulfinpyrazone, singly or in combination, was superior to placebo in preventing transient ischemic attacks, stroke, or death. The study showed that, although sulfinpyrazone had no statistically significant effect, aspirin reduced the risk of continuing transient ischemic attacks, stroke, or death by 19 percent and reduced the risk of stroke or death by 31 percent. Another aspirin study carried out in the United States with 178 patients, showed a statistically significant

number of "favorable outcomes," including reduced transient ischemic attacks, stroke, and death (2).

Precautions: Patients presenting with signs and symptoms of TIA's should have a complete medical and neurologic evaluation. Consideration should be given to other disorders that resemble TIA's. Attention should be given to risk factors: it is important to evaluate and treat, if appropriate, other diseases associated with TIA's and stroke, such as hypertension and diabetes.

Concurrent administration of absorbable antacids at therapeutic doses may increase the clearance of salicylates in some individuals. The concurrent administration of nonabsorbable antacids may alter the rate of absorption of aspirin, thereby resulting in a decreased acetylsalicylic acid/salicylate ratio in plasma. The clinical significance of these decreases in available aspirin is unknown. Aspirin at dosages of 1,000 milligrams per day has been associated with small increases in blood pressure, blood urea nitrogen, and serum uric acid levels. It is recommended that patients placed on long-term aspirin treatment be seen at regular intervals to assess changes in these measurements.

Adverse Reactions: At dosages of 1,000 milligrams or higher of aspirin per day, gastrointestinal side effects include stomach pain, heartburn, nausea and/or vomiting, as well as increased rates of gross gastrointestinal bleeding.

Dosage and Administration: Adult oral dosage for men is 1,300 milligrams a day, in divided doses of 650 milligrams twice a day or 325 milligrams four times a day.

References:
(1) The Canadian Cooperative Study Group. "A Randomized Trial of Aspirin and Sulfinpyrazone in Threatened Stroke," *New England Journal of Medicine,* 299:53–59, 1978.
(2) Fields, W.S., et al., "Controlled Trial of Aspirin in Cerebral Ischemia," *Stroke* 8:301–316, 1977.

2. BUFFERIN® FOR MYOCARDIAL INFARCTION

Indication: Aspirin is indicated to reduce the risk of death and/or nonfatal myocardial infarction in patients with a previous infarction or unstable angina pectoris.

Clinical Trials: The indication is supported by the results of six, large, randomized multicenter, placebo-controlled studies[1-7] involving 10,816, predominantly male, post-myocardial infarction (MI) patients and one randomized placebo-controlled study of 1,266 men with unstable angina. Therapy with aspirin was begun at intervals after the onset of acute MI varying from less than 3 days to more than 5 years and continued for periods of from less than one year to four years. In the unstable angina study, treatment was started within 1 month after the onset of unstable angina and continued for 12 weeks and complicating

conditions such as congestive heart failure were not included in the study.
Aspirin therapy in MI patients was associated with about a 20 percent reduction in the risk of subsequent death and/or nonfatal reinfarction, a median absolute decrease of 3 percent from the 12 to 22 percent event rates in the placebo groups. In the aspirin-treated unstable angina patients the reduction in risk was about 50 percent, a reduction in the event rate of 5% from the 10% rate in the placebo group over the 12 weeks of the study.
Daily dosage of aspirin in the post-myocardial infarction studies was 300 mg. in one study and 900 and 1500 mg. in five studies. A dose of 325 mg. was used in the study of unstable angina.

Adverse Reactions: Gastrointestinal Reactions: Doses of 1000 mg. per day of aspirin caused gastrointestinal symptoms and bleeding that in some cases were clinically significant. In the largest post-infarction study (The Aspirin Myocardial Infarection Study (AMIS) with 4,500 people), the percentage incidences of gastrointestinal symptoms for the aspirin (1000 mg. of a standard, solid-tablet formulation) and placebo-treated subjects, respectively, were: stomach pain (14.5%; 4.4%); heartburn (11.9%; 4.8%); nausea and/or vomiting (7.6%; 2.1%); hospitalization for gastrointestinal disorder (4.8%; 3.5%). In the AMIS and other trials, aspirin treated patients had increased rates of gross gastrointestinal bleeding. Symptoms and signs of gastrointestinal irritation were not significantly increased in subjects treated for unstable angina with buffered aspirin in solution.

Cardiovascular and Biochemical:
In the AMIS trial, the dosage of 1000 mg. per day of aspirin was associated with small increases in systolic blood pressure (BP) (average 1.5 to 2.1 mm) and diastolic BP (0.5 to 0.6 mm), depending upon whether maximal or last available readings were used. Blood urea nitrogen and uric acid levels were also increased, but by less than 1.0 mg%.
Subjects with marked hypertension or renal insufficiency had been excluded from the trial so that the clinical importance of these observations for such subjects or for any subjects treated over more prolonged periods is not known. It is recommended that patients placed on long-term aspirin treatment, even at doses of 300 mg. per day, be seen at regular intervals to assess changes in these measurements.

Administration and Dosage: Although most of the studies used dosages exceeding 300 mg., two trials used only 300 mg. and pharmacologic data indicate that this dose inhibits platelet function fully. Therefore, 300 mg. or a conventional 325 mg. aspirin dose is a reasonable, routine dose that would minimize gastrointestinal adverse reactions.

References: 1. Elwood P.C., et al., "A Randomized Controlled Trial of Acetylsalicylic Acid in the Secondary Prevention of Mortality from Myocardial Infarction," *British Medical Journal*, 1:436–440, 1974. 2. The Coronary Drug Project Research Group, "Aspirin in Coronary Heart Disease," *Journal of Chronic Disease*, 29:625–642, 1976. 3. Breddin K, et al., "Secondary Prevention of Myocardial Infarction; Comparison of Acetylsalicylic Acid Phenprocoumon and Placebo," *Thromb. Haemost.*, 41:225–236, 1979. 4. Aspirin Myocardial Infarction Study Research Group, "A Randomized, Controlled Trial of Aspirin in Persons Recovered from Myocardial Infarction," *Journal American Medical Association*, 243:661–669, 1980. 5. Elwood P.C., and Sweetnam, P.M., "Aspirin and Secondary Mortality after Myocardial Infarction," *Lancet*, pp. 1313–1315, December 22–29, 1979. 6. The Persantine-Aspirin Reinfarction Study Research Group. "Persantine and Aspirin in Coronary Heart Disease," *Circulation* 62;449–460, 1980. 7. Lewis H.D., et al., "Protective Effects of Aspirin Against Acute Myocardial Infarction and Death in Men with Unstable Angina, Results of a Veterans Administration Cooperative Study," *New England Journal of Medicine*, 309;396–403, 1983.

Shown in Product Identification Section, page 404

BUFFERIN® AF Nite Time

Composition:

Active Ingredients: Each caplet contains Acetaminophen 500 mg. and Diphenhydramine Citrate 38 mg.
Other Ingredients: Benzoic Acid, Carnauba Wax, Corn Starch, D&C Yellow No. 10, D&C Yellow No. 10 Aluminum Lake, FD&C Blue No. 1, FD&C Blue No. 1 Aluminum Lake, Hydroxypropyl Methylcellulose, Methylparaben, Magnesium Stearate, Propylene Glycol, Propylparaben, Simethicone Emulsion, Stearic Acid, Titanium Dioxide. Remove cotton and recap bottle.

Indications: For temporary relief of occasional minor aches and pains accompanied by sleeplessness.

Warnings: KEEP THIS AND ALL OTHER MEDICATIONS OUT OF THE REACH OF CHILDREN. IN CASE OF ACCIDENTAL OVERDOSE, SEEK PROFESSIONAL ASSISTANCE OR CONTACT A POISON CONTROL CENTER IMMEDIATELY. PROMPT MEDICAL ATTENTION IS CRITICAL FOR ADULTS AS WELL AS FOR CHILDREN EVEN IF YOU DO NOT NOTICE ANY SIGNS OR SYMPTOMS. As with any drug, if you are pregnant or nursing a baby, seek the advice of a health professional before using this product. Do not give this product to children under 12 years of age or use for more than 10 days unless directed by a doctor. Consult a doctor if symptoms persist or get worse or if new ones occur, or if sleeplessness persists continuously for more than 2 weeks because these may be symptoms of serious underlying medical illnesses. Do not take this product if you have asthma, glaucoma, emphysema, chronic pulmonary disease, shortness of breath, difficulty in breathing, or difficulty in urination due to enlargement of the prostate gland unless directed by a doctor. Avoid alcoholic beverages while taking this product. Do not take this product if you are taking sedatives or tranquilizers, without first consulting your doctor.

Directions: Adults: 2 caplets at bedtime if needed or as directed by a doctor.

Overdose: MUCOMYST (acetylcysteine) As An Antidote For Acetaminophen Overdose)
Acetaminophen is rapidly absorbed from the upper gastrointestinal tract with peak plasma levels occurring between 30 and 60 minutes after therapeutic doses and usually within 4 hours following an overdose. The parent compound, which is nontoxic, is extensively metabolized in the liver to form principally the sulfate and glucuronide conjugates which are also nontoxic and are rapidly excreted in the urine. A small fraction of an ingested dose is metabolized in the liver by the cytochrome P-450 mixed function oxidase enzyme system to form a reactive, potentially toxic, intermediate metabolite which preferentially conjugates with hepatic glutathione to form the nontoxic cysteine and mercapturic acid derivatives which are then excreted by the kidney. Therapeutic doses of acetaminophen do not saturate the glucuronide and sulfate conjugation pathways and do not result in the formation of sufficient reactive metabolite to deplete glutathione stores. However, following ingestion of a large overdose (150 mg/kg or greater) the glucuronide and sulfate conjugation pathways are saturated resulting in a larger fraction of the drug being metabolized via the P-450 pathway. The increased formation of reactive metabolite may deplete the hepatic stores of glutathione with subsequent binding of the metabolite to protein molecules within the hepatocyte resulting in cellular necrosis. Acetylcysteine has been shown to reduce the extent of liver injury following acetaminophen overdose. Early symptoms following a potentially hepatotoxic overdose may include: nausea, vomiting, diaphoresis and general malaise. Clinical and laboratory evidence of hepatic toxicity may not be apparent until 48 to 72 hours postingestion. In adults and adolescents, regardless of the quantity of acetaminophen reported to have been ingested, administer MUCOMYST® acetylcysteine immediately. MUCOMYST acetylcysteine therapy should be initiated and continued for a full course of therapy. Its effectiveness depends on early administration, with benefit seen principally in patients treated within 16 hours of the overdose. If acetaminophen plasma assay capability is not available, and the estimated acetaminophen ingestion exceeds 150 mg/kg, MUCOMYST acetylcysteine therapy should be initiated and continued for a full course of therapy. For full prescribing information, refer to the MUCOMYST package insert. Do not await the results of assays for acetaminophen level before initiating treatment with MUCOMYST acetylcysteine. The following additional procedures are recommended: The stomach should be emptied promptly by lavage or by induction of emesis with syrup of ipecac. A serum acetaminophen assay should be obtained as early as possible, but no sooner than four hours following ingestion. Liver function studies should be obtained initially and repeated at 24-hour intervals.
For additional emergency information call your regional poison center or toll-free (1-800-525-6115) to the Rocky Mountain Poison Center for assistance in diagnosis and for directions in the use of MUCOMYST acetylcysteine as an antidote.

How Supplied: BUFFERIN® A/F Nite Time is supplied as: Light blue coated caplets with "BUFFERIN® Nite Time" imprinted in dark blue on one side.
NDC 19810-0084-1 Bottles of 24's
NDC 19810-0084-2 Bottles of 50's
The 50 caplet size does not have a child resistant closure and is recommended for households without young children.
Store at room temperature.

Shown in Product Identification Section, page 404

Arthritis Strength BUFFERIN®
[bŭf'fĕr-ĭn]
Analgesic

Composition:
Active Ingredient: Aspirin (500 mg) in a formulation buffered with Calcium Carbonate, Magnesium Oxide and Magnesium Carbonate.
Other Ingredients: Benzoic Acid, Citric Acid, Corn Starch, FD&C Blue No. 1, Hydroxypropyl Methylcellulose, Magnesium Stearate, Mineral Oil, Polysorbate 20, Povidone, Propylene Glycol, Simethicone Emulsion, Sodium Phosphate, Sorbitan Monolaurate, Titanium Dioxide. May also contain: Carnauba Wax, Zinc Stearate.

Indications: For temporary relief of the minor aches and pains, stiffness, swelling and inflammation of arthritis.

Directions: Adults: 2 caplets with water every 6 hours while symptoms persist, not to exceed 8 caplets in 24 hours, or as directed by a doctor. Children under 12 years of age: Consult a doctor.

Warnings: Children and teenagers should not use this medicine for chicken pox or flu symptoms before a doctor is consulted about Reye syndrome, a rare but serious illness reported to be associated with aspirin. KEEP THIS AND ALL OTHER MEDICATIONS OUT OF THE REACH OF CHILDREN. IN CASE OF ACCIDENTAL OVERDOSE, SEEK PROFESSIONAL ASSISTANCE OR CONTACT A POISON CONTROL CENTER IMMEDIATELY. As with any drug, if you are pregnant or nursing a baby,

Continued on next page

Bristol-Myers—Cont.

seek the advice of a health professional before using this product.
IT IS ESPECIALLY IMPORTANT NOT TO USE ASPIRIN DURING THE LAST 3 MONTHS OF PREGNANCY UNLESS SPECIFICALLY DIRECTED TO DO SO BY A DOCTOR BECAUSE IT MAY CAUSE PROBLEMS IN THE UNBORN CHILD OR COMPLICATIONS DURING DELIVERY. Do not take this product for pain for more than 10 days or for fever for more than 3 days unless directed by a doctor. If pain or fever persists or gets worse, if new symptoms occur, or if redness or swelling is present, consult a doctor because these could be signs of a serious condition. Do not take this product if you are allergic to aspirin, have asthma, have stomach problems (such as heartburn, upset stomach or stomach pain) that persist or recur, or if you have ulcers or bleeding problems, unless directed by a doctor. If ringing in the ears or loss of hearing occurs, consult a doctor before taking any more of this product.

Drug Interaction Precaution: Do not take this product if you are taking a prescription drug for anticoagulation (thinning of blood), diabetes, gout or arthritis unless directed by a doctor.

How Supplied: Arthritis Strength BUFFERIN® is supplied as:
Plain white coated caplet "ASB" debossed on one side.
NDC 19810-0051-1 Bottle of 40's
NDC 19810-0051-2 Bottle of 100's
The 40 caplet size does not have a child resistant closure and is recommended for households without young children.
Store at room temperature.
Shown in Product Identification Section, page 404

Extra Strength BUFFERIN®
[bŭf'fĕr-ĭn]
Analgesic

Composition:
Active Ingredient: Aspirin (500 mg) in a formulation buffered with Calcium Carbonate, Magnesium Oxide and Magnesium Carbonate.
Other Ingredients: Benzoic Acid, Citric Acid, Corn Starch, FD&C Blue No. 1, Hydroxypropyl Methylcellulose, Magnesium Stearate, Mineral Oil, Polysorbate 20, Povidone, Propylene Glycol, Simethicone Emulsion, Sodium Phosphate, Sorbitan Monolaurate, Titanium Dioxide. May also contain: Carnauba Wax, Zinc Stearate.

Indications: For temporary relief of headaches, pain and fever of colds, muscle aches, arthritis pain and inflammation, menstrual pain and toothaches.

Directions: Adults: 2 tablets with water every 6 hours while symptoms persist, not to exceed 8 tablets in 24 hours, or as directed by a doctor. Children under 12 years of age: Consult a doctor.

Warnings: Children and teenagers should not use this medicine for chicken pox or flu symptoms before a doctor is consulted about Reye syndrome, a rare but serious illness reported to be associated with aspirin. KEEP THIS AND ALL OTHER MEDICATIONS OUT OF THE REACH OF CHILDREN. IN CASE OF ACCIDENTAL OVERDOSE, SEEK PROFESSIONAL ASSISTANCE OR CONTACT A POISON CONTROL CENTER IMMEDIATELY. As with any drug, if your are pregnant or nursing a baby, seek the advice of a health professional before using this product. IT IS ESPECIALLY IMPORTANT NOT TO USE ASPIRIN DURING THE LAST 3 MONTHS OF PREGNANCY UNLESS SPECIFICALLY DIRECTED TO DO SO BY A DOCTOR BECAUSE IT MAY CAUSE PROBLEMS IN THE UNBORN CHILD OR COMPLICATIONS DURING DELIVERY. Do not take this product for more than 10 days or for fever for more than 3 days unless directed by a doctor. If pain or fever persists or gets worse, if new symptoms occur, or if redness or swelling is present, consult a doctor because these could be signs of a serious condition. Consult a dentist promptly for toothache. Do not take this product if you are allergic to aspirin, have asthma, have stomach problems (such as heartburn, upset stomach or stomach pain) that persist or recur, or if you have ulcers or bleeding problems, unless directed by a doctor. If ringing in the ears or loss of hearing occurs, consult a doctor before taking any more of this product.

Drug Interaction Precaution: Do not take this product if you are taking a prescription drug for anticoagulation (thinning of blood), diabetes, gout or arthritis unless directed by a doctor.

How Supplied: Extra Strength BUFFERIN® is supplied as:
White elongated coated tablet with "ESB" debossed on one side.
NDC 19810-0074-1 Bottle of 30's
NDC 19810-0074-4 Bottle of 50's
NDC 19810-0074-3 Bottle of 100's
All sizes have child resistant closures except 50's which is recommended for households without young children.
Store at room temperature.
Shown in Product Identification Section, page 404

COMTREX®
[cŏm'trĕx]
Multi-Symptom Cold Reliever

Composition: Each tablet, caplet, liquigel and fluidounce (30 ml.) contains:
[See table next page.]

Indications: COMTREX® provides temporary relief of these major cold and flu symptoms: nasal and sinus congestion, runny nose, sneezing, coughing, minor sore throat pain, headache, fever, body aches and pain.

Directions:
Tablets or Caplets: Adults: 2 tablets or caplets every 4 hours while symptoms persist, not to exceed 8 tablets or caplets in 24 hours, or as directed by a doctor. Children 6 to under 12 years of age: One tablet or caplet every 4 hours while symptoms persist, not to exceed 4 tablets or caplets in 24 hours, or as directed by a doctor. Children under 6: Consult a doctor.
Liqui-Gel: Adults: 2 liqui-gels every 4 hours while symptoms persist, not to exceed 12 liqui-gels in 24 hours, or as directed by a doctor. Children 6 to under 12 years of age: 1 liqui-gel every 4 hours while symptoms persist, not to exceed 5 liqui-gels in 24 hours, or as directed by a doctor. Children under 6: Consult a doctor.
Liquid: Adults: One fluidounce (30 ml) in medicine cup provided or 2 tablespoons every 4 hours while symptoms persist, not to exceed 4 doses in 24 hours, or as directed by a doctor. Children 6 to under 12 years of age: ½ fluidounce (15 ml) or one tablespoon every 4 hours while symptoms persist, not to exceed 4 doses in 24 hours, or as directed by a doctor. Children under 6: Consult a doctor.

Warnings: KEEP THIS AND ALL OTHER MEDICATIONS OUT OF THE REACH OF CHILDREN. IN CASE OF ACCIDENTAL OVERDOSE, SEEK PROFESSIONAL ASSISTANCE OR CONTACT A POISON CONTROL CENTER IMMEDIATELY. PROMPT MEDICAL ATTENTION IS CRITICAL FOR ADULTS AS WELL AS FOR CHILDREN EVEN IF YOU DO NOT NOTICE ANY SIGNS OR SYMPTOMS. As with any drug, if you are pregnant or nursing a baby, seek the advice of a health professional before using this product. Do not take this product for more than 7 days (for adults) or 5 days (for children), unless directed by a doctor. If symptoms do not improve or are accompanied by a fever that lasts for more than 3 days, or if new symptoms occur, consult a doctor. Do not exceed recommended dosage because at higher doses nervousness, dizziness or sleeplessness may occur. May cause excitability especially in children. A persistent cough may be a sign of a serious condition. If cough persists for more than 7 days, tends to recur, or is accompanied by rash, persistent headache, fever that lasts for more than 3 days, or if new symptoms occur, consult a doctor. Do not take this product for persistent or chronic cough such as occurs with smoking, asthma or emphysema, or if cough is accompanied by excessive phlegm (mucus/sputum) unless directed by a doctor. If sore throat is severe, persists for more than 2 days, is accompanied or followed by a fever, headache, rash, nausea or vomiting, consult a doctor promptly. This product should not be taken by persons who have asthma, glaucoma, emphysema, chronic pulmonary disease, high blood pressure,

	COMTREX Per Tablet or Caplet	COMTREX Liquid-Gel per Liqui-Gel	COMTREX Liquid Per Fl. Ounce
Acetaminophen:	325 mg.	325 mg.	650 mg.
Pseudoephedrine HCl:	30 mg.	—	60 mg.
Phenylpropanolamine HCl:	—	12.5 mg.	—
Chlorpheniramine Maleate:	2 mg.	2 mg.	4 mg.
Dextromethorphan HBr:	10 mg.	10 mg.	20 mg.

Other Ingredients:

Tablet	Caplet	Liqui-Gels	Liquid
Corn Starch	Benzoic Acid	D&C Yellow No. 10	Alcohol (20% by volume)
D&C Yellow No. 10 Lake	Carnauba Wax	FD&C Red No. 40	Citric Acid
FD&C Red No. 40 Lake	Corn Starch	Gelatin	D&C Yellow No. 10
Magnesium Stearate	D&C Yellow No. 10 Lake	Glycerin	FD&C Blue No. 1
Methylparaben	FD&C Red No. 40 Lake	Polyethylene Glycol	FD&C Red No. 40
Propylparaben	Hydroxypropyl Methylcellulose	Povidone	Flavors
Stearic Acid	Magnesium Stearate	Propylene Glycol	Polyethylene Glycol
May also contain:	Methylparaben	Silicon Dioxide	Povidone
Povidone	Mineral Oil	Sorbitol	Sodium Citrate
	Polysorbate 20	Titanium Dioxide	Sucrose
	Povidone	Water	Water
	Propylene Glycol		
	Propylparaben		
	Simethicone Emulsion		
	Sorbitan Monolaurate		
	Stearic Acid		
	Titanium Dioxide		

heart disease, thyroid disease, diabetes, shortness of breath, difficulty in breathing or difficulty in urination due to enlargement of the prostate gland unless directed by a doctor. May cause marked drowsiness; alcohol may increase the drowsiness effect. Avoid alcoholic beverages, and do not take this product if you are taking sedatives or tranquilizers without first consulting your doctor. Use caution when driving a motor vehicle or operating machinery.

Drug Interaction Precaution: This product should not be taken by any adult or child who is taking a prescription medication for high blood pressure or depression without first consulting a doctor.

Overdose:
MUCOMYST (acetylcysteine) As An Antidote For Acetaminophen Overdose)
Acetaminophen is rapidly absorbed from the upper gastrointestinal tract with peak plasma levels occurring between 30 and 60 minutes after therapeutic doses and usually within 4 hours following an overdose. The parent compound, which is nontoxic, is extensively metabolized in the liver to form principally the sulfate and glucuronide conjugates which are also nontoxic and are rapidly excreted in the urine. A small fraction of an ingested dose is metabolized in the liver by the cytochrome P-450 mixed function oxidase enzyme system to form a reactive, potentially toxic, intermediate metabolite which preferentially conjugates with hepatic glutathione to form the nontoxic cysteine and mercapturic acid derivatives which are then excreted by the kidney. Therapeutic doses of acetaminophen do not saturate the glucuronide and sulfate conjugation pathways and do not result in the formation of sufficient reactive metabolite to deplete glutathione stores. However, following ingestion of a large overdose (150 mg/kg or greater) the glucuronide and sulfate conjugation pathways are saturated resulting in a

larger fraction of the drug being metabolized via the P-450 pathway. The increased formation of reactive metabolite may deplete the hepatic stores of glutathione with subsequent binding of the metabolite to protein molecules within the hepatocyte resulting in cellular necrosis. Acetylcysteine has been shown to reduce the extent of liver injury following acetaminophen overdose. Early symptoms following a potentially hepatotoxic overdose may include: nausea, vomiting, diaphoresis and general malaise. Clinical and laboratory evidence of hepatic toxicity may not be apparent until 48 to 72 hours postingestion. In adults and adolescents, regardless of the quantity of acetaminophen reported to have been ingested, administer MUCOMYST® acetylcysteine immediately. MUCOMYST acetylcysteine therapy should be initiated and continued for a full course of therapy. Its effectiveness depends on early administration, with benefit seen principally in patients treated within 16 hours of the overdose.

If acetaminophen plasma assay capability is not available, and the estimated acetaminophen ingestion exceeds 150 mg/kg, MUCOMYST acetylcysteine therapy should be initiated and continued for a full course of therapy.
For full prescribing information, refer to the MUCOMYST package insert. Do not await the results of assays for acetaminophen level before initiating treatment with MUCOMYST acetylcysteine. The following additional procedures are recommended: The stomach should be emptied promptly by lavage or by induction of emesis with syrup of ipecac. A serum acetaminophen assay should be obtained as early as possible, but no sooner than four hours following ingestion. Liver function studies should be obtained initially and repeated at 24-hour intervals.
For additional emergency information call your regional poison center or toll-free (1-800-525-6115) to the Rocky Mountain Poison Center for assistance in diag-

nosis and for directions in the use of MUCOMYST acetylcysteine as an antidote.

How Supplied:
COMTREX® is supplied as:
Yellow tablet with letter "C" debossed on one surface.
NDC 19810-0790-1 Blister packages of 24's
NDC 19810-0790-2 Bottles of 50's
NDC 19810-0790-3 Vials of 10's
Coated yellow caplet with "Comtrex" printed in red on one side.
NDC 19810-0792-3 Blister packages of 24's
NDC 19810-0792-4 Bottles of 50's
Yellow Liqui-Gel with "Comtrex" printed in red on one side.
NDC 19810-0561-1 Blister packages of 24's
NDC 19810-0561-2 Blister packages of 50's
Clear Red Cherry Flavored liquid:
NDC 19810-0791-1 6 oz. plastic bottles.
All sizes packaged in child resistant closures except for 24's for tablets, caplets and liqui-gels which are sizes recommended for households without young children. Store caplets, tablets and liquid at room temperature.
Store liqui-gels below 86° F. (30° C.). Keep from freezing.
Shown in Product Identification Section, page 404

ALLERGY–SINUS COMTREX
[cŏm 'trĕx]
Multi-Symptom Allergy/Sinus Formula

Composition:
Active Ingredients: Each coated tablet or caplet contains 500 mg acetaminophen, 30 mg pseudoephedrine HCl, 2 mg chlorpheniramine maleate.
Other Ingredients: Benzoic acid, carnauba wax, corn starch, D&C yellow No. 10 lake, FD&C blue No. 1 lake, FD&C Red No. 40 lake, hydroxypropyl methyl-

Continued on next page

Bristol-Myers—Cont.

cellulose, mineral oil, polysorbate 20, povidone, propylene glycol, simethicone emulsion, sodium citrate, sorbitan monolaurate, stearic acid, titanium dioxide. May also contain: crospovidone, D&C yellow No. 10, erythorbic acid, FD&C blue No. 1, magnesium stearate, methylparaben, microcrystalline cellulose, polysorbate 80, propylparaben, silicon dioxide, wood cellulose.

Indications:
ALLERGY-SINUS COMTREX provides temporary relief of these upper respiratory allergy, hay fever, and sinusitis symptoms: sneezing, itchy, watery eyes, runny nose, headache, nasal and sinus pressure and congestion.

Directions: Adults: 2 tablets or caplets every 6 hours while symptoms persist, not to exceed 8 tablets or caplets in 24 hours, or as directed by a doctor. Children under 12 years of age: Consult a doctor.

Warnings: KEEP THIS AND ALL OTHER MEDICATIONS OUT OF THE REACH OF CHILDREN. IN CASE OF ACCIDENTAL OVERDOSE, SEEK PROFESSIONAL ASSISTANCE OR CONTACT A POISON CONTROL CENTER IMMEDIATELY. PROMPT MEDICAL ATTENTION IS CRITICAL FOR ADULTS AS WELL AS FOR CHILDREN EVEN IF YOU DO NOT NOTICE ANY SIGNS OR SYMPTOMS. As with any drug, if you are pregnant or nursing a baby, seek the advice of a health professional before using this product. Do not take this product for more than 7 days unless directed by a doctor. If symptoms do not improve or are accompanied by a fever that lasts for more than 3 days, or if new symptoms occur, consult a doctor. Do not exceed recommended dosage because at higher doses nervousness, dizziness or sleeplessness may occur. May cause excitability especially in children. This product should not be taken by persons who have asthma, glaucoma, emphysema, chronic pulmonary disease, high blood pressure, heart disease, thyroid disease, diabetes, shortness of breath, difficulty in breathing or difficulty in urination due to enlargement of the prostate gland unless directed by a doctor. May cause drowsiness; alcohol may increase the drowsiness effect. Avoid alcoholic beverages, and do not take this product if you are taking sedatives or tranquilizers without first consulting your doctor. Use caution when driving a motor vehicle or operating machinery.

Drug Interaction Precaution: Do not take this product if you are presently taking a prescription drug for high blood pressure or depression, without first consulting your doctor.

Overdose:
MUCOMYST (acetylcysteine) As An Antidote For Acetaminophen Overdose)

Acetaminophen is rapidly absorbed from the upper gastrointestinal tract with peak plasma levels occurring between 30 and 60 minutes after therapeutic doses and usually within 4 hours following an overdose. The parent compound, which is nontoxic, is extensively metabolized in the liver to form principally the sulfate and glucuronide conjugates which are also nontoxic and are rapidly excreted in the urine. A small fraction of an ingested dose is metabolized in the liver by the cytochrome P-450 mixed function oxidase enzyme system to form a reactive, potentially toxic, intermediate metabolite which preferentially conjugates with hepatic glutathione to form the nontoxic cysteine and mercapturic acid derivatives which are then excreted by the kidney. Therapeutic doses of acetaminophen do not saturate the glucuronide and sulfate conjugation pathways and do not result in the formation of sufficient reactive metabolite to deplete glutathione stores. However, following ingestion of a large overdose (150 mg/kg or greater) the glucuronide and sulfate conjugation pathways are saturated resulting in a larger fraction of the drug being metabolized via the P-450 pathway. The increased formation of reactive metabolite may deplete the hepatic stores of glutathione with subsequent binding of the metabolite to protein molecules within the hepatocyte resulting in cellular necrosis. Acetylcysteine has been shown to reduce the extent of liver injury following acetaminophen overdose. Early symptoms following a potentially hepatotoxic overdose may include: nausea, vomiting, diaphoresis and general malaise. Clinical and laboratory evidence of hepatic toxicity may not be apparent until 48 to 72 hours postingestion. In adults and adolescents, regardless of the quantity of acetaminophen reported to have been ingested, administer MUCOMYST® acetylcysteine immediately. MUCOMYST acetylcysteine therapy should be initiated and continued for a full course of therapy. Its effectiveness depends on early administration, with benefit seen principally in patients treated within 16 hours of the overdose. If acetaminophen plasma assay capability is not available, and the estimated acetaminophen ingestion exceeds 150 mg/kg, MUCOMYST acetylcysteine therapy should be initiated and continued for a full course of therapy.
For full prescribing information, refer to the MUCOMYST package insert. Do not await the results of assays for acetaminophen level before initiating treatment with MUCOMYST acetylcysteine. The following additional procedures are recommended: The stomach should be emptied promptly by lavage or by induction of emesis with syrup of ipecac. A serum acetaminophen assay should be obtained as early as possible, but no sooner than four hours following ingestion. Liver function studies should be obtained initially and repeated at 24-hour intervals.
For additional emergency information call your regional poison center or toll-

free (1-800-525-6115) to the Rocky Mountain Poison Center for assistance in diagnosis and for directions in the use of MUCOMYST acetylcysteine as an antidote.

How Supplied: Allergy-Sinus COMTREX® is supplied as:
Coated green tablets with "Comtrex A/S" printed in black on one side.
NDC 19810-0774-1 Blister packages of 24's
NDC 19810-0774-2 Bottles of 50's
Coated green caplets with "A/S" debossed on one surface.
NDC 19810-0081-4 Blister packages of 24's
NDC 19810-0081-5 Bottles of 50's
All sizes packaged in child resistant closures except 24's for tablets and caplets which are sizes recommended for households without young children.
Store at room temperature.
Shown in Product Identification Section, page 404

Cough Formula COMTREX®
[cŏm 'trĕx]
Multi-Symptom Cough Formula

Composition:
Active Ingredients: Each 4 teaspoonfuls (⅔ fl. oz.) contains:
—EXPECTORANT—200 mg Guaifenesin
—COUGH SUPPRESSANT—20 mg Dextromethorphan HBr
—ANALGESIC—500 mg Acetaminophen
—DECONGESTANT—60 mg Pseudoephedrine HCl

Other Ingredients: Alcohol (20% by volume), Citric Acid, FD&C Red No. 40, Flavor, Menthol, Povidone, Saccharin Sodium, Sodium Citrate, Sucrose, Water.

Indications: For temporary relief of cough, nasal and upper chest congestion, minor sore throat pain, and fever and pain due to a chest cold.

Directions: Adults: ⅔ fluidounce (20 ml) in medicine cup provided or four teaspoons every 4 hours while symptoms persist, not to exceed 4 doses in 24 hours, or as directed by a doctor. Children 6 to under 12 years of age: ⅓ fluidounce (10 ml) in medicine cup provided or 2 teaspoons every 4 hours while symptoms persist, not to exceed 4 doses in 24 hours, or as directed by a doctor. Children under 6: Consult a doctor.

Warnings: KEEP THIS AND ALL OTHER MEDICATIONS OUT OF THE REACH OF CHILDREN. IN CASE OF ACCIDENTAL OVERDOSE, SEEK PROFESSIONAL ASSISTANCE OR CONTACT A POISON CONTROL CENTER IMMEDIATELY. PROMPT MEDICAL ATTENTION IS CRITICAL FOR ADULTS AS WELL AS FOR CHILDREN EVEN IF YOU DO NOT NOTICE ANY SIGNS OR SYMPTOMS. As with any drug, if you are pregnant or nursing a baby, seek the advice of a health professional before using this product. Do not take this product for more than 7 days (for adults) or 5 days (for children) unless directed by a doctor. If symptoms do not improve or are accompanied by a fever that lasts for more than 3 days, or if new symptoms occur, consult a doctor. Do not exceed recommended dosage because at higher doses nervousness, dizziness or sleeplessness may occur. A persistent cough may be a sign of a serious condition. If cough persists for more than 7 days, tends to recur or is accompanied by rash, persistent headache, fever that lasts for more than 3 days, or if new symptoms occur, consult a doctor. Do not take this product for persistent or chronic cough such as occurs with smoking, asthma, chronic bronchitis or emphysema or if cough is accompanied by excessive phlegm (mucus/sputum) unless directed by a doctor. If sore throat is severe, persists for more than two days, is accompanied or followed by a fever, headache, rash, nausea or vomiting, consult a doctor promptly. This product should not be taken by persons who have heart disease, high blood pressure, thyroid disease, diabetes or difficulty in urination due to enlargement of the prostate gland unless directed by a doctor.

Overdose:
MUCOMYST (acetylcysteine) As An Antidote For Acetaminophen Overdose)

Acetaminophen is rapidly absorbed from the upper gastrointestinal tract with peak plasma levels occurring between 30 and 60 minutes after therapeutic doses and usually within 4 hours following an overdose. The parent compound, which is nontoxic, is extensively metabolized in the liver to form principally the sulfate and glucuronide conjugates which are also nontoxic and are rapidly excreted in the urine. A small fraction of an ingested dose is metabolized in the liver by the cytochrome P-450 mixed function oxidase enzyme system to form a reactive, potentially toxic, intermediate metabolite which preferentially conjugates with hepatic glutathione to form the nontoxic cysteine and mercapturic acid derivatives which are then excreted by the kidney. Therapeutic doses of acetaminophen do not saturate the glucuronide and sulfate conjugation pathways and do not result in the formation of sufficient reactive metabolite to deplete glutathione stores. However, following ingestion of a large overdose (150 mg/kg or greater) the glucuronide and sulfate conjugation pathways are saturated resulting in a larger fraction of the drug being metabolized via the P-450 pathway. The increased formation of reactive metabolite may deplete the hepatic stores of glutathione with subsequent binding of the metabolite to protein molecules within the hepatocyte resulting in cellular necrosis. Acetylcysteine has been shown to reduce the extent of liver injury following acetaminophen overdose. Early symptoms following a potentially hepatotoxic overdose may include nausea, vomiting, diaphoresis and general malaise. Clinical and laboratory evidence of hepatic toxicity may not be apparent until 48 to 72 hours postingestion. In adults

and adolescents, regardless of the quantity of acetaminophen reported to have been ingested, administer MUCOMYST® acetylcysteine immediately. MUCOMYST acetylcysteine therapy should be initiated and continued for a full course of therapy. Its effectiveness depends on early administration, with benefit seen principally in patients treated within 16 hours of the overdose. If acetaminophen plasma assay capability is not available, and the estimated acetaminophen ingestion exceeds 150 mg/kg, MUCOMYST acetylcysteine therapy should be initiated and continued for a full course of therapy.

For full prescribing information, refer to the MUCOMYST package insert. Do not await the results of assays for acetaminophen level before initiating treatment with MUCOMYST acetylcysteine. The following additional procedures are recommended: The stomach should be emptied promptly by lavage or by induction of emesis with syrup of ipecac. A serum acetaminophen assay should be obtained as early as possible, but no sooner than four hours following ingestion. Liver function studies should be obtained initially and repeated at 24-hour intervals.

For additional emergency information call your regional poison center or toll-free (1-800-525-6115) to the Rocky Mountain Poison Center for assistance in diagnosis and for directions in the use of MUCOMYST acetylcysteine as an antidote.

How Supplied: Cough Formula COMTREX® is supplied as a clear red raspberry flavored liquid:
NDC 19810-0783-1 4 oz. plastic bottle
NDC 19810-0783-2 8 oz. plastic bottle
The 4 oz. size is not child resistant and is recommended for households without young children.
Store at room temperature.
Shown in Product Identification Section, page 405

DAY-NIGHT COMTREX®

Composition:
Active Ingredients: EACH DAYTIME CAPLET CONTAINS 325mg Acetaminophen, 30mg Pseudoephedrine HCl, 10mg Dextromethorphan HBr. EACH NIGHTTIME TABLET CONTAINS 325mg Acetaminophen, 30mg Pseudoephedrine HCl, 10mg Dextromethorphan HBr, 2mg Chlorpheniramine Maleate.
Other Ingredients: DAYTIME CAPLETS AND NIGHTTIME TABLETS BOTH CONTAIN: Corn Starch, D&C Yellow No. 10 Lake, FD&C Red No. 40 Lake, Magnesium Stearate, Methylparaben, Propylparaben, Stearic Acid. DAYTIME CAPLETS ALSO CONTAIN: Benzoic Acid, Carnauba Wax, Hydroxypropyl Methylcellulose, Mineral Oil, Polysorbate 20, Povidone, Propylene Glycol, Simethicone Emulsion, Sorbitan Monolaurate, Titanium Dioxide. NIGHTTIME TABLETS MAY ALSO CONTAIN: Povidone.

Indications: Day/Night COMTREX provides you with two different formulas. COMTREX Daytime Caplets (orange) and COMTREX Nighttime Tablets (yellow), for effective relief. COMTREX Daytime Caplets contain three ingredients for the temporary relief of these major cold and flu symptoms without causing drowsiness: a decongestant—to relieve stuffy nose and sinus congestion; a cough suppressant—to quiet cough; a non-aspirin analgesic—to relieve headache, fever, minor sore throat pain and body aches and pain. COMTREX Nighttime Tablets relieve all these symptoms plus they contain an antihistamine to temporarily relieve runny nose and sneezing.

Warnings for Daytime Caplets and Nighttime Tablets KEEP THESE AND ALL OTHER MEDICATIONS OUT OF THE REACH OF CHILDREN. IN CASE OF ACCIDENTAL OVERDOSE, SEEK PROFESSIONAL ASSISTANCE OR CONTACT A POISON CONTROL CENTER IMMEDIATELY. PROMPT MEDICAL ATTENTION IS CRITICAL FOR ADULTS AS WELL AS FOR CHILDREN EVEN IF YOU DO NOT NOTICE ANY SIGNS OR SYMPTOMS. As with any drug, if you are pregnant or nursing a baby, seek the advice of a health professional before using these products. Do not take these products for more than 7 days or for fever for more than 3 days unless directed by a doctor. If symptoms do not improve or are accompanied by a fever that lasts for more than 3 days, or if new symptoms occur, consult a doctor. Do not exceed recommended dosage because at higher doses nervousness, dizziness or sleeplessness may occur. A persistent cough may be a sign of a serious condition. If cough persists for more than 7 days, tends to recur or is accompanied by rash, persistent headache, fever that lasts for more than 3 days, or if new symptoms occur, consult a doctor. Do not take these products for persistent or chronic cough such as occurs with smoking, asthma or emphysema, or if cough is accompanied by excessive phlegm (mucus/sputum) unless directed by a doctor. If sore throat is severe, persists for more than 2 days, is accompanied or followed by a fever, headache, rash, nausea or vomiting, consult a doctor promptly. These products should not be taken by persons who have asthma, glaucoma, emphysema, chronic pulmonary disease, high blood pressure, heart disease, thyroid disease, diabetes, shortness of breath, difficulty in breathing, or difficulty in urination due to an enlargement of the prostate gland unless directed by a doctor.
Additional Warnings for Nighttime Tablets May cause marked drowsiness; alcohol may increase the drowsiness effect. Avoid alcoholic beverages, and do not take this product if you are taking sedatives or tranquilizers without first consulting your doctor. Use caution when driving a motor vehicle or operat-

Continued on next page

Bristol-Myers—Cont.

ing machinery. May cause excitability especially in children.

DRUG INTERACTION PRECAUTION: Do not take these products if you are presently taking a prescription for high blood pressure or depression without first consulting your doctor.

Directions: Adults: 2 Daytime Caplets every 4 hours while symptoms persist, not to exceed 6 Daytime Caplets in 24 hours, or as directed by a doctor. 2 Nighttime Tablets at bedtime, if needed, to be taken no sooner than 4 hours after the last Daytime Caplet dose, or as directed by a doctor. **Children under 12:** Consult a doctor.

Overdose: MUCOMYST (acetylcysteine) As An Antidote For Acetaminophen Overdose)

Acetaminophen is rapidly absorbed from the upper gastrointestinal tract with peak plasma levels occurring between 30 and 60 minutes after therapeutic doses and usually within 4 hours following an overdose. The parent compound, which is nontoxic, is extensively metabolized in the liver to form principally the sulfate and glucuronide conjugates which are also nontoxic and are rapidly excreted in the urine. A small fraction of an ingested dose is metabolized in the liver by the cytochrome P-450 mixed function oxidase enzyme system to form a reactive, potentially toxic, intermediate metabolite which preferentially conjugates with hepatic glutathione to form the nontoxic cysteine and mercapturic acid derivatives which are then excreted by the kidney. Therapeutic doses of acetaminophen do not saturate the glucuronide and sulfate conjugation pathways and do not result in the formation of sufficient reactive metabolite to deplete glutathione stores. However, following ingestion of a large overdose (150 mg/kg or greater) the glucuronide and sulfate conjugation pathways are saturated resulting in a larger fraction of the drug being metabolized via the P-450 pathway. The increased formation of reactive metabolite may deplete the hepatic stores of glutathione with subsequent binding of the metabolite to protein molecules within the hepatocyte resulting in cellular necrosis. Acetylcysteine has been shown to reduce the extent of liver injury following acetaminophen overdose. Early symptoms following a potentially hepatotoxic overdose may include: nausea, vomiting, diaphoresis and general malaise. Clinical and laboratory evidence of hepatic toxicity may not be apparent until 48 to 72 hours postingestion. In adults and adolescents, regardless of the quantity of acetaminophen reported to have been ingested, administer MUCOMYST® acetylcysteine immediately. MUCOMYST acetylcysteine therapy should be initiated and continued for a full course of therapy. Its effectiveness depends on early administration, with benefit seen principally in patients treated within 16 hours of the overdose.

If acetaminophen plasma assay capability is not available, and the estimated acetaminophen ingestion exceeds 150 mg/kg, MUCOMYST acetylcysteine therapy should be initiated and continued for a full course of therapy.

For full prescribing information, refer to the MUCOMYST package insert. Do not await the results of assays for acetaminophen level before initiating treatment with MUCOMYST acetylcysteine. The following additional procedures are recommended: The stomach should be emptied promptly by lavage or by induction of emesis with syrup of ipecac. A serum acetaminophen assay should be obtained as early as possible, but no sooner than four hours following ingestion. Liver function studies should be obtained initially and repeated at 24-hour intervals.

For additional emergency information call your regional poison center or toll-free (1-800-525-6115) to the Rocky Mountain Poison Center for assistance in diagnosis and for directions in the use of MUCOMYST acetylcysteine as an antidote.

How Supplied: DAY-NIGHT COMTREX® is supplied as:
Day-Coated orange caplet with letter "C" debossed on one surface.
Night-Coated yellow tablet with letter "C" debossed on one surface.
NDC 19810-0078-1 Blister packages of 24's (18 caplets/6 tablets)
Store at room temperature.

Shown in Product Identification Section, page 404

Non-Drowsy COMTREX®

Composition:

Active Ingredients: Each caplet contains 325mg Acetaminophen, 30 mg Pseudoephedrine HCl, 10mg Dextromethorphan HBr. Other Ingredients: Benzoic Acid, Carnauba Wax, Corn Starch, D&C Yellow No. 10 Lake, FD&C Red No. 40 Lake, Hydroxypropyl Methylcellulose, Magnesium Stearate, Methylparaben, Mineral Oil, Polysorbate 20, Povidone, Propylene Glycol, Propylparaben, Simethicone Emulsion, Sorbitan Monolaurate, Stearic Acid, Titanium Dioxide.

Indications: For temporary relief of nasal and sinus congestion, coughing, minor sore throat pain, headache, fever, body aches and pain.

Warnings: KEEP THIS AND ALL OTHER MEDICATIONS OUT OF THE REACH OF CHILDREN. IN CASE OF ACCIDENTAL OVERDOSE, SEEK PROFESSIONAL ASSISTANCE OR CONTACT A POISON CONTROL CENTER IMMEDIATELY. PROMPT MEDICAL ATTENTION IS CRITICAL FOR ADULTS AS WELL AS FOR CHILDREN EVEN IF YOU DO NOT NOTICE ANY SIGNS OR SYMPTOMS. As with any drug, if you are pregnant or nursing a baby, seek the advice of a health professional before using this product. Do not take this product for

more than 7 days (for adults) or 5 days (for children) or for fever for more than 3 days unless directed by a doctor. Do not exceed recommended dosage because at higher doses nervousness, dizziness or sleeplessness may occur. A persistent cough may be a sign of a serious condition. If cough persists for more than 7 days, tends to recur or is accompanied by rash, persistent headache, fever that lasts for more than 3 days, or if new symptoms occur, consult a doctor. Do not take this product for persistent or chronic cough such as occurs with smoking, asthma or emphysema, or if cough is accompanied by excessive phlegm (mucus/sputum) unless directed by a doctor. If sore throat is severe, persists for more than 2 days, is accompanied or followed by a fever, headache, rash, nausea or vomiting, consult a doctor promptly. This product should not be taken by persons who have high blood pressure, heart disease, thyroid disease, diabetes or difficulty in urination due to enlargement of the prostate gland unless directed by a doctor.

DRUG INTERACTION PRECAUTION: This product should not be taken by any adult or child who is taking a prescription medication for high blood pressure or depression without first consulting a doctor.

Directions: Adults: 2 caplets every 4 hours while symptoms persist, not to exceed 8 caplets in 24 hours, or as directed by doctor. **Children 6 to under 12 years of age:** One caplet every 4 hours while symptoms persist, not to exceed 4 caplets in 24 hours, or as directed by a doctor. **Children under 6:** Consult a doctor.

Overdose: MUCOMYST (acetylcysteine) As An Antidote For Acetaminophen Overdose)

Acetaminophen is rapidly absorbed from the upper gastrointestinal tract with peak plasma levels occurring between 30 and 60 minutes after therapeutic doses and usually within 4 hours following an overdose. The parent compound, which is nontoxic, is extensively metabolized in the liver to form principally the sulfate and glucuronide conjugates which are also nontoxic and are rapidly excreted in the urine. A small fraction of an ingested dose is metabolized in the liver by the cytochrome P-450 mixed function oxidase enzyme system to form a reactive, potentially toxic, intermediate metabolite which preferentially conjugates with hepatic glutathione to form the nontoxic cysteine and mercapturic acid derivatives which are then excreted by the kidney. Therapeutic doses of acetaminophen do not saturate the glucuronide and sulfate conjugation pathways and do not result in the formation of sufficient reactive metabolite to deplete glutathione stores. However, following ingestion of a large overdose (150 mg/kg or greater) the glucuronide and sulfate conjugation pathways are saturated resulting in a larger fraction of the drug being metabolized via the P-450 pathway. The increased formation of reactive metabolite may deplete the hepatic stores of glutathione with subsequent binding of the metabolite to protein molecules within the hepatocyte resulting in cellular necrosis. Acetylcysteine has been shown to reduce the extent of liver injury following acetaminophen overdose. Early symptoms following a potentially hepatotoxic overdose may include: nausea, vomiting, diaphoresis and general malaise. Clinical and laboratory evidence of hepatic toxicity may not be apparent until 48 to 72 hours postingestion. In adults and adolescents, regardless of the quantity of acetaminophen reported to have been ingested, administer MUCO-MYST® acetylcysteine immediately. MUCOMYST acetylcysteine therapy should be initiated and continued for a full course of therapy. Its effectiveness depends on early administration, with benefit seen principally in patients treated within 16 hours of the overdose. If acetaminophen plasma assay capability is not available, and the estimated acetaminophen ingestion exceeds 150 mg/kg, MUCOMYST acetylcysteine therapy should be initiated and continued for a full course of therapy.

For full prescribing information, refer to the MUCOMYST package insert. Do not await the results of assays for acetaminophen level before initiating treatment with MUCOMYST acetylcysteine. The following additional procedures are recommended: The stomach should be emptied promptly by lavage or by induction of emesis with syrup of ipecac. A serum acetaminophen assay should be obtained as early as possible, but no sooner than four hours following ingestion. Liver function studies should be obtained initially and repeated at 24-hour intervals.

For additional emergency information call your regional poison center or toll-free (1-800-525-6115) to the Rocky Mountain Poison Center for assistance in diagnosis and for directions in the use of MUCOMYST acetylcysteine as an antidote.

How Supplied: Non-Drowsy Comtrex® is supplied as:
Coated yellow caplet with letter "C" debossed on one surface.
NDC 19810-0041-1 Blister packages of 24's
NDC 19810-0041-2 Bottles of 50's
The 24 size does not have a child resistant closure and is recommended for households without young children.
Store at room temperature.
Shown in Product Identification Section, page 405

CONGESPIRIN® for Children
Aspirin Free
Chewable Cold Tablets
[cŏn "gĕs 'pir-in]

Composition: Each tablet contains acetaminophen 81 mg. (1¼ grains), phenylephrine hydrochloride 1¼ mg. Also Contains: Calcium Stearate, D&C Red No. 30 Aluminum Lake, D&C Yellow No. 10 Aluminum Lake, Ethyl Cellulose, Flavor, Mannitol, Microcrystalline Cel-

lulose, Polyethylene, Saccharin Calcium, Sucrose.

Indications: A non-aspirin analgesic/nasal decongestant that temporarily reduces fever and relieves aches, pains and nasal congestion associated with colds and "flu."

Warnings: KEEP THIS AND ALL MEDICINES OUT OF CHILDREN'S REACH. IN CASE OF ACCIDENTAL OVERDOSE, CONTACT A PHYSICIAN IMMEDIATELY.

Caution: If child is under medical care, do not administer without consulting physician. Do not exceed recommended dosage. Consult your physician if symptoms persist or if high blood pressure, heart disease, diabetes or thyroid disease is present. Do not administer for more than 10 days unless directed by physician.

Directions:
Under 2, consult your physician.
2–3 years ....2 tablets
4–5 years ....3 tablets
6–8 years ....4 tablets
9–10 years ....5 tablets
11–12 years ....6 tablets
over 12 years ....8 tablets
Repeat dose in four hours if necessary. Do not give more than four doses per day unless prescribed by your physician.

Overdose:
MUCOMYST (acetylcysteine) As An Antidote For Acetaminophen Overdose)
Acetaminophen is rapidly absorbed from the upper gastrointestinal tract with peak plasma levels occurring between 30 and 60 minutes after therapeutic doses and usually within 4 hours following an overdose. The parent compound, which is nontoxic, is extensively metabolized in the liver to form principally the sulfate and glucuronide conjugates which are also nontoxic and are rapidly excreted in the urine. A small fraction of an ingested dose is metabolized in the liver by the cytochrome P-450 mixed function oxidase enzyme system to form a reactive, potentially toxic, intermediate metabolite which preferentially conjugates with hepatic glutathione to form the nontoxic cysteine and mercapturic acid derivatives which are then excreted by the kidney. Therapeutic doses of acetaminophen do not saturate the glucuronide and sulfate conjugation pathways and do not result in the formation of sufficient reactive metabolite to deplete glutathione stores. However, following ingestion of a large overdose (150 mg/kg or greater) the glucuronide and sulfate conjugation pathways are saturated resulting in a larger fraction of the drug being metabolized via the P-450 pathway. The increased formation of reactive metabolite may deplete the hepatic stores of glutathione with subsequent binding of the metabolite to protein molecules within the hepatocyte resulting in cellular necrosis. Acetylcysteine has been shown to reduce the extent of liver injury following acetaminophen overdose. Early symptoms following a potentially hepa-

totoxic overdose may include nausea, vomiting, diaphoresis and general malaise. Clinical and laboratory evidence of hepatic toxicity may not be apparent until 48 to 72 hours postingestion. In adults and adolescents, regardless of the quantity of acetaminophen reported to have been ingested, administer MUCO-MYST® acetylcysteine immediately. MUCOMYST acetylcysteine therapy should be initiated and continued for a full course of therapy. Its effectiveness depends on early administration, with benefit seen principally in patients treated within 16 hours of the overdose. If acetaminophen plasma assay capability is not available, and the estimated acetaminophen ingestion exceeds 150 mg/kg, MUCOMYST acetylcysteine therapy should be initiated and continued for a full course of therapy.

For full prescribing information, refer to the MUCOMYST package insert. Do not await the result of assays for acetaminophen level before initiating treatment with MUCOMYST acetylcysteine. The following additional procedures are recommended: The stomach should be emptied promptly by lavage or by induction of emesis with syrup of ipecac. A serum acetaminophen assay should be obtained as early as possible, but no sooner than four hours following ingestion. Liver function studies should be obtained initially and repeated at 24-hour intervals.

For additional emergency information call your regional poison center or toll-free (1-800-525-6115) to the Rocky Mountain Poison Center for assistance in diagnosis and for directions in the use of MUCOMYST acetylcysteine as an antidote.

How Supplied: CONGESPIRIN Aspirin Free Chewable Cold Tablets are supplied as scored orange tablets with "C" on one side.
NDC 19810-0748-1 Bottles of 24's.
Bottles are child resistant.
Store at room temperature.
Shown in Product Identification Section, page 405

Extra–Strength DATRIL®
[dā 'trĭl]
Analgesic

Composition: Each tablet contains Acetaminophen 500 mg. Other ingredients: Corn Starch, Povidone, Stearic Acid. May also contain: Croscarmellose Sodium, Crospovidone, Erythorbic Acid, Methylparaben, Propylparaben, Wood Cellulose.

Indications: For temporary relief of the pain of headaches, sinusitis, colds or flu, muscular aches, menstrual discomfort, toothaches, and minor arthritis pain and to reduce fever.

Directions: Adults: 2 tablets every 6 hours while symptoms persist, not to exceed 8 tablets in 24 hours, or as directed

Continued on next page

Bristol-Myers—Cont.

by a doctor. Children under 12: Consult a doctor.

Warnings: KEEP THIS AND ALL OTHER MEDICATIONS OUT OF THE REACH OF CHILDREN. IN CASE OF ACCIDENTAL OVERDOSE, SEEK PROFESSIONAL ASSISTANCE OR CONTACT A POISON CONTROL CENTER IMMEDIATELY. PROMPT MEDICAL ATTENTION IS CRITICAL FOR ADULTS AS WELL AS FOR CHILDREN EVEN IF YOU DO NOT NOTICE ANY SIGNS OR SYMPTOMS. As with any drug, if you are pregnant or nursing a baby, seek the advice of a health professional before using this product. Do not take this product for pain for more than 10 days or for fever for more than 3 days unless directed by a doctor. If pain or fever persists or gets worse, if new symptoms occur, or if redness or swelling is present, consult a doctor because these could be signs of a serious condition. Consult a dentist promptly for toothache.

Overdose:
MUCOMYST (acetylcysteine) As An Antidote For Acetaminophen Overdose)
Acetaminophen is rapidly absorbed from the upper gastrointestinal tract with peak plasma levels occurring between 30 and 60 minutes after therapeutic doses and usually within 4 hours following an overdose. The parent compound, which is nontoxic, is extensively metabolized in the liver to form principally the sulfate and glucuronide conjugates which are also nontoxic and are rapidly excreted in the urine. A small fraction of an ingested dose is metabolized in the liver by the cytochrome P-450 mixed function oxidase enzyme system to form a reactive, potentially toxic, intermediate metabolite which preferentially conjugates with hepatic glutathione to form the nontoxic cysteine and mercapturic acid derivatives which are then excreted by the kidney. Therapeutic doses of acetaminophen do not saturate the glucuronide and sulfate conjugation pathways and do not result in the formation of sufficient reactive metabolite to deplete glutathione stores. However, following ingestion of a large overdose (150 mg/kg or greater) the glucuronide and sulfate conjugation pathways are saturated resulting in a larger fraction of the drug being metabolized via the P-450 pathway. The increased formation of reactive metabolite may deplete the hepatic stores of glutathione with subsequent binding of the metabolite to protein molecules within the hepatocyte resulting in cellular necrosis. Acetylcysteine has been shown to reduce the extent of liver injury following acetaminophen overdose. Early symptoms following a potentially hepatotoxic overdose may include: nausea, vomiting, diaphoresis and general malaise. Clinical and laboratory evidence of hepatic toxicity may not be apparent until 48 to 72 hours postingestion. In adults and adolescents, regardless of the quantity of acetaminophen reported to have been ingested, administer MUCOMYST® acetylcysteine immediately. MUCOMYST acetylcysteine therapy should be initiated and continued for a full course of therapy. Its effectiveness depends on early administration, with benefit seen principally in patients treated within 16 hours of the overdose. If acetaminophen plasma assay capability is not available, and the estimated acetaminophen ingestion exceeds 150 mg/kg, MUCOMYST acetylcysteine therapy should be initiated and continued for a full course of therapy.

For full prescribing information, refer to the MUCOMYST package insert. Do not await the results of assays for acetaminophen level before initiating treatment with MUCOMYST acetylcysteine. The following additional procedures are recommended: The stomach should be emptied promptly by lavage or by induction of emesis with syrup of ipecac. A serum acetaminophen assay should be obtained as early as possible, but no sooner than four hours following ingestion. Liver function studies should be obtained initially and repeated at 24-hour intervals.

For additional emergency information call your regional poison center or toll-free (1-800-525-6115) to the Rocky Mountain Poison Center for assistance in diagnosis and for directions in the use of MUCOMYST acetylcysteine as an antidote.

How Supplied: Extra Strength DATRIL® is supplied as:
White circular tablets with "DATRIL" debossed on one surface.
NDC 19810-0705-1 Bottles of 30's
Store at room temperature.
Shown in Product Identification Section, page 405

Aspirin Free EXCEDRIN®

Composition: Each caplet contains Acetaminophen 500 mg. and Caffeine 65 mg. Other Ingredients: Benzoic Acid, Carnauba Wax, Corn Starch, Croscarmellose Sodium, D&C Red No. 27 Lake, D&C Yellow No. 10 Lake, FD&C Blue No. 1 Lake, Hydroxypropyl Methylcellulose, Magnesium Stearate, Methylparaben, Microcrystalline Cellulose, Propylparaben, Saccharin Sodium, Simethicone Emulsion, Stearic Acid, Titanium Dioxide. May also contain: Erythorbic Acid, Mineral Oil, Polyethylene Glycol, Polysorbate 20, Polysorbate 80, Povidone, Propylene Glycol.

Indications: For temporary relief of the pain of headache, sinusitis, colds, muscular aches, menstrual discomfort, toothaches and minor arthritis pain.

Directions: Adults: 2 caplets every 6 hours while symptoms persist, not to exceed 8 caplets in 24 hours, or as directed by a doctor. Children under 12 years of age: Consult a doctor.

Warnings: KEEP THIS AND ALL OTHER MEDICATIONS OUT OF THE REACH OF CHILDREN. IN CASE OF ACCIDENTAL OVERDOSE, SEEK PROFESSIONAL ASSISTANCE OR CONTACT A POISON CONTROL CENTER IMMEDIATELY. PROMPT MEDICAL ATTENTION IS CRITICAL FOR ADULTS AS WELL AS FOR CHILDREN EVEN IF YOU DO NOT NOTICE ANY SIGNS OR SYMPTOMS. As with any drug, if you are pregnant or nursing a baby, seek the advice of a health professional before using this product. Do not take this product for pain for more than 10 days or for fever for more than 3 days unless directed by a doctor. If pain or fever persists or gets worse, if new symptoms occur, or if redness or swelling is present, consult a doctor because these could be signs of a serious condition. Consult a dentist promptly for toothache.

Overdose:
MUCOMYST (acetylcysteine) As An Antidote For Acetaminophen Overdose)
Acetaminophen is rapidly absorbed from the upper gastrointestinal tract with peak plasma levels occurring between 30 and 60 minutes after therapeutic doses and usually within 4 hours following an overdose. The parent compound, which is nontoxic, is extensively metabolized in the liver to form principally the sulfate and glucuronide conjugates which are also nontoxic and are rapidly excreted in the urine. A small fraction of an ingested dose is metabolized in the liver by the cytochrome P-450 mixed function oxidase enzyme system to form a reactive, potentially toxic, intermediate metabolite which preferentially conjugates with hepatic glutathione to form the nontoxic cysteine and mercapturic acid derivatives which are then excreted by the kidney. Therapeutic doses of acetaminophen do not saturate the glucuronide and sulfate conjugation pathways and do not result in the formation of sufficient reactive metabolite to deplete glutathione stores. However, following ingestion of a large overdose (150 mg/kg or greater) the glucuronide and sulfate conjugation pathways are saturated resulting in a larger fraction of the drug being metabolized via the P-450 pathway. The increased formation of reactive metabolite may deplete the hepatic stores of glutathione with subsequent binding of the metabolite to protein molecules within the hepatocyte resulting in cellular necrosis. Acetylcysteine has been shown to reduce the extent of liver injury following acetaminophen overdose. Early symptoms following a potentially hepatotoxic overdose may include: nausea, vomiting, diaphoresis and general malaise. Clinical and laboratory evidence of hepatic toxicity may not be apparent until 48 to 72 hours postingestion. In adults and adolescents, regardless of the quantity of acetaminophen reported to have been ingested, administer MUCOMYST® acetylcysteine immediately. MUCOMYST acetylcysteine therapy should be initiated and continued for a full course of therapy. Its effectiveness depends on early administration, with benefit seen principally in patients treated within 16 hours of the overdose.

If acetaminophen plasma assay capability is not available, and the estimated acetaminophen ingestion exceeds 150 mg/kg, MUCOMYST acetylcysteine therapy should be initiated and continued for a full course of therapy.

For full prescribing information, refer to the MUCOMYST package insert. Do not await the results of assays for acetaminophen level before initiating treatment with MUCOMYST acetylcysteine. The following additional procedures are recommended: The stomach should be emptied promptly by lavage or by induction of emesis with syrup of ipecac. A serum acetaminophen assay should be obtained as early as possible, but no sooner than four hours following ingestion. Liver function studies should be obtained initially and repeated at 24-hour intervals.

For additional emergency information call your regional poison center or toll-free (1-800-525-6115) to the Rocky Mountain Poison Center for assistance in diagnosis and for directions in the use of MUCOMYST acetylcysteine as an antidote.

How Supplied: Aspirin Free EXCEDRIN® is supplied as: Coated red caplets with "AF Excedrin" printed in white on one side.
NDC 19810-0089-1 Bottles of 24's
NDC 19810-0089-2 Bottles of 50's
NDC 19810-0089-3 Bottles of 100's
All sizes packaged in child resistant closures except 100's which is recommended for households without young children. Store at room temperature.
Shown in Product Identification Section, page 405

EXCEDRIN® Extra-Strength Analgesic
[ĕx "cĕd 'rĭn]

Composition:
Each tablet or caplet contains Acetaminophen 250 mg.: Aspirin 250 mg.; and Caffeine 65 mg.
Other Ingredients: (Tablets) Benzoic Acid, FD&C Blue No. 1, Hydroxypropyl Methylcellulose, Microcrystalline Cellulose, Mineral Oil, Polysorbate 20, Povidone, Propylene Glycol, Saccharin Sodium, Simethicone Emulsion, Sorbitan Monolaurate, Stearic Acid, Titanium Dioxide. May Also Contain: Carnauba Wax, Hydroxypropylcellulose. (Caplets) Benzoic Acid, FD&C Blue No. 1, Hydroxypropylcellulose, Hydroxypropyl Methylcellulose, Microcrystalline Cellulose, Mineral Oil, Polysorbate 20, Povidone, Propylene Glycol, Simethicone Emulsion, Sorbitan Monolaurate, Stearic Acid, Titanium Dioxide. Caplets may also contain: Carnauba wax.

Indications: For temporary relief of the pain of headache, sinusitis, colds, muscular aches, menstrual discomfort, toothaches and minor arthritis pain.

Directions: Adults: 2 tablets or caplets with water every 6 hours while symptoms persist, not to exceed 8 tablets or caplets in 24 hours, or as directed by a doctor. Children under 12 years of age: Consult a doctor.

Warnings: Children and teenagers should not use this medicine for chickenpox or flu symptoms before a doctor is consulted about Reye syndrome, a rare but serious illness reported to be associated with aspirin. KEEP THIS AND ALL OTHER MEDICATIONS OUT OF THE REACH OF CHILDREN. IN CASE OF ACCIDENTAL OVERDOSE, SEEK PROFESSIONAL ASSISTANCE OR CONTACT A POISON CONTROL CENTER IMMEDIATELY. PROMPT MEDICAL ATTENTION IS CRITICAL FOR ADULTS AS WELL AS FOR CHILDREN EVEN IF YOU DO NOT NOTICE ANY SIGNS OR SYMPTOMS. As with any drug, if you are pregnant or nursing a baby, seek the advice of a health professional before using this product. IT IS ESPECIALLY IMPORTANT NOT TO USE ASPIRIN DURING THE LAST 3 MONTHS OF PREGNANCY UNLESS SPECIFICALLY DIRECTED TO DO SO BY A DOCTOR BECAUSE IT MAY CAUSE PROBLEMS IN THE UNBORN CHILD OR COMPLICATIONS DURING DELIVERY. Do not take this product for pain for more than 10 days or for fever for more than 3 days unless directed by a doctor. If pain or fever persists or gets worse, if new symptoms occur, or if redness or swelling is present, consult a doctor because these could be signs of a serious condition. Consult a dentist promptly for toothache. Do not take this product if you are allergic to aspirin, have asthma, have stomach problems (such as heartburn, upset stomach or stomach pain) that persist or recur, or if you have ulcers or bleeding problems, unless directed by a doctor. If ringing in the ears or loss of hearing occurs, consult a doctor before taking any more of this product.

Drug Interaction Precaution: Do not take this product if you are taking a prescription drug for anticoagulation (thinning of blood), diabetes, gout or arthritis unless directed by a doctor.

Overdose:
MUCOMYST (acetylcysteine As An Antidote For Acetaminophen Overdose)
Acetaminophen is rapidly absorbed from the upper gastrointestinal tract with peak plasma levels occurring between 30 and 60 minutes after therapeutic doses and usually within 4 hours following an overdose. The parent compound, which is nontoxic, is extensively metabolized in the liver to form principally the sulfate and glucuronide conjugates which are also nontoxic and are rapidly excreted in the urine. A small fraction of an ingested dose is metabolized in the liver by the cytochrome P-450 mixed function oxidase enzyme system to form a reactive, potentially toxic, intermediate metabolite which preferentially conjugates with hepatic glutathione to form the nontoxic cysteine and mercapturic acid derivatives which are then excreted by the kidney. Therapeutic doses of acetaminophen do not saturate the glucuronide and sulfate conjugation pathways and do not result in the formation of sufficient reactive metabolite to deplete glutathione stores. However, following ingestion of a larger overdose (150 mg/kg or greater) the glucuronide and sulfate conjugation pathways are saturated resulting in larger fraction of the drug being metabolized via the P-450 pathway. The increased formation of reactive metabolite may deplete the hepatic stores of glutathione with subsequent binding of the metabolite to protein molecules within the hepatocyte resulting in cellular necrosis. Acetylcysteine has been shown to reduce the extent of liver injury following acetaminophen overdose. Early symptoms following a potentially hepatotoxic overdose may include nausea, vomiting, diaphoresis and general malaise. Clinical and laboratory evidence of hepatic toxicity may not be apparent until 48 to 72 hours postingestion. In adults and adolescents, regardless of the quantity of acetaminophen reported to have been ingested, administer MUCOMYST® acetylcysteine immediately. MUCOMYST acetylcysteine therapy should be initiated and continued for a full course of therapy. Its effectiveness depends on early administration, with benefit seen principally in patients treated within 16 hours of the overdose. If acetaminophen plasma assay capability is not available, and the estimated acetaminophen ingestion exceeds 150 mg/kg, MUCOMYST acetylcysteine therapy should be initiated and continued for a full course of therapy.

For full prescribing information, refer to the MUCOMYST package insert. Do not await the results of assays for acetaminophen level before initiating treatment with MUCOMYST acetylcysteine. The following additional procedures are recommended. The stomach should be emptied promptly by lavage or by induction of emesis with syrup of ipecac. A serum acetaminophen assay should be obtained as early as possible, but no sooner than four hours following ingestion. Liver function studies should be obtained initially and repeated at 24-hour intervals.

For additional emergency information call your regional poison center or toll-free (1-800-525-6115) to the Rocky Mountain Poison Center for assistance in diagnosis and for directions in the use of MUCOMYST acetylcysteine as an antidote.

How Supplied: Extra Strength EXCEDRIN® is supplied as:
White circular tablet with letter "E" debossed on one side.
NDC 19810-0700-2 Bottles of 12's
NDC 19810-0782-3 Bottles of 24's
NDC 19810-0782-4 Bottles of 50's
NDC 19810-0700-5 Bottles of 100's
NDC 19810-0782-5 Bottles of 150's
NDC 19810-0782-6 Bottles of 200's
NDC 19810-0782-2 Bottles of 275's
NDC 19810-0700-1 A metal tin of 12's
NDC 19810-0772-1 Vials of 10's
Coated white caplets with "Excedrin" printed in red on one side.

Continued on next page

Bristol-Myers—Cont.

NDC 19810-0002-1 Bottles of 24's
NDC 19810-0002-2 Bottles of 50's
NDC 19810-0002-8 Bottles of 100's
All sizes packaged in child resistant closures except 100's for tablets, 50's for caplets which are sizes recommended for households without young children.
Store at room temperature.

Shown in Product Identification Section, page 405

EXCEDRIN P.M.®
[ĕx″cĕd′rĭn]
Analgesic Sleeping Aid

Composition: Each tablet, caplet and fluidounce (30 ml.) contains:
[See table below.]

Indications: For temporary relief of occasional headaches and minor aches and pains with accompanying sleeplessness.

Directions:
Tablets or Caplets:
Adults, 2 tablets or caplets at bedtime if needed or as directed by a doctor.
Liquid:
Adults, 1 fluidounce (2 tablespoons) at bedtime if needed, or as directed by a doctor, using the dosage cup provided.

Warnings: KEEP THIS AND ALL OTHER MEDICATIONS OUT OF THE REACH OF CHILDREN. IN CASE OF ACCIDENTAL OVERDOSE, SEEK PROFESSIONAL ASSISTANCE OR CONTACT A POISON CONTROL CENTER IMMEDIATELY. PROMPT MEDICAL ATTENTION IS CRITICAL FOR ADULTS AS WELL AS FOR CHILDREN EVEN IF YOU DO NOT NOTICE ANY SIGNS OR SYMPTOMS. As with any drug, if you are pregnant or nursing a baby, seek the advice of a health professional before using this product. Do not give this product to children under 12 years of age or use for more than 10 days unless directed by a doctor. Consult a doctor if symptoms persist or get worse or if new ones occur, or if sleeplessness persists continuously for more than 2 weeks because these may be symptoms of serious underlying medical illnesses. Do not take this product if you have asthma, glaucoma, emphysema, chronic pulmonary disease, shortness of breath, difficulty in breathing, or difficulty in urination due to enlargement of the prostate gland unless directed by a doctor. Avoid alcoholic beverages while taking this product. Do not take this product if you are taking sedatives or tranquilizers, without first consulting your doctor.

Overdose:
MUCOMYST (acetylcysteine) As An Antidote For Acetaminophen Overdose)
Acetaminophen is rapidly absorbed from the upper gastrointestinal tract with peak plasma levels occurring between 30 and 60 minutes after therapeutic doses and usually within 4 hours following an overdose. The parent compound, which is nontoxic, is extensively metabolized in the liver to form principally the sulfate and glucuronide conjugates which are also nontoxic and are rapidly excreted in the urine. A small fraction of an ingested dose is metabolized in the liver by the cytochrome P-450 mixed function oxidase enzyme system to form a reactive, potentially toxic, intermediate metabolite which preferentially conjugates with hepatic glutathione to form the nontoxic cysteine and mercapturic acid derivatives which are then excreted by the kidney. Therapeutic doses of acetaminophen do not saturate the glucuronide and sulfate conjugation pathways and do not result in the formation of sufficient reactive metabolite to deplete glutathione stores. However, following ingestion of a large overdose (150 mg/kg or greater) the glucuronide and sulfate conjugation pathways are saturated resulting in a larger fraction of the drug being metabolized via the P-450 pathway. The increased formation of reactive metabolite may deplete the hepatic stores of glutathione with subsequent binding of the metabolite to protein molecules within the hepatocyte resulting in cellular necrosis. Acetylcysteine has been shown to reduce the extent of liver injury following acetaminophen overdose. Early symptoms following a potentially hepatotoxic overdose may include: nausea, vomiting, diaphoresis and general malaise. Clinical and laboratory evidence of hepatic toxicity may not be apparent until 48 to 72 hours postingestion. In adults and adolescents, regardless of the quantity of acetaminophen reported to have been ingested, administer MUCOMYST® acetylcysteine immediately. MUCOMYST acetylcysteine therapy should be initiated and continued for a full course of therapy. Its effectiveness depends on early administration, with benefit seen principally in patients treated within 16 hours of the overdose. If acetaminophen plasma assay capability is not available, and the estimated acetaminophen ingestion exceeds 150 mg/kg, MUCOMYST acetylcysteine therapy should be initiated and continued for a full course of therapy.
For full prescribing information, refer to the MUCOMYST package insert. Do not await the results of assays for acetaminophen level before initiating treatment with MUCOMYST acetylcysteine. The following additional procedures are recommended: The stomach should be emptied promptly by lavage or by induction of emesis with syrup of ipecac. A serum acetaminophen assay should be obtained as early as possible, but no sooner than four hours following ingestion. Liver function studies should be obtained initially and repeated at 24-hour intervals.
For additional emergency information call your regional poison center or toll-free (1-800-525-6115) to the Rocky Mountain Poison Center for assistance in diagnosis and for directions in the use of MUCOMYST acetylcysteine as an antidote.

How Supplied: EXCREDRIN P.M.® is supplied as:
Light blue circular tablets with "PM" debossed on one side.

	EXCEDRIN® PM Per Tablet or Caplet	EXCEDRIN® PM Per Fl. Ounce (30 ml.)
Acetaminophen	500 mg.	1000 mg.
Diphenhydramine Citrate:	38 mg.	—
Diphenhydramine HCl:	—	50 mg

Other Ingredients:

Tablet	Caplet	Liquid
Corn Starch	Benzoic Acid	Alcohol (10% by volume)
D&C Yellow No. 10	Carnauba Wax	Benzoic Acid
D&C Yellow No. 10 Aluminum Lake	Corn Starch	FD&C Blue No. 1
FD&C Blue No. 1	D&C Yellow No. 10	Flavor
FD&C Blue No. 1 Aluminum Lake	D&C Yellow No. 10 Aluminum Lake	Polyethylene Glycol
Magnesium Stearate	FD&C Blue No. 1	Povidone
Methylparaben	FD&C Blue No. 1 Aluminum Lake	Sodium Citrate
Propylparaben	Hydroxypropyl Methylcellulose	Sucrose
Stearic Acid	Methylparaben	Water
	Magnesium Stearate	
May Also Contain:	Propylene Glycol	
Microcrystalline Cellulose	Propylparaben	
Povidone	Simethicone Emulsion	
	Stearic Acid	
	Titanium Dioxide	

NDC 19810-0763-6 Bottles of 10's
NDC 19810-0763-3 Bottles of 30's
NDC 19810-0763-4 Bottles of 50's
NDC 19810-0763-5 Bottles of 80's
NDC 19810-0763-9 Vials of 10's
Light blue coated caplet with "Excedrin P.M." imprinted on one side.
NDC 19810-0032-2 Bottles of 30's
NDC 19810-0032-3 Bottles of 50's
Light blue wild berry flavored liquid.
NDC 19810-0060-1 6 oz. (177 ml) Plastic Bottle
All sizes packaged in child resistant closures except 50's tablets and caplets which are recommended for households without young children.
Store at room temperature
Shown in Product Identification Section, page 405

Sinus EXCEDRIN®
[ex ″cĕd ′rĭn]
Analgesic, Decongestant

Composition: Each coated tablet or caplet contains 500 mg Acetaminophen and 30 mg Pseudoephedrine HCl.

Other Ingredients: Corn Starch, D&C Yellow No. 10 Lake, FD&C Red No. 40 Lake, Hydroxypropyl Methylcellulose, Mineral Oil, Polysorbate 20, Povidone, Propylene Glycol, Simethicone Emulsion, Sorbitan Monolaurate, Stearic Acid, Titanium Dioxide. May also contain: Benzoic Acid, Carnauba Wax.

Indications: For temporary relief of headache, sinus pain and sinus pressure and congestion due to sinusitis or the common cold.

Directions: Adults: 2 tablets or caplets every 6 hours while symptoms persist, not to exceed 8 tablets or caplets in 24 hours, or as directed by a doctor. Children under 12 years of age: Consult a doctor.

Warnings: KEEP THIS AND ALL MEDICATIONS OUT OF THE REACH OF CHILDREN. IN CASE OF ACCIDENTAL OVERDOSE, SEEK PROFESSIONAL ASSISTANCE OR CONTACT A POISON CONTROL CENTER IMMEDIATELY. PROMPT MEDICAL ATTENTION IS CRITICAL FOR ADULTS AS WELL AS FOR CHILDREN EVEN IF YOU DO NOT NOTICE ANY SIGNS OR SYMPTOMS. As with any drug, if you are pregnant or nursing a baby, seek the advice of a health professional before using this product. Do not take this product for more than 10 days unless directed by a doctor. If symptoms do not improve or are accompanied by a fever that lasts for more than 3 days, or if new symptoms occur, consult a doctor. Do not exceed recommended dosage because at higher doses nervousness, dizziness or sleeplessness may occur. Do not take this product if you have heart disease, high blood pressure, thyroid disease, diabetes, or difficulty in urination due to enlargement of the prostate gland unless directed by a doctor.

Drug Interaction Precaution: Do not take this product if you are taking a pre-scription medication for high blood pressure or depression without first consulting a doctor.

Overdose:
MUCOMYST (acetylcysteine) As An Antidote for Acetaminophen Overdose)
Acetaminophen is rapidly absorbed from the upper gastrointestinal tract with peak plasma levels occurring between 30 and 60 minutes after therapeutic doses and usually within 4 hours following an overdose. The parent compound, which is nontoxic, is extensively metabolized in the liver to form principally the sulfate and glucuronide conjugates which are also nontoxic and are rapidly excreted in the urine. A small fraction of an ingested dose is metabolized in the liver by the cytochrome P-450 mixed function oxidase enzyme system to form a reactive, potentially toxic, intermediate metabolite which preferentially conjugates with hepatic glutathione to form the nontoxic cysteine and mercapturic acid derivatives which are then excreted by the kidney. Therapeutic doses of acetaminophen do not saturate the glucuronide and sulfate conjugation pathways and do not result in the formation of sufficient reactive metabolite to deplete glutathione stores. However, following ingestion of a large overdose (150 mg/kg or greater) the glucuronide and sulfate conjugation pathways are saturated resulting in a larger fraction of the drug being metabolized via the P-450 pathway. The increased formation of reactive metabolite may deplete the hepatic stores of glutathione with subsequent binding of the metabolite to protein molecules within the hepatocyte resulting in cellular necrosis. Acetylcysteine has been shown to reduce the extent of liver injury following acetaminophen overdose. Early symptoms following a potentially hepatotoxic overdose may include: nausea, vomiting, diaphoresis and general malaise. Clinical and laboratory evidence of hepatic toxicity may not be apparent until 48 to 72 hours postingestion. In adults and adolescents, regardless of the quantity of acetaminophen reported to have been ingested, administer MUCOMYST® acetylcysteine immediately. MUCOMYST acetylcysteine therapy should be initiated and continued for a full course of therapy. Its effectiveness depends on early administration, with benefit seen principally in patients treated within 16 hours of the overdose. If acetaminophen plasma assay capability is not available, and the estimated acetaminophen ingestion exceeds 150 mg/kg, MUCOMYST acetylcysteine therapy should be initiated and continued for a full course of therapy.
For full prescribing information, refer to the MUCOMYST package insert. Do not await the results of assays for acetaminophen level before initiating treatment with MUCOMYST acetylcysteine. The following additional procedures are recommended: The stomach should be emptied promptly by lavage or by induction of emesis with syrup of ipecac. A serum acetaminophen assay should be obtained as early as possible, but no sooner than four hours following ingestion. Liver function studies should be obtained initially and repeated at 24-hour intervals.
For additional emergency information call your regional poison center or toll-free (1-800-525-6115) to the Rocky Mountain Poison Center for assistance in diagnosis and for directions in the use of MUCOMYST acetylcysteine as an antidote.

How Supplied: Sinus EXCEDRIN® is supplied as:
Coated circular orange tablets with "Sinus Excedrin" imprinted in green on one side.
NDC 19810-0080-1 Blister packages of 24's
NDC 19810-0080-2 Bottles of 50's
Coated orange caplets with "Sinus Excedrin" imprinted in green on one side.
NDC 19810-0077-1 Blister packages of 24's
NDC 19810-0077-2 Bottles of 50's
All sizes have child resistant closures except 24's for tablets and caplets which are recommended for households without young children.
Store at room temperature.
Shown in Product Identification Section, page 405

4-WAY® Cold Tablets

Composition: Each tablet contains acetaminophen 325 mg., phenylpropanolamine HCl 12.5 mg., and chlorpheniramine maleate 2 mg. Other Ingredients: Corn Starch, Corn Starch Pregelatinized, Microcrystalline Cellulose, Sodium Starch Glycolate, Stearic Acid, Sucrose.

Indications: For temporary relief of nasal and sinus congestion, runny nose, sneezing, fever, minor sore throat pain, body aches and pain.

Directions:
Adults: 2 tablets every 4 hours while symptoms persist, not to exceed 12 tablets in 24 hours, or as directed by a doctor. Children 6 to under 12 years of age: One tablet every 4 hours while symptoms persist, not to exceed 5 tablets in 24 hours, or as directed by a doctor. Children under 6: Consult a doctor.

Warnings: KEEP THIS AND ALL OTHER MEDICATIONS OUT OF THE REACH OF CHILDREN. IN CASE OF ACCIDENTAL OVERDOSE, SEEK PROFESSIONAL ASSISTANCE OR CONTACT A POISON CONTROL CENTER IMMEDIATELY. PROMPT MEDICAL ATTENTION IS CRITICAL FOR ADULTS AS WELL AS FOR CHILDREN EVEN IF YOU DO NOT NOTICE ANY SIGNS OR SYMPTOMS. As with any drug, if you are pregnant or nursing a baby, seek the advice of a health professional before using this product. Do not take this product for more than 10 days (for adults) or 5 days (for children) unless directed by a doctor. If symptoms do not

Continued on next page

Bristol-Myers—Cont.

improve or are accompanied by a fever that lasts for more than 3 days, or if new symptoms occur, consult a doctor. Do not exceed recommended dosage because at higher doses nervousness, dizziness or sleeplessness may occur. May cause excitability especially in children. If sore throat is severe, persists for more than 2 days, is accompanied or followed by a fever, headache, rash, nausea or vomiting, consult a doctor promptly. This product should not be taken by persons who have asthma, glaucoma, emphysema, chronic pulmonary disease, high blood pressure, heart disease, thyroid disease, diabetes, shortness of breath, difficulty in breathing or difficulty in urination due to enlargement of the prostate gland unless directed by a doctor. May cause drowsiness; alcohol may increase the drowsiness effect. Avoid alcoholic beverages, and do not take this product if you are taking sedatives or tranquilizers without first consulting your doctor. Use caution when driving a motor vehicle or operating machinery.

Drug Interaction Precaution: This product should not be taken by any adult or child who is taking a prescription medication for high blood pressure or depression without first consulting a doctor.

Overdose:
MUCOMYST (acetylcysteine) As An Antidote For Acetaminophen Overdose)
Acetaminophen is rapidly absorbed from the upper gastrointestinal tract with peak plasma levels occurring between 30 and 60 minutes after therapeutic doses and usually within 4 hours following an overdose. The parent compound, which is nontoxic, is extensively metabolized in the liver to form principally the sulfate and glucuronide conjugates which are also nontoxic and are rapidly excreted in the urine. A small fraction of an ingested dose is metabolized in the liver by the cytochrome P-450 mixed function oxidase enzyme system to form a reactive, potentially toxic, intermediate metabolite which preferentially conjugates with hepatic glutathione to form the nontoxic cysteine and mercapturic acid derivatives which are then excreted by the kidney. Therapeutic doses of acetaminophen do not saturate the glucuronide and sulfate conjugation pathways and do not result in the formation of sufficient reactive metabolite to deplete glutathione stores. However, following ingestion of a large overdose (150 mg/kg or greater) the glucuronide and sulfate conjugation pathways are saturated resulting in a larger fraction of the drug being metabolized via the P-450 pathway. The increased formation of reactive metabolite may deplete the hepatic stores of glutathione with subsequent binding of the metabolite to protein molecules within the hepatocyte resulting in cellular necrosis. Acetylcysteine has been shown to reduce the extent of liver injury following acetaminophen overdose. Early symptoms following a potentially hepatotoxic overdose may include: nausea, vomiting, diaphoresis and general malaise. Clinical and laboratory evidence of hepatic toxicity may not be apparent until 48 to 72 hours postingestion. In adults and adolescents, regardless of the quantity of acetaminophen reported to have been ingested, administer MUCOMYST® acetylcysteine immediately. MUCOMYST acetylcysteine therapy should be initiated and continued for a full course of therapy. Its effectiveness depends on early administration, with benefit seen principally in patients treated within 16 hours of the overdose. If acetaminophen plasma assay capability is not available, and the estimated acetaminophen ingestion exceeds 150 mg/kg, MUCOMYST acetylcysteine therapy should be initiated and continued for a full course of therapy.
For full prescribing information, refer to the MUCOMYST package insert. Do not await the results of assays for acetaminophen level before initiating treatment with MUCOMYST acetylcysteine. The following additional procedures are recommended: The stomach should be emptied promptly by lavage or by induction of emesis with syrup of ipecac. A serum acetaminophen assay should be obtained as early as possible, but no sooner than four hours following ingestion. Liver function studies should be obtained initially and repeated at 24-hour intervals.
For additional emergency information call your regional poison center or toll-free (1-800-525-6115) to the Rocky Mountain Poison Center for assistance in diagnosis and for directions in the use of MUCOMYST acetylcysteine as an antidote.

How Supplied: 4-WAY Cold Tablets are supplied as a white tablet with the number "4" debossed on one surface.
NDC 19810-0040-1 Bottle of 36's
All sizes packaged in child resistant bottle closures.
Store at room temperature.
Shown in Product Identification Section, page 405

4-WAY® Fast Acting Nasal Spray

Composition:
Original Formula: Phenylephrine hydrochloride 0.5%, naphazoline hydrochloride 0.05%, pyrilamine maleate 0.2%, in a buffered isotonic aqueous solution with thimerosal 0.005% added as a preservative. Also Contains: Benzalkonium Chloride, Poloxamer 188, Potassium Phosphate, Sodium Chloride, Sodium Phosphate, Water. Also available in a mentholated formula containing Phenylephrine hydrochloride 0.5%, naphazoline hydrochloride 0.05%, pyrilamine maleate 0.2%, in a buffered isotonic aqueous solution with thimerosal 0.005% added as a preservative. Also Contains: Benzalkonium Chloride, Camphor, Eucalyptol, Menthol, Poloxamer 188, Polysorbate 80, Potassium Phosphate, Sodium Chloride, Sodium Phosphate, Water.

New Formula: Phenylephrine Hydrochloride 0.5% in a buffered isotonic solution. Also contains: Benzalkonium Chloride, Disodium EDTA, Potassium Phosphate, Sodium Chloride, Sodium Phosphate, Water. Also available in a mentholated formula containing Phenylephrine Hydrochloride 0.5% in a buffered isotonic solution. Also contains: Benzalkonium Chloride, Camphor, Disodium EDTA, Eucalyptol, Menthol, Poloxamer 188, Polysorbate 80, Potassium Phosphate, Sodium Chloride, Sodium Phosphate, Water.

Indications: For prompt, temporary relief of nasal congestion due to the common cold, sinusitis, hay fever or other upper respiratory allergies.

Directions and Use Instructions:
Directions: Adults: Spray twice into each nostril not more often than every 4 hours. Do not give to children under 12 years of age unless directed by a doctor. Use Instructions: For Metered Pump— Remove protective cap. Hold bottle with thumb at base and nozzle between first and second fingers. With head upright, insert metered pump spray nozzle into nostril. Depress pump all the way down, with a firm even stroke and sniff deeply. Repeat in other nostril. Do not tilt head backward while spraying. Wipe tip clean after each use. Note: This bottle is filled to correct level for proper pump action. Before using the first time, remove the protective cap from the tip and prime the metered pump by depressing pump firmly several times.
Use Instructions: For Atomizer— With head in a normal upright position, put atomizer tip into nostril. Squeeze bottle with firm, quick pressure while inhaling.

Warnings: KEEP THIS AND ALL OTHER MEDICATIONS OUT OF THE REACH OF CHILDREN. IN CASE OF ACCIDENTAL OVERDOSE OR INGESTION, SEEK PROFESSIONAL ASSISTANCE OR CONTACT A POISON CONTROL CENTER IMMEDIATELY. Do not exceed recommended dosage because burning, stinging, sneezing, or increase of nasal discharge may occur. The use of this container by more than one person may spread infection. Do not use this product for more than 3 days. If symptoms persist, consult a doctor. Adults and children who have heart disease, high blood pressure, thyroid disease, diabetes, or difficulty in urination due to enlargement of the prostate gland should not use this product unless directed by a doctor.

How Supplied:
4-WAY® Fast Acting Nasal Spray is supplied as:
Original Regular formula:
NDC 19810-0001-1 Atomizer of ½ fluid ounce.
NDC 19810-0001-2 Atomizer of 1 fluid ounce.
NDC 19810-0001-3 Metered pump of ½ fluid ounce.

Original Mentholated formula:
NDC 19810-0003-1 Atomizer of ½ fluid ounce.
NDC 19810-0003-2 Atomizer of 1 fluid ounce.
New Regular formula:
NDC 19810-0047-1 Atomizer of ½ fluid ounce.
NDC 19810-0047-2 Atomizer of 1 fluid ounce.
NDC 19810-0047-3 Metered pump of ½ fluid ounce.
New Mentholated formula:
NDC 19810-0049-1 Atomizer of ½ fluid ounce.
NDC 19810-0049-2 Atomizer of 1 fluid ounce.
Store at room temperature.
Shown in Product Identification Section, page 405

4–WAY® Long Lasting Nasal Spray

Composition: Oxymetazoline Hydrochloride 0.05% in a buffered isotonic aqueous solution. **Also Contains:** Benzalkonium Chloride, Glycine, Sorbitol, Water. May also contain: Disodium EDTA, Phenylmercuric Acetate, Sodium Hydroxide.

Indications: For prompt, temporary relief of nasal congestion due to the common cold, sinusitis, hay fever or other upper respiratory allergies.

Directions and Use Instructions:
Directions: Adults and children 6 to under 12 years of age (with adult supervision): 2 or 3 sprays in each nostril not more often than every 10 to 12 hours. Do not exceed 2 applications in any 24-hour period. Children under 6 years of age: Consult a doctor.
Use Instructions: For Metered Pump—Remove protective cap. Hold bottle with thumb at base and nozzle between first and second fingers. With head upright, insert metered pump spray nozzle into nostril. Depress pump all the way down, with a firm even stroke and sniff deeply. Repeat in other nostril. Do not tilt head backward while spraying. Wipe tip clean after each use. Note: This bottle is filled to correct level for proper pump action. Before using the first time, remove the protective cap from the tip and prime the metered pump by depressing pump firmly several times.
Use Instructions: For Atomizer—
With head in a normal, upright position, put atomizer tip into nostril. Squeeze bottle with firm, quick pressure while inhaling.

Warnings: KEEP THIS AND ALL OTHER MEDICATIONS OUT OF THE REACH OF CHILDREN. IN CASE OF ACCIDENTAL OVERDOSE OR INGESTION, SEEK PROFESSIONAL ASSISTANCE OR CONTACT A POISON CONTROL CENTER IMMEDIATELY. Do not exceed recommended dosage because burning, stinging, sneezing, or increase of nasal discharge may occur. The use of this container by more than one person may spread infection. Do not use this product for more than 3 days. If symp-

toms persist, consult a doctor. Adults and children who have heart disease, high blood pressure, thyroid disease, diabetes, or difficulty in urination due to enlargement of the prostate gland should not use this product unless directed by a doctor.

How Supplied: 4-WAY Long Lasting Nasal Spray is supplied as:
Atomizers and a metered pump:
NDC 19810-0728-1 Atomizers of ½ fluid ounce.
NDC 19810-0728-3 Metered pump of ½ fluid ounce.
NDC 19810-0048-1 Atomizer of ½ fluid ounce.
Store at room temperature.
Shown in Product Identification Section, page 405

KERI LOTION
Skin Lubricant—Moisturizer

Available in three formulations:
KERI Original—recommended for dry skin.

Composition: Mineral oil in water, propylene glycol, glyceryl stearate/PEG-100 stearate, PEG-40 stearate, PEG-4 dilaurate, laureth-4, lanolin oil, methylparaben, propylparaben, fragrance, carbomer-934, triethanolamine, dioctyl sodium sulfosuccinate, quaternium-15. Fresh Herbal scent: FD&C blue 1, D&C yellow 10.

KERI Silky Smooth—recommended for daily use on dry skin.

Composition: Water, petrolatum, glycerin, dimethicone, steareth-2, cetyl alcohol, benzyl alcohol, laureth-23, carbomer-934, MgAl silicate, fragrance, quaternium-15, sodium hydroxide.

KERI Silky Smooth Fragrance Free—recommended for daily use on dry skin.

Composition: Water, petrolatum, glycerin, dimethicone, steareth-2, cetyl alcohol, benzyl alcohol, laureth-23, MgAl silicate, carbomer-934, sodium hydroxide, quaternium-15.

Indications: KERI Lotion lubricates and helps hydrate the skin, making it soft and smooth. It relieves itching, helps maintain a normal moisture balance and supplements the protective action of skin lipids. Indicated for generalized dryness; detergent hands; chapped or chafed skin; "winter-itch," diaper rash; heat rash.

Directions for Use: Apply as often as needed. Use particularly after bathing and exposure to sun, water, soaps and detergents. For external use only.

How Supplied: KERI Lotion Original 6½ oz., 11 oz., 15 oz. and 20 oz. plastic bottles. KERI Silky Smooth 6½ oz. and 15 oz. plastic bottles. KERI Silky Smooth Fragrance Free 6½ oz., 11 oz. and 15 oz. plastic bottles.
Shown in Product Identification Section, page 405

NO DOZ® Tablets
[nō 'dōz]

Composition: Each tablet contains 100 mg. Caffeine. Other Ingredients: Cornstarch, Flavors, Mannitol, Microcrystalline Cellulose, Stearic Acid, Sucrose.

Indications: Helps restore mental alertness or wakefulness when experiencing fatigue or drowsiness.

Directions: Adults 1 or 2 tablets not more often than every 3 to 4 hours.

Warnings: KEEP THIS AND ALL OTHER MEDICATIONS OUT OF THE REACH OF CHILDREN. IN CASE OF ACCIDENTAL OVERDOSE, SEEK PROFESSIONAL ASSISTANCE OR CONTACT A POISON CONTROL CENTER IMMEDIATELY. As with any drug, if you are pregnant or nursing a baby, seek the advice of a health professional before using this product. Do not give to children under 12 years of age. For occasional use only. Not intended for use as a substitute for sleep. If fatigue or drowsiness persists or continues to occur, consult a doctor. The recommended dose of this product contains about as much caffeine as a cup of coffee. Limit the use of caffeine-containing medications, foods, or beverages while taking this product because too much caffeine may cause nervousness, irritability, sleeplessness and, occasionally, rapid heart beat.

How Supplied: NO DOZ® is supplied as:
A circular white tablet with "NoDoz" debossed on one side.
NDC 19810-0063-2 Blister pack of 16's
NDC 19810-0063-3 Blister pack of 36's
NDC 19810-0062-5 Bottle of 60's
NDC 19810-0063-1 Vials of 15's
Store at room temperature.
Shown in Product Identification Section, page 406

NO DOZ® Maximum Strength Caplets

Composition: Each caplet contains 200 mg. Caffeine. Other ingredients: Benzoic Acid, Corn Starch, FD&C Blue No. 1, Flavors, Hydroxypropyl Methylcellulose, Microcrystalline Cellulose, Propylene Glycol, Simethicone Emulsion, Stearic Acid, Sucrose, Titanium Dioxide. May also contain: Carnauba Wax, Mineral Oil, Polysorbate 20, Povidone, Sorbitan Monolaurate.

Indications: Helps restore mental alertness or wakefulness when experiencing fatigue or drowsiness.

Directions: Adults: one-half to one caplet not more often than every 3 to 4 hours.

Warnings: KEEP THIS AND ALL OTHER MEDICATIONS OUT OF THE REACH OF CHILDREN. IN CASE OF ACCIDENTAL OVERDOSE, SEEK PROFESSIONAL ASSISTANCE OR

Continued on next page

Bristol-Myers—Cont.

CONTACT A POISON CONTROL CEN-
TER IMMEDIATELY. As with any drug,
if you are pregnant or nursing a baby,
seek the advice of a health professional
before using this product. Do not give to
children under 12 years of age. For occasional use only. Not intended for use as a
substitute for sleep. If fatigue or drowsiness persists or continues to occur, consult a doctor. The recommended dose of
this product contains about as much caffeine as a cup of coffee. Limit the use of
caffeine-containing medications, foods,
or beverages while taking this product
because too much caffeine may cause
nervousness, irritability, sleeplessness
and, occasionally, rapid heart beat.

How Supplied: NO DOZ® Maximum
Strength is supplied as: White coated
caplets with "NO DOZ" debossed on one
side. The opposite side is scored.
NDC 19810-0064-1 Blister Packs of 12's
Store at room temperature.
*Shown in Product Identification
Section, page 405*

NUPRIN®
(ibuprofen)
Analgesic

Warning: ASPIRIN SENSITIVE PA-
TIENTS. Do not take this product if you
have had a severe allergic reaction to aspirin, e.g.—asthma, swelling, shock or
hives, because even though this product
contains no aspirin or salicylates, cross-
reactions may occur in patients allergic
to aspirin. (See ADDITIONAL WARN-
INGS BELOW)

Composition: Each tablet or caplet contains ibuprofen USP, 200 mg. **Other Ingredients:** Carnauba wax, cornstarch,
D&C Yellow No. 10, FD&C Yellow No. 6,
hydroxypropyl methylcellulose, propylene glycol, silicon dioxide, stearic acid,
titanium dioxide.

Indications: For the temporary relief
of minor aches and pains associated with
the common cold, headache, toothache,
muscular aches, backache, for the minor
pain of arthritis, for the pain of menstrual cramps and for reduction of fever.

Additional Warnings: The following
warnings are stated on the Nuprin label:
Do not take for pain for more than 10
days or for fever for more than 3 days unless directed by a doctor. If pain or fever
persists or gets worse, if new symptoms
occur, or if the painful area is red or
swollen, consult a doctor. These could be
signs of serious illness. If you are under a
doctor's care for any serious condition,
consult a doctor before taking this product. As with aspirin and acetaminophen,
if you have any condition which requires
you to take prescription drugs or if you
have had any problems or serious side
effects from taking any non-prescription
pain reliever, do not take NUPRIN without first discussing it with your doctor. If
you experience any symptoms which are
unusual or seem unrelated to the condi-

tion for which you took ibuprofen, consult a doctor before taking any more of it.
Although ibuprofen is indicated for the
same conditions as aspirin and acetaminophen, it should not be taken with them
except under a doctor's direction. Do not
combine this product with any other ibuprofen-containing product. As with any
drug, if you are pregnant or nursing a
baby, seek the advice of a health professional before using this product. IT IS
ESPECIALLY IMPORTANT NOT TO
USE IBUPROFEN DURING THE LAST
3 MONTHS OF PREGNANCY UNLESS
SPECIFICALLY DIRECTED TO DO SO
BY A DOCTOR BECAUSE IT MAY
CAUSE PROBLEMS IN THE UNBORN
CHILD OR COMPLICATIONS DURING
DELIVERY. Keep this and all drugs out
of the reach of children. In case of accidental overdose, seek professional assistance or contact a poison control center
immediately.

Caution: Store at room temperature.
Avoid excessive heat 40°C (104°F).

Directions: Adults: Take 1 tablet or
caplet every 4 to 6 hours while symptoms
persist. If pain or fever does not respond
to 1 tablet or caplet, 2 tablets or caplets
may be used but do not exceed 6 tablets
or caplets in 24 hours, unless directed by
a doctor. The smallest effective dose
should be used. Take with food or milk if
occasional and mild heartburn, upset
stomach, or stomach pain occurs with
use. Consult a doctor if these symptoms
are more than mild or if they persist.
Children: Do not give this product to children under 12 except under the advice
and supervision of a doctor.

How Supplied:
NUPRIN® is supplied as:
Golden yellow round tablets with "NU-
PRIN" printed in black on one side.
NDC 19810-0767-2 Bottles of 24's
NDC 19810-0767-3 Bottles of 50's
NDC 19810-0767-4 Bottles of 100's
NDC 19810-0767-7 Bottles of 150's
NDC 19810-0767-8 Bottles of 225's
NDC 19810-0767-9 Vials of 10's
Golden yellow caplets with "NUPRIN"
printed in black on one side.
NDC 19810-0796-1 Bottles of 24's
NDC 19810-0796-2 Bottles of 50's
NDC 19810-0796-3 Bottles of 100's
All sizes packaged in child resistant clo-
sures except 24's for tablets and 24's for
caplets, which are sizes recommended for
households without young children.
Store at room temperature. Avoid exces-
sive heat 40°C. (104°F.).
Distributed by Bristol-Myers Company
*Shown in Product Identification
Section, page 406*

PAZO® Hemorrhoid
Ointment/Suppositories

Composition:
Ointment: Active Ingredients: Cam-
phor, 2%; Ephedrine Sulfate, 0.2%; Zinc
Oxide, 5%. Other Ingredients: Lanolin,
Petrolatum.
Suppositories (per suppository): Ac-
tive Ingredients: Ephedrine Sulfate, 3.86

mg; Zinc Oxide, 96.5 mg. Other Ingredients: Hydrogenated Vegetable Oil.

Indications:
Ointment: For the temporary relief of
local pain, itching, and discomfort associated with inflamed hemorrhoidal tissues. Temporarily shrinks hemorrhoidal
tissue.
Suppositories: For the temporary relief of local itching and discomfort associated with inflamed hemorrhoidal tissues. Temporarily shrinks hemorrhoidal
tissue.

Directions:
Ointment — Adults: When practical,
cleanse the affected area with soap and
warm water and rinse thoroughly.
Gently dry by patting or blotting with
toilet tissue or a soft cloth before application of this product. Apply to the affected
area up to 4 times daily. Do not put this
product into the rectum by using fingers
or any mechanical device or applicator.
Children under 12 years of age: consult a
doctor.
Suppositories—Adults: When practical, cleanse the affected area with mild
soap and warm water and rinse thoroughly. Gently dry by patting or blotting
with toilet tissue or a soft cloth before
application of this product. Remove foil
wrapper and insert suppository into the
rectum. Use rectally up to 4 times daily.
Children under 12 years of age: consult a
doctor.

Warnings: KEEP THIS AND ALL
OTHER MEDICATIONS OUT OF THE
REACH OF CHILDREN. IN CASE OF
ACCIDENTAL INGESTION OR OVER-
DOSE, SEEK PROFESSIONAL ASSIS-
TANCE OR CONTACT A POISON CON-
TROL CENTER IMMEDIATELY. As
with any drug, if you are pregnant or
nursing a baby, seek the advice of a
health professional before using this
product. If condition worsens or does not
improve within 7 days, consult a doctor.
Do not exceed the recommended daily
dosage unless directed by a doctor. In
case of bleeding consult a doctor
promptly. Do not use this product if you
have heart disease, high blood pressure,
thyroid disease, diabetes, or difficulty in
urination due to enlargement of the prostate gland unless directed by a doctor.
Some users of this product may experience nervousness, tremor, sleeplessness,
nausea, and loss of appetite. If these
symptoms persist or become worse consult your doctor.
**DRUG   INTERACTION   PRECAU-
TION: Do not use this product if you
are taking a prescription drug for high
blood pressure or depression without
first consulting your doctor. Store at
room temperature.**

How Supplied: PAZO® ointment is
supplied with a plastic applicator as:
NDC 19810-0768-1 One ounce tubes
PAZO® suppositories are silver foil
wrapped and supplied as:
NDC 19810-0703-1 Box of 12's
*Shown in Product Identification
Section, page 406*

PRESUN® ACTIVE 15 AND 30
Clear Gel Sunscreens

Active Ingredients: Oxybenzone. Octyl Methoxycinnamate. Octyl Salicylate.
PRESUN® 15 Also contains: S.D. Alcohol 40, 71.5% PPG-15 Stearyl Ether, Acrylates/t-Ocylpropenamide Copolymer, Hydroxypropylcellulose.
PRESUN® 30 Also contains: S.D. Alcohol 40, 69% PPG-15 Stearyl Ether, Acrylates/t-Ocylpropenamide Copolymer, Hydroxypropylcellulose.

Indications: 15 OR 30 TIMES NATURAL UVB PROTECTION: Used liberally and regularly PreSun® 15 or 30 Active Clear Gel Sunscreens provide 15 or 30 times your natural UVB sunburn protection and may help reduce the chance of premature wrinkling of the skin caused by repeated and prolonged overexposure to the sun.
UVA/UVB PROTECTION: PreSun® 15 or 30 Active Clear Gel Sunscreens are formulated to provide protection from sunburn caused by both UVA and UVB rays.
CLEAR GEL FORMULA: PreSun® Active Sunscreens are cool refreshing Clear Gels that feel non-greasy. They are fragrance and PABA free, which fits your Active lifestyle.
WATERPROOF: PreSun® 15 or 30 Active Clear Gel Sunscreens maintain their degree of protection even after 80 minutes in the water.

Directions: Smooth evenly and liberally onto dry skin before sun exposure. Massage in gently. Reapply to dry skin after swimming, excessive perspiration or towel drying.

Warnings: For external use only. As with all sunscreens, avoid contact with eyes. Discontinue use if irritation or rash appears. Consult a physician before using on children under six months of age.

How Supplied: 4 oz. plastic bottles

PRESUN® FOR KIDS
Children's Sunscreen

Active Ingredients: Octyl methoxycinnamate, oxybenzone, octyl salicylate. Also contains: Carbomer-940, cetyl alcohol, diazolidinyl urea, dimethicone, methylchloroisothiazolinone and methylisothiazolinone, stearic acid, triethanolamine, water and other ingredients.

Indications: 29 TIMES NATURAL PROTECTION: Used as directed, PRESUN For Kids provides 29 times your child's natural sunburn protection and may help reduce the chance of premature aging and wrinkling of the skin.
NONSTINGING: A non-PABA, fragrance-free formula that is designed not to sting sensitive skin. (Avoid contact with eyes since all sunscreens can cause irritation and stinging of the eye.)
HYPOALLERGENIC: PRESUN For Kids is hypoallergenic and, because the

known sensitizers common to most sunscreens have been removed, is suitable for your child's sensitive skin.
WATERPROOF 29: PRESUN For Kids maintains its degree of protection (SPF 29) even after 80 minutes in the water.

Warnings: For external use only. Protect from freezing. *As with all sunscreens:* Apply to a small area; check after 24 hours. Discontinue use if irritation or rash appears. Avoid contact with eyes. In case of contact, flush eyes with water. Keep out of the reach of children. Use on children under six months of age only with the advice of a physician.

Directions for Use: For maximum protection, smooth evenly and liberally onto dry skin before sun exposure. Massage in gently. Reapplication to dry skin after prolonged swimming, excessive perspiration or towel drying is recommended for all-day protection.

How Supplied: 4 oz. plastic bottle.
Shown in Product Identification Section, page 406

PRESUN® 8, 15 AND 25 MOISTURIZING SUNSCREENS WITH KERI

PreSun® 8 and 15 Moisturizing Sunscreens

Active Ingredient: Oxybenzone, octyl dimethyl PABA. Also contains: Water, petrolatum, isopropyl myristate, PG dioctanoate, isodecyl neopentanoate, DEA cetyl phosphate, PVP/Eicosene copolymer, stearic acid, cetyl alcohol, dimethicone, diazolidinyl urea, Carbomer-940, triethanolamine, methylchloroisothiazolinone and methylisothiazolinone. May also contain fragrance.

PreSun® 25 Moisturizing Sunscreen

Active Ingredient: Octyl methoxycinnamate, oxybenzone, octyl salicylate. Also contains: Water, isopropyl myristate, isodecyl neopentanoate, propylene glycol dioctanoate, petrolatum, DEA-cetyl phosphate, PVP-Eicosene copolymer, stearic acid, cetyl alcohol, dimethicone, diazolidinyl urea, Carbomer-940, triethanolamine, methylchloroisothiazolinone and methylisothiazolinone.

Indications: 8, 15 or 25 TIMES NATURAL UVB PROTECTION: Used liberally and regularly, PreSun® Moisturizing Sunscreens provide 8, 15 or 25 times your natural UVB sunburn protection and may help reduce the chance of premature wrinkling of the skin caused by repeated and prolonged exposure to the sun. **UVA/UVB Protection:** PreSun® Moisturizing Sunscreens are formulated to provide protection from sunburn caused by both UVA nd UVB rays.
Moisturizing: PreSun® Moisturizing Sunscreen with Keri moisturizing is a moisture-rich formula that is absorbed in quickly to provide a high degree of UVB sunburn protection while helping to relieve the drying effects of the sun.

Waterproof: PreSun® Moisturizing Sunscreen maintains its degree of protection even after 80 minutes in the water.

Directions: Smooth evenly and liberally onto dry skin before sun exposure. Massage in gently. Reapply to dry skin after swimming, excessive perspiration or towel drying.

Warning: For external use only. As with all sunscreens, avoid contact with eyes. Discontinue use if irritation or rash appears. Consult a physician before using on children under six months of age.

How Supplied: 4 oz. plastic bottles

PRESUN® 23 and
PRESUN® FOR KIDS
Spray Mist Sunscreens

Active Ingredients: Octyl dimethyl PABA, octyl methoxycinnamate, oxybenzone, octyl salicylate. Also contains: C_{12-15} alcohols benzoate, cyclomethicone, PG dioctanoate, PVP hexadecene, copolymer, and 19% (w/w) SD alcohol 40.

Indications: 23 TIMES NATURAL PROTECTION: Used as directed, PRESUN 23 and PRESUN For Kids Spray Mist Sunscreens provide 23 times your natural sunburn protection and may help reduce the chance of premature aging and wrinkling of the skin.
WATERPROOF 23: PRESUN 23 and PRESUN For Kids Spray Mist Sunscreens maintain their degree of protection (SPF 23) even after 80 minutes in the water.
Convenience Spray: This revolutionary new spray bottle design is non-aerosol.

Directions for Use: For best results, hold bottle about ten inches away from body while spraying. Massage in gently. Reapplication to dry skin after prolonged swimming, excessive perspiration or towel drying is recommended for all-day protection.

Warnings: For external use only. Do not use if sensitive to *p*-aminobenzoic acid (PABA) or related compounds. Avoid flame. Do not expose to heat or store above 86°F. As with all sunscreens: Apply to a small area; check after 24 hours. Discontinue use if irritation or rash appears. Avoid spraying in the eyes. In case of contact, flush eyes with water. Keep out of reach of children. Use on children under six months of age only with the advice of a physician.

How Supplied: 23 Spray Mist Sunscreen: 3.5 oz. plastic bottle with non-aerosol spray. For Kids Spray Mist Sunscreen: 3.5 oz. plastic bottle with non-aerosol spray.
Shown in Product Identification Section, page 406

Continued on next page

Bristol-Myers—Cont.

PRESUN® 15 and 29 SENSITIVE SKIN SUNSCREENS
PABA-FREE Sunscreen Protection

Active Ingredients: Octyl methoxycinnamate, oxybenzone, octyl salicylate. Also contains: Carbomer-940, cetyl alcohol, diazolidinyl urea, dimethicone, methylchloroisothiazolinone and methylisothiazolinone, stearic acid, triethanolamine, water, and other ingredients.

Indications:
15 or 29 TIMES NATURAL PROTECTION: Used as directed, PRESUN 15 or 29 Sensitive Skin Sunscreen provides 15 or 29 times your natural *sunburn* protection and may help reduce the chance of premature aging and wrinkling of the skin as well as skin cancer caused by overexposure to the sun.
PABA-FREE FORMULAS: PABA- and fragrance-free formulas that provide a very high degree of sunburn protection and, because the known sensitizers common to most sunscreens have been removed, is suitable for sensitive skin.
WATERPROOF: PRESUN Sensitive Skin Sunscreen maintains its degree of protection even after 80 minutes in the water.

Directions for Use: For maximum protection, smooth evenly and liberally onto dry skin before sun exposure. Massage in gently. Reapplication to dry skin after prolonged swimming, excessive perspiration or towel drying is recommended for all-day protection.

Warnings: For external use only. Protect from freezing. *As with all sunscreens:* Apply to a small area; check after 24 hours. Discontinue use if irritation or rash appears. Avoid contact with eyes. In case of contact, flush eyes with water. Keep out of the reach of children. Use on children under six months of age only with the advice of a physician.

How Supplied: 29 Sensitive Skin: 4 oz. (NSN 6505-01-267-1483) plastic bottle. 15 Sensitive Skin: 4 oz. plastic bottle.
*Shown in Product Identification
Section, page 406*

PRESUN® 46 MOISTURIZING SUNSCREEN

Active Ingredient: Octyl dimethyl PABA, oxybenzone. Also contains: water, isopropyl myristate, PG dioctanoate, isodecyl neopentanoate, DEA cetyl phosphate, PVP/Elcosene copolymer, stearic acid, cetyl alcohol, dimethicone, diazolidinyl urea, carbomer-940, triethanolamine, methylchloroisothiazolinone and methylisothiazolinone. May also contain fragrance.

Indications: 46 TIMES NATURAL UVB PROTECTION: Used liberally and regularly, PreSun® 46 Moisturizing Sunscreen provides 46 times your natural UVB sunburn protection and may help reduce the chance of premature wrinkling of the skin caused by repeated and prolonged exposure to the sun.
UVA/UVB: PreSun 46 Moisturizing Sunscreen is formulated to provide protection from sunburn caused by both UVA nd UVB rays.
Moisturizing: A moisture-rich formula that is absorbed in quickly to provide a high degree of UVB sunburn protection while helping to relieve the drying effects of the sun.
Waterproof: PreSun® 46 Moisturizing Sunscreen maintains its degree of protection even after 80 minutes in the water.

Directions: Smooth evenly and liberally onto dry skin before sun exposure. Massage in gently. Reapply to dry skin after swimming, excessive perspiration or towel drying.

Warnings: For external use only. As with all sunscreens, avoid contact with eyes. Discontinue use if irritation or rash appears. Consult a physician before using on children under six months of age.

How Supplied: 4 oz. plastic bottle

THERAPEUTIC MINERAL ICE®

Composition:
Active Ingredient: Menthol 2%
Other Ingredients: Ammonium Hydroxide, Carbomer 934, Cupric Sulfate, FD&C Blue No. 1, Isopropyl Alcohol, Magnesium Sulfate, Sodium Hydroxide, Thymol, Water.

Indications: For the temporary relief of minor aches and pains of muscles and joints associated with arthritis, simple backache, strains, bruises, sprains and sports injuries. **USE ONLY AS DIRECTED. Read all warnings before use.**

Warnings: KEEP OUT OF THE REACH OF CHILDREN. For external use only. Not for internal use. Avoid contact with eyes and mucous membranes. Do not use with other ointments, creams, sprays, or liniments. **Do not use with Heating Pads or Heating Devices.** If condition worsens, or if symptoms persist for more than 7 days, or clear up and occur again within a few days, discontinue use of this product and consult your doctor. Do not apply to wounds or damaged skin. Do not bandage tightly. If you have sensitive skin, consult doctor before use. If skin irritation develops, discontinue use and consult your doctor. As with any drug, if you are pregnant or nursing a baby, seek the advice of a health professional before using this product. Keep cap tightly closed. Do not use, pour, spill or store near heat or open flame. **Note:** You can always use Mineral Ice as directed, but its use is never intended to replace your doctor's advice.

Directions: Adults and children 2 years of age and older: Clean skin of all other ointments, creams, sprays, or liniments. Apply to affected areas not more than 3 to 4 times daily. May be used with wet or dry bandages or with ice packs. No protective cover needed. Children under 2 years of age: Consult a doctor.

How Supplied:
NDC 19810-0034-4 3.5 oz.
NDC 19810-0034-2 8 oz.
NDC 19810-0034-3 16 oz.
Store at room temperature.
*Shown in Product Identification
Section, page 406*

THERAPEUTIC MINERAL ICE®
Exercise Formula, Pain Relieving Gel

Composition:
Active Ingredient: Menthol 4%.
Other Ingredients: Ammonium Hydroxide, Carbomer 934P or Carbomer 934, Cupric Sulfate, FD&C Blue No. 1, Fragrance, Isopropyl Alcohol, Magnesium Sulfate, Sodium Hydroxide, Thymol, Water.

Indications: For the temporary relief of minor aches and pains of muscles and joints associated with strains, sprains, bruises, sports injuries and simple backache. USE ONLY AS DIRECTED. Read all warnings before use.

Warnings: KEEP OUT OF REACH OF CHILDREN. For external use only. Not for internal use. Avoid contact with eyes and mucous membranes. Do not use with other ointments, creams, sprays, or liniments. DO NOT USE WITH HEATING PAD OR HEATING DEVICES. If condition worsens, or if symptoms persist for more than 7 days, or clear up and occur again within a few days, discontinue use of this product and consult your doctor. Do not apply to wounds or damaged skin. Do not bandage tightly. If you have sensitive skin, consult doctor BEFORE use. If skin irritation develops, discontinue use and consult your doctor. As with any drug, if you are pregnant or nursing a baby, seek the advice of a health professional before using this product. Do not use, pour, spill, or store near heat or open flame.
NOTE: You can always use MINERAL ICE® EXERCISE FORMULA as directed, but its use is never intended to replace your doctor's advice.

Directions: Adults and children 2 years of age and older: Clean skin of all other ointments, creams, sprays, or liniments. Apply to affected areas not more than 3 to 4 times daily. May be used with wet or dry bandages or with ice packs. Not greasy. No protective cover needed. Children: Do not use on children under 2 years of age, except under the advice and supervision of a doctor.

How Supplied: Available in 3 oz. tubes.
STORE AT ROOM TEMPERATURE.
KEEP CAP TIGHTLY CLOSED.
*Shown in Product Identification
Section, page 406*

Burroughs Wellcome Co.
3030 CORNWALLIS ROAD
RESEARCH TRIANGLE PARK,
NC 27709

ACTIFED® PLUS Caplets
[ăk 'tuh-fĕd]

Product Benefits: Each ACTIFED PLUS Caplet contains three important ingredients for maximum strength relief from symptoms of the common cold, seasonal allergies (hay fever) and sinus congestion.

The **ANTIHISTAMINE** (triprolidine) temporarily dries runny nose and relieves sneezing associated with the common cold, hay fever or other upper respiratory allergies. Also relieves itching of the nose or throat, and itchy, watery eyes due to hay fever.

The **DECONGESTANT** (pseudoephedrine) temporarily relieves nasal congestion due to the common cold, hay fever or other upper respiratory allergies, or associated with sinusitis. Temporarily relieves nasal stuffiness. Reduces the swelling of nasal passages; shrinks swollen membranes; and temporarily restores freer breathing through the nose. Also, helps to decongest sinus openings and passages; relieves sinus pressure.

The non-aspirin **ANALGESIC** (acetaminophen) temporarily relieves occasional minor aches, pains and headache, and reduces fever due to the common cold.

Each ACTIFED PLUS Caplet Contains: acetaminophen 500 mg, pseudoephedrine hydrochloride 30 mg and triprolidine hydrochloride 1.25 mg. Also contains: D&C Yellow No. 10 Lake, FD&C Blue No. 1 Lake, hydroxypropyl cellulose, magnesium stearate, microcrystalline cellulose, and povidone.

Directions: Adults and children 12 years and over, 2 caplets every 6 hours, not to exceed 8 caplets in a 24-hour period. Not recommended for children under 12 years of age.

Warnings: May cause excitability especially in children. May cause drowsiness. Do not exceed recommended dosage because at higher doses nervousness, dizziness, or sleeplessness may occur. If symptoms do not improve within 7 days or are accompanied by high fever, consult a physician before continuing use. Do not take this product for more than 10 days. Do not take this product if you have high blood pressure, heart disease, diabetes, thyroid disease, asthma, glaucoma, or difficulty in urination due to enlargement of the prostate gland except under the advice and supervision of a physician. As with any drug, if you are pregnant or nursing a baby, seek the advice of a health professional before using this product.

Drug Interaction Precaution: Do not take this product if you are presently taking a prescription antihypertensive or antidepressant drug containing a monoamine oxidase inhibitor except under the advice and supervision of a physician.

Caution: Avoid driving a motor vehicle, operating heavy machinery, or drinking alcoholic beverages while taking this product.

KEEP THIS AND ALL DRUGS OUT OF THE REACH OF CHILDREN. In case of accidental overdose, seek professional assistance or contact a Poison Control Center immediately.

Store at 15° to 25°C (59° to 77°F) in a dry place and protect from light.

How Supplied: Boxes of 20, 40.
Shown in Product Identification Section, page 406

ACTIFED® Syrup
[ăk 'tuh-fĕd]

Product Benefits: ACTIFED Syrup contains two important ingredients for relief from symptoms of the common cold, seasonal allergies (hay fever) and sinus congestion.

The **ANTIHISTAMINE** (triprolidine) temporarily dries runny nose and relieves sneezing associated with the common cold, hay fever, or other upper respiratory allergies. Also relieves itching of the nose or throat, and itchy, watery eyes due to hay fever.

The **DECONGESTANT** (pseudoephedrine) temporarily relieves nasal congestion due to the common cold, hay fever or other upper respiratory allergies, or associated with sinusitis. Temporarily relieves nasal stuffiness. Reduces the swelling of nasal passages; shrinks swollen membranes; and temporarily restores freer breathing through the nose. Also, helps to decongest sinus openings and passages; relieves sinus pressure.

Each 5 mL (1 teaspoonful) Actifed Syrup Contains: pseudoephedrine hydrochloride 30 mg and triprolidine hydrochloride 1.25 mg. Also contains: methylparaben 0.1% and sodium benzoate 0.1% (added as preservatives), D&C Yellow No. 10, glycerin, purified water, and sorbitol.

Directions: Adults and children 12 years of age and over, 2 teaspoonfuls every 4 to 6 hours. Children 6 to under 12 years of age, 1 teaspoonful every 4 to 6 hours. Children under 6 years of age, consult a physician. Do not exceed 4 doses in 24 hours.

Warnings: May cause excitability especially in children. Do not give this product to children under 6 years except under the advice and supervision of a physician. May cause drowsiness. Do not exceed recommended dosage because at higher doses nervousness, dizziness or sleeplessness may occur. If symptoms do not improve within 7 days or are accompanied by high fever, consult a physician before continuing use. Do not take this product if you have high blood pressure, heart disease, diabetes, thyroid disease, asthma, glaucoma or difficulty in urination due to enlargement of the prostate gland except under the advice and supervision of a physician. As with any drug, if you are pregnant or nursing a baby, seek the advice of a health professional before using this product.

Drug Interaction Precaution: Do not take this product if you are presently taking a prescription antihypertensive or antidepressant drug containing a monoamine oxidase inhibitor except under the advice and supervision of a physician.

Caution: Avoid driving a motor vehicle, operating heavy machinery, or drinking alcoholic beverages while taking this product.

KEEP THIS AND ALL DRUGS OUT OF THE REACH OF CHILDREN. In case of accidental overdose, seek professional assistance or contact a Poison Control Center immediately.

Store at 15° to 25°C (59° to 77°F) and protect from light.

How Supplied: Bottles of 4 fl oz and 1 pint.
Shown in Product Identification Section, page 406

ACTIFED® Tablets
[ăk 'tuh-fĕd]

Product Benefits: Each ACTIFED Tablet contains two important ingredients for relief from symptoms of the common cold, seasonal allergies (hay fever) and sinus congestion.

The **ANTIHISTAMINE** (triprolidine) temporarily dries runny nose and relieves sneezing associated with the common cold, hay fever or other upper respiratory allergies. Also relieves itching of the nose or throat, and itchy, watery eyes due to hay fever.

The **DECONGESTANT** (pseudoephedrine) temporarily relieves nasal congestion due to the common cold, hay fever or other upper respiratory allergies, or associated with sinusitis. Temporarily relieves nasal stuffiness. Reduces the swelling of nasal passages; shrinks swollen membranes; and temporarily restores freer breathing through the nose. Also, helps to decongest sinus openings and passages; relieves sinus pressure.

Each Actifed Tablet Contains: pseudoephedrine hydrochloride 60 mg and triprolidine hydrochloride 2.5 mg. Also contains: flavor, hydroxypropyl methylcellulose, lactose, magnesium stearate, polyethylene glycol, potato starch, povidone, sucrose, and titanium dioxide.

Directions: Adults and children 12 years of age and over, 1 tablet every 4 to 6 hours. Children 6 to under 12 years of age, ½ tablet every 4 to 6 hours. Children under 6 years of age, consult a physician. Do not exceed 4 doses in 24 hours.

Warnings: May cause excitability especially in children. Do not give this product to children under 6 years except under the advice and supervision of a physician. May cause drowsiness. Do not exceed recommended dosage because at higher doses nervousness, dizziness or

Continued on next page

Burroughs Wellcome—Cont.

sleeplessness may occur. If symptoms do not improve within 7 days or are accompanied by high fever, consult a physician before continuing use. Do not take this product if you have high blood pressure, heart disease, diabetes, thyroid disease, asthma, glaucoma or difficulty in urination due to enlargement of the prostate gland except under the advice and supervision of a physician. As with any drug, if you are pregnant or nursing a baby, seek the advice of a health professional before using this product.

Drug Interaction Precaution: Do not take this product if you are presently taking a prescription antihypertensive or antidepressant drug containing a monoamine oxidase inhibitor except under the advice and supervision of a physician.

Caution: Avoid driving a motor vehicle, operating heavy machinery, or drinking alcoholic beverages while taking this product.

KEEP THIS AND ALL DRUGS OUT OF THE REACH OF CHILDREN. In case of accidental overdose, seek professional assistance or contact a Poison Control Center immediately.

Store at 15° to 25°C (59° to 77°F) in a dry place and protect from light.

How Supplied: Boxes of 12, 24, 48 and bottles of 100 and 1000; unit dose pack box of 100.

Shown in Product Identification Section, page 406

ACTIFED® PLUS Tablets
[ăk 'tuh-fĕd]

Product Benefits: Each ACTIFED PLUS Tablet contains three important ingredients for maximum strength relief from symptoms of the common cold, seasonal allergies (hay fever) and sinus congestion.

The **ANTIHISTAMINE** (triprolidine) temporarily dries runny nose and relieves sneezing associated with the common cold, hay fever or other upper respiratory allergies. Also relieves itching of the nose or throat, and itchy, watery eyes due to hay fever.

The **DECONGESTANT** (pseudoephedrine) temporarily relieves nasal congestion due to the common cold, hay fever or other upper respiratory allergies, or associated with sinusitis. Temporarily relieves nasal stuffiness. Reduces the swelling of nasal passages; shrinks swollen membranes; and temporarily restores freer breathing through the nose. Also, helps to decongest sinus openings and passages; relieves sinus pressure.

The non-aspirin **ANALGESIC** (acetaminophen) temporarily relieves occasional minor aches, pains and headache, and reduces fever due to the common cold.

Each ACTIFED PLUS Tablet Contains: acetaminophen 500 mg, pseudoephedrine hydrochloride 30 mg and triprolidine hydrochloride 1.25 mg. Also

contains: D&C Yellow No. 10 Lake, FD&C Blue No. 1 Lake, hydroxypropyl cellulose, magnesium stearate, microcrystalline cellulose and povidone.

Directions: Adults and children 12 years and over, 2 tablets every 6 hours, not to exceed 8 tablets in a 24-hour period. Not recommended for children under 12 years of age.

Warnings: May cause excitability, especially in children. May cause drowsiness. Do not exceed recommended dosage because at higher doses nervousness, dizziness, or sleeplessness may occur. If symptoms do not improve within 7 days or are accompanied by high fever, consult a physician before continuing use. Do not take this product for more than 10 days. Do not take this product if you have high blood pressure, heart disease, diabetes, thyroid disease, asthma, glaucoma, or difficulty in urination due to enlargement of the prostate gland except under the advice and supervision of a physician. As with any drug, if you are pregnant or nursing a baby, seek the advice of a health professional before using this product.

Drug Interaction Precaution: Do not take this product if you are presently taking a prescription antihypertensive or antidepressant drug containing a monoamine oxidase inhibitor except under the advice and supervision of a physician.

Caution: Avoid driving a motor vehicle, operating heavy machinery, or drinking alcoholic beverages while taking this product.

KEEP THIS AND ALL DRUGS OUT OF THE REACH OF CHILDREN. In case of accidental overdose, seek professional assistance or contact a Poison Control Center immediately.

Store at 15° to 25°C (59° to 77°F) in a dry place and protect from light.

How Supplied: Boxes of 20, 40.
Shown in Product Identification Section, page 406

BOROFAX® Ointment
[bôr 'uh-făks]

Description: Contains boric acid 5% and lanolin.

Inactive Ingredients: fragrances, glycerin, mineral oil, purified water and sodium borate.

Indications: A soothing application for burns, abrasions, chafing, and for infants' tender skin.

Directions: Apply topically as required.

Keep this and all medicines out of children's reach.

Store at 15° to 25°C (59° to 77°F).

How Supplied: Tube, 1¾ oz.

EMPIRIN® ASPIRIN
[ĕm 'puh-rŭn]

For relief of headache, minor muscular aches and pains, toothache, discomfort and fever of colds and flu, pain of the premenstrual and menstrual periods, and temporary relief of minor arthritis pain (see CAUTION below).

Directions: Adults: 1 or 2 tablets with a full glass of water. Repeat every 4 hours as needed, up to 12 tablets a day. **Children:** Consult a physician (see WARNINGS).

Caution: In arthritic conditions, if pain persists for more than 10 days or redness is present, consult a physician immediately.

Warnings: Children and teenagers should not use this medicine for chicken pox or flu symptoms before a doctor is consulted about Reye syndrome, a rare but serious illness reported to be associated with aspirin. Keep this and all medicines out of children's reach. In case of accidental overdose, contact a physician immediately.

High or continued fever, severe or persistent sore throat especially when accompanied by high fever, headache, nausea or vomiting, may be serious. Consult your physician. Do not exceed dose unless directed by a physician. Do not take this product if you are allergic to aspirin, have asthma, a gastric ulcer or its symptoms, or are taking a medication that affects the clotting of blood, except under the advice of a physician. As with any drug, if you are pregnant or nursing a baby, seek the advice of a health professional before using this product.

IT IS ESPECIALLY IMPORTANT NOT TO USE ASPIRIN DURING THE LAST 3 MONTHS OF PREGNANCY UNLESS SPECIFICALLY DIRECTED TO DO SO BY A DOCTOR BECAUSE IT MAY CAUSE PROBLEMS IN THE UNBORN CHILD OR COMPLICATIONS DURING DELIVERY.

Active Ingredients: Each tablet contains aspirin 325 mg (5 gr).

Inactive Ingredients: microcrystalline cellulose and potato starch.

Store at 15° to 25°C (59° to 77°F) in a dry place.

How Supplied: Bottles of 50, 100, 250.
Shown in Product Identification Section, page 406

FILTERAY®
Broad Spectrum
Sunscreen Lotion

Indications: FILTERAY Broad Spectrum Sunscreen Lotion provides protection from acute and long-term risks associated with UVA and UVB light exposure. FILTERAY screens out the sun's burning rays to prevent sunburn. Overexposure to the sun may lead to premature aging of the skin and skin cancer. The liberal and regular use over the years of this product may help reduce the chance of these harmful effects.

Directions: Shake well before using.
Prior to sun exposure, apply liberally and evenly over areas to be protected. To maintain maximal protection, reapply after 40 minutes in the water or after excessive perspiration. There is no recommended dosage for children under six months of age except under the advice and supervision of a physician.

Warnings: Do not use if sensitive to benzocaine, sulfonamides, aniline dyes, aminobenzoic acid (PABA) or related compounds or any other ingredient in this product. Use on children under six months of age only with the advice of a physician.
For external use only. Avoid contact with eyes, eyelids and mouth. If contact with eyes occurs, rinse thoroughly with water. Should skin irritation or rash develop, discontinue use. If irritation or rash persists, consult a physician. Keep out of the reach of children. In case of accidental ingestion, seek professional assistance or contact a Poison Control Center immediately.

Caution: FILTERAY Sunscreen Lotion may stain some fabrics.

Contains: Avobenzone 3.0%, Padimate O (octyl dimethyl p-aminobenzoic acid) 7.0% with: benzyl alcohol; carbomer 934P; cetyl esters wax; edetate disodium; glycerin; imidurea; mineral oil (light); oleth-3 phosphate; purified water; stearyl alcohol (and) ceteareth-20 and white petrolatum. May contain sodium hydroxide or hydrochloric acid to adjust pH.

NOTE: Store at room temperature. Protect from freezing.

How Supplied: 4 oz bottle.
Shown in Product Identification Section, page 406

MAREZINE® Tablets
[*mâr'uh-zēn*]

FDA APPROVED USES

Indications: For the prevention and treatment of the nausea, vomiting or dizziness associated with motion sickness.

Directions: Adults and children 12 years of age and over: 1 tablet every 4 to 6 hours, not to exceed 4 tablets in 24 hours or as directed by a doctor. Children 6 to under 12 years of age: ½ tablet every 6 to 8 hours, not to exceed 1½ tablets in 24 hours or as directed by a doctor. For prevention, take the first dose one half-hour before departure.

Warnings: Do not take this product if you have asthma, glaucoma, emphysema, chronic pulmonary disease, shortness of breath, difficulty in breathing or difficulty in urination due to enlargement of the prostate gland unless directed by a doctor. Do not give to children under 6 years of age unless directed by a doctor. May cause drowsiness; alcohol, sedatives and tranquilizers may increase the drowsiness effect. Avoid alcoholic beverages while taking this product. Do not take this product if you are taking sedatives or tranquilizers without first consulting your doctor. Use caution when driving a motor vehicle or operating machinery. As with any drug, if you are pregnant or nursing a baby, seek the advice of a health professional before using this product. Keep this and all drugs out of the reach of children. Overdosage may cause severe agitation or psychosis; seek professional assistance or contact a Poison Control Center immediately.

Active Ingredients: Each scored tablet contains cyclizine hydrochloride 50 mg.

Inactive Ingredients: Corn and potato starch, dextrin, lactose, and magnesium stearate.

Store at 15° to 25°C (59° to 77°F) in a dry place and protect from light.

How Supplied: Box of 12, bottle of 100.
Shown in Product Identification Section, page 406

Maximum Strength NEOSPORIN® Ointment
[*nē'uh-spō'run*]

Indications: First aid to help prevent infection in minor cuts, scrapes and burns.

Directions: Clean the affected area. Apply a small amount of this product (an amount equal to the surface area of the tip of a finger) on the area 1 to 3 times daily. May be covered with a sterile bandage.

Warnings: For external use only. Do not use in the eyes or apply over large areas of the body. In case of deep or puncture wounds, animal bites, or serious burns, consult a physician. Stop use and consult a physician if the condition persists or gets worse. Do not use longer than 1 week unless directed by a physician. Keep this and all drugs out of the reach of children. In case of accidental ingestion, seek professional assistance or contact a Poison Control Center immediately.

Each Gram Contains: polymyxin B sulfate 10,000 units, bacitracin zinc 500 units and neomycin 3.5 mg in a special white petrolatum base.

Store at 15° to 25°C (59° to 77°F).

How Supplied: ½ oz tube (with applicator tip) and 1 oz tube.

Professional Labeling: Consult *1992 Physicians' Desk Reference®.*
Shown in Product Identification Section, page 406

NEOSPORIN® Cream
[*nē'uh-spō'run*]

Indications: First aid to help prevent infection in minor cuts, scrapes, and burns.

Directions: Clean the affected area. Apply a small amount of this product (an amount equal to the surface area of the tip of a finger) on the area 1 to 3 times daily. May be covered with sterile bandage.

Warnings: For external use only. Do not use in the eyes or apply over large areas of the body. In case of deep or puncture wounds, animal bites, or serious burns, consult a physician. Stop use and consult a physician if the condition persists or gets worse. Do not use longer than 1 week unless directed by a physician. Keep this and all drugs out of the reach of children. In case of accidental ingestion, seek professional assistance or contact a Poison Control Center immediately.

Each Gram Contains: polymyxin B sulfate 10,000 units and neomycin 3.5 mg. Also contains: methylparaben 0.25% (added as a preservative), emulsifying wax, mineral oil, polyoxyethylene polyoxypropylene compound, propylene glycol, purified water and white petrolatum.

Store at 15° to 25°C (59° to 77°F).

How Supplied: ½ oz tube (with applicator tip); 1/32 oz (approx.) foil packets packed 144 per carton.

Professional Labeling: Consult *1992 Physicians' Desk Reference®.*
Shown in Product Identification Section, page 406

NEOSPORIN® Ointment
[*nē'uh-spō'run*]

Indications: First aid to help prevent infection in minor cuts, scrapes and burns.

Directions: Clean the affected area. Apply a small amount of this product (an amount equal to the surface area of the tip of a finger) on the area 1 to 3 times daily. May be covered with a sterile bandage.

Warnings: For external use only. Do not use in the eyes or apply over large areas of the body. In case of deep or puncture wounds, animal bites, or serious burns, consult a physician. Stop use and consult a physician if the condition persists or gets worse. Do not use longer than 1 week unless directed by a physician. Keep this and all drugs out of the reach of children. In case of accidental ingestion, seek professional assistance or contact a Poison Control Center immediately.

Each Gram Contains: polymyxin B sulfate 5,000 units, bacitracin zinc 400 units and neomycin 3.5 mg in a special white petrolatum base.

Store at 15° to 25°C (59° to 77°F).

How Supplied: Tubes, ½ oz (with applicator tip), 1 oz; 1/32 oz (approx.) foil packets packed 144 per carton.

Continued on next page

Burroughs Wellcome—Cont.

Professional Labeling: Consult *1992 Physicians' Desk Reference®*.
Shown in Product Identification Section, page 406

NIX™
Permethrin
Lice Treatment

Product Benefits: Nix Creme Rinse kills lice and their unhatched eggs with only one application. Nix protects against head lice reinfestation for a full 14 days. The unique creme rinse formula leaves hair manageable and easy to comb.

Indications: For the treatment of head lice.

Directions for Use: Nix Creme Rinse should be used after hair has been washed with your regular shampoo, rinsed with water and towel dried. A sufficient amount should be applied to saturate hair and scalp (especially behind the ears and on the nape of the neck). Leave on hair for 10 minutes but no longer. Rinse with water. A single application is sufficient. Retreatment is required in less than 1% of patients. If live lice are observed seven days or more after the first application of this product, a second treatment should be given. For proper head lice management, remove nits with the nit comb provided.
Head lice live on the scalp and lay small white eggs (nits) on the hair shaft close to the scalp. The nits are most easily found on the nape of the neck or behind the ears. All personal headgear, scarfs, coats, and bed linen should be disinfected by machine washing in hot water and drying, using the hot cycle of a dryer for at least 20 minutes. Personal articles of clothing or bedding that cannot be washed may be dry-cleaned, sealed in a plastic bag for a period of about 2 weeks, or sprayed with a product specifically designed for this purpose. Personal combs and brushes may be disinfected by soaking in hot water (above 130°F) for 5 to 10 minutes. Thorough vacuuming of rooms inhabited by infected patients is recommended.

Warnings: For external use only. Itching, redness, or swelling of the scalp may occur. If skin irritation persists or infection is present or develops, discontinue use and consult a doctor. Do not use near the eyes or permit contact with mucous membranes. If product gets into the eyes, immediately flush with water. Consult a doctor if infestation of eyebrows or eyelashes occurs. This product may cause breathing difficulty or an asthmatic episode in susceptible persons. This product should not be used on children less than 2 months of age. As with any drug, if you are pregnant or nursing a baby, seek the advice of a health professional before using this product. Keep this and all drugs out of the reach of children. In case of accidental ingestion, seek professional as-

sistance or contact a Poison Control Center immediately.

Each Fluid Ounce Contains: permethrin 280 mg (1%). Inactive ingredients are: balsam canada, cetyl alcohol, citric acid, FD&C Yellow No. 6, fragrance, hydrolyzed animal protein, hydroxyethylcellulose, polyoxyethylene 10 cetyl ether, propylene glycol, and stearalkonium chloride. Also contains: isopropyl alcohol 5.6 g (20%) and added as preservatives, imidazolidinyl urea 56 mg (0.2%), methylparaben 56 mg (0.2%), and propylparaben 22 mg (0.08%). Store at 15° to 25°C (59° to 77°F).

How Supplied: Bottles of 2 fl oz with special comb and Family Pack of 2 bottles, 2 fl oz each, with special comb.
Shown in Product Identification Section, page 407

POLYSPORIN® Ointment
[pŏl 'ē-spō 'rŭn]

Indications: First aid to help prevent infection in minor cuts, scrapes and burns.

Directions: Clean the affected area. Apply a small amount of this product (an amount equal to the surface area of the tip of a finger) on the area 1 to 3 times daily. May be covered with a sterile bandage.

Warnings: For external use only. Do not use in the eyes or apply over large areas of the body. In case of deep or puncture wounds, animal bites, or serious burns, consult a physician. Stop use and consult a physician if the condition persists or gets worse. Do not use longer than 1 week unless directed by a physician. Keep this and all drugs out of the reach of children. In case of accidental ingestion, seek professional assistance or contact a Poison Control Center immediately.

Each Gram Contains: Aerosporin® (polymyxin B sulfate) 10,000 units and bacitracin zinc 500 units in a special white petrolatum base.

Store at 15° to 25°C (59° to 77°F).

How Supplied: Tubes, ½ oz with applicator tip, 1 oz; 1/32 oz (approx.) foil packets packed in cartons of 144.
Shown in Product Identification Section, page 407

POLYSPORIN® Powder
[pŏl 'ē-spō 'rŭn]

Indications: First aid to help prevent infection in minor cuts, scrapes and burns.

Directions: Clean the affected area. Apply a light dusting of the powder on the area 1 to 3 times daily. May be covered with a sterile bandage.

Warnings: For external use only. Do not use in the eyes or apply over large areas of the body. In case of deep or puncture wounds, animal bites, or serious

burns, consult a physician. Stop use and consult a physician if the condition persists or gets worse.
Do not use longer than 1 week unless directed by a physician. Keep this and all drugs out of the reach of children. In case of accidental ingestion, seek professional assistance or contact a Poison Control Center immediately.

Each Gram Contains: polymyxin B sulfate 10,000 units and bacitracin zinc 500 units in a lactose base.
Store at 15° to 25°C (59° to 77°F). Do not store under refrigeration.

How Supplied: 0.35 oz (10 g) shaker-vial.
Shown in Product Identification Section, page 407

Children's
SUDAFED® Liquid
[sū 'duh-fĕd]

Each 5 mL (1 teaspoonful) contains pseudoephedrine hydrochloride 30 mg. Also contains: methylparaben 0.1% and sodium benzoate 0.1% (added as preservatives), citric acid, FD&C Red No. 40, flavor, glycerin, purified water, sorbitol and sucrose.

Indications: For temporary relief of nasal congestion due to the common cold, hay fever or other upper respiratory allergies and nasal congestion associated with sinusitis; promotes nasal and/or sinus drainage.

Directions: To be given every 4 to 6 hours. Do not exceed 4 doses in 24 hours. Children 6 to under 12 years of age, 1 teaspoonful. Children 2 to under 6 years of age, ½ teaspoonful. For children under 2 years of age, consult a physician.

Warnings: Do not exceed recommended dosage because at higher doses nervousness, dizziness or sleeplessness may occur. Do not give this product to children for more than 7 days. If symptoms do not improve or are accompanied by high fever, consult a physician. Do not give this product to children who have heart disease, high blood pressure, thyroid disease, or diabetes unless directed by a physician.

Drug Interaction Precaution: Do not give this product to a child who is taking a prescription drug for high blood pressure or depression, without first consulting the child's physician.

KEEP THIS AND ALL MEDICINES OUT OF CHILDREN'S REACH. In case of accidental overdose, seek professional assistance or contact a Poison Control Center immediately.

Store at 15° to 25°C (59° to 77°F) and protect from light.

How Supplied: Bottles of 4 fl oz.
Shown in Product Identification Section, page 407

SUDAFED® Cough Syrup
[sū 'duh-fĕd]

Each 5 mL (1 teaspoonful) contains pseudoephedrine hydrochloride 15 mg, dextromethorphan hydrobromide 5 mg and guaifenesin 100 mg. Also contains: alcohol 2.4%, methylparaben 0.1% and sodium benzoate 0.1% (added as preservatives), citric acid, D&C Yellow No. 10, FD&C Blue No. 1, flavor, glycerin, purified water, saccharin sodium, sodium chloride and sucrose.

Indications: For temporary relief of cough due to minor throat and bronchial irritation as may occur with the common cold or inhaled irritants. For temporary relief of nasal congestion due to the common cold. Helps loosen phlegm (sputum) and thin bronchial secretions to rid the bronchial passageways of bothersome mucus.

Directions: To be given every 4 hours. Do not exceed 4 doses in 24 hours. Adults and children 12 years of age and over, 4 teaspoonfuls. Children 6 to under 12 years of age, 2 teaspoonfuls. Children 2 to under 6 years of age, 1 teaspoonful. For children under 2 years of age, consult a physician.

Warnings: Do not give this product to children under 2 years of age unless directed by a physician. Do not exceed recommended dosage because at higher doses nervousness, dizziness or sleeplessness may occur. Do not take this product for persistent or chronic cough such as occurs with smoking, asthma, chronic bronchitis, or emphysema, or where cough is accompanied by excessive phlegm (sputum) unless directed by a physician. A persistent cough may be a sign of a serious condition. If cough persists for more than 1 week, tends to recur, or is accompanied by fever, rash, or persistent headache, consult a physician. Do not take this preparation if you have high blood pressure, heart disease, diabetes, thyroid disease, or difficulty in urination due to enlargement of the prostate gland, except under the advice and supervision of a physician. As with any drug, if you are pregnant or nursing a baby, seek the advice of a health professional before using this product.

Drug Interaction Precaution: Do not take this product if you are presently taking a prescription antihypertensive or antidepressant drug containing a monoamine oxidase inhibitor except under the advice and supervision of a physician.

KEEP THIS AND ALL DRUGS OUT OF THE REACH OF CHILDREN. In case of accidental overdose, seek professional assistance or contact a Poison Control Center immediately.

Store at 15° to 25°C (59° to 77°F).
DO NOT REFRIGERATE.

How Supplied: Bottles of 4 fl oz and 8 fl oz.
Shown in Product Identification Section, page 407

SUDAFED® Tablets 30 mg
[sū 'duh-fĕd]

Each tablet contains pseudoephedrine hydrochloride 30 mg. Also contains: acacia, carnauba wax, dibasic calcium phosphate, FD&C Red No. 40 Lake and Yellow No. 6 Lake, magnesium stearate, polysorbate 60, potato starch, povidone, sodium benzoate, stearic acid, sucrose and titanium dioxide.

Indications: For temporary relief of nasal congestion due to the common cold, hay fever or other upper respiratory allergies, and nasal congestion associated with sinusitis; promotes nasal and/or sinus drainage.

Directions: To be given every 4 to 6 hours. Do not exceed 4 doses in 24 hours. Adults and children 12 years of age and over, 2 tablets. Children 6 to under 12 years of age, 1 tablet. Children 2 to under 6 years of age, use Children's Sudafed Liquid. For children under 2 years of age, consult a physician.

Warnings: Do not exceed recommended dosage because at higher doses nervousness, dizziness or sleeplessness may occur. If symptoms do not improve within 7 days, or are accompanied by a high fever, consult a physician before continuing use. Do not take this preparation if you have high blood pressure, heart disease, diabetes, thyroid disease, or difficulty in urination due to enlargement of the prostate gland, except under the advice and supervision of a physician. As with any drug, if you are pregnant or nursing a baby, seek the advice of a health professional before using this product.

Drug Interaction Precaution: Do not take this product if you are presently taking a prescription antihypertensive or antidepressant drug containing a monoamine oxidase inhibitor except under the advice and supervision of a physician.

KEEP THIS AND ALL MEDICINES OUT OF CHILDREN'S REACH. In case of accidental overdose, seek professional assistance or contact a Poison Control Center immediately.

Store at 15° to 25°C (59° to 77°F) in a dry place and protect from light.

How Supplied: Boxes of 24, 48. Bottles of 100. Institutional Pack, Carton of 500 x 2.
Shown in Product Identification Section, page 407

SUDAFED® Tablets 60 mg (Adult Strength)
[sū 'duh-fĕd]

Each tablet contains pseudoephedrine hydrochloride 60 mg. Also contains: acacia, carnauba wax, corn starch, dibasic calcium phosphate, hydroxypropyl methylcellulose, magnesium stearate, polysorbate 60, sodium starch glycolate, stearic acid, sucrose, titanium dioxide, and white shellac. Printed with edible red ink.

Indications: For temporary relief of nasal congestion due to the common cold, hay fever or other upper respiratory allergies, and nasal congestion associated with sinusitis; promotes nasal and/or sinus drainage.

Directions: To be given every 4 to 6 hours. Do not exceed 4 doses in 24 hours. Adults and children 12 years of age and over, 1 tablet. Children 6 to under 12 years of age, use Sudafed 30 mg Tablets. Children 2 to under 6 years of age, use Children's Sudafed Liquid. For children under 2 years of age, consult a physician.

Warnings: Do not exceed recommended dosage because at higher doses nervousness, dizziness or sleeplessness may occur. If symptoms do not improve within 7 days, or are accompanied by a high fever, consult a physician before continuing use. Do not take this preparation if you have high blood pressure, heart disease, diabetes, thyroid disease, or difficulty in urination due to enlargement of the prostate gland, except under the advice and supervision of a physician. As with any drug, if you are pregnant or nursing a baby, seek the advice of a health professional before using this product.

Drug Interaction Precaution: Do not take this product if you are presently taking a prescription antihypertensive or antidepressant drug containing a monoamine oxidase inhibitor, except under the advice and supervision of a physician.

KEEP THIS AND ALL MEDICINES OUT OF CHILDREN'S REACH. In case of accidental overdose, seek professional assistance or contact a Poison Control Center immediately.

Store at 15° to 25°C (59° to 77°F) in a dry place and protect from light.

How Supplied: Bottles of 100.
Shown in Product Identification Section, page 407

SUDAFED PLUS® Liquid
[sū 'duh-fĕd]

Each 5 mL (1 teaspoonful) contains pseudoephedrine hydrochloride 30 mg and chlorpheniramine maleate 2 mg. Also contains: methylparaben 0.1% and sodium benzoate 0.1% (added as preservatives), citric acid, D&C Yellow No. 10, FD&C Yellow No. 6, flavor, glycerin, purified water and sucrose.

Indications: For the temporary relief of nasal/sinus congestion associated with the common cold; also sneezing; watery, itchy eyes; runny nose and other hay fever/upper respiratory allergy symptoms.

Directions: To be given every 4 to 6 hours. Do not exceed 4 doses in 24 hours. Adults and children 12 years of age and over, 2 teaspoonfuls. Children 6 to under 12 years of age, 1 teaspoonful. Children under 6 years of age, consult a physician.

Continued on next page

Burroughs Wellcome—Cont.

Warnings: May cause excitability, especially in children. Do not give to children under 6 years except as directed by a physician. May cause drowsiness. Do not exceed recommended dosage because at higher doses nervousness, dizziness or sleeplessness may occur. If symptoms do not improve within 7 days, or are accompanied by a high fever, consult a physician before continuing use. Do not take this product if you have high blood pressure, heart disease, diabetes, thyroid disease, asthma, glaucoma or difficulty in urination due to enlargement of the prostate gland except under the advice and supervision of a physician. As with any drug, if you are pregnant or nursing a baby, seek the advice of a health professional before using this product.

Drug Interaction Precaution: Do not take this product if you are presently taking a prescription antihypertensive or antidepressant drug containing a monoamine oxidase inhibitor except under the advice and supervision of a physician.

Caution: Avoid driving a motor vehicle or operating heavy machinery. Avoid alcoholic beverages while taking this product.

KEEP THIS AND ALL MEDICINES OUT OF CHILDREN'S REACH. In case of accidental overdose, seek professional assistance or contact a Poison Control Center immediately.

Store at 15° to 25°C (59° to 77°F) and protect from light.

How Supplied: Bottles of 4 fl oz.
Shown in Product Identification Section, page 407

SUDAFED PLUS® Tablets
[sū 'duh-fĕd]

Each scored tablet contains pseudoephedrine hydrochloride 60 mg and chlorpheniramine maleate 4 mg. Also contains: lactose, magnesium stearate, potato starch and povidone.

Indications: For the temporary relief of nasal/sinus congestion associated with the common cold; also sneezing; watery, itchy eyes; runny nose and other hay fever/upper respiratory allergy symptoms.

Directions: To be given every 4 to 6 hours. Do not exceed 4 doses in 24 hours. Adults and children 12 years of age and over, 1 tablet. Children 6 to under 12 years of age, ½ tablet. Children under 6 years of age, consult a physician.

Warnings: May cause excitability, especially in children. Do not give to children under 6 years except as directed by a physician. May cause drowsiness. Do not exceed recommended dosage because at higher doses nervousness, dizziness or sleeplessness may occur. If symptoms do not improve within 7 days, or are accompanied by a high fever, consult a physician before continuing use. Do not take

this product if you have high blood pressure, heart disease, diabetes, thyroid disease, asthma, glaucoma or difficulty in urination due to enlargement of the prostate gland except under the advice and supervision of a physician. As with any drug, if you are pregnant or nursing a baby, seek the advice of a health professional before using this product.

Drug Interaction Precaution: Do not take this product if you are presently taking a prescription antihypertensive or antidepressant drug containing a monoamine oxidase inhibitor except under the advice and supervision of a physician.

Caution: Avoid driving a motor vehicle or operating heavy machinery. Avoid alcoholic beverages while taking this product.

KEEP THIS AND ALL MEDICINES OUT OF CHILDREN'S REACH. In case of accidental overdose, seek professional assistance or contact a Poison Control Center immediately.

Store at 15° to 25°C (59° to 77°F) in a dry place and protect from light.

How Supplied: Boxes of 24, 48.
Shown in Product Identification Section, page 407

SUDAFED® Severe Cold Formula Caplets
[sū' duh-fĕd]

Product Benefits: Maximum allowable levels of nasal decongestant, cough suppressant, and non-aspirin pain reliever/fever reducer provide temporary relief from symptoms of the common cold and flu. This product contains no ingredients that may cause drowsiness. The **DECONGESTANT** (pseudoephedrine) temporarily relieves nasal and sinus congestion due to the common cold. It temporarily relieves nasal stuffiness; reduces the swelling of nasal passages; shrinks swollen membranes; and temporarily restores freer breathing through the nose. The **COUGH SUPPRESSANT** (dextromethorphan) temporarily relieves cough due to the common cold. The non-aspirin **PAIN RELIEVER/FEVER REDUCER** (acetaminophen) temporarily relieves headache, body aches and pains, minor sore throat pain, and reduces fever due to the common cold.

Directions: Adults and children 12 years of age and over, 2 caplets every 6 hours, not to exceed 8 caplets in 24 hours. Not recommended for children under 12 years of age.

Each Caplet Contains: acetaminophen 500 mg, dextromethorphan hydrobromide 15 mg, and pseudoephedrine hydrochloride 30 mg. Also contains: crospovidone, magnesium stearate, microcrystalline cellulose, povidone, pregelatinized corn starch, sodium starch glycolate and stearic acid.

Warnings: Do not exceed recommended dosage because at higher doses nervousness, dizziness or sleeplessness may oc-

cur. Do not take this product for more than 10 days. A persistent cough may be a sign of a serious condition. If cough persists for more than 7 days, tends to recur, or is accompanied by rash, persistent headache, fever that lasts more than 3 days, or if new symptoms occur, consult a physician. Do not take this product for persistent or chronic cough such as occurs with smoking, asthma, emphysema, or if cough is accompanied by excessive phlegm (mucus) unless directed by a physician. If sore throat is severe, persists for more than 2 days, is accompanied or followed by fever, headache, rash, nausea, or vomiting, consult a physician promptly. Do not take this product if you have high blood pressure, heart disease, diabetes, thyroid disease, or difficulty in urination due to enlargement of the prostate gland except under the advice and supervision of a physician. As with any drug, if you are pregnant or nursing a baby, seek the advice of a health professional before using this product.

Drug Interaction Precaution: Do not take this product if you are presently taking a prescription antihypertensive or antidepressant drug containing a monoamine oxidase inhibitor except under the advice and supervision of a physician.

KEEP THIS AND ALL DRUGS OUT OF THE REACH OF CHILDREN. In case of accidental overdose, seek professional assistance or contact a Poison Control Center immediately. Prompt medical attention is critical for adults as well as for children even if you do not notice any signs or symptoms.

Store at 15° to 25°C (59° to 77°F) in a dry place.

How Supplied: Boxes of 10, 20.
Shown in Product Identification Section, page 407

SUDAFED® Severe Cold Formula Tablets
[sū' duh-fĕd]

Product Benefits: Maximum allowable levels of nasal decongestant, cough suppressant, and non-aspirin pain reliever/fever reducer provide temporary relief from symptoms of the common cold and flu. This product contains no ingredients that may cause drowsiness. The **DECONGESTANT** (pseudoephedrine) temporarily relieves nasal and sinus congestion due to the common cold. It temporarily relieves nasal stuffiness; reduces the swelling of nasal passages; shrinks swollen membranes; and temporarily restores freer breathing through the nose. The **COUGH SUPPRESSANT** (dextromethorphan) temporarily relieves cough due to the common cold. The non-aspirin **PAIN RELIEVER/FEVER REDUCER** (acetaminophen) temporarily relieves headache, body aches and pains, minor sore throat pain, and reduces fever due to the common cold.

Directions: Adults and children 12 years of age and over, 2 tablets every 6 hours, not to exceed 8 tablets in 24 hours.

Not recommended for children under 12 years of age.

Each Tablet Contains: acetaminophen 500 mg, dextromethorphan hydrobromide 15 mg, and pseudoephedrine hydrochloride 30 mg. Also contains: crospovidone, magnesium stearate, microcrystalline cellulose, povidone, pregelatinized corn starch, sodium starch glycolate and stearic acid.

Warnings: Do not exceed recommended dosage because at higher doses nervousness, dizziness or sleeplessness may occur. Do not take this product for more than 10 days. A persistent cough may be a sign of a serious condition. If cough persists for more than 7 days, tends to recur, or is accompanied by rash, persistent headache, fever that lasts more than 3 days, or if new symptoms occur, consult a physician. Do not take this product for persistent or chronic cough such as occurs with smoking, asthma, emphysema, or if cough is accompanied by excessive phlegm (mucus) unless directed by a physician. If sore throat is severe, persists for more than 2 days, is accompanied or followed by fever, headache, rash, nausea, or vomiting, consult a physician promptly. Do not take this product if you have high blood pressure, heart disease, diabetes, thyroid disease, or difficulty in urination due to enlargement of the prostate gland except under the advice and supervision of a physician. As with any drug, if you are pregnant or nursing a baby, seek the advice of a health professional before using this product.
Drug Interaction Precaution: Do not take this product if you are presently taking a prescription antihypertensive or antidepressant drug containing a monoamine oxidase inhibitor except under the advice and supervision of a physician.
KEEP THIS AND ALL DRUGS OUT OF THE REACH OF CHILDREN. In case of accidental overdose, seek professional assistance or contact a Poison Control Center immediately. Prompt medical attention is critical for adults as well as for chilren even if you do not notice any signs or symptoms.
Store at 15° to 25°C (59° to 77°F) in a dry place.

How Supplied: Boxes of 10, 20.
Shown in Product Identification Section, page 407

SUDAFED® SINUS Caplets
[sū′ duh-fĕd sī′ nəs]

Product Benefits:
● Maximum allowable levels of non-aspirin pain reliever and nasal decongestant provide temporary relief of sinus headache pain, pressure and nasal congestion due to colds and flu or hay fever and other allergies.
● Contains no ingredients which may cause drowsiness.

Directions: Adults and children 12 years and over, 2 caplets every 6 hours, not to exceed 8 caplets in a 24-hour pe-

riod. Not recommended for children under 12 years of age.

Each Caplet Contains: acetaminophen 500 mg and pseudoephedrine hydrochloride 30 mg. Also contains: crospovidone, FD&C Yellow No. 6 Lake, magnesium stearate, microcrystalline cellulose, povidone, pregelatinized corn starch, sodium starch glycolate and stearic acid.

Warnings: Do not exceed recommended dosage because at higher doses nervousness, dizziness, or sleeplessness may occur. Do not take this product for more than 10 days. If symptoms do not improve or are accompanied by fever that lasts for more than 3 days, or if new symptoms occur, consult a physician. Do not take this product if you have high blood pressure, heart disease, diabetes, thyroid disease, or difficulty in urination due to enlargement of the prostate gland except under the advice and supervision of a physician. As with any drug, if you are pregnant or nursing a baby, seek the advice of a health professional before using this product.
Drug Interaction Precaution: Do not take this product if you are presently taking a prescription antihypertensive or antidepressant drug containing a monoamine oxidase inhibitor except under the advice and supervision of a physician.
KEEP THIS AND ALL DRUGS OUT OF THE REACH OF CHILDREN. In case of accidental overdose, seek professional assistance or contact a Poison Control Center immediately. Prompt medical attention is critical for adults as well as children even if you do not notice any signs or symptoms.
Store at 15° to 25°C (59° to 77°F) in a dry place and protect from light.

How Supplied: Boxes of 24 and 48.
Shown in Product Identification Section, page 407

SUDAFED® SINUS Tablets
[sū′ duh-fĕd sī′ nəs]

Product Benefits:
● Maximum allowable levels of non-aspirin pain reliever and nasal decongestant provide temporary relief of sinus headache pain, pressure and nasal congestion due to colds and flu or hay fever and other allergies.
● Contains no ingredients which may cause drowsiness.

Directions: Adults and children 12 years and over, 2 tablets every 6 hours, not to exceed 8 tablets in a 24-hour period. Not recommended for children under 12 years of age.

Each Tablet Contains: Acetaminophen 500 mg and pseudoephedrine hydrochloride 30 mg. Also contains: crospovidone, FD&C Yellow No. 6 Lake, magnesium stearate, microcrystalline cellulose, povidone, pregelatinized corn starch, sodium starch glycolate and stearic acid.

Warnings: Do not exceed recommended dosage because at higher doses nervousness, dizziness, or sleeplessness may occur. Do not take this product for more than 10 days. If symptoms do not improve or are accompanied by fever that lasts for more than 3 days, or if new symptoms occur, consult a physician. Do not take this product if you have high blood pressure, heart disease, diabetes, thyroid disease, or difficulty in urination due to enlargement of the prostate gland except under the advice and supervision of a physician. As with any drug, if you are pregnant or nursing a baby, seek the advice of a health professional before using this product.
Drug Interaction Precaution: Do not take this product if you are presently taking a prescription antihypertensive or antidepressant drug containing a monoamine oxidase inhibitor except under the advice and supervision of a physician.
KEEP THIS AND ALL DRUGS OUT OF THE REACH OF CHILDREN. In case of accidental overdose, seek professional assistance or contact a Poison Control Center immediately. Prompt medical attention is critical for adults as well as children even if you do not notice any signs or symptoms.
Store at 15° to 25°C (59° to 77°F) in a dry place and protect from light.

How Supplied: Boxes of 24 and 48.
Shown in Product Identification Section, page 407

SUDAFED® 12 Hour Tablets
[sū′ duh-fĕd]

SUDAFED 12 HOUR Long-Acting Nasal Decongestant Tablets contain pseudoephedrine sulfate, a nasal decongestant, in a special timed-release tablet providing up to 12 hours of continuous relief. . . without drowsiness.

Indications: For temporary relief of nasal congestion due to the common cold, hay fever, or other upper respiratory allergies, and nasal congestion associated with sinusitis. Helps decongest sinus openings and sinus passages.

Directions: Adults and Children 12 Years and Over—One tablet every 12 hours. SUDAFED 12 HOUR is not recommended for children under 12 years of age.

Each Extended-Release Tablet Contains: 120 mg pseudoephedrine sulfate. Half the dose is released after the tablet is swallowed and the other half is released hours later, providing continuous relief for up to 12 hours.

Warnings: Do not exceed recommended dosage because at higher doses, nervousness, dizziness, or sleeplessness may occur. Do not take this product if you have heart disease, high blood pressure, thyroid disease, diabetes, or difficulty in urination due to enlargement of the prostate gland

Continued on next page

Burroughs Wellcome—Cont.

unless directed by a doctor. If symptoms do not improve within 7 days or are accompanied by fever, consult your doctor before continuing use. Keep this and all drugs out of the reach of children. In case of accidental overdose, seek professional assistance or contact a Poison Control Center immediately. As with any drug, if you are pregnant or nursing a baby, seek the advice of a health professional before using this product.

Drug Interaction Precautions: Do not take this product if you are presently taking a prescription drug for high blood pressure or depression, without first consulting your doctor.

Active Ingredient: Pseudoephedrine Sulfate

Also Contains: Acacia, Butylparaben, Calcium Sulfate, Carnauba Wax, Corn Starch, FD&C Blue No. 1, Gelatin, Lactose, Magnesium Stearate, Neutral Soap, Oleic Acid, Povidone, Rosin, Sugar, Talc, White Wax, Zein.
Store between 2° and 25°C (36° and 77°F). Protect from excessive moisture.

How Supplied: Boxes of 10, 20.
Shown in Product Identification Section, page 407

WELLCOME® brand LANOLINE
[lăn'ō-lŭn]

Description: Lanolin with solid and liquid petrolatum, fragrances, and glycerin.

Indications: A soothing and softening application for dry, rough skin and a protective application against the effects of harsh weather.

Directions: Apply topically to the hands and face as required.

Keep this and all medicines out of children's reach.

Store at 15°–25°C (59°–77°F).

How Supplied: Tubes, 1¾ oz.

Campbell Laboratories Inc.
300 EAST 51st STREET
P.O. BOX 812, FDR STATION
NEW YORK, NY 10150

HERPECIN–L® Cold Sore Lip Balm
[her"puh-sin-el"]

PRODUCT OVERVIEW

Key Facts: HERPECIN-L Lip Balm is a convenient, easy-to-use treatment for perioral herpes simplex infections. Sunscreens provide an SPF of 15.

Major Uses: HERPECIN-L not only treats cold sores, sun and fever blisters, but with prophylactic use, its sunscreens also protect to help prevent them. Users

report early use at the prodromal stages of an attack will often abort the lesions and prevent scabbing. Prescribe: Apply "early, often and liberally."

Safety Information: For topical use only. A rare sensitivity may occur.

PRESCRIBING INFORMATION

HERPECIN–L® Cold Sore Lip Balm

Composition: A soothing, emollient, lip balm incorporating allantoin, the sunscreen, octyl-dimethyl-PABA (Padimate O), in a balanced, slightly acidic lipid base that includes petrolatum and titanium dioxide at a cosmetically acceptable level. (No caines, antibiotics, phenol or camphor.) (NDC 38083-777-31)

Actions and Uses: HERPECIN-L® relieves dryness and chapping by providing a lipid barrier to help restore normal moisture balance to the lips. Skin protectants help to soften the crusts and scabs of "cold sores." The sunscreen is effective in 2900-3200 AU range while titanium dioxide, though at low levels, helps to block, scatter and reflect the sun's rays. Applied as a lip balm, SPF is 15. Frequent reapplication, however, is advised.

Administration: (1) *Recurrent "cold sores, sun and fever blisters":* Simply put, use **soon** and **often.** Frequent sufferers report that with *prophylactic* use (BID/PRN), attacks are fewer and less severe. Most recurrent herpes labialis patients are aware of the prodromal symptoms: tingling, itching, burning. At this stage, or if the lesion has already developed, HERPECIN-L should be applied liberally as often as convenient—at least *every hour.* (2) *Outdoor protection:* Apply before and during sun exposure, after swimming and again at bedtime (h.s.). (3) *Dry, chapped lips:* Apply as needed.

Adverse Reactions: If sensitive to any of the ingredients, discontinue use.

Contraindications: None.

How Supplied: 2.8 gm. swivel tubes.

Samples Available: Yes. (Request on professional letterhead or Rx pad.)

Caraco Pharmaceutical Laboratories, Ltd.
1150 ELIJAH McCOY DRIVE
DETROIT, MI 48202

SURELAC™
Lactase Enzyme Tablets

Ingredients: Each chewable tablet contains 3000 FCC Lactase Units. Other ingredients: dibasic calcium phosphate, sorbitol or mannitol, colloidal silicon dioxide, magnesium stearate.

Indications: Surelac Chewable Tablets are a pleasant tasting, natural nutritional supplement which permits enjoyment of dairy products and lactose-containing substances, without discomfort. Surelac Chewable Tablets are safe and non-habit forming. They are a natural

nutritional supplement which makes eating more enjoyable.

Warnings: Occasionally sensitive persons with allergy could experience gastric discomfort or nausea. Do not use this product for children under 12 years of age except under the supervision of a doctor.

Directions: In most cases, we suggest using 2 or 3 chewable tablets with or immediately following a meal containing dairy food. Store at room temperature or below. Keep away from heat.

How Supplied: Surelac is available in bottles of 60 tablets.
Caraco Pharmaceutical Laboratories, Ltd.
Detroit, Michigan 48202

Care-Tech Laboratories
Div. of Consolidated Chemical, Inc.
3224 SOUTH KINGSHIGHWAY BOULEVARD
ST. LOUIS, MO 63139

BARRI–CARE®

Composition: Active Ingredient: Chloroxylenol
Inactive Ingredients: Petrolatum, Water, Paraffin, Propylene Glycol, Milk Protein, Cod Liver Oil, Aloe Vera Gel, Fragrance, Potassium Hydroxide, Methyl Paraben, Propyl Paraben, Vitamin A & D_3, (E) dl Alpha-Tocopheryl Acetate, (E) dl-Alpha-Tocopherol, D&C Yellow #11 and D&C Red #17.

Actions and Uses: Barri-Care is an antimicrobial ointment formulated to provide a moisture proof barrier against urine, detergent irritants, feces and drainage from wounds or skin lesions. Proven antimicrobial action against E. coli, MRSA, S. aureus and Pseudomonas aeruginosa. Protects perineal area of the incontinent patient from painful skin rashes and relieves irritation around stoma sites. Utilize on Grades I–IV pressure ulcers to halt skin breakdown. Can be used also on minor burns. Will not melt under feverish conditions.

Precautions: External Use Only. Non-Toxic. Avoid eye contact.

Directions: Cleanse affected area with Satin thoroughly. Apply ointment topically to affected area. Reapply 2–3 times daily or as directed by physician.

How Supplied: 2 oz. jar, 4 oz. tubes, 8 oz. jar. NDC #46706-206

CARE CREME®

Composition: Active Ingredient: Chloroxylenol
Inactive Ingredients: Water, Cetyl Alcohol, Lanolin Oil, Cod Liver Oil, Sodium Laureth Sulfate, Triethanolamine, Propylene Glycol, Petrolatum, Lanolin Alcohol, Methyl Gluceth 20 Distearate, Beeswax, Citric Acid, Methyl Paraben, Fra-

grance, Propyl Paraben, Vitamins A, D_3 and E-dl Alpha-Tocopherol.

Actions and Uses: Care Creme is an antimicrobial skin care creme specially formulated for use on severely dry skin such as Sjogren's Syndrome, atopic dermatitis, psoriasis, minor burns, urine or fecal exposure, scaling and inter-tissue ammonia related rash. Extremely effective on oncology radiation burns. Use at first sign of reddened skin or initial breakdown. Vitamin and oil enriched to promote skin integrity. Contains no metallic ions.

Precautions: Non-toxic, External Use Only. Avoid use around eye area.

Directions: Cleanse affected area with Satin and gently massage Care Creme into skin until completely absorbed or as directed by physician.

How Supplied: 2 oz., 4 oz. tubes, 9 oz. jar. NDC #46706-205

CLINICAL CARE® WOUND CLEANSER

Composition: Active Ingredient: Benzethonium Chloride
Inactive Ingredients: Water, Amphoteric 2, Aloe Vera Gel, DMDM Hydantoin, Citric Acid.

Actions and Uses: Clinical Care is an antimicrobial, emulsifying solution which aids in removing debris and particulate matter from open, dermal wounds. Clinical Care inhibits the growth of pathogenic organisms. Proven effective at eliminating S. aureus, P. aeruginosa, S. typhimurium, Aspergillus, E. coli, MRSA, S. pyogenes and K. pneumonia. Will not produce dermal irritation.

Precautions: External Use Only. Non-Toxic. No contra-indicators.

Directions: Spray affected area as necessary to debride. Use sterile gauze to gently remove debris and necrotic tissue at dermal surface.

How Supplied: 4 oz. spray, 8 oz. spray

CONCEPT®

Composition: Active Ingredient: Chloroxylenol
Inactive Ingredients: Water, Amphoteric 9, Polysorbate 20, PEG-150 Distearate, Cocamide DEA, Cocoyl Sarcosine, Fragrance, D&C Green #5.

Actions and Uses: Concept is a geriatric shampoo and body wash for patients whose skin is irritated by soaps and harsh detergents. Concept is non-eye irritating and reduces bacteria on the skin. Excellent for replenishing moisture in dry, flaky dermal tissues and eliminating body odors. Utilize on children over 6 months of age to address rashing or atopic dermatitis.

Precautions: External Use Only. Non-Toxic.

Directions: Use in normal manner of bathing and shampooing. Rinse thoroughly.

How Supplied: 8 oz., Gallons

FORMULA MAGIC®

Composition: Active Ingredient: Benzethonium Chloride
Inactive Ingredients: Talc, Mineral Oil, Magnesium Carbonate, Fragrance, DMDM Hydantoin.

Actions and Uses: Formula Magic is primarily a geriatric care powder and nursing lubricant. Aids in preventing excoriation, friction chafing and eliminating odor. Antibacterial action proven effective at 99.9% inhibition where Formula Magic is applied. Excellent for use on diabetic patients, feet and under breasts to relieve redness and skin irritation.

Precautions: Non-irritating to skin, non-toxic, slightly irritating to eyes.

Directions: Apply liberally to body and rub gently into skin.

How Supplied: 4 oz. and 12 oz. NDC #46706-202

ORCHID FRESH II®
Perineal/Ostomy Cleanser

Composition: Active Ingredient: Benzethonium Chloride
Inactive Ingredients: Water, Amphoteric 2, DMDM Hydantoin, Fragrance, Citric Acid.

Actions and Uses: Orchid Fresh II is an amphoteric, topical antimicrobial cleansing solution which gently cleans and emulsifies feces and urine on the incontinent patient. Use also on stoma sites and ostomy bags to deodorize and eliminate odor. Outstanding antimicrobial action on Pseudomonas, E. coli, Staphylococcus aureus, MRSA, etc. Orchid Fresh II will aid in reducing skin breakdown.

Precautions: External Use Only, Non-Toxic—Non-Dermal Irritating

Directions: Spray topically and remove feces and urine with warm, moist washcloth. Spray directly on peristomal skin areas, clean gently and pat dry. Utilize Care Creme on reddened skin areas.

How Supplied: 4 oz., 8 oz. and Gallons NDC #46706-115

SATIN® ANTIMICROBIAL SKIN CLEANSER

Composition: Active Ingredient: Chloroxylenol
Inactive Ingredients: Water, Sodium Laureth Sulfate, Cocamidopropyl Betaine, PEG-8, Cocamide DEA, Glycol Stearate, Lanolin Oil, Tetrasodium EDTA, D&C Yellow #10.

Actions and Uses: Satin has been specially formulated for use on sensitive or aging dermal tissue, atopic dermatitis and psoriasis. Effective in eliminating gram-positive and gram-negative pathogens such as E. coli, S. aureus, Pseudomonas, etc. Contains emollients to replenish natural oils and proteins. Satin also eliminates skin odor and dry, itchy skin.

Precautions: No contra-indicators. External use only. Non-Toxic.

Directions: Use during shower, bath or regular cleansing or as directed by physician.

How Supplied: 4 oz., 8 oz., 12 oz. 16 oz., 1 Gallon NDC #46706-101

TECHNI–CARE® SURGICAL SCRUB

Composition: Active Ingredient: Chloroxylenol 3%
Inactive Ingredients: Water, Sodium Lauryl Sulfate, Cocamide DEA, Propylene Glycol, Cocamidopropyl Betaine, Cocamidopropyl PG-Dimonium Chloride Phosphate, Citric Acid, Tetrasodium EDTA, Aloe Vera Gel, Hydrolyzed Animal Protein, D&C Yellow #10, Fragrance.

Actions and Uses: Techni-Care represents entirely new technology in a broad-spectrum, topical, antiseptic microbicide for skin degerming. 99.99% Bacterial reduction in 30 second contact usage. Techni-Care may be used for disinfection of wounds, for pre-op and post-op along with surgical scrub applications. Non-staining and non-irritating to dermal tissue. Techni-Care conditions dermal tissue and promotes more rapid rate of healing.

Precautions: Non-Toxic, Non-Irritating, External Use Only. Can be used safely around ears and eyes or as directed by a physician.

Directions: Apply, lather and rinse well. For pre-op, apply and let dry, no rinsing required.

How Supplied: 4 oz. packets, 8 oz., 16 oz., 32 oz., Gallons

Chattem Consumer Products
Division of Chattem, Inc.
1715 WEST 38TH STREET
CHATTANOOGA, TN 37409

FLEX–ALL 454® PAIN RELIEVING GEL

Active Ingredient: Menthol 7%.

Inactive Ingredients: Alcohol, Allantoin, Aloe Vera Gel, Boric Acid Carbomer 940, Diazolidinyl Urea, Eucalyptus Oil, Glycerin, Iodine, Methylparaben, Methyl Salicylate, Peppermint Oil, Polysorbate 60, Potassium Iodide, Propylene Glycol, Propylparaben, Thyme Oil, Triethanolamine, Water, 97-116.

Continued on next page

Chattem—Cont.

Indications: To relieve the pain of minor arthritis, simple backache, strains, sprains, bruises, and cramps.

Actions: Flex-all is classified as a counterirritant which provides relief of deep-seated pain through cutaneous stimulation rather than through a direct analgesic effect.

Warnings: For external use only. Keep out of reach of children. If swallowed, call a physician or contact a poison control center. Keep away from eyes and mucous membranes, broken or irritated skin. Do not bandage tightly or use heating pad. If skin redness or irritation develops, or pain lasts more than 10 days, discontinue use and call a physician.

Dosage and Administration: Apply generously to painful muscles and joints and gently massage until Flex-all 454 disappears. Use before and after exercise. Repeat as needed for temporary relief of minor arthritis pain, simple backache, strains, sprains, bruises, and cramps.

How Supplied: Available in 2 oz., 4 oz. and 8 oz. bottles.

ICY HOT® Balm
[ī′see hot]
(topical analgesic balm)
ICY HOT® Cream
(topical analgesic cream)
ICY HOT® Stick
(topical analgesic stick)

Active Ingredients: Icy Hot Balm contains methyl salicylate 29%, menthol 7.6%. Icy Hot Cream contains methyl salicylate 30%, menthol 10%. Icy Hot Stick contains methyl salicylate 30%, menthol 10%.
Inactive ingredients of Icy Hot Balm include paraffin and white petrolatum. Inactive ingredients of Icy Hot Cream include carbomer, cetyl esters wax, emulsifying wax, oleth-3 phosphate, stearic acid, trolamine, and water. Inactive ingredients of Icy Hot Stick include ceresin, cyclomethicone, hydrogenated castor oil, microcrystalline wax, paraffin, PEG-150 distearate, propylene glycol, stearic acid, and stearyl alcohol.

Description: Icy Hot Balm, Icy Hot Cream, and Icy Hot Stick are topically applied analgesics containing two active ingredients, methyl salicylate and menthol. It is the particular concentration of these ingredients, in combination with inert ingredients, that results in the distinct, combined heating/cooling sensation of Icy Hot.

Actions: Icy Hot is classified as a counterirritant which, when rubbed into the intact skin, provides relief of deep-seated pain through a counterirritant action rather than through a direct analgesic effect. In acting as a counterirritant, Icy Hot replaces the perception of pain with another sensation that blocks deep pain temporarily by its action on or near the skin surface.

Indications: For the temporary relief of minor aches and pains of muscles and joints associated with arthritis, simple backache, strains, bruises, and sprains.

Directions: Adults and children 2 years of age and older: Apply to affected area not more than 3 to 4 times daily. Children under 2 years of age: Do not use, consult a doctor.
Stick: Twist base to raise Icy Hot approximately one quarter inch above container.
Adults and children 2 years of age and older: Apply to affected area not more than 3 to 4 times daily. Children under 2 years of age: Do not use, consult a doctor.

Warnings: For external use only. Do not use otherwise than as directed. Keep this and all drugs out of the reach of children. In case of accidental ingestion, seek professional assistance or contact a poison control center immediately. Avoid contact with eyes. Avoid contact with mouth, genitalia, and mucous membranes, irritated, or very sensitive skin. If you have diabetes or impaired circulation, use Icy Hot only upon the advice of a physician. Do not apply to wounds or damaged skin, Do not bandage tightly. Do not apply external heat or hot water. If condition worsens, or if symptoms persist for more than 7 days or clear up and occur again within a few days, discontinue use of this product and consult a doctor.
CAUTION: Discontinue use if excessive irritation of the skin develops.

Adverse Reactions: The most common adverse reactions that may occur with Icy Hot use are skin irritation and blistering. The most serious adverse reaction is severe toxicity that occurs if the product is ingested.

How Supplied: Icy Hot Balm is available in a 3½ oz jar. Icy Hot Cream is available in tubes in two sizes, 1¼ oz and 3 oz. Icy Hot Stick is available as a 1¾ oz stick.

NORWICH® MAXIMUM STRENGTH ASPIRIN
Aspirin (acetylsalicylic acid) tablets

Active Ingredient: Each tablet contains 500 mg (7.7 grains) of pure aspirin.

Inactive Ingredients: Starch, Hydroxypropyl Methylcellulose, Polyethylene Glycol.

Actions: Analgesic and antipyretic.

Indications: For fast, effective relief of headache, minor aches and pains, and for reduction of fever, as well as temporary relief of minor aches and pains of arthritis, muscular aches, colds and flu, and menstrual discomfort.

Warnings: Children and teenagers should not use this medicine for chicken pox or flu symptoms before a doctor is consulted about Reye syndrome, a rare but serious illness reported to be associated with aspirin. As with any drug, if you are pregnant or nursing a baby, seek the advice of a health professional before using this product. IT IS ESPECIALLY IMPORTANT NOT TO USE ASPIRIN DURING THE LAST 3 MONTHS OF PREGNANCY UNLESS SPECIFICALLY DIRECTED TO DO SO BY A DOCTOR BECAUSE IT MAY CAUSE PROBLEMS IN THE UNBORN CHILD OR COMPLICATIONS DURING DELIVERY. Keep this and all medicines out of reach of children. In case of accidental overdose, seek professional assistance or contact a poison control center immediately.

Caution: If pain persists for more than 10 days or if redness is present, or in conditions affecting children under 12, consult physician immediately. If asthmatic or taking medicines for anticoagulation (thinning the blood), diabetes, gout, or arthritis, consult physician before use. Discontinue if ringing in the ears occurs.

Treatment of Oral Overdosage: IN CASE OF ACCIDENTAL OVERDOSE, SEEK PROFESSIONAL ASSISTANCE OR CONTACT A POISON CONTROL CENTER IMMEDIATELY.

Dosage and Administration: Adults: Initial dose 2 tablets followed by 1 tablet every 3 hours or 2 tablets every 6 hours, not to exceed 8 tablets in any 24-hour period, or as directed by a physician. NOT RECOMMENDED FOR CHILDREN UNDER 12.

Professional Labeling: Same as outlined under Indications.

How Supplied: In child-resistant bottles of 150 tablets.

NORWICH® REGULAR STRENGTH ASPIRIN
Aspirin (acetylsalicylic acid) tablets

Active Ingredient: Each tablet contains 325 mg (5 grains) of pure aspirin.

Inactive Ingredients: Starch, Hydroxypropyl Methylcellulose, Polyethylene Glycol.

Actions: Analgesic and antipyretic.

Indications: For fast, effective relief of headache, minor aches and pains, and for reduction of fever, as well as temporary relief of minor aches and pains of arthritis, muscular aches, colds and flu, and menstrual discomfort.

Warnings: Children and teenagers should not use this medicine for chicken pox or flu symptoms before a doctor is consulted about Reye syndrome, a rare but serious illness reported to be associated with aspirin. As with any drug, if you are pregnant or nursing a baby, seek the advice of a health professional before using this product. IT IS ESPECIALLY IMPORTANT NOT TO USE ASPIRIN DURING THE LAST 3 MONTHS OF PREGNANCY UNLESS SPECIFICALLY DIRECTED TO DO SO BY A DOCTOR BECAUSE IT MAY CAUSE PROBLEMS IN THE UNBORN CHILD

OR COMPLICATIONS DURING DE-LIVERY. Keep this and all medicines out of reach of children. In case of accidental overdose, seek professional assistance or contact a poison control center immediately.

Caution: If pain persists for more than 10 days or if redness is present, or in conditions affecting children under 12, consult physician immediately. Do not take if you have ulcers, ulcer symptoms or bleeding problems. If asthmatic or taking medicines for anticoagulation (thinning the blood), diabetes, gout, or arthritis, consult physician before use. Discontinue if ringing in the ears occurs.

Treatment of Oral Overdosage: IN CASE OF ACCIDENTAL OVERDOSE, SEEK PROFESSIONAL ASSISTANCE OR CONTACT A POISON CONTROL CENTER IMMEDIATELY.

Dosage and Administration: Adults: 1 or 2 tablets every 3–4 hours up to 6 times a day. Children: under 3 years, consult physician; 3–6 years, ½–1 tablet; over 6 years, 1 tablet. May be taken every 3–4 hours up to 3 times a day.

Professional Labeling: Same as outlined under Indications.

How Supplied: In child-resistant bottles of 500 tablets, 250 tablets and 100 tablets.

**Extra Strength
PAMPRIN
Multi-Symptom Formula
Menstrual Relief Tablets/Caplets**

Active Ingredients: Each tablet/caplet contains acetaminophen 400 mg, pamabrom 25 mg, and pyrilamine maleate 15 mg.

Inactive Ingredients: Corn starch, croscarmellose sodium, hydrogenated vegetable oil, magnesium stearate, microcrystalline cellulose, and silica.

Indications: Clinically tested and found to be safe and effective in the relief of menstrual pain of cramps, backache, headache, water weight gain, premenstrual tension, and irritability.

Warning: Keep this and all drugs out of the reach of children. In case of accidental overdose, seek professional assistance or contact a poison control center immediately.

Precautions: IF DROWSINESS OCCURS, DO NOT DRIVE OR OPERATE MACHINERY. As with any drug, if you are pregnant or nursing a baby, seek the advice of a health professional before using this product.

Dosage and Administration: Two tablets (or caplets) and repeat every three to four hours as needed, not to exceed 8 tablets (or caplets) in a 24 hour period.

How Supplied: Non-child resistant packages of foil pouches containing 24 tablets or caplets and child resistant bot-

tles containing 12 or 48 tablets or 48 caplets.

Product Identification: White, round tablets with PAMPRIN debossed in the center of the tablet surrounded by three rosette shaped designs on the top and bottom of the word PAMPRIN **OR** white capsule shaped caplets with PAMPRIN debossed in the center of the caplet and faced on either end by a single rosette.

**Maximum Strength
PAMPRIN
Cramp Relief Formula
Menstrual Relief Caplets**

Active Ingredients: Each tablet/caplet contains acetaminophen 500 mg, pamabrom 25 mg, and pyrilamine maleate 15 mg.

Inactive Ingredients: Corn starch, croscarmellose sodium, hydrogenated vegetable oil, magnesium stearate, microcrystalline cellulose, and silica.

Indications: Clinically tested and found to provide safe and effective relief of menstrual pain of cramps, backache, and legaches that occur before and during the menstrual period.

Warning: Keep this and all drugs out of the reach of children. In case of accidental overdose, seek professional assistance or contact a poison control center immediately.

Precautions: IF DROWSINESS OCCURS, DO NOT DRIVE OR OPERATE MACHINERY. As with any drug, if you are pregnant or nursing a baby, seek the advice of a health professional before using this product.

Dosage and Administration: Two tablets (or caplets) and repeat every three to four hours as needed, not to exceed 8 tablets (or caplets) in a 24 hour period.

How Supplied: Non-child resistant foil pouches containing 16 caplets and child resistant bottles containing 32 caplets.

Product Identification: White capsule shaped caplets with PAMPRIN debossed in the center of the caplet.

PRĒMSYN PMS®
[*preem 'sin pms*]
Premenstrual Syndrome Caplets

Active Ingredients: Each caplet contains Acetaminophen 500 mg., Pamabrom 25 mg., and Pyrilamine Maleate 15 mg.

Indications: PRĒMSYN PMS® has been clinically proven to safely and effectively relieve premenstrual tension, irritability, nervousness, edema, backaches, legaches, and headaches that often accompany premenstrual syndrome.

Warning: KEEP THIS AND ALL DRUGS OUT OF THE REACH OF CHILDREN. In case of accidental overdose, seek professional assistance or contact a poison control center immediately.

Precautions: If drowsiness occurs, do not drive or operate machinery. As with any drug, if pregnant or nursing a baby, seek the advice of a health professional before using this product.

Dosage and Administration: Two caplets at first sign of premenstrual discomfort and repeat every three or four hours as needed, not to exceed 8 caplets in a 24-hour period.

How Supplied: Tamper-resistant bottles of 20 and 40 caplets.

Product Identification Marks: White caplet with PRĒMSYN PMS debossed on one surface.

EDUCATIONAL MATERIAL

PRĒMSYN PMS®
Pamabrom and Pyrilamine Maleate, Two of the Active Ingredients in PRĒMSYN PMS®
The 22-page booklet presents information about the ingredients in PRĒMSYN PMS®. The booklet includes results of basic pharmacology and clinical studies. Free to physicians and pharmacists.
PMS: Premenstrual Syndrome, A Review for Health Professionals
This 16-page booklet is directed to the health professional. It is a review of premenstrual syndrome, the mechanism, the varying symptoms, and modes of treatment, including dietary tips and a daily symptom diary. Free to physicians and pharmacists.
PMS, You 're Not Alone
(30-Minute Videotape)
Both are used by health professionals as instructional tools for educating either individual patients or groups of patients, other health professionals, and community groups. These can be obtained by writing Chattem, Inc.
PMS—Practical Advice for the Period Before Your Period
This booklet is written to the woman who suffers from PMS. It describes PMS, the various symptoms associated with the syndrome, a three-month symptom dairy and treatments including dietary tips, stress reduction and exercise. Free to physicians, pharmacists and other health professionals for distribution to patients.

IDENTIFICATION PROBLEM?
Consult the
Product Identification Section
where you'll find
products pictured
in full color.

Chesebrough-Pond's Inc.
33 BENEDICT PLACE
GREENWICH, CT 06830

VASELINE®
Pure Petroleum Jelly
Skin Protectant/Lip Therapy

Composition: White Petrolatum U.S.P.

Indication: A soothing protectant for minor skin irritations such as burns, scrapes, abrasions, chafing, detergent hands, dry or chapped skin, and sunburn. Provides temporary relief of external hemorrhoids and scaling due to psoriasis. Helps prevent diaper rash, soothes chapped skin and temporarily soothes minor sunburn due to its emollient and lubricant properties. Helps prevent and heal dry, chapped sun- and wind-burned lips. Vaseline products are non-comedogenic.

Directions: Cleanse affected areas with soap and water prior to application, then apply generously to provide a continuous protective film. For lips, apply as needed, before, during and following exposure to sun, wind, water, and cold weather.

Drug Interaction: No known drug interactions. Product is innocuous, physiologically inert with no known sensitization potential.

Warning: Not meant for puncture wounds, serious burns, or cuts.

How Supplied: 1 oz. and 2.5 oz. plastic tubes. (NDC 0521-8120-01,31). 1.75 oz., 3.75 oz., 7.5 oz., and 13 oz. plastic jars (NDC 0521-8120-24, -28, -29, -32). 4.25 gram tubes in regular, mint, cherry, and orange flavors (also available with SPF #15).

VASELINE® INTENSIVE CARE®
MOISTURIZING SUNBLOCK LOTION

Active Ingredients: Ethylhexyl p-methoxycinnamate, oxybenzone, 2-ethylhexyl salicylate.

Inactive Ingredients: Water, glycerin, stearic acid, aloe vera gel, PVP/Eicosene copolymer, dimethicone, triethanolamine, deacetyl phosphate, cetyl alcohol, petrolatum, tocopheryl acetate, magnesium aluminum silicate, carbomer 934, fragrance, methylparaben, propylparaben, disodium EDTA, DMDM hydantoin.

Indications/Actions: Vaseline Intensive Care Moisturizing Sunblock Lotion is a non-greasy, fragrance-free formula which provides broad-spectrum protection from the sun's harmful UVA and UVB rays. These effective moisturizers are hypo-allergenic, oil-free, non-comedogenic and will penetrate into the skin quickly to replenish moisture loss due to sun and wind exposure. Vaseline Intensive Care Moisturizing Sunblock Lotion is also PABA-free; gentle and non-stinging, and waterproof for 80 minutes.

Directions: Apply generously and evenly to exposed areas. Apply product liberally prior to exposure to sun. Re-apply after prolonged swimming or excessive perspiration or every two hours.

Warnings: Avoid contact with eyes. For external use only.

How Supplied: 4 oz., 6 oz., and 10 oz.

VASELINE® INTENSIVE CARE®
ULTRA VIOLET (UV) DAILY DEFENSE LOTION FOR HAND AND BODY—SPF 15

Active Ingredients: Ethylhexyl p-methoxycinnamate, oxybenzone.

Inactive Ingredients: Water, glycerin, stearic acid, C11–13 isoparaffin, glycol stearate, triethanolamine, tocopheryl acetate (Vitamin E acetate), cetyl acetate, glyceryl stearate, cetyl alcohol, dimethicone, deacetyl phosphate, magnesium aluminum silicate, acetylated lanolin alcohol, stearamide AMP, methylparaben, propylparaben, fragrance, carbomer 934, disodium EDTA, DMDM hydantoin.

Indications/Actions: Vaseline Intensive Care Ultra Violet Daily Defense Lotion is a light, non-greasy hand and body lotion that contains a UVA and UVB sunscreen to provide daily protection from the harmful burning rays which can cause premature aging and other long-term skin damage. It provides 15 times the natural sunburn protection. In addition, Vaseline Intensive Care UV Daily Defense Lotion has been formulated with a special blend of moisturizers to soften and smooth the skin without a greasy after feel. It is also dermatologist tested and PABA free.

Directions: Use every day. Apply liberally to all areas of the body, especially on the back of hands, arms, legs, and neck to guard against sun damage and to soften skin.

Warnings: For external use only. Avoid contact with eyes.

How Supplied: SPF #15 4 oz. and 10 oz.

Extra Strength
VASELINE® INTENSIVE CARE
Lotion

Active Ingredients: Glycerin, petrolatum, zinc oxide.

Inactive Ingredients: Water, stearic acid, C11–13 isoparaffin, glycol stearate, mineral oil, triethanolamine, cetyl acid, glyceryl stearate, magnesium aluminum silicate, dimethicone, deacetyl phosphate, cetyl alcohol, acetylated lanolin alcohol, fragrance, methylparaben, DMDM hydantoin, propylparaben, stearamide AMP, carbomer 934, disodium EDTA.

Indications: Extra Strength Vaseline Intensive Care Lotion is specially formulated to treat and prevent severe dry skin. Its clinically tested formula contains a unique blend of Vaseline Petroleum Jelly, glycerin, and silicone oil to treat rough, cracked, and irritated skin. Extra Strength Vaseline Intensive Care Lotion is clinically proven and is non-comedogenic.

Directions: Apply liberally to severely dry skin, particularly hands, elbows, and feet. Use to moisturize and treat skin after bathing/showering; under shaving cream, after shaving; overnight.

Warnings: For external use only. Avoid contact with eyes.

How Supplied: 4 oz., 6 oz., and 10 oz.

Church & Dwight Co., Inc.
469 N. HARRISON STREET
PRINCETON, NJ 08540

ARM & HAMMER®
Pure Baking Soda

Active Ingredient: Sodium Bicarbonate U.S.P.

Indications: For alleviation of acid indigestion, also known as heartburn or sour stomach. Not a remedy for other types of stomach complaints such as nausea, stomachache, abdominal cramps, gas pains, or stomach distention caused by overeating and/or overdrinking. In the latter case, one should not ingest solids, liquids or antacid but rather refrain from all physical activity and—if uncomfortable—call a physician.

Actions: ARM & HAMMER® Pure Baking Soda provides fast-acting, effective neutralization of stomach acids. Each level ½ teaspoon dose will neutralize 20.9 mEq of acid.

Warnings: Except under the advice and supervision of a physician: (1) do not administer to children under five years of age, (2) do not take more than eight level ½ teaspoons per person up to 60 years old or four level ½ teaspoons per person 60 years or older in a 24-hour period, (3) do not use this product if you are on a sodium restricted diet, (4) do not use the maximum dose for more than two weeks, (5) do not ingest food, liquid or any antacid when stomach is overly full to avoid possible injury to the stomach.

Dosage and Administration: Level ½ teaspoon in ½ glass (4 fl. oz.) of water every two hours up to maximum dosage or as directed by a physician. Accurately measure level ½ teaspoon. Each level ½ teaspoon contains 20.9 mEq (.476 gm) sodium.

How Supplied: Available in 8 oz., 16 oz., 32 oz., and 64 oz. boxes.

Products are indexed by
generic and chemical names in the
YELLOW SECTION.

CIBA Consumer Pharmaceuticals
Division of CIBA-GEIGY
Corporation
MACK WOODBRIDGE II
WOODBRIDGE, NJ 07095

ACUTRIM® 16 HOUR*
STEADY CONTROL
APPETITE SUPPRESSANT
TABLETS
Caffeine Free

ACUTRIM® II—MAXIMUM STRENGTH
APPETITE SUPPRESSANT
TABLETS
Caffeine Free

ACUTRIM LATE DAY®
STRENGTH*
APPETITE SUPPRESSANT
TABLETS
Caffeine Free

Description:
ACUTRIM® tablets deliver their maximum strength dosage of appetite suppressant at a precisely controlled, even rate.
This steady release is scientifically targeted to effectively distribute the appetite suppressant all day.
ACUTRIM makes it easier to follow the kind of reduced calorie diet needed for best weight control results.
A diet plan developed by an expert dietitian is included in the package for your personal use as a further aid.

Formula: Each ACUTRIM® tablet contains: Active Ingredient— phenylpropanolamine HCl 75 mg (appetite suppressant).
Inactive Ingredients—ACUTRIM® 16 HOUR Steady Control: Cellulose Acetate, Hydroxypropyl Methylcellulose, Stearic Acid—ACUTRIM® II MAXIMUM STRENGTH: Cellulose Acetate, D&C Yellow #10, FD&C Blue #1, FD&C Yellow #6, Hydroxypropyl Methylcellulose, Povidone, Propylene Glycol, Stearic Acid, Titanium Dioxide—ACUTRIM LATE DAY® Strength: Cellulose Acetate, FD&C Yellow #6, Hydroxypropyl Methylcellulose, Isopropyl Alcohol, Propylene Glycol, Riboflavin, Stearic Acid, Titanium Dioxide.

Dosage: For best results, take one tablet daily directly after breakfast. Do not take more than one tablet every 24 hours. Recommended dosage may be used up to three months.

Caution: Do not give this product to children under 12. Do not exceed recommended dosage. If nervousness, dizziness, or sleeplessness occurs, stop taking this medication and consult your physician. If you are being treated for high blood pressure or depression, or have heart disease, diabetes, or thyroid disease, do not take this product, except under the supervision of a physician. If you are taking a cough/cold allergy medication containing any form of phenylpropanolamine, do not take this product.

Warning: As with any drug, if you are pregnant or nursing a baby, seek the advice of a health professional before using this product.
KEEP THIS AND ALL MEDICATION OUT OF THE REACH OF CHILDREN. In case of accidental overdose, seek professional assistance or contact a poison control center immediately.

Drug Interaction Precaution: If you are taking any prescription drugs, or any type of nasal decongestant, antihypertensive or antidepressant drug, do not take this product, except under the supervision of a physician.

How Supplied: Tamper-evident blister packages of 20 and 40 tablets. Do not use if individual seals are broken.
DO NOT STORE ABOVE 86°F PROTECT FROM MOISTURE
12/86
Shown in Product Identification Section, page 407

EXTRA STRENGTH DOAN'S®
Analgesic Caplets

Indications: For temporary relief of occasional minor backache.

Directions: Adults—Two caplets 3 or 4 times daily, not to exceed 8 caplets during a 24-hour period or as directed by a physician. Not intended for use by children or teenagers except under the advice of a physician. If pain persists for more than 10 days, discontinue use and consult your physician.

Warning: Children and teenagers should not use this medicine for chicken pox or flu symptoms before a doctor is consulted about Reye's syndrome, a rare but serious illness. As with any drug, if you are pregnant or nursing a baby, seek the advice of a health professional before using this product. Do not use this product if you are under medical care or are allergic to aspirin or salicylates, except under the advice and supervision of your physician. **Keep this and all medicines out of the reach of children.** In case of accidental overdose, seek professional assistance or consult a Poison Control Center immediately.

Active Ingredient: Each caplet contains Magnesium Salicylate 500 mg. **Also Contains:** Hydroxypropyl methylcellulose, magnesium stearate, microcrystalline cellulose, polyethylene glycol, polysorbate 80, propylene glycol, stearic acid and titanium dioxide.

How Supplied: Tamper-evident blister packages of 24 and 48 caplets. Do not use if individual seals are broken. Store at 15°–30°C (59°–86°F). Protect from moisture.
Shown in Product Identification Section, page 407

Extra Strength
DOAN'S® P.M.
Magnesium Salicylate/ Diphenhydramine
Analgesic/Sleep Aid Caplets

Active Ingredients: Magnesium salicylate USP 500 mg, and Diphenhydramine HCl 25 mg. Also contains: Colloidal silicon dioxide, dibasic calcium phosphate, croscarmellose sodium, lactose, microcrystalline cellulose, magnesium stearate, stearic acid, Opadry blue color, Opadry clear.

Indications: For temporary relief of occasional minor back pain accompanied by sleeplessness.

Directions: Adults: Take 2 caplets at bedtime if needed, or as directed by a doctor.

Warnings: KEEP THIS AND ALL OTHER MEDICATIONS OUT OF THE REACH OF CHILDREN. IN CASE OF ACCIDENTAL OVERDOSE, SEEK PROFESSIONAL ASSISTANCE OR CONTACT A POISON CONTROL CENTER IMMEDIATELY. DO NOT GIVE THIS PRODUCT TO CHILDREN UNDER 12 YEARS OF AGE. As with any drug, if you are pregnant or nursing a baby, seek the advice of a health professional before using this product. If pain or sleeplessness persist continuously for more than 2 weeks, consult your doctor. Insomnia may be a symptom of a serious underlying medical illness. Do not take this product if you have asthma, glaucoma, emphysema, chronic pulmonary disease, shortness of breath, difficulty in breathing, or difficulty in urination due to enlargement of the prostate gland, or if you are allergic to aspirin or salicylates unless directed by a doctor. Avoid alcoholic beverages while taking this product. Do not take this product if you are taking sedatives or tranquilizers without first consulting your doctor. Children and teenagers should not use this medicine if chicken pox or flu symptoms exist before a doctor is consulted about Reye syndrome, a rare but serious disease.

How Supplied: Extra Strength Doan's P.M. is available in tamper resistant foil blister packages of 20 caplets. See back of blister pack and carton flap for lot number and expiration date. Store at room temperature. Protect from moisture.
NDC 0083-0245
Shown in Product Identification Section, page 407

REGULAR STRENGTH DOAN'S®
Analgesic Caplets

Indications: For temporary relief of occasional minor backache.

Continued on next page

The full prescribing information for each CIBA Consumer Pharmaceuticals product is contained herein and is that in effect as of December 1, 1991.

*Peak strength and duration claims relate solely to blood levels.

CIBA Consumer—Cont.

Directions: Adults—Two caplets every 4 hours as needed, not to exceed 12 caplets during a 24-hour period or as directed by a physician. Not intended for use by children or teenagers except under the advice of a physician. If pain persists for more than 10 days, discontinue use and consult your physician.

Warning: Children and teenagers should not use this medicine for chicken pox or flu symptoms before a doctor is consulted about Reye's syndrome, a rare but serious illness. As with any drug, if you are pregnant or nursing a baby, seek the advice of a health professional before using this product. Do not use this product if you are under medical care or are allergic to aspirin or salicylates, except under the advice and supervision of your physician. **Keep this and all medicines out of the reach of children.** In case of accidental overdose, seek professional assistance or consult a Poison Control Center immediately.

Active Ingredient: Each caplet contains Magnesium Salicylate 325 mg. **Also Contains:** Magnesium Stearate, Microcrystalline Cellulose, Opadry Olive Green, Polyethylene Glycol, Purified Water, Stearic Acid.

How Supplied: Tamper-evident blister packages of 24 and 48 caplets. Do not use if individual seals are broken. Store at 15°–30°C (59°–86°F). Protect from moisture.

Shown in Product Identification Section, page 407

DULCOLAX®
[dul'co-lax]
brand of bisacodyl USP
Tablets of 5 mg
Suppositories of 10 mg
Laxative

Ingredients: Each enteric coated tablet contains: Active: Bisacodyl USP 5 mg. Also contains: Acacia, acetylated monoglyceride, carnauba wax, cellulose acetate phthalate, corn starch, D&C Red No. 30 aluminum lake, D&C Yellow No. 10 aluminum lake, dibutyl phthalate, docusate sodium, gelatin, glycerin, iron oxides, kaolin, lactose, magnesium stearate, methylparaben, pharmaceutical glaze, polyethylene glycol, povidone, propylparaben, sodium benzoate, sorbitan monooleate, sucrose, talc, titanium dioxide, white wax.
Each suppository contains: Active: Bisacodyl USP 10 mg. Also contains: Hydrogenated vegetable oil.
SODIUM CONTENT: Tablets and suppositories contain less than 0.2 mg per dosage unit and are thus dietetically sodium free.

Indications: For the relief of occasional constipation and irregularity. Physicians should refer to the "Professional Labeling" section for additional indications and information.

Directions:
Tablets
Adults and children 12 years of age and over: Take 2 or 3 tablets (usually 2) in a single dose once daily.
Children 6 to under 12 years of age: Take 1 tablet once daily.
Children under 6 years of age: Consult a physician.
Expect results in 8–12 hours if taken at bedtime or within 6 hours if taken before breakfast.
Suppositories
Adults and children 12 years of age and over: 1 suppository once daily. Remove foil wrapper. Lie on your side and, with pointed end first, push suppository high into the rectum so it will not slip out. Retain it for 15 to 20 minutes. If you feel the suppository must come out immediately, it was not inserted high enough and should be pushed higher.
Children 6 to under 12 years of age: ½ suppository once daily.
Children under 6 years of age: Consult a physician.
If the suppository seems soft, hold in foil wrapper under cold water for one or two minutes. In the presence of anal fissures or hemorrhoids, suppository may be coated at the tip with petroleum jelly before insertion.

Warnings: Do not use laxative products when abdominal pain, nausea, or vomiting are present unless directed by a physician. Laxative products should not be used for a period longer than 1 week unless directed by a physician. Rectal bleeding or failure to have a bowel movement after use of a laxative may indicate a serious condition. If this occurs, discontinue use and consult your physician. As with any drug, if you are pregnant or nursing a baby, seek the advice of a health care professional before using this product. KEEP THIS AND ALL MEDICATION OUT OF THE REACH OF CHILDREN. In case of accidental overdose or ingestion, seek professional assistance or contact a poison control center immediately.
For tablets: Do not chew or crush. Do not give to children under 6 years of age unless directed by a physician. Do not take this product within 1 hour after taking an antacid or milk.

How Supplied: Dulcolax, brand of bisacodyl: Yellow, enteric-coated tablets of 5 mg in boxes of 10, 25, 50 and 100; suppositories of 10 mg in boxes of 4, 8, 16 and 50.
NDC 0083-6200 (tablets)
NDC 0083-6100 (suppositories)

Note: Store Dulcolax suppositories and tablets at temperatures below 77°F (25°C). Avoid excessive humidity.

Also Available: Dulcolax® Bowel Prep Kit. Each kit contains:
 1 Dulcolax suppository of 10 mg bisacodyl;
 4 Dulcolax tablets of 5 mg bisacodyl;
Complete patient instructions.

PROFESSIONAL LABELING:

Description and Clinical Pharmacology: Dulcolax is a contact stimulant laxative, administered either orally or rectally, which acts directly on the colonic mucosa to produce normal peristalsis throughout the large intestine. The active ingredient in Dulcolax, bisacodyl, is a colorless, tasteless compound that is practically insoluble in water or alkaline solution. Its chemical name is: bis(p-acetoxyphenyl)-2-pyridylmethane. Bisacodyl is very poorly absorbed, if at all, in the small intestine following oral administration, nor in the large intestine following rectal administration. On contact with the mucosa or submucosal plexi of the large intestine, bisacodyl stimulates sensory nerve endings to produce parasympathetic reflexes resulting in increased peristaltic contractions of the colon. It has also been shown to promote fluid and ion accumulation in the colon, which increases the laxative effect. A bowel movement is usually produced approximately 6 hours after oral administration (8–12 hours if taken at bedtime), and approximately 15 minutes to 1 hour after rectal administration, providing satisfactory cleansing of the bowel which may, under certain circumstances, obviate the need for colonic irrigation.

Indications and Usage: For use as part of a bowel cleansing regimen in preparing the patient for surgery or for preparing the colon for x-ray endoscopic examination. Dulcolax will not replace the colonic irrigations usually given patients before intracolonic surgery, but is useful in the preliminary emptying of the colon prior to these procedures.
Also for use as a laxative in postoperative care (i.e., restoration of normal bowel hygiene), antepartum care, postpartum care, and in preparation for delivery.

Contraindications: Stimulant laxatives, such as Dulcolax, are contraindicated for patients with acute surgical abdomen, appendicitis, rectal bleeding, or intestinal obstruction.

Precautions: Long-term administration of Dulcolax is not recommended in the treatment of chronic constipation.

Dosage and Administration:
Preparation for x-ray endoscopy: For barium enemas, no food should be given following oral administration to prevent reaccumulation of material in the cecum, and a suppository should be administered one to two hours prior to examination.
Children under 6 years of age: Oral administration is not recommended due to the requirement to swallow tablets whole. For rectal administration, the suppository dosage is 5 mg (½ of 10 mg suppository) in a single daily dose.

Shown in Product Identification Section, page 407

EUCALYPTAMINT®
100% All Natural Ointment
External Analgesic

Description: An all-natural, deep-penetrating topical analgesic that provides hours of soothing relief.

Active Ingredient: Natural Menthol (15%)

Inactive Ingredients: Lanolin and Eucalyptus Oil

Indications: For the temporary relief of minor aches and pains of muscles and joints associated with arthritis, backache, strains, bruises, and sprains.

Directions: Adults and children 2 years of age and older: Gently massage a conservative amount into affected area not more than 3 to 4 times daily. Children under 2 years of age: Consult a physician. For best results, gently massage ointment into affected area and loosely cover with a warm moist towel.

Warning: FOR EXTERNAL USE ONLY. Avoid contact with eyes. Do not apply to wounds or damaged skin. Do not bandage tightly. If condition worsens, or if symptoms persist for more than 7 days, discontinue use of this product and consult a physician. Keep this and all drugs out of the reach of children. In case of accidental ingestion, seek professional assistance or contact a Poison Control Center immediately.

How Supplied: Eucalyptamint is supplied in 2 oz. and 4 oz. bottles.
Shown in Product Identification Section, page 407

FIBERALL® Chewable Tablets
[fi'ber-all]
Lemon Creme Flavor

Description: Fiberall Chewable Tablets are a bulk-forming, nonirritant laxative which contain less than 1.5 grams of sugar per tablet. The active ingredient is calcium polycarbophil, a bulk-forming man-made fiber. The smooth gelatinous bulk formed by Fiberall Chewable Tablets encourages peristaltic activity and a more normal elimination of the bowel contents.
The recommended dose of one tablet contains the equivalent to 1 gram of polycarbophil.
Inactive Ingredients: Crospovidone, dextrose, flavors, magnesium stearate and yellow No. 10 aluminum lake. Each dose contains less than 1 mg of sodium, 225 mg of calcium and less than 6 calories.

Indications: Fiberall Chewable Tablets are indicated for the management of chronic constipation, temporary constipation caused by illness or pregnancy, irritable bowel syndrome, and for constipation related to duodenal ulcer or diverticulosis. Fiberall Chewable Tablets are also indicated for stool softening in patients with hemorrhoids or after anorectal surgery.

Actions: After the tablet is chewed it readily disperses and acts without irritants or stimulants. Polycarbophil absorbs water in the gastrointestinal tract to form a gelatinous bulk which encourages a more normal bowel movement.

Dosage and Administration: *Adults and children 12 years and older:* chew and swallow 1 tablet, 1–4 times a day. *Children 6 to under 12 years:* one-half the usual adult dose or as recommended by a physician. *Children under 6:* consult a physician. **Drink a full glass (8 fl oz) of liquid with each dose.** Drinking additional liquid helps Fiberall work even more effectively. Continued use for 2 to 3 days may be desired for maximum laxative benefits.

Contraindications: Fecal impaction or intestinal obstruction. Any disease state in which consumption of extra calcium is contraindicated.

Drug Interactions: This product contains calcium, which may interact with some forms of TETRACYCLINE if taken concomitantly. The tetracycline product should be taken 1 hour before or 2–3 hours after taking a Fiberall Chewable Tablet.

How Supplied: Boxes containing 18 tablets.

FIBERALL® Fiber Wafers
[fi'ber-all]
Fruit & Nut, Oatmeal Raisin

Description: Fiberall Fiber Wafers are a bulk-forming, nonirritant laxative. The active ingredient is psyllium hydrophilic mucilloid, a dietary fiber extracted from the seed husk of blond psyllium seed *(Plantago ovata)*. The smooth gelatinous bulk formed by Fiberall Wafers encourages peristaltic activity and a more normal elimination of the bowel contents.
One (1) Fiberall Fiber Wafer contains 3.4 g of psyllium hydrophilic mucilloid in a good-tasting wafer form, of which approximately 2.2 g is soluble fiber. One wafer is equivalent to one teaspoonful of Fiberall Powder.
Inactive Ingredients: Fruit & Nut Flavor: Baking powder, brown sugar, butter flavor, cinnamon, corn syrup, crisp rice, dried ground apricots, flour, glycerin, granulated sugar, granulated walnuts, lecithin, margarine, molasses, oats, salt, vegetable oil shortening (soybean and cottonseed oil), water and wheat bran. Fiberall Fruit & Nut Fiber Wafers contain approximately 79 calories and 110 mg of sodium per wafer.
Oatmeal Raisin Flavor: Baking powder, cinnamon, cinnamon flavor, cloves, corn syrup, flour, glycerin, granulated sugar, lecithin, molasses, oats, raisins, vegetable oil shortening (soybean and cottonseed oil), water and wheat bran. Fiberall Oatmeal Raisin Fiber Wafers contain approximately 78 calories and 30 mg of sodium per wafer.

Indications: Fiberall Fiber Wafers are indicated for the management of chronic constipation, temporary constipation caused by illness or pregnancy, irritable bowel syndrome, and for constipation related to duodenal ulcer or diverticulosis. Fiberall Wafers are also indicated for stool softening in patients with hemorrhoids or after anorectal surgery.

Actions: The homogenous high-fiber formula of Fiberall Fiber Wafers, eaten with 8 oz of a beverage of the patient's choice, acts without irritants or stimulants in the gastrointestinal tract.

Dosage and Administration: The recommended dosage for adults is one to two Fiberall Fiber Wafers 1 to 3 times daily, with a full 8 oz glass of water or other liquid with each wafer. The recommended daily dose for children 6 to under 12 years old is one-half the usual adult dose (with liquid), or as recommended by a physician. For children under 6, consult a physician. Drinking additional liquid is recommended and helps Fiberall work even more effectively. Two to three days' usage may be required for optimal laxative benefits.

Contraindications: Fecal impaction or intestinal obstruction.

Precaution: As with any grain product, inhaled or ingested psyllium powder may cause an allergic reaction in individuals sensitive to it.

How Supplied: Boxes containing 14 wafers.
Shown in Product Identification Section, page 407

FIBERALL® Powder, Orange or Natural Flavor
[fi'ber-all]

Description: Fiberall is a bulk-forming, nonirritant laxative which contains no sugar. The active ingredient is psyllium hydrophilic mucilloid, a dietary fiber extracted from the seed husk of blond psyllium seed *(Plantago ovata)*. The smooth gelatinous bulk formed by Fiberall encourages peristaltic activity and a more normal elimination of the bowel contents.
The recommended dose contains 3.4 g psyllium hydrophilic mucilloid, of which approximately 2.2 g is soluble fiber.

Inactive Ingredients: <u>Natural</u> <u>Flavor</u>: Citric acid, flavor, polysorbate 60 and wheat bran. <u>Orange</u> <u>Flavor</u>: Beta-carotene, citric acid, flavor, polysorbate 60, saccharin, wheat bran and yellow No. 6 lake. Each dose contains less than 10 mg of sodium, less than 60 mg of potassium,

Continued on next page

The full prescribing information for each CIBA Consumer Pharmaceuticals product is contained herein and is that in effect as of December 1, 1991.

CIBA Consumer—Cont.

and provides less than 6 calories (10 calories for Orange).

Indications: Fiberall is indicated for the management of chronic constipation, temporary constipation caused by illness or pregnancy, irritable bowel syndrome, and for constipation related to duodenal ulcer or diverticulosis. Fiberall is also indicated for stool softening in patients with hemorrhoids or after anorectal surgery.

Actions: The homogenous, high-fiber formula of Fiberall is readily dispersed in liquids and acts without irritants or stimulants in the gastro-intestinal tract.

Dosage and Administration:
Adults: Natural: Place one scoopful filled to the line (5 g) or one slightly rounded teaspoonful in a glass and add 8 oz. of cool water or other liquid. Stir to mix. Orange: Place one level scoopful (5.9 g) or one rounded teaspoonful in glass and add liquid as above. Take orally one to three times daily according to individual response.
Children 6 to under 12 years old: One-half the usual adult dose (with liquid) or as recommended by a physician. Drinking additional liquid is recommended and helps Fiberall work even more effectively. Two to three days' usage may be required for maximum laxative benefits. **New Users:** Start by taking 1 dose each day. Gradually increase to 3 doses per day if needed or recommended by doctor. If minor gas or bloating occurs, reduce the amount taken until system adjusts.

Contraindications: Fecal impaction or intestinal obstruction.

Precaution: As with any grain product, inhaled or ingested psyllium powder may cause an allergic reaction in individuals sensitive to it.

How Supplied: Powder, in 10 or 15 oz containers.
Shown in Product Identification Section, page 407

NŌSTRIL® Nasal Decongestant
[nō'stril]
phenylephrine HCl, USP

Active Ingredient: phenylephrine HCl 0.25% (¼% Mild strength) or phenylephrine HCl 0.5% (½% Regular strength). Also contains benzalkonium chloride 0.004% as a preservative, boric acid, sodium borate, water.

Indications: For temporary relief of nasal congestion due to the common cold, hay fever, other upper respiratory allergies, or associated with sinusitis.

Actions: NŌSTRIL metered pump spray for nasal decongestion delivers measured, uniform doses. The medication constricts the smaller arterioles of the nasal passages, producing a gentle, predictable, decongestant effect. Nōstril penetrates and shrinks swollen membranes, restoring freer breathing and

unclogs sinus passages, bringing the effective medication in contact with inflamed, swollen tissues. It will not hurt tender membranes since it is formulated to match the pH of normal nasal secretions. The one-way pump helps prevent draw-back contamination of the medication.

Warnings: Do not exceed recommended dosage because burning, stinging, sneezing, or increased nasal discharge may occur. Do not use for more than 3 days. If symptoms persist, consult a physician. Use of the dispenser by more than one person may spread infection. Do not use this product if you have heart disease, high blood pressure, thyroid disease, diabetes or difficulty in urination due to enlargement of the prostate gland, unless directed by a physician. Keep this and all drugs out of reach of children.

Symptoms and Treatment of Oral Overdosage: In case of accidental ingestion, seek professional assistance or consult a poison control center immediately.

Dosage and Administration:
¼% Mild—Adults and children 6 to under 12 years of age (with adult supervision): 2 or 3 sprays in each nostril not more often than every 4 hours. Children under 6 years of age: consult a doctor.
½% Regular—Adults: 2 or 3 sprays in each nostril not more often than every 4 hours. Do not give to children under 12 years of age unless directed by a doctor. Remove protective cap. Hold bottle with thumb at base and nozzle between first and second fingers. With head upright, insert nozzle into nostril. Depress pump 2 or 3 times, all the way down, and sniff deeply. Repeat in other nostril. Before using the first time, prime pump by depressing it firmly several times.

How Supplied: Metered nasal pump spray in white plastic bottles of ½ fl. oz. (15 ml) packaged in tamper-resistant outer cartons.
0.25% (¼% Mild strength) for children 6 years and over and adults who prefer a milder decongestant (NDC 0597-0083-85).
0.5% (½% Regular strength) for adults and children 12 years or older (NDC 0597-0084-85).
Shown in Product Identification Section, page 407

NŌSTRILLA® Long Acting
[nō-stril'a]
Nasal Decongestant
oxymetazoline HCl, USP

Active Ingredient: oxymetazoline HCl 0.05%. Also contains benzalkonium chloride 0.02% as a preservative, glycine, sorbitol solution, water. (Mercury preservatives are not used in this product.)

Indications: For temporary relief of nasal congestion due to the common cold, hay fever, other upper respiratory allergies, or associated with sinusitis.

Actions: NŌSTRILLA metered pump spray for nasal decongestion delivers measured, uniform doses. The medication constricts the smaller arterioles of the nasal passages, producing a prolonged (up to 12 hours), gentle, predictable, decongestant effect. Nōstrilla penetrates and shrinks swollen membranes, restoring freer breathing and unclogs sinus passages, bringing the effective medication in contact with inflamed, swollen tissues. It will not hurt tender membranes since it is formulated to match the pH of normal nasal secretions. Use at bedtime restores freer nasal breathing through the night. The one-way pump helps prevent draw-back contamination of the medication.

Warnings: Do not exceed recommended dosage because burning, stinging, sneezing or increased nasal discharge may occur. Do not use for more than 3 days. If symptoms persist, consult a physician. Use of the dispenser by more than one person may spread infection. Do not use this product if you have heart disease, high blood pressure, thyroid disease, diabetes or difficulty in urination due to enlargement of the prostate gland unless directed by a doctor. Keep this and all drugs out of reach of children.

Symptoms and Treatment of Oral Overdosage: In case of accidental ingestion, seek professional assistance or contact a poison control center immediately.

Dosage and Administration: Adults and children 6 to under 12 years of age (with adult supervision): 2 or 3 sprays in each nostril not more often than every 10 to 12 hours. Do not exceed 2 applications in any 24-hour period. Children under 6 years of age: consult a doctor. Remove protective cap. Hold bottle with thumb at base and nozzle between first and second fingers. With head upright, insert nozzle into nostril. Depress pump 2 or 3 times, all the way down, and sniff deeply. Repeat in other nostril. Before using the first time, prime pump by depressing it firmly several times.

How Supplied: Metered nasal pump spray in white plastic bottles of ½ fl. oz. (15 ml) packaged in tamper-resistant outer cartons (NDC 0597-0085-85).
Shown in Product Identification Section, page 407

NUPERCAINAL®
Dibucaine
Hemorrhoidal and Anesthetic
Ointment

Active Ingredient: 1% dibucaine USP. Also contains: acetone sodium bisulfite, lanolin, light mineral oil, purified water, and white petrolatum.

Indications: For prompt, temporary relief of pain, itching and burning due to hemorrhoids or other anorectal disorders. May also be used topically for temporary relief of pain and itching associated with sunburn, minor burns, cuts, scrapes, insect bites, or minor skin irritation.

Directions: Adults: When practical, cleanse the affected area with mild soap and water and rinse thoroughly. Gently dry by patting or blotting with toilet tissue or a soft cloth before application of this product. Apply externally to the affected area up to 3 or 4 times daily. Children 2–12: Do not use except under the advice and supervision of a physician. DO NOT USE IN INFANTS UNDER 2 YEARS OF AGE OR LESS THAN 35 LBS. WEIGHT.

Warnings: IF SWALLOWED, CONSULT A PHYSICIAN OR POISON CONTROL CENTER IMMEDIATELY. **Do not use in or near the eyes.** If condition worsens or does not improve within 7 days, consult a physician. Do not put this product into the rectum by using fingers or any mechanical device. Do not exceed recommended daily dosage unless directed by a physician. Certain persons can develop allergic reactions to ingredients in this product. If the symptom being treated does not subside or if redness, irritation, swelling, pain, bleeding or other symptoms develop or increase, discontinue use and consult a physician promptly. As with any drug, if you are pregnant or nursing a baby, seek the advice of a health care professional before using this product. KEEP THIS AND ALL MEDICATION OUT OF REACH OF CHILDREN.

How Supplied: Nupercainal Hemorrhoidal and Anesthetic Ointment is available in tamper-evident packaged tubes of 1 and 2 ounces. See crimp of tube for lot number and expiration date. Store between 59–86°. NDC 0083-5812.

Shown in Product Identification Section, page 408

NUPERCAINAL®
Pain Relief Cream

Active Ingredient: 0.5% dibucaine USP.
Also contains: acetone sodium bisulfite, fragrance, glycerin, potassium hydroxide, purified water, stearic acid, and trolamine.

Indications: For prompt, temporary relief of pain and itching due to sunburn, minor burns, cuts, scrapes, scratches, and nonpoisonous insect bites.

Directions: Apply to affected area, rub in gently. **Do not use in or near eyes.**

Caution: IF SWALLOWED, CONSULT A PHYSICIAN OR POISON CONTROL CENTER IMMEDIATELY. Not for prolonged use. Not more than ⅔ tube should be applied in 24 hours for adults or ⅙ tube to a child. If the symptom being treated does not subside or rash, irritation, swelling, pain, or other symptoms develop or increase, discontinue use and consult a physician.

How Supplied: Nupercainal Pain-Relief Cream is available in tamper-evident

packaged tubes of 1½ ounces. See crimp of tube for lot number and expiration date. NDC 0083-5830-91.

Shown in Product Identification Section, page 408

NUPERCAINAL®
Suppositories

Indications: Nupercainal Rectal Suppositories give temporary relief of itching, burning, and discomfort associated with hemorrhoids or other anorectal disorders.
Each suppository contains 2.1 gram cocoa butter and .25 gram zinc oxide. Also contains acetone sodium bisulfite and bismuth subgallate.

Directions: ADULTS—When practical, cleanse the affected area. Tear one suppository at the "V" cut, peel foil downward and remove foil wrapper before inserting into the rectum. Gently insert the suppository rectally, rounded end first. Use one suppository up to 6 times daily or after each bowel movement. CHILDREN UNDER 12 YEARS OF AGE—Consult a physician.

WARNING: IF ACCIDENTALLY SWALLOWED, CONSULT A PHYSICIAN OR POISON CONTROL CENTER IMMEDIATELY.
If condition worsens or does not improve within 7 days, consult a physician. Do not exceed the recommended daily dosage unless directed by a physician. In case of bleeding consult a physician promptly. As with any drug, if you are pregnant or nursing a baby, seek the advice of a health professional before using this product.
Keep this and all medications out of reach of children.
Nupercainal Suppositories are available in tamper-evident packages of 12 and 24. Do not store above 86 °F.

C86-42 (Rev. 9/86)
Shown in Product Identification Section, page 408

OTRIVIN®
xylometazoline hydrochloride USP
Nasal Spray and Nasal Drops 0.1%
Pediatric Nasal Drops 0.05%
Nasal Decongestant

One application provides rapid and long-lasting relief of nasal congestion for up to 10 hours.
Quickly clears stuffy noses due to common cold, sinusitis, hay fever.
Nasal congestion can make life miserable—you can't breathe, smell, taste, or sleep comfortably. That is why Otrivin is so helpful. It clears away that stuffy feeling.
Otrivin has been prescribed by doctors for many years. Here is how you use it:
Nasal Spray 0.1%—for adults and children 12 years and older. Spray 2 or 3 times into each nostril every 8–10 hours. With head upright, squeeze sharply and firmly while inhaling (sniffing) through the nose. For adult use only.

Nasal Drops 0.1%—for adults and children 12 years and older. Put 2 or 3 drops into each nostril every 8 to 10 hours. Tilt head as far back as possible. Immediately bend head forward toward knees, hold for a few seconds, then return to upright position.
Do not give Nasal Spray 0.1% or Nasal Drops 0.1% to children under 12 years except under the advice and supervision of a physician.
Pediatric Nasal Drops 0.05%—for children 2 to 12 years of age. Put 2 or 3 drops into each nostril every 8 to 10 hours. Tilt head as far back as possible. Immediately bend head forward toward knees, hold a few seconds, then return to upright position.
Do not give this product to children under 2 years except under the advice and supervision of a physician.
Otrivin Nasal Spray/Nasal Drops contain 0.1% xylometazoline hydrochloride, USP. Also contains benzalkonium chloride, dibasic sodium phosphate, disodium edetate, monobasic sodium phosphate, purified water and sodium chloride. They are available in an unbreakable plastic spray package of 0.66 fl oz (20 ml) and in a plastic dropper bottle of 0.83 fl oz (25 ml).

Otrivin Pediatric Nasal Drops contain 0.05% xylometazoline hydrochloride, USP. Also contains benzalkonium chloride, dibasic sodium phosphate, disodium edetate, monobasic sodium phosphate, purified water and sodium chloride. It is available in a plastic dropper bottle of 0.83 fl oz (25 ml).

Warnings: Do not exceed recommended dosage, because symptoms such as burning, stinging, sneezing, or increase of nasal discharge may occur. Do not use this product for more than 3 days. If symptoms persist, consult a physician. The use of this dispenser by more than one person may cause infection.

Keep this and all medicines out of the reach of children. Overdosage in young children may cause marked sedation. In case of accidental ingestion, seek professional assistance or contact a Poison Control Center immediately.

Caution: Do not use if the clear overwrap with the name Otrivin® or the printed band on the bottle is missing or damaged.
Store between 59°–86°F.
Shown in Product Identification Section, page 408

Continued on next page

The full prescribing information for each CIBA Consumer Pharmaceuticals product is contained herein and is that in effect as of December 1, 1991.

CIBA Consumer—Cont.

PRIVINE®
naphazoline hydrochloride, USP
0.05% Nasal Solution
0.05% Nasal Spray
Nasal Decongestant

Privine is a nasal decongestant that comes in three forms: Nasal Drops (in a bottle with a dropper), Nasal Spray (in a plastic squeeze bottle) and Nasal Solution (in a 16 fl oz bottle). All are for prompt, and prolonged relief of nasal congestion due to common colds, sinusitis, hay fever, etc.

Privine is an effective nasal decongestant **when you use it in the recommended dosage.** If you use too much, too long, or too often, Privine may be harmful to your nasal mucous membranes and cause burning, stinging, sneezing or an increased runny nose. Do not use Privine by mouth.

IF NASAL STUFFINESS PERSISTS AFTER 3 DAYS OF TREATMENT, DISCONTINUE USE AND CONSULT A DOCTOR.

Keep this and all medications out of the reach of children. Do not use Privine in children under 12 years of age, except with the advice and supervision of a doctor.

Caution: Do not use Privine if you have glaucoma.

OVERDOSAGE IN YOUNG CHILDREN MAY CAUSE MARKED SEDATION AND IF SEVERE, EMERGENCY TREATMENT MAY BE NECESSARY. IN CASE OF ACCIDENTAL INGESTION, SEEK PROFESSIONAL ASSISTANCE OR CONTACT A POISON CONTROL CENTER IMMEDIATELY.

How to use Nasal Drops.
Use only 1 to 2 drops in each nostril. Do not repeat this dosage more than every 6 hours. Squeeze rubber bulb to fill dropper with proper amount of medication. For best results, tilt head as far back as possible and put 1 to 2 drops of solution into your right nostril. Then lean head forward, inhaling and turning your head to the left. Refill dropper by squeezing bulb. Now tilt head as far back as possible and put 1 to 2 drops of solution into your left nostril. Then lean head forward, inhaling, and turning your head to the right.

The Privine dropper bottle is designed to make administration of the proper dosage easy. Privine will not cause sleeplessness, so you may use it before going to bed.

Important: After use, be sure to rinse the dropper with very hot water. This helps prevent contamination of the bottle with bacteria from nasal secretions. Use of the dispenser by more than one person may spread infection.

Note: Privine Nasal Solution may be used on contact with glass, plastic, stainless steel and specially treated metals used in atomizers. Do not let the solution come in contact with reactive metals, especially aluminum. If solution becomes discolored, it should be discarded.

How to use Nasal Spray.
Spray 1 or 2 times in each nostril, not more often than every 6 hours. Avoid overdosage. Follow directions for use carefully. For best results do **not** shake the plastic squeeze bottle.

Remove cap. With head held upright, spray twice into each nostril. Squeeze the bottle sharply and firmly while sniffing through the nose.

Privine Nasal Drops contain 0.05% naphazoline HCl, USP. It also contains benzalkonium chloride, dibasic sodium phosphate, disodium edetate, monobasic sodium phosphate, purified water and sodium chloride.

Privine Nasal Solution contains 0.05% naphazoline hydrochloride, USP. It also contains benzalkonium chloride, disodium edetate dihydrate, hydrochloric acid, purified water, sodium chloride, and trolamine. It is available in bottles of 16 fl. oz. (473 ml).

Privine Nasal Spray contains 0.05% naphazoline hydrochloride USP. It also contains benzalkonium chloride, dibasic sodium phosphate, disodium edetate, monobasic sodium phosphate, purified water, and sodium chloride. It is available in plastic squeeze bottles of 0.66 fl oz (20 ml).

Caution: Do not use if the clear overwrap on the box with the name Privine® or the printed band on the bottle is missing or damaged.

Store the nasal drops, nasal solution and nasal spray between 59°–86°F.

Shown in Product Identification Section, page 408

Q–VEL®
Muscle Relaxant Pain Reliever

Active Ingredient: Quinine Sulfate 1 gr. (64.8 mg).

Contains: Vitamin E (400 I.U. *dl*-alpha tocopheryl acetate) in a lecithin base.

Indications: For prevention and temporary relief of night leg cramps.

Warnings: Do not take if pregnant, nursing a baby or of childbearing potential, if sensitive to quinine, or under 12 years of age. Discontinue use and consult your physician if ringing in the ears, deafness, diarrhea, nausea, skin rash, bruising or visual disturbances occur. In case of accidental overdose, seek medical assistance or contact Poison Control Center at once. Keep this and all medicine out of reach of children.

Dosage: To prevent night leg cramps take 2 soft caplets after the evening meal plus 2 at bedtime. For relief in case of sudden attack, take 2 soft caplets at once plus 2 after ½ hour if needed. Do not exceed 4 soft caplets daily.

How Supplied: Bottles of 16, 30 and 50 softgels.
Store at 15°–30°C (59°–86°F) and protect from moisture.
Shown in Product Identification Section, page 408

SLOW FE®
Slow Release Iron Tablets

Description: SLOW FE supplies ferrous sulfate for the treatment of iron deficiency and iron deficiency anemia with a significant reduction in the incidence of the common side effects of oral iron preparations. The wax matrix delivery system of SLOW FE is designed to maximize the release of ferrous sulfate in the duodenum and the jejunum where it is best tolerated and absorbed. SLOW FE has been clinically shown to be associated with a lower incidence of constipation, diarrhea and abdominal discomfort when compared to regular iron tablets and the leading capsule.

Formula: Each tablet contains 160 mg. dried ferrous sulfate USP, equivalent to 50 mg. elemental iron. Also contains cetostearyl alcohol, colloidal silicon dioxide, hydroxypropyl methylcellulose, shellac, lactose, magnesium stearate, polyethylene glycol.

Dosage: ADULTS—one or two tablets daily or as recommended by a physician. A maximum of four tablets daily may be taken. CHILDREN—one tablet daily. Tablets must be swallowed whole.

Warning: The treatment of any anemic condition should be on the advice and under the supervision of a physician. As oral iron products interfere with absorption of oral tetracycline antibiotics, these products should not be taken within two hours of each other. As with any drug, if you are pregnant or nursing a baby, seek the advice of a health professional before using this product.

Keep this and all medicines out of reach of children. In case of accidental overdose, contact your physician or poison control center immediately.
Tamper-Evident Packaging.

How Supplied: Blister packages of 30, 60 and bottles of 100. Do Not Store Above 86°F. Protect From Moisture.
Shown in Product Identification Section, page 408

SUNKIST CHILDREN'S CHEWABLE MULTIVITAMINS—REGULAR

Vitamin Ingredients: Each tablet contains:
[See table on top of next page.]

Indication: Dietary supplementation.

Dosage and Administration: One chewable tablet daily for children two years and older.

Warning: Phenylketonurics: Contains Phenylalanine

How Supplied: SUNKIST Children's Multivitamins-Regular are supplied in bottles of 60 chewable tablets with child resistant caps.
Shown in Product Identification Section, page 408

VITAMINS	QUANTITY PER TABLET	PERCENT U.S. RDA	
		FOR CHILD. 2 TO 4 YRS OF AGE (1 TABLET)	FOR ADULTS & CHILD. OVER 4 YRS OF AGE (1 TABLET)
Vitamin A (as Palmitate + Beta Carotene)	2500 IU	100	50
Vitamin D-3	400 IU	100	100
Vitamin E	15 IU	150	50
Vitamin C	60 mg	150	100
Folic Acid	0.3 mg	150	75
Niacinamide	13.5 mg	150	68
Vitamin B-6	1.05 mg	150	53
Vitamin B-12	4.5 mcg	150	75
Vitamin B-1	1.05 mg	150	70
Vitamin B-2	1.20 mg	150	71
Vitamin K-1	5 mcg	*	*

*Recognized as essential in human nutrition, but no U.S. RDA established.

SUNKIST CHILDREN'S CHEWABLE MULTIVITAMINS—PLUS EXTRA C

Vitamin Ingredients: Each tablet contains the ingredients of the Regular vitamin product plus extra Vitamin C (a total of 250 mg).

Indication: Dietary supplementation.

Dosage and Administration: One chewable tablet daily for adults and children two years and older.

Warning: Phenylketonurics: Contains Phenylalanine.

How Supplied: SUNKIST Children's Multivitamins Plus Extra C are supplied in bottles of 60 chewable tablets with child resistant caps.

Shown in Product Identification Section, page 408

SUNKIST CHILDREN'S CHEWABLE MULTIVITAMINS—PLUS IRON

Vitamin Ingredients: Each tablet contains the vitamins of the Regular product plus 15 mg of Iron.

Indication: Dietary supplementation.

Dosage and Administration: One chewable tablet daily for children two years and older.

Warning: Phenylketonurics: Contains Phenylalanine.

Precaution: Contains iron, which can be harmful in large doses. Close tightly and keep out of reach of children. In case of overdose, contact a physician or poison control center immediately.

How Supplied: SUNKIST Children's Multivitamins Plus Iron are supplied in bottles of 60 chewable tablets with child resistant caps.

Shown in Product Identification Section, page 408

SUNKIST CHILDREN'S CHEWABLE MULTIVITAMINS—COMPLETE

Vitamin Ingredients: Each tablet contains the following ingredients: [See table below.]

Indication: Dietary supplementation.

Dosage and Administration: Children ages 2 to 4 one-half chewable tablet daily; One chewable tablet daily for children four years and older.

Warning: Phenylketonurics: Contains Phenylalanine.

Precautions: Contains iron, which can be harmful in large doses. Close tightly and keep out of reach of children. In case of overdose, contact a physician or poison control center immediately.

How Supplied: SUNKIST Children's Multivitamins Complete are supplied in bottles of 60 chewable tablets with child resistant caps.

Shown in Product Identification Section, page 408

SUNKIST® VITAMIN C
Citrus Complex
Chewable Tablets
Easy to Swallow Caplets

Description: All Sunkist Vitamin C chewable tablets have a delicious orange flavor unlike any other Vitamin C tablet. Each 60 mg chewable tablet contains 100% of the U.S. RDA* of Vitamin C. Each 250 mg chewable tablet contains 417% of the U.S. RDA* of Vitamin C. Each 500 mg chewable tablet contains 833% of the U.S. RDA* of Vitamin C.

Each 500 mg easy to swallow caplet contains 833% of the U.S. RDA* of Vitamin C.

Sunkist Vitamin C chewable tablets and easy to swallow caplets do not contain artificial flavors, colors or preservatives.

*U.S. Recommended Daily Allowance for adults and children over 4 years of age.

Indication: Dietary supplement.

How Supplied: 60 mg Chewable Tablets—Rolls of 11.
250 mg and 500 mg Chewable Tablets—Bottles of 60.
500 mg Easy to Swallow Caplets—Bottles of 60.

Store in a cool dry place.

Sunkist® is a registered trademark of Sunkist Growers, Inc., Sherman Oaks, CA 91423.©

(12/86)

Shown in Product Identification Section, page 408

VITAMINS	QUANTITY PER TABLET	PERCENT U.S. RDA	
		FOR CHILD. 2 TO 4 YRS OF AGE (½ TABLET)	FOR ADULTS & CHILD. OVER 4 YRS OF AGE (1 TABLET)
Vitamin A (as Palmitate + Beta Carotene)	5000 IU	100	100
Vitamin D-3	400 IU	50	100
Vitamin E	30 IU	150	100
Vitamin C	60 mg	75	100
Folic Acid	0.4 mg	100	100
Biotin	40 mcg	13	13
Pantothenic Acid	10 mg	100	100
Niacinamide	20 mg	111	100
Vitamin B-6	2 mg	143	100
Vitamin B-12	6 mcg	100	100
Vitamin B-1	1.5 mg	107	100
Vitamin B-2	1.7 mg	106	100
Vitamin K-1	10 mcg	*	*
MINERALS			
Iron	18 mg	90	100
Magnesium	20 mg	5	5
Iodine	150 mcg	107	100
Zinc	10 mg	63	67
Manganese	1 mg	*	*
Calcium	100 mg	6	10
Phosphorus	78 mg	5	8
Copper	2 mg	100	100

*Recognized as essential in human nutrition, but no U.S. RDA established.

The full prescribing information for each CIBA Consumer Pharmaceuticals product is contained herein and is that in effect as of December 1, 1991.

Columbia Laboratories, Inc.
4000 HOLLYWOOD BLVD.
HOLLYWOOD, FL 33021

DIASORB®
[dī'ă-zorb]
Activated Nonfibrous Attapulgite Liquid and Tablets

Description: Diasorb relieves cramps and pain associated with diarrhea. It is available as a pleasant-tasting cola-flavored liquid and as easy-to-swallow tablets. Diasorb is safe for children.

Active Ingredient: Each liquid teaspoonful and tablet contains 750 mg activated nonfibrous attapulgite.

Inactive Ingredients: *Liquid*—Benzoic acid, citric acid, flavor, glycerin, magnesium aluminum silicate, methylparaben, polysorbate, propylene glycol, propylparaben, saccharin, sodium hypochlorite solution, sorbitol, xanthan gum, and water. *Tablet*—D&C Red No. 30 Al Lake, Gelatin, Hydroxypropyl Cellulose, Hydroxypropyl Methylcellulose, Magnesium Stearate, Pharmaceutical Shellac, Polyethylene Glycol, Povidone, Propylene Glycol, Sorbitol, Titanium Dioxide, and Water.

Directions for Use: Take the full recommended starting dose at the first sign of diarrhea, and repeat after each subsequent bowel movement. Do not exceed maximum recommended dose per day. Shake liquid well before using. **Swallow tablets with water. Do not chew.**

Caution: Do not use if foil seal around tablet is broken.

Warning: Do not use for more than 2 days or in the presence of fever or in infants or children under 3, unless directed by a physician. In case of accidental overdose, seek professional assistance or contact a poison control center immediately. **Store at room temperature (59° to 86° F) in a dry place. KEEP THIS AND ALL MEDICATIONS OUT OF THE REACH OF CHILDREN.**

Dosage: See Table for recommended dosage for acute diarrhea.

How Supplied: *Liquid*—In plastic bottles of 4 fl oz (120 mL).
Tablets—Packaged in blister packs of 24.
Shown in Product Identification Section, page 408

LEGATRIN®
[leg'a-trin]

Active Ingredient: Quinine Sulfate, 162.5 mg per tablet.

Other Ingredients: Calcium phosphate dibasic, cellulose, croscarmellose sodium, FD&C blue No. 2 aluminum lake, FD&C red No. 40 aluminum lake, gelatin, hydroxypropyl cellulose, hydroxypropyl methylcellulose, magnesium stearate, polyethylene glycol 400, silica, starch, stearic acid, titanium dioxide.

Indications: For relief of night leg cramps, muscle spasms, restless legs.

Warnings: Discontinue use and consult a physician immediately if swelling, bruising, skin rash, skin discoloration or bleeding occurs. These symptoms may indicate a serious condition. Discontinue use if ringing in the ears, deafness, diarrhea, nausea or visual disturbances occur. In case of accidental overdose, seek medical assistance or contact Poison Control Center immediately. Do not take if pregnant, nursing a baby, allergic or sensitive to quinine or under 12 years of age. Keep this and all medication out of reach of children.

Caution: Do not use if Legatrin printed foil seal is damaged or missing.

Dosage: When a leg cramp occurs, take two tablets at once. To help prevent future night leg cramp attacks, take two tablets two hours before bedtime. Do not exceed two tablets daily. Consult a physician if symptoms persist longer than ten days.

How Supplied: Blister packages of 30 and 50 tablets.
Shown in Product Identification Section, page 408

LEGATRIN® RUB
[leg'a-trin]

Description: An external topical analgesic gel that aids in prompt temporary relief of muscular soreness and pain associated with arthritis, backache, strains, bruises and sprains.

Ingredients: Menthol 4%, Benzocaine 2%, in a Gel Base containing Isopropyl Alcohol 44%, Carbomer 940, FDC Blue #1, Methylparaben, Potassium Chloride, Propylparaben, Propylene Glycol, Sodium Chloride, Thymol, Trolamine, Water Deionized.

Indications: An external coolant gel. Aids in prompt, temporary relief of muscular soreness and pain.

Directions: Clean skin of all other ointments, creams, sprays, or liniments. Apply one or two liberal applications of Legatrin Rub. May be used 3 to 4 times daily, may be used with wet towels or with ice packs. Legatrin Rub will not burn or blister. Non-greasy. No protective cover needed. **Children: Do not use on children under 2 years of age, except under the advice and supervision of physician.**

Warning: KEEP THIS AND ALL MEDICATIONS OUT OF REACH OF CHILDREN. In case of accidental ingestion, contact a physician immediately.
For external use only. Avoid contact with eyes and mucous membranes. Do not apply to wounds or damaged skin. If condition worsens, or if symptoms persist for more than 7 days, or clear up and occur again within a few days, discontinue use of this product and consult a physician. Do not bandage tightly. Do not store near heat or expose to an open flame.

How Supplied: Legatrin Rub is available in 8 oz. jars.
Shown in Product Identification Section, page 408

Copley Pharmaceutical Inc.
25 JOHN RD
CANTON, MA 02021

LICE·ENZ® FOAM
Shampoo Aerosol
Lice Killing Shampoo Kit

Description: Lice·Enz® Foam shampoo is supplied as a metered aerosol delivery system for ease of application to the patient for the treatment of lice infestation.

Active Ingredients: Pyrethrins 0.3%, Piperonyl Butoxide, 3.0%; inert ingredients, 96.7%.

Indications: Lice·Enz® is indicated for the treatment of human pediculosis—head lice, body lice, pubic lice and their eggs. Lice·Enz® is specially formulated for head lice in children. The mousse application allows complete control of the amount of pesticide the child is exposed to; no messy shampoo to drip onto the child. Lice·Enz® is user friendly and easy to apply.

Age	Initial Dose	Maximum Dose per 24 hours
Adults and children over 12 years	4 tsp or 4 Tablets	12 tsp or 12 Tablets
Children 6–12 years	2 tsp or 2 Tablets	6 tsp or 6 Tablets
Children 3–6 years	1 tsp or 1 Tablet	3 tsp or 3 Tablets
Infants and children under 3 years	Only as directed by a physician	

Actions: Lice·Enz® is a pediculicide for control of head lice, pubic lice and body lice and their nits.
SHOULD NOT BE USED BY RAGWEED-SENSITIZED PERSONS.
KEEP THIS AND ALL DRUGS OUT OF THE REACH OF CHILDREN.
CAUTIONS: For external use only. Harmful if swallowed. Do not inhale. Keep out of eyes and avoid contact with mucous membranes.

First Aid: In case this product should get in eyes, flush immediately with water. In case of infection or skin irritation, discontinue use and consult a physician. Consult a physician if infestation of eyebrows and eyelashes occur. Avoid contamination of food or foodstuffs. Use only as directed. Intentional misuse by deliberately concentrating and inhaling the contents can be harmful or fatal.

Physical or Chemical Hazard: Contents under pressure. Do not use or store near heat or open flame. Do not puncture or incinerate container. Exposure to temperatures above 120°F may cause bursting.

Storage: Store away from heat, sparks and open flame in original container and in an area inaccessible to children.

Disposal: Do not reuse empty container. Replace cap and discard container in trash. Do not incinerate or puncture.

Directions for Use: It is a violation of Federal Law to use this product in a manner inconsistent with its labeling. 1. Shake well. Apply as much LICE·ENZ® FOAM as needed to the hair and scalp or any other infested areas until entirely wet. Do not use on eyelashes or eyebrows. 2. Massage LICE·ENZ® FOAM into scalp and allow it to remain for no more than 10 minutes. 3. Wash hair thoroughly with warm water and shampoo or soap. 4. If desired, apply creme rinse to ease the nit removal process. 5. Comb hair with special no-nit comb to remove dead lice and eggs. 6. After combing, rinse hair thoroughly. 7. Repeat treatment in 7–10 days if reinfestation has occurred. 8. Do not exceed two consecutive applications within 24 hours. To help eliminate infestation, it is important to sterilize all clothing and bedding of infested person at time of treatment.
Note: The manufacturer of this product endorses the National Pediculosis Association's "No Nit Policy."

How Supplied: LICE·ENZ® FOAM aerosol is supplied in a 2-ounce aerosol container (ozone-friendly propellant).

Literature Available: Additional patient literature available upon request.
Shown in Product Identification Section, page 408

Del Pharmaceuticals Inc.
A Subsidiary of Del Laboratories, Inc.
163 E. BETHPAGE ROAD
PLAINVIEW, NY 11805

BABY ORAJEL®

Active Ingredients: *Baby Orajel:* Benzocaine 7.5%.
Inactive Ingredients: *Baby Orajel:* FD&C Red No. 40, flavor, glycerin, polyethylene glycols, sodium saccharin, sorbic acid, sorbitol.
Indications: Baby Orajel is a soothing, cherry-flavored product which quickly relieves teething pain.
Actions: Benzocaine is a topical, local anesthetic commonly used for pain, discomfort, or pruritis associated with wounds, mucous membranes and skin irritations.
Warnings: Do not use if tube tip is out prior to opening. As with all products containing benzocaine, localized allergic reactions may occur after prolonged or repeated use. Keep this and all medications out of reach of children.
Precaution: For persistent or excessive teething pain, consult your physician.
Dosage and Administration: Wash hands. Cut open tip of tube on score mark. For infants 4 months of age and older, apply a *small* amount with fingertip or cotton applicator on affected area no more than four times daily.
How Supplied: Baby Orajel: Gel in ⅓ oz (9.45 g) tube.
Shown in Product Identification Section, page 408

Maximum Strength ORAJEL®
[ōr ʹah-jel]

Active Ingredient: Benzocaine 20% in a special base.
Inactive Ingredients: Clove oil, flavors, polyethylene glycols, sodium saccharin, sorbic acid.
Indications: Maximum Strength Orajel is formulated to provide faster relief from toothache pain for hours.
Actions: Benzocaine is a topical, local anesthetic commonly used for pain, discomfort, or pruritis associated with wounds, mucous membranes and skin irritation.
Warnings: Keep this and all drugs out of the reach of children. Do not use if tube tip is cut prior to opening.
Precaution: This preparation is intended for use in cases of toothache only as a temporary expedient until a dentist can be consulted. Do not use continuously.
Directions: Cut open tip of tube on score mark. Squeeze a small quantity of Maximum Strength Orajel directly into cavity and around gum surrounding the teeth.

How Supplied: Gel in two sizes— ³⁄₁₆ oz (5.3 g) and ⅓ oz (9.45 g) tubes.
Shown in Product Identification Section, page 408

ORAJEL® Mouth-Aid®
[ōr ʹah-jel]

Active Ingredients: Benzocaine 20%, benzalkonium chloride 0.12%, zinc chloride 0.1% in a special emollient base.

Inactive Ingredients: Allantoin, flavor, polyethylene glycols, propyl gallate, propylene glycol, purified water, sodium saccharin, sorbic acid, trisodium EDTA.

Indications: Orajel Mouth-Aid combines a fast-acting maximum strength pain reliever, soothing ingredients which aid healing, a germicide and an astringent to help provide relief of minor mouth and lip irritations.

Actions: Benzocaine is a topical, local anesthetic commonly used for pain, discomfort, or pruritis associated with wounds, mucous membranes and skin irritations. Benzalkonium chloride is a rapidly acting surface disinfectant and detergent. Zinc chloride provides an astringent effect.

Warnings: Keep this and all medications out of reach of children. Do not use if tube tip is cut prior to opening.

Precaution: If condition persists, discontinue use and consult your physician or dentist. Not for prolonged use.

Directions: Cut open tip of tube on score mark. Apply directly to affected area as needed.

How Supplied: Gel in a ⅓ oz (9.45 g) tube.
Shown in Product Identification Section, page 408

PRONTO® Lice Killing Shampoo Kit

Active Ingredients: Pyrethrins 0.33%, piperonyl butoxide technical 4.00% [equivalent to 3.2% butylcarbityl (6-propylpiperonyl) ether and 0.80% related compounds].

Indications: One treatment pediculicide shampoo kills head, body and pubic lice on contact.

Actions: Pronto Lice Killing Shampoo contains the maximum strength of pyrethrins and piperonyl butoxide. Pyrethrins act directly on the nervous system of insects and piperonyl butoxide enhances the neurotoxic effect of pyrethrins by inhibiting the oxidative breakdown of the pyrethrins by the insect's detoxification system. This results in a longer amount of time which the pyrethrins may exert their toxic effect on the insect.

Warnings: May cause eye injury. Do not use near eyes or permit contact with eyes or nose. May cause skin irritation.

Continued on next page

Del Pharm.—Cont.

Wash thoroughly with soap and water after handling. If product should get into eyes, immediately flush with water. Follow directions carefully.

Not to be used by persons allergic to ragweed. Harmful if swallowed. In case of infection or skin irritation, discontinue use and consult a physician. In order to prevent reinfestation with lice, all clothing and bedding must be sterilized or treated concurrent with the application of this preparation. Do not exceed two consecutive applications within 24 hours.

Precaution: If in eyes, flush with plenty of water and get medical attention.

Directions for Use: It is a violation of Federal Law to use this product in a manner inconsistent with its labeling.

Instruct child to close eyes and cover eyes with clean wet towel. Apply Pronto Shampoo Concentrate cautiously to dry hair, scalp or any affected areas. Add a generous amount of water to work Pronto Shampoo Concentrate into a rich lather. Allow the shampoo to remain on area for 10 minutes, but no longer. Rinse treated areas thoroughly with warm water. Rinse eyes out with water following use. A fine-toothed comb (included) may be used to help remove dead lice and their eggs (nits) from hair. Handy applicator gloves are provided for convenience in applying the shampoo to avoid contact with lice.

Storage and Disposal: Do not reuse empty container. Rinse thoroughly. Securely wrap original container in several layers of newspaper and discard in waste container.

How Supplied: Shampoo in two sizes:
2 fl oz plastic bottle
4 fl oz plastic bottle
Shown in Product Identification Section, page 408

EDUCATIONAL MATERIAL

Teething Booklet From Baby Orajel®
Facts parents should know about tooth development and the teething process. Free to physicians, pharmacists and patients

Fact and Fallacy Booklet From Pronto®
Answers questions about head lice control.
Free to physicians, pharmacists and patients.

Products are indexed
by product category
in the
BLUE SECTION.

Fisons
Consumer Health
Division
Fisons Corporation
P.O. BOX 1212
ROCHESTER, NY 14603

ALLEREST® MAXIMUM STRENGTH TABLETS, NO DROWSINESS TABLETS, HEADACHE STRENGTH TABLETS, SINUS PAIN FORMULA TABLETS, CHILDREN'S CHEWABLE TABLETS AND 12 HOUR CAPLETS

Active Ingredients:
Maximum Strength Tablets—Chlorpheniramine maleate 2 mg, pseudoephedrine HCl 30 mg.
No Drowsiness Tablets—Acetaminophen 325 mg, pseudoephedrine HCl 30 mg.
Headache Strength Tablets—Acetaminophen 325 mg, chlorpheniramine maleate 2 mg, pseudoephedrine HCl 30 mg.
Sinus Pain Formula Tablets—Acetaminophen 500 mg, chlorpheniramine maleate 2 mg, pseudoephedrine HCl 30 mg.
Children's Chewable Tablets—Chlorpheniramine maleate 1 mg, phenylpropanolamine HCl 9.4 mg.
12 Hour Caplets—Chlorpheniramine maleate 12 mg, phenylpropanolamine HCl 75 mg.

Other Ingredients:
Maximum Strength Tablets—Blue 1 lake, dibasic calcium phosphate, magnesium stearate, microcrystalline cellulose, povidone, pregelatinized starch, sodium starch glycolate. *No Drowsiness and Headache Strength Tablets*—Magnesium stearate, microcrystalline cellulose, povidone, pregelatinized starch. *Sinus Pain Formula Tablets*—Magnesium stearate, microcrystalline cellulose, povidone, pregelatinized starch, sodium starch glycolate. *Children's Chewable ·Tablets*—Calcium stearate, citric acid, flavor, magnesium trisilicate, mannitol, saccharin sodium, sorbitol. *12 Hour Caplets*—Carnauba wax, colloidal silicon dioxide, lactose, methylcellulose, polyethylene glycol, povidone, Red 30, stearic acid, titanium dioxide, Yellow 6.

Indications: *Maximum Strength, Headache Strength, Sinus Pain Formula, Children's Chewable Tablets and 12 Hour Caplets*—Temporarily relieves nasal congestion, runny nose, sneezing, itching of the nose or throat, and itchy, watery eyes due to hay fever or other upper respiratory allergies; also *Headache Strength and Sinus Pain Formula Tablets*—For the temporary relief of minor aches, pains, and headache; also *12 Hour Caplets*—For temporary relief of nasal congestion due to the common cold and associated with sinusitis.
No Drowsiness Tablets—Temporarily relieves nasal congestion due to hay fever or other upper respiratory allergies. For the temporary relief of minor aches, pains, and headache.

Warnings: *All Products*—Do not exceed recommended dosage because at higher doses, nervousness, dizziness, or sleeplessness may occur. Do not take this product if you have heart disease, high blood pressure, thyroid disease, diabetes, or difficulty in urination due to enlargement of the prostate gland, unless directed by a physician. As with any drug, if you are pregnant or nursing a baby, seek the advice of a health professional before using this product. **Keep this and all drugs out of the reach of children.** In case of accidental overdose, seek professional assistance or contact a Poison Control Center immediately. Prompt medical attention is critical for adults as well as children even if you do not notice any signs or symptoms. And, *All Products Except No Drowsiness Tablets*—Do not take this product if you have asthma, glaucoma, emphysema, chronic pulmonary disease, shortness of breath, or difficulty in breathing unless directed by a physician. May cause excitability, especially in children. May cause drowsiness; alcohol, sedatives, and tranquilizers may increase the drowsiness effect. Avoid alcoholic beverages while taking this product. Do not take this product if you are taking sedatives or tranquilizers, without first consulting your physician. Use caution when driving a motor vehicle or operating machinery.
Maximum Strength Tablets, Children's Chewable Tablets and 12 Hour Caplets—Do not take this product for more than 7 days. If symptoms do not improve or are accompanied by fever, consult a physician.
Headache Strength, Sinus Pain Formula, and No Drowsiness Tablets—Do not take this product for more than 10 days (for adults) or 5 days (for children). If symptoms do not improve or are accompanied by fever that lasts more than 3 days, or if new symptoms occur, consult a physician.

Drug Interaction Precaution: *All Products*—Do not take this product if you are presently taking a prescription drug for high blood pressure or depression, without first consulting your physician; and *Children's Chewable Tablets and 12 Hour Caplets*—Do not take this product if you are presently taking another medication containing phenylpropanolamine.

Directions: Dose as follows while symptoms persist, or as directed by a physician.
Maximum Strength, No Drowsiness and Headache Strength Tablets—Adults and children 12 years of age and older: 2 tablets every 4 hours, not to exceed 8 tablets in 24 hours. Children 6 to under 12 years of age: 1 tablet every 4 hours, not to exceed 4 tablets in 24 hours. Children under 6 years of age: Consult a physician.
Sinus Pain Formula Tablets—Adults and children 12 years of age and older: 2 tablets every 6 hours, not to exceed 8 tablets in 24 hours. Children under 12 years of age: Consult a physician.
Children's Chewable Tablets—Children 6 to under 12 years of age: 2 tablets every 4 hours, not to exceed 8 tablets in 24

hours. Children under 6 years of age: Consult a physician.

12 Hour Caplets —Adults and children over 12 years of age: 1 caplet swallowed whole every 12 hours, not to exceed 2 caplets in 24 hours.

How Supplied:
Maximum Strength Tablets —Boxes of 24, 48, and 72.
No Drowsiness Tablets —Boxes of 20.
Headache Strength Tablets —Boxes of 24.
Sinus Pain Formula Tablets —Boxes of 20.
Children's Chewable Tablets —Boxes of 24.
12 Hour Caplets —Boxes of 10.
ALLEREST is a registered trademark of Fisons BV.

Shown in Product Identification Section, page 408

AMERICAINE® HEMORRHOIDAL OINTMENT
[*a-mer 'i-kān*]

Active Ingredient: Benzocaine 20%.

Other Ingredients: Benzethonium chloride, polyethylene glycol 300, polyethylene glycol 3350.

Indications: For the temporary relief of local pain, itching and soreness associated with hemorrhoids and anorectal inflammation.

Warnings: If condition worsens, or does not improve within 7 days, consult a physician. Do not exceed the recommended daily dosage unless directed by a physician. In case of bleeding, consult a physician promptly. Do not put this product into the rectum by using fingers or any mechanical device or applicator. Certain persons can develop allergic reactions to ingredients in this product. If the symptom being treated does not subside or if redness, irritation, swelling, pain, or other symptoms develop or increase, discontinue use and consult a physician. **Keep this and all drugs out of the reach of children.** In case of accidental ingestion, seek professional assistance or contact a Poison Control Center immediately.

Directions: *Adults:* When practical, cleanse the affected area with mild soap and warm water and rinse thoroughly. Gently dry by patting or blotting with toilet tissue or a soft cloth before application of this product. Apply externally to the affected area up to 6 times daily. *Children under 12 years of age:* Consult a physician.

How Supplied: *Hemorrhoidal Ointment* —1 oz. tube.
AMERICAINE is a registered trademark of Fisons BV.

Shown in Product Identification Section, page 409

AMERICAINE® TOPICAL ANESTHETIC SPRAY AND FIRST AID OINTMENT
[*a-mer 'i-kān*]

Active Ingredient: Benzocaine 20%.

Other Ingredients: *Spray* —Butane (propellant), isobutane (propellant), polyethylene glycol 200, propane (propellant). *Ointment* —Benzethonium chloride, polyethylene glycol 300, polyethylene glycol 3350.

Indications: For the temporary relief of pain and itching associated with minor cuts, scrapes, burns, sunburn, insect bites, or minor skin irritations.

Warnings: For external use only. Avoid contact with the eyes. If condition worsens, or if symptoms persist for more than 7 days or clear up and occur again within a few days, discontinue use of this product and consult a physician. **Keep this and all drugs out of the reach of children.** In case of accidental ingestion, seek professional assistance or contact a Poison Control Center immediately. *For Spray only* —Contents under pressure. Do not puncture or incinerate. Flammable mixture; do not use near fire or flame. Do not store at temperature above 120°F. Use only as directed. Intentional misuse by deliberately concentrating and inhaling the contents can be harmful or fatal.

Directions: Adults and children 2 years of age and older: Apply liberally to affected area not more than 3 to 4 times daily. Children under 2 years of age: Consult a physician.

How Supplied: *Topical Anesthetic Spray* —²⁄₃ oz., 2 oz. and 4 oz. aerosol containers. *First Aid Ointment* —¾ oz. tube, which is a clear, fragrance-free gel formula that is nonstaining, easy to apply, and is easily removed with soap and water.
AMERICAINE is a registered trademark of Fisons BV.

Shown in Product Identification Section, page 409

CALDECORT® ANTI-ITCH CREAM AND SPRAY; CALDECORT LIGHT® CREAM
[*kal 'de-kort*]

Active Ingredient: *Cream* —Hydrocortisone acetate (equivalent to hydrocortisone 1%). *Light Cream* —Hydrocortisone acetate (equivalent to hydrocortisone ½%). *Spray* —Hydrocortisone 1%.

Other Ingredients: *Cream* —Isopropyl myristate, methylparaben, polysorbate 60, propylparaben, purified water, sorbitan monostearate, sorbitol solution, stearic acid. *Light Cream* —Aloe vera gel, isopropyl myristate, methylparaben, polysorbate 60, propylparaben, purified water, sorbitan monostearate, sorbitol solution, stearic acid. *Spray* —Isobutane (propellant), isopropyl myristate, SD alcohol 40-B 62.7% (w/w).

Indications: For the temporary relief of itching associated with minor skin irritations, inflammation, and rashes due to eczema, insect bites, poison ivy, poison oak, poison sumac, soaps, detergents, cosmetics, jewelry, seborrheic dermatitis, psoriasis, and external feminine itching. Other uses of this product should be only under the advice and supervision of a doctor.

Warnings: For external use only. Avoid contact with the eyes. If condition worsens, or if symptoms persist for more than 7 days or clear up and occur again within a few days, stop use of this product and do not begin use of any other hydrocortisone product unless you have consulted a doctor. Do not use for the treatment of diaper rash. Consult a doctor. Do not use if you have a vaginal discharge. Consult a doctor. **Keep this and all drugs out of the reach of children.** In case of accidental ingestion, seek professional assistance or contact a Poison Control Center immediately. *For Spray only* —Avoid contact with the eyes or on other mucous membranes. Contents under pressure. Do not puncture or incinerate. Flammable mixture, do not use near fire or flame. Do not store at temperature above 120°F. Use only as directed. Intentional misuse by deliberately concentrating and inhaling the contents can be harmful or fatal.

Directions: Adults and children 2 years of age and older: Apply to affected area not more than 3 or 4 times daily. Children under 2 years of age: Do not use, consult a doctor.

How Supplied: *Cream* —½ oz. and 1 oz. tubes. *Light Cream* —½ oz. tubes. *Spray* —1.5 oz. aerosol container.
CALDECORT and CALDECORT LIGHT are registered trademarks of Fisons BV.

Shown in Product Identification Section, page 409

CALDESENE® MEDICATED POWDER AND OINTMENT
[*kal 'de-sēn*]

Active Ingredients: *Powder* —Calcium undecylenate 10%. *Ointment* —Petrolatum 53.9%; zinc oxide 15%.

Other Ingredients: *Powder* —Fragrance, talc. *Ointment* —Cod liver oil, fragrance, lanolin oil, methylparaben, propylparaben, talc.

Indications: Caldesene Medicated Powder is indicated to help heal, relieve and prevent diaper rash, prickly heat and chafing. Caldesene Ointment helps treat and prevent diaper rash, protects against urine and other irritants, soothes chafed skin, and promotes healing.

Actions: Only Caldesene Medicated Powder contains calcium undecylenate, an antibacterial that inhibits growth of the organisms frequently associated with diaper rash (including *S aureus, S epidermidis, E coli, and P aeruginosa*). Also

Continued on next page

Fisons Consumer—Cont.

forms a protective coating to repel moisture, soothe and comfort minor skin irritations, help heal and prevent chafing and prickly heat. Caldesene Ointment forms a protective skin coating to repel moisture and promote healing of diaper rash, while its natural ingredients protect irritated skin against wetness and other irritants. Unlike other ointments containing zinc oxide, Caldesene Ointment has a mild fragrance and is easily removed from the diaper area with soap and water.

Warnings: For external use only. Avoid contact with eyes. If condition worsens or does not improve within 7 days, consult a doctor. **Keep this and all drugs out of the reach of children.** In case of accidental ingestion, seek professional assistance or contact a Poison Control Center immediately.
Powder only: Keep powder away from child's face to avoid inhalation, which can cause breathing problems.
Ointment only: Do not apply over deep puncture wounds, infections and lacerations.

Directions: Use on baby after every bath or diaper change as directed by a pediatrician. Cleanse and thoroughly dry baby's skin, then smooth on Caldesene. Powder only: Apply powder close to the body away from child's face.

How Supplied: *Medicated Powder —* 2 oz. and 4 oz. shaker containers. *Medicated Ointment —* 1.25 oz.
CALDESENE is a registered trademark of Fisons BV.
Shown in Product Identification Section, page 409

CRUEX® ANTIFUNGAL POWDER, SPRAY POWDER AND CREAM
[kru 'ex]

Active Ingredients: *Powder —* Calcium undecylenate 10%. *Spray Powder —* Total undecylenate 19%, as undecylenic acid and zinc undecylenate. *Cream —* Total undecylenate 20%, as undecylenic acid and zinc undecylenate.

Other Ingredients: *Powder —* Colloidal silicon dioxide, fragrance, isopropyl myristate, talc. *Spray Powder —* Fragrance, isobutane (propellant), isopropyl myristate, menthol, talc, trolamine. *Cream —* Fragrance, glycol stearate SE, lanolin, methylparaben, PEG-8 laurate, PEG-6 stearate, propylparaben, purified water, sorbitol solution, stearic acid, trolamine, white petrolatum.

Indications: For the treatment of jock itch (tinea cruris) and relief of itching, chafing, burning rash and irritation in the groin area. Cruex powders also absorb perspiration.

Warnings: Do not use on children under 2 years of age except under the advice and supervision of a doctor. For external use only. If irritation occurs, or if there is no improvement within 2 weeks,

discontinue use and consult a doctor or pharmacist. **Keep this and all drugs out of the reach of children.** In case of accidental ingestion, seek professional assistance or contact a Poison Control Center immediately. *For Spray Powder only—* Avoid spraying in eyes or on other mucous membranes. Contents under pressure. Do not puncture or incinerate. Flammable mixture, do not use near a fire or flame. Do not store at temperature above 120° F. Use only as directed. Intentional misuse by deliberately concentrating and inhaling the contents can be harmful or fatal.

Directions: Cleanse skin with soap and water and dry thoroughly. Apply Cruex to affected area morning and night, before and after athletic activity, or as directed by a doctor. Best results are usually obtained with 2 weeks' use of this product. If satisfactory results have not occurred within this time, consult a doctor or pharmacist. Children under 12 years of age should be supervised in the use of this product. This product is not effective on the scalp or nails.

How Supplied: *Powder —* 1.5 oz. plastic squeeze bottle. *Spray Powder —* 1.8 oz., 3.5 oz. and 5.5 oz. aerosol containers. *Cream —* ½ oz. tube.
CRUEX is a registered trademark of Fisons BV.
Shown in Product Identification Section, page 409

DESENEX® ANTIFUNGAL POWDER, SPRAY POWDER, CREAM, OINTMENT, AND PENETRATING FOAM
[dess 'i-nex]

Active Ingredients: *Cream, Ointment, Powder, and Spray Powder, —* Total undecylenate 25%, as undecylenic acid and zinc undecylenate. *Penetrating Foam —* Undecylenic acid 10%.

Other Ingredients: *Cream, Ointment —* Fragrance, glycol stearate SE, lanolin, methylparaben, PEG-8 laurate, PEG-6 stearate, propylparaben, purified water, sorbitol solution, stearic acid, trolamine, white petrolatum. *Powder —* Fragrance, talc. *Spray Powder —* Fragrance, isobutane (propellant), isopropyl myristate, menthol, talc, trolamine. *Penetrating Foam —* Emulsifying wax, fragrance, isobutane (propellant), isopropyl alcohol 35.2% by volume, purified water, sodium benzoate, trolamine.

Indications: Desenex Antifungal Products cure athlete's foot (tinea pedis) exclusive of the nails and scalp. Relieves itching, burning, and cracking.

Warnings: Do not use on children under 2 years of age except under the advice and supervision of a doctor. For external use only. Avoid contact with the eyes. If irritation occurs, or if there is no improvement within 4 weeks, discontinue use and consult a doctor. **Keep this and all drugs out of the reach of children.** In case of accidental ingestion, seek professional assistance or contact a

Poison Control Center immediately. *For Spray Powder and Penetrating Foam —* Avoid spraying in the eyes or on other mucous membranes. Contents under pressure. Do not puncture or incinerate. Flammable mixture, do not use near fire or flame. Do not store at temperature above 120° F. Use only as directed. Intentional misuse by deliberately concentrating and inhaling the contents can be harmful or fatal.

Directions: Cleanse skin with soap and water and dry thoroughly. Apply over affected area morning and night or as directed by a doctor, paying special attention to the spaces between the toes. It is also helpful to wear well-fitting, ventilated shoes and to change shoes and socks at least once daily. Best results are usually obtained with 4 weeks' use of this product. If satisfactory results have not occurred within this time, consult a doctor. Children under 12 years of age should be supervised in the use of this product. This product is not effective on the scalp or nails. For persistent cases of athlete's foot, use Desenex Ointment or Cream at night and Desenex Powder or Spray Powder during the day.

How Supplied: *Cream —* ½ oz. tube. *Ointment —* ½ oz. and 1 oz. tubes. *Powder —* 1.5 oz. and 3 oz. shaker containers. *Spray Powder —* 2.7 oz. and 5.5 oz. aerosol containers. *Penetrating Foam—* 1.5 oz. aerosol container.
DESENEX is a registered trademark of Fisons BV.
Shown in Product Identification Section, page 409

DESENEX® FOOT & SNEAKER DEODORANT SPRAY
[dess 'i-nex]

Ingredients: Isobutane (propellant), SD alcohol 40-B, talc, aluminum chlorohydrex, silica, diisopropyl adipate, fragrance, menthol, tartaric acid.

Description: Foot & Sneaker Deodorant Spray cools and comforts feet, helping them feel clean and refreshed, Helps foster good foot hygiene with regular use. Specially formulated to absorb wetness, deodorize and relieve the discomfort of hot, perspiring, active feet. Sprays on like a liquid—dries quickly to a fine powder.

Directions: **Shake well,** hold 6 inches from area and spray onto soles of your feet and between your toes daily. Also, spray liberally over entire area of shoes or sneakers before wearing.

Warnings: Avoid spraying in eyes. Contents under pressure. Do not puncture or incinerate. Flammable mixture, do not use near fire or flame. Do not store at temperature above 120° F. Use only as directed. Intentional misuse by deliberately concentrating and inhaling the contents can be harmful or fatal. **Keep out of reach of children.**

How Supplied: *Desenex Foot & Sneaker Powder —* 3 oz. aerosol container.

DESENEX is a registered trademark of Fisons BV.

Shown in Product Identification Section, page 409

ISOCLOR® TIMESULE® Capsules
[ĭs ʹŏ-klŏr]

Active Ingredients: Chlorphenira-mine maleate 8 mg and pseudoephedrine HCl 120 mg.

Other Ingredients: Castor wax, ethyl-cellulose, gelatin, mineral oil, silicone oil, sugar spheres, white petrolatum.

Indications: For temporary relief of nasal congestion due to the common cold, hay fever, or other upper respiratory allergies, or associated with sinusitis. Helps decongest sinus openings, sinus passages. Reduces swelling of nasal passages, shrinks swollen membranes, and temporarily restores freer breathing through the nose. Alleviates runny nose, sneezing, itching of the nose or throat, and itchy and watery eyes as may occur in allergic rhinitis (such as hay fever).

Warnings: Do not exceed recommended dosage because, at higher doses, nervousness, dizziness, or sleeplessness may occur. Do not give this product to children under 12 years except under the advice and supervision of a physician. Do not take this product if you have asthma, glaucoma, emphysema, chronic pulmonary disease, shortness of breath, difficulty in breathing, difficulty in urination due to enlargement of the prostate gland, high blood pressure, heart disease, diabetes, or thyroid disease except under the advice and supervision of a physician. If symptoms do not improve within seven days or are accompanied by a high fever, consult a physician before continuing use. May cause drowsiness; alcohol may increase the drowsiness effect. May cause excitability especially in children. As with any drug, if you are pregnant or nursing a baby, seek the advice of a health professional before using this product.
Avoid driving a motor vehicle or operating heavy machinery. Avoid alcoholic beverages while taking this product.
Keep this and all drugs out of the reach of children. In case of accidental overdose, seek professional assistance or contact a Poison Control Center immediately.

Drug Interaction Precaution: Do not take this product if you are currently taking a prescription drug for high blood pressure or depression without first consulting your physician.

Directions: Adults and children 12 years and older—one capsule every 12 hours. Do not exceed two capsules in 24 hours.

How Supplied: Packaged on blister cards in cartons of 10's and 20's, and bottles of 100.
ISOCLOR® and TIMESULE® are registered trademarks of Fisons Corporation.

Distributed by:
FISONS
Consumer Health
Rochester, NY 14623 USA
Shown in Product Identification Section, page 409

MYOFLEX® ANALGESIC CREME
[mī ʹŏ-flex]

Active Ingredient: Trolamine salicylate 10%.

Other Ingredients: Cetyl alcohol, disodium EDTA, fragrance, propylene glycol, purified water, sodium lauryl sulfate, stearyl alcohol, white wax.

Indications: For the temporary pain relief of minor backache, sore muscular and aching joints caused by arthritis, overexertion, muscle strain and rheumatism.

Warning: For external use only. Use only as directed. Do not apply to irritated skin or if excessive irritation develops. Avoid contact with eyes or mucous membranes. If pain persists for more than 10 days or redness is present, consult a physician. For children under 12, consult a physician. **Keep this and all other medication out of the reach of children.** In case of accidental ingestion, seek professional assistance or contact a Poison Control Center immediately. As with any drug, if you are pregnant or nursing a baby, seek the advice of a health professional before using this product.

Directions: Adults—Rub into areas of soreness two or three times daily. Affected areas may be wrapped loosely with two- or three-inch elastic bandage after liberal application.

How Supplied: As an odorless, stainless, non-burning creme in 2 oz. and 4 oz. tubes, and 8 oz. and 16 oz. jars.
MYOFLEX is a registered trademark of Fisons Corporation.
Shown in Product Identification Section, page 409

SINAREST® TABLETS, EXTRA STRENGTH TABLETS AND NO DROWSINESS TABLETS
[sĭn ʹa-rest]

Active Ingredients:
Tablets—Acetaminophen 325 mg, chlorpheniramine maleate 2 mg, pseudoephedrine HCl 30 mg.
Extra Strength Tablets—Acetaminophen 500 mg, chlorpheniramine maleate 2 mg, pseudoephedrine HCl 30 mg.
No Drowsiness Tablets—Acetaminophen 500 mg, pseudoephedrine HCl 30 mg.

Other Ingredients:
All Products—Magnesium stearate, microcrystalline cellulose, povidone, pregelatinized starch.
Extra Strength and No Drowsiness Tablets also contain—Sodium starch glycolate. *Tablets and Extra Strength Tablets* also contain—Yellow 6 lake, Yellow 10 lake.

Indications:
Tablets and Extra Strength Tablets—Temporarily relieves nasal congestion, runny nose, sneezing, itching of the nose and throat, and itchy, watery eyes due to hay fever or other upper respiratory allergies, or associated with sinusitis. For temporary relief of minor aches, pains, and headache.
No Drowsiness Tablets—Temporarily relieves nasal congestion due to hay fever or other upper respiratory allergies, or associated with sinusitis. For temporary relief of minor aches, pains, and headache.

Warnings: *All Products*—Do not exceed recommended dosage because at higher doses, nervousness, dizziness, or sleeplessness may occur. Do not take this product for more than 10 days (for adults) or 5 days (for children). If symptoms do not improve or are accompanied by fever that lasts more than 3 days, or if new symptoms occur, consult a physician. Do not take this product if you have heart disease, high blood pressure, thyroid disease, diabetes, or difficulty in urination due to enlargement of the prostate gland, unless directed by a physician. As with any drug, if you are pregnant or nursing a baby, seek the advice of a health professional before using this product. **Keep this and all drugs out of the reach of children.** In case of accidental overdose, seek professional assistance or contact a Poison Control Center immediately. Prompt medical attention is critical for adults as well as children even if you do not notice any signs or symptoms. Also, *Tablets and Extra Strength Tablets*—Do not take this product if you have asthma, glaucoma, emphysema, chronic pulmonary disease, shortness of breath, or difficulty in breathing unless directed by a physician. May cause excitability, especially in children. May cause drowsiness; alcohol, sedatives, and tranquilizers may increase the drowsiness effect. Avoid alcoholic beverages while taking this product. Do not take this product if you are taking sedatives or tranquilizers, without first consulting your physician. Use caution when driving a motor vehicle or operating machinery.

Drug Interaction Precautions: *All Products*—Do not take this product if you are presently taking a prescription drug for high blood pressure or depression, without first consulting your physician.

Directions: Dose as follows while symptoms persist, or as directed by a physician.
Tablets—Adults and children 12 years of age and older: 2 tablets every 4 hours, not to exceed 8 tablets in 24 hours. Children 6 to under 12 years of age: 1 tablet every 4 hours, not to exceed 4 tablets in 24 hours. Children under 6 years of age: Consult a physician.
Extra Strength and No Drowsiness Tablets — Adults and children 12 years of

Continued on next page

Fisons Consumer—Cont.

age and older: 2 tablets every 6 hours, not to exceed 8 tablets in 24 hours. Children under 12 years of age: Consult a physician.

How Supplied:
Tablets —Boxes of 20, 40, and 80.
Extra Strength Tablets —Boxes of 24.
No Drowsiness Tablets —Boxes of 20.
SINAREST is a registered trademark of Fisons BV.

TING® ANTIFUNGAL CREAM, POWDER, SPRAY LIQUID, and SPRAY POWDER

Active Ingredient: Tolnaftate, 1%.

Other Ingredients: *Cream* —BHT, fragrance, polyethylene glycol 400, polyethylene glycol 3350, titanium dioxide. *Powder* —Corn starch, fragrance, talc. *Spray Liquid* —BHT, fragrance, isobutane (propellant), polyethylene glycol 400, SD alcohol 40-B (41% w/w). *Spray Powder* —BHT, fragrance, isobutane (propellant), PPG-12-buteth-16, SD alcohol 40-B (14% w/w), talc.

Indications: Cures athlete's foot and jock itch with a clinically proven ingredient. Relieves itching and burning. Prevents recurrence of athlete's foot with daily use.

Warnings: Do not use on children under 2 years of age except under the advice and supervision of a doctor. For external use only. Avoid contact with the eyes. If irritation occurs, or if there is no improvement within 4 weeks for athlete's foot, or within 2 weeks for jock itch, discontinue use and consult a doctor or pharmacist. **Keep this and all drugs out of the reach of children.** In case of accidental ingestion, seek professional assistance or contact a Poison Control Center immediately. *For Spray Liquid and Spray Powder only* —Avoid spraying in eyes or on other mucous membranes. Contents under pressure; do not puncture or incinerate. Flammable mixture, do not use near fire or flame. Do not store at temperature above 120°F. Use only as directed. Intentional misuse by deliberately concentrating and inhaling contents can be harmful or fatal.

Directions: Cleanse skin with soap and water and dry thoroughly. Apply over affected area morning and night or as directed by a doctor. For athlete's foot pay special attention to the spaces between the toes. It is also helpful to wear well-fitting, ventilated shoes and to change shoes and socks at least once daily. Best results in athlete's foot are usually obtained within 4 weeks' use of this product, and in jock itch, with two weeks' use. If unsatisfactory results have not occurred within these times, consult a doctor or pharmacist. Children under 12 years of age should be supervised in the use of this product. This product is not effective on the scalp or nails. To prevent recurrence of athlete's foot, apply

Ting to feet once or twice daily following the above directions.

How Supplied: *Cream* —½ oz. tube, *Powder* —1.5 oz. shaker container, *Spray Liquid and Spray Powder* —3 oz. aerosol containers.
TING is a registered trademark of Fisons BV.

Shown in Product Identification Section, page 409

VITRON–C® TABLETS
[*vī'tron c*]

Active Ingredients: Ferrous fumarate, 200 mg (66 mg elemental iron), 365% U.S. RDA; Ascorbic acid, 125 mg, 200% U.S. RDA (present in part as sodium ascorbate).

Other Ingredients: Colloidal silicon dioxide, flavor, glycine, hydroxypropyl methylcellulose, iron oxides, magnesium stearate, microcrystalline cellulose, polyethylene glycol, polysorbate 80, povidone, saccharin sodium, talc, titanium dioxide.

Indications: For iron deficiency anemia.

Actions: Vitron-C contains ferrous fumarate with ascorbic acid to enhance iron absorption. Vitron-C, a well-tolerated formula, is especially useful when pregnancy, menstruation, or chronic blood loss increases iron needs. The chewable, fruit-flavored, sugar-free tablets are easy to take and help improve patient compliance.

Warnings: The treatment of any anemic condition should be under the advice and supervision of a physician. As with any drug, if you are pregnant or nursing a baby, seek the advice of a health professional before using this product. **Keep this and all drugs out of the reach of children.** In case of accidental overdose, seek professional assistance or contact a Poison Control Center immediately.

Directions: Adults—one or two tablets daily or as directed by a physician. Tablet is palatable, and may be swallowed whole, chewed or sucked like a lozenge.

How Supplied: Bottles of 100 and 1000 tablets.
VITRON-C is a registered trademark of Fisons Corporation.

EDUCATIONAL MATERIAL

Americaine® Hemorrhoidal Ointment
Comforting Facts On a Painful Subject
Booklet with cents-off coupon describing hemorrhoidal conditions, with instructions on self-treatment, and when to consult a doctor.
Samples
To order FREE booklets and Americaine® Hemorrhoidal patient samples, write to Fisons Consumer Health.

Americaine® Topical Anesthetic
Make It All Better
Booklet with cents-off coupon featuring basic information on child safety/accident prevention, with instructions on self-treatment of minor pain and itching, and when to consult a doctor. To order FREE booklet, write to Fisons Consumer Health.

Caldesene®
Health and Safety Tips
Booklets with cents-off coupon and basic information on prevention of diaper rash, with instructions on home treatment, and when to consult a doctor (English and Spanish).
Samples
To order FREE booklets and Caldesene® Medicated Powder and Caldesene® Ointment patient samples, write to Fisons Consumer Health.

Fisons Corporation
P.O. BOX 1710
ROCHESTER, NY 14603

DELSYM®
(dextromethorphan polistirex)
12-Hour Cough Relief
[*del'sim*]

Active Ingredients: Each teaspoonful (5 mL) contains dextromethorphan polistirex equivalent to 30 mg dextromethorphan hydrobromide.

Other Ingredients: Citric acid, ethylcellulose, FD&C Yellow No. 6, flavor, high fructose corn syrup, methylparaben, polyethylene glycol 3350, polysorbate 80, propylene glycol, propylparaben, purified water, sucrose, tragacanth, vegetable oil, xanthan gum.

Indications: Temporarily relieves cough due to minor throat and bronchial irritation as may occur with the common cold or inhaled irritants.

Warnings: Do not take this product for persistent or chronic cough such as occurs with smoking, asthma, emphysema, or if cough is accompanied by excessive phlegm (mucus) unless directed by a physician. A persistent cough may be a sign of a serious condition. If cough persists for more than 1 week, tends to recur, or is accompanied by fever, rash, or persistent headache, consult a physician. As with any drug, if you are pregnant or nursing a baby, seek the advice of a health professional before using this product. **Keep this and all drugs out of the reach of children.** In case of accidental overdose, seek professional assistance or contact a Poison Control Center immediately.

Directions: Shake Bottle Well Before Using. Dose as follows or as directed by a physician.
Adults and Children 12 years of age and over: 2 teaspoonfuls every 12 hours, not to exceed 4 teaspoonfuls in 24 hours.
Children 6 to under 12 years of age: 1 teaspoonful every 12 hours, not to exceed 2 teaspoonfuls in 24 hours.

Children 2 to under 6 years of age: ½ teaspoonful every 12 hours, not to exceed 1 teaspoonful in 24 hours.

Children under 2 years of age: Consult a physician.

How Supplied: 3 fl. oz. bottles NDC 0585-0842-61
Fisons Corporation
Rochester, NY 14623 USA
DELSYM is a registered trademark of Fisons Corporation.

Fleming & Company
1600 FENPARK DR.
FENTON, MO 63026

CHLOR–3
Medicinal Condiment

Active Ingredients: A troika of sodium chloride (50% 24.3 mEq/half tsp. iodized); potassium chloride (30% 11.5 mEq/half tsp.); magnesium chloride (20% 5.6 mEq/half tsp.).

Indications: The first medicinal condiment to restore needed K^+ & Mg^{++} lost during diuresis, at the expense of Na^+. To restore electrolytes lost by overcooking foods, or to add to diets that lack green vegetables, bananas, etc. And to replace conventional salting of foods in culinary and gourmet arts.

Symptoms and Treatment of Oral Overdosage: Hyperkalemia and hypermagnesemia are not end-stage results of usage.

How Supplied: In 8-oz plastic shaker, tamper-evident bottles.

IMPREGON Concentrate

Active Ingredient: Tetrachlorosalicylanilide 2%

Indications: Diaper Rash Relief, 'Staph' control, Mold inhibitor.

Actions: This is a bacteriostatic/fungistatic agent for home usage and hospital usage.

Warnings: Impregon should not be exposed to direct sunlight for long periods after applications.

Precaution: Addition of bleach prior to diaper treatment negates application effects.

Dosage and Administration: One capful (5ml) per gallon of water to impregnate diapers in the diaper pail. Dilutions for many home areas accompany the full package.

Note: For disposable-type diapers, add one teaspoonful to 8 oz of water to a 'Windex-type' sprayer. Spray middle half area of diapers until damp, and allow to dry before using, to prevent rashes.

How Supplied: Four ounce amber plastic bottles.

MAGONATE TABLETS
MAGONATE LIQUID
Magnesium Gluconate (Dihydrate)

Active Ingredients: Each tablet contains magnesium gluconate (dihydrate) 500mg (27mg of Mg^{++}). Each 5cc of Magonate Liquid contains magnesium gluconate (dihydrate) 1000mg (54mg of Mg^{++}).

Indications: For all patients in negative magnesium balance.

Precaution: Excessive dosage may cause loose stools.

Dosage and Administration: Magonate is recommended during and for three weeks after a course in chemotherapy, then monitored regularly.
Adults and children over 12 yrs.—one or two tablets or ½ to 1 teaspoon of liquid t.i.d. Under 12 yrs.—one tablet or ½ teaspoon of liquid t.i.d. Dosage may be increased in severe cases.

How Supplied: Magonate Tablets are supplied in bottles of 100 and 1000 tablets. Magonate Liquid is supplied in pints and gallons.

MARBLEN Suspensions and Tablet

Composition: A modified 'Sippy Powder' antacid containing magnesium and calcium carbonates.

Action and Uses: The peach/apricot (pink) or unflavored (green) antacid suspensions are sugar-free and neutralize 18 mEq acid per teaspoonful with a low sodium content of 18mg per fl. oz. Each pink tablet consumes 18.0 mEq acid.

Administration and Dosage: One teaspoonful rather than a tablespoonful or one tablet to reduce patient cost by ⅔.

How Supplied: Plastic pints and bottles of 100 and 1000.

NEPHROX SUSPENSION
(aluminum hydroxide)
Antacid Suspension

Composition: A watermelon flavored aluminum hydroxide (320mg as gel)/ mineral oil (10% by volume) antacid per teaspoonful.

Action and Uses: A sugar-free/saccharin-free pink suspension containing no magnesium and low sodium (19mg/oz). Extremely palatable and especially indicated in renal patients. Each teaspoon consumes 9 mEq acid.

Administration and Dosage: Two teaspoonfuls or as directed by a physician.

Caution: To be taken only at bedtime. Do not use at any other time or administer to infants, expectant women, and nursing mothers except upon the advice of a physician as this product contains mineral oil.

How Supplied: Plastic pints and gallons.

NICOTINEX Elixir
nicotinic acid

Composition: Contains niacin 50 mg./tsp. in a sherry wine base (amber color).

Action and Uses: Produces flushing when tablets fail. To increase micro-circulation of inner-ear in Meniere's, tinnitus and labyrinthine syndromes. For 'cold hands & feet', and as a vehicle for additives.

Administration and Dosage: One or two teaspoonsful on fasting stomach.

Side Effects: Patients should be warned of dermal flush. Ulcer and gout patients may be affected by 14% alcoholic content.

Contraindications: Severe hypotension and hemorrhage.

How Supplied: Plastic pints and gallons.

OCEAN MIST
(buffered saline)

Composition: Special isotonic saline, buffered with sodium bicarbonate to proper pH so as not to irritate the nose.

Action and Uses: Rhinitis medicamentosa, rhinitis sicca and atrophic rhinitis. For patients 'hooked on nose drops' and glaucoma patients on diuretics having dry nasal capillaries. OCEAN may be used as a mist or drop.

Administration and Dosage: One or two squeezes in each nostril.

Supplied: Plastic 45cc spray bottles and pints.

PURGE
(flavored castor oil)

Composition: Contains 95% castor oil (USP) in a sweetened lemon flavored base that completely masks the odor and taste of the oil.

Indications: Preparation of the bowel for x-ray, surgery and proctological procedures, IVPs, and constipation.

Dosage: Infants—1–2 teaspoonfuls. Children—adjust between infant and adult dose. Adult—2–4 tablespoonfuls.

Precaution: Not indicated when nausea, vomiting, abdominal pain or symptoms of appendicitis occur. Pregnancy, use only on advice of physician.

Supplied: Plastic 1 oz. & 2 oz. bottles.

Products are indexed by
generic and chemical names
in the
YELLOW SECTION.

Gebauer Company
9410 ST. CATHERINE AVENUE
CLEVELAND, OH 44104

SALIVART®
[sal 'ĭ-vart]
Saliva Substitute

Description: Prompt, lasting relief of dryness of the mouth or throat (hyposalivation, xerostomia).

Active Ingredients:

	%W/W
Sodium carboxymethyl-cellulose	1.000
Sorbitol	3.000
Sodium chloride	0.084
Potassium chloride	0.120
Calcium chloride, dihydrate	0.015
Magnesium chloride, hexahydrate	0.005
Potassium phosphate, dibasic	0.034

Inactive Ingredients:

Purified water	95.742
	100.000

No preservatives
Propellant: Nitrogen

Indications: For reduced salivary flow, caused by medications, radiation therapy near the mouth or throat, salivary gland infection, mouth or throat inflammation, dental or oral surgery, fever, emotional factors. Also for relieving nasal crusting and bad taste.

Actions: Moistens and lubricates the oral cavity like natural saliva to allow normal eating, swallowing, and talking. Improves adherence of dentures.

Warnings: Avoid spraying in eyes. Keep out of reach of children. Contents under pressure. Do not puncture or incinerate. Protect from direct sunlight and from heat above 50°C (120°F).

Dosage and Administration: Spray Salivart directly into the mouth or throat, for 1 or 2 seconds, using it as often as needed to maintain moistness, or as instructed by physician. Nasal crusting can be relieved by applying Salivart with a cotton swab.

How Supplied:
75 Gram	NDC 0386-0009-75
25 Gram	NDC 0386-0009-25

IDENTIFICATION PROBLEM?
Consult the
Product Identification Section
where you'll find
products pictured
in full color.

Herald Pharmacal, Inc.
6503 WARWICK ROAD
RICHMOND, VA 23225

AQUA GLYCOLIC LOTION

Description: Aqua Glycolic lotion is a high-potency moisturizer containing 12 per cent partially neutralized Glycolic Acid in an unscented lanolin-free lotion base.

How Supplied: 4 oz. bottles and 8 oz. bottles

AQUA GLYCOLIC SHAMPOO®

Description: Cosmetically elegant shampoo, non-irritating, containing Glycolic Acid, leaves hair soft, manageable, helps eliminate itching, leaves scalp free from scale.

How Supplied: 8 oz. bottles and 16 oz. bottles

AQUA GLYDE CLEANSER®

Description: A cleanser for acne and other oily skin conditions. Contains special denatured alcohol #40, purified water, and Glycolic Acid.

How Supplied: 8 oz. plastic bottles.

AQUARAY® 20 SUNSCREEN

Description: AQUARAY Sunscreen is free of the sensitizing ingredients PABA, Padimate O, fragrance, lanolin, alcohol and parabens. It offers a wide range of protection from both UVA and UVB sun rays.

How Supplied: 4 fl. oz. bottles.

CAM LOTION®

Description: Lipid-free, soap-free skin cleanser for atopic dermatitis and other diseases aggravated by oily, greasy substances of animal and vegetable origin.

How Supplied: 8 and 16 oz. bottles.

ICN Pharmaceuticals, Inc.
ICN PLAZA
3300 HYLAND AVENUE
COSTA MESA, CA 92626

INSTA–GLUCOSE
[n-sta glū-cose]
Liquid Glucose

Active Ingredient: Liquid Glucose NF, 30 grams. Each 31 g tube contains 24 g carbohydrate.

Indications: For quick relief from insulin reaction/hypoglycemia, Insta-Glucose is readily absorbed into the bloodstream from the digestive tract. The cherry flavored liquid gel is pleasant tasting and easy to swallow.

Dosage and Administration: The recommended dosage is one entire 31 g unit dose tube of Insta-Glucose (24 g carbohydrate). One tube will usually treat a mild to moderate insulin reaction. Notify your physician or diabetes specialist immediately to report occurrence of hypoglycemia.

How Supplied: Three 31 g unit dose tubes in a Tri-Pak container. 5-year shelf life.   NDC #0187-0746-33
Shown in Product Identification Section, page 409

EDUCATIONAL MATERIAL

STAYING IN CONTROL
A guide to insulin reaction and hypoglycemia. This pamphlet describes common causes of hypoglycemia as well as stages, symptoms and treatment as recommended by the American Diabetes Assn.

Inter-Cal Corporation
421 MILLER VALLEY RD.
PRESCOTT, AZ 86301

ESTER–C®
(Calcium Ascorbate)

Description: Each Ester-C tablet contains 500 mg Vitamin C in the form of Calcium Ascorbate 550 mg, vegetable-derived cellulose, stearic acid, and magnesium stearate. Ester-C contains no preservatives, sugars, artificial colorings, or flavorings.
As the calcium salt of L-ascorbic acid, Ester-C has an empirical formula of $CaC_{12}H_{14}O_{12}$ and a formula weight of 390.3.

Actions: Vitamin C has been found to be essential for the prevention of scurvy. In humans, an exogenous source of the vitamin is required for collagen formation and tissue repair. Ascorbate ion is reversibly oxidized to dehydroascorbate ion in the body. Both of these are active forms of the vitamin and are considered to play important roles in biochemical oxidation-reduction reactions. The vitamin is involved in tyrosine metabolism, carbohydrate metabolism, iron metabolism, folic acid-folinic acid conversion, synthesis of lipids and proteins, resistance to infections, and cellular respiration.

Indications and Usage: Vitamin C and its salts, such as Calcium Ascorbate, are recommended as nutritional supplements in the prevention of scurvy. In scurvy, collagenous structures are primarily affected, and lesions develop in blood vessels and bones. Symptoms of mild deficiency may include faulty development of teeth and bones, bleeding gums, gingivitis, and loose teeth. An increased need for the vitamin exists in febrile states, chronic illness and infection, e.g., rheumatic fever, pneumonia, tuberculosis, whooping cough, diphtheria, sinusitis, etc. Additional increases in the daily intake of ascorbate are indicated in burns, delayed healing of bone fractures and wounds, and hemovascular disorders. Immature and premature infants require relatively larger amounts of Vitamin C.

Contraindications: Because of its calcium content, Ester-C is contraindicated in hypercalcemic states, e.g., from dosing with parathyroid hormone or overdosage of Vitamin D.

Adverse Reactions: There are no known adverse reactions following ingestion of Ester-C tablets. The gastric disturbances characteristic of large doses of ascorbic acid are absent or greatly diminished when the pH-neutral form of calcium ascorbate present in Ester-C tablets is utilized as the source of Vitamin C supplementation.

Dosage and Administration: The minimum U.S. Recommended Daily Allowance for Vitamin C for the prevention of diseases such as scurvy is 60 mg per day. Optimum daily allowances, e.g., for the maintenance of increased plasma and cellular reserves, are significantly greater. For adults, the recommended average preventative dose of the vitamin is 70 to 150 mg daily. The recommended average optimum dose of Ester-C is 550 to 1650 mg (1 to 3 tablets) daily.
For frank scurvy, doses of 300 mg to one gram of Vitamin C daily have been recommended. Normal adults, however, have received as much as six grams of the vitamin without evidence of toxicity.
For enhancement of wound healing, doses of the vitamin approximating two Ester-C tablets daily for a week or ten days both preoperatively and postoperatively are generally considered adequate, although considerably larger amounts may be recommended. In the treatment of burns, the daily number of Ester-C tablets recommended is governed by the extent of tissue injury. For severe burns, daily doses of 2 to 4 tablets (approximately one to two grams of Vitamin C) are recommended.
In other conditions in which the need for increased Vitamin C is recognized, three to five times the optimum allowance appears to be adequate.

How Supplied: 550 mg tablets of Ester-C in plastic bottles of 100, 250, 90, and 225's. 4 oz. and 8 oz. powders, 275 mg tablet also available.
Store at room temperature.
U.S. Patent granted April 18, 1989; No. 4,822,816.

Literature revised: December, 1989.
Mfd. by Inter-Cal Corp.
Prescott, AZ 86301

Products are indexed by generic and chemical names in the **YELLOW SECTION.**

Johnson&Johnson ●
MERCK
Consumer Pharmaceuticals Co.
CAMP HILL ROAD
FORT WASHINGTON, PA 19034

ALternaGEL™
[al-tern 'a-jel]
Liquid
High-Potency Aluminum Hydroxide Antacid

Description: ALternaGEL is available as a white, pleasant-tasting, high-potency aluminum hydroxide liquid antacid.

Ingredients: Each 5 mL teaspoonful contains: Active: 600 mg aluminum hydroxide (equivalent to dried gel, USP) providing 16 milliequivalents (mEq) of acid-neutralizing capacity (ANC), and less than 2.5 mg (0.109 mEq) of sodium and no sugar. Inactive: butylparaben, flavors, propylparaben, purified water, simethicone, and other ingredients.

Indications: ALternaGEL is indicated for the symptomatic relief of hyperacidity associated with peptic ulcer, gastritis, peptic esophagitis, gastric hyperacidity, hiatal hernia, and heartburn.
ALternaGEL will be of special value to those patients for whom magnesium-containing antacids are undesirable, such as patients with renal insufficiency, patients requiring control of attendant G.I. complications resulting from steroid or other drug therapy, and patients experiencing the laxation which may result from magnesium or combination antacid regimens.

Directions: One to two teaspoonfuls, as needed, between meals and at bedtime, or as directed by a physician: May be followed by a sip of water if desired. Concentrated product. Shake well before using. Keep tightly closed.

Warnings: Keep this and all drugs out of the reach of children. ALternaGEL may cause constipation.
Except under the advice and supervision of a physician: do not take more than 18 teaspoonfuls in a 24-hour period, or use the maximum dose of ALternaGEL for more than two weeks. ALternaGEL may cause constipation.
Prolonged use of aluminum-containing antacids in patients with renal failure may result in or worsen dialysis osteomalacia. Elevated tissue aluminum levels contribute to the development of the dialysis encephalopathy and osteomalacia syndromes. Small amounts of aluminum are absorbed from the gastrointestinal tract and renal excretion of aluminum is impaired in renal failure. Aluminum is not well removed by dialysis because it is bound to albumin and transferrin, which do not cross dialysis membranes. As a result, aluminum is deposited in bone, and dialysis osteomalacia may develop when large amounts of aluminum are ingested orally by patients with impaired renal function.
Aluminum forms insoluble complexes with phosphate in the gastrointestinal

tract, thus decreasing phosphate absorption. Prolonged use of aluminum-containing antacids by normophosphatemic patients may result in hypophosphatemia if phosphate intake is not adequate. In its more severe forms, hypophosphatemia can lead to anorexia, malaise, muscle weakness, and osteomalacia.

Drug Interaction Precaution: Do not use this product for any patient receiving a prescription antibiotic containing any form of tetracycline.

How Supplied: ALternaGEL is available in bottles of 12 fluid ounces and 5 fluid ounces, and 1 fluid ounce hospital unit doses. NDC 16837-860
Shown in Product Identification Section, page 409

DIALOSE® Tablets
[di 'a-lose]
Stool Softener Laxative

Description: DIALOSE is a very low sodium, nonhabit forming, stool softener containing 100 mg docusate sodium per tablet.
The docusate in DIALOSE is a highly efficient surfactant which facilitates absorption of water by the stool to form a soft, easily evacuated mass. Unlike stimulant laxatives, DIALOSE does not interfere with normal peristalsis, neither does it cause griping nor sensations of urgency.

Ingredients: Active: docusate sodium, 100 mg per tablet
Inactive: Acacia, Calcium Carbonate, Calcium Sulfate, Carnauba Wax, Powdered Cellulose, Croscarmellose Sodium, D & C Red #27 Al. Lake, Diacetylated Monoglycerides, FD & C Yellow #6 Al. Lake, Gelatin, Hydroxypropyl Methylcellulose, Kaolin, Lactose, Magnesium Stearate, Pharmaceutical Glaze, Povidone, Colloidal Silicon Dioxide, Sodium Benzoate, Sodium Starch Glycolate, Pregelatinized Starch, Stearic Acid, Sugar, Talc, Titanium Dioxide, White Wax.

Indications: DIALOSE is indicated for the relief of occasional constipation (irregularity).
DIALOSE is an effective aid to soften or prevent formation of hard stools in a wide range of conditions that may lead to constipation. DIALOSE helps to eliminate straining associated with obstetric, geriatric, cardiac, surgical, anorectal, or proctologic conditions. In cases of mild constipation, the fecal softening action of DIALOSE can prevent constipation from progressing and relieve painful defecation.

Directions: *Adults:* One tablet, one to three times daily: adjust dosage as needed.
Children 6 to under 12 years: One tablet daily or as directed by physician.
Children under 6 years: As directed by physician.

Continued on next page

J&J • Merck—Cont.

It is helpful to increase the daily intake of fluids by taking a glass of water with each dose.

Warnings: Unless directed by a physician: Do not use when abdominal pain, nausea, or vomiting are present. Do not use for a period longer than one week. Do not take this product if you are presently taking a prescription drug or mineral oil. As with any drug, if you are pregnant or nursing a baby, seek the advice of a health professional before using this product.
Keep out of the reach of children.

How Supplied: Bottles of 36 and 100 pink tablets. Also available in 100 tablet unit dose boxes (10 strips of 10 tablets each). NDC 16837-870.

Shown in Product Identification Section, page 409

DIALOSE® PLUS Tablets
[di'a-lose Plus]
Stool Softener/Stimulant Laxative

Description: DIALOSE PLUS provides a very low sodium tablet formulation of 100 mg docusate sodium and 65 mg yellow phenolphthalein.

Ingredients: Each tablet contains: Actives: docusate sodium, 100 mg., yellow phenolphthalein, 65 mg.
Inactives: Acacia, Calcium Carbonate, Calcium Sulfate, Carnauba Wax, Powdered Cellulose, Croscarmellose Sodium, D & C Yellow #10 Al. Lake, Diacetylated Monoglycerides, FD & C Yellow #6 Al. Lake, Gelatin, Hydroxypropyl Methylcellulose, Kaolin, Magnesium Stearate, Pharmaceutical Glaze, Povidone, Colloidal Silicon Dioxide, Sodium Benzoate, Sodium Starch Glycolate, Pregelatinized Starch, Stearic Acid, Sugar, Talc, Titanium Dioxide, White Wax.

Indications: DIALOSE PLUS is indicated for the treatment of constipation characterized by lack of moisture in the intestinal contents, resulting in hardness of stool and decreased intestinal motility. DIALOSE PLUS combines the advantages of the stool softener, docusate sodium, with the peristaltic activating effect of yellow phenolphthalein.

Directions: *Adults:* One or two tablets daily as needed, at bedtime or on arising. *Children 6 to under 12 years:* One tablet daily as needed
Children under 6 years: As directed by physician.
It is helpful to increase the daily intake of fluids by taking a glass of water with each dose.

Warnings: Unless directed by a physician: Do not use when abdominal pain, nausea, or vomiting are present. Do not use for a period longer than one week. If skin rash appears do not use this product or any other preparation containing phenolphthalein. Frequent or prolonged use may result in dependence on laxatives. Do not take this product if you are pres-

ently taking a prescription drug or mineral oil.
As with any drug, if you are pregnant or nursing a baby, seek the advice of a health professional before using this. Keep out of the reach of children.

How Supplied: Bottles of 36 and 100 yellow tablets. Also available in 100 capsule unit dose boxes (10 strips of 10 capsules each). NDC 16837-871.

Shown in Product Identification Section, page 409

EFFER-SYLLIUM®
[ef'fer-sil'lium]
Natural Fiber Bulking Agent

Description: EFFER-SYLLIUM is a tan, granular powder. Each rounded teaspoonful, or individual packet (7 g) contains psyllium hydrocolloid, 3 g.

Ingredients: Active: psyllium hydrocolloid. Inactive: citric acid, ethyl vanillin, lemon and lime flavors, potassium bicarbonate, potassium citrate, saccharin calcium, starch, sucrose.
EFFER-SYLLIUM contains less than 5 mg sodium per rounded teaspoonful and is considered dietetically sodium free.

Indications: EFFER-SYLLIUM is indicated to restore normal bowel habits in chronic constipation, to promote normal elimination in irritable bowel syndrome, and to ease passage of stools in presence of anorectal disorders. EFFER-SYLLIUM produces a soft, lubricating bulk which promotes natural elimination.
EFFER-SYLLIUM is not a one-dose, fast-acting bowel regulator. Administration for several days may be needed to establish regularity.

Directions:
Adults: One rounded teaspoonful, or one packet, in a glass of water one to three times a day, or as directed by physician. *Children, 6 years and over:* One level teaspoonful, or one-half packet (3.5 g) in one-half glass of water at bedtime, or as directed by physician. *Children, under 6 years:* As directed by physician.

Instructions: Pour EFFER-SYLLIUM into a *dry* glass, add water and stir briskly. Drink immediately. To avoid caking, always use a *dry* spoon to remove EFFER-SYLLIUM from its container. Replace cap tightly. Keep in a dry place.

Warning: Avoid inhalation. May cause a potentially severe reaction when inhaled by persons sensitive to psyllium powder or suffering from respiratory disorders. As with all medications, keep out of the reach of children.

How Supplied: Bottles of 9 oz and 16 oz, and individual convenience packets (7 g each) packaged in boxes of 24. NDC 16837-440.

Shown in Product Identification Section, page 409

FERANCEE®
[fer'an-see]
Chewable Hematinic

Two Tablets Daily Provide:

	US RDA*	
Iron	744%	134 mg
Vitamin C	500%	300 mg

*Percentage of US Recommended Daily Allowances for adults and children 4 or more years of age.

Ingredients: Active: ferrous fumarate, sodium ascorbate, ascorbic acid. Inactive: confectioner's sugar, flavors, magnesium stearate, mannitol, povidone, saccharin calcium, starch, Yellow 5 (tartrazine), Yellow 6.

Indications: A pleasant-tasting hematinic for iron deficiency anemias, well-tolerated FERANCEE is particularly useful when chronic blood loss, onset of menses, or pregnancy create additional demands for iron supplementation. Available information indicates a low incidence of staining of the teeth by ferrous fumarate, alone or in combination with ascorbic acid. The peach-cherry flavored chewable tablets dissolve quickly in the mouth and may be either chewed or swallowed.

Directions:
Adults: Two tablets daily, or as directed by physician.
Chidren over 6 years of age: One tablet daily, or as directed by physician.
Children under 6 years of age: As directed by physician.

Warnings: As with any drug, if you are pregnant or nursing a baby, seek the advice of a health professional before using this product. Keep out of the reach of children. In case of accidental overdose, seek professional assistance or contact a Poison Control Center immediately.

How Supplied: FERANCEE is supplied in bottles of 100 brown and yellow, two-layer tablets. A child-resistant cap is standard on each bottle as a safeguard against accidental ingestion by children. Keep in a dry place. Replace cap tightly. NDC 16837-650.

FERANCEE®-HP Tablets
[fer-an-see hp]
High Potency Hematinic

One Tablet Daily Provides:

	US RDA*	
Iron	611%	110 mg
Vitamin C	1000%	600 mg

*Percentage of US Recommended Daily Allowances for adults and children 4 or more years of age.

Ingredients: Active: ferrous fumarate, sodium ascorbate, ascorbic acid. Inactive: flavor, hydrogenated vegetable oil, microcrystalline cellulose, povidone, Red 40, and other ingredients.

Indications: FERANCEE-HP is a high potency formulation of iron and vitamin C and is intended for use as either:
(1)   a maintenance hematinic for those patients needing a daily iron sup-

plement to maintain normal hemoglobin levels, or

(2) intensive therapy for the acute and/or severe iron deficiency anemia where a high intake of elemental iron is required.

The use of well-tolerated ferrous fumarate provides high levels of elemental iron with a low incidence of gastric distress. The inclusion of 600 mg of vitamin C per tablet serves to maintain more of the iron in the absorbable ferrous state.

Precautions: Because FERANCEE-HP contains 110 mg of elemental iron per tablet, it is recommended that its use be limited to adults, ie over 12 years of age.

Directions: One tablet per day after a meal or as directed by a physician. Should be sufficient to maintain normal hemoglobin levels in most patients with a history of recurring iron deficiency anemia. Not recommended for children under 12 years of age.

For acute and/or severe iron deficiency anemia, two or three tablets per day taken one tablet per dose after meals. (Each tablet provides 110 mg elemental iron).

Warnings: As with all medications, keep out of the reach of children. In case of accidental overdose, seek professional assistance or contact a Poison Control Center immediately.

How Supplied: FERANCEE-HP is supplied in bottles of 60 red, film coated, oval shaped tablets.
NDC 16837-863.
Note: A child-resistant safety cap is standard on each bottle of 60 tablets as a safeguard against accidental ingestion by children.

Shown in Product Identification Section, page 409

MYLANTA®
[*my-lan 'ta*]
Alumina, Magnesia and Simethicone Liquid and Tablets
Antacid/Anti-Gas

Description: MYLANTA is a well-balanced, pleasant-tasting antacid/anti-gas medication that provides consistent, effective relief of symptoms associated with gastric hyperacidity and excess gas. Non-constipating and dietetically sodium-free, MYLANTA contains two proven antacids, magnesium hydroxide and aluminum hydroxide, plus simethicone for gas relief.

Ingredients: Each 5mL (one teaspoonful) of liquid suspension or each chewable tablet contains: **Active:** Magnesium hydroxide 200 mg, Aluminum hydroxide (Dried Gel, USP in tablet and equiv. to Dried Gel USP in liquid) 200 mg and Simethicone 20 mg. **Inactive:** Tablets: Dextrates, flavors, magnesium stearate, mannitol, sorbitol, Yellow 10, colloidal silicon dioxide, sodium saccharin, Blue 1 or Red 27. Liquid: Butylparaben, carboxymethylcellulose sodium, flavors, hydroxypropyl methylcellulose, microcrys-

talline cellulose, propylparaben, purified water, saccharin sodium and sorbitol.

Sodium Content: MYLANTA contains an insignificant amount of sodium per daily dose and is considered dietetically sodium-free. Typical values are 0.68 mg (0.03 mEq) sodium per 5 mL teaspoonful of liquid and 0.77 mg (0.03 mEq) per tablet.

Acid Neutralizing Capacity: Two teaspoonfuls of MYLANTA liquid has an acid neutralizing capacity, as measured in laboratory testing, of 25.4 mEq. Two MYLANTA tablets have an acid neutralizing capacity of 23.0 mEq.

Indications: As an antacid for symptomatic relief of hyperacidity associated with the diagnosis of peptic ulcer, gastritis, peptic esophagitis, heartburn and hiatal hernia. As an antiflatulent to alleviate the symptoms of mucus-entrapped gas, including postoperative gas pain.

Advantages: MYLANTA is homogenized for a smooth, creamy taste. The choice of two pleasant-tasting liquid flavors and the non-constipating formula encourage patient acceptance, thereby minimizing the skipping of prescribed doses. MYLANTA is also available in equipotent tablets, and both the liquid and tablet forms are sodium-free. MYLANTA provides consistent relief in patients suffering from distress associated with hyperacidity, mucus-entrapped gas, or swallowed air.

Directions:
Liquid: Shake well. 2–4 teaspoonfuls between meals and at bedtime or as directed by a physician.
Tablets: 2–4 tablets, well chewed, between meals and at bedtime or as directed by a physician.

Warnings: Keep this and all other drugs out of the reach of children. Do not take more than 24 tsps/tablets in a 24 hour period or use the maximum dose of this product for more than two weeks, except under the advice and supervision of a physician. Do not use this product if you have kidney disease.

Prolonged use of aluminum-containing antacids in patients with renal failure may result in or worsen dialysis osteomalacia. Elevated tissue aluminum levels contribute to the development of the dialysis encephalopathy and osteomalacia syndromes. Small amounts of aluminum are absorbed from the gastrointestinal tract and renal excretion of aluminum is impaired in renal failure. Aluminum is not well removed by dialysis because it is bound to albumin and transferrin, which do not cross dialysis membranes. As a result, aluminum is deposited in bone, and dialysis osteomalacia may develop when large amounts of aluminum are ingested orally by patients with impaired renal function.

Aluminum forms insoluble complexes with phosphate in the gastrointestinal tract, thus decreasing phosphate absorption. Prolonged use of aluminum-containing antacids by normophosphatemic patients may result in hypophosphatemia if phosphate intake is not adequate.

In its more severe forms, hypophosphatemia can lead to anorexia, malaise, muscle weakness, and osteomalacia.

Drug Interaction Precaution: Do not use this product for any patient receiving a prescription antibiotic containing any form of tetracycline.

How Supplied: MYLANTA is available as a white liquid suspension in two pleasant-tasting flavors, Original and Cherry Creme, and in a two-layer green and white chewable Cool Mint Creme flavored tablet, as well as a two-layer pink and white Cherry Creme flavored tablet, identified on white layer "Mylanta." Liquid supplied in bottles of 5 oz, 12 oz, and 24 oz. Tablets supplied in bottles of 48 and 100 count sizes and in 12 tablet rollpacks. Also available for hospital use in liquid unit dose bottles of 1 oz, and bottles of 5 oz.
NDC 16837-610 (original liquid). NDC 16837-620 (cool mint creme tablets). NDC 16837-621 (cherry creme liquid). NDC 16837-628 (cherry creme tablets).
Shown in Product Identification Section, page 410

MYLANTA® DOUBLE STRENGTH
[*my-lan 'ta*]
Alumina, Magnesia and Simethicone Liquid and Tablets
Double-Strength Antacid/Anti-Gas

Description: MYLANTA DOUBLE STRENGTH is a well-balanced, high-potency antacid/anti-gas medication that provides rapid, effective, and long-lasting relief of symptoms associated with gastric hyperacidity and excess gas. Pleasant-tasting, non-constipating and dietetically sodium-free, MYLANTA DOUBLE STRENGTH contains two proven antacids, magnesium hydroxide and aluminum hydroxide, plus simethicone for gas relief.

Ingredients: Each 5mL (one teaspoonful) of liquid suspension or each chewable tablet contains: Active: Magnesium hydroxide 400 mg, Aluminum hydroxide (Dried Gel, USP in tablet and equiv. to Dried Gel USP in liquid) 400 mg and Simethicone 40 mg. Inactive: Tablets: Colloidal silicon dioxide, dextrose, flavors, magnesium stearate, mannitol, sodium saccharin, sorbitol, Yellow 10; Cherry: Citric acid, Red 27; Mint: Blue 1. Liquid: Butylparaben, carboxymethylcellulose sodium, flavors, hydroxypropyl methylcellulose, microcrystalline cellulose, potassium citrate, propylparaben, purified water, saccharin sodium and sorbitol.

Sodium Content: MYLANTA DOUBLE STRENGTH contains an insignificant amount of sodium per daily dose. Typical values are 1.14 mg (0.05 mEq) sodium per 5 mL teaspoonful of liquid and 1.3 mg (0.06 mEq) per tablet.

Acid Neutralizing Capacity: Two teaspoonfuls of MYLANTA DOUBLE STRENGTH liquid has an acid neutralizing capacity of 50.8 mEq, as measured in

Continued on next page

J&J • Merck—Cont.

laboratory testing. Two MYLANTA DOUBLE STRENGTH tablets have an acid neutralizing capacity of 46.0 mEq.

Indications: As an antacid for symptomatic relief of hyperacidity associated with the diagnosis of peptic ulcer, gastritis, peptic esophagitis, heartburn and hiatal hernia. As an antiflatulent to alleviate the symptoms of mucus-entrapped gas, including postoperative gas pain.

Advantages: MYLANTA DOUBLE STRENGTH is homogenized for a smooth, creamy taste. The choice of three pleasant-tasting liquid flavors and the non-constipating formula encourage patient acceptance, thereby minimizing the skipping of prescribed doses. MYLANTA DOUBLE STRENGTH is also available in equipotent tablets, and both the liquid and tablet forms are sodium-free. The high potency of MYLANTA DOUBLE STRENGTH is achieved through greater concentration of two proven antacid ingredients, plus simethicone. MYLANTA DOUBLE STRENGTH provides rapid, consistent and long-lasting relief in patients suffering from distress associated with hyperacidity, mucus-entrapped gas, or swallowed air.

Directions:
Liquid: Shake well. 2–4 teaspoonfuls between meals and at bedtime, or as directed by a physician.
Tablets: 2–4 tablets, well chewed, between meals and at bedtime, or as directed by a physician.
Because patients with peptic ulcer vary greatly in both acid output and gastric emptying time, the amount and schedule of dosages should be varied accordingly.

Warnings: Keep this an all drugs out of the reach of children. Do not take more than 12 tsps/tablets in a 24-hour period or use the maximum dose of this product for more than two weeks, except under advice and supervision of a physician. Do not use this product if you have kidney disease.
Prolonged use of aluminum-containing antacids in patients with renal failure may result in or worsen dialysis osteomalacia. Elevated tissue aluminum levels contribute to the development of the dialysis encephalopahty and osteomalacia syndromes. Small amounts of aluminum are absorbed from the gastrointestinal tract and renal excretion of aluminum is impaired in renal failure. Aluminum is not well removed by dialysis because it is bound to albumin and transferrin, which do not cross dialysis membranes. As a result, aluminum is deposited in bone, and dialysis osteomalacia may develop when large amounts of aluminum are ingested orally by patients with impaired renal function.
Aluminum forms insoluble complexes with phosphate in the gastrointestinal tract, thus decreasing phosphate absorption. Prolonged use of aluminum-containing antacids by normophosphatemic patients may result in hypophosphate-

mia if phosphate intake is not adequate. In its more severe forms, hypophosphatemia can lead to anorexia, malaise, muscle weakness, and osteomalacia.

Drug Interaction Precaution: Do not use this product for any patient receiving a prescription antibiotic containing any form of tetracycline.

How Supplied: MYLANTA DOUBLE STRENGTH is available as a white liquid suspension in three pleasant-tasting flavors, Original, Cherry Creme, and Cool Mint Creme, and in a two-layer, green and white chewable Cool Mint Creme flavored tablet, as well as a two-layer pink and white Cherry Creme flavored tablet identified on white layer "Mylanta DS". Liquid supplied in 5 oz, 12 oz and 24 oz bottles. Tablets supplied in bottles of 30 and 60 count sizes, and 8 tablet roll packs. Also available for hospital use in liquid unit dose bottles of 1 oz, and bottles of 5 oz.
NDC 16837-652 (original liquid). NDC 16837-651 (cool mint creme tablets).
NDC 16837-624 (cool mint creme liquid)
NDC 16837-622 (cherry creme liquid)
NDC 16837-627 (cherry creme tablets).

Professional Labeling

Indications: Stress-induced upper gastrointestinal hemorrhage: MYLANTA DOUBLE STRENGTH is indicated for the prevention of stress-induced upper gatrointestinal hemorrhage.
Hyperacidic conditions: As an antacid, for the symptomatic relief of hyperacidity associated with the diagnosis of peptic ulcer and other gastrointestinal conditions where a high degree of acid neutralization is desired.

Directions: Prevention of stress-induced upper gastrointestinal hemorrhage: 1) Aspirate stomach via nasogastric tube* and record pH. 2) Instill 10 mL of MYLANTA DOUBLE STRENGTH followed by 30 mL of water via nasogastric tube. Clamp tube. 3) Wait one hour. Aspirate stomach and record pH. 4a) If pH equals or exceeds 4.0, apply drainage or intermittent suction for one hour, then repeat the cycle. 4b) If pH is less than 4.0, instill double (20 mL) MYLANTA DOUBLE STRENGTH followed by 30 mL of water. Clamp tube. 5) Wait one hour. If pH equals or exceeds 4.0, see number 7, if pH is still less than 4.0, instill double (40 mL) MYLANTA DOUBLE STRENGTH followed by 30 mL of water. Clamp tube. 6) Wait one hour. If pH equals or exceeds 4.0, see number 7. If pH is still less than 4.0, instill double (80 mL)† MYLANTA DOUBLE STRENGTH followed by 30 mL of water. 7) Drain for one hour and repeat cycle with the effective dosage of MYLANTA DOUBLE STRENGTH.
*If nasogastric tube is not in place, administer 20 mL of MYLANTA DOUBLE STRENGTH orally q2h.
†In a recent clinical study[1] 20 mL of MYLANTA DOUBLE STRENGTH, q2h, was sufficient in more than 85 percent of the patients. No patient studied required more than 80 mL of MYLANTA DOUBLE STRENGTH q2h.

In hyperacid states for symptomatic relief: One or two teaspoonfuls as needed between meals and at bedtime or as directed by a physician. Higher dosage regimens may be employed under the direct supervision of a physician in the treatment of active peptic ulcer disease.

Precaution: Aluminum-magnesium hydroxide containing antacids should be used with caution in patients with renal impairment.

Adverse Effects: Occasional regurgitation and mild diarrhea have been reported with the dosage recommended for the prevention of stress-induced upper gastrointestinal hemorrhage.

References: 1. Zinner MJ, Zuidema GD, Smigh PL, Mignosa M: The prevention of upper gastrointestinal tract bleeding in patients in an intensive care unit. *Surg Gynecol Obster* 153:214–220, 1981. 2. Lucas CE, Sugawa C, Riddle J, et al.: Natural history and surgical dilemma of "stress" gastric bleeding. *Arch Surg* 102:266–273, 1971. 3. Hastings PR, Skillman JJ, Bushnell LS, Silen W: Antacid titration in the prevention of acute gastrointestinal bleeding: a controlled, randomized trial in 100 critically ill patients. *N Engl J Med* 298:1042–1045, 1978. 4. Day SB, MacMillan BG, Altemeier WA: *Curling's Ulcer, An Experience of Nature.* Springfield, IL, Charles C Thomas Co., 1972, p. 205. 5. Skillman JJ, Bushnell LS, Goldman H, Silen W: Respiratory failure, hypotension, sepsis, and jaundice. A clinical syndrome associated with lethal hemorrhage from acute stress ulceration of the stomach. *Am J Surg* 117:523–530, 1969. 6. Priebe HJ, Skillman J, Bushnell LS, et al. Antacid versus cimetidine in preventing acute gastrointestinal bleeding. *N Engl J Med* 302:426–430, 1980. 7. Silen W: The prevention and management of stress ulcers. *Hosp Pract* 15:93–97, 1980. 8. Herrmann V, Kaminski DL: Evaluation of intragastric pH in acutely ill patients. *Arch Surg* 114:511–514, 1979. 9. Martin LF, Staloch DK, Simonowitz DA, et al.: Failure of cimetidine prophylaxis in the critically ill. *Arch Surg* 114:492–496, 1979. 10. Zinner MJ, Turtinen L, Gurll NJ, Reynolds DG: The effect of metiamide on gastric mucosal injury in rat restraint. *Clin Res* 23:484A, 1975. 11. Zinner M, Turtinen BA, Gurll NJ: The role of acid and ischemia in production of stress ulcers during canine hemorrhagic shock. *Surgery* 77:807–816, 1975. 12. Winans CS: Prevention and treatment of stress ulcer bleeding: Antacids or cimetidine? *Drug Ther Bull* (hospital) 12:37–45, 1981.

Shown in Product Identification Section, page 410

MYLANTA® GAS—40 mg Tablets
MYLICON® Drops
[*my'li-con*]
Antiflatulent

Ingredients: Each tablet or 0.6 mL of drops contains: Active: simethicone, 40 mg. Inactive: Tablets: calcium silicate, lactose, povidone, saccharin calcium. Drops: carbomer 934P, citric acid, flavors, hydroxypropyl methylcellulose, purified water, Red 3, saccharin calcium, sodium benzoate, sodium citrate.

Indications: Adults and children: For relief of the painful symptoms of excess gas in the digestive tract. Such gas is frequently caused by excessive swallowing of air or by eating foods that disagree. MYLANTA Gas-40 mg is a valuable adjunct in the treatment of many conditions in which the retention of gas may be a problem, such as: postoperative gaseous distention, air swallowing, functional dyspepsia, peptic ulcer, spastic or irritable colon, diverticulosis. If condition persists, consult your physician.

Infants: MYLICON drops are also useful for relief of the painful symptoms of excess gas associated with excessive swallowing of air or food intolerance. The defoaming action of MYLICON relieves flatulence by dispersing and preventing the formation of mucus-surrounded gas pockets in the gastrointestinal tract. MYLICON acts in the stomach and intestines to change the surface tension of gas bubbles enabling them to coalesce; thus the gas is freed and is eliminated more easily by belching or passing flatus.

Directions:
Tablets—One or two tablets four times daily after meals and at bedtime. May also be taken as needed up to 12 tablets daily or as directed by a physician. TABLETS SHOULD BE CHEWED THOROUGHLY.

Drops—Adults and Children: 0.6 mL four times daily after meals and at bedtime or as directed by a physician. Shake well before using.
Infants (under 2 years): Initially, 0.3 mL four times daily, after meals and at bedtime, or as directed by a physician. The dosage can also be mixed with 1 oz of cool water, infant formula, or other suitable liquids to ease administration.

Warnings: Do not exceed 12 doses per day except under the advice and supervision of a physician. Keep this and all drugs out of the reach of children.

How Supplied: Bottles of 100 white, scored, chewable tablets, identified MYL GAS 40, and dropper bottles of 15 mL (0.5 fl. oz) and 30 mL (1 fl oz) pink, pleasant tasting liquid. Also available in 100 tablet unit dose boxes (10 strips of 10 tablets each).
NDC 16837-450 (tablets).
NDC 16837-630 (drops).
Shown in Product Identification Section, page 410

MYLANTA® GAS Tablets
[my'li-con]
High-Capacity Antiflatulent

Ingredients: Each tablet contains:
Active: simethicone, 80 mg.
Inactive: dextrates, flavor, sorbitol, stearic acid, tricalcium phosphate.

Indications: For relief of the painful symptoms of excess gas in the digestive tract. Such gas is frequently caused by excessive swallowing of air or by eating foods that disagree. MYLANTA® GAS is a high capacity antiflatulent for adjunctive treatment of many conditions in which the retention of gas may be a problem, such as the following: air swallowing, functional dyspepsia, postoperative gaseous distention, peptic ulcer, spastic or irritable colon, diverticulosis. If condition persists, consult your physician. MYLANTA® GAS has a defoaming action that relieves flatulence by dispersing and preventing the formation of mucus-surrounded gas pockets in the gastrointestinal tract. MYLANTA® GAS acts in the stomach and intestines to change the surface tension of gas bubbles enabling them to coalesce; thus, the gas is freed and is eliminated more easily by belching or passing flatus.

Directions: One tablet four times daily after meals and at bedtime. May also be taken as needed up to 6 tablets daily or as directed by a physician. TABLETS SHOULD BE CHEWED THOROUGHLY.

Warnings: Keep this and all drugs out of the reach of children.

How Supplied: Economical bottles of 100 and convenience packages of individually wrapped 12 and 48 pink, scored, chewable tablets identified MYL GAS 80. Also available in 100 tablet unit dose boxes (10 strips of 10 tablets each).
NDC 16837-858.
Shown in Product Identification Section, page 410

Maximum Strength
MYLANTA® GAS Tablets
[my'li-con]
Maximum Strength Antiflatulent

Ingredients: Each tablet contains:
Active: simethicone, 125 mg.
Inactive: dextrates, flavor, sorbitol, stearic acid, tricalcium phosphate.

Indications: Maximum Strength MYLANTA® GAS is useful for relief of the painful symptoms of excess gas in the digestive tract. Such gas is frequently caused by excessive swallowing of air or by eating foods that disagree. Maximum Strength MYLANTA® GAS is the strongest possible antiflatulent for adjunctive treatment of many conditions in which the retention of gas may be a problem, such as the following: air swallowing, functional dyspepsia, postoperative gaseous distention, peptic ulcer, spastic or irritable colon, diverticulosis. If condition persists, consult your physician. Maximum Strength MYLANTA® GAS has a defoaming action that relieves flatulence by dispersing and preventing the formation of mucus-surrounded gas pockets in the gastrointestinal tract. Maximum Strength MYLANTA® GAS acts in the stomach and intestines to change the surface tension of gas bubbles enabling them to coalesce; thus, the gas is freed and is eliminated more easily by belching or passing flatus.

Directions: One tablet four times daily after meals and at bedtime or as directed by physician. TABLETS SHOULD BE CHEWED THOROUGHLY.

Warnings: Keep this and all drugs out of the reach of children.

How Supplied: Convenience packages of individually wrapped 12 and 60 white, scored chewable tablets identified MYL GAS 125. NDC 16837-455.
Shown in Product Identification Section, page 410

THE STUART FORMULA® Tablets
Multivitamin/Multimineral Supplement

One Tablet Daily Provides:

VITAMINS:	US RDA*	
A	100%	5,000 IU
D	100%	400 IU
E	50%	15 IU
C	100%	60 mg
Folic Acid	100%	0.4 mg
B₁ (thiamin)	80%	1.2 mg
B₂ (riboflavin)	100%	1.7 mg
Niacin	100%	20 mg
B₆ (pyridoxine hydrochloride)	100%	2 mg
B₁₂ (cyanocobalamin)	100%	6 mcg
MINERALS:	**US RDA**	
Calcium	16%	160 mg
Phosphorus	12%	125 mg
Iodine	100%	150 mcg
Iron	100%	18 mg
Magnesium	25%	100 mg

*Percentage of US Recommended Daily Allowances for adults and children 4 or more years of age.

Ingredients: Each tablet contains: Active: dibasic calcium phosphate, magnesium oxide, ascorbic acid, ferrous fumarate, dl-alpha tocopheryl acetate, folic acid, niacinamide, vitamin A palmitate, cyanocobalamin, pyridoxine hydrochloride, riboflavin, thiamin mononitrate, ergocalciferol, potassium iodide. Inactive: calcium sulfate, carnauba wax, pharmaceutical glaze, povidone, sodium starch glycolate, starch, sucrose, titanium dioxide, white wax.

Indications: The STUART FORMULA tablet provides a well-balanced multivitamin/multimineral formula intended for use as a daily dietary supplement for adults and children over age four.

Directions: One tablet daily or as directed by physician.

Warnings: Keep this and all drugs out of the reach of children. In case of accidental overdose, seek professional assistance or contact a Poison Control Center immediately.

How Supplied: Bottles of 100 and 250 white round tablets. Child-resistant safety caps are standard on both bottles

Continued on next page

J&J • Merck—Cont.

as a safeguard against accidental ingestion by children.
NDC 16837-866.

*Shown in Product Identification
Section, page 410*

STUARTINIC® Tablets
[*stu "are-tin 'ic*]
Hematinic

One Tablet Daily Provides:
US RDA*

Iron	556%	100 mg
VITAMINS:		
C	833%	500 mg
B$_1$	327%	4.9 mg
(thiamin)		
B$_2$	353%	6 mg
(riboflavin)		
Niacin	100%	20 mg
B$_6$	40%	0.8 mg
(pyridoxine hydrochloride)		
B$_{12}$	417%	25 mcg
(cyanocobalamin)		
Pantothenic		
Acid	92%	9.2 mg

*Percentage of US Recommended Daily Allowances for adults and children 4 or more years of age.

Ingredients: Active: ferrous fumarate, ascorbic acid, sodium ascorbate, niacinamide, calcium pantothenate, thiamin mononitrate, riboflavin, pyridoxine hydrochloride, cyanocobalamin. Inactive: flavor, hydrogenated vegetable oil, microcrystalline cellulose, povidone, Yellow 6, Yellow 10, and other ingredients.

Indications: STUARTINIC is a complete hematinic for patients with history of iron deficiency anemia who also lack proper amounts of vitamin C and B-complex vitamins due to inadequate diet. The use of well-tolerated ferrous fumarate in STUARTINIC provides a high level of elemental iron with a low incidence of gastric distress. The inclusion of 500 mg of Vitamin C per tablet serves to maintain more of the iron in the absorbable ferrous state. The B-complex vitamins improve nutrition where B-complex deficient diets contribute to the anemia.

Warnings: As with any drug, if you are pregnant or nursing a baby, seek the advice of a health professional before using this product. Keep out of the reach of children. In case of accidental overdose, seek professional assistance or contact a Poison Control Center immediately.

Dosage: One tablet daily taken after a meal or as directed by physician. Because of the high amount of iron per tablet, STUARTINIC is not recommended for children under 12 years of age.

How Supplied: STUARTINIC is supplied in bottles of 60 yellow, film coated, oval shaped tablets. NDC 16837-862.
Note: A child-resistant safety cap is standard on each 60 tablet bottle as a safeguard against accidental ingestion by children.

*Shown in Product Identification
Section, page 410*

Kramer Laboratories
8778 S.W. 8 STREET
MIAMI, FLA 33174

HALFPRIN™
PRODUCT OVERVIEW

Halfprin is a low strength (165 mg.) enteric coated aspirin of special interest to men and women who take low doses of aspirin on a continuous basis. Low strength allows for flexible dosing because there is usually no need to break a regular aspirin in half or alternate the daily dose to achieve individualized dosing. The enteric coating minimizes gastric distress.

Indication: Aspirin is indicated to reduce the risk of death and/or non-fatal myocardial infarction in patients with a previous infarction or unstable angina pectoris.

Clinical Trials: The indication is supported by the results of six large, randomized multicenter, placebo-controlled studies involving 10,816 predominantly male, post-myocardial infarction (MI) patients and one randomized placebo-controlled study of 1,266 men with unstable angina (1–7). Therapy with aspirin was begun at intervals after the onset of acute MI varying from less than 3 days to more than 5 years and continued for periods of from less than 1 year to 4 years. In the unstable angina study, treatment was started within 1 month after the onset of unstable angina and continued for 12 weeks, and patients with complicating conditions such as congestive heart failure were not included in the study.
Aspirin therapy in MI patients was associated with about a 20-percent reduction in the risk of subsequent death and/or non-fatal reinfarction, a median absolute decrease of 3 percent from the 12- to 22-percent event rates in the placebo groups. In aspirin-treated unstable angina patients the reduction in risk was about 50 percent, a reduction in the event rate of 5 percent from the 10-percent rate in the placebo group during the 12 weeks of the study.
Daily dosage of aspirin in the post-myocardial infarction studies was 300 milligrams in one study and 900 to 1,500 milligrams in 5 studies. A dose of 325 milligrams was used in the study of unstable angina.

Adverse Reactions: Gastrointestinal Reactions—Doses of 1,000 milligrams per day of aspirin caused gastrointestinal symptoms and bleeding that in some cases were clinically significant. In the largest post-infarction study (the Aspirin Myocardial Infarction Study (AMIS) with 4,500 people), the percentage incidences of gastrointestinal symptoms for the aspirin (1,000 milligrams of a standard, solid-tablet formulation) and placebo-treated subjects, respectively, were: stomach pain (14.5 percent; 4.4 percent); heartburn (11.9 percent; 4.8 percent); nausea and/or vomiting (7.6 percent; 2.1

percent); hospitalization for gastrointestinal disorder (4.8 percent; 3.5 percent). In the AMIS and other trials, aspirin-treated patients had increased rates of gross gastrointestinal bleeding. Symptoms and signs of gastrointestinal irritation were not significantly increased in subjects treated for unstable angina with buffered aspirin in solution.

Cardiovascular and Biochemical —
In the AMIS trial, the dosage of 1,000 milligrams per day of aspirin was associated with small increases in systolic blood pressure (BP) (average 1.5 to 2.1 millimeters) and diastolic BP (0.5 to 0.6 millimeters), depending upon whether maximal or last available readings were used. Blood urea nitrogen and uric acid levels were also increased, but by less than 1.0 milligram percent.
Subjects with marked hypertension or renal insufficiency had been excluded from the trial so that the clinical importance of these observations for such subjects or for any subjects treated over more prolonged periods is not known. It is recommended that patients placed on long-term aspirin treatment, even at doses of 300 milligrams per day, be seen at regular intervals to assess changes in these measurements.

Dosage and Administration: Although most of the studies used dosages exceeding 300 milligrams, 2 trials used only 300 milligrams and pharmacologic data indicate that this dose inhibits platelet function fully. Therefore, 300 milligrams or a conventional 325 milligram aspirin dose is a reasonable, routine dose that would minimize gastrointestinal adverse reactions. This use of aspirin applies to both solid, oral dosage forms (buffered and plain aspirin) and buffered aspirin in solution.

References:
(1) Elwood, P.C., et al., "A Randomized Controlled Trial of Acetylsalicylic Acid in the Secondary Prevention of Mortality from Myocardial Infarction." British Medical Journal 1:436–440, 1974.
(2) The Coronary Drug Project Research Group, "Aspirin in Coronary Heart Diseases," Journal of Chronic Diseases, 29:625–642, 1976.
(3) Breddin, K., et al., "Secondary Prevention of Myocardial Infarction: A Comparison of Acetylsalicylic Acid, Phenprocoumon or Placebo," Homeostasis, 470:263–268, 1979.
(4) Aspirin Myocardial Infarction Study Research Group, "A Randomized, Controlled Trial of Aspirin in Persons Recovered from Myocardial Infarction," Journal of the American Medical Association, 243:661–669, 1980.
(5) Elwood, P.C., and P.M. Sweetnam, "Aspirin and Secondary Mortality after Myocardial Infarction," Lancet, II:1313–1315, December 22–29, 1979.
(6) The Persantine-Aspirin Reinfarction Study Research Group, "Persantine and Aspirin in Coronary Heart Disease," Circulation 62:449–461, 1980.

(7) Lewis, H.D., et al, "Protective Effects of Aspirin Against Acute Myocardial Infarction and Death in Men with Unstable Angina, Results of a Veterans Administration Cooperative Study," New England Journal of Medicine, 309:396–403, 1983.

(8) "1984 Report of the Joint National Committee on Detection, Evaluation, and Treatment of High Blood Pressure," United States Department of Health and Human Services and United States Public Health Service, National Institutes of Health., Publication No. NIH 84–1088, 1984.

Shown in Product Identification Section, page 410

EDUCATIONAL MATERIAL

Questions and Answers on Halfprin™
Free booklet — Information for physicians, pharmacists and other health care professionals on Halfprin, low strength 165 mg enteric coated aspirin, for patients who use aspirin to reduce the risk of recurrent myocardial infarction and unstable angina.

Lactaid Inc.
PLEASANTVILLE, NJ 08232

LACTAID®
Lactaid Drops
and
Lactaid Caplets
(lactase enzyme)

PRODUCT OVERVIEW

Key Facts: Lactaid® lactase enzyme hydrolyzes lactose into digestible simple sugars: glucose and galactose. Lactaid Drops are added to milk for *in vitro* hydrolysis of lactose; Lactaid Caplets are taken orally for *in vivo* hydrolysis of lactose.

Major Uses: Lactaid lactase enzyme (liquid and caplets) have proven to be clinically effective in preventing the GI symptoms associated with lactose intolerance, which include abdominal pain, cramps, bloating, flatulence, and diarrhea.

PRESCRIBING INFORMATION

LACTAID®
Lactaid Drops
and
Lactaid Caplets
(lactase enzyme)

Description:
DROPS: Each 5 drop dosage contains 1250 NLU (Neutral Lactase Units) of lactase enzyme derived from *Kluyveromyces lactis.*
CAPLETS: Each caplet contains 3300 FCC (Food Chemical Codex) units of lactose enzyme (derived from *Aspergillus oryzae*) per caplet.

Action: The lactase enzyme hydrolyzes the lactose sugar (a double sugar) found in milk and all dairy products into two digestible single sugars, glucose and galactose.

Indications: Indicated for patients with lactose intolerance who experience related GI symptoms such as abdominal pain, cramps, bloating, flatulence, and/or diarrhea, after the ingestion of milk or other lactose containing products.

Precautions: Do not use if you have had an allergic reaction to Lactaid products. Diabetics should be aware that the lactose sugar will now be metabolically available as glucose and galactose.

Usual Dosage:
DROPS: Put 5 drops of Lactaid in a quart of milk, shake gently, and refrigerate for 24 hours. This makes 70% of the lactose digestible. For greater lactose reduction: Use 10 drops per quart of milk for 90% reduction or 15 drops for 99+% lactose removal.
CAPLETS: Lactose intolerance varies: Start with two caplets and work up or down to find your own level of comfort. Use no more than 6 caplets at one time. If symptoms persist, consult a physician.

Inactive Ingredients:
DROPS: Glycerin, Water
CAPLETS: Calcium Phosphate, Corn Starch, Hydrogenated Vegetable Oil Croscarmellose Sodium, Dextrose, Microcrystalline Cellulose.

How Supplied:
DROPS: 3 ml, 7 ml, and 19 ml dropper bottles
CAPLETS: Bottles of 12, 50, and 100
Shown in Product Identification Section, page 414

Lavoptik Company, Inc.
**661 WESTERN AVENUE N.
ST. PAUL, MN 55103**

LAVOPTIK® Eye Wash

Description: Isotonic LAVOPTIK Eye Wash is a buffered solution designed to help physically remove contaminants from the surface of the eye and lids. Formulated to buffer contaminants toward the safe range and help restore normal salts and water ratios in the tears.

Contents: Each 100 ml

Sodium Chloride	0.49	gram
Sodium Biphosphate	0.40	gram
Sodium Phosphate	0.45	gram
Preservative Agent		
Benzalkonium Chloride	0.005	gram

Precautions: If you experience severe eye pain, headache, rapid change in vision (side or straight ahead); sudden appearance of floating objects, acute redness of the eyes, pain on exposure to light or double vision consult a physician at once. If symptoms persist or worsen after use of this product, consult a physician. If solution changes color or becomes cloudy do not use. Keep this and all medicines out of reach of children. Keep container

tightly closed. Do not use if safety seal is broken at time of purchase.

Administration: 6 ounce size with Eye Cup.
Rinse cup with clean water immediately before and after each use, avoid contamination of rim and inside surfaces of cup. Apply cup, half-filled with LAVOPTIK Eye Wash tightly to the eye. Tilt head backward. Open eyelids wide, rotate eyeball and blink several times to insure thorough washing. Discard washings. Repeat other eye. Tightly cap bottle.
32 ounce size.
Break seal as you remove cap and pour directly on contaminated area.

How Supplied: 6 ounce bottle with eyecup, NDC 10651-01040.
32 ounce bottle, NDC 10651-01019.

Lederle Laboratories
A Division of American Cyanamid Co.
**ONE CYANAMID PLAZA
WAYNE, NJ 07470**

LEDERMARK®
Product Identification Code

Many Lederle tablets and capsules bear an identification code. A current listing appears in the Product Information Section of the 1992 PDR for prescription drugs.

CALTRATE® 600
[*căl-trāte*]
**High Potency Calcium Supplement
Nature's Most Concentrated Form of Calcium**™
No Sugar, No Salt, No Lactose, No Cholesterol, No Preservatives, Film-Coated for Easy Swallowing

Inactive Ingredients: Croscarmellose Sodium, Hydroxypropyl Methylcellulose, Magnesium Stearate, Microcrystalline Cellulose, PVPP, Sodium Lauryl Sulfate, and Titanium Dioxide.
TWO TABLETS DAILY PROVIDE:

	For Adults— Percentage of U.S. Recommended Daily Allowance (U.S. RDA)
3000 mg Calcium Carbonate which provides 1200 mg elemental calcium	120%

Recommended Intake: One or two tablets daily or as directed by the physician.

Warnings: Keep this and all medications out of the reach of children.

How Supplied: Bottle of 60— NDC 0005-5510-19
Store at Room Temperature.

26276
D14

Shown in Product Identification Section, page 410

Continued on next page

Lederle—Cont.

CALTRATE® 600+Iron & Vitamin D

[căl-trāte]

High Potency Calcium Supplement
Nature's Most Concentrated Form of Calcium™
No Sugar, No Salt, No Lactose, No Cholesterol, Film-Coated for Easy Swallowing

ONE TABLET DAILY CONTAINS:

	For Adults— Percentage of U.S. Recommended Daily Allowance (RDA)
1500 mg Calcium Carbonate which provides 600 mg elemental calcium	60%
18 mg elemental Iron in the Optisorb® Time-Release System (as ferrous fumarate)	100%
125 I.U. Vitamin D	31%

Inactive Ingredients: Blue 2, Croscarmellose Sodium, Hydroxypropyl Cellulose, Magnesium Stearate, Microcrystalline Cellulose, Polysorbate 80, Povidone, PVPP, Red 40, Sodium Lauryl Sulfate, Titanium Dioxide, and Triethyl Citrate.

- CALTRATE + Iron contains pure calcium and time-release iron for diets deficient in both minerals.
- Plus Vitamin D to help absorb calcium.

Recommended Intake: One or two tablets daily or as directed by the physician.

Warnings: Keep out of the reach of children.

How Supplied: Bottle of 60—NDC 0005-5523-19
Store at Room Temperature.

27466
D8

Shown in Product Identification Section, page 410

CALTRATE® 600 + Vitamin D

[căl-trāte]

High Potency Calcium Supplement
Nature's Most Concentrated Form of Calcium™
No Sugar, No Salt, No Lactose, No Cholesterol, Film-Coated for Easy Swallowing

Inactive Ingredients: Blue 2, Croscarmellose Sodium, FD&C Yellow No. 6, Hydroxypropyl Methylcellulose, Magnesium Stearate, Microcrystalline Cellulose, Povidone, PVPP, Red 40, Sodium Lauryl Sulfate, and Titanium Dioxide.

TWO TABLETS DAILY PROVIDE:

	For Adults— Percentage of U.S. Recommended Daily Allowance (RDA)
3000 mg Calcium Carbonate which provides 1200 mg elemental calcium	120%
250 I.U. Vitamin D	62%

Recommended Intake: One or two tablets daily or as directed by the physician.

Warnings: Keep out of the reach of children.

How Supplied: Bottle of 60—NDC-0005-5509-19
Store at Room Temperature.

26277
D11

Shown in Product Identification Section, page 410

CENTRUM®

[sĕn-trŭm]

High Potency
Multivitamin/Multimineral Formula,
Advanced Formula
From A to Zinc®

Each tablet contains:

	For Adults— Percentage of U.S. Recommended Daily Allowance (U.S. RDA)
Vitamin A (as Acetate and Beta Carotene)	5000 I.U. (100%)
Vitamin E (as dl-Alpha Tocopheryl Acetate)	30 I.U. (100%)
Vitamin C (as Ascorbic Acid)	60 mg (100%)
Folic Acid	400 mcg (100%)
Vitamin B$_1$ (as Thiamine Mononitrate)	1.5 mg (100%)
Vitamin B$_2$ (as Riboflavin)	1.7 mg (100%)
Niacinamide	20 mg (100%)
Vitamin B$_6$ (as Pyridoxine Hydrochloride)	2 mg (100%)
Vitamin B$_{12}$ (as Cyanocobalamin)	6 mcg (100%)
Vitamin D	400 I.U. (100%)
Biotin	30 mcg (10%)
Pantothenic Acid (as Calcium Pantothenate)	10 mg (100%)
Calcium (as Dibasic Calcium Phosphate)	162 mg (16%)
Phosphorus (as Dibasic Calcium Phosphate)	125 mg (13%)
Iodine (as Potassium Iodide)	150 mcg (100%)
Iron (as Ferrous Fumarate)	18 mg (100%)
Magnesium (as Magnesium Oxide)	100 mg (25%)
Copper (as Cupric Oxide)	2 mg (100%)
Zinc (as Zinc Oxide)	15 mg (100%)
Manganese (as Manganese Sulfate)	2.5 mg*
Potassium (as Potassium Chloride)	40 mg*
Chloride (as Potassium Chloride)	36.3 mg*
Chromium (as Chromium Chloride)	25 mcg*
Molybdenum (as Sodium Molybdate)	25 mcg*
Selenium (as Sodium Selenate)	25 mcg*
Vitamin K$_1$ (as Phytonadione)	25 mcg*
Nickel (as Nickelous Sulfate)	5 mcg*
Tin (as Stannous Chloride)	10 mcg*
Silicon (as Metasilicates and Oxides)	2 mg*
Vanadium (as Sodium Metavanadate)	10 mcg*
Boron (as Borates)	150 mcg*

*No U.S. RDA established.

Inactive Ingredients: Acacia Gum, Dextrose, FD&C Yellow No. 6, Hydroxypropyl Methylcellulose, Lactose, Magnesium Stearate, Methylparaben, Microcrystalline Cellulose, Modified Food Starch, Mono- and Di-glycerides, Potassium Sorbate, Propylparaben, PVPP, Silica Gel, Sodium Benzoate, Sorbic Acid, Stearic Acid, and Sucrose.

Recommended Intake: Adults, 1 tablet daily.

How Supplied:
Light peach, engraved CENTRUM C1.
Bottle of 60—NDC 0005-4239-19
Combopack*—NDC 0005-4239-30
*Bottles of 100 plus 30
Store at Room Temperature.

26287
D33

Shown in Product Identification Section, page 410

CENTRUM® Liquid

High Potency
Multivitamin-Multimineral Formula

Each 15 mL (1 tablespoon) contains:

	For Adults— Percentage of U.S. Recommended Daily Allowance (U.S. RDA)
Vitamin A (as Palmitate)	2500 I.U. (50%)
Vitamin E (as dl-Alpha Tocopheryl Acetate)	30 I.U. (100%)
Vitamin C (as Ascorbic Acid)	60 mg (100%)
Vitamin B$_1$ (as Thiamine Hydrochloride)	1.5 mg (100%)
Vitamin B$_2$ (as Riboflavin)	1.7 mg (100%)
Niacinamide	20 mg (100%)
Vitamin B$_6$ (as Pyridoxine Hydrochloride)	2 mg (100%)
Vitamin B$_{12}$ (as Cyanocobalamin)	6 mcg (100%)
Vitamin D$_2$	400 I.U. (100%)
Biotin	300 mcg (100%)
Pantothenic Acid (as Panthenol)	10 mg (100%)
Iodine (as Potassium Iodide)	150 mcg (100%)
Iron (as Ferrous Gluconate)	9 mg (50%)
Zinc (as Zinc Gluconate)	3 mg (20%)
Manganese (as Manganese Chloride)	2.5 mg *
Chromium (as Chromium Chloride)	25 mcg *
Molybdenum (as Sodium Molybdate)	25 mcg *

*No U.S. RDA established.

Inactive Ingredients: Alcohol 6.6%, Artificial and Natural Flavors, Citric Acid, Glycerin, Polysorbate 80, Sodium Benzoate, and Sucrose.

Recommended Intake: Adults, 1 tablespoonful (15 mL) daily.

Warnings: Keep this and all medication out of the reach of children.

How Supplied: 8 oz Bottle— NDC 0005-4343-61 Store at Controlled Room Temperature 15°–30°C (59°–86°F). PROTECT FROM FREEZING.

23317 D3

Shown in Product Identification Section, page 411

CENTRUM, JR.®
[sĕn-trŭm]
Children's Chewable Vitamin/Mineral Formula+Extra C Tablets
Nutritional Support From Head to Toe®

[See table below.]

Inactive Ingredients: Acacia, Artificial Flavorings, Blue 1, Blue 2, Colloidal Silicon Dioxide, Dextrins, Dextrose, Gelatin, Hydrogenated Vegetable Oil, Hydrolyzed Protein, Lactose, Magnesium Stearate, Methylparaben, Microcrystalline Cellulose, Modified Food Starch,

Mono- and Di-glycerides, Potassium Sorbate, Povidone, Propylparaben, Red 40, Sodium Benzoate, Sorbic Acid, Stearic Acid, Sucrose, Yellow 6.

Warnings: CONTAINS IRON, WHICH CAN BE HARMFUL IN LARGE DOSES. CLOSE TIGHTLY AND KEEP OUT OF THE REACH OF CHILDREN. IN CASE OF ACCIDENTAL OVERDOSE, CONTACT A PHYSICIAN OR POISON CONTROL CENTER IMMEDIATELY.

How Supplied: Bottle of 60— NDC 0005-4249-19 Store at Room Temperature.

27120 D8

Shown in Product Identification Section, page 410

CENTRUM, JR.®
[sĕn-trŭm]
Children's Chewable Vitamin/Mineral Formula+Extra Calcium
Nutritional Support From Head to Toe®

[See table on next page.]

Inactive Ingredients:
Acacia, Artificial Flavorings, Colloidal Silicon Dioxide, Dextrins, Dextrose, Gelatin, Hydrogenated Vegetable Oil, Hydrolyzed Protein, Lactose, Magnesium Stearate, Methylparaben, Microcrystal-

line Cellulose, Modified Food Starch, Mono- and Di-glycerides, Potassium Sorbate, Propylparaben, Red 40, Sodium Benzoate, Sodium Starch Glycolate, Sorbic Acid, Stearic Acid, Sucrose.

Warnings: CONTAINS IRON, WHICH CAN BE HARMFUL IN LARGE DOSES. CLOSE TIGHTLY AND KEEP OUT OF THE REACH OF CHILDREN. IN CASE OF ACCIDENTAL OVERDOSE, CONTACT A PHYSICIAN OR POISON CONTROL CENTER IMMEDIATELY.

Recommended Intake: 2 to 4 years of age: chew one-half tablet daily. Over 4 years of age: chew one tablet daily.

How Supplied: Bottle of 60— NDC 0005-4222-19 Store at Room Temperature.

D3 21340

Shown in Product Identification Section, page 411

CENTRUM, JR.®
[sĕn-trŭm]
Children's Chewable Vitamin/Mineral Formula + Iron Tablets
Nutritional Support From Head to Toe®

[See table on next page.]

Inactive Ingredients: Acacia, Artificial Flavorings, Blue 1, Blue 2, Colloidal Silicon Dioxide, Dextrins, Dextrose, Gelatin, Hydrogenated Vegetable Oil, Hydrolyzed Protein, Lactose, Magnesium Stearate, Methylparaben, Microcrystalline Cellulose, Modified Food Starch,

Mono- and Di-glycerides, Potassium Sorbate, Propylparaben, Red 40, Sodium Benzoate, Sodium Starch Glycolate, Sorbic Acid, Stearic Acid, Sucrose, Yellow 6.

Recommended Intake: 2 to 4 years of age: Chew one-half tablet daily. Over 4 years of age: Chew one tablet daily.

Warnings: CONTAINS IRON, WHICH CAN BE HARMFUL IN LARGE DOSES. CLOSE TIGHTLY AND KEEP OUT OF THE REACH OF CHILDREN. IN CASE OF ACCIDENTAL OVERDOSE, CONTACT A PHYSICIAN OR POISON CONTROL CENTER IMMEDIATELY.

How Supplied: Assorted Flavors— Uncoated Tablet—Partially Scored —Engraved Lederle C2 and CENTRUM, JR. Bottle of 60—NDC 0005-4234-19 Store at Room Temperature.

27118 D9

Shown in Product Identification Section, page 410

Continued on next page

CENTRUM, JR.®
Children's Chewable
Vitamin/Mineral Formula+Extra C

	Quantity per tablet	Percentage of U.S. Recommended Daily Allowance (U.S. RDA)	
		For Children 2 to 4 (½ tablet)	For Children Over 4 (1 tablet)
EACH TABLET CONTAINS:			
VITAMINS			
Vitamin A (as Acetate)	5,000 I.U.	(100%)	(100%)
Vitamin D	400 I.U.	(50%)	(100%)
Vitamin E (as Acetate)	30 I.U.	(150%)	(100%)
Vitamin C (as Ascorbic Acid and Sodium Ascorbate)	300 mg	(375%)	(500%)
Folic Acid	400 mcg	(100%)	(100%)
Biotin	45 mcg	(15%)	(15%)
Thiamine (as Thiamine Mononitrate)	1.5 mg	(107%)	(100%)
Pantothenic Acid (as Calcium Pantothenate)	10 mg	(100%)	(100%)
Riboflavin	1.7 mg	(107%)	(100%)
Niacinamide	20 mg	(111%)	(100%)
Vitamin B$_6$ (as Pyridoxine Hydrochloride)	2 mg	(143%)	(100%)
Vitamin B$_{12}$ (as Cyanocobalamin)	6 mcg	(100%)	(100%)
Vitamin K$_1$ (as Phytonadione)	10 mcg*		
MINERALS			
Iron (as Ferrous Fumarate)	18 mg	(90%)	(100%)
Magnesium (as Magnesium Oxide)	40 mg	(10%)	(10%)
Iodine (as Potassium Iodide)	150 mcg	(107%)	(100%)
Copper (as Cupric Oxide)	2 mg	(100%)	(100%)
Phosphorus (as Tribasic Calcium Phosphate)	50 mg	(3.12%)	(5.0%)
Calcium (as Tribasic Calcium Phosphate)	108 mg	(6.75%)	(10.8%)
Zinc (as Zinc Oxide)	15 mg	(93%)	(100%)
Manganese (as Manganese Sulfate)	1 mg*		
Molybdenum (as Sodium Molybdate)	20 mcg*		
Chromium (as Chromium Chloride)	20 mcg*		

*Recognized as essential in human nutrition but no U.S. RDA established.

Lederle—Cont.

CENTRUM, JR.®
Children's Chewable
Vitamin/Mineral Formula + Extra Calcium

EACH TABLET CONTAINS:	Quantity per tablet	Percentage of U.S. Recommended Daily Allowance (U.S. RDA)	
		For Children 2 to 4 (½ tablet)	For Children Over 4 (1 tablet)
VITAMINS			
Vitamin A (as Acetate)	5,000 I.U.	(100%)	(100%)
Vitamin D	400 I.U.	(50%)	(100%)
Vitamin E (as Acetate)	30 I.U.	(150%)	(100%)
Vitamin C (as Ascorbic Acid)	60 mg	(75%)	(100%)
Folic Acid	400 mcg	(100%)	(100%)
Biotin	45 mcg	(15%)	(15%)
Thiamine (as Thiamine Mononitrate)	1.5 mg	(107%)	(100%)
Pantothenic Acid (as Calcium Pantothenate)	10 mg	(100%)	(100%)
Riboflavin	1.7 mg	(107%)	(100%)
Niacinamide	20 mg	(111%)	(100%)
Vitamin B_6 (as Pyridoxine Hydrochloride)	2 mg	(143%)	(100%)
Vitamin B_{12} (as Cyanocobalamin)	6 mcg	(100%)	(100%)
Vitamin K_1 (as Phytonadione)	10 mcg*		
MINERALS			
Iron (as Ferrous Fumarate)	18 mg	(90%)	(100%)
Magnesium (as Magnesium Oxide)	40 mg	(10%)	(10%)
Iodine (as Potassium Iodide)	150 mcg	(107%)	(100%)
Copper (as Cupric Oxide)	2 mg	(100%)	(100%)
Phosphorus (as Dibasic Calcium Phosphate)	50 mg	(3.12%)	(5.0%)
Calcium (as Dibasic Calcium Phosphate and Calcium Carbonate)	160 mg	(10%)	(16%)
Zinc (as Zinc Oxide)	15 mg	(93%)	(100%)
Manganese (as Manganese Sulfate)	1 mg*		
Molybdenum (as Sodium Molybdate)	20 mcg*		
Chromium (as Chromium Chloride)	20 mcg*		

*Recognized as essential in human nutrition but no U.S. RDA established.

CENTRUM, JR.®
Children's Chewable
Vitamin/Mineral Formula + Iron

EACH TABLET CONTAINS:	Quantity per tablet	Percentage of U.S. Recommended Daily Allowance (U.S. RDA)	
		For Children 2 to 4 (½ tablet)	For Children Over 4 (1 tablet)
VITAMINS			
Vitamin A (as Acetate)	5,000 I.U.	(100%)	(100%)
Vitamin D	400 I.U.	(50%)	(100%)
Vitamin E (as Acetate)	30 I.U.	(150%)	(100%)
Vitamin C (as Ascorbic Acid)	60 mg	(75%)	(100%)
Folic Acid	400 mcg	(100%)	(100%)
Biotin	45 mcg	(15%)	(15%)
Thiamine (as Thiamine Mononitrate)	1.5 mg	(107%)	(100%)
Pantothenic Acid (as Calcium Pantothenate)	10 mg	(100%)	(100%)
Riboflavin	1.7 mg	(107%)	(100%)
Niacinamide	20 mg	(111%)	(100%)
Vitamin B_6 (as Pyridoxine Hydrochloride)	2 mg	(143%)	(100%)
Vitamin B_{12} (as Cyanocobalamin)	6 mcg	(100%)	(100%)
Vitamin K_1 (as Phytonadione)	10 mcg*		
MINERALS			
Iron (as Ferrous Fumarate)	18 mg	(90%)	(100%)
Magnesium (as Magnesium Oxide)	40 mg	(10%)	(10%)
Iodine (as Potassium Iodide)	150 mcg	(107%)	(100%)
Copper (as Cupric Oxide)	2 mg	(100%)	(100%)
Phosphorus (as Dibasic Calcium Phosphate)	50 mg	(3.12%)	(5.0%)
Calcium (as Dibasic Calcium Phosphate and Calcium Carbonate)	108 mg	(6.75%)	(10.8%)
Zinc (as Zinc Oxide)	15 mg	(93%)	(100%)
Manganese (as Manganese Sulfate)	1 mg*		
Molybdenum (as Sodium Molybdate)	20 mcg*		
Chromium (as Chromium Chloride)	20 mcg*		

*Recognized as essential in human nutrition but no U.S. RDA established.

CENTRUM SILVER®
Specially Formulated
Multivitamin-Multimineral for Adults
50+

Each tablet contains:

	For Adults— Percentage of U.S. Recommended Daily Allowance (U.S. RDA)	
Vitamin A	6000 I.U.	(120%)
(as Acetate and Beta Carotene)		
Vitamin B₁	1.5 mg	(100%)
Vitamin B₂	1.7 mg	(100%)
Vitamin B₆	3 mg	(150%)
Vitamin B₁₂	25 mcg	(416%)
Biotin	30 mcg	(10%)
Folic Acid	200 mcg	(50%)
Niacinamide	20 mg	(100%)
Pantothenic Acid	10 mg	(100%)
Vitamin C	60 mg	(100%)
Vitamin D	400 I.U.	(100%)
Vitamin E	45 I.U.	(150%)
Vitamin K₁	10 mcg*	
Calcium	200 mg	(20%)
Copper	2 mg	(100%)
Iodine	150 mcg	(100%)
Iron	9 mg	(50%)
Magnesium	100 mg	(25%)
Phosphorus	48 mg	(5%)
Zinc	15 mg	(100%)
Chloride	72 mg*	
Chromium	100 mcg*	
Manganese	2.5 mg*	
Molybdenum	25 mcg*	
Nickel	5 mcg*	
Potassium	80 mg*	
Selenium	25 mcg*	
Silicon	10 mcg*	
Vanadium	10 mcg*	

*No U.S. RDA established.

Inactive Ingredients: Blue 2, Crospovidone, FD&C Yellow #6, Gelatin, Hydroxypropyl Methylcellulose, Lactose, Magnesium Stearate, Microcrystalline Cellulose, Polyethylene Glycol, Polysorbate 80, Red 40, Silica Gel, Stearic Acid, and Titanium Dioxide.

Gel-Tabs™ —Specially coated supplement to assure ease of swallowing.

Recommended Intake:
Adults, 1 tablet daily.

How Supplied: Bottle of 60—
NDC 0005-4177-19
Store at Room Temperature.
10225-91
D2

*Shown in Product Identification
Section, page 411*

Dual Action
FERRO–SEQUELS®
[fĕrrō-sēquals]
High Potency Iron Supplement
Time-Release Iron Plus
Clinically Proven Anticonstipant
Easy-to-Swallow Tablets
Low Sodium, No Sugar

Active Ingredients: Each tablet contains 150 mg of ferrous fumarate equivalent to 50 mg of elemental iron and 100 mg of docusate sodium (DSS).

Inactive Ingredients: Blue 1, Corn Starch, Crospovidone, Hydroxypropyl Methylcellulose, Lactose, Magnesium Stearate, Microcrystalline Cellulose, Modified Food Starch, Povidone, Silica Gel, Sodium Lauryl Sulfate, Titanium Dioxide, and Yellow 10.

Warning: As with any drug, if you are pregnant or nursing a baby, seek the advice of a health professional before using this product. Keep this and all medications out of the reach of children. In case of accidental overdose, seek professional assistance or contact a Poison Control Center immediately.

Recommended Intake: One tablet, once or twice daily or as prescribed by a physician.

How Supplied: Boxes of 30—
NDC 0005-5267-68
Bottle of 30—NDC 0005-5267-13
Bottle of 100—NDC 0005-5267-23
Unit Dose Pack 10×10—
NDC 0005-5267-60
Green, capsule-shaped, film-coated tablets engraved LL and F2.
Store at Room Temperature.
27533
D3

*Shown in Product Identification
Section, page 411*

FIBERCON®
[fĭ-bĕr-cŏn]
Calcium Polycarbophil
Bulk-Forming Fiber Laxative

Safe and effective, Less than one calorie per tablet, Sodium- and Preservative-free, Film-coated for easy swallowing, Calcium rich, No chemical stimulants.

Active Ingredient: Each tablet contains 625 mg calcium polycarbophil equivalent to 500 mg polycarbophil.

Inactive Ingredients: Calcium Carbonate, Caramel, Crospovidone, Hydroxypropyl Methylcellulose, Magnesium Stearate, Microcrystalline Cellulose, Povidone, and Silica Gel.

Indications: Relief of constipation (irregularity).

Actions: Increases bulk volume and water content of the stool.

Warnings: If you have noticed a sudden change in bowel habits that persists over a period of 2 weeks, consult a physician before using a laxative. If the recommended use of this product for 1 week has no effect, discontinue use and consult a physician.
Do not use laxative products when abdominal pain, nausea or vomiting is present except under the direction of a physician. Discontinue use and consult a physician if rectal bleeding occurs after use of any laxative product.
For chronic or continued constipation consult your physician.

Interaction Precaution: Contains calcium. Take this product at least 1 hour before or 2 hours after taking an oral dose of a prescription antibiotic containing any form of tetracycline.

KEEP THIS AND ALL MEDICINES OUT OF THE REACH OF CHILDREN. STORE AT CONTROLLED ROOM TEMPERATURE 15°–30°C (59°–86°F). PROTECT CONTENTS FROM MOISTURE.

Recommended Intake: Adults and children 12 years and older: swallow two tablets one to four times a day. Children 6 to 12 years: swallow one tablet one to three times a day. Children under 6 years: consult a physician. See package insert for additional information.
A FULL GLASS (8 fl oz) OF LIQUID SHOULD BE TAKEN WITH EACH DOSE.

How Supplied:
Film coated tablets, scored, engraved LL and F66.
Package of 36 tablets, NDC 0005-2500-02
Package of 60 tablets, NDC 0005-2500-86
Package of 90 tablets, NDC 0005-2500-33
Bottle of 500 tablets, NDC 0005-2500-31
Unit Dose Pkg, NDC 0005-2500-28
27982
D7

*Shown in Product Identification
Section, page 411*

FILIBON®
[fĭ-lĭ-bŏn]
Multivitamin-Multimineral
Supplement for Pregnant or
Lactating Women
Prenatal Tablets

Each tablet contains:

	For Pregnant or Lactating Women Percentage of U.S. Recommended Daily Allowance (U.S. RDA)	
Vitamin A (as Acetate)	5000 I.U.	(63%)
Vitamin D₂	400 I.U.	(100%)
Vitamin E (as dl-Alpha Tocopheryl Acetate)	30 I.U.	(100%)
Vitamin C (as Ascorbic Acid)	60 mg	(100%)
Folic Acid	0.4 mg	(50%)
Vitamin B₁ (as Thiamine Mononitrate)	1.5 mg	(88%)
Vitamin B₂ (as Riboflavin)	1.7 mg	(85%)
Niacinamide	20 mg	(100%)
Vitamin B₆	2 mg	(80%)
Vitamin B₁₂ (as Cyanocobalamin)	6 mcg	(75%)
Calcium (as Calcium Carbonate)	125 mg	(10%)
Iodine (as Potassium Iodide)	150 mcg	(100%)
Iron (as Ferrous Fumarate)	18 mg	(100%)
Magnesium (as Magnesium Oxide)	100 mg	(22%)

Inactive Ingredients: Ethylcellulose, Hydroxypropyl Methylcellulose, Lactose, Magnesium Stearate, Microcrystalline Cellulose, Povidone, Pregelatinized Starch, Red 40, Silicon Dioxide, Sodium

Continued on next page

Lederle—Cont.

Lauryl Sulfate, Sodium Starch Glycolate, Titanium Dioxide, and Stearic Acid.

Recommended Intake: 1 daily, or as prescribed by the physician.

How Supplied: Capsule-shaped tablets (film-coated, pink) engraved LL and F4.
Bottle of 100—NDC-0005-4294-23
Store at Room Temperature.

10999-91
D12

GEVRABON®
[jĕv-ra băn]
Vitamin-Mineral Supplement

Composition: Each fluid ounce (30 mL) contains:

For Adults—
Percentage of U.S.
Recommended Daily
Allowance (U.S. RDA)

Vitamin B_1 (as Thiamine
  Hydrochloride) ....5 mg (333%)
Vitamin B_2 (as Riboflavin-
  5-Phosphate Sodium) ....2.5 mg (147%)
Niacinamide ....50 mg (250%)
Vitamin B_6 (Pyridox-
  ine Hydrochloride) ....1 mg (50%)
Vitamin B_{12} (as
  Cyanocobalamin)...............1 mcg (17%)
Pantothenic Acid (as D-
  Pantothenyl Alcohol).....10 mg (100%)
Iodine (as Potassium
  Iodide) ....100 mcg (67%)
Iron (as Ferrous
  Gluconate) ....15 mg (83%)
Magnesium (as Magne-
  sium Chloride)....................2 mg (0.5%)
Zinc (as Zinc Chloride)..........2 mg (13%)
Choline (as Tricholine
  Citrate)..100 mg*
Manganese (as Manga-
  nese Chloride)..............................2 mg*
*Recognized as essential in human nutrition but no U.S. RDA established.
Alcohol 18%

Inactive Ingredients: Alcohol, Citric Acid, Glycerin, Sherry Wine, Sucrose.

Indications: For use as a nutritional supplement. Shake well.

Warning: As with any drug, if you are pregnant or nursing a baby, seek the advice of a health professional before using this product. Keep this preparation out of the reach of children.

Administration and Dosage: Adult: One ounce (30 mL) daily or as prescribed by the physician as a nutritional supplement.

Important Note: In time a slight natural deposit, characteristic of the sherry wine base, may occur. This does not indicate in any way a loss of quality.

How Supplied: Syrup (sherry flavor) decanters of 16 fl oz—NDC 0005-5250-35
Keep Out of Direct Sunlight.
Store at Room Temperature, 15°–30°C (59°–86°F).
DO NOT FREEZE.

16520
D4

GEVRAL®
[jĕv-ral]
Multivitamin and Multimineral Supplement Tablets

Composition: Each tablet contains:
For Adults—
Percentage of U.S.
Recommended Daily
Allowance (U.S. RDA)

Vitamin A (as
  Acetate) .... 5000 I.U. (100%)
Vitamin E (as dl-Alpha
  Tocopheryl Acetate)... 30 I.U. (100%)
Vitamin C (as Ascorbic
  Acid).............................. 60 mg (100%)
Folic Acid .... 0.4 mg (100%)
Vitamin B_1 (as Thia-
  mine Mononitrate)..... 1.5 mg (100%)
Vitamin B_2 (as
  Riboflavin) .... 1.7 mg (100%)
Niacinamide................... 20 mg (100%)
Vitamin B_6 (as Pyridoxine
  Hydrochloride)............ 2 mg (100%)
Vitamin B_{12} (as
  Cyanocobalamin)........ 6 mcg (100%)
Calcium (as Dibasic
  Calcium Phosphate)... 162 mg (16%)
Phosphorus (as Dibasic
  Calcium Phosphate)... 125 mg (13%)
Iodine (as Potassium
  Iodide)..........................150 mcg (100%)
Iron (as Ferrous
  Fumarate)................... 18 mg (100%)
Magnesium (as
  Magnesium Oxide)..... 100 mg (25%)

Inactive Ingredients: Blue 2, Ethylcellulose, Gelatin, Hydrolyzed Protein, Hydroxypropyl Methylcellulose, Lactose, Magnesium Stearate, Methylparaben, Microcrystalline Cellulose, Modified Food Starch, Mono- and Di-glycerides, Polacrilin, Potassium Sorbate, Propylparaben, PVPP, Red 30, Silica Gel, Sodium Benzoate, Sorbic Acid, Stearic Acid, Sucrose, Titanium Dioxide, and Yellow 6.

Indications: Supplementation of the diet.

Recommended Intake: One tablet daily or as prescribed by the physician.

Warnings: Keep this and all medications out of the reach of children.

How Supplied: Capsule-shaped tablets (film-coated, brown) engraved LL and G1.
Bottle of 100—NDC 0005-4289-23
Store at Room Temperature.
A SPECTRUM® Product

22788
D15

GEVRAL® T
[jĕv-ral t]
High Potency Multivitamin and Multimineral Supplement Tablets

Each tablet contains:
For Adults—
Percentage of U.S.
Recommended Daily
Allowance (U.S. RDA)

Vitamin A (as
  Acetate).......................5000 I.U. (100%)
Vitamin E (as dl-Alpha
  Tocopheryl Acetate)... 45 I.U. (150%)
Vitamin C (as Ascorbic
  Acid).............................. 90 mg (150%)
Folic Acid .... 0.4 mg (100%)
Vitamin B_1 (as Thiamine
  Mononitrate) .... 2.25 mg (150%)
Vitamin B_2 (as
  Riboflavin)................... 2.6 mg (153%)
Niacinamide...................... 30 mg (150%)
Vitamin B_6 (as Pyridoxine
  Hydrochloride)............ 3 mg (150%)
Vitamin B_{12} (as
  Cyanocobalamin)........ 9 mcg (150%)
Vitamin D_2.....................400 I.U. (100%)
Calcium (as Dibasic
  Calcium Phosphate)... 162 mg (16%)
Phosphorus (as Dibasic
  Calcium Phosphate)... 125 mg (13%)
Iodine (as Potassium
  Iodide)..........................225 mcg (150%)
Iron (as Ferrous
  Fumarate)................... 27 mg (150%)
Magnesium (as
  Magnesium Oxide)..... 100 mg (25%)
Copper (as Cupric Oxide) 1.5 mg (75%)
Zinc (as Zinc Oxide)....... 22.5 mg (150%)

Inactive Ingredients: BHA, BHT, Blue 2, Gelatin, Hydrolyzed Protein, Hydroxypropyl Methylcellulose, Lactose, Magnesium Stearate, Methylparaben, Microcrystalline Cellulose, Modified Food Starch, Mono- and Di-glycerides, Polacrilin, Polysorbate 60, Potassium Sorbate, Propylparaben, PVPP, Red 40, Silica Gel, Sodium Benzoate, Sodium Lauryl Sulfate, Sorbic Acid, Stearic Acid, Sucrose, Titanium Dioxide, and other ingredients.

Indications: For the treatment of vitamin and mineral deficiencies.

Recommended Intake: 1 tablet daily or as prescribed by physician.

Warnings: Keep this and all medications out of the reach of children.
Store at Room Temperature.

How Supplied: Tablets (film coated, maroon). Engraved LL and G2.
Bottle of 100—NDC 0005-4286-23
A SPECTRUM® Product

D7
14170

INCREMIN®
[in-cre-min]
WITH IRON SYRUP
Vitamins + Iron
DIETARY SUPPLEMENT
(Cherry Flavored)

Composition: Each teaspoonful (5 mL) supplies the following Minimum Daily Requirements:

	Child under 6	Child over 6	Adults
Vitamin B_1	20 MDR	13⅓ MDR	10 MDR
Iron	4 MDR	3 MDR	3 MDR

Each teaspoonful (5 mL) contains: Elemental Iron (as Ferric Pyrophosphate) 30 mg; L-Lysine HCl 300 mg; Thiamine HCl (B_1) 10 mg; Pyridoxine HCl (B_6) 5 mg; Vitamin B_{12} (Cyanocobalamin) 25 mcg; Sorbitol 3.50 gm; Alcohol 0.75%.

Inactive Ingredients: Alcohol, Flavorings, Red 33, Sodium Benzoate, Sorbic Acid.

Indications: For the prevention and treatment of iron deficiency anemia in children and adults.

Warning: As with any drug, if you are pregnant or nursing a baby, seek the advice of a health professional before using this product.

Keep this and all medications out of the reach of children.

Recommended Intake: or as prescribed by a physician.
Children: One teaspoonful (5 mL) daily for the prevention of iron deficiency anemia.
Adults: One teaspoonful (5 mL) daily for the prevention of iron deficiency anemia.

Notice: To protect from light always dispense in this container or in an amber bottle.

Store at Room Temperature.

How Supplied: Syrup (cherry flavor)—Bottles of 4 fl oz—NDC 0005-5604-58
16 fl oz—NDC 0005-5604-65

22835
D13

NEOLOID®
[*nēē-o-loid*]
Emulsified Castor Oil
Peppermint Flavored

Indications: For the treatment of isolated bouts of constipation.

SHAKE WELL.

Composition: Castor Oil USP 36.4% (w/w) with 0.1% (w/w) Sodium Benzoate and 0.2% (w/w) Potassium Sorbate added as preservatives, emulsifying and flavoring agents in water. Also contains the following inactive ingredients: Citric Acid, Glyceryl Monostearate, Polysorbate 80, Propylene Glycol, Sodium Alginate, Sodium Saccharin, Stearic Acid, Tenox II. NEOLOID is an emulsion with an exceptionally bland, pleasant taste.

Recommended Intake:
Infants —½ to 1½ teaspoonfuls
Children —Adjust between infant and adult dose.
Adult —Average dose, 2 to 4 tablespoonfuls or as prescribed by a physician.

Precautions: Not to be used when abdominal pain, nausea, vomiting, or other symptoms of appendicitis are present. Frequent or continued use of this preparation may result in dependence on laxatives. Do not use during pregnancy except on a physician's advice. Keep this and all drugs out of the reach of children.

Warning: As with any drug, if you are pregnant or nursing a baby, seek the ad-

vice of a health professional before using this product. In case of accidental overdose, seek professional assistance or contact a Poison Control Center immediately.

How Supplied: Bottles of 4 fl oz (118 mL) (peppermint flavor)—NDC-0005-5442-58
Store at Room Temperature.
DO NOT FREEZE.

16838
D4

STRESSTABS® Advanced Formula
[*strĕss-tăbs*]
High Potency
Stress Formula Vitamins

Each tablet contains:

	For Adults—Percentage of U.S. Recommended Daily Allowance (U.S. RDA)	
Vitamin E (as *dl*-Alpha Tocopheryl Acetate)...	30 I.U.	(100%)
Vitamin C (as Ascorbic Acid)	500 mg	(833%)
B VITAMINS		
Folic Acid	400 mcg	(100%)
Vitamin B_1 (as Thiamine Mononitrate)	10 mg	(667%)
Vitamin B_2 (as Riboflavin)	10 mg	(588%)
Niacinamide	100 mg	(500%)
Vitamin B_6 (as Pyridoxine Hydrochloride)	5 mg	(250%)
Vitamin B_{12} (as Cyanocobalamin)	12 mcg	(200%)
Biotin	45 mcg	(15%)
Pantothenic Acid (as Calcium Pantothenate USP) ...	20 mg	(200%)

Inactive Ingredients: Calcium Carbonate, Magnesium Stearate, Microcrystalline Cellulose, Modified Food Starch, Silica Gel, Stearic Acid, and Yellow 6.

Recommended Intake: Adults, 1 tablet daily or as directed by the physician.

How Supplied:
Bottle of 30—NDC 0005-4124-13
Bottle of 60—NDC 0005-4124-19
Unit Dose Pack 10 × 10s—NDC 0005-4124-60
Store at Room Temperature.

27196
D17

Shown in Product Identification Section, page 411

STRESSTABS® + IRON
Advanced Formula
[*strĕss-tăbs*]
High Potency
Stress Formula Vitamins

Each tablet contains:

	For Adults—Percentage of U.S. Recommended Daily Allowance (U.S. RDA)	
Vitamin E (as *dl*-Alpha Tocopheryl Acetate)....	30 I.U.	(100%)
Vitamin C (as Ascorbic Acid)	500 mg	(833%)

B VITAMINS

Folic Acid	400 mcg	(100%)
Vitamin B_1 (as Thiamine Mononitrate)	10 mg	(667%)
Vitamin B_2 (as Riboflavin)	10 mg	(588%)
Niacinamide	100 mg	(500%)
Vitamin B_6 (as Pyridoxine Hydrochloride)	5 mg	(250%)
Vitamin B_{12} (as Cyanocobalamin)	12 mcg	(200%)
Biotin	45 mcg	(15%)
Pantothenic Acid (as Calcium Pantothenate USP) ...	20 mg	(200%)
Iron (as Ferrous Fumarate)	27 mg	(150%)

Inactive Ingredients: Calcium Carbonate, Magnesium Stearate, Microcrystalline Cellulose, Modified Food Starch, Red 40, Silica Gel, Stearic Acid, and Yellow 6.

Recommended Intake: Adults, 1 tablet daily or as directed by physician.

How Supplied: Capsule-shaped tablets (film-coated, orange-red, scored). Engraved LL and S2.
Bottle of 30—NDC 0005-4126-13
Bottle of 60—NDC 0005-4126-19
Store at Room Temperature.

27403
D15

Shown in Product Identification Section, page 411

STRESSTABS® + ZINC
Advanced Formula
[*strĕss-tăbs*]
High Potency
Stress Formula Vitamins

Each tablet contains:

	For Adults—Percentage of U.S. Recommended Daily Allowance (U.S. RDA)	
Vitamin E (as *dl*-Alpha Tocopheryl Acetate)....	30 I.U.	(100%)
Vitamin C (as Ascorbic Acid)	500 mg	(833%)
B VITAMINS		
Folic Acid	400 mcg	(100%)
Vitamin B_1 (as Thiamine Mononitrate)	10 mg	(667%)
Vitamin B_2 (as Riboflavin)	10 mg	(588%)
Niacinamide	100 mg	(500%)
Vitamin B_6 (as Pyridoxine Hydrochloride)	5 mg	(250%)
Vitamin B_{12} (as Cyanocobalamin)	12 mcg	(200%)
Biotin	45 mcg	(15%)
Pantothenic Acid (as Calcium Pantothenate USP)	20 mg	(200%)
Copper (as Cupric Oxide)	3 mg	(150%)
Zinc (as Zinc Sulfate)	23.9 mg	(159%)

Inactive Ingredients: Calcium Carbonate, Magnesium Stearate, Microcrystalline Cellulose, Modified Food Starch, Silica Gel, Stearic Acid, and Yellow 6.

Continued on next page

Lederle—Cont.

Recommended Intake: Adults, 1 tablet daily or as directed by the physician.

How Supplied: Capsule-shaped tablet (film coated, peach color). Engraved LL and S3.
Bottle of 30—NDC 0005-4125-13
Bottle of 60—NDC 0005-4125-19
Store at Room Temperature.

27402
D17

Shown in Product Identification Section, page 411

ZINCON®
[*zinc-ŏn*]
Dandruff Shampoo

Contains: Pyrithione Zinc (1%), Water, Sodium Methyl Cocoyl Taurate, Cocamide MEA, Sodium Chloride, Magnesium Aluminum Silicate, Sodium Cocoyl Isethionate, Fragrance, Glutaraldehyde, D&C Green #5, Citric Acid or Sodium Hydroxide to adjust pH if necessary.

Indications: Relieves the itching and scalp flaking associated with dandruff. Relieves the itching, irritation, and skin flaking associated with seborrheic dermatitis of the scalp.

Directions: For best results use twice a week. Wet hair, apply to scalp and massage vigorously. Rinse and repeat. SHAKE WELL BEFORE USING.

Warnings: Keep this and all drugs out of the reach of children. For external use only. Avoid contact with the eyes—if this happens, rinse thoroughly with water. If condition worsens or does not improve after regular use of this product as directed, consult a doctor. Do not use on children under 2 years of age except as directed by a doctor.

How Supplied:
4 oz Bottle—NDC 0005-5455-58
8 oz Bottle—NDC 0005-5455-61

13918
D4

Shown in Product Identification Section, page 411

If desired, additional information on any Lederle product will be provided by contacting Lederle Professional Services Dept.

EDUCATIONAL MATERIAL

Calcium Supplements: The Differences Are Real
8-page pamphlet describing why today's women need to supplement their diet with calcium.
Write to: Lederle Promotional Center
2200 Bradley Hill Road
Blauvelt, NY 10913

Lever Brothers Company
390 PARK AVENUE
NEW YORK, NY 10022

DOVE® BAR

Active Ingredients: Sodium Cocoyl Isethionate, Stearic Acid, Sodium Tallowate, Water, Sodium Isethionate, Coconut Acid, Sodium Stearate, Sodium Dodecylbenzenesulfonate, Sodium Cocoate, Fragrance, Sodium Chloride, Titanium Dioxide.

Actions and Uses: Dove is specially formulated to be predictably gentle to all kinds of skin—dry, oily, normal skin, as well as sensitive pediatric or senescent skin. Dove is not a soap but a neutral cleansing bar with a pH of 7 that leaves skin soft, moist, and healthy looking.

Directions: Instruct patients to use Dove Bar as they would any other cleansing bar or soap.

How Supplied: Original Dove 3.5 oz. and 4.75 bars; Unscented Dove 4.75 oz.; 8 oz. pump dispenser—Liquid Dove Beauty Wash.

LEVER 2000®

Active Ingredients: Sodium tallowate, sodium cocoyl, isethionate, water, sodium cocoate, stearic acid, sodium isethionate, coconut fatty acid, fragrance, titanium dioxide, sodium chloride, triclosan tetrasodium EDTA, disodium phosphate, trisodium etidronate, BHT.

Actions and Uses: Lever 2000® is the mildest antibacterial bar soap available. Lever 2000® offers the broadest spectrum of gram-negative and gram-positive antibacterial efficacy. It is a useful adjunct to any therapeutic regimen that fights topical bacterial infection. It is also milder to the skin than any other antibacterial or deodorant bar soap. Lever 2000® has been proven mild enough for children's tender skin as young as 18 months and can also be used by adolescents and adults.

Directions: Instruct patients to use Lever 2000® as they would any other mild antibacterial or deodorant soap.

How Supplied: 3.5 oz., 5 oz., and 7 oz. bars.

IDENTIFICATION PROBLEM?
Consult the
Product Identification Section
where you'll find
products pictured
in full color.

Luyties Pharmacal
Company
P.O. BOX 8080
ST. LOUIS, MO 63156

YELLOLAX
[*yel'o-laks*]

Description: YELLOLAX is a combination of time proven Yellow-phenolphthalein, and the Homeopathic ingredients, Bryonia and Hydrastis. Clinically YELLOLAX is an oral laxative. Each tablet contains two grains of yellow phenolphthalein and the Bryonia and Hydrastis approximately one fortieth grain each.

Action: Yellow-phenolphthalein is an effective and safe laxative, which is not contraindicated in pregnancy. Homeopathic Bryonia is used to treat constipation and the pain associated with constipation. Homeopathic Bryonia tends to increase mucous membrane moisture. Homeopathic Hydrastis is also included in the treatment of constipation because the Homeopathic Hydrastis provides some relief of constipation and the associated pain and headaches by relaxing mucous membranes and encouraging their secretion. YELLOLAX has been safely used in pregnancy, children, and as conjunctive treatment with hemorrhoidal complications.

Indications: YELLOLAX is indicated in the management of simple constipation. YELLOLAX is also indicated in those conditions which require a gentle laxative.

Contraindications: YELLOLAX and all laxatives are contraindicated in appendicitis. All laxatives containing phenolphthalein are contraindicated in patients who have hypersensitivity to phenolphthalein.

Warnings: Do not use laxatives in cases of severe colic, nausea and other symptoms of appendicitis. Do not use laxatives habitually nor continually. If condition persists consult physician. Keep this and all medication out of the reach of children. DO NOT exceed the recommended dosage.

Caution: Frequent or prolonged use may result in laxative dependence. If skin rash appears, discontinue use.

Side Effects: The phenolphthalein may impart a red color to the urine, (phenolphthalein is also used as a pH indicator), this is normal.

Dosage: For adults one or two tablets chewed before retiring. For children over six a quarter tablet to half tablet before retiring. Tablets should be well chewed. For younger children consult physician.

Supplied: Compressed tablets packed in glass bottles of 36 (NDC 0618-0832-55) and 100 (NDC 0618-0832-12), and in repackers of 1000 tablets.

Homoeopathic
Luyties also manufactures a complete line of homoeopathic products. If more

information is needed contact them direct.

Macsil, Inc.
**1326 FRANKFORD AVENUE
PHILADELPHIA, PA 19125**

BALMEX® BABY POWDER

Composition: Contains: Active Ingredient—zinc oxide; Inactive Ingredients—corn starch, calcium carbonate, BALSAN® (especially purified balsam Peru).

Action and Uses: Absorbent, emollient, soothing—for diaper irritation, intertrigo, and other common dermatological conditions. In acute, simple miliaria, itching ceases in minutes and lesions dry promptly. For routine use after bathing and each diaper change.

How Supplied: 8 oz. shaker-top plastic containers.

BALMEX® EMOLLIENT LOTION

Gentle and effective scientifically compounded infant's skin conditioner.

Composition: Contains a special lanolin oil (non-sensitizing, dewaxed, moisturizing fraction of lanolin), BALSAN® (specially purified balsam Peru) and silicone.

Action and Uses: The special Lanolin Oil aids nature lubricate baby's skin to keep it smooth and supple. Balmex Emollient Lotion is also highly effective as a physiologic conditioner on adult's skin.

How Supplied: Available in 6 oz. dispenser-top plastic bottles.

BALMEX® OINTMENT

Composition: Contains: Active Ingredients—Bismuth Subnitrate, Zinc Oxide; Inactive Ingredients—Balsan (Specially Purified Balsam Peru), Benzoic Acid, Beeswax, Mineral Oil, Silicone, Synthetic White Wax, Purified Water, and other ingredients.

Action and Uses: Emollient, protective, anti-inflammatory, promotes healing—for diaper rash, minor burns, sunburn, and other simple skin conditions; also decubitus ulcers, skin irritations associated with ileostomy and colostomy drainage. Nonstaining, readily washes out of diapers and clothing.

How Supplied: 1, 2, 4 oz. tubes; 1 lb. plastic jars (½ oz. tubes for Hospitals only). Balmex Ointment-All Commercial Sizes-Safety Sealed.

Marion Merrell Dow Inc.
**Consumer Products Division
10123 ALLIANCE ROAD
P.O. BOX 429553
CINCINNATI, OHIO 45242-9553**

CĒPACOL®/CĒPACOL MINT
[sē'pə-cŏl]
Mouthwash/Gargle

Description: Cēpacol Mouthwash contains: Ceepryn® (cetylpyridinium chloride) 0.05%. Also contains: Alcohol 14%, Edetate Disodium, FD&C Yellow No. 5 (tartrazine) as a color additive, Flavors, Glycerin, Polysorbate 80, Saccharin, Sodium Biphosphate, Sodium Phosphate, and Water.
Cēpacol Mint Mouthwash contains: Ceepryn® (cetylpyridinium chloride) 0.05%. Also contains: Alcohol 14.5%, D&C Yellow No. 10, FD&C Green No. 3, Flavor, Glucono Delta-Lactone, Glycerin, Poloxamer 407, Saccharin Sodium, Sodium Gluconate, and Water.

Actions: Cēpacol/Cēpacol Mint is a soothing, pleasant-tasting mouthwash/gargle. It kills germs that cause bad breath for a fresher, cleaner mouth.
Cēpacol/Cēpacol Mint has a low surface tension, approximately ½ that of water. This property is the basis of the spreading action in the oral cavity as well as its foaming action. Cēpacol/Cēpacol Mint leaves the mouth feeling fresh and clean and helps provide soothing, temporary relief of dryness and minor mouth irritations.

Uses: Recommended as a mouthwash and gargle for daily oral care; as an aromatic mouth freshener to provide a clean feeling in the mouth; as a soothing, foaming rinse to freshen the mouth.
Used routinely before dental procedures, helps give patient confidence of not offending with mouth odor. Often employed as a foaming and refreshing rinse before, during, and after instrumentation and dental prophylaxis. Convenient as a mouth-freshening agent after taking dental impressions. Helpful in reducing the unpleasant taste and odor in the mouth following gingivectomy.
Used in hospitals as a mouthwash and gargle for daily oral care. Also used to refresh and soothe the mouth following emesis, inhalation therapy, and intubations, and for swabbing the mouths of patients incapable of personal care.

Warning: Keep out of the reach of children.

Directions for Use: Rinse vigorously before or after brushing or any time to freshen the mouth. Particularly useful after meals or before social engagements. Cēpacol/Cēpacol Mint leaves the mouth feeling refreshingly clean.
Use full strength every two or three hours as a soothing, foaming gargle, or as directed by a physician or dentist. May also be mixed with warm water.
Product label directions are as follows: Use full strength. Rinse mouth thoroughly before or after brushing or whenever desired or use as directed by a physician or dentist.

How Supplied:
Cēpacol Mouthwash: 12 oz, 18 oz, 24 oz, and 32 oz. 4 oz trial size.
Shown in Product Identification Section, page 411

CĒPACOL®
[sē'pə-cŏl]
**Dry Throat Lozenges
Cherry Flavor**

Description: Each lozenge contains Menthol 3.6 mg. Also contains: Benzyl Alcohol, Cetylpyridinium Chloride, D&C Red No. 33, FD&C Red No. 40, Flavor, Liquid Glucose, and Sucrose.

Actions: Menthol provides a cooling sensation to aid in symptomatic relief of minor throat irritations.

Indications: Cēpacol Cherry Flavor Lozenges provide temporary relief of occasional dry, scratchy throat.

Warnings: If sore throat is severe, persists for more than 2 days, is accompanied or followed by fever, headache, rash, nausea, or vomiting, consult a physician promptly. If sore mouth symptoms do not improve in 7 days, see your dentist or physician promptly. Do not administer to children under 6 years of age unless directed by physician or dentist. Keep this and all drugs out of the reach of children. In case of accidental overdose, seek professional assistance or contact a Poison Control Center immediately. As with any drug, if you are pregnant or nursing a baby, seek the advice of a health professional before using this product.

Dosage and Administration: Adults and children 6 years of age and older: Allow product to dissolve slowly in the mouth. May be repeated every 2 hours as needed or as directed by a dentist or physician. Do not exceed 10 lozenges per day.

How Supplied:
18 lozenges in 2 pocket packs of 9 each. Store at room temperature, below 86°F (30°C). Protect contents from humidity.
Shown in Product Identification Section, page 411

CĒPACOL®
[sē-pə-cŏl]
**Dry Throat Lozenges
Honey-Lemon Flavor**

Description: Each lozenge contains Menthol 3.6 mg. Also contains: Benzyl Alcohol, Caramel, Cetylpyridinium Chloride, FD&C Yellow No. 6, D&C Yellow No. 10, Flavors, Liquid Glucose, and Sucrose.

Actions: Menthol provides a cooling sensation to aid in symptomatic relief of minor throat irritations.

Continued on next page

Marion Merrell Dow—Cont.

Indications: Cēpacol Honey-Lemon Flavor Lozenges provide temporary relief of occasional dry, scratchy throat.

Warnings: If sore throat is severe, persists for more than 2 days, is accompanied or followed by fever, headache, rash, nausea, or vomiting, consult a physician promptly. If sore mouth symptoms do not improve in 7 days, see your dentist or physician promptly. Do not administer to children under 6 years of age unless directed by physician or dentist. Keep this and all drugs out of the reach of children. In case of accidental overdose, seek professional assistance or contact a Poison Control Center immediately. As with any drug, if you are pregnant or nursing a baby, seek the advice of a health professional before using this product.

Dosage and Administration: Adults and children 6 years of age and older: Allow product to dissolve slowly in the mouth. May be repeated every 2 hours as needed or as directed by a dentist or physician.

How Supplied:
18 lozenges in 2 pocket packs of 9 each. Store at room temperature, below 86°F (30°C). Protect contents from humidity.
Shown in Product Identification Section, page 411

CĒPACOL®
[sē-pə-cŏl]
Dry Throat Lozenges
Menthol-Eucalyptus Flavor

Description: Each lozenge contains Menthol 5.0 mg. Also contains: Benzyl Alcohol, Cetylpyridinium Chloride, Eucalyptol, Liquid Glucose, and Sucrose.

Actions: Menthol provides a cooling sensation to aid in symptomatic relief of minor throat irritations.

Indications: Cēpacol Menthol-Eucalyptus Flavor Lozenges provide temporary relief of occasional dry, scratchy throat.

Warnings: If sore throat is severe, persists for more than 2 days, is accompanied or followed by fever, headache, rash, nausea, or vomiting, consult a physician promptly. If sore mouth symptoms do not improve in 7 days, see your dentist or physician promptly. Do not administer to children under 6 years of age unless directed by physician or dentist. Keep this and all drugs out of the reach of children. In case of accidental overdose, seek professional assistance or contact a Poison Control Center immediately. As with any drug, if you are pregnant or nursing a baby, seek the advice of a health professional before using this product.

Dosage and Administration: Adults and children 6 years of age and older: Allow product to dissolve slowly in the mouth. May be repeated every 2 hours as needed or as directed by a dentist or physician.

How Supplied:
18 lozenges in 2 pocket packs of 9 each. Store at room temperature, below 86°F (30°C). Protect contents from humidity.
Shown in Product Identification Section, page 411

CĒPACOL®
[sē'pə-cŏl]
Dry Throat Lozenges
Original Flavor

Description: Each lozenge contains Ceepryn® (cetylpyridinium chloride) 0.07%, Benzyl Alcohol 0.3%. Also contains: FD&C Yellow No. 5 (tartrazine) as a color additive, Flavor, Glucose, and Sucrose.

Actions: Cetylpyridinium chloride (Ceepryn) is a cationic quaternary ammonium compound, which is a surface-active agent. Aqueous solutions of cetylpyridinium chloride have a surface tension lower than that of water.
Cetylpyridinium chloride in the concentration used in Cēpacol is nonirritating to tissues.

Indications: For soothing, temporary relief of dryness of the mouth and throat.

Warnings: Severe sore throat or sore throat accompanied by high fever, headache, nausea, or vomiting, or any sore throat or mouth irritations persisting more than 2 days may be serious. Consult a physician promptly. Persons with a high fever or persistent cough should not use this preparation unless directed by a physician. Do not administer to children under 6 years of age unless directed by a physician or dentist. If sensitive to any of the ingredients, do not use. Keep this and all drugs out of the reach of children. In case of accidental overdose, seek professional assistance or contact a Poison Control Center immediately. As with any drug, if you are pregnant or nursing a baby, seek the advice of a health professional before using this product.

Dosage and Administration: Adults and children 6 years and older, dissolve 1 lozenge in the mouth every 2 hours, if needed. For children under 6 years, consult a physician or dentist.

How Supplied:
Trade Package: 18 lozenges in 2 pocket packs of 9 each.
Professional Package: 648 lozenges in 72 blisters of 9 each.
Store at room temperature, below 86°F (30°C). Protect contents from humidity.
Shown in Product Identification Section, page 411

CĒPACOL®
[sē'pə-cŏl]
Anesthetic Lozenges (Troches)

Description: Each lozenge contains Benzocaine 10 mg, Ceepryn® (cetylpyridinium chloride) 0.07%. Also contains: FD&C Blue No. 1, FD&C Yellow No. 5

(tartrazine) as a color additive, Flavors, Glucose, and Sucrose.

Actions: Cetylpyridinium chloride (Ceepryn) is a cationic quaternary ammonium compound, which is a surface-active agent. Aqueous solutions of cetylpyridinium chloride have a surface tension lower than that of water.
Cetylpyridinium chloride in the concentration used in Cēpacol is nonirritating to tissues.
Cēpacol Anesthetic Lozenges stimulate salivation to relieve dryness of the mouth and provide a mild anesthetic effect for pain relief.

Indications: For fast, temporary relief of minor sore throat pain. For temporary relief of minor pain and discomfort associated with tonsillitis and pharyngitis.

Warnings: If sore throat is severe, persists for more than 2 days, is accompanied or followed by fever, headache, rash, nausea, or vomiting, consult a physician promptly. Keep this and all drugs out of the reach of children. In case of accidental overdose, seek professional assistance or contact a Poison Control Center immediately. As with any drug, if you are pregnant or nursing a baby, seek the advice of a health professional before using this product.

Dosage and Administration: Adults and children 6 years and older, dissolve 1 lozenge in the mouth every 2 hours, if needed. For children under 6 years, consult a physician or dentist.

How Supplied:
Trade Package: 18 lozenges in 2 pocket packs of 9 each.
Professional Package: 324 lozenges in 36 blisters of 9 each.
Store at room temperature, below 86°F (30°C). Protect contents from humidity.
Shown in Product Identification Section, page 411

CĒPASTAT®
[sē'pə-stăt]
Sore Throat Lozenges
Cherry Flavor and Extra Strength

Description: Each Cherry Flavor lozenge contains: Phenol 14.5 mg. Also contains: Antifoam Emulsion, D&C Red No. 33, FD&C Yellow No. 6, Flavor, Gum Crystal, Mannitol, Menthol, Saccharin Sodium, and Sorbitol.
Each Extra Strength lozenge contains: Phenol 29 mg. Also contains: Antifoam Emulsion, Caramel, Eucalyptus Oil, Gum Crystal, Mannitol, Menthol, Saccharin Sodium, and Sorbitol.

Actions: Phenol is a recognized topical anesthetic. The sugar-free formula should not promote tooth decay as sugar-based lozenges can.

Indications: For fast, temporary relief of minor sore throat pain.

Warnings: If sore throat is severe, persists for more than 2 days, is accompanied or followed by fever, headache, rash, nausea, or vomiting, consult a physician promptly. If sore mouth symptoms do not improve in 7 days, see your dentist or physician promptly. Keep this and all drugs out of the reach of children. In case of accidental overdose, seek professional assistance or contact a Poison Control Center immediately. As with any drug, if you are pregnant or nursing a baby, seek the advice of a health professional before using this product.

Note to Diabetics: Each lozenge contributes approximately 8 calories from 2 grams of sorbitol.

Dosage and Administration:
Lozenges–Cherry Flavor
Adults and children 12 years of age and older: Allow the lozenge to dissolve slowly in the mouth. May be repeated every 2 hours, or as directed by a dentist or physician. Children 6 to under 12 years of age: Allow lozenge to dissolve slowly in the mouth. May be repeated every 2 hours, not to exceed 10 lozenges per day, or as directed by a dentist or physician. Children under 6 years of age: Consult a dentist or physician.
Lozenges–Extra Strength
Adults and children 12 years of age and older: Allow the lozenge to dissolve slowly in the mouth. May be repeated every 2 hours, or as directed by a dentist or physician. Children 6 to under 12 years of age: Allow lozenge to dissolve slowly in the mouth. May be repeated every 2 hours, not to exceed 10 lozenges per day, or as directed by a dentist or physician. Children under 6 years of age: Consult a dentist or physician.

How Supplied:
Lozenges–Cherry Flavor
Trade package: Boxes of 18 lozenges as 2 pocket packs of 9 lozenges each. Professional package: 648 lozenges in 72 blisters of 9 lozenges each.
Lozenges–Extra Strength
Trade package: Boxes of 18 lozenges as 2 pocket packs of 9 lozenges each. Professional package: 648 lozenges in 72 blisters of 9 lozenges each.
Store at room temperature, below 86°F (30°C). Protect contents from humidity.
Shown in Product Identification Section, page 411

Orange Flavor
CITRUCEL®
[sĭt 'rə-sĕl]
(Methylcellulose)
Bulk-forming Fiber Laxative

Description: Each 19 g adult dose (approximately one heaping measuring tablespoonful) contains Methylcellulose 2 g. Each 9.5 g child's dose (one-half the adult dose) contains Methylcellulose 1 g. Methylcellulose is a nonallergenic fiber. Also contains: Citric Acid, FD&C Yellow No. 6, Orange Flavors (natural and artificial), Potassium Citrate, Riboflavin, Sucrose, and other ingredients. Each adult dose contains approximately 3 mg of sodium, 105 mg of potassium, and contributes 60 calories from Sucrose.

Actions: Promotes elimination by providing additional fiber (bulk) to the diet.

This product generally produces bowel movement in 12 to 72 hours.

Indications: For relief of constipation (irregularity). May also be used for relief of constipation associated with other bowel disorders such as irritable bowel syndrome, diverticular disease, and hemorrhoids as well as for bowel management during postpartum, postsurgical, and convalescent periods when recommended by a physician.

Contraindications: Intestinal obstruction, fecal impaction, known hypersensitivity to formula ingredients.

Precautions: Patients should be instructed to consult their physician before using any laxative if they have noticed a sudden change in bowel habits which persists for two weeks. Unless directed by a physician, patients should be advised not to use laxative products when abdominal pain, nausea, or vomiting is present. Patients should also be advised to discontinue use and consult a physician if rectal bleeding or failure to have a bowel movement occurs after use of any laxative product.

Dosage and Administration: Adults and children older than 12 years of age: *one heaping measuring* tablespoonful stirred briskly into 8 ounces of cold water one to three times a day at the first sign of constipation. Children 6 to under 12 years: *one-half the adult dose stirred briskly into 4 ounces of cold water, one to three times a day. The mixture should be administered promptly and drinking additional water is helpful. Children under 6 years: use only as directed by a physician.* Continued use for two or three days may be necessary for full benefit.

How Supplied:
16 oz, 24 oz, and 30 oz containers.
Boxes of 20 single-dose packets.
Store below 86°F (30°C). Protect contents from humidity; keep tightly closed.
Shown in Product Identification Section, page 411

Sugar Free Orange Flavor
CITRUCEL®
[sĭt 'rə-sĕl]
(Methylcellulose)
Bulk-forming Fiber Laxative

Description: Each 10.2 g adult dose (approximately one rounded measuring tablespoonful) contains Methylcellulose 2 g. Each 5.1 g child's dose (one-half the adult dose) contains Methylcellulose 1 g. Methylcellulose is a nonallergenic fiber. Also contains: Aspartame*, Dibasic Calcium Phosphate, FD&C Yellow No. 6, Malic Acid, Maltodextrin, Orange Flavors (natural and artificial), Potassium Citrate and Riboflavin. Each 10.2 g dose contributes 24 calories from Maltodextrin.

---

*NutraSweet and the NutraSweet symbol are trademarks of the NutraSweet Company.

Actions: Promotes elimination by providing additional fiber (bulk) to the diet. This product generally produces bowel movement in 12 to 72 hours.

Indications: For relief of constipation (irregularity). May also be used for relief of constipation associated with other bowel disorders such as irritable bowel syndrome, diverticular disease, and hemorrhoids as well as for bowel management during postpartum, postsurgical, and convalescent periods when recommended by a physician.

Contraindications: Intestinal obstruction, fecal impaction, known hypersensitivity to formula ingredients.

Warning: Individuals with phenylketonuria and other individuals who must restrict their intake of phenylalanine should be warned that each 10.2 g adult dose contains aspartame which provides 52 mg of phenylalanine.

Precautions: Patients should be instructed to consult their physician before using any laxative if they have noticed a sudden change in bowel habits which persists for two weeks. Unless directed by a physician, patients should be advised not to use laxative products when abdominal pain, nausea, or vomiting is present. Patients should also be advised to discontinue use and consult a physician if rectal bleeding or failure to have a bowel movement occurs after use of any laxative product.

Dosage and Administration: Adults and children older than 12 years of age: one rounded measuring tablespoonful stirred briskly into 8 ounces of cold water, one to three times a day at the first sign of constipation. Children 6 to 12 years of age: one-half the adult dose stirred briskly into 4 ounces of cold water one to three times a day. The mixture should be administered promptly and drinking additional water is helpful. Continued use for two or more days may be necessary for full benefit.

How Supplied:
8.6 oz and 16.9 oz containers.
Store below 86°F (30°C). Protect contents from humidity; keep tightly closed.
Shown in Product Identification Section, page 411

DEBROX® Drops
[dē 'brŏx]

Description: Carbamide peroxide 6.5%. Also contains citric acid, glycerin, propylene glycol, sodium stannate, water, and other ingredients.

Actions: DEBROX®, used as directed, cleanses the ear with sustained microfoam. DEBROX Drops foam on contact with earwax due to the release of oxygen.

Indications: DEBROX Drops provide a safe, nonirritating method of softening and removing earwax.

Continued on next page

Marion Merrell Dow—Cont.

Directions: FOR USE IN THE EAR ONLY. Adults and children over 12 years of age: tilt head sideways and place 5 to 10 drops into ear. Tip of applicator should not enter ear canal. Keep drops in ear for several minutes by keeping head tilted or placing cotton in the ear. Use twice daily for up to four days if needed, or as directed by a doctor. Any wax remaining after treatment may be removed by gently flushing the ear with warm water, using a soft rubber bulb ear syringe. Children under 12 years of age: consult a doctor.

Warnings: Do not use if you have ear drainage or discharge, ear pain, irritation or rash in the ear, or are dizzy, unless directed by a physician. Do not use if you have an injury or perforation (hole) of the eardrum or after ear surgery unless directed by a physician. Do not use for more than four consecutive days. If excessive earwax remains after use of this product, consult a physician. Consult a physician prior to use in children under 12.

Cautions: Avoid exposing bottle to excessive heat and direct sunlight. Keep tip on bottle when not in use. Avoid contact with eyes. Keep this and all drugs out of the reach of children. In case of accidental ingestion, seek professional assistance or contact a poison control center immediately.

How Supplied: DEBROX Drops are available in ½- or 1-fl-oz plastic squeeze bottles with applicator spouts.

Issued 1/89

Shown in Product Identification Section, page 411

GAVISCON® Antacid Tablets
[gǎv 'ĭs-kǒn]

Composition: Each chewable tablet contains the following active ingredients:
Aluminum hydroxide dried gel... 80 mg
Magnesium trisilicate .... 20 mg
and the following inactive ingredients: alginic acid, calcium stearate, flavor, sodium bicarbonate, starch (may contain cornstarch), and sucrose.

Actions: Unique formulation produces soothing foam which floats on stomach contents. Foam containing antacid precedes stomach contents into the esophagus when reflux occurs to help protect the sensitive mucosa from further irritation. GAVISCON® acts locally without neutralizing entire stomach contents to help maintain integrity of the digestive process. Endoscopic studies indicate that GAVISCON Antacid Tablets are equally as effective in the erect or supine patient.

Indications: GAVISCON is specifically formulated for the temporary relief of heartburn (acid indigestion) due to acid reflux. GAVISCON is not indicated for the treatment of peptic ulcers.

Directions: Chew two to four tablets four times a day or as directed by a physician. Tablets should be taken after meals and at bedtime or as needed. For best results follow by a half glass of water or other liquid. DO NOT SWALLOW WHOLE.

Warnings: Do not take more than 16 tablets in a 24-hour period or 16 tablets daily for more than 2 weeks, except under the advice and supervision of a physician. Do not use this product except under the advice and supervision of a physician if you are on a sodium-restricted diet. Each GAVISCON Tablet contains approximately 0.8 mEq sodium.

Drug Interaction Precautions: Do not take this product if you are presently taking a prescription antibiotic drug containing any form of tetracycline.
Store at a controlled room temperature in a dry place.
Keep this and all drugs out of the reach of children. In case of accidental overdose, seek professional assistance or contact a poison control center immediately.

How Supplied: Available in bottles of 100 tablets and in foil-wrapped 2s in boxes of 30 tablets.

Issued 2/87

Shown in Product Identification Section, page 412

GAVISCON® EXTRA STRENGTH RELIEF FORMULA Antacid Tablets
[gǎv 'ĭs-kǒn]

Composition: Each chewable tablet contains the following active ingredients:
Aluminum hydroxide .... 160 mg
Magnesium carbonate .... 105 mg
and the following inactive ingredients: alginic acid, calcium stearate, flavor, mannitol, sodium bicarbonate, stearic acid, and sucrose.

Directions: Chew 2 to 4 tablets four times a day or as directed by a physician. Tablets should be taken after meals and at bedtime or as needed. For best results follow by a half glass of water or other liquid. DO NOT SWALLOW WHOLE.

> **FDA Approved Uses:** For the relief of heartburn, sour stomach, and/or acid indigestion, and upset stomach associated with heartburn, sour stomach, and/or acid indigestion.

Warnings: Do not take more than 16 tablets in a 24-hour period or 16 tablets daily for more than 2 weeks, except under the advice and supervision of a physician. Do not use this product except under the advice and supervision of a physician if you are on a sodium-restricted diet. Each tablet contains approximately 1.3 mEq sodium.

Drug Interaction Precautions: Do not take this product if you are presently taking a prescription antibiotic drug containing any form of tetracycline.
Store at a controlled room temperature in a dry place.
Keep this and all drugs out of the reach of children.
In case of accidental overdose, seek professional assistance or contact a poison control center immediately.

How Supplied: Available in bottles of 100 tablets and in foil-wrapped 2s in boxes of 30.

Shown in Product Identification Section, page 412

GAVISCON® EXTRA STRENGTH RELIEF FORMULA
Liquid Antacid
[gǎv 'ĭs-kǒn]

Composition: Each 2 teaspoonfuls (10 mL) contains the following active ingredients:
Aluminum hydroxide .... 508 mg
Magnesium carbonate .... 475 mg
And the following inactive ingredients: butylparaben, edetate disodium, flavor, glycerin, propylparaben, saccharin sodium, simethicone emulsion, sodium alginate, sorbitol solution, water, and xanthan gum.

> **FDA Approved Uses:** For the relief of heartburn, sour stomach and/or acid indigestion, and upset stomach associated with heartburn, sour stomach and/or acid indigestion.

Directions: SHAKE WELL BEFORE USING. Take 2 to 4 teaspoonfuls four times a day or as directed by a physician. GAVISCON Extra Strength Relief Formula Liquid should be taken after meals and at bedtime, followed by half a glass of water. Dispense product only by spoon or other measuring device.

Warnings: Except under the advice and supervision of a physician, do not take more than 16 teaspoonfuls in a 24-hour period or 16 teaspoonfuls daily for more than 2 weeks. May have laxative effect. Do not use this product if you have a kidney disease; do not use this product if you are on a sodium-restricted diet. Each teaspoonful contains approximately 0.9 mEq sodium.

Drug Interaction Precautions: Do not take this product if you are presently taking a prescription antibiotic drug containing any form of tetracycline.
Keep tightly closed. Avoid freezing. Store at a controlled room temperature.
Keep this and all drugs out of the reach of children.
In case of accidental overdose, seek professional assistance or contact a poison control center immediately.

How Supplied: Available in 12 fl oz (355 mL) bottles.

Shown in Product Identification Section, page 412

GAVISCON® Liquid Antacid
[găv 'ĭs-kŏn]

Composition: Each tablespoonful (15 ml) contains the following active ingredients:
Aluminum hydroxide .... 95 mg
Magnesium carbonate .... 358 mg
And the following inactive ingredients: D&C Yellow #10, edetate disodium, FD&C Blue #1, flavor, glycerin, paraben preservatives, saccharin sodium, sodium alginate, sorbitol solution, water, and xanthan gum.

> **FDA Approved Uses:** For the relief of heartburn, sour stomach and/or acid indigestion, and upset stomach associated with heartburn, sour stomach and/or acid indigestion.

Directions: SHAKE WELL BEFORE USING. Take 1 or 2 tablespoonfuls four times a day or as directed by a physician. GAVISCON Liquid should be taken after meals and at bedtime, followed by half a glass of water. Dispense product only by spoon or other measuring device.

Warnings: Except under the advice and supervision of a physician, do not take more than 8 tablespoonfuls in a 24-hour period or 8 tablespoonfuls daily for more than 2 weeks. May have laxative effect. Do not use this product if you have a kidney disease; do not use this product if you are on a sodium-restricted diet. Each tablespoonful of GAVISCON Liquid contains approximately 1.7 mEq sodium.

Drug Interaction Precautions: Do not take this product if you are presently taking a prescription antibiotic drug containing any form of tetracycline. Keep tightly closed. Avoid freezing. Store at a controlled room temperature. Keep this and all drugs out of the reach of children.
In case of accidental overdose, seek professional assistance or contact a poison control center immediately.

How Supplied: Bottles of 12 fluid ounce (355 ml) and 6 fluid ounce (177 ml).
Shown in Product Identification Section, page 412

GAVISCON®-2 Antacid Tablets
[găv 'ĭs-kŏn]

Composition: Each chewable tablet contains the following active ingredients:
Aluminum hydroxide dried gel...160 mg
Magnesium trisilicate .... 40 mg
and the following inactive ingredients: alginic acid, calcium stearate, flavor, sodium bicarbonate, starch (may contain cornstarch), and sucrose.

Indications: GAVISCON® is specifically formulated for the temporary relief of heartburn (acid indigestion) due to acid reflux. GAVISCON is not indicated for the treatment of peptic ulcers.

Directions: Chew one to two tablets four times a day or as directed by a physician. Tablets should be taken after meals and at bedtime or as needed. For best results follow by a half glass of water or other liquid. DO NOT SWALLOW WHOLE.

Warnings: Do not take more than eight tablets in a 24-hour period or eight tablets daily for more than 2 weeks, except under the advice and supervision of a physician. Do not use this product except under the advice and supervision of a physician if you are on a sodium-restricted diet. Each GAVISCON-2 Tablet contains approximately 1.6 mEq sodium.

Drug Interaction Precautions: Do not take this product if you are presently taking a prescription antibiotic drug containing any form of tetracycline.
Store at a controlled room temperature in a dry place.
Keep this and all drugs out of the reach of children. In case of accidental overdose, seek professional assistance or contact a poison control center immediately.

How Supplied: Boxes of 48 foil-wrapped tablets.
Issued 2/87
Shown in Product Identification Section, page 412

GLY–OXIDE® Liquid
[glī-ok 'sīd]

Description: GLY-OXIDE® Liquid contains carbamide peroxide 10%. Also contains citric acid, flavor, glycerin, propylene glycol, sodium stannate, water, and other ingredients.

Actions: GLY-OXIDE® Liquid has an oxygen-rich formula that works to relieve the pain of canker sores by cleaning and debriding damaged tissue so natural healing can occur.

Administration: Do not dilute. Apply directly from bottle. Replace tip on bottle when not in use.

Indications: For local treatment and hygienic prevention of minor oral inflammation such as canker sores, denture irritation, and postdental procedure irritation. Place several drops on affected area four times daily, after meals and at bedtime, or as directed by a dentist or physician; expectorate after two or three minutes. Or place 10 drops onto tongue, mix with saliva, swish for several minutes, and expectorate.
As an adjunct to oral hygiene (orthodontics, dental appliances) after regular brushing, swish 10 or more drops vigorously. Continue for two to three minutes; expectorate.
When normal oral hygiene is inadequate or impossible (total care geriatrics, etc), swish 10 or more drops vigorously after meals and expectorate.

Precautions: Severe or persistent oral inflammation, denture irritation, or gingivitis may be serious. If these conditions or unexpected side effects occur, consult a dentist or physician immediately. Avoid contact with eyes. Protect from heat and direct light. Keep this and all drugs out of the reach of children. In case of accidental overdose, seek professional assistance or contact a poison control center immediately.

How Supplied: GLY-OXIDE® Liquid is available in ½-fl-oz and 2-fl-oz non-spill, plastic squeeze bottles with applicator spouts.
Issued 2/89
Shown in Product Identification Section, page 412

NOVAHISTINE® DMX
[nō "vă-hĭs 'tēn]
Cough/Cold Formula & Decongestant

Description: Each 5 mL teaspoonful of NOVAHISTINE DMX contains: Dextromethorphan Hydrobromide 10 mg, Guaifenesin 100 mg, Pseudoephedrine Hydrochloride 30 mg. Also contains: Alcohol 10%, FD&C Red No. 40, FD&C Yellow No. 6, Flavors, Glycerin, Hydrochloric Acid, Invert Sugar, Saccharin Sodium, Sodium Chloride, Sorbitol, and Water. Dextromethorphan hydrobromide, a synthetic nonnarcotic antitussive, is the dextrorotatory isomer of 3-methoxy-N-methylmorphinan. Guaifenesin is the glyceryl ether of guaiacol. Pseudoephedrine hydrochloride is the salt of a pharmacologically active stereoisomer of ephedrine (1-phenyl-2-methylamino-1-propanol).

Actions: Dextromethorphan hydrobromide suppresses the cough reflex by a direct effect on the cough center in the medulla of the brain. Although it is chemically related to morphine, it produces no analgesia or addiction. Its antitussive activity is about equal to that of codeine.
Pseudoephedrine hydrochloride is an orally effective nasal decongestant. It is a sympathomimetic amine with peripheral effects similar to epinephrine and central effects similar to, but less intense than, amphetamines. Therefore, it has the potential for excitatory side effects. Pseudoephedrine hydrochloride at the recommended oral dosage has little or no pressor effect in normotensive adults. Patients taking pseudoephedrine orally have not been reported to experience the rebound congestion sometimes experienced with frequent, repeated use of topical decongestants. Pseudoephedrine is not known to produce drowsiness.
Guaifenesin acts as an expectorant by increasing respiratory tract fluid which reduces the viscosity of tenacious secretions, thus making expectoration easier.

Indications: NOVAHISTINE DMX is indicated for temporary relief of cough and nasal congestion; helps loosen phlegm and bronchial secretions. It is useful when exhausting, nonproductive cough accompanies respiratory tract congestion and in the symptomatic relief of upper respiratory congestion associated with the common cold, influenza, bronchitis, and sinusitis.

Continued on next page

Marion Merrell Dow—Cont.

Contraindications: NOVAHISTINE DMX is contraindicated in patients with severe hypertension, severe coronary artery disease, and in patients on MAO inhibitor therapy. Patient idiosyncrasy to adrenergic agents may be manifested by insomnia, dizziness, weakness, tremor, or arrhythmias.

Nursing mothers: Pseudoephedrine is contraindicated in nursing mothers because of the higher than usual risk for infants from sympathomimetic amines.

Hypersensitivity: NOVAHISTINE DMX is contraindicated in patients with hypersensitivity or idiosyncrasy to sympathomimetic amines, dextromethorphan, or to other formula ingredients.

Warnings: At dosages higher than the recommended dose, nervousness, dizziness, sleeplessness, nausea, or headache may occur. Do not take for more than 7 days. A persistent cough may be a sign of a serious condition. If symptoms do not improve, recur, or are accompanied by fever, rash, or persistent headache, patients should be advised to consult their physician before continuing use. Do not use for persistent or chronic cough such as occurs with smoking, asthma, chronic bronchitis or emphysema, or where cough is accompanied by excessive phlegm (sputum) unless directed by a physician. Sympathomimetic amines should be used judiciously and sparingly in patients with hypertension, diabetes mellitus, cardiovascular disease (e.g. ischemic heart disease), increased intraocular pressure, hyperthyroidism, or prostatic hypertrophy. Sympathomimetics may produce central nervous system stimulation with convulsions or cardiovascular collapse with accompanying hypotension. See Contraindications.

Use in elderly: The elderly (60 years and older) are more likely to have adverse reactions to sympathomimetics. Overdosage of sympathomimetics in this age group may cause hallucinations, convulsions, CNS depression, and death.

Use in children: NOVAHISTINE DMX should not be used in children under 2 years except under the advice and supervision of a physician.

Use in pregnancy: Safety for use during pregnancy has not been established. As with any drug, if you are pregnant or nursing a baby, seek the advice of a health professional before using this product.

If sensitive to any of the ingredients, do not use.

Keep this and all drugs out of the reach of children. In case of accidental overdose, seek professional assistance or contact a Poison Control Center immediately.

Adverse Reactions: Adverse reactions occur infrequently with usual oral doses of NOVAHISTINE DMX. When they occur, adverse reactions may include gastrointestinal upset and nausea.

Because of the pseudoephedrine in NOVAHISTINE DMX, hyperreactive individuals may display ephedrine-like reactions such as tachycardia, palpitations, headache, dizziness or nausea. Sympathomimetic drugs have been associated with certain untoward reactions including fear, anxiety, tenseness, restlessness, tremor, weakness, pallor, respiratory difficulty, dysuria, insomnia, hallucinations, convulsions, CNS depression, arrhythmias, and cardiovascular collapse with hypotension.

Note: Guaifenesin interferes with the colorimetric determination of 5-hydroxyindoleacetic acid (5-HIAA) and vanillylmandelic acid (VMA).

Drug Interactions: NOVAHISTINE DMX should not be used in patients taking a prescription drug for hypertension or depression without the advice of a physician. MAO inhibitors and beta-adrenergic blockers increase the effects of pseudoephedrine (sympathomimetics). Sympathomimetics may reduce the antihypertensive effects of methyldopa, mecamylamine, reserpine, and veratrum alkaloids.

Dosage and Administration: Adults and children 12 years and over, 2 teaspoonfuls every 4 hours. Children 6 to under 12 years, 1 teaspoonful every 4 hours. Children 2 to under 6 years, ½ teaspoonful every 4 hours. Not more than 4 doses every 24 hours. For children under 2 years of age, give only as directed by a physician.

How Supplied: As a red syrup in 4 fluid ounce bottles.
Keep tightly closed. Protect from excessive heat and light. Avoid freezing.
Shown in Product Identification Section, page 412

NOVAHISTINE® Elixir
[nō″vă-hĭs′tēn]
Cold & Hay Fever Formula

Description: Each 5 mL teaspoonful of NOVAHISTINE Elixir contains: Chlorpheniramine Maleate 2 mg, Phenylephrine Hydrochloride 5 mg. Also contains: Alcohol 5%, D&C Yellow No. 10, FD&C Blue No. 1, Flavors, Glycerin, Sodium Chloride, Sorbitol, and Water. Although considered sugar-free, each 5 mL contributes approximately 7 calories from sorbitol.

Actions: Phenylephrine is a nasal decongestant. Its effects are similar to epinephrine, but it is less potent on a weight basis, and has a longer duration of action. Phenylephrine produces peripheral effects similar to epinephrine, but has little or no central nervous system stimulation. After oral administration, nasal decongestion may occur within 15 or 20 minutes and persist for 2 to 4 hours. Chlorpheniramine maleate, an antihistaminic effective for the symptomatic relief of allergic rhinitis, possesses anticholinergic and sedative effects. Chlorpheniramine antagonizes many of the pharmacologic actions of histamine. It

prevents released histamine from dilating capillaries and causing edema of the respiratory mucosa.

Indications: For the temporary relief of nasal congestion and eustachian tube congestion associated with the common cold, sinusitis, and hay fever (allergic rhinitis). Also provides temporary relief of runny nose, sneezing, itching of nose or throat, and itchy, watery eyes due to the common cold, hay fever (allergic rhinitis) or other upper respiratory allergies. May be given concomitantly, when indicated, with analgesics and antibiotics.

Contraindications: NOVAHISTINE Elixir is contraindicated in patients with severe hypertension, severe coronary artery disease, and in patients on MAO inhibitor therapy. Patient idiosyncrasy to adrenergic agents may be manifested by insomnia, dizziness, weakness, tremor, or arrhythmias.
NOVAHISTINE Elixir is also contraindicated in patients with narrow-angle glaucoma, urinary retention, peptic ulcer, asthma, emphysema, chronic pulmonary disease, shortness of breath, or difficulty in breathing.
Nursing mothers: Phenylephrine is contraindicated in nursing mothers.
Hypersensitivity: NOVAHISTINE Elixir is also contraindicated in patients with hypersensitivity or idiosyncrasy to sympathomimetic amines, antihistamines or to other formula ingredients.

Warnings: At dosages higher than the recommended dose, nervousness, dizziness, or sleeplessness may occur. If symptoms do not improve within 7 days or are accompanied by high fever, patients should be advised to consult their physician before continuing use. Sympathomimetic amines should be used judiciously and sparingly in patients with hypertension, diabetes mellitus, cardiovascular disease (e.g. ischemic heart disease), increased intraocular pressure, hyperthyroidism, or prostatic hypertrophy. Sympathomimetics may produce central nervous system stimulation with convulsions or cardiovascular collapse with accompanying hypotension. See Contraindications.

Use in elderly: The elderly (60 years and older) are more likely to have adverse reactions to sympathomimetics. Overdosage of sympathomimetics in this age group may cause hallucinations, convulsions, CNS depression, and death.

Use in children: May cause excitability. NOVAHISTINE Elixir should not be used in children under 6 years except under the advice and supervision of a physician.

Use in pregnancy: Safety for use during pregnancy has not been established. As with any drug, if you are pregnant or nursing a baby, seek the advice of a health professional before using this product.

If sensitive to any of the ingredients, do not use.

Keep this and all drugs out of the reach of children. In case of accidental overdose, seek professional assistance or contact a Poison Control Center immediately.

Precautions: The antihistamine may cause drowsiness, and ambulatory patients who operate machinery or motor vehicles should be cautioned accordingly.

Adverse Reactions: Drugs containing sympathomimetic amines have been associated with certain untoward reactions, including fear, anxiety, tenseness, restlessness, tremor, weakness, pallor, respiratory difficulty, dysuria, insomnia, hallucinations, convulsions, CNS depression, arrhythmias, and cardiovascular collapse with hypotension. Individuals hyperreactive to phenylephrine may display ephedrine-like reactions such as tachycardia, palpitation, headache, dizziness, or nausea.

Phenylephrine is considered safe and relatively free of unpleasant side effects when taken at recommended dosage. Patients sensitive to antihistamine drugs may experience mild sedation. Other side effects from antihistamines may include dry mouth, dizziness, weakness, anorexia, nausea, vomiting, headache, nervousness, polyuria, heartburn, diplopia, dysuria, and, very rarely, dermatitis.

Drug Interactions: NOVAHISTINE Elixir should not be used in patients taking a prescription drug for hypertension or depression without the advice of a physician. MAO inhibitors and beta-adrenergic blockers increase the effects of sympathomimetics. Sympathomimetics may reduce the antihypertensive effects of methyldopa, mecamylamine, reserpine, and veratrum alkaloids. Antihistamines have been shown to enhance one or more of the effects of tricyclic antidepressants, barbiturates, alcohol, and other central nervous system depressants.

Dosage and Administration: Adults and children 12 years and older, 2 teaspoonfuls every 4 hours; children 6 to under 12 years, 1 teaspoonful every 4 hours; children 2 to under 6 years, ½ teaspoonful every 4 hours.

For children under 2 years, at the discretion of the physician.

Product label dosage is as follows: Adults and children 12 years and older, 2 teaspoonfuls every 4 hours. Children 6 to under 12 years, 1 teaspoonful every 4 hours. Not more than 6 doses every 24 hours. For children under 6 years, give only as directed by a physician.

How Supplied: NOVAHISTINE Elixir, as a green liquid in 4 fluid ounce bottles. Keep tightly closed. Protect from excessive heat and light. Avoid freezing.

Shown in Product Identification Section, page 412

OS-CAL® 500 Chewable Tablets
[ăhs 'kăl]
(calcium supplement)

Each Tablet Contains: 1,250 mg of calcium carbonate.
Elemental calcium........................ 500 mg
Ingredients: calcium carbonate, dextrose monohydrate, maltodextrin, micro-crystalline cellulose, magnesium stearate, Bavarian cream flavor, sodium chloride, and coconut cream flavor.

Directions: One tablet two to three times a day with meals, or as recommended by your physician.

Two Tablets Provide: 1,000 mg calcium, 100% of U.S. RDA for adults and children 12 or more years of age.

Three Tablets Provide: 1,500 mg calcium, 115% of U.S. RDA for pregnant and lactating women.

Store at room temperature. Keep out of reach of children.

How Supplied: OS-CAL® 500 Chewable Tablets is available in bottles of 60 tablets.

Issued 5/91
Shown in Product Identification Section, page 412

OS-CAL® 500 Tablets
[ăhs 'kăl]
(calcium supplement)

Each Tablet Contains: 1,250 mg of calcium carbonate from oyster shell, an organic calcium source.
Elemental calcium .... 500 mg
Ingredients: oyster shell powder, corn syrup solids, talc, hydroxypropyl methylcellulose, cornstarch, sodium starch glycolate, calcium stearate, polysorbate 80, pharmaceutical glaze, titanium dioxide, methyl propyl paraben, polyethylene glycol, polyvinylpyrrolidone, carnauba wax, D&C Yellow #10, acetylated monoglyceride, edetate disodium, FD&C Blue #1, and simethicone emulsion.

Directions: One tablet two or three times a day with meals, or as recommended by your physician.

Two Tablets Provide: 1,000 mg calcium, 100% of U.S. RDA for adults and children 12 or more years of age.

Three Tablets Provide: 1,500 mg calcium, 115% of U.S. RDA for pregnant and lactating women.

Store at room temperature. Keep out of reach of children.

How Supplied: OS-CAL® 500 is available in bottles of 60 and 120 tablets.

Issued 10/87
Shown in Product Identification Section, page 412

OS-CAL® 250+D Tablets
[ăhs 'kăl]
(calcium supplement with vitamin D)

Each Tablet Contains: 625 mg of calcium carbonate from oyster shell, an organic calcium source.
Elemental calcium .... 250 mg
Vitamin D .... 125 USP Units

Ingredients: oyster shell powder, corn syrup solids, talc, cornstarch, hydroxypropyl methylcellulose, calcium stearate, polysorbate 80, titanium dioxide, methyl propyl paraben, polyethylene glycol, pharmaceutical glaze, vitamin D, polyvinylpyrrolidone, carnauba wax, D&C Yellow #10, acetylated monoglyceride, edetate disodium, FD&C Blue #1, simethicone emulsion, and edible gray ink.

Directions: One tablet three times a day with meals, or as recommended by your physician.

Three Tablets Provide:

		% U.S. RDA for Adults
Calcium	750 mg	.... 75%
Vitamin D	375 Units	.... 94%

Store at room temperature. Keep out of reach of children.

How Supplied: OS-CAL® 250+D is available in bottles of 100 and 240.

Issued 10/87
Shown in Product Identification Section, page 412

OS-CAL® 500+D Tablets
[ăhs 'kăl]
(calcium supplement with vitamin D)

Each Tablet Contains: 1,250 mg of calcium carbonate from oyster shell, an organic calcium source.
Elemental calcium .... 500 mg
Vitamin D .... 125 USP Units

Ingredients: oyster shell powder, corn syrup solids, talc, hydroxypropyl methylcellulose, cornstarch, sodium starch glycolate, calcium stearate, polysorbate 80, pharmaceutical glaze, titanium dioxide, methyl propyl paraben, polyc+hylene glycol, polyvinylpyrrolidone, vitamin D, carnauba wax, D&C Yellow #10, acetylated monoglyceride, edetate disodium, FD&C Blue #1, and simethicone emulsion.

Directions: One tablet two or three times a day with meals, or as recommended by your physician.

Two Tablets Provide: 1,000 mg calcium, 100% of U.S. RDA for adults and children 12 or more years of age and 64% of vitamin D.

Three Tablets Provide: 1,500 mg calcium, 115% of U.S. RDA for pregnant and lactating women and 94% of vitamin D.

Store at room temperature. Keep out of reach of children.

How Supplied: OS-CAL® 500+D is available in bottles of 60 and 120.

Issued 10/87
Shown in Product Identification Section, page 412

OS-CAL® FORTIFIED Tablets
[ăhs 'kăl]
(multivitamin and minerals supplement with added calcium)

Each Tablet Contains:
[See top of next page]

Continued on next page

Marion Merrell Dow—Cont.

Vitamin A (palmitate)	1668 USP Units
Vitamin D	125 USP Units
Thiamine mononitrate (vitamin B_1)	1.7 mg
Riboflavin (vitamin B_2)	1.7 mg
Pyridoxine hydrochloride (vitamin B_6)	2.0 mg
Ascorbic acid (vitamin C)	50.0 mg
dl-alpha-tocopherol acetate (vitamin E)	0.8 IU
Niacinamide	15.0 mg
Calcium (from oyster shell)	250.0 mg
Iron (as ferrous fumarate)	5.0 mg
Magnesium (as oxide)	1.6 mg
Manganese (as sulfate)	0.3 mg
Zinc (as sulfate)	0.5 mg

Ingredients: oyster shell powder, ascorbic acid, corn syrup solids, niacinamide, D&C Yellow #10 Aluminum Lake, ferrous fumarate, calcium stearate, FD&C Blue #1 Aluminum Lake, cornstarch, vitamin A palmitate, polysorbate 80, magnesium oxide, pyridoxine, thiamine, riboflavin, vitamin E, pharmaceutical glaze, methyl paraben, zinc sulfate, manganese sulfate, propylparaben, povidone, vitamin D, hydroxypropyl methylcellulose, carnauba wax, titanium dioxide, ethylcellulose, and acetylated monoglyceride.

Indication: Multivitamin and mineral supplement with added calcium.

Dosage: One tablet three times daily with meals or as directed by physician. In case of accidental overdose, seek professional assistance or contact a poison control center immediately.

Keep out of reach of children.
Store at room temperature.

How Supplied: Bottles of 100 tablets.
Issued 6/89

Shown in Product Identification Section, page 412

OS-CAL® PLUS Tablets
[ăhs ′kăl]
(multivitamin and multimineral supplement)

Each Tablet Contains:

Elemental calcium (from oyster shell)	250	mg
Vitamin D	125 USP	Units
Vitamin A (palmitate)	1666 USP	Units
Vitamin C (ascorbic acid)	33.0	mg
Vitamin B_2 (riboflavin)	0.66	mg
Vitamin B_1 (thiamine mononitrate)	0.5	mg
Vitamin B_6 (pyridoxine HCl)	0.5	mg
Niacinamide	3.33	mg
Iron (as ferrous fumarate)	16.6	mg
Zinc (as the sulfate)	0.75	mg
Manganese (as the sulfate)	0.75	mg

Ingredients: oyster shell powder, corn syrup solids, ferrous fumarate, ascorbic acid, calcium stearate, cornstarch, hydroxypropyl methylcellulose, polysorbate 80, titanium dioxide, vitamin A palmitate, niacinamide, ethylcellulose, manganese sulfate, methyl propyl paraben, zinc sulfate, pharmaceutical glaze, acetylated monoglyceride, ribofla-

vin, thiamine mononitrate, pyridoxine hydrochloride, povidone, vitamin D, carnauba wax, and D&C Red #33.

Indications: As a multivitamin and multimineral supplement.

Dosage: One (1) tablet three times a day before meals or as directed by a physician. For children under 4 years of age, consult a physician.
Store at room temperature.
Keep out of reach of children. In case of accidental overdose, seek professional assistance or contact a poison control center immediately.

How Supplied: Bottles of 100 tablets.
Issued 1/91

Shown in Product Identification Section, page 412

SINGLET® For Adults
[sĭng-lət]
Decongestant/Antihistamine/ Analgesic (pain reliever)/Antipyretic (fever reducer)

Description: Each pink Singlet tablet contains Pseudoephedrine Hydrochloride 60 mg, Chlorpheniramine Maleate 4 mg, and Acetaminophen 650 mg. Also contains: D&C Red No. 27, D&C Yellow No. 10, FD&C Blue No. 1, Hydroxypropyl Cellulose, Hydroxypropyl Methylcellulose 2910, Magnesium Stearate, Microcrystalline Cellulose, Polyethylene Glycol 8000, Pregelatinized Corn Starch, Sodium Starch Glycolate, Sucrose, and Titanium Dioxide.

Indications: For the temporary relief of nasal congestion, runny nose, occasional sinus headache, fever, sneezing, watery eyes or itching of the nose, throat, and eyes due to colds, hay fever, or other upper respiratory allergies.

Warnings: Do not take this product for more than 7 days. Unless directed by a physician, do not take this product if you have asthma, glaucoma, emphysema, chronic pulmonary disease, heart disease, high blood pressure, thyroid disease, diabetes, shortness of breath, difficulty in breathing, difficulty in urination due to enlargement of the prostate gland, or if you are presently taking a prescription drug for high blood pressure or depression. Do not exceed recommended dosage because severe liver damage, nervousness, dizziness, or sleeplessness may occur. May cause excitability. Consult your physician if symptoms persist, if new symptoms occur, or if redness or swelling is present, because these could be signs of a serious condition. Consult your physician if fever persists for more than 3 days (72 hours) or recurs. May cause drowsiness; alcohol, sedatives, and tranquilizers may increase the drowsiness effect. Avoid alcoholic beverages while taking this product. Do not take this product if you are taking sedatives or tranquilizers without first consulting your physician. Use caution when driving a motor vehicle or operating machinery. If sensitive to any of the ingredients, do not use.

As with any drug, if you are pregnant or nursing a baby, seek the advice of a health professional before using this product. KEEP THIS AND ALL DRUGS OUT OF THE REACH OF CHILDREN. In case of accidental overdose, seek professional assistance or contact a Poison Control Center immediately. Prompt medical attention is critical for adults as well as for children even if you do not notice any signs or symptoms.

Dosage and Administration: Adults and children 12 years and older: one tablet 3 to 4 times a day, taken with water, while symptoms persist. Do not take more than 1 tablet within a 4-hour period. Do not exceed 4 tablets in 24 hours. Children under 12 years of age: consult a physician.

Storage: Protect from excessive heat and moisture.

How Supplied: Bottles of 100.

THROAT DISCS® Throat Lozenges
[thrōt dĭsks]

Description: Each lozenge contains sucrose, starch (may contain cornstarch), acacia, glycyrrhiza extract (licorice), gum tragacanth, anethole, linseed, cubeb oleoresin, anise oil, peppermint oil, capsicum, and mineral oil.

Indications: Effective for soothing, temporary relief of minor throat irritations from hoarseness and coughs due to colds.

Precautions: For severe or persistent cough or sore throat, or sore throat accompanied by high fever, headache, nausea, and vomiting, consult physician promptly. Not recommended for children under 3 years of age.

Directions: Allow lozenge to dissolve slowly in mouth. One or two should give the desired relief.

How Supplied: Boxes of 60 lozenges.
Issued 9/88

Shown in Product Identification Section, page 412

Marlyn Health Care
14810 N. 73RD ST
SCOTTSDALE, AZ 85260

MARLYN FORMULA 50®

PRODUCT OVERVIEW

Key Facts: MARLYN FORMULA 50 is a combination of amino acids and B6 in a gelatin capsule which provides protein "building blocks" important to growth and development of all protein containing tissue including nails, hair and skin.

Major Uses: Dermatologists recommend Formula 50 not only for splitting, peeling nails but also prescribe it in conjunction with their favorite topical cream for control of nail fungus. OB-Gyn's recommend it for help in controlling excessive hair fall-out after child birth.

The recommended daily dose is six capsules daily.

Safety Information: There are no known contraindications or adverse reactions.

PRESCRIBING INFORMATION

MARLYN FORMULA 50®

Composition: Each capsule contains:
Amino Acids..................................0.3 Gm*
Vitamin B6 (pyridoxine HCl)......1.0 mg.
*Approximate analysis of the amino acids: indispensable amino acids (lysine, tryptophan, phenylalanine, methionine, threonine, leucine, isoleucine, valine), 35.30%; semi-dispensable amino acids (arginine, histidine, tyrosine, cystine, glycine), 19.18%; dispensable amino acids (glutamic acid, alanine, aspartic acid, serine, proline), 45.56%.
Amino acids: Protein "building blocks" important to growth and development of all protein containing tissue including nails, hair, and skin.

Dosage and Administration: The recommended daily dose is 6 capsules daily.

Supply: Bottles of 100, 250 and 1000 capsules.

MARLYN FORMULA 50 MEGA FORTE

PRODUCT OVERVIEW

Key Facts: MARLYN FORMULA 50 MEGA FORTE is a combination of amino acids and B6 in a gelatin capsule which provides protein "building blocks" important to growth and development of all protein containing tissues including nails, hair, and skin. In addition FORMULA 50 MEGA FORTE has the added advantages of Silicon, L-Cysteine and natural Mucopolysaccharides (from bovine cartilage.)

Major Uses: Dermatologists recommend FORMULA 50 MEGA FORTE not only for splitting, peeling nails but also prescribe it in conjunction with their favorite topical cream for control of nail fungus. OB-Gyn's recommend it for help in controlling excessive hair fall-out after child birth.
The recommended daily dose is six capsules daily.

Safety Information: There are no known contraindications or adverse reactions.

PRESCRIBING INFORMATION

MARLYN FORMULA 50 MEGA FORTE

Each 6 capsules contain:
Amino Acids .... 1980 mg
Vitamin B6 .... 6 mg
Silicon
(from Amino Acid Chelate).......... 90 mg
L-Cysteine HCl .... 120 mg
(Natural Extract)
Mucopolysaccharides..................... 60 mg
(from Bovine cartilage extract)

Approximate analysis of amino acids: indispensable amino acids: (lysine, tryptophan, phenylalanine, methionine, threonine, leucine, isoleucine, valine) 35.30%; semi-dispensable amino acids; (arginine, histidine, tyrosine, cystine, glycine, 19.18%; dispensable amino acids (glutamic acids, alanine, aspartic acid, serine, proline), 45.56%.
Amino Acids; Protein "building blocks" important to growth and development of all protein containing tissue including nails, hair, and skin.

Dosage and Administration: The recommended daily dose is 6 capsules daily.

Supply: Bottles of 100, 240, 500 and 1000.

McNeil Consumer Products Company
Division of McNeil-PPC, Inc.
FORT WASHINGTON, PA 19034

IMODIUM® A–D
(loperamide hydrochloride)

Description: Each 5 ml (teaspoon) of Imodium A-D liquid contains loperamide hydrochloride 1 mg. Imodium A-D liquid is stable, cherry flavored, and clear in color.
Each caplet of Imodium AD contains 2 mg of loperamide and is scored and colored green.

Actions: Imodium A-D contains a clinically proven antidiarrheal medication. Loperamide HCl acts by slowing intestinal motility and by affecting water and electrolyte movement through the bowel.

Indication: Imodium A-D is indicated for the control and symptomatic relief of acute nonspecific diarrhea.

Usual Dosage: Adults: Take four teaspoonfuls or two caplets after first loose bowel movement. If needed, take two teaspoonfuls or one caplet after each subsequent loose bowel movement. Do not exceed eight teaspoonfuls or four caplets in any 24 hour period, unless directed by a physician.
9–11 years old (60–95 lbs.): Two teaspoonfuls or one caplet after first loose bowel movement, followed by one teaspoonful or one-half caplet after each subsequent loose bowel movement. Do not exceed six teaspoonfuls or three caplets a day.
6–8 years old (48–59 lbs.): Two teaspoonfuls or one caplet after first loose bowel movement, followed by one teaspoonful or one-half caplet after each subsequent loose bowel movement. Do not exceed four teaspoonfuls or two caplets a day.
Professional Dosage Schedule for children two-five years old (24–47 lbs): one teaspoon after first loose bowel movement, followed by one after each subsequent loose bowel movement. Do not exceed three teaspoonfuls a day.
Warnings: DO NOT USE FOR MORE THAN TWO DAYS UNLESS DI-RECTED BY A PHYSICIAN. Do not use if diarrhea is accompanied by high fever (greater than 101°F), or if blood is present in the stool, or if you have had a rash or other allergic reaction to loperamide HCl. If you are taking antibiotics or have a history of liver disease, consult a physician before using this product. As with any drug, if you are pregnant or nursing a baby, seek the advice of a physician before using this product. Keep this and all drugs out of the reach of children. In case of accidental overdose, seek professional assistance or contact a poison control center immediately. Store at room temperature.

Overdosage: Overdosage of loperamide HCl in man may result in constipation, CNS depression and nausea. A slurry of activated charcoal administered promptly after ingestion of loperamide hydrochloride can reduce the amount of drug which is absorbed. If vomiting occurs spontaneously upon ingestion, a slurry of 100 grams of activated charcoal should be administered orally as soon as fluids can be retained. If vomiting has not occurred, and CNS depression is evident, gastric lavage should be performed followed by administration of 100 gms of the activated charcoal slurry through the gastric tube. In the event of overdosage, patients should be monitored for signs of CNS depression for at least 24 hours. Children may be more sensitive to central nervous system effects than adults. If CNS depression is observed, naloxone may be administered. If responsive to naloxone, vital signs must be monitored carefully for recurrence of symptoms of drug overdose for at least 24 hours after the last dose of naloxone.

Inactive Ingredients:
Liquid: Alcohol (5.25%), citric acid, flavors, glycerin, methylparaben, propylparaben and purified water.
Caplets: Corn starch, lactose, magnesium stearate, microcrystalline cellulose, FD&C Blue #1 and D&C yellow #10.

How Supplied: Cherry flavored liquid (clear) 2 fl. oz., 3 fl. oz., and 4 fl. oz. tamper resistant bottles with child resistant safety caps and special dosage cups. Green Scored caplets in 6's and 12's blister packaging which is tamper resistant and child resistant.
Shown in Product Identification Section, page 414

MEDIPREN®
Ibuprofen Caplets and Tablets
Pain Reliever/Fever Reducer

Warning: ASPIRIN SENSITIVE PATIENTS. Do not take this product if you have had a severe allergic reaction to aspirin (e.g., asthma, swelling, shock or hives) because even though this product contains no aspirin or salicylates, cross-reactions may occur in patients allergic to aspirin.

Continued on next page

McNeil Consumer—Cont.

Description: Each MEDIPREN Caplet or Tablet contains ibuprofen 200 mg.

Indications: For the temporary relief of minor aches and pains associated with the common cold, headache, toothaches, muscular aches, backache, for the minor pain of arthritis, for the pain of menstrual cramps, and for reduction of fever.

Usual Dosage:
Adults: One Caplet or Tablet every 4 to 6 hours while symptoms persist. If pain or fever does not respond to 1 Caplet or Tablet, 2 Caplets or Tablets may be used but do not exceed 6 Caplets or Tablets in 24 hours, unless directed by a doctor. The smallest effective dose should be used. Take with food or milk if occasional and mild heartburn, upset stomach, or stomach pain occurs with use. Consult a doctor if these symptoms are more than mild or if they persist.
Children: Do not give this product to children under 12 except under the advice and supervision of a doctor.
WARNINGS: Do not take for pain for more than 10 days or for fever for more than 3 days unless directed by a doctor. If pain or fever persists or gets worse, if new symptoms occur, or if the painful area is red or swollen, consult a doctor. These could be signs of serious illness. If you are under a doctor's care for any serious condition, consult a doctor before taking this product. As with aspirin and acetaminophen, if you have any condition which requires you to take prescription drugs or if you have had any problems or serious side effects from taking any non-prescription pain reliever, do not take this product without first discussing it with your doctor. If you experience any symptoms which are unusual or seem unrelated to the condition for which you took ibuprofen, consult a doctor before taking any more of it. Although ibuprofen is indicated for the same conditions as aspirin and acetaminophen, it should not be taken with them except under a doctor's direction. Do not combine this product with any other ibuprofen containing product. As with any drug, if you are pregnant or nursing a baby, seek the advice of a health professional before using this product. IT IS ESPECIALLY IMPORTANT NOT TO USE IBUPROFEN DURING THE LAST 3 MONTHS OF PREGNANCY UNLESS SPECIFICALLY DIRECTED TO DO SO BY A DOCTOR BECAUSE IT MAY CAUSE PROBLEMS IN THE UNBORN CHILD OR COMPLICATIONS DURING DELIVERY. Keep this and all drugs out of the reach of children.

Overdosage: In case of accidental overdose, contact a physician or poison control center.

Storage: Store at room temperature; avoid excessive heat 40°C (104°F).

Inactive Ingredients: Colloidal silicon dioxide, glyceryl triacetate, hydroxypropyl methylcellulose, microcrystalline cellulose, pregelatinized starch, sodium lauryl sulfate, sodium starch glycolate, titanium dioxide, Red # 40.

How Supplied: Coated Caplets (colored white, imprinted "MEDIPREN")—bottles of 24's, 50's, 125's. Coated Tablets (colored white, imprinted "MEDIPREN")—bottles of 24's and 50's.
Shown in Product Identification Section, page 414

PEDIACARE® Allergy Formula
PEDIACARE® Cough-Cold Formula Liquid and 6–12 Cough-Cold Formula Chewable Tablets
PEDIACARE® NightRest Cough-Cold Formula Liquid
PEDIACARE® Infants' Oral Decongestant Drops

Description: Each 5 ml of PEDIACARE Allergy Formula contains chlorpheniramine maleate 1 mg. Each 5 ml of PEDIACARE Cough-Cold Formula Liquid contains pseudoephedrine hydrochloride 15 mg, chlorpheniramine maleate 1 mg and dextromethorphan hydrobromide 5 mg. Each PEDIACARE 6–12 Cough-Cold Formula Chewable Tablet contains pseudoephedrine hydrochloride 15 mg, chlorpheniramine maleate 1 mg and dextromethorphan hydrobromide 5 mg. Each 0.8 ml oral dropper of PEDIACARE Infants' Oral Decongestant Drops contains pseudoephedrine hydrochloride 7.5 mg. PEDIACARE NightRest contains pseudoephedrine hydrochloride 15 mg, chlorpheniramine maleate 1 mg and dextromethorphan hydrobromide 7.5 mg per 5 ml. PEDIACARE Cough-Cold Formula Liquid and Infants' Drops are stable, cherry flavored and red in color. PEDIACARE Allergy Formula Liquid is grape flavored and purple in color. PEDIACARE Cough-Cold Formula Chewable Tablets are fruit flavored and pink in color.

Actions: PEDIACARE Products are available in four different formulas, allowing you to select the ideal product to temporarily relieve the patient's symptoms. PEDIACARE Allergy Formula contains an antihistamine to relieve children's allergy symptoms. PEDIACARE Cough-Cold Formula liquid and 6–12 Chewable Tablets contain both of the above ingredients plus a cough suppressant, dextromethorphan hydrobromide, to provide temporary relief of nasal congestion, runny nose, sneezing and coughing due to the common cold, hay fever or other upper respiratory allergies. PEDIACARE NightRest Cough-Cold Formula Liquid contains a decongestant, pseudoephedrine hydrochloride, an antihistamine, chlorpheniramine maleate, and a cough suppressant, dextromethorphan hydrobromide, to provide temporary relief of coughs, nasal congestion, runny nose and sneezing due to the common cold. PEDIACARE NightRest may be used day or night to relieve cough and cold symptoms. PEDIACARE Infants' Oral Decongestant Drops contain a decongestant, pseudoephedrine hydrochlo-

ride, to provide temporary relief of nasal congestion due to the common cold, hay fever or other upper respiratory allergies.

Professional Dosage: A calibrated dosage cup is provided for accurate dosing of the PEDIACARE Liquid formulas. A calibrated oral dropper is provided for accurate dosing of PEDIACARE Infants' Drops. All doses of PEDIACARE Allergy Formula Liquid, PEDIACARE Cough-Cold Formula Liquid and 6–12 Chewable Tablets and PEDIACARE Infants' Drops may be repeated every 4–6 hours, not to exceed 4 doses in 24 hours. PEDIACARE NightRest Liquid may be repeated every 6–8 hrs, not to exceed 4 doses in 24 hours. [See table top of next page.]

"**WARNINGS:** Do not use if carton is opened, or if printed plastic bottle wrap or foil inner seal is broken. Keep this and all medication out of the reach of children. In case of accidental overdosage, contact a physician or poison control center immediately."

The following information appears on the appropriate package labels:

PEDIACARE Allergy Formula Liquid: May cause drowsiness. May cause excitability, especially in children. Do not give this product to children who have asthma or glaucoma unless directed by a doctor.

PEDIACARE Cough-Cold Formula Liquid, NightRest Cough-Cold Formula and 6–12 Chewable Tablets: Do not exceed the recommended dosage because nervousness, dizziness or sleeplessness may occur. Do not give this product to children for more than 7 days. If symptoms do not improve, or are accompanied by fever, consult a doctor. A persistent cough may be a sign of a serious condition. If cough persists for more than one week, tends to recur or is accompanied by fever, rash, or persistent headache, consult a doctor. Do not give this product for persistent or chronic cough such as occurs with asthma or if cough is accompanied by excessive phlegm (mucus) unless directed by a doctor. This preparation may cause drowsiness or, in some cases, excitability. Do not give this product to children who have heart disease, high blood pressure, thyroid disease, glaucoma or asthma unless directed by a doctor.

DRUG INTERACTION PRECAUTION: Do not give this product to a child who is taking a prescription drug for high blood pressure or depression, without first consulting the child's doctor.

PEDIACARE Infants' Oral Decongestant Drops: "Do not exceed the recommended dosage because at higher doses nervousness, dizziness or sleeplessness may occur. Do not give this product to children who have heart disease, high blood pressure, thyroid disease or diabetes unless directed by a physician. Do not give this product to children for more than seven days. If symptoms do not improve or are accompanied by fever, consult a physician. Do not give this product to children who are taking a prescription drug for high blood pressure or depres-

Age Group	0–3 mos	4–11 mos	12–23 mos	2–3 yrs	4–5 yrs	6–8 yrs	9–10 yrs	11 yrs	Dosage
Weight (lbs)	6–11 lb	12–17 lb	18–23 lb	24–35 lb	36–47 lb	48–59 lb	60–71 lb	72–95 lb	
PEDIACARE Infants' Drops*	½ dropper (0.4 ml)	1 dropper (0.8 ml)	1½ droppers (1.2 ml)	2 droppers (1.6 ml)					q4–6h
PEDIACARE Allergy Formula Liquid**				1 tsp	1½ tsp	2 tsp	2½ tsp	3 tsp	q4–6h
PEDIACARE 6–12 Cough-Cold Formula Liquid**				1 tsp	1½ tsp	2 tsp	2½ tsp	3 tsp	q4–6h
and Chewable Tablets**				1 tabs	1½ tabs	2 tabs	2½ tabs	3 tabs	q4–6h
PEDIACARE NightRest Liquid**				1 tsp	1½ tsp	2 tsp	2½ tsp	3 tsp	q6–8h

*Administer to children under 2 years only on the advice of a physician.
**Administer to children under 6 years only on the advice of a physician.

sion without first consulting a physician. Take by mouth only. Not for nasal use."
PEDIACARE Cough-Cold Formula Liquid: Inactive Ingredients: Benzoic acid, citric acid, flavors, glycerin, polyethylene glycol, propylene glycol, sodium benzoate, sorbitol, sucrose, purified water, Red #33, Blue #1 and Red #40.
PEDIACARE NightRest Cough-Cold Formula Liquid: Inactive ingredients: Benzoic acid, citric acid, flavors, glycerin, polyethylene glycol, proplene glycol, sodium benzoate, sorbitol, sucrose, purified water, Red #33, Blue #1 and Red #40.
PEDIACARE 6–12 Cough-Cold Formula Chewable Tablets also contain the warning, "Phenylketonurics: contains phenylalanine 3 mg per tablet", and the inactive ingredient listing, "Inactive Ingredients: Aspartame, cellulose, citric acid, flavors, magnesium stearate, magnesium trisilicate, mannitol, starch and Red #7."
PEDIACARE Infants' Oral Decongestant Drops: "Inactive Ingredients: Benzoic acid, citric acid, flavors, glycerin, polyethylene glycol, propylene glycol, purified water, sodium benzoate, sorbitol, sucrose and Red #40."

Overdosage: Acute dextromethorphan overdose usually does not result in serious signs and symptoms unless massive amounts have been ingested. Signs and symptoms of a substantial overdose may include nausea and vomiting, visual disturbances, CNS disturbances, and urinary retention. Symptoms from pseudoephedrine overdose consist most often of mild anxiety, tachycardia and/or mild hypertension. Symptoms usually appear within 4 to 8 hours of ingestion and are transient, usually requiring no treatment. Chlorpheniramine toxicity should be treated as you would an antihistamine/anticholinergic overdose and is likely to be present within a few hours after acute ingestion.

How Supplied: PEDIACARE Cough-Cold Liquid and NightRest Cough-Cold Formula Liquid (colored red)—bottles of 4 fl. oz. with child-resistant safety cap and calibrated dosage cup. PEDIACARE Allergy Liquid (colored purple)—bottles of 4 fl. oz. with child resistant safety cap and calibrated dosage cup. PEDIACARE 6–12 Cough-Cold Formula Chewable Tablets (pink, scored)—blister packs of 16. PEDIACARE Infants' Drops (colored red)—bottles of ½ fl. oz with calibrated dropper.

Shown in Product Identification Section, page 414

MAXIMUM STRENGTH SINE-AID® Sinus Headache Gelcaps, Caplets and Tablets

Description: Each MAXIMUM STRENGTH SINE-AID® Gelcap, Caplet or Tablet contains acetaminophen 500 mg and pseudoephedrine hydrochloride 30 mg.

Actions: MAXIMUM STRENGTH SINE-AID® Gelcaps, Caplets and Tablets contain a clinically proven analgesic-antipyretic and a decongestant. Maximum allowable non-prescription levels of acetaminophen and pseudophedrine provide temporary relief of sinus congestion and pain. Acetaminophen is equal to aspirin in analgesic and antipyretic effectiveness and it is unlikely to produce many of the side effects associated with aspirin and aspirin-containing products. Acetaminophen produces analgesia by elevation of the pain threshold and antipyresis through action on the hypothalamic heat-regulating center. Pseudoephedrine hydrochloride is a sympathomimetic amine that promotes sinus cavity drainage by reducing nasopharyngeal mucosal congestion.

Indications: MAXIMUM STRENGTH SINE-AID® Gelcaps, Caplets and Tablets provide effective symptomatic relief from sinus headache pain and congestion. SINE-AID® is particularly well-suited in patients with aspirin allergy, hemostatic disturbances (including anticoagulant therapy), and bleeding diatheses (e.g. hemophilia) and upper gastrointestinal disease (e.g. ulcer, gastritis, hiatus hernia).

Precautions: If a rare sensitivity occurs, the drug should be discontinued. Although pseudoephedrine is virtually without pressor effect in normotensive patients, it should be used with caution in hypertensives.

Usual Dosage:
Adult dosage: Two gelcaps, caplets or tablets every four to six hours. Do not exceed eight gelcaps, caplets or tablets in any 24 hour period. **Warning:** Do not ad-

minister to children under 12 or exceed the recommended dosage because at higher doses nervousness, dizziness or sleeplessness may occur. Do not take this product for more than 7 days. If symptoms do not improve or are accompanied by a fever, consult a physician. Do not take this product if you have heart disease, high blood pressure, thyroid disease, diabetes or difficulty in urination due to enlargement of the prostate gland unless directed by a doctor.

Drug Interaction Precaution: Do not take this product if you are presently taking a prescription drug for high blood pressure or depression without first consulting your doctor.

Do not use if carton is open or if blister unit is broken, or if printed neck wrap or printed foil inner seal is broken. Keep this and all medication out of the reach of children. As with any drug, if you are pregnant or nursing a baby, seek the advice of a health professional before using this product. In case of accidental overdosage, contact a physician or poison control center immediately.

Overdosage: Acetaminophen in massive overdosage may cause hepatic toxicity in some patients. In adults and adolescents, hepatic toxicity has rarely been reported following ingestion of acute overdoses of less than 10 grams. Fatalities are infrequent (less than 3–4% of untreated cases) and have rarely been reported with overdoses of less than 15 grams. In children, an acute overdosage of less than 150 mg/kg has not been associated with hepatic toxicity.
Early symptoms following a potentially hepatotoxic overdose may include: nausea, vomiting, diaphoresis and general malaise. Clinical and laboratory evidence of hepatic toxicity may not be apparent until 48 to 72 hours postingestion. In adults and adolescents, regardless of the quantity of acetaminophen reported to have been ingested, administer MUCOMYST® acetylcysteine immediately if 24 hours or less have elapsed from the reported time of ingestion. For full prescribing information, refer to the MUCOMYST package insert. Do not await results of assays for acetaminophen level before initiating treatment with MUCOMYST acetylcysteine. The

Continued on next page

McNeil Consumer—Cont.

following additional procedures are recommended: The stomach should be emptied promptly by lavage or by induction of emesis with syrup of ipecac. A serum acetaminophen assay should be obtained as early as possible, but no sooner than four hours following ingestion. Liver function studies should be obtained initially and repeated at 24-hour intervals.

Serious toxicity or fatalities are extremely infrequent in children, possibly due to differences in the way they metabolize acetaminophen. In children, the maximum potential amount ingested can be more easily estimated. If more than 150 mg/kg or an unknown amount was ingested, obtain an acetaminophen plasma level. The acetaminophen plasma level should be obtained as soon as possible, but no sooner than 4 hours following the ingestion. Induce emesis using syrup of ipecac. If the plasma level is obtained and falls above the broken line on the acetaminophen overdose nomogram, the MUCOMYST acetylcysteine therapy should be initiated and continued for a full course of therapy. If acetaminophen plasma assay capability is not available, and the estimated acetaminophen ingestion exceeds 150 mg/kg, MUCOMYST acetylcysteine therapy should be initiated and continued for a full course of therapy.

For additional emergency information, call your regional poison center or call the Rocky Mountain Poison Center toll-free, (1-800-525-6115).

Symptoms from pseudoephedrine overdose consist most often of mild anxiety, tachycardia and/or mild hypertension. Symptoms usually appear within 4 to 8 hours of ingestion and are transient, usually requiring no treatment.

Inactive Ingredients: Gelcaps: Benzyl Alcohol, Butylparaben, Castor Oil, Cellulose, Corn Starch, Edetate Calcium Disodium, Gelatin, Hydroxypropyl Methylcellulose, Iron Oxide Black, Magnesium Stearate, Methylparaben, Propylparaben, Sodium Lauryl Sulfate, Sodium Propionate, Sodium Starch Glycolate, Titanium Dioxide, FD&C Red #40.
Caplets: Cellulose, Corn Starch, Hydroxypropyl Methylcellulose, Magnesium Stearate, Polyethylene Glycol, Sodium Starch Glycolate, Titanium Dioxide, Blue #1 and Red #40.
Tablets: Cellulose, Corn Starch, Magnesium Stearate and Sodium Starch Glycolate.

How Supplied:
Gelcaps (colored red and white imprinted "SINE-AID")—blister package of 20 and tamper resistant bottle of 40.
Caplets (colored white imprinted "Maximum SINE-AID")—blister package of 24 and tamper resistant bottle of 50.
Tablets (colored white embossed "Sine-Aid")—blister package of 24 and tamper resistant bottle of 50.

Shown in Product Identification Section, page 414

CHILDREN'S TYLENOL®
acetaminophen
Chewable Tablets, Elixir, Drops

Description: Infants' TYLENOL acetaminophen Drops are stable, alcohol-free, fruit-flavored and orange in color. Each 0.8 ml (one calibrated dropperful) contains 80 mg acetaminophen. Children's TYLENOL Elixir is stable and alcohol-free, cherry-flavored, and red in color or grape-flavored, and purple in color. Each 5 ml contains 160 mg acetaminophen. Each Children's TYLENOL Chewable Tablet contains 80 mg acetaminophen in a grape- or fruit-flavored tablet.

Actions: Acetaminophen is a clinically proven analgesic/antipyretic. Acetaminophen produces analgesia by elevation of the pain threshold and antipyresis through action on the hypothalamic heat regulating center. Acetaminophen is equal to aspirin in analgesic and antipyretic effectiveness and it is unlikely to produce many of the side effects associated with aspirin and aspirin containing products.

Indications: Children's TYLENOL Chewable Tablets, Elixir and Drops are designed for treatment of infants and children with conditions requiring temporary relief of fever and discomfort due to colds and "flu," and of simple pain and discomfort due to teething, immunizations and tonsillectomy.

Precautions: If a rare sensitivity reaction occurs, the drug should be stopped.

Usual Dosage: All dosages may be repeated every 4 hours, but not more than 5 times daily. Administer to children under 2 years only on the advice of a physician. Children's TYLENOL Chewable Tablets: 2–3 years: two tablets. 4–5 years: three tablets, 6–8 years: four tablets. 9–10 years: five tablets. 11–12 years: six tablets.
Children's TYLENOL Elixir: (special cup for measuring dosage is provided) 4–11 months: one-half teaspoon. 12–23 months: three-quarters teaspoon, 2–3 years: one teaspoon. 4–5 years: one and one-half teaspoons. 6–8 years: 2 teaspoons. 9–10 years: two and one-half teaspoons. 11–12 years: three teaspoons.
Infants' TYLENOL Drops: 0–3 months: 0.4 ml. 4–11 months: 0.8 ml. 12–23 months: 1.2 ml. 2–3 years: 1.6 ml. 4–5 years: 2.4 ml.
Warning: Keep this and all medication out of reach of children. In case of accidental overdose, contact a physician or poison control center immediately. Consult your physician if fever persists for more than 3 days or if pain continues for more than 5 days. Store at room temperature.
NOTE: In addition to the above:
Children's TYLENOL® Drops—Do not use if printed carton overwrap or printed plastic bottle wrap is broken or missing or if carton is opened.
Children's TYLENOL Elixir—Do not use if printed carton overwrap is broken or missing or if carton is opened. Do not use if printed plastic bottle wrap or printed

foil inner seal is broken. Not a USP elixir.
Children's TYLENOL Chewables—Do not use if carton is opened or if printed plastic bottle wrap or printed foil inner seal is broken. Phenylketonurics: contains phenylalanine 3mg per tablet.

Overdosage: Acetaminophen in massive overdosage may cause hepatic toxicity in some patients. In adults and adolescents, hepatic toxicity has rarely been reported following ingestion of acute overdoses of less than 10 grams. Fatalities are infrequent (less than 3–4% of untreated cases) and have rarely been reported with overdoses of less than 15 grams. In children, an acute overdosage of less than 150 mg/kg has not been associated with hepatic toxicity.

Early symptoms following a potentially hepatotoxic overdose may include: nausea, vomiting, diaphoresis and general malaise. Clinical and laboratory evidence of hepatic toxicity may not be apparent until 48 to 72 hours postingestion. In adults and adolescents, regardless of the quantity of acetaminophen reported to have been ingested, administer MUCOMYST® acetylcysteine immediately if 24 hours or less have elapsed from the reported time of ingestion. For full prescribing information, refer to the MUCOMYST package insert. Do not await results of assays for acetaminophen level before initiating treatment with MUCOMYST acetylcysteine. The following additional procedures are recommended: The stomach should be emptied promptly by lavage or by induction of emesis with syrup of ipecac. A serum acetaminophen assay should be obtained as early as possible, but no sooner than four hours following ingestion. Liver function studies should be obtained initially and repeated at 24-hour intervals.

Serious toxicity or fatalities are extremely infrequent in children, possibly due to differences in the way they metabolize acetaminophen. In children, the maximum potential amount ingested can be more easily estimated. If more than 150 mg/kg or an unknown amount was ingested, obtain an acetaminophen plasma level. The acetaminophen plasma level should be obtained as soon as possible, but no sooner than 4 hours following the ingestion. Induce emesis using syrup of ipecac. If the plasma level is obtained and falls above the broken line on the acetaminophen overdose nomogram, the MUCOMYST acetylcysteine therapy should be initiated and continued for a full course of therapy. If acetaminophen plasma assay capability is not available, and the estimated acetaminophen ingestion exceeds 150 mg/kg, MUCOMYST acetylcysteine therapy should be initiated and continued for a full course of therapy.

For additional emergency information, call your regional poison center or call the Rocky Mountain Poison Center toll free, (1-800-525-6115).

Inactive Ingredients: Children's Tylenol Chewable Tablets—Aspartame, Cellulose, Citric Acid, Ethylcellulose, Flavors, Hydroxypropyl Methylcellulose, Mannitol, Starch, Magnesium Stearate, Red #7 and Blue #1 (Grape only).

Children's Tylenol Elixir—Benzoic Acid, Citric Acid, Flavors, Glycerin, Polyethylene Glycol, Propylene Glycol, Sodium Benzoate, Sorbitol, Sucrose, Purified Water, Red #40. In addition to the above ingredients cherry flavored elixir contains Red #33 and grape flavored elixir contains malic acid and Blue #1.

Infant's Tylenol Drops—Butylparaben, Citric Acid, Glycerin, Polyethylene Glycol, Propylene Glycol, Saccharin, Sodium Citrate, purified water and yellow #6.

How Supplied: Chewable Tablets (pink colored fruit, purple colored grape, scored, imprinted "TYLENOL")—Bottles of 30 and child resistant blister packs of 48 (fruit only). Elixir (cherry colored red and grape colored purple)—bottles of 2 and 4 fl. oz. Drops (colored orange)—bottles of 1/2 oz. (15 ml.) and 1 oz. (30 ml.) with calibrated plastic dropper.

All packages listed above have child-resistant safety caps.

Shown in Product Identification
Section, page 413

Junior Strength TYLENOL®
acetaminophen
Coated Caplets and Chewable Tablets

Description: Each Junior Strength Caplet or Chewable tablet contains 160 mg acetaminophen in a small, coated, capsule shaped tablet or grape or fruit chewable tablet.

Actions: Acetaminophen is a clinically proven analgesic/antipyretic. Acetaminophen produces analgesia by elevation of the pain threshold and antipyresis through action on the hypothalamic heat-regulating center. Acetaminophen is equal to aspirin in analgesic and antipyretic effectiveness and it is unlikely to produce many of the side effects associated with aspirin and aspirin-containing products.

Indications: Junior Strength TYLENOL Caplets are designed for easy swallowability in older children and young adults. Both Junior Strength TYLENOL Caplets and Junior Strength Chewable Tablets provide fast, effective temporary relief of fever and discomfort due to colds and "flu," and pain and discomfort due to simple headaches, minor muscle aches, sprains and overexertion.

Precautions: If a rare sensitivity reaction occurs, the drug should be stopped.

Usual Dosage: Caplets should be taken with liquid. Chewable tablets should be well chewed. All dosages may be repeated every 4 hours, but not more than 5 times daily. For ages: 6–8 years: two Caplets or tablets, 9–10 years: two and one-half Caplets or tablets, 11 years: three Caplets or tablets, 12 years: four Caplets or tablets.

Warning: Do not use if carton is opened or if a blister unit is broken.

Keep this and all medications out of the reach of children. In case of accidental overdosage, contact a physician or poison control center immediately. Consult your physician if fever persists for more than three days or if pain continues for more than five days. As with any drug, if you are pregnant or nursing a baby, seek the advice of a health professional before using this product. In addition the caplet package states: Not for children who have difficulty swallowing tablets. In addition the chewable tablet package states: Phenylketonurics: contains phenylalanine 5 mg per tablet.

Overdosage: Acetaminophen in massive overdosage may cause hepatic toxicity in some patients. In adults and adolescents, hepatic toxicity has rarely been reported following ingestion of acute overdosage of less than 10 grams. Fatalities are infrequent (less than 3–4% of untreated cases) and have rarely been reported with overdoses of less than 15 grams. In children, an acute overdosage of less than 150 mg/kg has not been associated with hepatic toxicity.

Early symptoms following a potentially hepatotoxic overdose may include: nausea, vomiting, diaphoresis and general malaise. Clinical and laboratory evidence of hepatic toxicity may not be apparent until 48 to 72 hours postingestion. In adults and adolescents, regardless of the quantity of acetaminophen reported to have been ingested, administer MUCOMYST® acetylcysteine immediately if 24 hours or less have elapsed from the reported time of ingestion. For full prescribing information, refer to the MUCOMYST package insert. Do not await the results of assays for acetaminophen level before initiating treatment with MUCOMYST acetylcysteine. The following additional procedures are recommended: The stomach should be emptied promptly by lavage or by induction of emesis with syrup of ipecac. A serum acetaminophen assay should be obtained as early as possible, but no sooner than four hours following ingestion. Liver function studies should be obtained initially and repeated at 24-hour intervals.

Serious toxicity or fatalities are extremely infrequent in children, possibly due to differences in the way they metabolize acetaminophen. In children, the maximum potential amount ingested can be more easily estimated. If more than 150 mg/kg or an unknown amount was ingested, obtain an acetaminophen plasma level. The acetaminophen plasma level should be obtained as soon as possible, but no sooner than 4 hours following the ingestion. Induce emesis using syrup of ipecac. If the plasma level is obtained and falls above the broken line on the acetaminophen overdose nomogram, the MUCOMYST acetylcysteine therapy should be initiated and continued for a full course of therapy. If acetaminophen plasma assay capability is not available, and the estimated acetaminophen ingestion exceeds 150 mg/kg, MUCOMYST acetylcysteine therapy

should be initiated and continued for a full course of therapy.

For additional emergency information, call your regional poison center or call the Rocky Mountain Poison Center toll-free (1-800-525-6115).

Inactive Ingredients: Caplets: Cellulose, Ethylcellulose, Magnesium Stearate, Sodium Lauryl Sulfate, Sodium Starch Glycolate, Starch.

Tablets: Aspartame, Cellulose, Citric Acid, Ethylcellulose, Flavors, Magnesium Stearate, Mannitol, Starch, Blue #1 and Red #7.

How Supplied: Coated Caplets, (colored white, coated, scored, imprinted "TYLENOL 160") Package of 30.

Chewable tablets (colored purple or pink, imprinted "TYLENOL 160") Package of 24. All packages are safety sealed and use child resistant blister packaging.

Shown in Product Identification
Section, pages 413 and 414

Regular Strength
TYLENOL® acetaminophen Tablets and Caplets

Description: Each Regular Strength TYLENOL Tablet or Caplet contains acetaminophen 325 mg.

Actions: Acetaminophen is a clinically proven analgesic and antipyretic. Acetaminophen produces analgesia by elevation of the pain threshold and antipyresis through action on the hypothalamic heat-regulating center. Acetaminophen is equal to aspirin in analgesic and antipyretic effectiveness and it is unlikely to produce many of the side effects associated with aspirin and aspirin-containing products.

Indications: Acetaminophen acts safely and quickly to provide temporary relief from: simple headache; minor muscular aches; the minor aches and pains associated with bursitis, neuralgia, sprains, overexertion, menstrual cramps; and from the discomfort of fever due to colds and "flu". Also for temporary relief of minor aches and pains of arthritis and rheumatism.

Precautions: If a rare sensitivity reaction occurs, the drug should be discontinued.

Usual Dosage: Adults and Children 12 years of Age and Older: 1 to 2 tablets 3 or 4 times daily. Children (6-12): 1/2 to 1 tablet 3 or 4 times daily. Consult a physician for use by children under 6.

WARNING: DO NOT USE IF PRINTED RED NECK WRAP IS BROKEN OR MISSING. DO NOT TAKE FOR PAIN FOR MORE THAN 10 DAYS OR FOR FEVER FOR MORE THAN 3 DAYS UNLESS DIRECTED BY A PHYSICIAN. SEVERE OR RECURRENT PAIN OR HIGH OR CONTINUED FEVER MAY BE INDICATIVE OF SERIOUS ILLNESS. UNDER THESE CONDITIONS, CONSULT A PHYSICIAN. KEEP THIS AND ALL MEDICATION

Continued on next page

McNeil Consumer—Cont.

OUT OF THE REACH OF CHILDREN. AS WITH ANY DRUG, IF YOU ARE PREGNANT OR NURSING A BABY, SEEK THE ADVICE OF A HEALTH PROFESSIONAL BEFORE USING THIS PRODUCT. IN THE CASE OF ACCIDENTAL OVERDOSAGE, CONTACT A PHYSICIAN OR POISON CONTROL CENTER IMMEDIATELY.

Overdosage: Acetaminophen in massive overdosage may cause hepatic toxicity in some patients. In adults and adolescents, hepatic toxicity has rarely been reported following ingestion of acute overdoses of less than 10 grams. Fatalities are infrequent (less than 3–4% of untreated cases) and have rarely been reported with overdoses of less than 15 grams. In children, an acute overdosage of less than 150 mg/kg has not been associated with hepatic toxicity.

Early symptoms following a potentially hepatotoxic overdose may include: nausea, vomiting, diaphoresis and general malaise. Clinical and laboratory evidence of hepatic toxicity may not be apparent until 48 to 72 hours postingestion. In adults and adolescents, regardless of the quantity of acetaminophen reported to have been ingested, administer MUCOMYST® acetylcysteine immediately if 24 hours or less have elapsed from the reported time of ingestion. For full prescribing information, refer to the MUCOMYST package insert. Do not await results of assays for acetaminophen level before initiating treatment with MUCOMYST acetylcysteine. The following additional procedures are recommended: The stomach should be emptied promptly by lavage or by induction of emesis with syrup of ipecac. A serum acetaminophen assay should be obtained as early as possible, but no sooner than four hours following ingestion. Liver function studies should be obtained initially and repeated at 24-hour intervals.

Serious toxicity or fatalities are extremely infrequent in children, possibly due to differences in the way they metabolize acetaminophen. In children, the maximum potential amount ingested can be more easily estimated. If more than 150 mg/kg or an unknown amount was ingested, obtain an acetaminophen plasma level. The acetaminophen plasma level should be obtained as soon as possible, but no sooner than 4 hours following the ingestion. Induce emesis using syrup of ipecac. If the plasma level is obtained and falls above the broken line on the acetaminophen overdose nomogram, the MUCOMYST acetylcysteine therapy should be initiated and continued for a full course of therapy. If acetaminophen plasma assay capability is not available, and the estimated acetaminophen ingestion exceeds 150 mg/kg, MUCOMYST acetylcysteine therapy should be initiated and continued for a full course of therapy.

For additional emergency information, call your regional poison center or call the Rocky Mountain Poison Center toll-free (1-800-525-6115).

Inactive Ingredients: Tablets—Magnesium Stearate, Cellulose, Sodium Starch Glycolate, and Starch. Caplets—Cellulose, Hydroxpropyl Methylcellulose, Magnesium Stearate, Polyethylene Glycol, Sodium Starch Glycolate and Starch and Red #40 .

How Supplied: Tablets (colored white, scored, imprinted "TYLENOL")—tins of 12, and tamper-resistant bottles of 24, 50, 100 and 200. Caplets (colored white, "TYLENOL")—tamper-resistant bottles of 24, 50, 100. For additional pain relief, Extra-Strength TYLENOL® Tablets and Caplets, 500 mg, and Extra-Strength TYLENOL® Adult Liquid Pain Reliever are available (colored green; 1 fl. oz. = 1000 mg.)

Shown in Product Identification Section, page 412

Extra Strength
TYLENOL® acetaminophen
Caplets, Gelcaps, Tablets

Description: Each Extra Strength TYLENOL Caplet, Gelcap or Tablet contains acetaminophen 500 mg.

Actions: Acetaminophen is a clinically proven analgesic and antipyretic. Acetaminophen produces analgesia by elevation of the pain threshold and antipyresis through action on the hypothalamic heat-regulating center. Acetaminophen is equal to aspirin in analgesic and antipyretic effectiveness and it is unlikely to produce many of the side effects associated with aspirin and aspirin-containing products.

Indications: For the temporary relief of minor aches, pains, headaches and fever.

Precautions: If a rare sensitivity reaction occurs, the drug should be discontinued.

Usual Dosage: Adults and children 12 years of Age and Older: Two Caplets, Gelcaps or Tablets 3 or 4 times daily. No more than a total of 8 Caplets, Gelcaps or Tablets in any 24-hour period.

Warning: Do not take for more than 10 days or for fever for more than 3 days unless directed by a doctor. Severe or recurrent pain or high or continued fever may be indicative of serious illness. Under these conditions, consult a doctor. **Do not use if printed red neck wrap or printed foil inner seal is broken. Keep this and all medication out of the reach of children. As with any drug, if you are pregnant or nursing a baby, seek the advice of a health professional before using this product. In case of accidental overdosage, contact a doctor or poison control center immediately.**

Overdosage: Acetaminophen in massive overdosage may cause hepatic toxicity in some patients. In adults and adolescents, hepatic toxicity has rarely been reported following ingestion of acute overdosage of less than 10 grams. Fatalities are infrequent (less than 3–4% of untreated cases) and have rarely been reported with overdoses of less than 15 grams. In children, an acute overdosage of less than 150 mg/kg has not been associated with hepatic toxicity.

Early symptoms following a potentially hepatotoxic overdose may include: nausea, vomiting, diaphoresis and general malaise. Clinical and laboratory evidence of hepatic toxicity may not be apparent until 48 to 72 hours postingestion. In adults and adolescents, regardless of the quantity of acetaminophen reported to have been ingested, administer MUCOMYST® acetylcysteine immediately if 24 hours or less have elapsed from the reported time of ingestion. For full prescribing information, refer to the MUCOMYST package insert. Do not await the results of assays for acetaminophen level before initiating treatment with MUCOMYST acetylcysteine. The following additional procedures are recommended: The stomach should be emptied promptly by lavage or by induction of emesis with syrup of ipecac. A serum acetaminophen assay should be obtained as early as possible, but no sooner than four hours following ingestion. Liver function studies should be obtained initially and repeated at 24-hour intervals.

Serious toxicity or fatalities are extremely infrequent in children, possibly due to differences in the way they metabolize acetaminophen. In children, the maximum potential amount ingested can be more easily estimated. If more than 150 mg/kg or an unknown amount was ingested, obtain an acetaminophen plasma level. The acetaminophen plasma level should be obtained as soon as possible, but no sooner than 4 hours following the ingestion. Induce emesis using syrup of ipecac. If the plasma level is obtained and falls above the broken line on the acetaminophen overdose nomogram, the MUCOMYST acetylcysteine therapy should be initiated and continued for a full course of therapy. If acetaminophen plasma assay capability is not available, and the estimated acetaminophen ingestion exceeds 150 mg/kg, MUCOMYST acetylcysteine therapy should be initiated and continued for a full course of therapy.

For additional emergency information, call your regional poison center or call the Rocky Mountain Poison Center toll-free, (1-800-525-6115).

Inactive Ingredients: Tablets—Magnesium Stearate, Cellulose, Sodium Starch Glycolate and Starch. Caplets—Cellulose, Hydroxypropyl Methylcellulose, Magnesium Stearate, Polyethylene Glycol, Sodium Starch Glycolate, Starch and Red #40.

Gelcaps—Benzyl Alcohol, Butylparaben, Castor Oil, Cellulose, Edetate Calcium Disodium, Gelatin, Hydroxypropyl Methylcellulose, Magnesium Stearate, Methylparaben, Propylparaben, Sodium Lauryl Sulfate, Sodium Propionate, Sodium Starch Glycolate, Starch, Titanium Dioxide, Blue #1 and #2, Red #40 and Yellow #10.

How Supplied: Tablets (colored white, imprinted "TYLENOL" and "500")—vials of 10 and tamper-resistant bottles of 30, 60, 100, and 200. Caplets (colored white, imprinted "TYLENOL 500 mg")—vials of 10 and tamper-resistant bottles of 24, 50, 100, 175, and 250's. Gelcaps (colored yellow and red, imprinted "Tylenol 500") tamper-resistant bottles of 24, 50, 100, and 150. For adults who prefer liquids or can't swallow solid medication, Extra Strength TYLENOL® Adult Liquid Pain Reliever, mint flavored, is also available (colored green; 1 fl. oz. = 1000 mg.).

Shown in Product Identification Section, pages 412 and 413

**Extra Strength
TYLENOL® acetaminophen
Adult Liquid Pain Reliever**

Description: Each 15 ml. (½ fl. oz. or one tablespoonful) contains 500 mg. acetaminophen (alcohol 7%).

Actions: TYLENOL acetaminophen is a clinically proven analgesic and antipyretic. Acetaminophen produces analgesia by elevation of the pain threshold and antipyresis through action on the hypothalamic heat-regulating center. Acetaminophen is equal to aspirin in analgesic and antipyretic effectiveness and it is unlikely to produce many of the side effects associated with aspirin and aspirin-containing products.

Indications: Acetaminophen provides temporary relief of minor aches, pains, headaches and fevers.

Precautions: If a rare sensitivity reaction occurs, the drug should be discontinued.

Usual Dosage: Extra Strength TYLENOL Adult Liquid Pain Reliever is an adult preparation for those adults who prefer liquids or can't swallow solid medication. Not for use in children under 12. Measuring cup is marked for accurate dosage. Extra Strength Dose—1 fl. oz. (30 ml or 2 tablespoonsful, 1000 mg), which is equivalent to two 500 mg Extra Strength TYLENOL Tablets, Caplets or Gelcaps. Take every 4–6 hours, no more than 4 doses in any 24-hour period.

"Warning: Do not take for more than 10 days or for fever for more than 3 days unless directed by a doctor. Severe or recurrent pain or high or continued fever may be indicative of serious illness. Under these conditions, consult a physician. Do not use if printed plastic overwrap or printed foil inner seal is broken. Keep this and all medication out of the reach of children. As with any drug, if you are pregnant or nursing a baby, seek the advice of a health professional before using this product. In case of accidental overdosage, contact a doctor or poison control center immediately."

Overdosage: Acetaminophen in massive overdosage may cause hepatic toxicity in some patients. In adults and adoles-cents, hepatic toxicity has rarely been reported following ingestion of acute overdosage of less than 10 grams. Fatalities are infrequent (less than 3–4% of untreated cases) and have rarely been reported with overdoses of less than 15 grams. In children, an acute overdosage of less than 150 mg/kg has not been associated with hepatic toxicity.

Early symptoms following a potentially hepatotoxic overdose may include: nausea, vomiting, diaphoresis and general malaise. Clinical and laboratory evidence of hepatic toxicity may not be apparent until 48 to 72 hours postingestion. In adults and adolescents, regardless of the quantity of acetaminophen reported to have been ingested, administer MUCOMYST® acetylcysteine immediately if 24 hours or less have elapsed from the reported time of ingestion. For full prescribing information, refer to the MUCOMYST package insert. Do not await the results of assays for acetaminophen level before initiating treatment with MUCOMYST acetylcysteine. The following additional procedures are recommended: The stomach should be emptied promptly by lavage or by induction of emesis with syrup of ipecac. A serum acetaminophen assay should be obtained as early as possible, but no sooner than four hours following ingestion. Liver function studies should be obtained initially and repeated at 24-hour intervals.

Serious toxicity or fatalities are extremely infrequent in children, possibly due to differences in the way they metabolize acetaminophen. In children, the maximum potential amount ingested can be more easily estimated. If more than 150 mg/kg or an unknown amount was ingested, obtain an acetaminophen plasma level. The acetaminophen plasma level should be obtained as soon as possible, but no sooner than 4 hours following the ingestion. Induce emesis using syrup of ipecac. If the plasma level is obtained and falls above the broken line on the acetaminophen overdose nomogram, the MUCOMYST acetylcysteine therapy should be initiated and continued for a full course of therapy. If acetaminophen plasma assay capability is not available, and the estimated acetaminophen ingestion exceeds 150 mg/kg, MUCOMYST acetylcysteine therapy should be initiated and continued for a full course of therapy.

For additional emergency information, call your regional poison center or call the Rocky Mountain Poison Center toll-free, (1-800-525-6115).

Inactive Ingredients: Alcohol, Citric Acid, Flavors, Glycerin, Polyethylene Glycol, Purified Water, Sodium Benzoate, Sorbitol, Sucrose, Yellow #6 (Sunset Yellow), Yellow #10 and Blue #1.

How Supplied: Mint-flavored liquid (colored green), 8 fl. oz. tamper-resistant bottle with child resistant safety cap and special dosage cup.

Shown in Product Identification Section, page 413

**EXTRA STRENGTH TYLENOL® PM
Pain Reliever/Sleep Aid Caplets and
Tablets**

Description: Each EXTRA STRENGTH TYLENOL® PM Caplet or Tablet contains acetaminophen 500 mg and diphenhydramine HCl 25 mg.

Actions: EXTRA STRENGTH TYLENOL® PM caplets and tablets contain a clinically proven analgesic-antipyretic and an antihistamine. Maximum allowable non-prescription levels of acetaminophen and diphenhydramine provide temporary relief of occasional headaches and minor aches and pains accompanying sleeplessness. Acetaminophen is equal to aspirin in analgesic and antipyretic effectiveness and it is unlikely to produce many of the side effects associated with aspirin containing products. Acetaminophen produces analgesia by elevation of the pain threshold. Diphenhydramine HCl is an antihistamine with sedative properties.

Indications: EXTRA STRENGTH TYLENOL® PM caplets and tablets provide effective symptomatic relief from occasional headaches and minor aches and pains with accompanying sleeplessness.

Precautions: If a rare sensitivity occurs, the drug should be discontinued.

Usual Dosage: Adults and Children 12 years of Age and Older: Two caplets at bedtime or as directed by physician. Do not exceed recommended dosage.

"WARNING: Do not give to children under 12 years of age or use for more than 10 days unless directed by a physician. Consult your physician if symptoms persist or new ones occur, or if fever persists for more than 3 days, or if sleeplessness persists continuously for more than 2 weeks. Insomnia may be a symptom of a serious underlying medical illness. Do not take this product if you have asthma, glaucoma, emphysema, chronic pulmonary disease, shortness of breath, difficulty in breathing or difficulty in urination due to enlargement of the prostate gland unless directed by a physician. Avoid alcoholic beverages while taking this product. Do not take if you are taking sedatives or tranquilizers without first consulting your physician. **Do not use if carton is open or if printed plastic foil inner seal is broken. Keep this and all medications out of the reach of children. In case of accidental overdose, contact a physician or poison control center immediately. As with any drug, if you are pregnant or nursing a baby, seek the advice of a health professional before using this product.**

Caution: This product will cause drowsiness. Do not drive a motor vehicle or operate machinery after use.

Overdosage: Acetaminophen in massive overdosage may cause hepatic toxicity in some patients. In adults and adolescents, hepatic toxicity has rarely been

Continued on next page

McNeil Consumer—Cont.

reported following ingestion of acute overdosage of less than 10 grams. Fatalities are infrequent (less than 3–4% of untreated cases) and have rarely been reported with overdoses of less than 15 grams. In children, an acute overdosage of less than 150 mg/kg has not been associated with hepatic toxicity.

Early symptoms following a potentially hepatotoxic overdose may include: nausea, vomiting, diaphoresis and general malaise. Clinical and laboratory evidence of hepatic toxicity may not be apparent until 48 to 72 hours postingestion. In adults and adolescents, regardless of the quantity of acetaminophen reported to have been ingested, administer MUCOMYST® acetylcysteine immediately if 24 hours or less have elapsed from the reported time of ingestion. For full prescribing information, refer to the MUCOMYST package insert. Do not await results of assays for acetaminophen level before initiating treatment with MUCOMYST acetylcysteine. The following additional procedures are recommended: The stomach should be emptied promptly by lavage or by induction of emesis with syrup of ipecac. A serum acetaminophen assay should be obtained as early as possible, but no sooner than four hours following ingestion. Liver function studies should be obtained initially and repeated at 24-hour intervals. Serious toxicity or fatalities are extremely infrequent in children, possibly due to differences in the way they metabolize acetaminophen. In children, the maximum potential amount ingested can be more easily estimated. If more than 150 mg/kg or an unknown amount was ingested, obtain an acetaminophen plasma level. The acetaminophen plasma level should be obtained as soon as possible, but no sooner than 4 hours following the ingestion. Induce emesis using syrup of ipecac. If the plasma level is obtained and falls above the broken line on the acetaminophen overdose nomogram, the MUCOMYST acetylcysteine therapy should be initiated and continued for a full course of therapy. If acetaminophen plasma assay capability is not available, and the estimated acetaminophen ingestion exceeds 150 mg/kg, MUCOMYST acetylcysteine therapy should be initiated and continued for a full course of therapy.

For additional emergency information, call your regional poison center or call the Rocky Mountain Poison Center toll-free, (1-800-525-6115).

Diphenhydramine toxicity should be treated as you would an antihistamine/anticholinergic overdose and is likely to be present within a few hours after acute ingestion.

Inactive Ingredients: Tablets: Cellulose, colloidal silicon dioxide, corn starch, sodium citrate, sodium starch glycolate, stearic acid, and Blue #1. Caplets: Cellulose, colloidal silicon dioxide, corn starch, hydroxypropyl methylcellulose, polyethylene glycol, sodium citrate, sodium

starch glycolate, stearic acid, titanium dioxide, Blue #1 and Blue #2.

How Supplied: Caplets (colored light blue imprinted "Tylenol PM") tamper-resistant bottles of 24 and 50. Tablets (colored light blue embossed with "Tylenol" on one side and "PM" on the other) tamper-resistant bottles of 24 and 50.
Shown in Product Identification Section, page 414

CHILDREN'S TYLENOL COLD®
Multi Symptom Chewable Tablets and Liquid

Description: Each Children's Tylenol Cold Chewable Grape-Flavored Tablet contains acetaminophen 80 mg, chlorpheniramine maleate 0.5 mg and pseudoephedrine hydrochloride 7.5 mg. Children's Tylenol Cold Liquid is grape flavored and contains no alcohol. Each teaspoon (5 ml) contains acetaminophen 160 mg, chlorpheniramine maleate 1 mg, and pseudoephedrine hydrochloride 15 mg.

Actions: Children's Tylenol Cold Chewable Tablets and Liquid combine the analgesic-antipyretic acetaminophen with the decongestant pseudoephedrine hydrochloride and the antihistamine chlorpheniramine maleate to help relieve nasal congestion, dry runny noses and prevent sneezing as well as to relieve the fever, aches, pains and general discomfort associated with colds and upper respiratory infections.

Acetaminophen is equal to aspirin in analgesic and antipyretic effectiveness and it is unlikely to produce the side effects often associated with aspirin or aspirin-containing products.

Indications: Provides fast, effective temporary relief of nasal congestion, runny nose, sneezing, minor aches and pains, headaches and fever due to the common cold, hay fever or other upper respiratory allergies.

Usual Dosage: Administer to children under 6 years only on the advice of a physician. Children's Tylenol Cold Chewable Tablets: 2–5 years—2 tablets, 6–11 years—4 tablets.
Children's Tylenol Cold Liquid Formula: 2–5 years—1 teaspoonful; 6–11 years—2 teaspoonsful. Measuring cup is provided and marked for accurate dosing.
Doses may be repeated every 4-6 hours as needed, not to exceed 4 doses in 24 hours. The Warnings are identical for the two dosage forms except the Liquid Cold Formula does not contain the phenylketonurics statement since the product does not contain aspartame.

Warning: Do not use if carton is opened, or if printed plastic bottle wrap or printed foil inner seal is broken.

Keep this and all medication out of the reach of children. In case of accidental overdosage, contact a physician or poison control center immediately. Phenylketonurics: contains phenylalanine, 4 mg per tablet. Do not exceed the recommended dosage because nervousness, dizziness or sleeplessness

may occur. Do not take this product for more than 7 days. If fever persists for more than three days, or if symptoms do not improve or new ones occur within five days or are accompanied by high fever, consult a physician before continuing use. This preparation may cause drowsiness, or in some cases, excitability. Do not give this product to children who have heart disease, high blood pressure, thyroid disease, diabetes, glaucoma or asthma or are taking a prescription drug for high blood pressure or depression, except under the advice and supervision of a physician.

Overdosage: Acetaminophen in massive overdosage may cause hepatic toxicity in some patients. In adults and adolescents, hepatic toxicity has rarely been reported following ingestion of acute overdosage of less than 10 grams. Fatalities are infrequent (less than 3–4% of untreated cases) and have rarely been reported with overdoses of less than 15 grams. In children, an acute overdosage of less than 150 mg/kg has not been associated with hepatic toxicity.

Early symptoms following a potentially hepatotoxic overdose may include: nausea, vomiting, diaphoresis and general malaise. Clinical and laboratory evidence of hepatic toxicity may not be apparent until 48 to 72 hours postingestion. In adults and adolescents, regardless of the quantity of acetaminophen reported to have been ingested, administer MUCOMYST® acetylcysteine immediately if 24 hours or less have elapsed from the reported time of ingestion. For full prescribing information, refer to the MUCOMYST package insert. Do not await the results of assays for acetaminophen level before initiating treatment with MUCOMYST acetylcysteine. The following additional procedures are recommended: The stomach should be emptied promptly by lavage or by induction of emesis with syrup of ipecac. A serum acetaminophen assay should be obtained as early as possible, but no sooner than four hours following ingestion. Liver function studies should be obtained initially and repeated at 24-hour intervals.

Serious toxicity or fatalities are extremely infrequent in children, possibly due to differences in the way they metabolize acetaminophen. In children, the maximum potential amount ingested can be more easily estimated. If more than 150 mg/kg or an unknown amount was ingested, obtain an acetaminophen plasma level. The acetaminophen plasma level should be obtained as soon as possible, but no sooner than 4 hours following the ingestion. Induce emesis using syrup of ipecac. If the plasma level is obtained and falls above the broken line on the acetaminophen overdose nomogram, the MUCOMYST acetylcysteine therapy should be initiated and continued for a full course of therapy. If acetaminophen plasma assay capability is not available, and the estimated acetaminophen ingestion exceeds 150 mg/kg, MUCOMYST acetylcysteine therapy should be initiated and continued for a full course of therapy.

For additional emergency information, call your regional poison center or call the Rocky Mountain Poison Center toll-free, (1-800-525-6115).

Chlorpheniramine toxicity should be treated as you would an antihistamine/anticholinergic overdose and is likely to be present within a few hours after acute ingestion.

Symptoms from pseudoephedrine overdose consist most often of mild anxiety, tachycardia and/or mild hypertension. Symptoms usually appear within 4 to 8 hours of ingestion and are transient, usually requiring no treatment.

Inactive Ingredients: Chewable Tablets—Aspartame, citric acid, ethylcellulose, flavors, magnesium stearate, mannitol, microcrystalline cellulose, pregelatinized starch, sucrose, Blue #1 and Red #7.
Liquid—Benzoic acid, citric acid, flavors, glycerin, malic acid, polyethylene glycol, propylene glycol, sodium benzoate, sorbitol, sucrose, purified water, Blue #1 and Red #40.

How Supplied: Chewable Tablets (colored purple, scored, imprinted "Tylenol Cold") on one side and "TC" on opposite side—bottles of 24. Cold Formula—bottles (colored purple) of 4 fl. oz.
Shown in Product Identification Section, page 413

**Effervescent Formula
TYLENOL® Cold Medication Tablets**

Description: Each Effervescent TYLENOL Cold Tablet contains acetaminophen 325 mg., chlorpheniramine maleate 2 mg., and phenylpropanolamine hydrochloride 12.5 mg.

Actions: TYLENOL Cold Medication Tablets contain a clinically proven analgesic-antipyretic, decongestant and antihistamine. Acetaminophen produces analgesia by elevation of the pain threshold and antipyresis through action on the hypothalamic heat-regulating center. Acetaminophen is equal to aspirin in analgesic and antipyretic effectiveness and it is unlikely to produce many of the side effects associated with aspirin and aspirin-containing products. Phenylpropanolamine is a sympathomimetic amine which provides temporary relief of nasal congestion. Chlorpheniramine is an antihistamine which helps provide temporary relief of runny nose, sneezing and watery and itchy eyes.

Indications: TYLENOL Cold Medication provides effective temporary relief of runny nose, sneezing, watery and itchy eyes, nasal congestion, and aches, pains, sore throat and fever due to a cold or "flu."

Precautions: If a rare sensitivity reaction occurs, the drug should be stopped. Although phenylpropanolamine is virtually without pressor effect in normoten-

sive patients, it should be used with caution in hypertensives.

Usual Dosage: Effervescent TYLENOL® Cold must be dissolved in water before taking.
ADULTS (12 years and over): 2 tablets every 4 hours, not to exceed 12 tablets in 24 hours.
CHILDREN (6–11): 1 tablet every 4 hours, not to exceed 6 tablets in 24 hours.
"WARNINGS: Do not administer to children under 6. Do not take this product for more than 7 days (Adults) or 5 days (Children) or for fever for more than 3 days unless directed by a doctor. Do not exceed recommended dosage because at higher doses nervousness, dizziness or sleeplessness may occur. May cause excitability, especially in children. May cause drowsiness; alcohol may increase the drowsiness effect. Avoid alcoholic beverages while taking this product. Use caution when driving a motor vehicle or operating machinery. Do not take this product if you have asthma, glaucoma, emphysema, chronic pulmonary disease, shortness of breath, difficulty in breathing, heart disease, high blood pressure, thyroid disease, diabetes or difficulty in urination due to enlargement of the prostate gland unless directed by a doctor. DO NOT USE IF GLUED CARTON FLAP IS OPENED OR IF FOIL PACK IS TORN OR BROKEN. **KEEP THIS AND ALL MEDICATION OUT OF THE REACH OF CHILDREN. AS WITH ANY DRUG, IF YOU ARE PREGNANT OR NURSING A BABY, SEEK THE ADVICE OF A HEALTH PROFESSIONAL BEFORE USING THIS PRODUCT. IN CASE OF ACCIDENTAL OVERDOSAGE, CONTACT A PHYSICIAN OR POISON CONTROL CENTER IMMEDIATELY. DO NOT TAKE THIS PRODUCT IF YOU ARE ON A SODIUM RESTRICTED DIET, EXCEPT UNDER THE ADVICE AND SUPERVISION OF A DOCTOR. EACH TABLET CONTAINS 525 MG. OF SODIUM.**
DRUG INTERACTION PRECAUTION: Do not take this product if you are presently taking a prescription drug for high blood pressure or depression without first consulting your doctor."

Overdosage: Acetaminophen in massive overdosage may cause hepatic toxicity in some patients. In adults and adolescents, hepatic toxicity has rarely been reported following ingestion of acute overdosage of less than 10 grams. Fatalities are infrequent (less than 3–4% of untreated cases) and have rarely been reported with overdoses of less than 15 grams. In children, an acute overdosage of less than 150 mg/kg has not been associated with hepatic toxicity.

Early symptoms following a potentially hepatotoxic overdose may include: nausea, vomiting, diaphoresis and general malaise. Clinical and laboratory evidence of hepatic toxicity may not be apparent until 48 to 72 hours postingestion. In adults and adolescents, regardless of the quantity of acetaminophen reported to have been ingested, administer

MUCOMYST® acetylcysteine immediately if 24 hours or less have elapsed from the reported time of ingestion. For full prescribing information, refer to the MUCOMYST package insert. Do not await results of assays for acetaminophen level before initiating treatment with MUCOMYST acetylcysteine. The following additional procedures are recommended: The stomach should be emptied promptly by lavage or by induction of emesis with syrup of ipecac. A serum acetaminophen assay should be obtained as early as possible, but no sooner than four hours following ingestion. Liver function studies should be obtained initially and repeated at 24-hour intervals.

Serious toxicity or fatalities are extremely infrequent in children, possibly due to differences in the way they metabolize acetaminophen. In children, the maximum potential amount ingested can be more easily estimated. If more than 150 mg/kg or an unknown amount was ingested, obtain an acetaminophen plasma level. The acetaminophen plasma level should be obtained as soon as possible, but no sooner than 4 hours following the ingestion. Induce emesis using syrup of ipecac. If the plasma level is obtained and falls above the broken line on the acetaminophen overdose nomogram, the MUCOMYST acetylcysteine therapy should be initiated and continued for a full course of therapy. If acetaminophen plasma assay capability is not available, and the estimated acetaminophen ingestion exceeds 150 mg/kg, MUCOMYST acetylcysteine therapy should be initiated and continued for a full course of therapy.

For additional emergency information, call your regional poison center or call the Rocky Mountain Poison Center toll-free, (1-800-525-6115).

Symptoms from phenylpropanolamine overdose consist most often of mild anxiety, tachycardia and/or mild hypertension. Symptoms usually appear within 4 to 8 hours of ingestion and are transient, usually requiring no treatment.

Inactive Ingredients: Citric Acid, Flavor, Potassium Benzoate, Povidone, Saccharin, Sodium Bicarbonate, Sodium Carbonate, Sodium Docusate, Sorbitol.

How Supplied: Tablets: carton of 20 tablets in 10 foil twin packs; carton of 36 tablets in 18 foil twin packs.
Shown in Product Identification Section, page 413

**Hot Medication
TYLENOL® Cold & Flu Medication Packets**

Description: Each packet of TYLENOL Cold & Flu contains acetaminophen 650 mg., chlorpheniramine maleate 4 mg., pseudoephedrine hydrochloride 60 mg. and dextromethorphan hydrobromide 30 mg.

Continued on next page

McNeil Consumer—Cont.

Actions: TYLENOL Cold and Flu Medication contains a clinically proven analgesic-antipyretic, decongestant, cough suppressant and antihistamine. Acetaminophen produces analgesia by elevation of the pain threshold and antipyresis through action on the hypothalamic heat-regulating center. Acetaminophen is equal to aspirin in analgesic and antipyretic effectiveness and it is unlikely to produce many of the side effects associated with aspirin and aspirin-containing products. Pseudoephedrine hydrochloride is a sympathomimetic amine which provides temporary relief of nasal congestion. Dextromethorphan is a cough suppressant which provides temporary relief of coughs due to minor throat irritations that may occur with the common cold. Chlorpheniramine is an antihistamine which helps provide temporary relief of runny nose, sneezing and watery and itchy eyes.

Indications: TYLENOL Cold and Flu Medication provides effective temporary relief of runny nose, sneezing, watery and itchy eyes, nasal congestion, coughing, and aches, pains, sore throat and fever due to a cold or "flu."

Precautions: If a rare sensitivity reaction occurs, the drug should be stopped. Although pseudoephedrine is virtually without pressor effect in normotensive patients, it should be used with caution in hypertensives.

Usual Dosage: Adults (12 years and over): Dissolve one packet in 6 oz. cup of hot water. Sip while hot. Sweeten to taste, if desired. May repeat every 6 hours, not to exceed 4 doses in 24 hours. "**WARNINGS:** Not recommended for children under 12. Do not take this product for more than 7 days or for fever for more than 3 days unless directed by a doctor. If symptoms do not improve or are accompanied by fever, consult a doctor. A persistent cough may be a sign of a serious condition. If cough persists for more than 1 week, tends to recur or is accompanied by fever, rash or persistent headache, consult a doctor. Do not take this product for persistent or chronic cough such as occurs with smoking, asthma, emphysema, or if cough is accompanied by excessive phlegm (mucus) unless directed by a doctor. Do not exceed recommended dosage because at higher doses nervousness, dizziness, or sleeplessness may occur. May cause excitability, expecially in children. Do not take this product if you have asthma, glaucoma, heart disease, high blood pressure, emphysema, chronic pulmonary disease, shortness of breath, difficulty in breathing, diabetes, thyroid disease or difficulty in urination due to enlargement of the prostate gland unless directed by a doctor. May cause drowsiness, alcohol may increase the drowsiness effect. Avoid alcoholic beverages while taking this product. Use caution when driving a motor vehicle or operating machinery.

DO NOT USE IF GLUED CARTON FLAP IS OPENED OR IF FOIL PACKET IS TORN OR BROKEN. KEEP THIS AND ALL MEDICATION OUT OF THE REACH OF CHILDREN. AS WITH ANY DRUG, IF YOU ARE PREGNANT OR NURSING A BABY, SEEK THE ADVICE OF A HEALTH PROFESSIONAL BEFORE USING THIS PRODUCT. IN CASE OF ACCIDENTAL OVERDOSAGE, CONTACT A PHYSICIAN OR POISON CONTROL CENTER IMMEDIATELY. PHENYLKETONURICS: CONTAINS PHENYLALANINE 11 MG PER PACKET. DRUG INTERACTION PRECAUTION: Do not take this product if you are presently taking a prescription drug for high blood pressure or depression without first consulting your doctor."

Overdosage: Acetaminophen in massive overdosage may cause hepatic toxicity in some patients. In adults and adolescents, hepatic toxicity has rarely been reported following ingestion of acute overdosage of less than 10 grams. Fatalities are infrequent (less than 3–4% of untreated cases) and have rarely been reported with overdoses of less than 15 grams. In children, an acute overdosage of less than 150 mg/kg has not been associated with hepatic toxicity.

Early symptoms following a potentially hepatotoxic overdose may include: nausea, vomiting, diaphoresis and general malaise. Clinical and laboratory evidence of hepatic toxicity may not be apparent until 48 to 72 hours postingestion. In adults and adolescents, regardless of the quantity of acetaminophen reported to have been ingested, administer MUCOMYST® acetylcysteine immediately if 24 hours or less have elapsed from the reported time of ingestion. For full prescribing information, refer to the MUCOMYST package insert. Do not await results of assays for acetaminophen level before initiating treatment with MUCOMYST acetylcysteine. The following additional procedures are recommended: The stomach should be emptied promptly by lavage or by induction of emesis with syrup of ipecac. A serum acetaminophen assay should be obtained as early as possible, but no sooner than four hours following ingestion. Liver function studies should be obtained initially and repeated at 24-hour intervals.

Serious toxicity or fatalities are extremely infrequent in children, possibly due to differences in the way they metabolize acetaminophen. In children, the maximum potential amount ingested can be more easily estimated. If more than 150 mg/kg or an unknown amount was ingested, obtain an acetaminophen plasma level. The acetaminophen plasma level should be obtained as soon as possible, but no sooner than 4 hours following the ingestion. Induce emesis using syrup of ipecac. If the plasma level is obtained and falls above the broken line on the acetaminophen overdose nomogram, the MUCOMYST acetylcysteine therapy should be initiated and con-

tinued for a full course of therapy. If acetaminophen plasma assay capability is not available, and the estimated acetaminophen ingestion exceeds 150 mg/kg, MUCOMYST acetylcysteine therapy should be initiated and continued for a full course of therapy.

For additional emergency information, call your regional poison center or call the Rocky Mountain Poison Center toll-free, (1-800-525-6115).

Symptoms from pseudoephedrine overdose consist most often of mild anxiety, tachycardia and/or mild hypertension. Symptoms usually appear within 4 to 8 hours of ingestion and are transient, usually requiring no treatment.

Acute dextromethorphan overdose usually does not result in serious signs and symptoms unless massive amounts have been ingested. Signs and symptoms of a substantial overdose may include nausea and vomiting, visual disturbances, CNS disturbances, and urinary retention.

Chlorpheniramine toxicity should be treated as you would an antihistamine/anticholinergic overdose and is likely to be present within a few hours after acute ingestion.

Inactive Ingredients: Aspartame, Citric Acid, Flavors, Sodium Citrate, Starch, Sucrose, Tribasic Calcium Phosphate, Red #40 and Yellow #10.

How Supplied: Packets of powder (yellow colored) cartons of 6 foil packets and cartons of 12 tamper-resistant foil cartons.

Shown in Product Identification Section, page 413

Multisymptom TYLENOL® Cold Medication Tablets and Caplets

Description: Each TYLENOL Cold Tablet or Caplet contains acetaminophen 325 mg., chlorpheniramine maleate 2 mg., pseudoephedrine hydrochloride 30 mg. and dextromethorphan hydrobromide 15 mg.

Actions: TYLENOL Cold Medication Tablets and Caplets contain a clinically proven analgesic-antipyretic, decongestant, cough suppressant and antihistamine. Acetaminophen produces analgesia by elevation of the pain threshold and antipyresis through action on the hypothalamic heat-regulating center. Acetaminophen is equal to aspirin in analgesic and antipyretic effectiveness and it is unlikely to produce many of the side effects associated with aspirin and aspirin-containing products. Pseudoephedrine hydrochloride is a sympathomimetic amine which provides temporary relief of nasal congestion. Dextromethorphan is a cough suppressant which provides temporary relief of coughs due to minor throat irritations that may occur with the common cold. Chlorpheniramine is an antihistamine which helps provide temporary relief of runny nose, sneezing and watery and itchy eyes.

Indications: TYLENOL Cold Medication provides effective temporary relief of runny nose, sneezing, watery and itchy eyes, nasal congestion, coughing, and aches, pains and fever due to a cold or "flu."

Precautions: If a rare sensitivity reaction occurs, the drug should be stopped. Although pseudoephedrine is virtually without pressor effect in normotensive patients, it should be used with caution in hypertensives.

Usual Dosage: Adults: Two tablets or caplets every 6 hours, not to exceed 8 tablets or caplets in 24 hours. Children (6–12 years): One caplet or tablet every 6 hours, not to exceed 4 tablets or caplets in 24 hours for 5 days.
WARNING: Do not administer to children under 6 or exceed the recommended dosage because nervousness, dizziness or sleeplessness may occur. May cause excitability especially in children. Do not take this product for more than 7 days. If fever persists for more than three days, or if symptoms do not improve or are accompanied by high fever, consult a physician. A persistent cough may be a sign of a serious condition. If cough persists for more than 1 week, tends to recur or is accompanied by fever, rash or persistent headache, consult a physician. Do not take this product for persistent or chronic cough such as occurs with smoking, asthma, emphysema or if cough is accompanied by excessive phlegm (mucus) unless directed by a physician. This preparation may cause drowsiness, alcohol may increase the drowsiness effect. Avoid alcoholic beverages while taking this product. Use caution when driving a motor vehicle or operating machinery. Do not take this product if you have heart disease, high blood pressure, thyroid disease, diabetes, asthma, glaucoma, emphysema, chronic pulmonary disease, shortness of breath, difficulty in breathing or difficulty in urination due to enlargement of the prostate gland unless directed by a physician.
DO NOT USE IF CARTON IS OPENED OR IF A BLISTER UNIT IS BROKEN. KEEP THIS AND ALL MEDICATION OUT OF THE REACH OF CHILDREN. AS WITH ANY DRUG, IF YOU ARE PREGNANT OR NURSING A BABY, SEEK THE ADVICE OF A HEALTH PROFESSIONAL BEFORE USING THIS PRODUCT. IN THE CASE OF ACCIDENTAL OVER-DOSAGE CONTACT A PHYSICIAN OR POISON CONTROL CENTER IMMEDIATELY. DRUG INTERACTION PRECAUTION: Do not take this product if you are presently taking a prescription drug for high blood pressure or depression without first consulting your physician.

Overdosage: Acetaminophen in massive overdosage may cause hepatic toxicity in some patients. In adults and adolescents, hepatic toxicity has rarely been reported following ingestion of acute overdosage of less than 10 grams. Fatalities are infrequent (less than 3–4% of untreated cases) and have rarely been re-

ported with overdoses of less than 15 grams. In children, an acute overdosage of less than 150 mg/kg has not been associated with hepatic toxicity.
Early symptoms following a potentially hepatotoxic overdose may include: nausea, vomiting, diaphoresis and general malaise. Clinical and laboratory evidence of hepatic toxicity may not be apparent until 48 to 72 hours postingestion. In adults and adolescents, regardless of the quantity of acetaminophen reported to have been ingested, administer MUCOMYST® acetylcysteine immediately if 24 hours or less have elapsed from the reported time of ingestion. For full prescribing information, refer to the MUCOMYST package insert. Do not await results of assays for acetaminophen level before initiating treatment with MUCOMYST acetylcysteine. The following additional procedures are recommended: The stomach should be emptied promptly by lavage or by induction of emesis with syrup of ipecac. A serum acetaminophen assay should be obtained as early as possible, but no sooner than four hours following ingestion. Liver function studies should be obtained initially and repeated at 24-hour intervals.
Serious toxicity or fatalities are extremely infrequent in children, possibly due to differences in the way they metabolize acetaminophen. In children, the maximum potential amount ingested can be more easily estimated. If more than 150 mg/kg or an unknown amount was ingested, obtain an acetaminophen plasma level. The acetaminophen plasma level should be obtained as soon as possible, but no sooner than 4 hours following the ingestion. Induce emesis using syrup of ipecac. If the plasma level is obtained and falls above the broken line on the acetaminophen overdose nomogram, the MUCOMYST acetylcysteine therapy should be initiated and continued for a full course of therapy. If acetaminophen plasma assay capability is not available, and the estimated acetaminophen ingestion exceeds 150 mg/kg, MUCOMYST acetylcysteine therapy should be initiated and continued for a full course of therapy.
For additional emergency information, call your regional poison center or call the Rocky Mountain Poison Center toll-free, (1-800-525-6115).
Chlorpheniramine toxicity should be treated as you would an antihistamine/anticholinergic overdose and is likely to be present within a few hours after acute ingestion.
Symptoms from pseudoephedrine overdose consist most often of mild anxiety, tachycardia and/or mild hypertension. Symptoms usually appear within 4 to 8 hours of ingestion and are transient, usually requiring no treatment.
Acute dextromethorphan overdose usually does not result in serious signs and symptoms unless massive amounts have been ingested. Signs and symptoms of a substantial overdose may include nausea and vomiting, visual disturbances, CNS disturbances, and urinary retention.

Inactive Ingredients: Tablets: Cellulose, Starch, Magnesium Stearate, Yellow #6 and Yellow #10. Caplets: Cellulose, Glyceryl Triacetate, Hydroxypropyl Methylcellulose, Magnesium Stearate, Sodium Starch Glycolate, Starch, Titanium Dioxide, Blue #1 and Yellow #6 & #10.

How Supplied: Tablets (colored yellow, imprinted "TYLENOL Cold")—blister packs of 24 and tamper-resistant bottles of 50. Caplets (light yellow, imprinted "TYLENOL Cold")—blister packs of 24 and tamper-resistant bottles of 50.
Shown in Product Identification Section, page 413

TYLENOL® Cold Medication No Drowsiness Formula Caplets

Description: Each TYLENOL Cold Medication No Drowsiness Formula Caplet contains acetaminophen 325 mg., pseudoephedrine hydrochloride 30 mg. and dextromethorphan hydrobromide 15 mg.

Actions: TYLENOL Cold Medication No Drowsiness Formula Caplets contain a clinically proven analgesic-antipyretic, decongestant and cough suppressant. Acetaminophen produces analgesia by elevation of the pain threshold and antipyresis through action on the hypothalamic heat-regulating center. Acetaminophen is equal to aspirin in analgesic and antipyretic effectiveness and it is unlikely to produce many of the side effects associated with aspirin and aspirin-containing products. Pseudoephedrine hydrochloride is a sympathomimetic amine which provides temporary relief of nasal congestion. Dextromethorphan is a cough suppressant which provides temporary relief of coughs due to minor throat irritations that may occur with the common cold.

Indications: TYLENOL Cold Medication No Drowsiness Formula provides effective temporary relief of the nasal congestion, coughing, and aches, pains and fever due to a cold or "flu."

Precautions: If a rare sensitivity reaction occurs, the drug should be stopped. Although pseudoephedrine is virtually without pressor effect in normotensive patients, it should be used with caution in hypertensives.

Usual Dosage: Adults: Two caplets every 6 hours, not to exceed 8 caplets in 24 hours. Children (6–12 years): One caplet every 6 hours, not to exceed 4 tablets or caplets in 24 hours for 5 days.
WARNING: Do not administer to children under 6 or exceed the recommended dosage because nervousness, dizziness or sleeplessness may occur. Do not take this product for more than 7 days. If fever persists for more than three days, or if symptoms do not improve or are accompanied by high fever, consult a physician. A persistent cough may be a sign of a serious condition. If cough persists for

Continued on next page

McNeil Consumer—Cont.

more than 1 week, tends to recur or is accompanied by fever, rash or persistent headache, consult a physician. Do not take this product for persistent or chronic cough such as occurs with smoking, asthma, emphysema or if cough is accompanied by excessive phlegm (mucus) unless directed by a physician. Do not take this product if you have heart disease, high blood pressure, thyroid disease, diabetes, or difficulty in urination due to enlargement of the prostate gland unless directed by a physician.

DO NOT USE IF CARTON IS OPENED OR IF A BLISTER UNIT IS BROKEN. KEEP THIS AND ALL MEDICATION OUT OF THE REACH OF CHILDREN. AS WITH ANY DRUG, IF YOU ARE PREGNANT OR NURSING A BABY, SEEK THE ADVICE OF HEALTH PROFESSIONAL BEFORE USING THIS PRODUCT. IN THE CASE OF ACCIDENTAL OVERDOSAGE CONTACT A PHYSICIAN OR POISON CONTROL CENTER IMMEDIATELY.

DRUG INTERACTION PRECAUTION: Do not take this product if you are presently taking a prescription drug for high blood pressure or depression without first consulting your physician.

Overdosage: Acetaminophen in massive overdosage may cause hepatic toxicity in some patients. In adults and adolescents, hepatic toxicity has rarely been reported following ingestion of acute overdosage of less than 10 grams. Fatalities are infrequent (less than 3–4% of untreated cases) and have rarely been reported with overdosage of less than 15 grams. In children, an acute overdosage of less than 150 mg/kg has not been associated with hepatic toxicity.

Early symptoms following a potentially hepatotoxic overdose may include: nausea, vomiting, diaphoresis and general malaise. Clinical and laboratory evidence of hepatic toxicity may not be apparent until 48 to 72 hours postingestion. In adults and adolescents, regardless of the quantity of acetaminophen reported to have been ingested, administer MUCOMYST® acetylcysteine immediately if 24 hours or less have elapsed from the reported time of ingestion. For full prescribing information, refer to the MUCOMYST package insert. Do not await results of assays for acetaminophen level before initiating treatment with MUCOMYST acetylcysteine. The following additional procedures are recommended: The stomach should be emptied promptly by lavage or by induction of emesis with syrup of ipecac. A serum acetaminophen assay should be obtained as early as possible, but no sooner than four hours following ingestion. Liver function studies should be obtained initially and repeated at 24–hour intervals.

Serious toxicity or fatalities are extremely infrequent in children, possibly due to differences in the way they metabolize acetaminophen. In children, the maximum potential amount ingested

can be more easily estimated. If more than 150 mg/kg or an unknown amount was ingested, obtain an acetaminophen plasma level. The acetaminophen plasma level should be obtained as soon as possible, but no sooner than 4 hours following the ingestion. Induce emesis using syrup of ipecac. If the plasma level is obtained and falls above the broken line on the acetaminophen overdose nomogram, the MUCOMYST acetylcysteine therapy should be initiated and continued for a full course of therapy. If acetaminophen plasma assay capability is not available, and the estimated acetaminophen ingestion exceeds 150 mg/kg. MUCOMYST acetylcysteine therapy should be initiated and continued for a full course of therapy.

For additional emergency information, call your regional poison center or call the Rocky Mountain Poison Center toll-free, (1-800-525-6115).

Symptoms from pseudoephedrine overdose consist most often of mild anxiety, tachycardia and/or mild hypertension. Symptoms usually appear within 4 to 8 hours of ingestion and are transient, usually requiring no treatment.

Acute dextromethorphan overdose usually does not result in serious signs and symptoms unless massive amounts have been ingested. Signs and symptoms of a substantial overdose may include nausea and vomiting, visual disturbances, CNS disturbances, and urinary retention.

Inactive Ingredients: Cellulose, Glyceryl Triacetate, Hydroxypropyl Methylcellulose, Magnesium Stearate, Sodium Starch Glycolate, Starch, Titanium Dioxide, Blue #1 and Yellow #10.

How Supplied: Caplets (colored white, imprinted TYLENOL "cold")—blister packs of 24 and tamper-resistant bottles of 50.

Shown in Product Identification Section, page 413

No Drowsiness Formula TYLENOL® Cold & Flu Hot Medication Packets

Description: Each packet of No Drowsiness TYLENOL Cold & Flu contains acetaminophen 650 mg., pseudoephedrine hydrochloride 60 mg and dextromethorphan hydrobromide 30 mg.

Actions: No Drowsiness TYLENOL Cold and Flu Hot Medication contains a clinically proven analgesic-antipyretic, decongestant, and cough suppressant. Acetaminophen produces analgesia by elevation of the pain threshold and antipyresis through action on the hypothalamic heat-regulating center. Acetaminophen is equal to aspirin in analgesic and antipyretic effectiveness and it is unlikely to produce many of the side effects associated with aspirin and aspirin-containing products. Pseudoephedrine hydrochloride is a sympathomimetic amine which provides temporary relief of nasal congestion. Dextromethorphan is a cough suppressant which provides temporary

relief of coughs due to minor throat irritations that may occur with the common cold.

Indications: No Drowsiness TYLENOL Cold and Flu Hot Medication provides effective temporary relief of nasal congestion, coughing, and aches, pains, sore throat and fever due to a cold or "flu."

Precautions: If a rare sensitivity reaction occurs, the drug should be stopped. Although pseudoephedrine is virtually without pressor effect in normotensive patients, it should be used with caution in hypertensives.

Usual Dosage: Adults (12 years and over): Dissolve one packet in 6 oz. cup of hot water. Sip while hot. Sweeten to taste, if desired. May repeat every 6 hours, not to exceed 4 doses in 24 hours. "**WARNING:** Not recommended for children under 12. Do not take this product for more than 7 days or for fever for more than 3 days unless directed by a doctor. If symptoms do not improve or are accompanied by fever, consult a doctor. A persistent cough may be a sign of a serious condition. If cough persists for more than 1 week, tends to recur or is accompanied by fever, rash or persistent headache, consult a doctor. Do not take this product for persistent or chronic cough such as occurs with smoking, asthma, emphysema, or if cough is accompanied by excessive phlegm (mucus) unless directed by a doctor. Do not exceed recommended dosage because at higher doses nervousness, dizziness, or sleeplessness may occur. May cause excitability, especially in children. Do not take this product if you have asthma, glaucoma, heart disease, high blood pressure, emphysema, chronic pulmonary disease, shortness of breath, difficulty in breathing, diabetes, thyroid disease or difficulty in urination due to enlargement of the prostate gland unless directed by a doctor. May cause drowsiness, alcohol may increase the drowsiness effect. Avoid alcoholic beverages while taking this product. Use caution when driving a motor vehicle or operating machinery.

DO NOT USE IF GLUED CARTON FLAP IS OPENED OR IF FOIL PACKET IS TORN OR BROKEN. KEEP THIS AND ALL MEDICATION OUT OF THE REACH OF CHILDREN. AS WITH ANY DRUG, IF YOU ARE PREGNANT OR NURSING A BABY, SEEK THE ADVICE OF A HEALTH PROFESSIONAL BEFORE USING THIS PRODUCT. IN CASE OF ACCIDENTAL OVERDOSAGE, CONTACT A PHYSICIAN OR POISON CONTROL CENTER IMMEDIATELY. PHENYLKETONURICS: CONTAINS PHENYLALANINE 11 MG PER PACKET.

DRUG INTERACTION PRECAUTION: Do not take this product if you are presently taking a prescription drug for high blood pressure or depression without first consulting your doctor."

Overdosage: Acetaminophen in massive overdosage may cause hepatic toxicity in some patients. In adults and adolescents, hepatic toxicity has rarely been reported following ingestion of acute overdosage of less than 10 grams. Fatalities are infrequent (less than 3–4% of untreated cases) and have rarely been reported with overdoses of less than 15 grams. In children, an acute overdosage of less than 150 mg/kg has not been associated with hepatic toxicity.

Early symptoms following a potentially hepatotoxic overdose may include: nausea, vomiting, diaphoresis and general malaise. Clinical and laboratory evidence of hepatic toxicity may not be apparent until 48 to 72 hours postingestion. In adults and adolescents, regardless of the quantity of acetaminophen reported to have been ingested, administer MUCOMYST® acetylcysteine immediately if 24 hours or less have elapsed from the reported time of ingestion. For full prescribing information, refer to the MUCOMYST package insert. Do not await results of assays for acetaminophen level before initiating treatment with MUCOMYST acetylcysteine. The following additional procedures are recommended. The stomach should be emptied promptly by lavage or by induction of emesis with syrup of ipecac. A serum acetaminophen assay should be obtained as early as possible, but no sooner than four hours following ingestion. Liver function studies should be obtained initially and repeated at 24-hour intervals.

Serious toxicity or fatalities are extremely infrequent in children, possibly due to differences in the way they metabolize acetaminophen. In children, the maximum potential amount ingested can be more easily estimated. If more than 150 mg/kg or an unknown amount was ingested, obtain an acetaminophen plasma level. The acetaminophen plasma level should be obtained as soon as possible, but not sooner than 4 hours following the ingestion. Induce emesis using syrup of ipecac. If the plasma level is obtained and falls above the broken line on the acetaminophen overdose nomogram, the MUCOMYST acetylcysteine therapy should be initiated and continued for a full course of therapy. If acetaminophen plasma assay capability is not available, and the estimated acetaminophen ingestion exceeds 150 mg/kg, MUCOMYST acetylcysteine therapy should be initiated and continued for a full course of therapy.

For additional emergency information, call your regional poison center or call the Rocky Mountain Poison Control toll-free, (1-800-525-6115).

Symptoms from pseudoephedrine overdose consist most often of mild anxiety, tachycardia and/or mild hypertension. Symptoms usually appear within 4 to 8 hours of ingestion and are transient, usually requiring no treatment.

Acute dextromethorphan overdose usually does not result in serious signs and symptoms unless massive amounts have been ingested. Signs and symptoms of a substantial overdose may include nausea and vomiting, visual disturbances. CNS disturbances and urinary retention.

Inactive Ingredients: Aspartame, Citric Acid, Flavors, Sodium Citrate, Starch, Sucrose, Tribasic Calcium Phosphate, Red #40 and Yellow #10.

How Supplied: Packets of powder (yellow colored) cartons of 6 foil packets and cartons of 12 tamper-resistant foil cartons.

Shown in Product Identification Section, page 413

TYLENOL® Cold Night Time Medication Liquid

Description: Each 30 ml (1 fl. oz.) contains acetaminophen 650 mg., diphenhydramine hydrochloride 50 mg., pseudoephedrine hydrochloride 60 mg., and dextromethorphan hydrobromide 30 mg. (alcohol 10%).

Actions: TYLENOL Cold Night Time Medication Liquid contains a clinically proven analgesic-antipyretic, decongestant, cough suppressant and antihistamine. Acetaminophen produces analgesia by elevation of the pain threshold and antipyresis through action on the hypothalamic heat-regulating center. Acetaminophen is equal to aspirin in analgesic and antipyretic effectiveness and it is unlikely to produce many of the side effects associated with aspirin and aspirin-containing products. Pseudoephedrine hydrochloride is a sympathomimetic amine which provides temporary relief of nasal congestion. Dextromethorphan is a cough suppressant which provides temporary relief of coughs due to minor throat irritations that may occur with the common cold. Diphenhydramine is an antihistamine which helps provide temporary relief of runny nose, sneezing and watery and itchy eyes.

Indications: TYLENOL Cold Night Time Medication Liquid provides effective temporary relief of runny nose, sneezing, watery and itchy eyes, nasal congestion, coughing, and aches, pains, sore throat and fevers due to a cold or "flu."

Precautions: If a rare sensitivity reaction occurs, the drug should be stopped. Although pseudoephedrine is virtually without pressor effect in normotensive patients, it should be used with caution in hypertensives.

Usual Dosage: Measuring cup is provided and marked for accurate dosing. Adults (12 years and over): 1 fluid ounce (2 tbsp.) in measuring cup provided every 6 hours, not to exceed 4 doses in 24 hours. Not recommended for children.

WARNINGS: Do not take this product for more than 7 days or for fever for more than 3 days unless directed by a doctor. If symptoms do not improve or are accompanied by fever, consult a doctor. A persistent cough may be a sign of a serious condition. If cough persists for more than 1 week, tends to recur or is accompanied by fever, rash or persistent headache, consult a doctor. Do not take this product for persistent or chronic cough such as

occurs with smoking, asthma, emphysema, or if cough is accompanied by excessive phlegm (mucus) unless directed by a doctor. Do not exceed recommended dosage because at higher doses nervousness, dizziness or sleeplessness may occur. May cause excitability, especially in children. Do not take this product if you have asthma, glaucoma, heart disease, high blood pressure, emphysema, chronic pulmonary disease, shortness of breath, difficulty in breathing, diabetes, thyroid disease or difficulty in urination due to enlargement of the prostate gland, or if you are taking sedatives or tranquilizers, unless directed by a doctor. May cause marked drowsiness; alcohol, sedatives and tranquilizers may increase the drowsiness effect. Avoid alcoholic beverages while taking this product. Use caution when driving a motor vehicle or operating machinery.

DO NOT USE IF CARTON IS OPENED OR IF PRINTED PLASTIC WRAP OR PRINTED FOIL INNER SEAL IS BROKEN. KEEP THIS AND ALL MEDICATION OUT OF THE REACH OF CHILDREN. AS WITH ANY DRUG, IF YOU ARE PREGNANT OR NURSING A BABY, SEEK THE ADVICE OF A HEALTH PROFESSIONAL BEFORE USING THIS PRODUCT. IN CASE OF ACCIDENTAL OVERDOSAGE, CONTACT A PHYSICIAN OR POISON CONTROL CENTER IMMEDIATELY. DRUG INTERACTION PRECAUTION: Do not take this product if you are presently taking a prescription drug for high blood pressure or depression without first consulting your doctor.

Overdosage: Acetaminophen in massive overdosage may cause hepatic toxicity in some patients. In adults and adolescents, hepatic toxicity has rarely been reported following ingestion of acute overdosage of less than 10 grams. Fatalities are infrequent (less than 3–4% of untreated cases) and have rarely been reported with overdoses of less than 15 grams. In children, an acute overdosage of less than 150 mg/kg has not been associated with hepatic toxicity.

Early symptoms following a potentially hepatotoxic overdose may include: nausea, vomiting, diaphoresis and general malaise. Clinical and laboratory evidence of hepatic toxicity may not be apparent until 48 to 72 hours postingestion. In adults and adolescents, regardless of the quantity of acetaminophen reported to have been ingested, administer MUCOMYST® acetylcysteine immediately if 24 hours or less have elapsed from the reported time of ingestion. For full prescribing information, refer to the MUCOMYST package insert. Do not await results of assays for acetaminophen level before initiating treatment with MUCOMYST acetylcysteine. The following additional procedures are recommended: The stomach should be emptied promptly by lavage or by induction of emesis with syrup of ipecac. A serum acetaminophen assay should be obtained as early as possible, but no

Continued on next page

McNeil Consumer—Cont.

sooner than four hours following ingestion. Liver function studies should be obtained initially and repeated at 24-hour intervals.

Serious toxicity or fatalities are extremely infrequent in children, possibly due to differences in the way they metabolize acetaminophen. In children, the maximum potential amount ingested can be more easily estimated. If more than 150 mg/kg or an unknown amount was ingested, obtain an acetaminophen plasma level. The acetaminophen plasma level should be obtained as soon as possible, but no sooner than 4 hours following the ingestion. Induce emesis using syrup of ipecac. If the plasma level is obtained and falls above the broken line on the acetaminophen overdose nomogram, the MUCOMYST acetylcysteine therapy should be initiated and continued for a full course of therapy. If acetaminophen plasma assay capability is not available, and the estimated acetaminophen ingestion exceeds 150 mg/kg, MUCOMYST acetylcysteine therapy should be initiated and continued for a full course of therapy.

For additional emergency information, call your regional poison center or call the Rocky Mountain Poison Center toll-free, (1-800-525-6115).

Diphenhydramine toxicity should be treated as you would an antihistamine/anticholinergic overdose and is likely to be present within a few hours after acute ingestion.

Symptoms from pseudoephedrine overdose consist most often of mild anxiety, tachycardia and/or mild hypertension. Symptoms usually appear within 4 to 8 hours of ingestion and are transient, usually requiring no treatment.

Acute dextromethorphan overdose usually does not result in serious signs and symptoms unless massive amounts have been ingested. Signs and symptoms of a substantial overdose may include nausea and vomiting, visual disturbances, CNS disturbances, and urinary retention.

Inactive Ingredients: Alcohol (10%), Citric Acid, Flavors, Glycerin, Polyethylene Glycol, Purified Water, Sodium Benzoate, Sucrose, Red #40, Red #33 and Blue #1.

How Supplied: Cherry flavored (colored red) in 5 oz. bottles with child-resistant safety cap, special dosage cup graded in ounces and tablespoons, and tamper-resistant packaging.

*Shown in Product Identification
Section, page 413*

Maximum-Strength
TYLENOL® Allergy Sinus
Medication Caplets, Gelcaps

Description: Each TYLENOL® Allergy Sinus Caplet or Gelcap contains acetaminophen 500 mg, chlorpheniramine maleate 2 mg, and pseudoephedrine hydrochloride 30 mg.

Actions: TYLENOL® Allergy Sinus Caplets or Gelcaps contain a clinically proven analgesic-antipyretic, decongestant, and antihistamine. Acetaminophen produces analgesia by elevation of the pain threshold and antipyresis through action on the hypothalamic heat-regulating center. Acetaminophen is equal to aspirin in analgesic and antipyretic effectiveness, and it is unlikely to produce many of the side effects associated with aspirin and aspirin-containing products. Pseudoephedrine hydrochloride is a sympathomimetic amine which provides temporary relief of nasal congestion. Chlorpheniramine is an antihistamine which helps provide temporary relief of runny nose, sneezing and watery and itchy eyes.

Indications: TYLENOL® Allergy Sinus provides effective temporary relief of these upper respiratory allergy, hay fever and sinusitis symptoms: sneezing, itchy, watery eyes, runny nose, itching of the nose or throat, nasal and sinus congestion and sinus pain and headaches.

Precautions: If a rare sensitivity reaction occurs, the drug should be stopped. Although pseudoephedrine is virtually without pressor effect in normotensive patients, it should be used with caution in hypertensives.

Usual Dosage: Adults: Two caplets or gelcaps every 6 hours, not to exceed 8 caplets or gelcaps in 24 hours.

"WARNING: Do not administer to children under 12 or exceed the recommended dosage because nervousness, dizziness, or sleeplessness may occur. May cause excitability, especially in children. This preparation may cause drowsiness; alcohol may increase the drowsiness effect. Avoid alcoholic beverages when taking this product. Use caution when driving a motor vehicle or operating machinery. Do not take this product if you have heart disease, high blood pressure, thyroid disease, diabetes, glaucoma, asthma, emphysema, chronic pulmonary disease, shortness of breath, difficulty in breathing or difficulty in urination due to enlargement of prostate gland unless directed by a doctor. Do not take this product for more than 7 days. If symptoms do not improve or are accompanied by a high fever, consult a physician." **DO NOT USE IF CARTON IS OPEN OR IF A BLISTER UNIT IS BROKEN. KEEP THIS AND ALL MEDICATION OUT OF THE REACH OF CHILDREN. AS WITH ANY DRUG, IF YOU ARE PREGNANT OR NURSING A BABY, SEEK THE ADVICE OF A HEALTH PROFESSIONAL BEFORE USING THIS PRODUCT. IN THE CASE OF ACCIDENTAL OVERDOSE, CONTACT A PHYSICIAN OR POISON CONTROL CENTER IMMEDIATELY. DRUG INTERACTION PRECAUTION:** Do not take this product if you are presently taking a prescription drug for high blood pressure or depression without first consulting your doctor.

Overdosage: Acetaminophen in massive overdosage may cause hepatic toxicity in some patients. In adults and adolescents, hepatic toxicity has rarely been reported following ingestion of acute overdosage of less than 10 grams. Fatalities are infrequent (less than 3–4% of untreated cases) and have rarely been reported with overdoses of less than 15 grams. In children, an acute overdosage of less than 150 mg/kg has not been associated with hepatic toxicity.

Early symptoms following a potentially hepatotoxic overdose may include: nausea, vomiting, diaphoresis and general malaise. Clinical and laboratory evidence of hepatic toxicity may not be apparent until 48 to 72 hours postingestion. In adults and adolescents, regardless of the quantity of acetaminophen reported to have been ingested, administer MUCOMYST® acetylcysteine immediately if 24 hours or less have elapsed from the reported time of ingestion. For full prescribing information, refer to the MUCOMYST package insert. Do not await results of assays for acetaminophen level before initiating treatment with MUCOMYST acetylcysteine. The following additional procedures are recommended: The stomach should be emptied promptly by lavage or by induction of emesis with syrup of ipecac. A serum acetaminophen assay should be obtained as early as possible, but no sooner than four hours following ingestion. Liver function studies should be obtained initially and repeated at 24-hour intervals.

Several toxicity or fatalities are extremely infrequent in children, possibly due to differences in the way they metabolize acetaminophen. In children, the maximum potential amount ingested can be easily estimated. If more than 150 mg/kg or an unknown amount was ingested, obtain an acetaminophen plasma level. The acetaminophen plasma level should be obtained as soon as possible, but no sooner than 4 hours following ingestion. Induce emesis using syrup of ipecac. If the plasma level is obtained and falls above the broken line on the acetaminophen overdose nomogram, the MUCOMYST acetylcysteine therapy should be initiated and continued for a full course of therapy. If acetaminophen plasma assay capability is not available, and the estimated acetaminophen ingestion exceeds 150 mg/kg, MUCOMYST acetylcysteine therapy should be initiated and continued for a full course of therapy.

For additional emergency information, call your regional poison center or call the Rocky Mountain Poison Control Center toll-free, (1-800-525-6115).

Chlorpheniramine toxicity should be treated as you would an antihistamine/anticholinergic overdose and is likely to be present within a few hours after acute ingestion.

Symptoms from pseudophedrine overdose consist most often of mild anxiety, tachycardia and/or hypertension. Symptoms usually appear within 4 to 8 hours of ingestion and are transient, usually requiring no treatment.

Inactive Ingredients: CAPLET: Cellulose, hydroxypropyl cellulose, hydroxypropyl methylcellulose, magnesium stearate, polyethylene glycol, sodium starch glycolate, starch, titanium dioxide, blue #1, yellow #6, yellow #10.
GELCAP: Benzyl Alcohol, Butylparaben, Castor oil, Cellulose, Edetate Calcium Disodium, Gelatin, Hydroxypropyl Methylcellulose, Magnesium Stearate, Methylparaben, Propylparaben, Sodium Lauryl Sulfate, Sodium Propionate, Sodium Starch Glycolate, Starch, Titanium Dioxide Blue #1 and #2 and Yellow #10.

How Supplied: Caplets: (dark yellow, imprinted "TYLENOL Allergy Sinus")—Blister packs of 24 and tamper-resistant bottles of 50.
Gelcaps: (dark green and dark yellow, imprinted "TYLENOL A/S")—Blister packs of 24 and tamper-resistant bottles of 50.
Shown in Product Identification Section, page 413

MAXIMUM STRENGTH TYLENOL® COUGH MEDICATION

Description: Each 20 ml (4 tsp.) adult dose contains dextromethorphan HBr 30 mg., and acetaminophen 1,000mg.

Actions: MAXIMUM STRENGTH TYLENOL® COUGH Medication Liquid contains a clinically proven cough suppressant and analgesic-antipyretic. Acetaminophen produces analgesia by elevation of the pain threshold and antipyresis through action on the hypothalamic heat-regulating center. Dextromethorphan is a cough suppressant which provides temporary relief of coughs due to minor throat irritations that may occur with the common cold.

Indications: MAXIMUM STRENGTH TYLENOL® COUGH Medication provides effective, temporary relief of coughing, and the aches, pains and sore throat that may accompany a cough due to a cold.

Usual Dosage: A specially marked cup is provided for accurate dosing. Adults: (12 years and older) 4 teaspoons and 20ml as marked on cup every 6–8 hours, not to exceed 4 doses in 24 hours. Children: (ages 6–11) 1¼ teaspoons or 6.25ml as marked on cup every 4 hours, not to exceed 5 doses in 24 hours. Not recommended for children under 6 years.

"WARNING: Do not take this product for more than 10 days or for fever for more than 3 days unless directed by a physician. Severe or recurrent pain or high or continued fever may be indicative of serious illness. Under these conditions, consult a physician. A persistent cough may be a sign of a serious condition. If cough persists for more than 1 week, tends to recur or is accompanied by fever, rash or persistent headache, consult a doctor. Do not take this product for persistent or chronic cough such as occurs with smoking, asthma, emphysema,

or if cough is accompanied by excessive phlegm (mucus) unless directed by a doctor. Keep this and all medication out of the reach of children. As with any drug, if you are pregnant or nursing a baby, seek the advice of a health professional before using this product. In case of accidental overdosage, contact a doctor or poison control center immediately."

Overdosage: Acetaminophen in massive dosage may cause hepatic toxicity in some patients. In adults and adolescents, hepatic toxicity has rarely been reported following ingestion of acute overdosage of less than 10 grams. Fatalities are infrequent (less than 3–4% of untreated cases) and have rarely been reported with overdoses of less than 15 grams. In children, an acute overdosage of less than 150mg/kg has not been associated with hepatic toxicity.
Early symptoms following a potentially hepatotoxic overdose may include: nausea, vomiting, diaphoresis and general malaise. Clinical and laboratory evidence of hepatic toxicity may not be apparent until 48 to 72 hours postingestion. In adults and adolescents, regardless of the quantity of acetaminophen reported to have been ingested, administer MUCOMYST® acetylcysteine immediately if 24 hours or less have elapsed from the reported time of ingestion. For full prescribing information, refer to the MUCOMYST package insert. Do not await results of assays for acetaminophen level before initiating treatment with MUCOMYST acetylcysteine. The following additional procedures are recommended: The stomach should be emptied by lavage or by induction of emesis with syrup of ipecac. A serum acetaminophen assay should be obtained as early as possible, but no sooner than four hours following ingestion. Liver function studies should be obtained initially and repeated at 24-hour intervals.
Serious toxicity or fatalities are extremely infrequent in children, possibly due to differences in the way they metabolize acetaminophen. In children, the maximum potential amount ingested can be more easily estimated. If more than 150mg/kg or an unknown amount was ingested, obtain an acetaminophen plasma level. The acetaminophen plasma level should be obtained as soon as possible, but no sooner than 4 hours following the ingestion. Induce emesis using syrup of ipecac. If the plasma level is obtained and falls above the broken line on the acetaminophen overdose nomogram, the MUCOMYST acetylcysteine therapy should be initiated and continued for a full course of therapy. If acetaminophen plasma assay capability is not available, and the estimated acetaminophen ingestion exceeds 150mg/kg, MUCOMYST acetycysteine therapy should be initiated and continued for a full course of therapy.
For additional emergency information, call your regional poison center or call the Rocky Mountain Poison Center toll free (1-800-526-6115).
Acute dextromethorphan overdose usually does not result in serious signs and

symptoms unless massive amounts have been ingested. Signs and symptoms of a substantial overdose may include nausea and vomiting, visual disturbances, CNS disturbances, and urinary retention.

Inactive Ingredients: Alcohol (10%), Citric Acid, Flavors, Glycerin, Polyethylene Glycol, Purified Water, Sodium Benzoate, Sodium Carboxymethylcellulose, Sodium Saccharin, Sorbitol, Sucrose, Red #33, and Red #40.

How Supplied: MAXIMUM STRENGTH TYLENOL® COUGH is available in a 4 oz. bottle with child-resistant safety cap, special dosing cup marked in ml, and tamper resistant packaging.
Shown in Product Identification Section, page 414

MAXIMUM STRENGTH TYLENOL® COUGH MEDICATION WITH DECONGESTANT

Description: Each 20 ml (4 tsp.) adult dose contains dextromethorphan HBr 30 mg., and acetaminophen 1,000mg, and pseudoephedrine HCl 60mg.

Actions: MAXIMUM STRENGTH TYLENOL® COUGH Medication Liquid with Decongestant contains a clinically proven cough suppressant, an analgesic-antipyretic, and decongestant. Acetaminophen produces analgesia by elevation of the pain threshold and antipyresis through action on the hypothalamic heat-regulating center. Dextromethorphan is a cough suppressant which provides temporary relief of coughs due to minor throat irritations that may occur with the common cold. Pseudoephedrine hydrochloride is a sympathomimetic amine which provides temporary relief of nasal congestion.

Indications: MAXIMUM STRENGTH TYLENOL® COUGH Medication provides effective, temporary relief of coughing, and the aches, pains and sore throat that may accompany a cough due to a cold.

Usual Dosage: A specially marked cup is provided for accurate dosing. Adults: (12 years and older) 4 teaspoons and 20ml as marked on cup every 6–8 hours, not to exceed 4 doses in 24 hours. Children: (ages 6–11) 1¼ teaspoons or 6.25ml as marked on cup every 4 hours, not to exceed 5 doses in 24 hours. Not recommended for children under 6 years.

"WARNING: Do not take this product for more than 7 days or for fever for more than 3 days unless directed by a doctor. If symptoms do not improve or are accompanied by fever, consult a physician. A persistent cough may be a sign of a serious condition. If cough persists for more than 1 week, tends to recur or is accompanied by fever, rash or persistent headache, consult a doctor. Do not take this product for persistent or chronic cough such as occurs with smoking, asthma,

Continued on next page

McNeil Consumer—Cont.

emphysema, or if cough is accompanied by excessive phlegm (mucus) unless directed by a doctor. Do not exceed the recommended dosage because at higher doses nervousness, dizziness or sleeplessness may occur. Do not take this product if you have heart disease, high blood pressure, thyroid disease, diabetes or difficulty in urination due to enlargement of the prostate gland unless directed by a doctor. Keep this and all medication out of the reach of children. As with any drug, if you are pregnant or nursing a baby, seek the advice of a health professional before using this product. In case of accidental overdosage, contact a doctor or poison control center immediately."

Drug Interaction Precaution: Do not take this product if you are presently taking a prescription drug for high blood pressure or depression, without first consulting your doctor.

Overdosage: Acetaminophen in massive dosage may cause hepatic toxicity in some patients. In adults and adolescents, hepatic toxicity has rarely been reported following ingestion of acute overdosage of less than 10 grams. Fatalities are infrequent (less than 3–4% of untreated cases) and have rarely been reported with overdoses of less than 15 grams. In children, an acute overdosage of less than 150mg/kg has not been associated with hepatic toxicity.

Early symptoms following a potentially hepatotoxic overdose may include: nausea, vomiting, diaphoresis and general malaise. Clinical and laboratory evidence of hepatic toxicity may not be apparent until 48 to 72 hours postingestion. In adults and adolescents, regardless of the quantity of acetaminophen reported to have been ingested, administer MUCOMYST® acetylcysteine immediately if 24 hours or less have elapsed from the reported time of ingestion. For full prescribing information, refer to the MUCOMYST package insert. Do not await results of assays for acetaminophen level before initiating treatment with MUCOMYST acetylcysteine. The following additional procedures are recommended: The stomach should be emptied by lavage or by induction of emesis with syrup of ipecac. A serum acetaminophen assay should be obtained as early as possible, but no sooner than four hours following ingestion. Liver function studies should be obtained initially and repeated at 24-hour intervals.

Serious toxicity or fatalities are extremely infrequent in children, possibly due to differences in the way they metabolize acetaminophen. In children, the maximum potential amount ingested can be more easily estimated. If more than 150mg/kg or an unknown amount was ingested, obtain an acetaminophen plasma level. The acetaminophen plasma level should be obtained as soon as possible, but no sooner than 4 hours following the ingestion. Induce emesis using syrup of ipecac. If the plasma level

is obtained and falls above the broken line on the acetaminophen overdose nomogram, the MUCOMYST acetylcysteine therapy should be initiated and continued for a full course of therapy. If acetaminophen plasma assay capability is not available, and the estimated acetaminophen ingestion exceeds 150mg/kg, MUCOMYST acetycysteine therapy should be initiated and continued for a full course of therapy. For additional emergency information, call your regional poison center or call the Rocky Mountain Poison Center toll free (1-800-526-6115).

Acute dextromethorphan overdose usually does not result in serious signs and symptoms unless massive amounts have been ingested. Signs and symptoms of a substantial overdose may include nausea and vomiting, visual disturbances, CNS disturbances, and urinary retention.

Symptoms from pseudoephedrine overdose consist most often of mild anxiety, tachycardia and/or mild hypertension. Symptoms usually appear witin 4 to 8 hours of ingestion and are transient, usually requiring no treatment.

Inactive Ingredients: Alcohol (10%), Citric Acid, Flavors, Glycerin, Polyethylene Glycol, Purified Water, Sodium Benzoate, Sodium Carboxymethylcellulose, Sodium Saccharin, Sorbitol, Sucrose, Red #33, Red #40 and Blue #1.

How Supplied: MAXIMUM STRENGTH TYLENOL COUGH with Decongestant is available in a 4 oz. and 8 oz. bottles with child-resistant safety cap, special dosing cup marked in ml, and tamper resistant packaging.
Shown in Product Identification Section, page 414

Maximum-Strength TYLENOL® Sinus Medication Tablets, Caplets and Gelcaps

Description: Each Maximum-Strength TYLENOL® Sinus Medication tablet, caplet or gelcap contains acetaminophen 500 mg and pseudoephedrine hydrochloride 30 mg.

Actions: TYLENOL Sinus Medication contains a clinically proven analgesic-antipyretic and a decongestant. Maximum allowable non-prescription levels of acetaminophen and pseudoephedrine provide temporary relief of sinus headache and congestion. Acetaminophen is equal to aspirin in analgesic and antipyretic effectiveness and it is unlikely to produce many of the side effects associated with aspirin and aspirin-containing products.

Acetaminophen produces analgesia by elevation of the pain threshold and antipyresis through action on the hypothalamic heat-regulating center. Pseudoephedrine hydrochloride is a sympathomimetic amine which promotes sinus cavity drainage by reducing nasopharyngeal mucosal congestion.

Indications: Maximum-Strength TYLENOL Sinus Medication provides effective

symptomatic relief from sinus headache pain and congestion. Maximum-Strength TYLENOL Sinus Medication is particularly well-suited in patients with aspirin allergy, hemostatic disturbances (including anticoagulant therapy), and bleeding diatheses (e.g., hemophilia) and upper gastrointestinal disease (e.g., ulcer, gastritis, hiatus hernia).

Precautions: If a rare sensitivity occurs, the drug should be discontinued. Although pseudoephedrine is virtually without pressor effect in normotensive patients, it should be used with caution in hypertensives.

Usual Dosage: Adults and Children 12 years of Age and Older: Two Tablets, Caplets or Gelcaps every 4–6 hours. Do not exceed eight Tablets, Caplets or Gelcaps in any 24-hour period. WARNING: Do not administer to children under 12 or exceed the recommended dosage because at higher doses nervousness, dizziness, or sleeplessness may occur. Do not take this product for more than 7 days. If symptoms do not improve or are accompanied by fever, consult a physician. Do not take this product if you have heart disease, high blood pressure, thyroid disease, diabetes, or difficulty in urination due to enlargement of the prostate gland unless directed by a doctor.

DRUG INTERACTION PRECAUTION: Do not take this product if you are presently taking a prescription drug for high blood pressure or depression without first consulting your doctor. **Do not use if carton is opened or if blister unit is broken or if printed green neck wrap or printed foil inner seal is broken. Keep this and all medication out of the reach of children. As with any drug, if you are pregnant or nursing a baby, seek the advice of a health professional before using this product. In case of accidental overdosage, contact a physician or poison control center immediately.**

Overdosage: Acetaminophen in massive overdosage may cause hepatic toxicity in some patients. In adults and adolescents, hepatic toxicity has rarely been reported following ingestion of acute overdosage of less than 10 grams. Fatalities are infrequent (less than 3–4% of untreated cases) and have rarely been reported with overdoses of less than 15 grams. In children, an acute overdosage of less than 150 mg/kg has not been associated with hepatic toxicity.

Early symptoms following a potentially hepatotoxic overdose may include: nausea, vomiting, diaphoresis and general malaise. Clinical and laboratory evidence of hepatic toxicity may not be apparent until 48 to 72 hours postingestion. In adults and adolescents, regardless of the quantity of acetaminophen reported to have been ingested, administer MUCOMYST® acetylcysteine immediately if 24 hours or less have elapsed from the reported time of ingestion. For full prescribing information, refer to the MUCOMYST package insert. Do not await the results of assays for acetaminophen level before initiating treatment with MUCOMYST acetylcysteine. The following additional procedures are recommended: The stomach should be emptied promptly by lavage or by induction of emesis with syrup of ipecac. A serum acetaminophen assay should be obtained as early as possible, but no sooner than four hours following ingestion. Liver function studies should be obtained initially and repeated at 24-hour intervals.

Serious toxicity or fatalities are extremely infrequent in children, possibly due to differences in the way they metabolize acetaminophen. In children, the maximum potential amount ingested can be more easily estimated. If more than 150 mg/kg or an unknown amount was ingested, obtain an acetaminophen plasma level. The acetaminophen plasma level should be obtained as soon as possible, but no sooner than 4 hours following the ingestion. Induce emesis using syrup of ipecac. If the plasma level is obtained and falls above the broken line on the acetaminophen overdose nomogram, the MUCOMYST acetylcysteine therapy should be initiated and continued for a full course of therapy. If acetaminophen plasma assay capability is not available, and the estimated acetaminophen ingestion exceeds 150 mg/kg, MUCOMYST acetylcysteine therapy should be initiated and continued for a full course of therapy.

For additional emergency information, call your regional poison center or call the Rocky Mountain Poison Center toll-free, (1-800-525-6115).

Symptoms from pseudoephedrine overdose consist most often of mild anxiety, tachycardia and/or mild hypertension. Symptoms usually appear within 4 to 8 hours of ingestion and are transient, usually requiring no treatment.

Inactive Ingredients: Caplets—Cellulose, Hydroxypropyl Methylcellulose, Magnesium Stearate, Polyethylene Glycol, Polysorbate 80, Sodium Starch Glycolate, Starch, Titanium Dioxide, Blue #1, Red #40 and Yellow #10. Tablets—Cellulose, Magnesium Stearate, Sodium Lauryl Sulfate, Starch, Yellow #6, Yellow #10, and Blue #1. Gelcaps—Benzyl alcohol, butylparaben, castor oil, cellulose, edetate calcium disodium, gelatin, hydroxypropyl methylcellulose, iron oxide black, magnesium stearate, methylparaben, propylparaben, sodium lauryl sulfate, sodium propionate, sodium starch glycolate, starch, titanium dioxide, Blue #1 and Yellow #10.

How Supplied: Tablets (colored light green, imprinted "Maximum-Strength TYLENOL Sinus")—tamper-resistant bottles of 24 and 50. Caplets (light green coating, printed "TYLENOL Sinus" in dark green) tamper-resistant bottles of 24 and 50.

Gelcaps (colored green and white), imprinted "TYLENOL Sinus" in tamper-resistant packages of 20 and 40.

Shown in Product Identification Section, page 413

Mead Johnson Nutritionals
A Bristol-Myers Squibb Company
2400 W. LLOYD EXPRESSWAY
EVANSVILLE, IN 47721

Casec® Calcium Caseinate Powder
Ce-Vi-Sol® Vitamin C Supplement Drops for Infants
Criticare HN® Ready-To-Use High Nitrogen Elemental Diet
Enfamil® Infant Formula[1]
Enfamil® With Iron Infant Formula[1]
Enfamil Infant Formula Nursette®
Enfamil Premature Formula
Enfamil Premature Formula With Iron
Enfamil Human Milk Fortifier
Fer-In-Sol® Iron Supplement Drops, Syrup, Capsules
Isocal® Nutritionally Complete Liquid Tube-Feeding Formula
Isocal® HCN High Calorie and Nitrogen Nutritionally Complete Liquid Tube-Feeding Formula
Isocal® HN High Nitrogen, Nutritionally Complete Liquid Tube-Feeding Formula
Lipisorb™ MCT Formulation for Improved Fat Absorption
Lonalac® Powder, Low-Sodium, High-Protein Beverage Mix
MCT Oil, Medium Chain Triglycerides
Moducal® Dietary Carbohydrate
Nutramigen® Hypoallergenic Protein Hydrolysate Formula[1]
Portagen® Iron-Fortified Nutritionally Complete Powder with Medium Chain Triglycerides
ProSobee® Soy Isolate Formula[1]
ProSobee® Soy Isolate Formula Nursette®[1]

Special Metabolic Diets:
Lofenalac® Iron Fortified Low Phenylalanine Diet Powder
Low Methionine Diet Powder (Product 3200K)
Low PHE-TYR Diet Powder (Product 3200AB)
Mono- and Disaccharide-Free Diet Powder (Product 3232A)
MSUD Diet Powder
Phenyl-Free® Phenylalanine-Free Diet Powder

[1]Concentrated liquid, powder, and ready to use

Pregestimil® Iron Fortified Protein Hydrolysate Formula with Medium Chain Triglycerides

Special Metabolic Modules:
HIST 1
HIST 2
HOM 1
HOM 2
LYS 1
LYS 2
MSUD 1
MSUD 2
OS 1
OS 2
PKU 1
PKU 2
PKU 3
Protein-Free Diet Powder (Product 80056)
TYR 1
TYR 2
UCD 1
UCD 2
Sustacal® Nutritionally Complete Liquid, Powder, Pudding
Sustacal® with Fiber Nutritionally Complete Liquid Food with Soy Fiber
Sustacal® 8.8 Nutritionally Complete Liquid Food
Sustacal® Plus High-Calorie, Nutritionally Complete Food
Sustagen® High-Calorie, High-Protein Nutritional Supplement
TraumaCal® High-Nitrogen, Nutritionally Complete Formula for Metabolically Stressed Patients
Trind® Liquid, Antihistamine, Nasal Decongestant, Sugar-Free
Trind-DM® Liquid, Cough Suppressant, Antihistamine, Nasal Decongestant, Sugar-Free
Ultracal® High-Nitrogen, Nutritionally Complete Liquid Tube-Feeding Formula with Dietary Fiber

Detailed information may be obtained by contacting Mead Johnson Nutritionals Medical Affairs Department at (812) 429-6437.

POLY–VI–SOL®
[pahl-ē-vī-sahl″]
Vitamin drops • chewable tablets

Composition: Usual daily doses supply: [See table below.]

POLY-VI-SOL® Vitamin drops, chewable tablets	Drops 1.0 mL	% U.S. RDA for Infants	Chewable Tablets 1 tablet	% U.S. RDA	
				Children Age 2–3 Years	Adults and Children Age 4 Years or More
Vitamin A, IU	1500	100	2500	100	50
Vitamin D, IU	400	100	400	100	100
Vitamin E, IU	5	100	15	150	50
Vitamin C, mg	35	100	60	150	100
Folic acid, mg	—	—	0.3	150	75
Thiamine, mg	0.5	100	1.05	150	70
Riboflavin, mg	0.6	100	1.2	150	70
Niacin, mg	8	100	13.5	150	68
Vitamin B$_6$, mg	0.4	100	1.05	150	53
Vitamin B$_{12}$, µg	2	100	4.5	150	75

Continued on next page

Mead Johnson Nutr.—Cont.

Action and Uses: Daily vitamin supplementation for infants and children. Chewable tablets useful also for adults.

Administration and Dosage: Usual doses or as indicated.

How Supplied: Poly-Vi-Sol® vitamin drops: (with 'Safti-Dropper' marked to deliver 1.0 mL)
   0087-0402-02 Bottles of 1 fl oz (30 mL)
   0087-0402-03 Bottles of 1⅔ fl oz (50 mL)
   6505-00-104-8433 (50 mL) (Defense)
Poly-Vi-Sol® chewable vitamins tablets:
   0087-0412-03 Bottles of 100
Poly-Vi-Sol® chewable vitamins tablets in Circus Shapes:
   0087-0414-02 Bottles of 100
   0087-0414-06 Bottles of 60
   Shown in Product Identification Section, page 414

POLY–VI–SOL® with Iron
[pahl-ē-vī-sahl ″]
Chewable vitamins and minerals

Composition: Each tablet supplies same vitamins as Poly-Vi-Sol tablets plus 12 mg iron, 8 mg zinc, and 0.8 mg copper.

Action and Uses: Daily vitamin and mineral supplement for adults and children.

Administration and Dosage: 1 tablet daily.

How Supplied: Poly-Vi-Sol® chewable vitamins with Iron tablets.
   0087-0455-02 Bottles of 100
Poly-Vi-Sol® chewable vitamins with Iron tablets in Circus Shapes.
   0087-0456-02 Bottles of 100
   0087-0456-06 Bottles of 60
[See table above.]
   Shown in Product Identification Section, page 414

POLY–VI–SOL® with Iron
[pahl-ē-vī'sahl ″]
Vitamin and Iron drops

Composition: Each 1.0 mL supplies:

		% U.S. RDA Infants
Vitamin A, IU	1500	100
Vitamin D, IU	400	100
Vitamin E, IU	5	100
Vitamin C, mg	35	100
Thiamine, mg	0.5	100
Riboflavin, mg	0.6	100
Niacin, mg	8	100
Vitamin B₆, mg	0.4	100
Iron, mg	10	67

Action and Uses: Daily vitamin and iron supplement for infants.

Administration and Dosage: Drop into mouth with 'Safti-Dropper.' Dose: 1.0 mL daily, or as indicated.

POLY-VI-SOL® with Iron Chewable Tablets	Chewable Tablets 1 tablet	% U.S. RDA Children Age 2–3 Years	Adults and Children Age 4 Years or More
Vitamin A, IU	2500	100	50
Vitamin D, IU	400	100	100
Vitamin E, IU	15	150	50
Vitamin C, mg	60	150	100
Folic acid, mg	0.3	150	75
Thiamine, mg	1.05	150	70
Riboflavin, mg	1.2	150	70
Niacin, mg	13.5	150	68
Vitamin B₆, mg	1.05	150	53
Vitamin B₁₂, μg	4.5	150	75
Iron, mg	12	120	67
Copper, mg	0.8	80	40
Zinc, mg	8	100	53

When an infant or child is taking iron, stools may appear darker in color. This is to be expected and should be no cause for concern. When drops containing iron are given to infants or young children, some darkening of the plaque on the teeth may occur. This is not serious or permanent as it does not affect the enamel. The stains can be removed or prevented by rubbing the teeth with a little baking soda or powder on a toothbrush or small cloth once or twice a week.

How Supplied: Poly-Vi-Sol® vitamin and iron drops (with dropper marked to deliver 1 mL)
   0087-0405-01 Bottles of 1⅔ fl oz (50 mL)
   Shown in Product Identification Section, page 414

RICELYTE™
[rīs 'līt]
Rice-based oral electrolyte maintenance solution

Ricelyte rapidly replenishes fluid and electrolytes lost in diarrhea. It is designed for oral administration and provides electrolytes and rice carbohydrate in a balanced formulation.

Composition: Water, rice syrup solids, natural fruit flavors, sodium chloride, potassium citrate, sodium citrate, citric acid.

Concentrations of Electrolytes:

	Per liter
Sodium (mEq)	50
Potassium (mEq)	25
Chloride (mEq)	45
Citrate (mEq)	34
Rice Syrup Solids (g)	30
Calories	126

Indications: Oral feedings of Ricelyte may be used to supply water and electrolytes for maintenance during diarrhea; and to replace mild to moderate fluid losses.

Intake and Administration: Feed by nursing bottle, cup, straw, or spoon. Ricelyte should be initiated as soon as diarrhea is recognized and continued until after the last soft, watery stool. Intake should approximate the normal fluid intake plus 4 to 8 fluid ounces for each watery stool. Recommended approximate intakes by weight of the infant or child are shown in the accompanying table. [See table on top of next page]

For older children and adults two or more quarts per day may be necessary. Intake should be adjusted on the basis of clinical findings, amount of fluid loss, patient's usual fluid intake, and other relevant factors such as thirst.

Contraindications: Ricelyte should not be used:
—in the presence of severe, continuing diarrhea or other critical fluid losses requiring parenteral fluid therapy
—in intractable vomiting, adynamic ileus, intestinal obstruction, or perforated bowel
—when renal function is depressed (anuria, oliguria) or homeostatic mechanisms are impaired

Precautions: Urgent needs in severe fluid imbalances must be met parenterally. Ricelyte should be used on a doctor's orders and should be discontinued when the diarrhea has ceased. Ricelyte does not meet the caloric requirements of infants and children. Additional food or formula should be given as instructed by the doctor.
Opened bottles of Ricelyte should be resealed, refrigerated, and used within 48 hours.

Features: Ricelyte is ready to use—no mixing or dilution is necessary.
—Ricelyte is balanced to provide the necessary electrolytes and fluid
—Natural fruit flavor
—No artificial colors or flavors
—No fruit juice

How Supplied: Ricelyte is available in one-liter plastic bottles. It is also available in the Hospital Feeding System in 8 fl oz Nursette® Disposable Bottles.

Ricelyte™ ADMINISTRATION GUIDE
For Maintenance Therapy*

Weight lb	Ricelyte fl oz	Weight kg	Ricelyte mL
7	11–16	3.2	320– 480
13	20–30	5.9	590– 885
17	26–39	7.7	770–1155
20	30–46	9.1	910–1365
23	35–53	10.5	1050–1575
25	38–58	11.4	1140–1710
28	42–64	12.7	1270–1905
32	48–74	14.5	1450–2175
38	57–87	17.3	1730–2595

1.5–2.3 fl oz/lb Per Day   or 100–150 mL/kg Per Day

* *Ongoing Loss Replacement:* For every diarrheal stool, the caregiver should give an additional 4 to 8 fl oz (120 to 240 mL).
• For breast-fed infants, allow breast milk *ad lib.* For formula-fed infants, alternate Ricelyte with equal amounts of lactose-free formula, like ProSobee®, or half-strength lactose-containing formula, like Enfamil®.
• Avoid products such as carbonated or fruit-flavored drinks which have a high carbohydrate content.

Reference: Adapted from Santosham M., et al, *Ped Rev.* 1987; 8:273 as presented in The Harriet Lane Handbook, ed 12, 1990:274.
Shown in Product Identification Section, page 415

TEMPRA®
[tem 'prah]
Acetaminophen
Drops • syrup • chewable tablets
For infants and children

Description: Tempra is acetaminophen, a safe and effective analgesic-antipyretic. It is not a salicylate. It contains no phenacetin or caffeine. It has no effect on prothrombin time. Tempra offers prompt, non-irritating therapy. Because it provides significant freedom from side effects, it is particularly valuable for patients who do not tolerate aspirin well. Tempra drops contain no alcohol. Tempra syrup contains no alcohol. Tempra chewable tablets are sugar-free.

Indications and Usage: Tempra 1 Infant Drops, Tempra 2 Toddlers Syrup, and Tempra 3 Chewable Tablets (regular and double-strength forms) are useful for reducing fever and for the temporary relief of minor aches, pains and discomfort associated with the common cold or "flu," inoculations or vaccination. Tempra syrup is valuable in reducing pain following tonsillectomy and adenoidectomy. When Tempra is used by pregnant or nursing women, there are no known adverse effects upon fetal development or nursing infants.

Note: A prescription is not required for Tempra 1 Infant Drops, Tempra 2 Toddlers Syrup, or Tempra 3 Chewable Tablets (regular and double-strength forms) as an analgesic. To prevent its misuse by the layman, the following information appears on the package label:

Warnings: If fever persists for more than 3 days (72 hours) or if pain continues for more than 5 days, consult your physician.
Phenylketonurics: Each 80 mg tablet of Tempra 3 contains 3.3 mg phenylalanine. Each 160 mg tablet contains 6.6 mg phenylalanine.

Precaution: Acetaminophen has been reported to potentiate the effect of orally administered anticoagulants and may enhance the elimination of chloramphenicol. Therapeutic drug monitoring should be considered whenever these drugs are used concurrently.

Adverse Reactions: Infrequent, non-specific side effects have been reported with the therapeutic use of acetaminophen.

Overdosage: Acetaminophen in massive overdosage may cause hepatic toxicity in some patients. In adults and adolescents, hepatic toxicity has rarely been reported following ingestion of acute overdoses of less than 10 grams. Fatalities are infrequent (less than 3–4% of untreated cases) and have rarely been reported with overdoses of less than 15 grams. In children, an acute overdosage of less than 150 mg/kg has not been associated with hepatic toxicity.
Early symptoms following a potentially hepatotoxic overdose may include: nausea, vomiting, diaphoresis and general malaise. Clinical and laboratory evidence of hepatic toxicity may not be apparent until 48 to 72 hours postingestion. In adults and adolescents, regardless of the quantity of acetaminophen reported to have been ingested, administer MUCOMYST® acetylcysteine immediately if 24 hours or less have elapsed from the reported time of ingestion. For full prescribing information, refer to the MUCOMYST package insert. Do not await results of assays for acetaminophen level before initiating treatment with MUCOMYST acetylcysteine. The following additional procedures are recommended: The stomach should be emptied promptly by lavage or by induction of emesis with syrup of ipecac. A serum acetaminophen assay should be obtained as early as possible, but no sooner than four hours following ingestion. Liver function studies should be obtained initially and repeated at 24-hour intervals.
Serious toxicity or fatalities are extremely infrequent in children, possibly due to differences in the way they metabolize acetaminophen. In children, the maximum potential amount ingested can be more easily estimated. If more than 150 mg/kg or an unknown amount was ingested, obtain an acetaminophen plasma level. The acetaminophen plasma level should be obtained as soon as possible, but no sooner than 4 hours following the ingestion. Induce emesis using syrup of ipecac. If the plasma level is obtained and falls above the broken line on the nomogram, the MUCOMYST acetylcysteine therapy should be initiated and continued for a full course of therapy. If acetaminophen plasma assay capability is not available, and the estimated acetaminophen ingestion exceeds 150 mg/kg, MUCOMYST acetylcysteine therapy should be initiated and continued for a full course of therapy.
For additional emergency information, call your regional poison center or toll-free (1-800-525-6115) to the Rocky Mountain Poison Center for assistance in diagnosis and for directions on the use of MUCOMYST acetylcysteine as an antidote.

Dosage and Administration: Dosage may be given every 4 hours as needed but not more than 5 times daily. [See table.]
DROPS: Drops are given with calibrated 'Safti-Dropper' or mixed with water or fruit juices. Each 0.8 mL dropper contains 80 mg acetaminophen.
SYRUP: Syrup is given by teaspoon. Each 5 mL teaspoon contains 160 mg acetaminophen.

TEMPRA®

Age	Approximate Weight Range*	Tempra 1 Infant Drops	Tempra 2 Toddlers Syrup	Tempra 3 Regular Strength Chewables 80 mg	Tempra 3 Double Strength Chewables 160 mg
†Under 4 mo	Under 12 lb	½ dropper	¼ tsp	—	—
†4 to 11 mo	12–17 lb	1 dropper	½ tsp	—	—
†12 to 23 mo	18–23 lb	1½ droppers	¾ tsp	—	—
2 to 3 yr	24–35 lb	2 droppers	1 tsp	2 tablets	—
4 to 5 yr	36–47 lb	3 droppers	1½ tsp	3 tablets	—
6 to 8 yr	48–59 lb	—	2 tsp	4 tablets	2 tablets
9 to 10 yr	60–71 lb	—	2½ tsp	5 tablets	2½ tablets
11 yr	72–95 lb	—	3 tsp	6 tablets	3 tablets
12 yr & older	96 lb & over	—	4 tsp	8 tablets	4 tablets

*If child is significantly under- or overweight, dosage may need to be adjusted accordingly.
†Ask your doctor before administering to children under the age of 2 years.

Continued on next page

Mead Johnson Nutr.—Cont.

CHEWABLES: Each Regular tablet contains 80 mg acetaminophen. Each Double Strength tablet contains 160 mg acetaminophen.

How Supplied: Tempra® 1 (acetaminophen) Infant Drops: (with calibrated 'Safti-Dropper') grape-flavored
NDC 0087-0730-01 Bottles of 15 mL
Tempra® 2 (acetaminophen) Toddlers Syrup: grape-flavored
NDC 0087-0733-04 Bottles of 4 fl oz
NDC 0087-0733-03 Bottles of 16 fl oz
Tempra® 3 (acetaminophen) Chewable Tablets, Regular Strength: grape-flavored, no sucrose
NDC 0087-0738-01 Bottles of 30 (80 mg) tablets
Tempra® 3 (acetaminophen) Chewable Tablets, Double Strength: grape-flavored, no sucrose
NDC 0087-0749-01 Bottles of 30 (160 mg) tablets
No Rx required.
Shown in Product Identification Section, page 415

TRI-VI-SOL®
[*trī-vī-sahl"*]
Vitamins A, D and C drops

	Drops 1.0 mL	% U.S. RDA for Infants
Vitamin A, IU	1500	100
Vitamin D, IU	400	100
Vitamin C, mg	35	100

Action and Uses: Tri-Vi-Sol drops provide vitamins A, D and C.

How Supplied: Tri-Vi-Sol® drops: (with 'Safti-Dropper' marked to deliver 1 mL)
0087-0403-02 Bottles of 1 fl oz (30 mL)
0087-0403-03 Bottles of 1⅔ fl oz (50 mL)
Shown in Product Identification Section, page 415

TRI-VI-SOL® with Iron
[*trī-vī-sahl"*]
Vitamins A, D, C and Iron drops

Composition: Each 1.0 mL supplies same vitamins as in Tri-Vi-Sol® vitamin drops (see above) plus 10 mg iron.

Action and Uses: Tri-Vi-Sol with Iron vitamins A, D, C and Iron for infants and children.

Administration and Dosage: Drop into mouth with 'Safti-Dropper.' Dose: 1.0 mL daily, or as indicated.

How Supplied: Tri-Vi-Sol® vitamin drops with Iron (with dropper marked to deliver 1 mL)
0087-0453-03 Bottles of 1⅔ fl oz (50 mL)
Shown in Product Identification Section, page 415

Mead Johnson Pharmaceuticals
A Bristol-Myers Squibb Company
2400 W. LLOYD EXPRESSWAY
EVANSVILLE, IN 47721-0001

COLACE®
[*kōlās*]
docusate sodium, Mead Johnson capsules • syrup • liquid (drops)

Description: Colace (docusate sodium) is a stool softener.
Colace Capsules, 50 mg, contain the following inactive ingredients: citric acid, D&C Red No. 33, FD&C Red No. 40, nonporcine gelatin, edible ink, polyethylene glycol, propylene glycol, and purified water.
Colace Capsules, 100 mg, contain the following inactive ingredients: citric acid, D&C Red No. 33, FD&C Red No. 40, FD&C Yellow No. 6, nonporcine gelatin, edible ink, polyethylene glycol, propylene glycol, titanium dioxide, and purified water.
Colace Liquid, 1%, contains the following inactive ingredients: citric acid, D&C Red No. 33, methylparaben, poloxamer, polyethylene glycol, propylene glycol, propylparaben, sodium citrate, vanillin, and purified water.
Colace Syrup, 20 mg/5 mL, contains the following inactive ingredients: alcohol (not more than 1%), citric acid, D&C Red No. 33, FD&C Red No. 40, flavor (natural), menthol, methylparaben, peppermint oil, poloxamer, polyethylene glycol, propylparaben, sodium citrate, sucrose, and purified water.

Actions and Uses: Colace, a surface-active agent, helps to keep stools soft for easy, natural passage and is not a laxative, thus, not habit forming. Useful in constipation due to hard stools, in painful anorectal conditions, in cardiac and other conditions in which maximum ease of passage is desirable to avoid difficult or painful defecation, and when peristaltic stimulants are contraindicated.
Note: When peristaltic stimulation is needed due to inadequate bowel motility, see Peri-Colace® (laxative and stool softener).

Contraindications: There are no known contraindications to Colace.

Warning: As with any drug, if you are pregnant or nursing a baby, seek the advice of a health professional before using this product.

Side Effects: The incidence of side effects—none of a serious nature—is exceedingly small. Bitter taste, throat irritation, and nausea (primarily associated with the use of the syrup and liquid) are the main side effects reported. Rash has occurred.

Administration and Dosage: *Orally*—Suggested daily Dosage: *Adults and older children:* 50 to 200 mg *Children 6 to 12:* 40 to 120 mg *Children 3 to 6:* 20 to 60 mg. *Infants and children under 3:* 10 to 40 mg. The higher doses are recommended for initial therapy. Dosage should be ad-

justed to individual response. The effect on stools is usually apparent 1 to 3 days after the first dose. Give Colace liquid in half a glass of milk or fruit juice or in infant formula, to mask bitter taste. *In enemas*—Add 50 to 100 mg Colace (5 to 10 mL Colace liquid) to a retention or flushing enema.

How Supplied: Colace capsules, 50 mg
NDC 0087-0713-01 Bottles of 30
NDC 0087-0713-02 Bottles of 60
NDC 0087-0713-03 Bottles of 250
NDC 0087-0713-05 Bottles of 1000
NDC 0087-0713-07 Cartons of 100 single unit packs
Colace capsules, 100 mg
NDC 0087-0714-01 Bottles of 30
NDC 0087-0714-02 Bottles of 60
NDC 0087-0714-03 Bottles of 250
NDC 0087-0714-05 Bottles of 1000
NDC 0087-0714-07 Cartons of 100 single unit packs
Note: Colace capsules should be stored at controlled room temperature (59°–86°F or 15°–30°C)
Colace liquid, 1% solution; 10 mg/mL (with calibrated dropper)
NDC 0087-0717-04 Bottles of 16 fl oz
NDC 0087-0717-02 Bottles of 30 mL
NSN 6505-00-045-7786 Bottles of 30 mL (M)
Colace syrup, 20 mg/5-mL teaspoon; contains not more than 1% alcohol
NDC 0087-0720-01 Bottles of 8 fl oz
NDC 0087-0720-02 Bottles of 16 fl oz
Shown in Product Identification Section, page 415

PERI-COLACE® capsules • syrup
(casanthranol and docusate sodium)

Description: Peri-Colace is a combination of the mild stimulant laxative casanthranol, and the stool-softener Colace® (docusate sodium). Each capsule contains 30 mg of casanthranol and 100 mg of Colace; the syrup contains 30 mg of casanthranol and 60 mg of Colace per 15-mL tablespoon (10 mg of casanthranol and 20 mg of Colace per 5-mL teaspoon) and 10% alcohol.
Peri-Colace Capsules contain the following inactive ingredients: D&C Red No. 33, FD&C Red No. 40, nonporcine gelatin, edible ink, polyethylene glycol, propylene glycol, titanium dioxide, and purified water.
Peri-Colace Syrup contains the following inactive ingredients: alcohol (10% v/v), citric acid, flavors, methyl salicylate, methylparaben, poloxamer, polyethylene glycol, propylparaben, sodium citrate, sorbitol solution, sucrose, and purified water.

Action and Uses: Peri-Colace provides gentle peristaltic stimulation and helps to keep stools soft for easier passage. Bowel movement is induced gently—usually overnight or in 8 to 12 hours. Nausea, griping, abnormally loose stools, and constipation rebound are minimized. Useful in management of chronic or temporary constipation.
Note: To prevent hard stools when laxative stimulation is not needed or undesirable, see Colace (stool softener).

Warnings: Do not use when abdominal pain, nausea, or vomiting are present. Frequent or prolonged use of this preparation may result in dependence on laxatives.

As with any drug, if you are pregnant or nursing a baby, seek the advice of a health professional before using this product.

Side Effects: The incidence of side effects—none of a serious nature—is exceedingly small. Nausea, abdominal cramping or discomfort, diarrhea, and rash are the main side effects reported.

Administration and Dosage:
Adults—1 or 2 capsules, or 1 or 2 tablespoons syrup at bedtime, or as indicated. In severe cases, dosage may be increased to 2 capsules or 2 tablespoons twice daily, or 3 capsules at bedtime. *Children*—1 to 3 teaspoons of syrup at bedtime, or as indicated.

Overdosage: In addition to symptomatic treatment, gastric lavage, if timely, is recommended in cases of large overdosage.

How Supplied: Peri-Colace® Capsules
NDC 0087-0715-01 Bottles of 30
NDC 0087-0715-02 Bottles of 60
NDC 0087-0715-03 Bottles of 250
NDC 0087-0715-05 Bottles of 1000
NDC 0087-0715-07 Cartons of 100 single unit packs
Note: Peri-Colace capsules should be stored at controlled room temperatures (59°–86°F or 15°–30°C).
Peri-Colace® Syrup
NDC 0087-0721-01 Bottles of 8 fl oz
NDC 0087-0721-02 Bottles of 16 fl oz
Shown in Product Identification Section, page 415

Menley & James Laboratories, Inc.
COMMONWEALTH
CORPORATE CENTER
100 TOURNAMENT DRIVE,
SUITE 310
HORSHAM, PA 19044-3697

A.R.M.® Allergy Relief Medicine Maximum Strength Caplets

Product Information: A.R.M. combines two important medicines in one safe, fast-acting caplet:
● The highest level of antihistamine available without prescription—for better relief of sneezing, runny nose and itchy, weepy eyes.
● A clinically proven sinus decongestant to help ease breathing and drain sinus congestion for hours.

Active Ingredients: Each caplet contains Chlorpheniramine Maleate, 4 mg, Phenylpropanolamine Hydrochloride, 25 mg. **Inactive Ingredients:** Carnauba Wax, D&C Yellow 10, FD&C Yellow 6, Gelatin, Hydroxypropyl Methylcellulose, Lactose, Magnesium Stearate, Polyethylene Glycol, Sodium Starch Glycolate, Starch and trace amounts of other ingredients.

Directions: One caplet every 4 hours, not to exceed 6 caplets in 24 hours.

Children (6–12 years): one-half the adult dose. Children under 6 years use only as directed by physician.
TAMPER-RESISTANT PACKAGE FEATURES FOR YOUR PROTECTION:
● The carton has been sealed at the factory with a clear overwrap printed with "safety sealed."
● Each caplet is encased in a clear plastic cell with a foil back.
● The name A.R.M. appears on each caplet (see product illustration on front of carton).
● **DO NOT USE THIS PRODUCT IF ANY OF THESE TAMPER-RESISTANT FEATURES IS MISSING OR BROKEN. IF YOU HAVE ANY QUESTIONS, PLEASE CALL 1-800-321-1834 TOLL FREE.**

Warning: Do not exceed recommended dosage. If symptoms do not improve within 7 days, or are accompanied by high fever, consult a physician before continuing use. Stop use if dizziness, sleeplessness or nervousness occurs. If you have or are being treated for depression, high blood pressure, glaucoma, diabetes, asthma, heart disease, thyroid disease or difficulty in urination due to enlargement of the prostate gland, use only as directed by a physician. Do not take this product if you are taking another medication containing phenylpropanolamine.
Avoid alcoholic beverages while taking this product. Do not drive or operate heavy machinery. May cause drowsiness. May cause excitability, especially in children. **Keep this and all medication out of reach of children.** In case of accidental overdose, seek professional assistance or contact a Poison Control Center immediately. As with any drug, if you are pregnant or nursing a baby, seek the advice of a health professional before using this product.
Store at controlled room temperature (59°–86°F.).

How Supplied: Consumer packages of 20 and 40 caplets.
Shown in Product Identification Section, page 415

ACNOMEL® CREAM
Acne Therapy

Description: Cream—non-greasy, dries oily skin, easy to apply.

Active Ingredients: Resorcinol 2%, Sulfur 8%. **Inactive Ingredients:** Alcohol 11% (w/w), Bentonite, Fragrance, Iron Oxides, Potassium Hydroxide, Propylene Glycol, Titanium Dioxide, Purified Water.

Indications: ACNOMEL CREAM is effective in the treatment of pimples and blemishes due to acne.

Directions: Wash and dry affected areas thoroughly. Apply a thin coating of AC-NOMEL CREAM once or twice daily, making sure it does not get into the eyes or on eyelids. Do not rub in. If a marked

chapping effect occurs, discontinue use temporarily.

Warning: ACNOMEL CREAM should not be applied to acutely inflamed area. If undue skin irritation develops or increases, discontinue use and consult physician. **Keep this and all medication out of reach of children.** In case of accidental ingestion, seek professional assistance or contact a Poison Control Center immediately. Keep tube tightly closed to prevent drying.
Store at controlled room temperature (59°–86°F).

How Supplied: Cream—in specially lined 1 oz. tubes.
Shown in Product Identification Section, page 415

AQUA CARE® CREAM
With 10% Urea
Effective Medication for Dry Skin Relief

Product Information: AQUA CARE, with 10% urea, is a topical cream formulated to restore nature's moisture balance to rough, dry skin. The special urea ingredient penetrates the surface of the skin to both restore lost moisture and soften dry, rough skin.

Active Ingredient: Urea 10%. **Also Contains:** Purified Water, Cetyl Esters, DEA-Oleth-3 Phosphate, Petrolatum, Triethanolamine, Carbomer 934, Glycerin, Lanolin Oil, Mineral Oil and Lanolin Alcohol, Benzyl Alcohol, and Fragrance.

Directions: Apply two or three times daily to areas of need or as directed by a physician.

Warning: Discontinue use if irritation occurs.
Store at controlled room temperature (59°–86°F).
FOR EXTERNAL USE ONLY

How Supplied: Available in 2.5 oz. tubes.
Shown in Product Identification Section, page 415

AQUA CARE® LOTION
With 10% Urea
Effective Medication for Dry Skin Relief

Product Information: AQUA CARE, with 10% urea, is a topical lotion formulated to restore nature's moisture balance to rough, dry skin. The special urea ingredient penetrates the surface of the skin to both restore lost moisture and soften dry, rough skin.

Active Ingredient: Urea 10%. **Also Contains:** Purified Water, Mineral Oil, Petrolatum, Propylene Glycol Monostearate, Sorbitan Monostearate, Cetyl Alcohol, Sodium Lauryl Sulfate, Lactic Acid, Magnesium Aluminum Silicate, Methyl-

Continued on next page

Menley & James—Cont.

paraben, Propylparaben, may also contain Sodium Hydroxide.

Directions: Apply two or three times daily to areas of need or as directed by a physician.

Warning: Discontinue use if irritation occurs.

Store at controlled room temperature (59°–86°F).

FOR EXTERNAL USE ONLY

How Supplied: Available in 8 oz. bottles.

Shown in Product Identification Section, page 415

ASTHMAHALER® Mist
Epinephrine Bitartrate
Bronchodilator
Alcohol Free Formula

Active Ingredients: Contains Epinephrine Bitartrate 7 mg per ml in inert propellant. **Inactive Ingredients:** Cetylpyridinium Chloride, Propellants 11, 12, & 114, Sorbitan Trioleate.

Indications: For temporary relief of shortness of breath, tightness of chest, and wheezing due to bronchial asthma.

Warnings: Do not use this product unless a diagnosis of asthma has been made by a physician. Do not use this product if you have heart disease, high blood pressure, thyroid disease, diabetes, or difficulty in urination due to enlargement of the prostate gland unless directed by a physician. Do not use this product if you have ever been hospitalized for asthma or if you are taking any prescription drug for asthma unless directed by a physician.
DO NOT USE THIS PRODUCT MORE FREQUENTLY OR AT HIGHER DOSES THAN RECOMMENDED UNLESS DIRECTED BY A PHYSICIAN.
Excessive use may cause nervousness and rapid heart beat, and possibly, adverse effects on the heart.
DO NOT CONTINUE TO USE THIS PRODUCT, BUT SEEK MEDICAL ASSISTANCE IMMEDIATELY IF SYMPTOMS ARE NOT RELIEVED WITHIN 20 MINUTES OR BECOME WORSE.

Drug Interaction Precaution: Do not use this product if you are presently taking a prescription drug for high blood pressure or depression, without first consulting your physician.

Contents under pressure. Do not puncture or incinerate container. Do not expose to heat or store at temperature above 120°F.

As with any drug, if you are pregnant or nursing a baby, seek the advice of a health professional before using this product.
Keep this and all medication out of the reach of children. In case of accidental overdose, consult a physician immediately.

Dosage and Administration: For oral inhalation only. Each inhalation contains the equivalent of 0.16 milligram of epinephrine base.
Dosage: Inhalation dosage for adults and children 4 years of age and older: Start with one inhalation, then wait at least 1 minute. If not relieved, use once more. Do not use again for at least 3 hours. Use of this product by children should be supervised by an adult. Children under 4 years of age: consult a physician.

Directions: Shake well before each use.
1. Remove plastic dust cap, take mouthpiece off metal vial and fit other end of mouthpiece onto top of vial, turn vial upside down. Shake well.
2. Breathe out fully and place mouthpiece well into mouth, aimed at the back of the throat.
3. As you begin to breathe in deeply, press the vial firmly down into the adapter with the index finger. This releases one dose.
4. Release pressure on vial and remove unit from mouth. Hold the breath as long as possible, then breathe out slowly.
The plastic mouthpiece should be cleaned daily. Remove metal vial and wash adapter with soap and hot water and rinse thoroughly. Dry and replace with vial.

How Supplied: ½ fl. oz. (15 ml). Available as combination package metal vial plus plastic mouthpiece, or as refill metal vial only.

ASTHMANEFRIN®
Solution "A" Bronchodilator

Active Ingredients: Racepinephrine Hydrochloride Equivalent to 2.25% Epinephrine base. **Inactive Ingredients:** Benzoic Acid, Chlorobutanol, Glycerin, Hydrochloric Acid, Sodium Bisulfite, Sodium Chloride, Water.

Indications: For temporary relief of shortness of breath, tightness of chest, and wheezing due to bronchial asthma.

Warnings: Do not use this product unless a diagnosis of asthma has been made by a physician. Do not use this product if you have heart disease, high blood pressure, thyroid disease, diabetes, or difficulty in urination due to enlargement of the prostate gland unless directed by a physician. Do not use this product if you have ever been hospitalized for asthma or if you are taking any prescription drug for asthma unless directed by a physician.
DO NOT USE THIS PRODUCT MORE FREQUENTLY OR AT HIGHER DOSES THAN RECOMMENDED UNLESS DIRECTED BY A PHYSICIAN.
Excessive use may cause nervousness and rapid heart beat, and possibly, adverse effects on the heart. **DO NOT CONTINUE TO USE THIS PRODUCT, BUT SEEK MEDICAL ASSISTANCE IMMEDIATELY IF SYMPTOMS ARE NOT RELIEVED WITHIN 20 MINUTES OR BECOME WORSE.**
Do not use this product if it is pinkish or darker than slightly yellow or if it contains a precipitate.

Drug Interaction Precaution: Do not use this product if you are presently taking a prescription drug for high blood pressure or depression, without first consulting your physician.
As with any drug, if you are pregnant or nursing a baby, seek the advice of a physician before using this product.
Keep this and all medication out of the reach of children.
Store at 59° to 75° F. Avoid excessive heat.

Dosage and Administration: Inhalation dosage for adults and children 4 years of age and older: 1 to 3 inhalations not more often than every 3 hours. The use of this product by children should be supervised by an adult. Children under 4 years of age: consult a physician.

Directions: For use in hand-held rubber bulb nebulizer. Pour at least 8 drops of solution into ASTHMANEFRIN NEBULIZER.
Care of Solution: Refrigerate once bottle has been opened.

How Supplied: ½ fl. oz. (15 ml) and 1 fl. oz. (30 ml) Solutions. FOR USE WITH ASTHMANEFRIN® NEBULIZER.

BENZEDREX® INHALER
Nasal Decongestant

Active Ingredient: Propylhexedrine, 250 mg. **Inactive Ingredients:** Lavender Oil, Menthol.

Indications: For the temporary relief of nasal congestion due to the common cold, hay fever, or associated with sinusitis.

Directions: This product delivers in each 800 milliliters of air 0.04 to 0.50 milligrams of propylhexedrine. Adults and children 6 to 12 years of age (with adult supervision): 2 inhalations in each nostril not more often than every 2 hours. Children under 6 years of age: consult a physician.
This inhaler is effective for a minimum of 3 months after first use.

Warnings: Do not use this product continuously for more than 3 days. If symptoms persist, consult a physician. Do not exceed recommended dosage because burning, stinging, sneezing, or increase of nasal discharge may occur. The use of this container by more than one person may spread infection. **Keep this and all medication out of the reach of children.** Ill effects may result if taken internally. In case of accidental overdose or ingestion of contents, seek professional assistance or contact a Poison Control Center immediately. As with any drug, if you are pregnant or nursing a baby, seek the advice of a health professional before using this product.
Store at controlled room temperature (59°–86°F).

Keep inhaler tightly closed.

TAMPER-RESISTANT PACKAGE FEATURE FOR YOUR PROTECTION:

- Inhaler sealed with imprinted cellophane.
- **DO NOT USE THIS PRODUCT IF TAMPER-RESISTANT FEATURE IS MISSING OR BROKEN. IF YOU HAVE ANY QUESTIONS, PLEASE CALL 1-800-321-1834 TOLL FREE.**

How Supplied: In single plastic tubes.

Shown in Product Identification Section, page 415

CONGESTAC®
Congestion Relief Medicine
Nasal Decongestant/Expectorant Caplets

Product Information: Helps you breathe easier by temporarily relieving nasal congestion associated with the common cold, sinusitis, hay fever and allergies. Also helps relieve chest congestion by loosening phlegm and clearing bronchial passages of excess mucus. Contains no antihistamines which may overdry or make you drowsy.

Active Ingredients: Each caplet contains Guaifenesin 400 mg, Pseudoephedrine Hydrochloride 60 mg. **Inactive Ingredients:** Cellulose, Croscarmellose Sodium, Hydroxypropyl Methylcellulose, Magnesium Stearate, Polyethylene Glycol, Povidone, Silica Gel, Starch and trace amounts of other ingredients.

Directions: One caplet every 4 hours not to exceed 4 caplets in 24 hours. Children (6 to 12 years): one-half the adult dose (break caplet in half). Children under 6 years use only as directed by physician.

TAMPER-RESISTANT PACKAGE FEATURES FOR YOUR PROTECTION:

- The carton has been sealed at the factory with a clear overwrap printed with "safety sealed."
- Each caplet is encased in a clear plastic cell with a foil back.
- The letter "C" appears on each caplet (see product illustration on front of carton).
- **DO NOT USE THIS PRODUCT IF ANY OF THESE TAMPER-RESIST-ANT FEATURES IS MISSING OR BROKEN. IF YOU HAVE ANY QUESTIONS, PLEASE CALL 1-800-321-1834 TOLL FREE.**

Warning: Do not exceed recommended dosage. If symptoms do not improve within 7 days or are accompanied by high fever, rash, shortness of breath or persistent headache, consult a physician before continuing use. If you have or are being treated for high blood pressure, heart disease, diabetes, thyroid disease, persistent or chronic cough, or difficulty in urination due to enlargment of the prostate gland, use only as directed by a physician. **Keep this and all medication out of reach of children.**In case of accidental overdose, seek professional assistance or contact a Poison Control Center imme-diately. As with any drug, if you are pregnant or nursing a baby, seek the advice of a health professional before using this product.

Drug Interaction Precaution: Do not take this product if you are presently taking a prescription antihypertensive or antidepressant drug containing a monoamine oxidase inhibitor except under the advice and supervision of a physician.

Store at controlled room temperature (59°–86°F).

The CONGESTAC horizontal color bar is a trademark.

How Supplied: In consumer packages of 12 and 24 caplets.

Shown in Product Identification Section, page 415

FEMIRON® MultiVitamins and Iron
[fem 'i 'ern]

Each Tablet Contains:

	Quantity	% of U.S. RDA
Vitamin A	5,000 I.U.	100
Vitamin D	400 I.U.	100
Vitamin E	15 I.U.	50
Vitamin C	60 mg	100
Folic Acid	0.4 mg	100
Vitamin B$_1$	1.5 mg	100
Vitamin B$_2$	1.7 mg	100
Niacinamide	20 mg	100
Vitamin B$_6$	2 mg	100
Vitamin B$_{12}$	6 mcg	100
Pantothenic Acid	10 mg	100
Iron	**20 mg**	**111**

Ingredients: Calcium Carbonate, Ferrous Fumarate, Ascorbic Acid, Gelatin, Niacinamide, Vitamin E Acetate, Starch, Calcium Pantothenate, Microcrystalline Cellulose, Calcium Silicate, Alginic Acid, Hydroxypropyl Methylcellulose, Crospovidone, Stearic Acid, Sodium Lauryl Sulfate, Vitamin A Acetate, Pyridoxine Hydrochloride, FD&C Red 40, FD&C Blue 2, Riboflavin, Thiamine Mononitrate, Polyethylene Glycol. Magnesium Stearate, Folic Acid, Polysorbate 80, Vitamin D, Cyanocobalamin.

Indications: For use as an iron and vitamin supplement.

Actions: Helps ensure adequate intake of iron and vitamins.

Warning: Keep this and all medication out of the reach of children.

Precaution: Alcoholics and individuals with chronic liver or pancreatic disease may have enhanced iron absorption with the potential for iron overload. NOTE: Unabsorbed iron may cause some darkening of the stool.

Symptoms and Treatment of Oral Overdosage: Toxicity and symptoms are primarily due to iron overdose. Abdominal pain, nausea, vomiting and diarrhea may occur, with possible subsequent acidosis and cardiovascular collapse with severe poisoning. **Treatment:** Induce vomiting immediately. Administer milk, eggs to reduce gastric irritation. Contact a physician immediately.

Dosage and Administration: Women: One tablet daily.

TAMPER-RESISTANT PACKAGE FEATURE:

- Bottle has imprinted seal under cap.
- **DO NOT USE IF SEAL IS BROKEN OR MISSING. IF YOU HAVE ANY QUESTIONS, PLEASE CALL 1-800-321-1834 TOLL FREE.**

Store at controlled room temperature (59°–86°F).

How Supplied: Bottles of 35, 60, and 90 tablets. Femiron Iron Supplement (no added vitamins) is also available.

Shown in Product Identification Section, page 415

HOLD®
4 Hour Cough Suppressant Lozenge

Active Ingredient: Each lozenge contains Dextromethorphan Hydrobromide 5 mg. **Inactive Ingredients:** Original Flavor—Corn Syrup, D&C Yellow 10, Flavors, Sucrose, Vegetable Oil and trace amounts of other ingredients.
Cherry Flavor—Corn Syrup, FD&C Blue 1, FD&C Red 40, Imitation Flavor, Sucrose, Vegetable Oil and trace amounts of other ingredients.

Indications: Temporarily suppresses coughs due to minor sore throat and bronchial irritation associated with a cold or inhaled irritants.

Actions: Dextromethorphan is the most widely used, non-narcotic/non-habit forming antitussive. A 10-20 mg dose has been recognized as being effective in relieving the discomfort of coughs up to 4 hours by reducing cough intensity and frequency.

Warnings: Do not take this product for persistent or chronic cough such as occurs with smoking, asthma, chronic bronchitis, or emphysema, or where cough is accompanied by excessive phlegm (mucus), unless directed by a physician. A persistent cough may be a sign of a serious condition. If cough persists for more than one week, tends to recur, or is accompanied by fever, rash or persistent headache, consult a physician. Do not give this product to children under 6 years of age unless directed by a physician. As with any drug, if you are pregnant or nursing a baby, seek the advice of a health professional before using this product. **Keep this and all medication out of the reach of children.**In case of accidental overdose, seek professional assistance or contact a Poison Control Center immediately.

Dosage and Administration: Adults (12 years and older): Take two lozenges one after the other, every 4 hours as needed. **Children** (6-12 years): Take one lozenge every 4 hours as needed. Let dissolve fully.

Continued on next page

Menley & James—Cont.

How Supplied: Available in Original Flavor and Cherry Flavor. 10 individually wrapped lozenges come packaged in a plastic tube container.

Shown in Product Identification Section, page 415

LIQUIPRIN®
Infants' Drops
(acetaminophen)

Description: LIQUIPRIN is a nonsalicylate analgesic and antipyretic particularly suitable for infants and children. LIQUIPRIN Drops is a raspberry-flavored, reddish pink solution. It contains no alcohol.

Active Ingredient: Acetaminophen 80 mg per 1.66 ml (top mark on dropper).
Inactive Ingredients: Artificial Raspberry and other artificial and natural flavors, Citric Acid, D&C Red 33, Dextrose, FD&C Red 40, Fructose, Glycerin, Methylparaben, Polyethylene Glycol, Propylene Glycol, Propylparaben, Sodium Citrate, Sodium Gluconate, Sucrose, Water.

Actions: LIQUIPRIN safely and effectively reduces fever and pain in infants and children without the hazards of salicylate therapy (e.g., gastric mucosal irritation).

Warnings: Do not give this product for pain for more than 5 days or for fever for more than 3 days unless directed by a physician. If pain or fever persists or gets worse, if new symptoms occur, or if redness or swelling is present, consult a physician because these could be signs of a serious condition.

Indications: LIQUIPRIN is indicated for use in the treatment of infants and children with conditions requiring reduction of fever and/or relief of pain such as mild upper respiratory infections (tonsillitis, common cold, flu), teething, headache, myalgia, postimmunization reactions, posttonsillectomy discomfort and gastroenteritis. As adjunctive therapy with antibiotics or sulfonamides, LIQUIPRIN may be useful as an analgesic and antipyretic in bacterial or viral infections, such as bronchitis, pharyngitis, tracheobronchitis, sinusitis, pneumonia, otitis media and cervical adenitis.

Precautions and Adverse Reactions: If a sensitivity reaction occurs, the drug should be discontinued. LIQUIPRIN has rarely been found to produce side effects. It is usually well tolerated by patients who are sensitive to products containing aspirin.

Usual Dosage: LIQUIPRIN may be given alone or mixed with milk, juices, applesauce or other beverages and foods. All dosages may be repeated every 4 hours, if pain and fever persist, but not to exceed 5 times daily or as directed by physician.

LIQUIPRIN should be administered in the following dosages:
0–3 months: 40 mg—½ dropperful
4–11 months: 80 mg—1 dropperful
12–23 months: 120 mg—1½ droppersful
2–3 years, 24–35 lbs.: 160 mg—2 droppersful
4–5 years, 36–47 lbs.: 240 mg—3 droppersful
Store at controlled room temperature. Avoid excessive heat.

How Supplied: LIQUIPRIN is available in a 1.16 fl. oz. (35 ml) plastic bottle with a calibrated dropper and child-resistant cap, and safety-sealed package.
Shown in Product Identification Section, page 415

ORNEX®
Decongestant/Analgesic
Caplets

Product Information: For temporary relief of nasal congestion, headache, aches, pains and fever due to colds, sinusitis and flu.

NO ANTIHISTAMINE DROWSINESS

Active Ingredients: Each caplet contains Acetaminophen 325 mg, Pseudoephedrine Hydrochloride 30 mg. **Inactive Ingredients:** Cellulose, Crospovidone, FD&C Blue 1, Hydroxypropyl Methylcellulose, Magnesium Stearate, Polyethylene Glycol, Polysorbate 80, Povidone, Starch, Titanium Dioxide and trace amounts of other inactive ingredients.

Directions: Adults—TWO CAPLETS every 4 hours, not to exceed 8 caplets in any 24-hour period. Children (6 to 12 years)—ONE CAPLET every 4 hours, not to exceed 4 caplets in 24 hours.
TAMPER-RESISTANT PACKAGE FEATURES FOR YOUR PROTECTION:
● The carton has been sealed at the factory with a clear overwrap printed with "safety sealed."
● Each caplet is encased in a clear plastic cell with a foil back.
● The name ORNEX appears on each caplet (see product illustration on front of carton).
● DO NOT USE THIS PRODUCT IF ANY OF THESE TAMPER-RESISTANT FEATURES IS MISSING OR BROKEN. IF YOU HAVE ANY QUESTIONS, PLEASE CALL 1-800-321-1834 TOLL FREE.

Warnings: Do not exceed recommended dosage. Do not use for more than 10 days or give to children under 6, unless directed by a physician. If you have, or are being treated for depression, high blood pressure, diabetes, heart disease, thyroid disease, or difficulty in urination due to enlargement of the prostate gland, use only as directed by a physician. Stop use if dizziness, sleeplessness or nervousness occurs. **Keep this and all medication out of reach of children.** In case of accidental overdose, seek professional assistance or contact a Poison Control Center immediately. As with any drug, if you are pregnant or nursing a baby, seek

the advice of a health professional before using this product.
Store at controlled room temperature (59°–86°F.).

How Supplied: In consumer packages of 24 and 48 caplets. Also, Dispensary Packages of 792 caplets for industrial dispensaries and student health clinics only.
Shown in Product Identification Section, page 415

MAXIMUM STRENGTH
ORNEX®
Decongestant/Analgesic
Caplets

Product Information: For temporary relief of nasal congestion, headache, aches, pains and fever due to colds, sinusitis and flu.

NO ANTIHISTAMINE DROWSINESS

Active Ingredients: Each caplet contains Acetaminophen 500 mg, Pseudoephedrine Hydrochloride 30 mg. **Inactive Ingredients:** Cellulose, Crospovidone, Hydroxypropyl Methylcellulose, Magnesium Stearate, Polyethylene Glycol, Polysorbate 80, Povidone, Starch, Titanium Dioxide and trace amounts of other ingredients.

Directions: Adults—TWO CAPLETS every 4 hours, not to exceed 8 caplets in any 24-hour period. Children (6 to 12 years)—ONE CAPLET every 4 hours, not to exceed 4 caplets in 24 hours.
TAMPER-RESISTANT PACKAGE FEATURES FOR YOUR PROTECTION:
● The carton has been sealed at the factory with a clear overwrap printed with "safety sealed."
● Each caplet is encased in a clear plastic cell with a foil back.
● The name ORNEX MAX appears on each caplet (see product illustration on front of carton).
● DO NOT USE THIS PRODUCT IF ANY OF THESE TAMPER-RESISTANT FEATURES IS MISSING OR BROKEN. IF YOU HAVE ANY QUESTIONS, PLEASE CALL 1-800-321-1834 TOLL FREE.

Warnings: Do not exceed recommended dosage. Do not use for more than 10 days or give to children under 6, unless directed by a physician. If you have, or are being treated for depression, high blood pressure, diabetes, heart disease, thyroid disease, or difficulty in urination due to enlargement of the prostate gland, use only as directed by a physician. Stop use if dizziness, sleeplessness or nervousness occurs. **Keep this and all medication out of reach of children.** In case of accidental overdose, seek professional assistance or contact a Poison Control Center immediately. As with any drug, if you are pregnant or nursing a baby, seek the advice of a health professional before using this product.
Store at controlled room temperature (59°–86°F.).

How Supplied: In consumer packages of 24 and 48 caplets.

Shown in Product Identification Section, page 415

S.T.37®
Antiseptic Solution

Active Ingredients: Hexylresorcinol 0.10%, Glycerin 28.2%. **Inactive Ingredients:** Sodium Bisulfite and Water.

Indications: For use as a soothing antiseptic and anesthetic solution on minor cuts, abrasions, and burns.
For temporary relief of occasional minor irritation or pain associated with sore mouth or sore throat.
May also be used to cleanse cuts and scrapes.

Directions: Adults and children 2 years of age and older:
For external use: Use full strength. Apply liberally as often as necessary.
For the mouth: Dilute with 2 parts water. Gargle or rinse for about 15 seconds, then spit out. May be repeated up to 4 times daily, if necessary.

Warnings: Do not use S.T.37 to treat deep or puncture wounds, wild or domestic animal bites, or infections. Instead, consult your physician immediately. If redness, irritation, swelling or pain persists or increases, or if infection occurs, discontinue use and consult a physician. If sore throat is severe or persists for more than 2 days, or worsens, is accompanied or followed by fever, headache, rash, nausea, or vomiting, consult your physician promptly. If sore mouth symptoms do not improve in 7 days, see your dentist or physician. Do not administer to children under 2 years of age, unless directed by your physician. Avoid contact with the eyes. **Keep this and all medicines out of the reach of children.** As with any drug, if you are pregnant or nursing a baby, seek the advice of a health professional before using.

How Supplied:
5.5 and 12 fl. oz. bottles.

SERUTAN®
Toasted Granules
(brand of psyllium hydrophilic mucilloid)

Description: SERUTAN TOASTED GRANULES are an effective, natural way to restore or maintain regularity. They contain psyllium, one of the richest natural sources of soluble dietary fiber available. Unlike other psyllium products that are powdered, SERUTAN GRANULES need no mixing. Crunchy and lightly sweetened, they can be sprinkled on everday foods like cereal or oatmeal, salads, applesauce, casseroles, yogurt and desserts, accompanied by an 8 oz. beverage. SERUTAN GRANULES contain no chemical stimulants, are not habit forming, and can be used daily to maintain regularity by those who may not otherwise get enough fiber in their diets.

Action: SERUTAN GRANULES promotes normal elimination and regularity by increasing bulk volume and water content of the stool.

Indications: For the management of chronic constipation, irritable bowel syndrome and constipation due to pregnancy, convalescence or senility. Also for stool softening in hemorrhoid patients.

Directions: Adults: One to three heaping teaspoons 1 to 3 times daily sprinkled on food (cereals, salads, casseroles, desserts, etc.) Be sure to drink at least 8 oz. of liquid (a full glass) with your food each time you use SERUTAN GRANULES. SERUTAN GRANULES should always be put on food, not taken directly from a spoon. Children 6–12: give half the adult dose with 8 oz. of liquid. Do not exceed 9 teaspoons per day or five teaspoons per day for children 6–12. Note: it may require two to three days' therapy to produce full effectiveness.

Contraindications: Fecal impaction or intestinal obstruction.

Tamper resistant feature for your protection: Imprinted neck seal under cap. Do not use if seal is missing or broken. If you have any questions, please call 1-800-321-1834 toll free.

Warning: Keep this and all medications out of reach of children. May cause allergic reaction in those individuals sensitive to psyllium.

Active Ingredient: Psyllium Hydrophilic Mucilloid, 2.5 grams per heaping teaspoon. **Inactive Ingredients:** Acacia, BHA, Calcium Propionate, Caramel Color, Carboxymethylcellulose Sodium, Corn Starch, Invert Sugar, Magnesium Stearate, Oat Flour, Sodium Benzoate, Sodium Saccharin, Sucrose, Vegetable Oil, Wheat Germ.
Low sodium—less than 0.03 grams per teaspoon.

How Supplied: Available in 6 oz. and 18 oz. plastic jars. SERUTAN is also available in two other formulas: Regular Powder (in 7 oz., 14 oz. and 21 oz. sizes) and Fruit Flavored Powder (in 6 oz., 12 oz. and 18 oz. sizes).
Store at controlled room temperature (59°–86°F).

Shown in Product Identification Section, page 415

THERMOTABS®
[*ther 'mo-tabs*]
Buffered Salt Tablets

Active Ingredients: Each tablet contains Sodium Chloride 450 mg, Potassium Chloride 30 mg. **Inactive Ingredients:** Acacia, Calcium Carbonate, Calcium Stearate, Dextrose.

Indications: To minimize fatigue and prevent muscle cramps and heat prostration due to excessive perspiration.

Actions: THERMOTABS are designed for tennis players, joggers, golfers and other athletes who experience excessive perspiration. Also for use in steel mills, industrial plants, kitchens, stores, or other locations where high temperatures cause heat fatigue, cramps or heat prostration.

Warnings: If you have or are being treated for heart disease or high blood pressure, consult your physician before using this product. **Keep this and all medication out of the reach of children.** As with any drug, if you are pregnant or nursing a baby, seek the advice of a health professional before using this product.

Precaution: Individuals on a salt-restricted diet should use THERMOTABS only under the advice and supervision of a physician.

Symptoms and Treatment of Oral Overdosage: Signs of salt overdose include diarrhea and muscular twitching. If an overdose is suspected, contact a physician, the local Poison Control Center, or call the Rocky Mt. Poison Control Center at 303-592-1710 (Collect), 24 hours a day.

Dosage and Administration: One tablet with a full glass of water, 5 to 10 times a day depending on temperature and conditions.

How Supplied: 100 tablet bottles.

TROPH–IRON®
Vitamins B₁, B₁₂ and Iron

Indications: For deficiencies of vitamins B_1, B_{12} and iron.

Active Ingredients: Each 5 ml. (1 teaspoonful) contains Thiamine Hydrochloride (vitamin B_1), 10 mg.; Cyanocobalamin (vitamin B_{12}), 25 mcg.; Iron, 20 mg., present as soluble ferric pyrophosphate. **Inactive Ingredients:** Citric Acid, FD&C Red 40, Flavor, Glucose, Glycerin, Methyl and Propyl Paraben, Saccharin Sodium, Sodium Citrate, Purified Water.

Directions: One teaspoonful daily, or as directed by physician. While its effectiveness is in no way affected, TROPH-IRON Liquid may darken as it ages.

TAMPER-RESISTANT PACKAGE FEATURE: Sealed, imprinted bottle cap; do not use if broken.

Warning: The treatment of any anemic condition should be under the advice and supervision of a physician. Since oral iron products interfere with absorption of oral tetracycline antibiotics, these products should not be taken within two hours of each other.
Iron-containing medications may occasionally cause gastrointestinal discomfort, such as nausea, constipation or diarrhea.
Keep this and all medication out of reach of children. In case of accidental overdose, seek professional assistance or contact a Poison Control Center immediately.
As with any drug, if you are pregnant or nursing a baby, seek the advice of a

Continued on next page

Menley & James—Cont.

health professional before using this product.

Store at controlled room temperature (59°–86°F).

How Supplied: 4 fl. oz. (118 ml) bottles.

TROPHITE®
Vitamins B₁ and B₁₂

Indications: For deficiencies of vitamins B_1 and B_{12}.

Active Ingredients: Each 5 ml. (1 teaspoonful) contains Thiamine Hydrochloride (vitamin B_1), 10 mg.; and Cyanocobalamin (vitamin B_{12}), 25 mcg. **Inactive Ingredients:** D&C Red 33, D&C Yellow 10, Dextrose, FD&C Blue 1, Flavor, Glycerin, Methyl and Propyl Paraben, Sodium Tartrate, Tartaric Acid, Purified Water.

Directions: One 5 ml. teaspoonful or as directed by physician.

Important: Dispense liquid only in original bottle or an amber bottle. This product is light-sensitive. Never dispense in a flint, green, or blue bottle.
TROPHITE Liquid may be mixed with water, milk, or fruit or vegetable juices immediately before taking.
TAMPER-RESISTANT PACKAGE FEATURE: Sealed, imprinted bottle cap; do not use if broken.

Warning: Keep this and all medication out of reach of children. In case of accidental overdose, seek professional assistance or contact a Poison Control Center immediately.
As with any drug, if you are pregnant or nursing a baby, seek the advice of a health professional before using this product.
Store at controlled room temperature (59°–86°F).

How Supplied: 4 fl. oz. (118 ml.) bottles.

Miles Inc.
P. O. BOX 340
ELKHART, IN 46515

ALKA–MINTS® Chewable Antacid Rich in Calcium

Active Ingredient: Each ALKA-MINTS Chewable Antacid tablet contains calcium carbonate 850 mg. (340 mg of elemental calcium). Each tablet contains less than .5 mg sodium per tablet, and is dietarily sodium free.

Inactive Ingredients: Dioctyl sodium sulfosuccinate, flavor, hydrolyzed cereal solids, magnesium stearate, polyethylene glycol, sorbitol, sugar (compressible)

Indications: ALKA-MINTS is an antacid for occasional use for relief of acid indigestion, heartburn and sour stomach.

Actions: ALKA-MINTS has a natural, clean, spearmint taste that leaves the mouth feeling refreshed. Measured by the in-vitro standard established by the Food and Drug Administration, one ALKA-MINTS tablet neutralizes 15.9 mEq of acid.

Warnings: Do not take more than 9 tablets in a 24 hour period, or use the maximum dosage of this product for more than 2 weeks, except under the advice and supervision of a physician. May cause constipation. As with any drug, if you are pregnant or nursing a baby, seek the advice of a health professional before using this product. Keep this and all drugs out of the reach of children.

Dosage and Administration: Chew 1 tablet every 2 hours or as directed by a physician.

How Supplied: Cartons of 30's. Each carton contains convenient pocket-sized packs with individually sealed tablets so ALKA-MINTS stay fresh wherever you go.

Product Identification Mark:
ALKA-MINTS embossed on each tablet.
Shown in Product Identification Section, page 416

ALKA–SELTZER® Effervescent Antacid & Pain Reliever With Specially Buffered Aspirin

Active Ingredients: Each tablet contains: aspirin 325 mg., heat treated sodium bicarbonate 1916 mg., citric acid 1000 mg. ALKA-SELTZER® in water contains principally the antacid sodium citrate and the analgesic sodium acetylsalicylate. Buffered pH is between 6 and 7.

Inactive Ingredients: None.

Indications: ALKA-SELTZER® Effervescent Antacid & Pain Reliever is an analgesic and an antacid and is indicated for relief of sour stomach, acid indigestion or heartburn with headache or body aches and pains. Also for fast relief of upset stomach with headache from overindulgence in food and drink—especially recommended for taking before bed and again on arising. Effective for pain relief alone: headache or body or muscular aches and pains.

Actions: When the ALKA-SELTZER® Effervescent Antacid & Pain Reliever tablet is dissolved in water, the acetylsalicylate ion differs from acetylsalicylic acid chemically, physically and pharmacologically. Being fat insoluble, it is not absorbed by the gastric mucosal cells. Studies and observations in animals and man including radiochrome determinations of fecal blood loss, measurement of ion fluxes and direct visualization with gastrocamera, have shown that, as contrasted with acetylsalicylic acid, the acetylsalicylate ion delivered in the solution does not alter gastric mucosal permeability to permit back-diffusion of hydrogen ion, and gastric damage and acute gastric

mucosal lesions are therefore not seen after administration of the product. ALKA-SELTZER® Effervescent Antacid & Pain Reliever has the capacity to neutralize gastric hydrochloric acid quickly and effectively. In-vitro, 154 ml. of 0.1 N hydrochloric acid are required to decrease the pH of one tablet of ALKA-SELTZER® Effervescent Antacid & Pain Reliever in solution to 4.0. Measured against the in vitro standard established by the Food and Drug Administration one tablet neutralizes 17.2 mEq of acid. In vivo, the antacid activity of two ALKA-SELTZER® Antacid & Pain Reliever tablets is comparable to that of 10 ml. of milk of magnesia. ALKA-SELTZER® Effervescent Antacid & Pain Reliever is able to resist pH changes caused by the continuing secretion of acid in the normal individual and to maintain an elevated pH until emptying occurs.
ALKA-SELTZER® Effervescent Antacid & Pain Reliever provides highly water soluble acetylsalicylate ions which are fat insoluble. Acetylsalicylate ions are not absorbed from the stomach. They empty from the stomach and thereby become available for absorption from the duodenum. Thus, fast drug absorption and high plasma acetylsalicylate levels are achieved. Plasma levels of salicylate following the administration of ALKA-SELTZER® Effervescent Antacid & Pain Reliever solution (acetylsalicylate ion equivalent to 648 mg. acetylsalicylic acid) can reach 29 mg./liter in 10 minutes and rise to peak levels as high as 55 mg./liter within 30 minutes.

Warnings: Children and teenagers should not use this medicine for chicken pox or flu symptoms before a doctor is consulted about Reye syndrome, a rare but serious illness reported to be associated with aspirin. As with any drug, if you are pregnant or nursing a baby, seek the advice of a health professional before using this product. IT IS ESPECIALLY IMPORTANT NOT TO USE ASPIRIN DURING THE LAST 3 MONTHS OF PREGNANCY UNLESS SPECIFICALLY DIRECTED TO DO SO BY A DOCTOR BECAUSE IT MAY CAUSE PROBLEMS IN THE UNBORN CHILD OR COMPLICATIONS DURING DELIVERY. Except under the advice and supervision of a physician, do not take more than, Adults: 8 tablets in a 24 hour period. (60 years of age or older: 4 tablets in a 24 hour period), or use the maximum dosage for more than 10 days. Do not use if you are allergic to aspirin or have asthma, if you have a coagulation (bleeding) disease, or if you are on a sodium restricted diet. Each tablet contains 567 mg. of sodium.
Keep this and all drugs out of the reach of children.

Dosage and Administration:
ALKA-SELTZER® must be dissolved in water before taking.
Adults: 2 tablets every 4 hours.
CAUTION: If symptoms persist or recur frequently, or if you are under treatment for ulcer, consult your physician.

Professional Labeling:

ASPIRIN FOR MYOCARDIAL INFARCTION

Indication: The Aspirin contained in ALKA-SELTZER® is indicated to reduce the risk of death and/or non-fatal myocardial infarction in patients with a previous infarction or unstable angina pectoris.

Clinical Trials: The indication is supported by the results of six, large, randomized multicenter, placebo-controlled studies[1-7] involving 10,816, predominantly male, post-myocardial infarction (MI) patients and one randomized placebo-controlled study of 1,266 men with unstable angina. Therapy with aspirin was begun at intervals after the onset of acute MI varying from less than 3 days to more than 5 years and continued for periods of from less than one year to four years. In the unstable angina study, treatment was started within 1 month after the onset of unstable angina and continued for 12 weeks and complicating conditions such as congestive heart failure were not included in the study.

Aspirin therapy in MI patients was associated with about a 20 percent reduction in the risk of subsequent death and/or non-fatal reinfarction, a median absolute decrease of 3 percent from the 12 to 22 percent event rates in the placebo groups. In aspirin-treated unstable angina patients the reduction in risk was about 50 percent, a reduction in event rate of 5 percent from the 10 percent rate in the placebo group over the 12 weeks of the study.

Daily dosage of aspirin in the post-myocardial infarction studies was 300 mg in one study and 900 to 1500 mg in five studies. A dose of 325 mg was used in the study of unstable angina.

Adverse Reactions: Gastrointestinal Reactions: Symptoms and signs of gastrointestinal irritation were not significantly increased in subjects treated for unstable angina with buffered aspirin in solution (ALKA-SELZER®.) Doses of 1000 mg per day of aspirin tablets caused gastrointestinal symptoms and bleeding that in some cases were clinically significant. In the largest post-infarction study (the Aspirin Myocardial Infarction Study (AMIS) with 4,500 people), the percentage incidences of gastrointestinal symptoms for the aspirin (1000 mg of a standard, solid-tablet formulation) and placebo-treated subjects, respectively, were: stomach pain (14.5%; 4.4%); heartburn (11.9%; 4.8%); nausea and/or vomiting (7.6%; 2.1%); hospitalization for gastrointestinal disorder (4.9%; 3.5%). In the AMIS and other trials, aspirin treated patients had increased rates of gross gastrointestinal bleeding. As with all aspirin products ALKA-SELTZER is contraindicated in patients with aspirin sensitivity, with asthma, or with coagulation disease.

Cardiovascular and Biochemical: In the AMIS trial, the dosage of 1000 mg per day of aspirin was associated with small increases in systolic blood pressure (BP) (average 1.5 to 2.1 mm) and diastolic BP (0.5 to 0.6 mm), depending upon whether maximal or last available readings were used. Blood urea nitrogen and uric acid levels were also increased, but by less than 1.0 mg%. Subjects with marked hypertension or renal insufficiency had been excluded from the trial so that the clinical importance of these observations for such subjects or for any subjects treated over more prolonged periods is not known. It is recommended that patients placed on long-term aspirin treatment, even at doses of 300 mg per day, be seen at regular intervals to assess changes in these measurements.

Sodium in Buffered Aspirin for Solution Formulations: One tablet daily of buffered aspirin in solution adds 567 mg of sodium to that in the diet and may not be tolerated by patients with active sodium-retaining states such as congestive heart or renal failure. This amount of sodium adds about 30 percent to the 70 to 90 meq intake suggested as appropriate for dietary treatment of essential hypertension in the 1984 Report of the Joint National Committee on Detection, Evaluation, and Treatment of High Blood Pressure.[8]

Dosage and Administration: Although most of the studies used dosages exceeding 300 mg daily, two trials used only 300 mg and pharmacologic data indicate that this dose inhibits platelet function fully. Therefore, 300 mg or a conventional 325 mg aspirin dose daily is a reasonable, routine dose that would minimize gastrointestinal adverse reactions. This use of aspirin applies to both solid, oral dosage forms (buffered and plain aspirin) and buffered aspirin in solution.

References:
(1) Elwood, P. C., et al., A Randomized Controlled Trial of Acetysalicylic Acid in the Secondary Prevention of Mortality from Myocardial Infarction," *British Medical Journal* 1:436–440, 1974.
(2) The Coronary Drug Project Research Group, "Aspirin in Coronary Heart Disease," *Journal of Chronic Diseases,* 29:625–642, 1976.
(3) Breddin K., et al., "Secondary Prevention of Myocardial Infarction: A Comparison of Acetylsalicylic Acid, Phenprocoumon or Placebo," *International Congress Series* 470:263–268, 1979.
(4) Aspirin Myocardial Infarction Study Research Group, "A Randomized, Controlled Trial of Aspirin in Persons Recovered from Myocardial Infarction," *Journal American Medical Association* 245:661–669, 1980.
(5) Elwood, P. C., and P. M. Sweetnam, "Aspirin and Secondary Mortality after Myocardial Infarction," *Lancet* pp. 1313–1315, December 22–29, 1979.
(6) The Persantine-Aspirin Reinfarction Study Research Group, "Persantine and Aspirin in Coronary Heart Disease," *Circulation,* 62: 449–460, 1980.
(7) Lewis, H. D., et al., "Protective Effects of Aspirin Against Acute Myocardial Infarction and Death in Men with Unstable Angina, Results of a Veterans Administration Cooperative Study," *New England Journal of Medicine* 309:396–403, 1983.
(8) "1984 Report of the Joint National Committee on Detection, Evaluation, Treatment of High Blood Pressure," U.S. Department of Health and Human Services and United States Public Health Service, National Institutes of Health.

How Supplied: Tablets: foil sealed; box of 12 in 6 foil twin packs; box of 24 in 12 foil twin packs; box of 36 tablets in 18 foil twin packs; 100 tablets in 50 foil twin packs; carton of 72 tablets in 36 foil twin packs. Product Identification Mark: "ALKA-SELTZER" embossed on each tablet.

Shown in Product Identification Section, page 416

Flavored ALKA-SELTZER®
Effervescent Antacid & Pain Reliever

Active Ingredients: Each tablet contains: Aspirin 325 mg, heat treated sodium bicarbonate 1710 mg, citric acid 1220 mg. Alka-Seltzer in water contains principally the antacid sodium citrate and the analgesic sodium acetylsalicylate.

Inactive Ingredients: Flavors, Saccharin Sodium.

Indications: For fast relief of ACID INDIGESTION, SOUR STOMACH or HEARTBURN with HEADACHE, or BODY ACHES AND PAINS. Also for fast relief of UPSET STOMACH with HEADACHE from overindulgence in food and drink—especially recommended for taking before bed and again on arising. EFFECTIVE FOR PAIN RELIEF ALONE: HEADACHE or BODY and MUSCULAR ACHES and PAINS.

Warnings: Children and teenagers should not use this medicine for chicken pox or flu symptoms before a doctor is consulted about Reye syndrome, a rare but serious illness reported to be associated with aspirin.

As with any drug, if you are pregnant or nursing a baby, seek the advice of a health professional before using this product. IT IS ESPECIALLY IMPORTANT NOT TO USE ASPIRIN DURING THE LAST 3 MONTHS OF PREGNANCY UNLESS SPECIFICALLY DIRECTED TO DO SO BY A DOCTOR BECAUSE IT MAY CAUSE PROBLEMS IN THE UNBORN CHILD OR COMPLICATIONS DURING DELIVERY.

Except under the advice and supervision of a physician: Do not take more than, ADULTS: 6 tablets in a 24-hour period, (60 years of age or older: 4 tablets in a 24-hour period), or use the daily maximum dosage for more than 10 days. Do not use if you are allergic to aspirin or have

Continued on next page

Miles—Cont.

asthma, if you have a coagulation (bleeding) disease, or if you are on a sodium restricted diet. Each tablet contains 506 mg of sodium.

Keep this and all drugs out of the reach of children.

Directions: Alka-Seltzer must be dissolved in water before taking. ADULTS: 2 tablets every 4 hours. CAUTION: If symptoms persist or recur frequently or if you are under treatment for ulcer, consult your physician.

Professional Labeling:

ASPIRIN FOR MYOCARDIAL INFARCTION

Indication: The Aspirin contained in Alka-Seltzer is indicated to reduce the risk of death and/or non-fatal myocardial infarction in patients with a previous infarction or unstable angina pectoris.

Clinical Trials: The indication is supported by the results of six, large, randomized multicenter, placebo-controlled studies[1-7] involving 10,816, predominantly male, post-myocardial infarction (MI) patients and one randomized placebo-controlled study of 1,266 men with unstable angina. Therapy with aspirin was begun at intervals after the onset of acute MI varying from less than 3 days to more than 5 years and continued for periods of from less than one year to four years. In the unstable angina study, treatment was started within 1 month after the onset of unstable angina and continued for 12 weeks and complicating conditions such as congestive heart failure were not included in the study.

Aspirin therapy in MI patients was associated with about a 20 percent reduction in the risk of subsequent death and/or non-fatal reinfarction, a median absolute decrease of 3 percent from the 12 to 22 percent event rates in the placebo groups. In aspirin-treated unstable angina patients the reduction in risk was about 50 percent, a reduction in event rate of 5 percent from the 10 percent rate in the placebo group over the 12 weeks of the study.

Daily dosage of aspirin in the post-myocardial infarction studies was 300 mg in one study and 900 to 1500 mg in five studies. A dose of 325 mg was used in the study of unstable angina.

Adverse Reactions: Gastrointestinal Reactions: Symptoms and signs of gastrointestinal irritation were not significantly increased in subjects treated for unstable angina with buffered aspirin in solution (ALKA-SELZER®). Doses of 1000 mg per day of aspirin tablets caused gastrointestinal symptoms and bleeding that in some cases were clinically significant. In the largest post-infarction study (the Aspirin Myocardial Infarction Study (AMIS) with 4,500 people), the percentage incidences of gastrointestinal symptoms for the aspirin (1000 mg of a standard, solid-tablet formulation) and placebo-treated subjects, respectively, were:

stomach pain (14.5%; 4.4%); heartburn (11.9%; 4.8%); nausea and/or vomiting (7.6%; 2.1%); hospitalization for gastrointestinal disorder (4.9%; 3.5%). In the AMIS and other trials, aspirin treated patients had increased rates of gross gastrointestinal bleeding. As with all aspirin products Alka-Seltzer is contraindicated in patients with aspirin sensitivity, with asthma, or with coagulation disease.

Cardiovascular and Biochemical: In the AMIS trial, the dosage of 1000 mg per day of aspirin was associated with small increases in systolic blood pressure (BP) (average 1.5 to 2.1 mm) and diastolic BP (0.5 to 0.6 mm), depending upon whether maximal or last available readings were used. Blood urea nitrogen and uric acid levels were also increased, but by less than 1.0 mg%. Subjects with marked hypertension or renal insufficiency had been excluded from the trial so that the clinical importance of these observations for such subjects or for any subjects treated over more prolonged periods is not known. It is recommended that patients placed on long-term aspirin treatment, even at doses of 300 mg per day, be seen at regular intervals to assess changes in these measurements.

Sodium in Buffered Aspirin for Solution Formulations: One tablet daily of flavored buffered aspirin in solution adds 506 mg of sodium to that in the diet and may not be tolerated by patients with active sodium-retaining states such as congestive heart or renal failure. This amount of sodium adds about 30 percent to the 70 to 90 meq intake suggested as appropriate for dietary treatment of essential hypertension in the 1984 Report of the Joint National Committee on Detection, Evaluation, and Treatment of High Blood Pressure.[8]

Dosage and Administration: Although most of the studies used dosages exceeding 300 mg, daily, two trials used only 300 mg and pharmacologic data indicate that this dose inhibits platelet function fully. Therefore, 300 mg or a conventional 325 mg aspirin dose daily is a reasonable, routine dose that would minimize gastrointestinal adverse reactions. This use of aspirin applies to both solid, oral dosage forms (buffered and plain aspirin) and buffered aspirin in solution.

References:

(1) Elwood, P. C., et al., A Randomized Controlled Trial of Acetysalicylic Acid in the Secondary Prevention of Mortality from Myocardial Infarction," *British Medical Journal* 1:436–440, 1974.

(2) The Coronary Drug Project Research Group, "Aspirin in Coronary Heart Disease," *Journal of Chronic Diseases,* 29:625–642, 1976.

(3) Breddin K., et al., "Secondary Prevention of Myocardial Infarction: A Comparison of Acetylsalicylic Acid, Phenprocoumon or Placebo," *International Congress Series* 470:263–268, 1979.

(4) Aspirin Myocardial Infarction Study Research Group, "A Randomized, Controlled Trial of Aspirin in Persons Recovered from Myocardial Infarction," *Journal American Medical Association* 245:661–669, 1980.

(5) Elwood, P. C., and P. M. Sweetnam, "Aspirin and Secondary Mortality after Myocardial Infarction," *Lancet* pp. 1313–1315, December 22–29, 1979.

(6) The Persantine-Aspirin Reinfarction Study Research Group, "Persantine and Aspirin in Coronary Heart Disease," *Circulation*, 62: 449–460, 1980.

(7) Lewis, H. D., et al., "Protective Effects of Aspirin Against Acute Myocardial Infarction and Death in Men with Unstable Angina, Results of a Veterans Administration Cooperative Study," *New England Journal of Medicine* 309:396–403, 1983.

(8) "1984 Report of the Joint National Committee on Detection, Evaluation, Treatment of High Blood Pressure," U.S. Department of Health and Human Services and United States Public Health Service, National Institutes of Health.

How Supplied: Foil sealed effervescent tablets in cartons of 12's in 6 foil twin packs; 24's in 12 foil twin packs; 36's in 18 foil twin packs.

Shown in Product Identification Section, page 416

ALKA–SELTZER® Effervescent Antacid

Active Ingredients: Each tablet contains heat treated sodium bicarbonate 958 mg., citric acid 832 mg., potassium bicarbonate 312 mg. ALKA-SELTZER® Effervescent Antacid in water contains principally the antacids sodium citrate and potassium citrate.

Inactive Ingredients: A tableting aid.

Indications: ALKA-SELTZER® Effervescent Antacid is indicated for relief of acid indigestion, sour stomach or heartburn.

Actions: The ALKA-SELTZER® Effervescent Antacid solution provides quick and effective neutralization of gastric acid. Measured by the in vitro standard established by the Food and Drug Administration one tablet will neutralize 10.6 mEq of acid.

Warnings: Except under the advice and supervision of a physician, do not take more than: Adults: 8 tablets in a 24 hour period (60 years of age or older: 7 tablets in a 24 hour period), Children: 4 tablets in a 24 hour period; or use the maximum dosage of this product for more than 2 weeks.

Do not use this product if you are on a sodium restricted diet. Each tablet contains 311 mg. of sodium.

Keep this and all drugs out of the reach of children. As with any drug, if you are pregnant or nursing a baby, seek the advice of a health professional before using this product.

Dosage and Administration: Adults: Take 1 or 2 tablets fully dissolved in water every 4 hours. Children: ½ the adult dosage.

How Supplied: Boxes of 20 tablets in 10 foil twin packs; 36 tablets in 18 foil twin packs.

Shown in Product Identification Section, page 416

ALKA–SELTZER® Extra Strength Antacid & Pain Reliever

Active Ingredients: Each tablet contains: Aspirin 500mg, heat treated sodium bicarbonate 1985mg, citric acid 1000mg. Alka-Seltzer in water contains principally the antacid sodium citrate and the analgesic sodium acetylsalicylate.

Inactive Ingredients: Flavors

Indications: For fast relief of acid indigestion, sour stomach or heartburn with headache or body aches and pains. Also, for fast relief of upset stomach with headache from overindulgence in food and drink—especially recommended for taking before bed and again on arising. Effective for pain relief alone: headache or body and muscular aches and pains.

Warnings: Children and teenagers should not use this medicine for chicken pox or flu symptoms before a doctor is consulted about Reye syndrome, a rare but serious illness reported to be associated with aspirin. As with any drug, if you are pregnant or nursing a baby, seek the advice of a health professional before using this product. IT IS ESPECIALLY IMPORTANT NOT TO USE ASPIRIN DURING THE LAST 3 MONTHS OF PREGNANCY UNLESS SPECIFICALLY DIRECTED TO DO SO BY A DOCTOR BECAUSE IT MAY CAUSE PROBLEMS IN THE UNBORN CHILD OR COMPLICATIONS DURING DELIVERY. Except under the advice and supervision of a physician, do not take more than, Adults: 7 tablets in a 24-hour period (60 years of age or older, 4 tablets in a 24-hour period), or use the daily maximum dosage for more than 10 days. Do not use if you are allergic to aspirin or have asthma, if you have a coagulation (bleeding) disease, or if you are on a sodium restricted diet. Each tablet contains 588mg of sodium. Keep this and all drugs out of the reach of children.

Dosage and Administration: Extra Strength Alka-Seltzer must be dissolved in water before taking. Adults: 2 tablets every 4 hours. Caution: If symptoms persist, or recur frequently, or if you are under treatment for ulcer, consult your physician.

How Supplied: Foil sealed effervescent tablets in cartons of 12's in 6 foil twin packs; 24's in 12 foil twin packs.

Shown in Product Identification Section, page 416

ALKA-SELTZER PLUS®
Cold Medicine

Active Ingredients:
Each dry ALKA-SELTZER PLUS® Cold Tablet contains the following active ingredients: Phenylpropanolamine bitartrate 24.08 mg., chlorpheniramine maleate 2 mg., aspirin 325 mg. The product is dissolved in water prior to ingestion and the aspirin is converted into its soluble ionic form, sodium acetylsalicylate.

Inactive Ingredients: Citric acid, flavors, sodium bicarbonate.

Indications: For relief of the symptoms of common colds and flu.

Actions: Provides temporary relief of these major cold and flu symptoms: nasal and sinus congestion, runny nose, sneezing, headache, sore throat, fever, body aches and pains.

Warnings: Children and teenagers should not use this medicine for chicken pox or flu symptoms before a doctor is consulted about Reye syndrome, a rare but serious illness reported to be associated with aspirin. Do not exceed recommended dosage because at higher doses nervousness, dizziness or sleeplessness may occur. May cause excitability, especially in children. Do not take this product if you are allergic to aspirin or have asthma, glaucoma, bleeding problems, emphysema, chronic pulmonary disease, shortness of breath, difficulty in breathing, heart disease, high blood pressure, thyroid disease, diabetes or difficulty in urination due to enlargement of the prostate gland or on a sodium-restricted diet unless directed by a doctor. Each tablet contains 506 mg of sodium. May cause drowsiness; alcohol, sedatives and tranquilizers may increase drowsiness effect. Avoid alcoholic beverages while taking this product. Do not take this product if you are taking sedatives or tranquilizers without first consulting your doctor. Use caution when driving a motor vehicle or operating machinery. If sore throat is severe, persists for more than 2 days, is accompanied by a high fever, headache, nausea or vomiting, consult a physician promptly. Do not take this product for more than 7 days. If symptoms do not improve or are accompanied by fever or if fever persists for more than 3 days, consult a doctor. As with any drug, if you are pregnant or nursing a baby, seek the advice of a health professional before using this product. IT IS ESPECIALLY IMPORTANT NOT TO USE ASPIRIN DURING THE LAST 3 MONTHS OF PREGNANCY UNLESS SPECIFICALLY DIRECTED TO DO SO BY A DOCTOR BECAUSE IT MAY CAUSE PROBLEMS IN THE UNBORN CHILD OR COMPLICATIONS DURING DELIVERY. Keep this and all drugs out of the reach of children.

Drug Interaction Precaution: Do not take this product if you are presently taking a prescription drug for anticoagulation (thinning the blood), high blood pressure or depression without first consulting your doctor.

Dosage and Administration:
ALKA-SELTZER PLUS® is taken in solution; 2 tablets dissolved in approximately 4 ounces of water. Adults: two tablets every 4 hours up to 8 tablets in 24 hours.

How Supplied: Tablets: carton of 12 tablets in 6 foil twin packs; 20 tablets in 10 foil twin packs; carton of 36 tablets in 18 foil twin packs; carton of 48 tablets in 24 foil twin packs.
Product Identification Mark:
"Alka-Seltzer Plus" embossed on each tablet.

Shown in Product Identification Section, page 416

ALKA–SELTZER PLUS®
Night-Time Cold Medicine

Active Ingredients: Each tablet contains phenylpropanolamine bitartrate 24.08 mg, diphenhydramine citrate 38 mg, aspirin 325 mg. In water the aspirin is converted into its soluble ionic form, sodium acetylsalicylate.

Inactive Ingredients: Citric acid, flavors, heat-treated sodium bicarbonate, tableting aids.

Indications: For relief of the symptoms of common colds and flu, to help you get the rest you need.

Actions: Provides temporary relief of these major cold and flu symptoms: nasal and sinus congestion, runny nose, sneezing, headache, sore throat, fever, body aches and pains.

Warnings: Children and teenagers should not use this medicine for chicken pox or flu symptoms before a doctor is consulted about Reye syndrome, a rare but serious illness reported to be associated with aspirin. Do not exceed recommended dosage because at higher doses nervousness, dizziness or sleeplessness may occur. May cause excitability, especially in children. Do not take this product if you are allergic to aspirin or have asthma, glaucoma, bleeding problems, emphysema, chronic pulmonary disease, shortness of breath, difficulty in breathing, heart disease, high blood pressure, thyroid disease, diabetes or difficulty in urination due to enlargement of the prostate gland or on a sodium-restricted diet unless directed by a doctor. Each tablet contains 506 mg of sodium. May cause marked drowsiness; alcohol, sedatives and tranquilizers may increase drowsiness effect. Avoid alcoholic beverages while taking this product. Do not take this product if you are taking sedatives or tranquilizers without first consulting your doctor. Use caution when driving a motor vehicle or operating machinery. If sore throat is severe, persists for more than 2 days, is accompanied by high fever, headache, nausea or vomiting, consult a physician promptly. Do not take this product for more than 7 days. If symptoms do not improve or are accompanied by fever or if fever persists for

Continued on next page

Miles—Cont.

more than 3 days, consult a doctor. As with any drug, if you are pregnant or nursing a baby, seek the advice of a health professional before using this product. IT IS ESPECIALLY IMPORTANT NOT TO USE ASPIRIN DURING THE LAST 3 MONTHS OF PREGNANCY UNLESS SPECIFICALLY DIRECTED TO DO SO BY A DOCTOR BECAUSE IT MAY CAUSE PROBLEMS IN THE UNBORN CHILD OR COMPLICATIONS DURING DELIVERY. Keep this and all drugs out of the reach of children.

Drug Interaction Precaution: Do not take this product if you are presently taking a prescription drug for anticoagulation (thinning the blood), high blood pressure or depression without first consulting your doctor.

Dosage and Administration: Adults: Take 2 tablets dissolved in 4 ounces of water every 4 to 6 hours, not to exceed 8 tablets daily.

How Supplied: Tablets: carton of 12 tablets in 6 child-resistant foil twin packs; carton of 20 tablets in 10 child-resistant foil twin packs; carton of 36 tablets in 18 child-resistant foil twin packs.

Product Identification Mark: "A/S PLUS NIGHT-TIME" etched on each tablet

Shown in Product Identification Section, page 416

ALKA–SELTZER PLUS®
Sinus Allergy Medicine

Active Ingredients: Phenylpropanolamine bitartrate 24.08 mg, brompheniramine maleate 2 mg, aspirin 500 mg. In water the aspirin is converted into its soluble ionic form, sodium acetylsalicylate.

Inactive Ingredients: Aspartame, citric acid, flavors, heat-treated sodium bicarbonate, tableting aids

Indications: For the temporary relief of nasal congestion, sinus pain and pressure headache, runny nose, sneezing and itchy, watery eyes due to sinusitis, allergic rhinitis, hay fever or other upper respiratory allergies.

Warnings: Children and teenagers should not use this medicine for chicken pox or flu symptoms before a doctor is consulted about Reye syndrome, a rare but serious illness reported to be associated with aspirin. Do not exceed recommended dosage because at higher doses nervousness, dizziness or sleeplessness may occur. Adults: Do not take this product for more than 7 days. If symptoms do not improve or are accompanied by fever or if fever persists for more than 3 days, consult a doctor. May cause excitability, especially in children. Do not take this product if you have thyroid or heart disease, diabetes, high blood pressure, asthma, glaucoma, emphysema, chronic pulmonary disease, shortness of breath, difficulty in breathing, difficulty in uri-

nation due to enlargement of the prostate gland, bleeding problems, allergy to aspirin or are on a sodium restricted diet, unless directed by a doctor. Each tablet contains 506 mg of sodium. May cause drowsiness. Alcohol, sedatives and tranquilizers may increase the drowsiness effect. Avoid alcoholic beverages while taking this product. Do not take this product if you are taking sedatives or tranquilizers without first consulting your doctor. Use caution when driving a motor vehicle or operating machinery. As with any drug, if you are pregnant or nursing a baby, seek the advice of a health professional before using this product. IT IS ESPECIALLY IMPORTANT NOT TO USE ASPIRIN DURING THE LAST 3 MONTHS OF PREGNANCY UNLESS SPECIFICALLY DIRECTED TO DO SO BY A DOCTOR BECAUSE IT MAY CAUSE PROBLEMS IN THE UNBORN CHILD OR COMPLICATIONS DURING DELIVERY. Keep this and all drugs out of the reach of children.

Drug Interaction: Do not take this product if you are presently taking a prescription drug for anticoagulation (thinning of the blood), high blood pressure or depression without first consulting your doctor.

PHENYLKETONURICS: Contains 8.98 mg phenylalanine per tablet.

Directions: Adults: Take 2 tablets dissolved in approximately 4 ounces (½ glass) of water every 4 hours. Do not exceed 8 tablets in any 24-hour period.

How Supplied: Boxes of 32 tablets in 16 foil twin packs; 16 tablets in 8 foil twin packs

Shown in Product Identification Section, page 416

ALKA-SELTZER PLUS® COLD & COUGH MEDICINE

Active Ingredients: Each ALKA-SELTZER PLUS® COLD AND COUGH tablet contains the following active ingredients: Aspirin 500 mg, Chlorpheniramine Maleate 2 mg, Phenylpropanolamine Bitartrate 24.08 mg, Dextromethorphan Hydrobromide 10 mg. In water the aspirin is converted into its soluble ionic form, sodium acetylsalicylate.

Inactive Ingredients: Aspartame, Citric Acid, Flavor, Sodium Bicarbonate, Tableting Aids.

Indications: Provides temporary relief of the major symptoms of colds and flu with cough.

Actions: Provides temporary relief of these major symptoms of colds and flu with cough: nasal and sinus congestion, body aches and pains, runny nose, coughing, headache, scratchy sore throat, sneezing, fever.

Warnings: Children and teenagers should not use this medicine for chicken pox or flu symptoms before a doctor is consulted about Reye syndrome, a rare but serious illness reported to be associ-

ated with aspirin. If sore throat is severe, persists for more than 2 days, is accompanied by high fever, headache, nausea or vomiting, consult a physician promptly. As with any drug, if you are pregnant or nursing a baby, seek the advice of a health professional before using this product. **IT IS ESPECIALLY IMPORTANT NOT TO USE ASPIRIN DURING THE LAST 3 MONTHS OF PREGNANCY UNLESS SPECIFICALLY DIRECTED TO DO SO BY A DOCTOR BECAUSE IT MAY CAUSE PROBLEMS IN THE UNBORN CHILD OR COMPLICATIONS DURING DELIVERY.** Do not exceed recommended dosage because at higher doses nervousness, dizziness or sleeplessness may occur. May cause excitability, especially in children. Do not take this product unless directed by a doctor if you are allergic to aspirin, have chronic pulmonary disease, glaucoma, asthma, shortness of breath, bleeding problems, difficulty in breathing, thyroid disease, diabetes, emphysema, high blood pressure or difficulty in urination due to enlargement of the prostate gland or on a sodium restricted diet. Each tablet contains 506 mg of sodium. May cause drowsiness; alcohol, sedatives, and tranquilizers may increase drowsiness effect. Avoid alcoholic beverages while taking this product. Do not take this product if you are taking sedatives or tranquilizers without first consulting your doctor. Use caution when driving a motor vehicle or operating machinery. Do not take this product for persistent or chronic cough such as occurs with smoking, asthma, emphysema, or if cough is accompanied by excessive phlegm (mucus) unless directed by a doctor. A persistent cough may be a sign of a serious condition. If cough persists for more than 1 week, tends to recur or is accompanied by fever, rash, or persistent headache, consult a doctor. Do not take this product for more than 7 days. If symptoms do not improve or are accompanied by fever or if fever persists for more than 3 days, consult a doctor. Keep this and all drugs out of the reach of children.

PHENYLKETONURICS: Contains Phenylalanine 7 mg per tablet.

Drug Interaction Precaution: Do not take this product if you are presently taking a prescription drug for anticoagulation (thinning the blood), diabetes, gout, arthritis, high blood pressure or depression without first consulting your doctor.

Dosage and Administration: ALKA-SELTZER PLUS® COLD & COUGH MEDICINE is taken in solution; approximately 4 ounces of water. Additional fluid intake is encouraged for cold sufferers. Adults: 2 tablets every 4 hours up to 8 tablets in 24 hours.

How Supplied: Tablets: carton of 36 tablets in 18 foil twin packs: carton of 20 tablets in 10 foil twin packs.

Product Identification Mark: "AS Plus Cold Cough" embossed on each tablet.

Shown in Product Identification Section, page 416

BACTINE® Antiseptic·Anesthetic First Aid Liquid

Active Ingredients: Benzalkonium Chloride 0.13% w/w, Lidocaine HCl 2.5% w/w.

Inactive Ingredients: Edetate Disodium, Fragrances, Octoxynol 9, Propylene Glycol, Purified Water, Alcohol 3.17% w/w.

Indications: Antiseptic/anesthetic for helping prevent infection, cleanse wounds, and for the temporary relief of pain and itching due to insect bites, minor burns, sunburn, minor cuts and minor skin irritations.

Warnings: For external use only. Do not use in large quantities, particularly over raw surfaces or blistered areas. Avoid spraying in eyes, mouth, ears or on sensitive areas of the body. This product is not for use on wild or domestic animal bites. If you have an animal bite or puncture wound, consult your physician immediately. If condition worsens or if symptoms persist for more than 7 days, discontinue use of this product and consult a physician. Do not bandage tightly. Keep this and all drugs out of reach of children. In case of accidental ingestion, seek professional assistance or contact a Poison Control Center immediately.

Dosage and Administration: For adults and children 2 years of age or older. For superficial skin wounds, cuts, scratches, scrapes, cleanse affected area thoroughly.

Directions: To apply, hold bottle 2 to 3 inches from injured area and squeeze repeatedly. To aid in removing foreign particles, dab injured area with clean gauze saturated with product. For sunburn, minor burns, insect bites, and minor skin irritations, apply to affected area of skin for temporary relief. Product can be applied to affected area with clean gauze saturated with product.

How Supplied: 2 oz., 4 oz. and 16 oz. liquid, and 3.5 oz. pump spray.
Shown in Product Identification Section, page 416

BACTINE® First Aid Antibiotic Plus Anesthetic Ointment

Active Ingredients: Each gram contains Polymyxin B Sulfate 5000 units; Bacitracin 400 units; Neomycin Sulfate 5 mg (equivalent to 3.5 mg Neomycin base); Diperodon HCl 10 mg (pain reliever).

Inactive Ingredients: Mineral Oil, White Petrolatum.

Indications: First aid to help prevent infection, guard against bacterial contamination, relieve pain and itching in minor cuts, scrapes and burns.

Warning: For external use only. Do not use in the eyes or apply over large areas of the body. In case of deep or puncture wounds, animal bites or serious burns, consult a physician. Stop use and consult a physician if the condition persists or gets worse. Do not use longer than one (1) week unless directed by a physician. Keep this and all medicines out of children's reach. In case of accidental ingestion, seek professional assistance or contact a Poison Control Center immediately.

Directions: Clean the affected area. Apply a small amount of this product (an amount equal to the surface area of the tip of a finger) one to three times daily. May be covered with a sterile bandage.

How Supplied: ½ oz. tube.
Shown in Product Identification Section, page 416

BACTINE® Brand Hydrocortisone Anti-Itch Cream

Active Ingredient: Hydrocortisone 0.5%.

Inactive Ingredients: Butylated Hydroxyanisole, Butylated Hydroxytoluene, Butylparaben, Carbomer, Cetyl Alcohol, Colloidal Silicon Dioxide, Corn oil (and) Gylceryl Oleate (and) Propylene Glycol (and) (BHA) (and) BHT (and) Propyl Gallate (and) Citric Acid, DEA-Oleth-3 Phosphate, Diisopropyl Sebacate, Edetate Disodium, Glycerin, Hydroxypropyl Methylcellulose 2906, Lanolin Alcohol, Methylparaben, Mineral Oil (and) Lanolin Alcohol, Propylene Glycol Stearate SE, Propylparaben, Purified Water.

Indications: For the temporary relief of minor skin irritations, itching, and rashes due to eczema, insect bites, poison ivy, poison oak, poison sumac, soaps, detergents, cosmetics, and jewelry.

Warnings: For external use only. Avoid contact with the eyes. If condition worsens or if symptoms persist for more than seven days, discontinue use and consult a physician.

Do not use on children under 2 years of age except under the advice and supervision of a physician.
Keep this and all drugs out of the reach of children. In case of accidental ingestion, seek professional assistance or contact a Poison Control Center immediately.

Directions: For adults and children 2 years of age and older. Gently massage into affected skin area not more than 3 or 4 times daily.

How Supplied: ½ oz. plastic tube.
Shown in Product Identification Section, page 416

BUGS BUNNY™ Children's Chewable Vitamins (Sugar Free)
BUGS BUNNY™ Children's Chewable Vitamins Plus Iron (Sugar Free)
FLINTSTONES™ Children's Chewable Vitamins
FLINTSTONES™ Children's Chewable Vitamins Plus Iron

Vitamin Ingredients: Each multivitamin supplement with iron contains the ingredients listed in the chart below.
BUGS BUNNY™ Children's Chewable Vitamins and FLINTSTONES™ Children's Chewable Vitamins provide the same quantities of vitamins, but do not provide iron.

Indication: Dietary supplementation.

Dosage and Administration: One chewable tablet daily. For adults and children two years and older; tablet must be chewed.

Warning For Bugs Bunny Only: Phenylketonurics: Contains Phenylalanine.

Precaution:
IRON SUPPLEMENTS ONLY.
Contains iron, which can be harmful in large doses. Close tightly and keep out of reach of children. In case of overdose contact a Poison Control Center immediately.

BUGS BUNNY™ Children's Chewable Vitamins Plus Iron (Sugar Free)
FLINTSTONES™ Children's Chewable Vitamins Plus Iron
One Tablet Provides

Vitamins	Quantity	% of U.S. RDA For Children 2 to 4 Years of Age	For Adults and Children over 4 Years of Age
Vitamin A (as Acetate and Beta Carotene)	2500 I.U.	100	50
Vitamin D	400 I.U.	100	100
Vitamin E	15 I.U.	150	50
Vitamin C	60 mg.	150	100
Folic Acid	0.3 mg.	150	75
Thiamine	1.05 mg.	150	70
Riboflavin	1.20 mg.	150	70
Niacin	13.50 mg.	150	67
Vitamin B_6	1.05 mg.	150	52
Vitamin B_{12}	4.5 mcg.	150	75
Mineral: Iron (Elemental)	15 mg.	150	83

Continued on next page

Miles—Cont.

How Supplied: Flintstones are supplied in bottles of 60 and 100, Bugs Bunny in bottles of 60 with child-resistant caps.

*Shown in Product Identification
Section, page 416*

FLINTSTONES™ With Extra C
Children's Chewable Vitamins
BUGS BUNNY™ With Extra C
Children's Chewable Vitamins
(Sugar Free)

Vitamin Ingredients: Each multivitamin supplement contains the ingredients listed in the chart .
[See table immediately below.]

Indication: Dietary supplementation.

BUGS BUNNY™ With Extra C
Children's Chewable Vitamins
(Sugar Free)
FLINTSTONES™ With Extra C
Children's Chewable Vitamins

One Tablet Provides Vitamins	Quantity	% of U.S. RDA	
		For Children 2 To 4 Years of Age	For Adults and Children Over 4 Years of Age
Vitamin A (as Acetate and Beta Carotene)	2500 I.U.	100	50
Vitamin D	400 I.U.	100	100
Vitamin E	15 I.U.	150	50
Vitamin C	250 mg.	625	417
Folic Acid	0.3 mg.	150	75
Thiamine	1.05 mg.	150	70
Riboflavin	1.20 mg.	150	70
Niacin	13.50 mg.	150	67
Vitamin B_6	1.05 mg.	150	52
Vitamin B_{12}	4.5 mcg.	150	75

FLINTSTONES™ COMPLETE
Children's Chewable Vitamins
BUGS BUNNY™
Children's Chewable
Vitamins + Minerals
(Sugar Free)

Vitamins	Quantity Per Tablet	Percentage of U.S. Recommended Daily Allowance (U.S. RDA)	
		For Children 2 to 4 Years of Age (½ tablet)	For Adults & Children Over 4 Years of Age (1 tablet)
Vitamin A (as Acetate and Beta Carotene)	5000 I.U.	100	100
Vitamin D	400 I.U.	50	100
Vitamin E	30 I.U.	150	100
Vitamin C	60 mg.	75	100
Folic Acid	0.4 mg.	100	100
Vitamin B-1 (Thiamine)	1.5 mg.	107	100
Vitamin B-2 (Riboflavin)	1.7 mg.	106	100
Niacin	20 mg.	111	100
Vitamin B-6 (Pyridoxine)	2 mg.	143	100
Vitamin B-12 (Cyanocobalamin)	6 mcg.	100	100
Biotin	40 mcg.	13	13
Pantothenic Acid	10 mg.	100	100
Minerals	Quantity	Percent U.S. RDA	
Iron (elemental)	18 mg.	90	100
Calcium	100 mg.	6	10
Copper	2 mg.	100	100
Phosphorus	100 mg.	6	10
Iodine	150 mcg.	107	100
Magnesium	20 mg.	5	5
Zinc	15 mg.	94	100

Dosage and Administration: One tablet daily for adults and children two years and older; tablet must be chewed.

Warning For Bugs Bunny Only: Phenylketonurics: Contains Phenylalanine.

How Supplied: Flintstones in bottles of 60's & 100's, Bugs Bunny in bottles of 60 with child-resistant caps.

*Shown in Product Identification
Section, page 416*

FLINTSTONES™ COMPLETE
With Iron, Calcium & Minerals
Children's Chewable Vitamins
BUGS BUNNY™ Children's
Chewable Vitamins + Minerals
With Iron and Calcium
(Sugar Free)

Ingredients: Each supplement provides the ingredients listed in the chart below: [See table at bottom .]

Indication: Dietary Supplementation.

Dosage and Administration: 2–4 years of age: Chew one-half tablet daily. Over 4 years of age: Chew one tablet daily.

Warning: Phenylketonurics: Contains Phenylalanine.

Precaution: Contains iron, which can be harmful in large doses. Close tightly and keep out of reach of children. In case of overdose, contact a physician or Poison Control Center immediately.

How Supplied: Bottles of 60's with child-resistant caps.

*Shown in Product Identification
Section, page 416*

DOMEBORO® Astringent Solution Powder Packets

Active Ingredients: Each powder packet contains aluminum sulfate 1191 mg and calcium acetate 938 mg. DOMEBORO in water contains principally, the astringent aluminum acetate buffered to an acid pH.

Inactive Ingredient: Dextrin

Indications: For temporary relief of minor skin irritations due to poison ivy, poison oak, poison sumac, insect bites, athlete's foot or rashes caused by soaps, detergents, cosmetics or jewelry.

Actions: DOMEBORO provides soothing, effective relief of minor skin irritations. For over 50 years, doctors have been recommending DOMEBORO ASTRINGENT SOLUTION to help relieve minor skin irritations.

Warnings: If condition worsens or symptoms persist for more than 7 days, discontinue use of the product and consult a doctor. For external use only. Avoid contact with the eyes. Do not cover compress or wet dressing with plastic to prevent evaporation. Keep this and all drugs out of the reach of children. In case of accidental ingestion, seek professional assistance or contact a Poison Control Center immediately.

Directions: One packet dissolved in 16 ounces of water makes a modified Burow's Solution approximately equivalent to a 1:40 dilution; two packets, a 1:20 dilution; and four packets, a 1:10 dilution. Dissolve one or two packets in water and stir the solution until fully dissolved. Do not strain or filter the solution. Can be used as a compress, wet dressing or as a soak. AS A COMPRESS OR WET DRESSING: Saturate a clean, soft, white cloth or gauze in the solution; gently squeeze and apply loosely to the affected area. Saturate the cloth in the solution every 15 to 30 minutes and apply to the affected area. Repeat as often as necessary. Discard remaining solution after use. AS A SOAK: Soak affected area in the solution for 15 to 30 minutes. Repeat 3 times a day. Discard remaining solution after use.

How Supplied: Boxes of 12 or 100 powder packets.

Shown in Product Identification Section, page 417

DOMEBORO® Astringent Solution Effervescent Tablets

Active Ingredients: Aluminum sulfate 878 mg and calcium acetate 604 mg. DOMEBORO in water contains principally the astringent aluminum acetate buffered to an acid pH.

Inactive Ingredients: Dextrin, polyethylene glycol, sodium bicarbonate

Indications: For temporary relief of minor skin irritations due to poison ivy, poison oak, poison sumac, insect bites, athlete's foot or rashes caused by soaps, detergents, cosmetics or jewelry.

Actions: DOMEBORO provides soothing, effective relief of minor skin irritations. For over 50 years doctors have been recommending DOMEBORO ASTRINGENT SOLUTION to help relieve minor skin irritations.

Warnings: If conditions worsens or symptoms persist for more than 7 days, discontinue use of the product and consult a doctor. For external use only. Avoid contact with the eyes. Do not cover compress or wet dressing with plastic to prevent evaporation. Keep this and all drugs out of the reach of children. In case of accidental ingestion, seek professional assistance or contact a Poison Control Center immediately.

Directions: One tablet dissolved in 12 ounces of water makes a modified Burow's Solution approximately equivalent to a 1:40 dilution; two tablets, a 1:20 dilution; and four tablets, a 1:10 dilution. Dissolve one or two tablets in water and stir the solution until fully dissolved. Do not strain or filter the solution. Can be used as a compress, wet dressing or as a soak. AS A COMPRESS OR WET DRESSING: Saturate a clean, soft, white cloth or gauze in the solution; gently squeeze and apply loosely to the affected area. Saturate the cloth in the solution every 15 to 30 minutes and apply to the affected area. Repeat as often as necessary. Discard remaining solution after use. AS A SOAK: Soak affected area in the solution for 15 to 30 minutes. Repeat 3 times a day. Discard remaining solution after use.

How Supplied: Boxes of 12 or 100 effervescent tablets

MILES® Nervine
Nighttime Sleep–Aid

Active Ingredient: Each capsule-shaped tablet contains diphenhydramine HCl 25 mg.

Inactive Ingredients: Calcium Phosphate Dibasic, Calcium Sulfate, Carboxymethylcellulose Sodium, Corn Starch, Magnesium Stearate, Microcrystalline Cellulose.

Indications: Miles® Nervine helps you fall asleep and relieves occasional sleeplessness.

Actions: Antihistamines act on the central nervous system and produce drowsiness.

Warnings: Do not give to children under 12 years of age. Avoid alcoholic beverages while taking this product. Do not take this product if you are taking sedatives or tranquilizers without first consulting your doctor. If sleeplessness persists continuously for more than 2 weeks, consult your doctor. Insomnia may be a symptom of serious underlying medical illness. Do not take this product if you have asthma, glaucoma, emphysema, chronic pulmonary disease, shortness of breath, difficulty in breathing or difficulty in urination due to enlargement of the prostate gland unless directed by a doctor. As with any drug, if you are pregnant or nursing a baby, seek the advice of a health professional before using this product. Keep this and all drugs out of the reach of children. In case of accidental overdose, seek professional assistance or contact a poison control center immediately.

Dosage and Administration: Two caplets once daily at bedtime or as directed by a physician.

How Supplied: Blister pack 12's, bottle of 30's with a child-resistant cap.

Shown in Product Identification Section, page 417

MYCELEX® OTC
CREAM ANTIFUNGAL

Active Ingredient: Clotrimazole 1%

Inactive Ingredients: Benzyl alcohol (1%) as a preservative, cetostearyl alcohol, cetyl esters wax, octyldodecanol, polysorbate 60, purified water, sorbitan monostearate.
Store between 2°–30°C (36°–86°F).

Indications: Cures athlete's foot (tinea pedis), jock itch (tinea cruris), and ringworm (tinea corporis). For effective relief of the itching, cracking, burning and discomfort which can accompany these conditions.

Warnings: For external use only. Do not use on children under 2 years of age except under the advice and supervision of a doctor. If irritation occurs or if there is no improvement within 4 weeks (for athlete's foot or ringworm) or within 2 weeks (for jock itch) discontinue use and consult a doctor or pharmacist. Keep this and all drugs out of the reach of children. In case of accidental ingestion seek professional assistance or contact a Poison Control Center immediately. Use only as directed.

Directions: Cleanse skin with soap and water and dry thoroughly. Apply a thin layer and gently massage over affected area morning and evening or as directed by a doctor. For athlete's foot, pay special attention to the spaces between the toes. It is also helpful to wear well-fitting, ventilated shoes and to change shoes and socks at least once daily. Best results in athlete's foot and ringworm are usually obtained with 4 weeks' use of this product and in jock itch with 2 weeks' use. If satisfactory results have not occurred within these times, consult a doctor or pharmacist. Children under 12 years of age should be supervised in the use of this product. This product is not effective on the scalp or nails.
FOR BEST RESULTS, FOLLOW DIRECTIONS AND CONTINUE TREATMENT FOR LENGTH OF TIME INDICATED.

How Supplied: Cream Tube 15 g
Shown in Product Identification Section, page 417

MYCELEX® OTC
SOLUTION ANTIFUNGAL

Active Ingredient: Clotrimazole 1%

Inactive Ingredient: Polyethylene glycol 400
Store between 2°–30°C (36°–86°T).

Indications: Cures athlete's foot (tinea pedis), jock itch (tinea cruris), and ringworm (tinea corporis). For effective relief of the itching, cracking, burning and discomfort which can accompany these conditions.

Warnings: For external use only. Do not use on children under 2 years of age except under the advice and supervision of a doctor. If irritation occurs or if there is no improvement within 4 weeks (for athlete's foot or ringworm) or within 2 weeks (for jock itch) discontinue use and consult a doctor or pharmacist. Keep this and all drugs out of the reach of children. In case of accidental ingestion seek professional assistance or contact a Poison Control Center immediately. Use only as directed.

Directions: Cleanse skin with soap and water and dry thoroughly. Apply a thin layer and gently massage over affected area morning and evening as directed by a doctor. For athlete's foot, pay special attention to the spaces between the toes. It is also helpful to wear well-fitting, ventilated shoes and to change shoes and socks at least once daily. Best results in athlete's foot and ringworm are usually obtained with 4 weeks' use of this product and in jock itch with 2 weeks' use. If satisfactory results have not occurred within these times, consult a doctor or pharmacist. Children under 12 years of age should be supervised in the use of this product. This product is not effective on the scalp or nails.
FOR BEST RESULTS, FOLLOW DIRECTIONS AND CONTINUE TREAT-

Continued on next page

Miles—Cont.

MENT FOR LENGTH OF TIME INDI-
CATED.

How Supplied: Solution Bottle 10 mL

*Shown in Product Identification
Section, page 417*

ONE–A–DAY® Essential Vitamins
11 Essential Vitamins

Ingredients: One tablet daily of
ONE-A-DAY® Essential provides:

Vitamins	Quantity	U.S. RDA
Vitamin A (as Acetate and Beta Carotene)	5000 I. U.	100
Vitamin C	60 mg.	100
Thiamine (B_1)	1.5 mg.	100
Riboflavin (B_2)	1.7 mg.	100
Niacin	20 mg.	100
Vitamin D	400 I.U.	100
Vitamin E	30 I.U.	100
Vitamin B_6	2 mg.	100
Folic Acid	0.4 mg.	100
Vitamin B_{12}	6 mcg.	100
Pantothenic Acid	10 mg.	100

Indication: Dietary supplementation.

Dosage and Administration: One
tablet daily for adults and teens.

How Supplied: ONE-A-DAY® Essential, bottles of 60 and 100.

*Shown in Product Identification
Section, page 417*

ONE-A-DAY® Maximum Formula
Vitamins and Minerals
Supplement for adults and teens
The most complete ONE-A-DAY®
brand.

Ingredients:
One tablet daily of ONE-A-DAY® Maximum Formula provides:

Vitamins	Quantity	% of U.S. RDA
Vitamin A (as Acetate and Beta Carotene)	5000 I.U.	100
Vitamin C	60 mg.	100
Thiamine (B_1)	1.5 mg.	100
Riboflavin (B_2)	1.7 mg.	100
Niacin	20 mg.	100
Vitamin D	400 I.U.	100
Vitamin E	30 I.U.	100
Vitamin B_6	2 mg.	100
Folic Acid	0.4 mg.	100
Vitamin B_{12}	6 mcg.	100
Biotin	30 mcg.	10
Pantothenic Acid	10 mg.	100

Minerals	Quantity	% of U.S. RDA
Iron (Elemental)	18 mg.	100
Calcium	130 mg.	13
Phosphorus	100 mg.	10
Iodine	150 mcg.	100
Magnesium	100 mg.	25
Copper	2 mg.	100
Zinc	15 mg.	100
Chromium	10 mcg.	*

Mineral	Quantity	% of U.S. RDA
Selenium	10 mcg.	*
Molybdenum	10 mcg.	*
Manganese	2.5 mg.	*
Potassium	37.5 mg.	*
Chloride	34 mg.	*

*No U.S. RDA established

Indication: Dietary supplementation.

Dosage and Administration: One
tablet daily for adults and teens.

Precaution: Contains iron, which can
be harmful in large doses. Close tightly
and keep out of reach of children. In case
of overdose, contact a physician or Poison
Control Center immediately.

How Supplied: Bottles of 30, 60, and
130 with child-resistant caps.

*Shown in Product Identification
Section, page 417*

ONE-A-DAY® Plus Extra C
Vitamins. For adults and teens.

Vitamin ingredients: One tablet daily
of ONE-A-DAY® Plus Extra C provides:

Vitamins	Quantity	% of U.S. RDA
Vitamin A (as Acetate and Beta Carotene)	5000 I.U.	100
Vitamin C	300 mg.	500
Thiamine (B_1)	1.5 mg.	100
Riboflavin (B_2)	1.7 mg.	100
Niacin	20 mg.	100
Vitamin D	400 I.U.	100
Vitamin E	30 I.U.	100
Vitamin B_6	2 mg.	100
Folic Acid	0.4 mg.	100
Vitamin B_{12}	6 mcg.	100
Pantothenic Acid	10 mg.	100

Indication: Dietary supplementation.

Dosage and Administration: One tablet daily.

How Supplied: Bottles of 60's with child
resistant caps.

*Shown in Product Identification
Section, page 417*

ONE-A-DAY
STRESSGARD® FORMULA
High Potency B Complex and C plus
A, D, E, Iron and Zinc
Multivitamin/Multimineral
Supplement For Adults

Ingredients:

Vitamins	Quantity	% of U.S. RDA
Vitamin A (as Acetate and Beta Carotene)	5000 I.U.	100
Vitamin C	600 mg.	1000
Thiamine (B_1)	15 mg.	1000
Riboflavin (B_2)	10 mg.	588
Niacin	100 mg.	500
Vitamin D	400 I.U.	100
Vitamin E	30 I.U.	100
Vitamin B_6	5 mg.	250
Folic Acid	400 mcg.	100
Vitamin B_{12}	12 mcg.	200
Pantothenic Acid	20 mg.	200

Minerals	Quantity	% of U.S. RDA
Iron (Elemental)	18 mg.	100
Zinc	15 mg.	100
Copper	2 mg.	100

Indication: Dietary supplementation.

Dosage and Administration: Adults
—one tablet daily with food.

Precaution: Contains iron, which can
be harmful in large doses. Close tightly
and keep out of reach of children. In case
of overdose, contact a physician or Poison
Control Center immediately.

How Supplied: Bottles of 60 with
child-resistant caps.

*Shown in Product Identification
Section, page 417*

ONE-A-DAY® WOMEN'S
FORMULA
Advanced Multivitamin Formula
with Calcium, Extra Iron, Zinc and
Beta Carotene.
Provides calcium and extra iron
Plus the daily nutritional support of
11 essential vitamins.

Ingredients: One tablet daily of ONE-
A-DAY® WOMEN'S FORMULA pro-
vides:

Vitamins	Quantity	% of U.S. RDA
Vitamin A (as Acetate and Beta Carotene)	5000 I.U.	100
Vitamin C	60 mg.	100
Thiamine (B_1)	1.5 mg.	100
Riboflavin (B_2)	1.7 mg.	100
Niacin	20 mg.	100
Vitamin D	400 I.U.	100
Vitamin E	30 I.U.	100
Vitamin B_6	2 mg.	100
Folic Acid	0.4 mg.	100
Vitamin B_{12}	6 mcg.	100
Pantothenic Acid	10 mg.	100

Mineral	Quantity	% of U.S. RDA
Iron (Elemental)	27 mg.	150
Calcium (Elemental)	450 mg.	45
Zinc	15 mg.	100

Indication: Dietary supplementation.

Dosage and Administration: One tablet daily.

Precaution: Contains iron, which can
be harmful in large doses. Close tightly
and keep out of reach of children. In case
of overdose, contact a physician or Poison
Control Center immediately.

How Supplied: Bottles of 60 and 130
with child-resistant caps.

*Shown in Product Identification
Section, page 417*

Muro Pharmaceutical, Inc.
890 EAST STREET
TEWKSBURY, MA 01876-9987

BROMFED® SYRUP
Antihistamine-Decongestant
(alcohol free)
ORANGE-LEMON FLAVOR

Each 5 mL (1 teaspoonful) contains: 2 mg brompheniramine maleate and 30 mg pseudoephedrine hydrochloride; also contains citric acid, FD & C Yellow #6, flavor, glycerin, methyl paraben, sodium benzoate, sodium citrate, sodium saccharin, sorbitol, sucrose, purified water.

Indications: For temporary relief of nasal congestion, sneezing, itchy and watery eyes and running nose due to common cold, hay fever or other upper respiratory allergies.

Directions: Adults and children 12 years of age and over: 2 teaspoonfuls every 4–6 hours. Children 6 to 12 years of age: 1 teaspoonful every 4–6 hours. Do not exceed 4 doses in 24 hours. Children under 6 years of age, consult a physician.

Warnings: If symptoms do not improve within 7 days or are accompanied by high fever, consult a physician before continuing use. May cause drowsiness. May cause excitability especially in children. DO NOT exceed recommended daily dosage because at higher doses nervousness, dizziness, or sleeplessness may occur. **Except under the advice and supervision of a physician:** DO NOT give this product to children under 6 years. DO NOT take this product if you have asthma, glaucoma, difficulty in urination due to enlargement of the prostate gland, high blood pressure, heart disease, diabetes, or thyroid disease. As with any drug, if you are pregnant or nursing a baby, seek the advice of a health professional before using this product.

Caution: Avoid operating a motor vehicle or heavy machinery and alcoholic beverages while taking this product. Keep this and all drugs out of the reach of children.

Drug Interaction Precaution: Do not take this product if you are presently taking a prescription antihypertensive or antidepressant drug containing a monoamine oxidase inhibitor except under the advice and supervision of a physician.

Overdosage: In case of accidental overdose, seek professional assistance or contact a Poison Control Center immediately.

Store between 15° and 30°C (59° and 86°F). Dispense in tight, light resistant containers as defined in USP.

How Supplied: NDC 0451-4201-16 —16 fl. oz. (480 mL), NDC 0451-4201-04—4 fl. oz. (120 mL).

GUAIFED® SYRUP
Expectorant/Decongestant

A red colored, berry citrus flavored syrup.
Each 5mL (teaspoonful) contains:
Pseudoephedrine HCl   30mg
Guaifenesin   200mg
CONTAINS NO ANTIHISTAMINE which may cause drowsiness or excessive drying.
Guaifed® Syrup also contains inactive ingredients:
Benzoic Acid, Berry Citrus Flavor, Citric Acid, FD&C Red #40, Glycerin, Propylene Glycol, Purified Water, Saccharin Sodium, Sorbitol, Sucrose. "ALCOHOL FREE"

GUAITAB™ TABLETS
Expectorant/Decongestant

A purple layered tablet
Each tablet contains:
Pseudoephedrine HCl   60mg
Guaifenesin   400mg
GUAITAB™ TABLET also contains inactive ingredients: colloidal silicon dioxide, lactose, magnesium stearate, microcrystalline cellulose, pharmaceutical glaze, sodium starch glycolate, starch, talc, FD&C Blue #2, D&C Red #27.

Indications: For the temporary relief of nasal congestion associated with the common cold, sinusitis, hay fever or other upper respiratory allergies. Also helps loosen phlegm (sputum) and thin bronchial secretions to rid the bronchial passageways of bothersome mucus, drain bronchial tubes, and make coughs more productive.

Warnings: Do not exceed recommended dosage because at higher doses nervousness, dizziness or sleeplessness may occur. Do not use if you have high blood pressure, heart disease, diabetes, thyroid disease or a persistent chronic cough, except under the advice and supervision of a physician. Do not take this product for persistent or chronic cough such as occurs with smoking, asthma, chronic bronchitis, or emphysema, or where cough is accompanied by excessive phlegm (sputum) unless directed by a doctor. A persistent cough may be a sign of a serious condition. If cough persists for more than 1 week, tends to recur, or is accompanied by a fever, rash or persistent headache, consult a doctor.

Contraindications: Hypersensitivity to guaifenesin or sympathomimetic amines; marked hypertension, hyperthyroidism; or in patients receiving monoamine oxidase (MAO) inhibitors.

Adverse Reactions: Possible side effects include nausea, vomiting, nervousness, restlessness, rash (including urticaria), headache, or dry mouth.

Drug Interaction Precautions: Do not take this medication if you are presently taking a prescription antihypertensive or antidepressant drug containing a monoamine oxidase inhibitor except under the advice and supervision of a physician.

Geriatrics: Pseudoephedrine should be used with caution in the elderly because they may be more sensitive to the effect of the sympathomimetics.

Note: As with any drug, if you are pregnant or nursing a baby, seek the advice of a health professional before using this product.
In the case of accidental overdose, seek professional assistance or contact a Poison Control Center immediately.
Guaifenesin has been shown to produce a color interference with certain clinical laboratory determinations of 5-hydroxyindoleacetic acid (5-HIAA) and vanillylmandelic acid (VMA).

Directions: Guaifed® Syrup—Adults and Children 12 years of age and over: Two teaspoonfuls every 4–6 hours, not to exceed eight teaspoonfuls in 24 hours. Children 6 to under 12 years of age: One teaspoonful every 4–6 hours, not to exceed four teaspoonfuls in 24 hours. Children 2 to under 6 years of age: ½ teaspoonful every 4–6 hours, not to exceed two teaspoonfuls in 24 hours. Children under 2 years of age: consult a physician.
GUAITAB™ TABLETS—Adults and Children 12 years of age and over: One Tablet every 4–6 hours, not to exceed four tablets in 24 hours. Children 6 to under 12 years of age: ½ the adult dosage (break tablet in half): ½ tablet every 4–6 hours, not to exceed two tablets in 24 hours.

How Supplied: Guaifed® Syrup is a red colored, berry citrus flavored syrup supplied in 480 mL bottles (NDC #0451-2600-16) and 120 mL bottles (NDC #0451-2600-04).
Store at controlled room temperature between 15°C and 30°C (59°F and 86°F). Dispense in Child Resistant, tight and light resistant containers.
GUAITAB™ TABLET is a purple layered Tablet in bottles of 100's. Each scored Tablet is coded "60/400" on one side and "Muro" on the other side. NDC 0451-4600-50.

SALINEX NASAL MIST AND DROPS
Buffered Isotonic Saline Solutions

Ingredients: Sodium Chloride 0.4%. Also contains disodium phosphate, edetate disodium, hydroxypropyl methylcellulose, monosodium phosphate, polyethylene glycol, propylene glycol and purified water. Preservative used is benzalkonium chloride 0.01%.

Indications: Rhinitis Medicamentosa and Rhinitis Sicca. For relief of nasal congestion associated with overuse of nasal sprays, drops and inhalers.
To alleviate crusting due to nose bleeds; to compensate for nasal stuffiness and dryness due to lack of humidity.

Continued on next page

Muro—Cont.

Directions: Squeeze twice in each nostril as needed.

How Supplied: SPRAY: 50 ml plastic spray bottle. DROPS: 15 ml plastic dropper bottle.

Nature's Bounty, Inc.
**90 ORVILLE DRIVE
BOHEMIA, NY 11716**

**ENER–B®
Vitamin B-12 Nasal Gel
Dietary Supplement**

Description: ENER-B™ is the first intra-nasal application for Vitamin B-12. Each delivery supplies 400 mcg. of Vitamin B-12. This method of delivery provides the highest Vitamin B-12 blood levels that can be obtained without a prescription. Clinical tests show that ENER-B produced 8.4 to 10 times more Vitamin B-12 in the blood than tablets.

Measured Vitamin B-12 Increase in Blood Levels

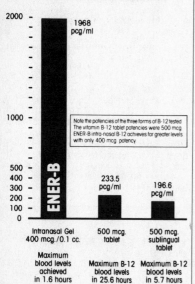

Note the potencies of the three forms of B-12 tested. The vitamin B-12 tablet potencies were 500 mcg. ENER-B intra-nasal B-12 achieves far greater levels with only 400 mcg. potency.

Intranasal Gel 400 mcg./0.1 cc.	500 mcg. tablet	500 mcg. sublingual tablet
Maximum blood levels achieved in 1.6 hours	Maximum B-12 blood levels in 25.6 hours	Maximum B-12 blood levels in 5.7 hours

Clinical Tests results are available by writing Nature's Bounty.

Potency and Administration: Each nasal applicator delivers $\frac{1}{10}$ cc of gel into the nose which adheres to the mucous membranes providing 400 mcg. of Vitamin B-12. Odorless and non-irritating to the nose.

Directions: As a dietary supplement, one unit every two to three days.

How Supplied: Packages of 12 unit doses. Supplies 400 mcg. of B-12 each.
*Shown in Product Identification
Section, page 417*

Neutrin Drug, Inc.
**1800 NORTH CHARLES STREET
BALTIMORE, MD 21201**

ANTICON

**Each Capsule Contains
Active Ingredients:**

Docusate Sodium (USP)	100mg
Casanthranol (USP)	30mg

Excipients:

Soybean Oil (USP)	94mg
Lecithin (NF)	52mg
Yellow Wax (NF)	24mg

Shell:

Gelatin (NF)	115mg
Glycerin (USP)	66mg
Methylparaben (USP)	0.24mg
Propylparaben (USP)	0.19mg
Titanium dioxide (USP)	Q.S.

Useful in the management of chronic and acute constipation.

Indications: Anticon is a combination of the mild stimulant laxative casanthranol and the stool softener Docusate Sodium. Bowel movement is induced gently—usually overnight or in 8 to 12 hours.

Warnings: Not to be taken in case of nausea, vomiting, or abdominal pain. Frequent or continued use of this preparation may result in dependence on laxatives. As with any drug, if you are pregnant or nursing a baby, seek the advice of a health professional before using this product.

Dosage and Administration:
Adults—1 or 2 capsules at bed time, or as indicated. In severe cases, dosage may be increased to 2 capsules two times daily.

How Supplied: Anticon capsule
NDC 57655-315-01 Bottles of 60
*Shown in Product Identification
Section, page 417*

**NATURAL BEST VITAMIN E
1000 I.U.
400 I.U.**

Active Ingredient:
1000 I.U.—d-Alpha-Tocopheryl Acetate 1000 I.U.
400 I.U.—d-Alpha-Tocopheryl Acetate 400 I.U.

100% Natural Vitamin E
No Artificial Colors, No Artificial Flavors, No Preservatives, Sodium Free.

Indications:
Vitamin E deficiency
Progressive muscular dystrophy
Recurrent abortion
Cardiovascular disease
Disturbance in peripheral circulation

Side Effect: The incidence of side effects—none of a serious nature.

Safety Information: Keep out of the reach of children.

Storage: Natural Best Vitamin E should be stored at controlled room temperature (59°–86°F or 15°–30°C).

Period of Validity: Valid until 5 years from the date of manufacturing.

Dosage and Administration:

Adults:	1000 I.U.	one capsule daily
	400 I.U.	one capsule two times daily

How Supplied:
Natural Best Vitamin E 1000 I.U.
  NDC 57655-715-01   Bottle of 100, 50
Natural Best Vitamin E 400 I.U.
  NDC 57655-715-02   Bottle of 200, 100
*Shown in Product Identification
Section, page 417*

Neutrogena Corporation
**5760 W. 96TH ST.
LOS ANGELES, CA 90045**

NEUTROGENA® CLEANSING WASH

Inactive Ingredients: Purified water, glycerin, sodium oleate, sodium cocoate, lauroamphocarboxyl glycinate (and) sodium trideceth sulfate, cocamidopropyl betaine, lauramide DEA, triethanolamine, BHA, BHT, citric acid, trisodium HEDTA.

Indications: A mild-lather cleanser especially formulated for dry, sensitive skin, for skin irritated by drying medications, or for use in conjunction with dermabrasions, chemical peels or facial surgery.

Actions: Neutrogena Cleansing Wash is a gentle, glycerin-enriched formula designed to effectively cleanse skin, extremely sensitive skin or skin made hyperirritable by drying medications or facial procedures. It is residue-free so as not to interfere with skin treatments. It is fragrance-free, contains no color and is noncomedogenic.

Dosage and Administration: Use twice daily, or as directed by physician. Mix with water, work Neutrogena Cleansing Wash into a creamy lather and apply to face. Gently massage in a circular motion. Rinse completely.

How Supplied: Available in 6 oz pump dispenser bottle.
*Shown in Product Identification
Section, page 417*

NEUTROGENA MOISTURE®

Active Ingredient: Octyl methoxycinnamate (SPF 5).

Inactive Ingredients: Purified water, glycerin, glyceryl stearate and PEG-100 stearate, petrolatum, isopropyl isostearate, octyl palmitate, soya sterol, cetyl alcohol, PEG-10 soya sterol, carbomer 954, methylparaben, imidazolidinyl urea, sodium hydroxide, tetrasodium EDTA, propylparaben, tocopherol.

Actions: Neutrogena Moisture is an extremely effective facial moisturizer for even the most fragile complexions. It is noncomedogenic, fragrance-free, and contains no color. Hypoallergenic. Provides an SPF 5 protection for the skin.

Dosage and Administration: Apply Neutrogena Moisture over face and throat morning and night, after thoroughly cleansing the skin.

How Supplied: 2 oz and 4 oz bottle.
Shown in Product Identification Section, page 417

NEUTROGENA MOISTURE®
SPF 15 UNTINTED

Active Ingredients: Octyl methoxycinnamate and benzophenone-3.

Inactive Ingredients: Purified water, PPG-1 isoceteth-3 acetate, glycerin, emulsifying wax NF, glyceryl stearate, PEG-100 stearate, dimethicone, PEG-6000 monostearate, triethanolamine, methylparaben, diazolidinyl urea, carbomer 954, ethylparaben, propylparaben.

Actions: Effective 8 hours' moisturization with maximum sunblock protection (SPF 15) in a noncomedogenic facial moisturizer. Fragrance-free, hypoallergenic.

Dosage and Administration: Use daily after thorough cleansing of skin, alone or under makeup.

How Supplied: 4 oz bottle.
Shown in Product Identification Section, page 417

NEUTROGENA MOISTURE®
SPF 15 WITH SHEER TINT

Active Ingredients: Octyl methoxycinnamate and benzophenone-3.

Inactive Ingredients: Purified water, PPG-1 Isoceteth-3 acetate, glycerin, emulsifying wax NF, glyceryl stearate, PEG-100 stearate, dimethicone, PEG-6000 monostearate, triethanolamine, methylparaben, diazolidinyl urea, carbomer 954, ethylparaben, propylparaben, iron oxides.

Actions: A PABA-free, noncomedogenic facial moisturizer that provides maximum sunblock protection (SPF 15). Fragrance-free, hypoallergenic. Moisturizes for 8 hours with just a hint of color.

Dosage and Administration: Use during the day with or without makeup.

How Supplied: 4 oz bottle.

NEUTROGENA® NORWEGIAN
FORMULA® EMULSION

Inactive Ingredients: Purified Water, Glycerin, Caprylic/Capric Triglyceride, Dimethicone, Octyldodecanol, Petrolatum, Cetyl Alcohol, Glyceryl Laurate, Stearic Acid, Stearyl Alcohol, Hydrogenated Lanolin, Triethanolamine, Fragrance (scented only), Dimethicone Copolyol, Methylparaben, Imidazolidinyl Urea, Steapyrium Chloride, Sodium

Cetearyl Sulfate, Propylparaben, BHA, BHT, Sodium Sulfate.

Indications: Neutrogena® Norwegian Formula® Emulsion has a glycerin-enriched formula that provides eight hours of moisturizing relief for dry hands and skin.

Dosage and Administration: Apply liberally to arms, legs, and body as needed or as directed by a physician.

How Supplied: Available in 5.25 fl. oz. and 10.5 fl. oz. pump bottles, scented and fragrance-free.
Shown in Product Identification Section, page 417

NEUTROGENA® NORWEGIAN
FORMULA® HAND CREAM

Inactive Ingredients: Purified Water, Glycerin, Cetearyl Alcohol, Sodium Cetearyl Sulfate, Fragrance (scented only), Stearic Acid, Methylparaben, Propylparaben, Sodium Sulfate, Dilauryl Thiodipropionate.

Indications: Neutrogena® Norwegian Formula® Hand Cream is a concentrated, emollient-rich cream for localized topical application. The non-comedogenic, cosmetically acceptable formula is effective for a wide range of dry skin conditions, including chronic hand dermatoses, xeroses and other conditions responsive to adjunctive hydration.

Dosage and Administration: Apply a small amount to affected area as needed or as directed by a physician.

How Supplied: Available in 2 oz. tube, scented and fragrance-free.
Shown in Product Identification Section, page 417

NEUTROGENA® SUNBLOCK

Active Ingredients: Octyl methoxycinnamate, Octyl salicylate, and Menthyl anthranilate (SPF 15).

Inactive Ingredients: Mineral oil, aluminum starch octenylsuccinate, silica, PVP/eicosene copolymer, glyceryl tribenate and calcium behenate, phenyltrimethicone, cyclomethicone and dimethiconol, titanium dioxide, C_{18}–C_{36} acid triglyceride, propylparaben.

Indications: Neutrogena Sunblock provides broad spectrum protection (UVA/UVB/IR) from the damaging rays of the sun.

Actions: Provides broad spectrum protection with a SPF 15 effective in preventing sun damage. Liberal and regular use of Neutrogena Sunblock may help reduce the chance of premature aging of the skin and protects against the cancer-causing rays of the sun.

Waterproof: Stays on the skin even after long exposure in the water. Excellent for children above the age of 6 months. Remove with soap and water.

Rubproof/Sweatproof: Abrasion-resistant. Stays on even after rubbing or towel drying. Lower potential to run into eyes and cause stinging.

PABA-Free/Noncomedogenic: Suitable for those sensitive to PABA and its related compounds; won't clog pores. Fragrance-free. Hypoallergenic.

Warnings: For external use only, not to be swallowed. Avoid contact with eyes. Discontinue use if irritation or rash develops.

Dosage and Administration: For best results, apply to face and body 15 minutes before sun exposure. Reapply after rigorous swimming or exercise.

How Supplied: 2¼ oz tube.
Shown in Product Identification Section, page 417

NEUTROGENA® T/DERM® TAR
EMOLLIENT

Ingredients: Neutar® Solubilized Coal Tar Extract 5% in a soothing, emollient oil base.

Indications: Neutrogena® T/Derm® is the cosmetically acceptable liquid tar preparation for soothing relief of psoriasis and other chronic, crusted, pruritic skin conditions.

Actions: Neutar® Solubilized Coal Tar Extract is biologically equivalent to crude coal tar and proven to reduce hyper-keratotic cell turnover by inhibiting DNA synthesis.

Dosage and Administration: Gently rub into affected areas of the skin once or twice a day. Allow 15–20 minutes to dry. Any excess may be removed by gently patting the area dry with a soft cloth or tissue.

Caution: Avoid exposure to sunlight for 24 hours unless otherwise directed by a physician. Do not use on broken or inflamed skin. If irritation develops, discontinue use and consult physician. Avoid contact with eyes. Temporary discoloration of light colored hair may occur. This is not uncommon with tar medications. Slight staining of clothing may occur. Standard laundry procedures will remove most stains. Keep out of the reach of children.

How Supplied: 4 fl. oz. bottle.

NEUTROGENA® T/GEL®
THERAPEUTIC SHAMPOO

Ingredients: Neutar® Solubilized Coal Tar Extract 2% in a bland shampoo base.

Indications: The clear amber formula of Neutrogena® T/Gel® Therapeutic Shampoo provides significant relief for serious scalp conditions such as psoriasis, seborrheic dermatitis and dandruff, leaving hair clean and fresh smelling, with no residual tar odor.

Continued on next page

Neutrogena—Cont.

Actions: Neutar® Solubilized Coal Tar Extract is biologically equivalent to crude coal tar and proven to reduce hyper-keratotic cell turnover by inhibiting DNA synthesis.

Dosage and Administration: Use daily or as directed by a physician. Wet hair thoroughly. Massage a liberal amount of T/Gel® into scalp and leave on for several minutes. Rinse thoroughly and repeat.

Caution: For external use only. If irritation develops, discontinue use and consult physician. May temporarily discolor gray, blond, bleached or tinted hair. Store away from direct sunlight. Avoid contact with eyes. Keep out of the reach of children.

How Supplied: 4.4 fl. oz., 8.5 fl. oz and 16 fl. oz. bottles.
Shown in Product Identification Section, page 417

NEUTROGENA® T/SAL® THERAPEUTIC SHAMPOO

Ingredients: Neutar® Solubilized Coal Tar Extract 2% and Salicylic Acid 2% in a bland shampoo base.

Indications: The clear amber formula of Neutrogena® T/Sal® Therapeutic Shampoo provides dual action for significant relief for serious scalp conditions requiring keratolytic action, such as psoriasis and seborrheic dermatitis, leaving hair clean and fresh smelling, with no residual tar odor.

Actions: Neutar® Solubilized Coal Tar Extract is biologically equivalent to crude coal tar and proven to reduce hyper-keratotic cell turnover by inhibiting DNA synthesis. The keratolytic activity of salicyclic acid reduces hyperkeratotic lesions.

Dosage and Administration: Use daily or as directed by a physician. Wet hair thoroughly. Massage a liberal amount of T/Sal® into scalp and leave on for several minutes. Rinse thoroughly and repeat.

Caution: For external use only. Do not apply to acutely inflamed or broken skin. If irritation develops, discontinue use and consult physician. In rare instances, discoloration of gray, blond, bleached or tinted hair may occur. Avoid contact with eyes. If contact occurs rinse thoroughly with water. Keep out of the reach of children.

How Supplied: 4.5 fl. oz. bottle.
Shown in Product Identification Section, page 417

Products are indexed by generic and chemical names in the **YELLOW SECTION.**

Niché Pharmaceuticals, Inc.
300 TROPHY CLUB DRIVE #400
ROANOKE, TX 76262

MAGTAB® SR
[măg-tăb]
(Magnesium Lactate)
Sustained release Magnesium Supplement

Description: MagTab® SR is a sustained release oral magnesium supplement. Each pale yellow caplet contains 7mEq (84 Mg) magnesium as magnesium lactate in a wax matrix.

Ingredients: Each caplet contains 7mEq (84 MG) elemental magnesium as magnesium L.Lactate dihydrate (835 Mg) in a sustained release wax matrix formulation. Inactive ingredients: polyethylene glycol, microcrystalline cellulose, carnauba wax, stearic acid, calcium stearate, and D & C yellow No. 10 aluminum lake.

Indications/Uses: As a dietary supplement, MagTab® SR is indicated for patients with, or at risk for, magnesium deficiency. Hypomagnesemia and/or magesium deficiency can result from inadequate nutritional intake or absorption, magnesium depleting drugs such as diuretics, or alcoholism.

Warnings: Patients with renal disease should not take magnesium supplements without the advice and direct supervision of a physician.

Side Effects: Excessive dosage of magnesium can cause loose stools or diarrhea.

Dosage: As a dietary supplement, take 1 or 2 caplets b.i.d. or as directed by a physician. Four caplets of MagTab® SR will meet the USRDA range for average adult males and females (300–350 mg) where magnesium depleting drugs are being used, supplementation with higher dosages may be required and should be considered.

How Supplied: MagTab® SR is available for oral administration as uncoated yellow caplets, coded Niche/420. Caplets are supplied as follows:
59016-42016   Bottles of 60
59016-42017   Bottles of 100
Store at 15°–30°C (59°–86°F)
U.S. Patent Number: 5,002,774

IDENTIFICATION PROBLEM?
Consult the
Product Identification Section
where you'll find products pictured in full color.

Ohm Laboratories, Inc.
P. O. BOX 279
FRANKLIN PARK, NJ 08823

CRAMP END
Ibuprofen Tablets, USP, 200 mg
Menstrual Pain & Cramp Reliever

WARNING: ASPIRIN-SENSITIVE PATIENTS: Do not take this product if you have had a severe allergic reaction to aspirin, e.g., asthma, swelling, shock or hives, because even though this product contains no aspirin or salicylates, cross-reactions may occur in patients allergic to aspirin.

Indications: For the temporary relief of painful menstrual cramps (Dysmenorrhea); also headaches, backaches and muscular aches and pains associated with Premenstrual Syndrome.

Directions: Adults: Take 1 tablet every 4 to 6 hours at the onset of menstrual symptoms and while pain persists. If pain does not respond to 1 tablet, 2 tablets may be used but do not exceed 6 tablets in 24 hours, unless directed by a doctor. The smallest effective dose should be used. Take with food or milk if occasional and mild heartburn, upset stomach, or stomach pain occurs with use. Consult a doctor if these symptoms are more than mild or if they persist.
Children: Do not give this product to children under 12 except under the advice and supervision of a doctor.

Warnings: Do not take for pain for more than 10 days unless directed by a doctor. If pain persists or gets worse, or if new symptoms occur, consult a doctor. These could be signs of serious illness. If you are under a doctor's care for any serious condition, consult a doctor before taking this product. As with aspirin and acetaminophen, if you have any condition which requires you to take prescription drugs or if you have had any problems or serious side effects from taking any non-prescription pain reliever, do not take this product without first discussing it with your doctor. If you experience any symptoms which are unusual or seem unrelated to the condition for which you took ibuprofen, consult a doctor before taking any more of it. Although ibuprofen is indicated for the same conditions as aspirin and acetaminophen, it should not be taken with them except under a doctor's direction. Do not combine this product with any other ibuprofen-containing product. As with any drug, if you are pregnant or nursing a baby, seek the advice of a health professional before using this product. **IT IS ESPECIALLY IMPORTANT NOT TO USE IBUPROFEN DURING THE LAST 3 MONTHS OF PREGNANCY UNLESS SPECIFICALLY DIRECTED TO DO SO BY A DOCTOR BECAUSE IT MAY CAUSE PROBLEMS IN THE UNBORN CHILD OR COMPLICATIONS DURING DELIVERY.** Keep this and all drugs out of the reach of children. In case of accidental overdose, seek professional assistance or contact a poison control center immediately.

How Supplied: Coated tablets in blister packs of 12's
Store at room temperature; avoid excessive heat 40°C (104°F).

Active Ingredient: Each tablet contains Ibuprofen 200 mg.
Manufactured by OHM LABORATORIES, INC, Franklin Park, NJ 08823
Shown in Product Identification Section, page 418

IBUPROHM®
Ibuprofen Tablets, USP
Ibuprofen Caplets, USP

Active Ingredient: Each tablet contains Ibuprofen USP, 200 mg.

Warning: ASPIRIN SENSITIVE PATIENTS: Do not take this product if you have had a severe allergic reaction to aspirin, e.g., asthma, swelling, shock or hives, because even though this product contains no aspirin or salicylates, cross-reactions may occur in patients allergic to aspirin.

Indications: For the temporary relief of minor aches and pains associated with the common cold, headache, toothache, muscular aches, backache, for the minor pain of arthritis, for the pain of menstrual cramps, and for reduction of fever.

Directions: *Adults:* Take 1 tablet every 4 to 6 hours while symptoms persist. If pain or fever does not respond to 1 tablet, 2 tablets may be used but do not exceed 6 tablets in 24 hours, unless directed by a doctor. The smallest effective dose should be used. Take with food or milk if occasional and mild heartburn, upset stomach, or stomach pain occurs with use. Consult a doctor if these symptoms are more than mild or if they persist. Children: Do not give this product to children under 12 except under the advice and supervision of a doctor.

Warnings: Do not take for pain for more than 10 days or for fever for more than 3 days unless directed by a doctor. If pain or fever persists or gets worse, if new symptoms occur, or if the painful area is red or swollen, consult a doctor. These could be signs of serious illness. If you are under a doctor's care for any serious condition, consult a doctor before taking this product. As with aspirin and acetaminophen, if you have any condition which requires you to take prescription drugs or if you have had any problems or serious side effects from taking any nonprescription pain reliever, do not take this product without first discussing it with your doctor. If you experience any symptoms which are unusual or seem unrelated to the condition for which you took ibuprofen, consult a doctor before taking any more of it. Although ibuprofen is indicated for the same conditions as aspirin and acetaminophen, it should not be taken with them except under a doctor's direction. Do not combine the product with any other ibu-

profen-containing product. As with any drug, if you are pregnant or nursing a baby, seek the advice of a health professional before using this product. IT IS ESPECIALLY IMPORTANT NOT TO USE IBUPROFEN DURING THE LAST 3 MONTHS OF PREGNANCY UNLESS SPECIFICALLY DIRECTED TO DO SO BY A DOCTOR BECAUSE IT MAY CAUSE PROBLEMS IN THE UNBORN CHILD OR COMPLICATIONS DURING DELIVERY. Keep this and all drugs out of the reach of children. In case of accidental overdose, seek professional assistance or contact a poison control center immediately.

How Supplied: Coated tablets in bottles of 24, 50, 100, 165, 250, 500 and 1000. Coated caplets in bottles of 24, 50, 100 and 250.

Storage: Store at room temperature; avoid excessive heat 40° (104°F).
Shown in Product Identification Section, page 418

Ortho Pharmaceutical Corporation
Advanced Care Products
RARITAN, NJ 08869

CONCEPTROL®
Contraceptive Gel/Inserts

Description: CONCEPTROL Contraceptive Gel: An unscented, unflavored, colorless, greaseless and non-staining gel in convenient, easy-to-use disposable plastic applicators. Each applicator is filled with a single, pre-measured dose containing the active spermicide Nonoxynol-9—4.0%, (100 mg per application) at pH 4.5.
CONCEPTROL Contraceptive Inserts: A non-foaming, single dose vaginal contraceptive containing the active spermicide Nonoxynol-9-8.34% (150 mg per insert).

Indication: Contraception.

Actions and Uses: Spermicidal products for use whenever control of conception is desirable.

Warning: Occasional burning and/or irritation of the vagina or penis have been reported. If this occurs, discontinue use and consult a physician as necessary. Not effective if taken orally. Keep out of reach of children. When pregnancy is contraindicated, the contraceptive program should be discussed with a health care professional.

Dosage and Administration:
CONCEPTROL Contraceptive Gel: One applicatorful of CONCEPTROL Contraceptive Gel should be inserted deeply into the vagina just before intercourse. An additional applicatorful is required each time intercourse is repeated.
CONCEPTROL Contraceptive Inserts: One insert should be placed into the vagina at least ten minutes prior to male penetration to insure proper dispersion. An additional insert is required each time intercourse is repeated.

CONCEPTROL Contraceptive Gel/Inserts:
If intercourse has not occurred within one hour after the application of CONCEPTROL, repeat application. Add a new application each time intercourse is repeated. Douching after use of CONCEPTROL is not recommended; however should you desire to do so, wait at least six hours to avoid interfering with contraceptive protection.
CONCEPTROL is an effective method of contraception. While no method of birth control can provide an absolute guarantee against becoming pregnant, for maximum protection, CONCEPTROL must be used according to directions.

How Supplied:
CONCEPTROL Contraceptive Gel is available in packages of 6 or 10 easy-to-use single-dose applicators.
CONCEPTROL Contraceptive Inserts are available in packages containing 10 inserts.

Inactive Ingredients:
CONCEPTROL Contraceptive Gel:
Lactic Acid, Methylparaben, Povidone, Propylene Glycol, Purified Water, Sodium Carboxymethylcellulose, Sorbic Acid, Sorbitol Solution.
CONCEPTROL Contraceptive Inserts:
Lauroamphodiacetate Sodium Trideceth Sulfate, Polyethylene Glycol 1000, Polyethylene Glycol 1450, Povidone.

Storage: Avoid excessive heat (over 86°F or 30°C).
Shown in Product Identification Section, page 418

DELFEN®
Contraceptive Foam

Description: A contraceptive foam in an aerosol dosage formulation containing 12.5% Nonoxynol-9 (100 mg. per application) and buffered to normal vaginal pH 4.5.

Indication: Contraception.

Action and Uses: A spermicidal foam for intravaginal contraception.

Warning: Occasional burning and/or irritation of the vagina or penis have been reported. In such cases, the use of the product should be discontinued and a physician consulted as necessary. Not effective if taken orally. Keep out of reach of children.
When pregnancy is contraindicated, the contraceptive program should be discussed with a health care professional.

Dosage and Administration: Insert DELFEN Contraceptive Foam just prior to each act of intercourse. You may have intercourse any time up to one hour after you have inserted the foam. If you repeat intercourse, insert another applicatorful of DELFEN Foam. After shaking the can, remove cap and place can upright on a level surface. Place the measured-dose (5cc) applicator on top of the can, then press applicator down very gently to fill.

Continued on next page

Ortho Pharm.—Cont.

Fill to the top of the ribbed section of the applicator. Remove applicator from can to stop flow of foam. Insert the filled applicator well into the vagina and depress the plunger. Remove the applicator with the plunger in depressed position. Douching is not recommended after using DELFEN Foam. However, if douching is desired for cleansing purposes, wait at least six hours after intercourse. Refer to direction circular in package for diagrams and detailed instructions. While no method of contraception can provide an absolute guarantee against becoming pregnant, for maximum protection, DELFEN Foam must be used according to directions.

How Supplied: DELFEN Contraceptive Foam 0.60 oz. Starter can with applicator. Also 1.40 oz. refill can without applicator.

Inactive Ingredients: Benzoic Acid, Cetyl Alcohol, Cellulose Gum, Glacial Acetic Acid, Methylparaben, Perfume, Phosphoric Acid, Polyvinyl Alcohol, Propellant A-31, Propylene Glycol, Purified Water, Stearamidoethyl Diethylamine, Sorbic Acid, Stearic Acid.

Storage: Contents under pressure. Do not puncture or incinerate container. Do not expose to heat or store at temperatures above 120°F.

Shown in Product Identification Section, page 418

GYNOL II® Original Formula ORTHO-GYNOL® Contraceptive Jelly

Description:
GYNOL II Original Formula:
A colorless, unscented, unflavored, greaseless and non-staining contraceptive jelly containing the active spermicide Nonoxynol-9 (2%, 100 mg. per application) and having a pH of 4.5.
ORTHO-GYNOL: Is a water-dispersible spermicidal jelly having a pH of 4.5 and contains the active spermicide Octoxynol-9 (1%).

Indication: Contraception.

Actions and Uses: An aesthetically pleasing spermicidal vaginal jelly for use with a vaginal diaphragm whenever the control of conception is desired.

Warning: Occasional burning and/or irritation of the vagina or penis have been reported. In such cases, use of the product should be discontinued and a physician consulted as necessary. Not effective if taken orally. Keep out of reach of children. When pregnancy is contraindicated, the contraceptive program should be discussed with a health care professional.

Dosage and Administration: Used in conjunction with a vaginal diaphragm. Prior to insertion, put about a teaspoonful of contraceptive jelly into the cup of the dome of the diaphragm and spread a

small amount around the edge with your fingertip. This will aid in insertion and provide protection.
It is also important to remember that if intercourse occurs more than six hours after insertion, or if repeated intercourse takes place, an additional application of contraceptive jelly is necessary. DO NOT REMOVE THE DIAPHRAGM—simply add more contraceptive jelly with an applicator, being careful not to dislodge the diaphragm. Remember, another application of contraceptive jelly is required each time intercourse is repeated, regardless of how little time has transpired since the diaphragm has been in place.
IMPORTANT—For contraceptive effectiveness, the diaphragm should remain in place for six hours after intercourse and should be removed as soon as possible thereafter. Continuous wearing of the diaphragm for more than 24 hours is not recommended. Retention of the diaphragm for prolonged periods may encourage the growth of certain bacteria in the vaginal tract. It has been suggested that under certain as yet unestablished conditions overgrowth of these bacteria may lead to symptoms of toxic shock syndrome (TSS). For further information, consult your physician.
If a douche is desired for cleansing purposes, wait at least six hours after intercourse. While no method of contraception can provide an absolute guarantee against becoming pregnant, for maximum protection, the contraceptive jelly must be used according to directions. Refer to direction circular enclosed in the package for diagrams and complete instructions.

Inactive Ingredients:
GYNOL II Original Formula:
Lactic Acid, Methylparaben, Povidone, Propylene Glycol, Purified Water, Sodium Carboxymethylcellulose, Sorbic acid, Sorbitol Solution.
ORTHO-GYNOL:
Benzoic Acid, Castor Oil, Fragrance, Glacial Acetic Acid, Methylparaben, Potassium Hydroxide, Propylene Glycol, Purified Water, Sodium Carboxymethylcellulose, Sorbic Acid.

How Supplied: 2.5 oz and 3.8 oz tube packages.
Storage: Should be stored at room temperature.
Shown in Product Identification Section, page 418

GYNOL II EXTRA STRENGTH CONTRACEPTIVE JELLY

Description: GYNOL II Extra Strength Contraceptive Jelly is a clear, unscented, water-soluble, greaseless gel. It is mildly lubricating and non-staining. Each applicatorful contains 150 mg of nonoxynol-9 (3%), a potent spermicide which provides effective protection against pregnancy when used with a diaphragm or a condom or alone. A diaphragm alone is not effective protection against pregnancy.

Indication: Contraception.

Actions and Uses: An aesthetically pleasing spermicidal jelly for use alone, with a condom or a diaphragm whenever control of contraception is desired.

Warning: Occasional burning and/or irritation of the vagina or penis have been reported. In such cases, the medication should be discontinued and a physician consulted as necessary. Not effective if taken orally. Keep out of reach of children. When pregnancy is contraindicated, the contraceptive program should be discussed with a health care professional.

Dosage and Administration: When used in conjunction with a vaginal diaphragm. Prior to insertion, put about a teaspoonful of GYNOL II Extra Strength Contraceptive Jelly into the cup of the dome of the diaphragm and spread a small amount around the edge with your fingertip then insert.
It is also important to remember that if intercourse occurs more than six hours after insertion, or if repeated intercourse takes place, an additional application of GYNOL II Extra Strength is necessary. DO NOT REMOVE THE DIAPHRAGM, simply add more GYNOL II Extra Strength with the applicator provided in the applicator package, being careful not to dislodge the diaphragm. Remember, another application of GYNOL II Extra Strength is required each time intercourse is repeated, regardless of how little time has transpired since the diaphragm has been in place.
IMPORTANT—For contraceptive effectiveness, the diaphragm should remain in place for six hours after intercourse and should be removed as soon as possible thereafter. Continuous wearing of the diaphragm for more than 24 hours is not recommended. Retention of the diaphragm for prolonged periods may encourage the growth of certain bacteria in the vaginal tract. It has been suggested that under certain as yet unestablished conditions overgrowth of these bacteria may lead to symptoms of toxic shock syndrome (TSS). For further information, consult your physician.

Dosage and Administration: For use with a condom or as a use-alone product. Insert an applicatorful of GYNOL II Extra Strength into the vagina as shown in the illustration. Intercourse should occur within one hour after GYNOL II Extra Strength has been inserted. An additional application must be used prior to each additional act of intercourse. This method of contraception must be used each and every time intercourse takes place, regardless of the time of the month.

Inactive Ingredients: Lactic Acid, Methylparaben, Povidone, Propylene Glycol, Purified Water, Sodium Carboxymethylcellulose, Sorbic Acid, Sorbitol Solution.
Shown in Product Identification Section, page 418

MICATIN®
['mī-kə-tin]
Antifungal For Athlete's Foot

Description: An antifungal containing the active ingredient miconazole nitrate 2%, clinically proven to cure athlete's foot, jock itch and ringworm.

Indications: Athlete's foot (tinea pedis), jock itch (tinea cruris), and ringworm (tinea corporis).

Actions and Uses: Proven clinically effective in the treatment of athlete's foot (tinea pedis), jock itch (tinea cruris), and ringworm (tinea corporis). For effective relief of the itching, scaling, burning and discomfort that can accompany these conditions.

Directions: Cleanse skin with soap and water and dry thoroughly. Apply a thin layer of MICATIN over affected area morning and night or as directed by a doctor. For athlete's foot, pay special attention to the spaces between the toes. It is also helpful to wear well-fitting, ventilated shoes and to change shoes and socks at least once daily. Best results in athlete's foot and ringworm are usually obtained with 4 weeks' use of this product and in jock itch with 2 weeks' use. If satisfactory results have not occurred within these times, consult a doctor or pharmacist. Children under 12 years of age should be supervised in the use of this product. This product is not effective on the scalp or nails.
Do not use on children under 2 years of age except under the advice and supervision of a doctor. For external use only. If irritation occurs, or if there is no improvement within 4 weeks (for athlete's foot or ringworm) or within 2 weeks (for jock itch), discontinue use and consult a doctor or pharmacist. Keep this and all drugs out of the reach of children. In case of accidental ingestion, seek professional assistance or contact a Poison Control Center immediately.

How Supplied:
MICATIN® Antifungal Cream is available in a 0.5 oz. tube and a 1.0 oz. tube.
MICATIN Antifungal Spray Powder is available in a 3.0 oz. aerosol can.
MICATIN Antifungal Deodorant Spray Powder is available in a 3.0 oz. aerosol can.
MICATIN Antifungal Powder is available in a 3.0 oz. plastic bottle.
MICATIN Antifungal Spray Liquid is available in a 3.5 oz. aerosol can.

Inactive Ingredients:
MICATIN Antifungal Cream: Benzoic Acid, BHA, Mineral Oil, Peglicol 5 Oleate, Pegoxol 7 Stearate, Purified Water.
MICATIN Antifungal Spray Powder: Alcohol, Propellant A-46, Sorbitan Sesquioleate, Stearalkonium Hectorite, Talc.
MICATIN Antifungal Deodorant Spray Powder: Alcohol, Propellant A-46, Talc, Stearalkonium Hectorite, Sorbitan Sesquioleate, Fragrance.
MICATIN Antifungal Powder: Talc.
MICATIN Antifungal Spray Liquid: Alcohol, Benzyl Alcohol, Cocamide DEA, Propellant A-46, Sorbitan Sesquioleate, Tocopherol.

Storage: Store at room temerature.
Shown in Product Identification Section, page 418

MICATIN®
['mī-kə-tin]
Antifungal For Jock Itch

Description: An antifungal containing the active ingredient miconazole nitrate 2%, clinically proven to cure jock itch.

Indications: Jock itch (tinea cruris).

Actions and Uses: Proven clinically effective in the treatment of jock itch (tinea cruris). For effective relief of the itching, scaling, burning and discomfort that can accompany this condition.

Directions: Cleanse skin with soap and water and dry thoroughly. Apply a thin layer of product over affected area morning and night or as directed by a doctor. Best results are usually obtained within 2 weeks' use of this product. If satisfactory results have not occurred within this time, consult a doctor or pharmacist. Children under 12 years of age should be supervised in the use of this product. This product is not effective on the scalp or nails.

Warnings: Do not use on children under 2 years of age except under the advice and supervision of a doctor. For external use only. If irritation occurs, or if there is no improvement of jock itch within 2 weeks, discontinue use and consult a doctor or pharmacist. Keep this and all drugs out of the reach of children. In case of accidental ingestion, seek professional assistance or contact a Poison Control Center immediately.

How Supplied:
MICATIN® Jock Itch Cream is available in a 0.5 oz. tube.
MICATIN Jock Itch Spray Powder is available in a 3.0 oz. aerosol can.

Inactive Ingredients:
MICATIN Jock Itch Cream: Benzoic Acid, BHA, Mineral Oil, Peglicol 5 Oleate, Pegoxol 7 Stearate, Purified Water.
MICATIN Jock Itch Spray Powder: Alcohol, Propellant A-46, Sorbitan Sesquioleate, Stearalkonium Hectorite, Talc.

Storage: Store at room temperature.

MONISTAT® 7
(miconazole nitrate)
Vaginal Cream, Suppositories

PRODUCT OVERVIEW

Key Facts: Monistat 7 is a vaginal antifungal. Monistat 7 is available in two forms: cream; and soft, emollient vaginal suppositories.

Major Uses: 1. For the treatment of **RECURRENT** vulvovaginal candidiasis (moniliasis) when the patient is treating herself, i.e. for women who have been diagnosed by a doctor in the past with vulvovaginal candidiasis, and who recognize the symptoms.
2. For the treatment of vulvovaginal candidiasis (moniliasis) for first-time sufferers **ONLY WHEN THE CONDITION IS DIAGNOSED BY A PHYSICIAN AND THE PHYSICIAN RECOMMENDATION CALLS FOR AN OTC PRODUCT.**

Safety Information:
● Do not use Monistat 7 if the following signs and symptoms are present. If they occur while using Monistat 7, STOP using the product and contact a doctor right away.
—Fever (Above 100°F orally)
—Pain in the lower abdomen, back or either shoulder
—A vaginal discharge that smells bad
● If there is not improvement or if the infection worsens within three days, or complete relief is not felt within seven days, or your symptoms return within two months, then you may have something other than a yeast infection. You should consult your doctor.
● If your doctor has told you that you are sensitive or allergic to any Monistat product, do not use Monistat 7 without talking to your doctor first.
● Do not use in girls less than 12 years of age.
● If you are pregnant or think you may be, do not use this product except under the advice and supervision of a doctor.

PRODUCT INFORMATION

Active Ingredients: miconazole nitrate (vaginal cream, 2%; vaginal suppositories, 100 mg each)

Inactive Ingredients: Cream: benzoic acid, BHA, mineral oil, peglicol 5 oleate, pegoxol 7 stearate, purified water. Suppository: hydrogenated vegetable oil base.

Indications:
1. For the treatment of **RECURRENT** vulvovaginal candidiasis (moniliasis) when the patient is treating herself, i.e. for women who have been diagnosed by a doctor in the past with vulvovaginal candidiasis, and who recognize the symptoms.
2. For the treatment of vulvovaginal candidiasis (moniliasis) for first-time sufferers **ONLY WHEN THE CONDITION IS DIAGNOSED BY A PHYSICIAN AND THE PHYSICIAN RECOMMENDATION CALLS FOR AN OTC PRODUCT.**
As Monistat 7 is effective only for candidal vulvovaginitis, the physician diagnosis should be confirmed by KOH smears and/or cultures. Other pathogens commonly associated with vulvovaginitis (*Trichomonas* and *Haemophilus vaginalis* [*Gardnerella*]) should be ruled out by appropriate laboratory methods.

Actions: Monistat 7 exhibits fungicidal activity *in vitro* against the species of the genus *Candida*. The pharmacological mode of action is unknown.

Continued on next page

Ortho Pharm.—Cont.

Warnings/Precautions:
- This product is only effective in treating vaginal yeast infection caused by yeast. Do not use in eyes or take by mouth.
- **Do not use Monistat 7 vaginal cream or suppositories if you have any of the following signs and symptoms. Also, if they occur while using Monistat 7, <u>STOP</u> using the product and contact a doctor right away. You may have a more serious illness.**
  Fever (Above 100°F orally)
  Pain in the lower abdomen, back or either shoulder
  A vaginal discharge that smells bad
- If there is no improvement or if the infection worsens within 3 days, or complete relief is not felt within 7 days, or your symptoms return within two months, then you may have something other than a yeast infection. You should consult your doctor.
- Monistat 7 cream contains mineral oil. Monistat 7 suppositories contain hydrogenated vegetable oil. Mineral oil and hydrogenated vegetable oil may weaken latex condoms or diaphragms. Do not rely on condoms or diaphragms to prevent sexually transmitted diseases or pregnancy while using Monistat 7 vaginal cream or suppositories.
- If your doctor has previously told you that you are sensitive or allergic to any Monistat product, do not use Monistat 7 vaginal cream or suppositories without talking to your doctor first.
- Do not use tampons while using this medication.
- Do not use in girls less than 12 years of age.
- If you are pregnant or think you may be, do not use this product except under the advice and supervision of a doctor.
- Keep this and all drugs out of the reach of children.
- In case of accidental ingestion, seek professional assistance or contact a poison control center immediately.

Dosage and Administration: One applicatorful of cream or one suppository is administered intravaginally once daily at bedtime for seven days. Course of therapy may be repeated after other pathogens have been ruled out by appropriate smears and cultures.

How Supplied: Monistat 7 vaginal cream is available in 1.59 oz. (45 g) tube (NDC/UPC 0062-5426-01) with applicator. Monistat 7 vaginal suppositories are available as 100 mg per dose, elliptically-shaped white to off-white suppositories in packages of seven (NDC/UPC 0062-5427-01).

Shown in Product Identification Section, page 418

P & S Laboratories
**210 WEST 131st STREET
LOS ANGELES, CA 90061**

See Standard Homeopathic Company.

Paddock Laboratories, Inc.
**3101 LOUISIANA AVE. NORTH
MINNEAPOLIS, MN 55427**

ACTIDOSE–AQUA™
(Highly Activated Charcoal Suspension)

Each milliliter contains 208 mg of highly activated charcoal.

How Supplied:
15 Grams/72 ml　　NDC 0574-0121-25
25 Grams/120 ml　　NDC 0574-0121-04
50 Grams/240 ml　　NDC 0574-0121-08
See PDR for full information.

ACTIDOSE with SORBITOL™
(Highly Activated Charcoal Suspension with Sorbitol)

Each milliliter contains 208 mg of highly activated charcoal and 400 mg of sorbitol.

How Supplied:
25 Grams/120 ml　　NDC 0574-0120-04
50 Grams/240 ml　　NDC 0574-0120-08
See PDR for full information.

GLUTOSE®
Oral Glucose Gel

Active Ingredient: Dextrose (D-Glucose) 40%. Each 25-gram unit-of-use tube contains 10 grams of glucose. Each 80-gram package contains 32 grams of glucose.

Indications: Glutose is a dye-free oral glucose gel for treatment of insulin reaction or hypoglycemia.

Dosage and Administration: Recommended dose is one 25-gram tube or ⅓ of an 80-gram package, delivering 10 grams of glucose. Inform your physician or healthcare provider immediately of any insulin reaction or hypoglycemic episode. Glutose is not recommended for use in children under 2 years of age or persons who are unconscious or unable to swallow.

How Supplied: Three unit-of use 25-gram tubes　　NDC 0574-0069-25
Multi-dose 80-gram package
　　　　　　　　　NDC 0574-0069-06

IPECAC SYRUP

Active Ingredients: Ipecac Syrup, USP contains in each 30 ml, not less than 36.9 and not more than 47.1 mg total ether soluble alkaloids of ipecac. The content of emetine and cephaeline together

is not less than 90% of the total ether soluble alkaloids.

Indications: Ipecac Syrup is indicated to induce vomiting in poisoning emergencies.

Warning: Do not use in unconscious persons. Ordinarily, this drug should not be used if strychnine, corrosives such as alkalies, lye and strong acids, or petroleum distillates such as kerosene, gasoline, coal oil, fuel oil, paint thinners, or cleaning fluids have been ingested.

Dosage and Administration: Usual Dosage (1 year of age and older): One tablespoon (15 ml) followed by one to two glasses of water. Repeat dosage in 20 minutes if vomiting does not occur.

How Supplied: 1 fl. oz. bottle (12 per case) NDC 0574-0012-01

Parke-Davis
**Consumer Health Products Group
Division of Warner-Lambert
　　Company
201 TABOR ROAD
MORRIS PLAINS, NJ 07950
(See also Warner-Lambert)**

AGORAL® Raspberry
AGORAL® Marshmallow
[ă'gō-răl"]

Description: Each tablespoonful (15 mL) of Agoral Raspberry (pink) or of Agoral Marshmallow (white) contains 4.2 grams mineral oil and 0.2 gram phenolphthalein in a thoroughly homogenized emulsion.
Also contains acacia; agar; benzoic acid; egg albumin; flavors; glycerin; saccharin sodium; sodium benzoate; tragacanth; citric acid or sodium hydroxide to adjust pH; water. Agoral Raspberry Flavor also contains D&C Red No. 30 Lake.

Actions: Agoral, containing mineral oil, facilitates defecation by lubricating the fecal mass and softening the stool. More effective than nonemulsified oil in penetrating the feces, Agoral thereby greatly reduces the possibility of oil leakage at the anal sphincter. Phenolphthalein gently stimulates motor activity of the lower intestinal tract. Agoral's combined lubricating-softening and peristaltic actions can help to restore a normal pattern of evacuation.

Indications: Relief of constipation. Agoral may be especially required when straining at stool is a hazard, as in hernia, cardiac, or hypertensive patients; during convalescence from surgery; before and after surgery for hemorrhoids or other painful anorectal disorders; for patients confined to bed.
The management of chronic constipation should also include attention to fluid intake, diet and bowel habits.

Contraindication: Sensitivity to phenolphthalein.

Warning: Do not use laxative products when abdominal pain, nausea, or vomiting are present unless directed by a physician. If you have noticed a sudden change in bowel habits that persists over a period of 2 weeks, consult a physician before using a laxative. Laxative products should not be used for a period longer than 1 week unless directed by a physician. Rectal bleeding or failure to have a bowel movement after use of a laxative may indicate a serious condition. Discontinue use and consult your physician. Do not administer to children under 6 years of age, to pregnant women, to bedridden patients or to persons with difficulty swallowing. As with any drug, if you are nursing a baby, seek the advice of a health professional before using this product. Do not take with meals. If skin rash appears, do not use this product or any other preparation containing phenolphthalein. Keep this and all drugs out of the reach of children. In case of accidental overdose, seek professional assistance or contact a Poison Control Center immediately. Drug interaction precaution: Do not take this product if you are presently taking a stool softener laxative.

Dosage: Agoral Raspberry and Marshmallow—Adults—½ to 1 tablespoonful at bedtime only, unless other time is advised by physician. Children—Over 6 years, ½ to ¾ teaspoonfuls at bedtime only, unless other time is advised by physician. This product generally produces bowel movement in 6 to 8 hours.

Supplied: Agoral (raspberry flavor), plastic bottles of 16 fl oz. Agoral (marshmallow flavor), plastic bottles of 16 fl oz. **Store between 15°–30° C (59°–86° F). Keep this and all drugs out of the reach of children.**
In case of accidental overdose, seek professional assistance or contact a Poison Control Center immediately.

ANUSOL®
[ă′nū-sŏl″]
Suppositories/Ointment

Description:
Anusol Suppositories: Active Ingredients: Phenylephrine HCl 0.25% and Hard Fat 88.7%. Also contains: Corn Starch, Methylparaben and Propylparaben.
Anusol Ointment: Active ingredients: Pramoxine HCl 1%, Mineral Oil 46.7% and Zinc Oxide 12.5%. Also contains: Benzyl Benzoate, Calcium Phosphate Dibasic, Cocoa Butter, Glyceryl Monostearate, Kaolin, Peruvian Balsam and Polyethylene Wax.

Actions: Anusol Suppositories and Anusol Ointment help to relieve pain, itching and discomfort arising from irritated anorectal tissues. They have a soothing, lubricant action on mucous membranes. Pramoxine Hydrochloride in Anusol Ointment is a rapidly acting local anesthetic for the skin and mucous membranes of the anus and rectum. Pramoxine HCl is also chemically distinct from procaine, cocaine, and dibucaine and can often be used in the patient previously sensitized to other surface anesthetics. Surface analgesia lasts for several hours.

Indications: Anusol Ointment: Temporarily relieves the pain, soreness, and burning of hemorrhoids and other anorectal disorders while it forms a temporary protective coating over inflamed tissues. Anusol Suppositories: Temporarily shrinks the swelling associated with irritated hemorrhoidal tissues, and gives temporary relief from the itching, burning and discomfort of hemorrhoids and other anorectal disorders.

Contraindications: Anusol Suppositories and Anusol Ointment are contraindicated in those patients with a history of hypersensitivity to any of the components of the preparations.

Warnings: Anusol Ointment: Certain persons can develop allergic reactions to ingredients in this product. If the symptom being treated does not subside, if condition worsens or does not improve within 7 days, if redness, irritation, swelling, pain, or other symptoms develop or increase, discontinue use and consult a physician promptly. Do not exceed the recommended daily dosage unless directed by a physician. Do not put this product into the rectum by using fingers or any mechanical device or applicator. Keep this and all drugs out of the reach of children. In case of accidental ingestion seek professional advice or contact a Poison Control Center immediately. Suppositories : Do not exceed recommended daily dosage unless directed by a physician. Do not use this product if you have heart disease, high blood pressure, thyroid disease, diabetes, or difficulty in urination due to enlargement of the prostate gland unless directed by a physician. It condition worsens or does not improve within 7 days, consult a physician. In case of bleeding, consult a doctor. Keep this and all drugs out of the reach of children. In case of accidental ingestion seek professional advice or contact a Poison Control Center immediately.

Adverse Reactions: Upon application of Anusol Ointment, which contains Pramoxine HCl, a patient may occasionally experience burning, especially if the anoderm is not intact. Sensitivity reactions have been rare; discontinue medication if suspected. Certain persons can develop allergic reactions to ingredients in this product.

Drug Interaction Precaution: Anusol Suppositories: Do not use this product if you are presently taking a prescription drug for high blood pressure or depression without consulting a physician

Directions: Anusol Suppositories: Adults: When practical, cleanse the affected area with Tucks Hemorrhoidal Pads or mild soap and warm water and rinse thoroughly. Gently dry by patting or blotting with toilet tissue or soft cloth before application of this product. Remove foil wrapper and insert suppository into the anus. Insert one suppository rectally up to four times daily: one in the morning, one in the evening, and one after each bowel movement. Children under 12 years of age: consult a physician. Anusol Ointment: Adults: When practical, cleanse the affected area with Tucks Hemorrhoidal Pads or mild soap and warm water and rinse thoroughly. Gently dry by patting or blotting with toilet tissue or soft cloth before application of this product. Apply ointment externally to the affected area up to five (5) times daily. To use dispensing cap, attach it to tube, lubricate well, then gently insert part way into the anus. Squeeze tube to deliver medication. Thoroughly cleanse dispensing cap after use. Children under 12 years of age: Consult a physician.
NOTE: If staining from either of the above products occurs, the stain may be removed from fabric by hand or machine washing with household detergent.

How Supplied: Anusol Suppositories—boxes of 12, 24 and 48; in silver foil strips. Anusol Ointment—1-oz tubes and 2-oz tubes with plastic applicator.
Store between 15° and 30°C (59° and 86°F).
Shown in Product Identification Section, page 418

BENADRYL Anti-Itch Cream, Regular Strength, 1%
BENADRYL Anti-Itch Cream, Maximum Strength, 2%

Active Ingredients: Regular Strength contains Benadryl® (diphenhydramine hydrochloride USP) 1%; Maximum Strength contains Benadryl® (diphenhydramine hydrochloride USP) 2%.

Inactive Ingredients: Cetyl Alcohol, Methylparaben, Polyethylene Glycol Monostearate, Propylene Glycol and Water, Purified.

Indications: For the temporary relief of ITCHING and PAIN associated with insect bites, rashes, poison oak, poison sumac, allergic itches, and minor skin irritations.

Actions: Benadryl is the most prescribed topical antihistamine available. It stops the itch at the source by blocking the action of histamine that causes the itch. Benadryl also provides local anesthetic action to soothe the pain. Benadryl gives you the kind of itch and pain relief that you can't get from hydrocortisone. Benadryl cream is soothing and greaseless.

Warnings: For external use only. Do not apply to blistered, raw or oozing areas of the skin. Do not use on chicken

Continued on next page

This product information was prepared in November 1991. On these and other Parke-Davis Products, detailed information may be obtained by addressing PARKE-DAVIS, Consumer Health Products Group, Division of Warner-Lambert Company, Morris Plains, NJ 07950.

Parke-Davis—Cont.

pox or measles unless supervised by a physician. Do not use on extensive areas of the skin or for longer than 7 days except as directed by a physician. Avoid contact with the eyes or other mucous membranes. If condition worsens, or if symptoms persist for more than 7 days, or clear up and occur again within a few days, discontinue use of this product and consult a physician. Do not use any other drugs containing diphenhydramine while using this product. KEEP THIS AND ALL DRUGS OUT OF THE REACH OF CHILDREN. In case of accidental ingestion, seek professional assistance or contact a Poison Control Center immediately.

Dosage and Administration: Regular Strength 1%—For adults and children 6 years of age and older: Apply to affected area not more than three to four times daily, or as directed by a physician. For children under 6 years of age: consult a physician.
Maximum Strength 2%—For adults and children 12 years of age and older: Apply to affected area not more than three to four times daily, or as directed by a physician. For children under 12 years of age: consult a physician.

How Supplied: Benadryl Anti-Itch Cream is available in ½ oz. Regular Strength and ½ oz. Maximum Strength tubes.
Shown in Product Identification Section, page 418

BENADRYL®
[bě'nă-drĭl]
Decongestant Elixir

Description: Each teaspoonful (5 mL) contains: Benadryl (diphenhydramine hydrochloride) 12.5 mg; pseudoephedrine hydrochloride 30 mg; alcohol 5%. Also contains: FD&C Yellow No. 6; glucose, liquid; glycerin, USP; flavors; menthol, USP; saccharin sodium, USP; sodium citrate, USP; sucrose, NF; water, purified, USP.

Indications: Temporarily relieves nasal congestion, runny nose, sneezing, itching of the nose or throat, itchy, watery eyes due to hay fever or other upper respiratory allergies, and runny nose, sneezing and nasal congestion of the common cold.

Warnings: Do not exceed recommended dosage because at higher doses nervousness, dizziness, or sleeplessness may occur. Do not take this product for more than 7 days. If symptoms do not improve or are accompanied by fever, consult a physician. Do not take this product if you have high blood pressure, heart disease, diabetes, thyroid disease, asthma, glaucoma, emphysema, chronic pulmonary disease, shortness of breath, difficulty in breathing or difficulty in urination due to enlargement of the prostate gland unless directed by a physician. May cause excitability, especially in chil-

dren. May cause marked drowsiness: alcohol may increase the drowsiness effect. Avoid alcoholic beverages while taking this product. Use caution when driving a motor vehicle or operating machinery. As with any drug, if you are pregnant or nursing a baby seek the advice of a health professional before using this product. Keep this and all drugs out of the reach of children. In case of accidental overdose, seek professional assistance or contact a Poison Control Center immediately.

Drug Interaction Precaution: Do not take this product if you are presently taking a prescription drug for high blood pressure or depression without first consulting your physician.

Directions: Children 6 to under 12 years oral dosage is one teaspoonful every 4 to 6 hours not to exceed 4 teaspoonfuls in 24 hours, or as directed by a physician. For children under 6 years of age, consult a physician. Adult oral dosage is two teaspoonfuls every 4 to 6 hours not to exceed 8 teaspoonfuls in 24 hours, or as directed by a physician.

How Supplied: Benadryl Decongestant Elixir is supplied in 4-oz bottles. Store below 30° C (86°F). Protect from freezing.
Shown in Product Identification Section, page 419

BENADRYL® Decongestant
[bě'nă-drĭl]
Decongestant Tablets and Kapseals®

Active Ingredients: Each tablet/Kapseal® contains: Benadryl® (diphenhydramine hydrochloride USP) 25 mg. and pseudoephedrine hydrochloride 60 mg.

Inactive Ingredients: Each tablet contains: Corn Starch, Croscarmellose Sodium, Dibasic Calcium Phosphate Dihydrate, FD&C Blue No. 1 Aluminum Lake, Hydroxypropyl Methylcellulose, Microcrystalline Cellulose, Polyethylene Glycol, Polysorbate 80, Stearic Acid, Titanium Dioxide and Zinc Stearate.
Each Kapseals® capsule contains: Calcium Stearate, Lactose (Hydrous), Syloid Silica Gel. The Kapseals® capsule shell contains: D&C Red No. 28, FD&C Blue No. 1 and Red No. 3, Gelatin, Glyceryl Monooleate, PEG-200 Ricinoleate and Titanium Dioxide.

Indications: Temporarily relieves nasal congestion, runny nose, sneezing, itching of the nose or throat, itchy, watery eyes due to hay fever or other upper respiratory allergies, and runny nose, sneezing and nasal congestion of the common cold.

Warning: Do not exceed recommended dosage because at higher doses nervousness, dizziness, or sleeplessness may occur. Do not take this product for more than 7 days. If symptoms do not improve or are accompanied by fever, consult a physician. Do not take this product if you have high blood pressure, heart disease,

diabetes, thyroid disease, asthma, glaucoma, emphysema, chronic pulmonary disease, shortness of breath, difficulty in breathing or difficulty in urination due to enlargement of the prostate gland unless directed by a physician. May cause excitability, especially in children. May cause marked drowsiness: alcohol may increase the drowsiness effect. Avoid alcoholic beverages while taking this product. Use caution when driving a motor vehicle or operating machinery. Do not give this product to children under 12 years except under the advice and supervision of a physician. As with any drug, if you are pregnant or nursing a baby seek the advice of a health professional before using this product. Keep this and all drugs out of the reach of children. In case of accidental overdose, seek professional assistance or contact a Poison Control Center immediately.

Drug Interaction Precaution: Do not take this product if you are presently taking a prescription drug for high blood pressure or depression without first consulting your physician.

Directions: Adults and children over 12 years of age: 1 tablet/Kapseal® every 4 to 6 hours not to exceed 4 tablets/Kapseals® in 24 hours. Benadryl Decongestant is not recommended for children under 12 years of age.

How Supplied: Benadryl Decongestant Tablets and Kapseals® are supplied in boxes of 24.
Store at room temperature 15°–30° C (59°–86° F).
Protect from moisture.
Shown in Product Identification Section, page 418

BENADRYL® Elixir

Active Ingredients: Each teaspoonful (5 mL) contains: Benadryl® (diphenhydramine hydrochloride USP) 12.5 mg. and Alcohol 5.6%.

Inactive Ingredients: Also contains: Citric Acid, D&C Red No. 33, EDTA, FD&C Red No. 40, Flavors, Glycerin, Mono Ammonium Glycyrrhizinate, Propyl Gallate, Sodium Citrate, Sodium Saccharin, Sugar, Purified Water.

Indications: Temporarily relieves runny nose, sneezing, itching of the nose or throat and itchy, watery eyes due to hay fever or other upper respiratory allergies and runny nose and sneezing associated with the common cold.

Warnings: Do not take this product if you have asthma, glaucoma, emphysema, chronic pulmonary disease, shortness of breath, difficulty in breathing or difficulty in urination due to enlargement of the prostate gland unless directed by a physician. May cause excitability especially in children. May cause marked drowsiness; alcohol may increase the drowsiness effect. Avoid alcoholic beverages while taking this product. Use caution when driving a motor vehicle or operating machinery. As with any drug if you are pregnant or nursing a baby seek the advice of a health professional before using this product. Keep this and all drugs out of the reach of children. In case of accidental overdose, seek professional assistance or contact a Poison Control Center immediately.

Dosage and Administration: Children 6 to under 12 years of age oral dosage is 12.5 to 25 mg. (1 to 2 teaspoonfuls) every 4 to 6 hours not to exceed 12 teaspoonfuls in 24 hours, or as directed by a physician. For children under 6 years your physician should be contacted for the recommended dosage. Adult oral dosage is 25 mg. (2 teaspoonfuls) to 50 mg. (4 teaspoonfuls) every 4 to 6 hours not to exceed 24 teaspoonfuls in 24 hours, or as directed by a physician.

How Supplied: Benadryl Elixir is supplied in 4 oz. and 8 oz. bottles.

Shown in Product Identification Section, page 419

BENADRYL® 25
[bĕ'nă-dril]
Tablets and Kapseals®

Active Ingredient: Each tablet/Kapseal® contains: Benadryl® (diphenhydramine hydrochloride USP) 25 mg.

Inactive Ingredients: Each tablet contains: Corn Starch, Croscarmellose Sodium, Dibasic Calcium Phosphate Dihydrate, D&C Red No. 27 Aluminum Lake, Hydroxypropyl Methylcellulose, Microcrystalline Cellulose, Polyethylene Glycol, Polysorbate 80, Stearic Acid, Titanium Dioxide and Zinc Stearate. Each Kapseal capsule contains: Lactose (Hydrous) and Magnesium Stearate. The Kapseal capsule shell contains: Artificial Colors, Gelatin, Glyceryl Mono-oleate, PEG-200 Ricinoleate and Titanium Dioxide.

Indications: Temporarily relieves runny nose, sneezing, itching of the nose or throat, itchy, watery eyes due to hay fever or other upper respiratory allergies and runny nose and sneezing of the common cold.

Warnings: Do not take this product if you have asthma, glaucoma, emphysema, chronic pulmonary disease, shortness of breath, difficulty in urination due to enlargement of the prostate gland unless directed by physician. May cause excitability, especially in children. May cause marked drowsiness: alcohol may increase the drowsiness effect. Avoid alcoholic beverages while taking this product. Use caution when driving a motor vehicle or operating machinery. As with any drug if you are pregnant or nursing a baby seek the advice of a health professional before using this product. Keep this and all drugs out of the reach of children. In case of accidental overdose, seek professional assistance or contact a Poison Control Center immediately.

Directions: Adult oral dosage is 25–50 mg (1 to 2 tablets/Kapseals®) every 4 to

6 hours not to exceed 12 tablets/Kapseals® in 24 hours, or as directed by a physician.

Children 6 to under 12 years oral dosage is 12.5 mg* to 25 mg (1 tablet/Kapseal®) every 4 to 6 hours, not to exceed 6 tablets/Kapseals® in 24 hours, or as directed by a physician. For children under 6 years your physician should be contacted for the recommended dosage.

How Supplied: Benadryl 25 Tablets and Kapseals® are supplied in boxes of 24 and 48.

Store at room temperature 15°–30° C (59°–86° F). Protect from moisture.

* This dosage strength is not available in this package. Do not attempt to break tablets/Kapseals®. This dosage is available in pleasant tasting Benadryl Elixir.

Shown in Product Identification Section, page 418

BENADRYL® COLD
Tablets

Active Ingredients: Each tablet contains: Benadryl® (diphenhydramine hydrochloride USP) 12.5 mg., pseudoephedrine hydrochloride 30 mg., and acetaminophen 500 mg.

Inactive Ingredients: Each tablet contains: Carboxymethylcellulose, Croscarmellose Sodium, Hydroxypropyl Cellulose, Hydroxypropyl Methylcellulose, Magnesium Stearate, Microcrystalline Cellulose, Polyethylene Glycol, Propylene Glycol, Starch, Stearic Acid, Titanium Dioxide, and Zinc Stearate.

Indications: Temporarily relieves sneezing, running nose, nasal and sinus congestion, fever, minor sore throat pain, headache, sinus pressure, body aches and pain due to the common cold, and sneezing, runny nose, itching of the nose or throat, and itchy, watery eyes due to hay fever or other upper respiratory allergies.

Warnings: Do not exceed recommended dosage because at higher doses nervousness, dizziness, or sleeplessness may occur. Do not take this product if you have high blood pressure, heart disease, diabetes, thyroid disease, asthma, glaucoma, emphysema, chronic pulmonary disease, shortness of breath, difficulty in breathing, or difficulty in urination due to enlargement of the prostate gland unless directed by a physician. May cause excitability especially in children. May cause marked drowsiness; alcohol may increase the drowsiness effect. Avoid alcoholic beverages while taking this product. Use caution when driving a motor vehicle or operating machinery. If fever persists for more than 3 days (72 hours) or recurs, consult your physician. If sore throat persists for more than 2 days, is accompanied or followed by fever, headache, rash, nausea or vomiting, consult a physician promptly. As with any drug if you are pregnant or nursing a baby seek the advice of a health professional before using this product. Keep

this and all drugs out of the reach of children. In case of accidental overdose, seek professional assistance or contact a Poison Control Center immediately. Do not give this product to children under 12 years except under the advice and supervision of a physician.

Drug Interaction Precaution: Do not take this product if you are presently taking a prescription drug for high blood pressure or depression without consulting your physician.

Directions: Adults (12 years and over): Two tablets every 6 hours, not to exceed 8 tablets in a 24-hour period. Benadryl Cold is not recommended for children under 12 years of age.

How Supplied: Benadryl Cold Tablets are supplied in boxes of 24 and 48. Store at room temperature 15°–30°C (59°–86°F). Protect from moisture.

Shown in Product Identification Section, page 418

BENADRYL® COLD NIGHTTIME FORMULA

Active Ingredients: Each fluid ounce or 2 tablespoons contains: Acetaminophen 1000 mg., diphenhydramine hydrochloride 50 mg., and pseudoephedrine hydrochloride 60 mg.

Inactive Ingredients: Alcohol 10%, citric acid, D&C Yellow No. 10, FD&C Red No. 40, FD&C Green No. 3, disodium edetate, flavoring, glycerin, polyethylene glycol, potassium sorbate, propyl gallate, propylene glycol, sodium benzoate, sodium citrate, sodium saccharin and purified water.

Indications: Benadryl Cold Nighttime Formula provides temporary relief of sneezing, runny nose, nasal and sinus congestion, fever, minor sore throat pain, headache, sinus pressure, body aches and pain due to the common cold, and sneezing, runny nose, itching of the nose or throat, and itchy, watery eyes due to hay fever and other respiratory allergies.

Warnings: Do not exceed recommended dosage because at higher doses nervousness, dizziness, or sleeplessness may occur. Do not take this product for more than 7 days. If symptoms do not improve or are accompanied by fever, consult a physician. Do not take this product if you have high blood pressure, heart disease, diabetes, thyroid disease, asthma, glaucoma, emphysema, chronic pulmonary disease, shortness of breath, difficulty in breathing, or difficulty in urination due to enlargement of the pros-

Continued on next page

This product information was prepared in November 1991. On these and other Parke-Davis Products, detailed information may be obtained by addressing PARKE-DAVIS, Consumer Health Products Group, Division of Warner-Lambert Company, Morris Plains, NJ 07950.

Parke-Davis—Cont.

tate gland unless directed by a physician. If fever persists for more than 3 days (72 hours) or recurs, consult your physician. If sore throat is severe, persists for more than 2 days, is accompanied or followed by fever, headache, rash, nausea or vomiting, consult a physician promptly. As with any drug if you are pregnant or nursing a baby seek the advice of a health professional before using this product. Keep this and all drugs out of the reach of children. In case of accidental ingestion, seek professional assistance or contact a Poison Control Center immediately. May cause marked drowsiness; alcohol may increase the drowsiness effect. Do not give this product to children under 12 years except under the advice of a physician.

Caution: Avoid alcoholic beverages while taking this product. Use caution when driving a motor vehicle or operating heavy machinery.

Drug Interaction Precaution: Do not take this product if you are presently taking a prescription drug for high blood pressure or depression without first consulting your physician.

Directions for Use: Adults take one fluid ounce using dosage cup or two (2) tablespoons at bedtime for nighttime relief. Dosage may be repeated every six (6) hours or as directed by a physician. Do not exceed 4 fluid ounces or eight (8) tablespoons in any 24-hour period. Children under 12 should use only as directed by a physician.

How Supplied: Benadryl Cold Nighttime Formula is supplied in 6 ounce bottles. Store at room temperature, 15°–30°C (59°–86°F).

Questions about Benadryl® Cold Nighttime Formula?
Call us toll free 9 AM to 5 PM EST. Weekdays at 1-800-524-2624. In New Jersey call 1-800-338-0326.

Shown in Product Identification Section, page 419

BENADRYL® Spray Regular Strength 1%
BENADRYL® Spray Maximum Strength 2%

Active Ingredients: Regular Strength contains Benadryl® (diphenhydramine hydrochloride USP) 1%; Maximum Strength contains Benadryl® (diphenhydramine hydrochloride USP) 2%.

Inactive Ingredients: Alcohol, Glycerin, Povidone, Tromethamine, and Water, Purified.

Indications: For the temporary relief of ITCHING and PAIN associated with insect bites, rashes, poison oak, poison sumac, allergic itches, and minor skin irritations.

Actions: Benadryl Spray forms a clear, anti-itch "bandage" to protect and relieve affected areas. Benadryl stops the itch at the source by blocking the action of histamine that causes the itch. Benadryl also provides an anesthetic action to soothe the pain. The spray feature allows soothing relief without touching or rubbing the affected area. Benadryl spray is clear, won't stain clothing and won't rinse off (can be easily removed with soap and water).

Warnings: FOR EXTERNAL USE ONLY. Do not apply to blistered, raw or oozing areas of the skin. Do not use on chicken pox or measles unless supervised by a physician. Do not use on extensive areas of the skin for longer than 7 days except as directed by a physician. Avoid contact with the eyes or other mucous membranes. If condition worsens or if symptoms persist for more than 7 days or clear up and occur again within a few days, discontinue use of this product and consult a physician. Do not use any other drugs containing diphenhydramine while using this product. KEEP THIS AND ALL DRUGS OUT OF THE REACH OF CHILDREN. In case of accidental ingestion, seek professional assistance or contact a Poison Control Center immediately. Flammable, keep away from fire or flame.

Dosage and Administration: Regular Strength 1%—For adults and children 6 years of age and older: Spray on affected area not more than three to four times daily, or as directed by a physician. For children under 6 years of age: consult a physician. **Maximum Strength 2%**—For adults and children 12 years of age or older: Spray on affected area not more than three to four times daily, or as directed by a physician. For children under 12 years of age: consult a physician.

How Supplied: Benadryl® Spray is available in a 2 oz. pump spray bottle.
Shown in Product Identification Section, page 418

BENYLIN®
Cough Syrup

Description: Each teaspoonful (5 mL) contains:
Diphenhydramine
　Hydrochloride　　　　　　12.5 mg
Also contains: Alcohol 5%; Ammonium Chloride; Caramel; Citric Acid; D&C Red No. 33; FD&C Red No. 40; Flavor; Glucose Liquid; Glycerin; Menthol; Purified Water; Sodium Citrate; Sodium Saccharin; Sucrose.

Indications: For the temporary relief of cough due to minor throat and bronchial irritation as may occur with the common cold or with inhaled irritants.

Warnings: A persistent cough may be a sign of a serious condition. Do not take this product for persistent or chronic cough such as occurs with smoking, asthma, emphysema, or when cough is accompanied by excessive phlegm (mu-

cus). If cough persists for more than one (1) week, tends to recur, or is accompanied by fever, rash, or persistent headache, consult a physician. May cause excitability, especially in children. Do not take this product if you have glaucoma, or difficulty in urination due to enlargement of the prostate gland except under the advice of a physician. May cause marked drowsiness. Avoid driving a motor vehicle or operating heavy machinery, or drinking alcoholic beverages. Do not give to children under six (6) years of age except under the advice and supervision of a physician. Keep this and all drugs out of the reach of children. In case of accidental overdose, seek professional assistance or contact a Poison Control Center immediately. As with any drug, if you are pregnant or nursing a baby, seek the advice of a health professional before using this product.

Directions for Use:
Adults: (12 years and older): Take 2 teaspoonfuls every 4 hours. Do not exceed 12 teaspoonfuls in 24 hours.
Children (6–12 years): Take 1 teaspoonful every 4 hours. Do not exceed 6 teaspoonfuls in 24 hours.
Children (under 6 years): Consult physician for recommended dosage.

How Supplied: Benylin Cough Syrup is supplied in 4-oz and 8-oz bottles. Store at 59°–86°F.
Shown in Product Identification Section, page 419

BENYLIN® DM®
Pediatric Cough Formula

Description: Each teaspoonful (5 mL) contains:
Dextromethorphan
　Hydrobromide　　　　　　10 mg
Also contains: Alcohol 5%; Ammonium Chloride; Caramel; Citric Acid; D&C Red No. 33; Flavor; Glucose Liquid; Glycerin; Menthol; Purified Water; Sodium Citrate; Sucrose.

Indications: Nonnarcotic cough suppressant for the temporary relief of coughs due to minor bronchial irritation as may occur with the common cold or inhaled irritants.

Warnings: A persistent cough may be a sign of a serious condition. If cough persists for more than one week, tends to recur, or is accompanied by fever, rash, or persistent headache, consult a physician. Do not take this product for persistent or chronic cough such as occurs with smoking, asthma, emphysema, or if cough is accompanied by excessive phlegm (mucus) unless directed by a physician. As with any drug, if you are pregnant or nursing a baby, seek the advice of a health professional before using this product. Keep this and all drugs out of reach of children. In case of accidental overdose, seek professional assistance or contact a Poison Control Center immediately.

Directions for Use:
Adults (12 years and older): Take 1 to 2 teaspoonfuls every 4 hours or 3 teaspoonfuls every 6 to 8 hours. Do not exceed 12 teaspoonfuls in 24 hours.
Children (6–12 years): Take ½–1 teaspoonful every 4 hours or 1½ teaspoonfuls every 6 to 8 hours. Do not exceed 6 teaspoonfuls in 24 hours.
Children (2–6 years): Take ¼ to ½ teaspoonful every 4 hours or ¾ teaspoonful every 6 to 8 hours. Do not exceed 3 teaspoonfuls in 24 hours.
Children (under 2 years): Consult physician for recommended dosage.

How Supplied: 4-oz bottles. Store at 59°–86°F.
Shown in Product Identification Section, page 419

BENYLIN® Decongestant

Description: Each teaspoonful (5 mL) contains:
Diphenhydramine
    Hydrochloride   12.5 mg
Pseudoephedrine
    Hydrochloride   30.0 mg
Also contains: Alcohol 5%; FD&C Yellow No. 6 (Sunset Yellow); Flavors; Glucose Liquid; Glycerin; Menthol; Purified Water; Saccharin Sodium; Sodium Citrate; Sucrose.

Indications: For the temporary relief of cough due to minor throat and bronchial irritations as may occur with the common cold or with inhaled irritants; and nasal congestion due to the common cold, hay fever, or other upper respiratory allergies.

Warnings: A persistent cough may be a sign of a serious condition. Do not take this product for persistent or chronic cough such as occurs with smoking, asthma, emphysema, or when cough is accompanied by excessive phlegm (mucus). If cough persists for more than one (1) week, tends to recur, or is accompanied by fever, rash, or persistent headache, consult a physician. May cause excitability, especially in children. Do not take this product if you have high blood pressure, heart disease, diabetes, thyroid disease, glaucoma, or difficulty in urination due to enlargement of the prostate gland except under the advice and supervision of a physician. Do not exceed recommended dosage because at higher doses nervousness, dizziness, or sleeplessness may occur. Do not give to children under six (6) years of age except under the advice and supervision of a physician. May cause marked drowsiness. Avoid driving a motor vehicle or operating heavy machinery, or drinking alcoholic beverages. Keep this and all drugs out of the reach of children. In case of accidental overdose, seek professional assistance or contact a Poison Control Center immediately. As with any drug, if you are pregnant or nursing a baby, seek the advice of a health professional before using this product.

Drug Interaction Precaution: Do not take this product if you are presently taking a prescription drug for high blood pressure or depression without first consulting your doctor.

Directions for Use:
Adults (12 years and older): Take 2 teaspoonfuls every 4 hours. Do not exceed 8 teaspoonfuls in 24 hours.
Children (6–12 years): Take 1 teaspoonful every 4 hours. Do not exceed 4 teaspoonfuls in 24 hours.
Children (under 6 years): Consult physician for recommended dosage.

How Supplied: 4-oz. bottles. Store at 59°–86°F.
Shown in Product Identification Section, page 419

BENYLIN® Expectorant

Description: Each teaspoonful (5 mL) contains:
Dextromethorphan
    Hydrobromide   5.0 mg
Guaifenesin   100.0 mg
Also contains: Alcohol 5%; Citric Acid; FD&C Red No. 40; Flavors; Glycerin; Purified Water; Saccharin Sodium, Sodium Benzoate, Sodium Citrate; Sucrose.

Indications: Nonnarcotic cough suppressant for the temporary relief of coughs plus an expectorant to relieve upper chest congestion due to minor bronchial irritations as may occur with the common cold, or inhaled irritants. Helps loosen phlegm (sputum) and thin bronchial secretions to rid the bronchial passageways of bothersome mucus.

Warnings: Do not take this product for persistent or chronic cough such as occurs with smoking, asthma, chronic bronchitis, or emphysema, or where cough is accompanied by excessive phlegm (mucus or sputum) unless directed by a physician. A persistent cough may be a sign of a serious condition. If cough persists for more than one week, tends to recur, or is accompanied by fever, rash, or persistent headache, consult a physician. Do not give to children under 2 years of age unless directed by a physician. As with any drug, if you are pregnant or nursing a baby, seek the advice of a health professional before using this product. Keep this and all drugs out of the reach of children. In case of accidental overdose, seek professional assistance or contact a Poison Control Center immediately.

Directions for Use:
Adults (12 years and older): Take 2–4 teaspoonfuls every 4 hours (or fill dosage cup to the corresponding teaspoon level indicated). Do not exceed 24 teaspoonfuls in 24 hours.
Children (6–12 years): Take 1–2 teaspoonfuls every 4 hours (or fill dosage cup to the corresponding teaspoon level indicated). Do not exceed 12 teaspoonfuls in 24 hours.
Children (2–6 years): Take ½–1 teaspoonful every 4 hours (or fill dosage cup

to the corresponding teaspoon level indicated). Do not exceed 6 teaspoonfuls in 24 hours.
Children (under 2 years): Consult your physician for recommended dosage.

How Supplied: Benylin Expectorant is supplied in 4-oz and 8-oz bottles. Store at 59°–86°F.
Shown in Product Identification Section, page 419

CALADRYL® Lotion
[că 'lă drĭl "]
CALADRYL Cream
CALADRYL Spray
CALADRYL Clear Lotion

Description: Caladryl Lotion—A drying, calamine-antihistamine lotion containing Calamine 8%, Benadryl® (diphenhydramine hydrochloride), 1%. Also contains: Alcohol 2%; Camphor; Fragrances; Glycerin; Sodium Carboxymethylcellulose; and Water, Purified.
Caladryl Cream—Calamine 8%, Benadryl (diphenhydramine hydrochloride) 1%. Also contains: Camphor; Cetyl Alcohol; Cresin White; Fragrance; Propylene Glycol; Propylparaben; Polysorbate 60; Sorbitan Stearate; Water, Purified.
Caladryl Spray—Calamine 8%, Benadryl (diphenhydramine hydrochloride) 1%. Also contains: Alcohol 9%, Camphor, FD&C Red #40, Fragrance, Isobutane, Quarternium-18 Hectorite, Sorbitan Sesquioleate, and Talc.
Caladryl Clear Lotion—Benadryl (diphenhydramine hydrochloride) 1%, Zinc Oxide 2%. Also contains: Alcohol 2%, Camphor, Chlorophyllin Sodium, Diazolidinyl Urea, Fragrance, Glycerin, Hydroxypropyl Methylcellulose, Methylparaben, Polysorbate 40, Propylene Glycol, Propylparaben, and Water.

Indications: For relief of itching due to mild poison ivy or oak, insect bites, or other minor skin irritations.

Warnings: For external use only. Do not apply to blistered, raw or oozing areas of the skin. Do not use on chicken pox or measles, unless supervised by a doctor. Do not use on extensive areas of the skin or for longer than 7 days except as directed by a doctor. Avoid contact with the eyes or other mucous membranes. Discontinue use if burning sensation or rash develops or condition persists. Remove by washing with soap and water. Do not use any other drugs containing diphenhydramine while using this product. Additional spray warnings: Flammable. Do not use while smoking or near an open flame. Contents under pres-

Continued on next page

This product information was prepared in November 1991. On these and other Parke-Davis Products, detailed information may be obtained by addressing PARKE-DAVIS, Consumer Health Products Group, Division of Warner-Lambert Company, Morris Plains, NJ 07950.

Parke-Davis—Cont.

sure. Do not puncture or incinerate. Do not store at temperatures above 120°F. Intentional misuse by deliberately concentrating and inhaling the contents can be harmful or fatal.
KEEP THIS AND ALL DRUGS OUT OF THE REACH OF CHILDREN. In case of accidental ingestion seek professional assistance or contact a Poison Control Center immediately.

Directions: For adults and children 6 years of age and older: Apply sparingly to the affected area three to four times daily. Before each application cleanse skin with soap and water and dry affected area. Children under 6 years of age: Consult a doctor.

How Supplied: Caladryl Cream—1½-oz tubes.
Caladryl Lotion—2½ fl.-oz. (75 ml) squeeze bottles and 6 fl.-oz. bottles.
Caladryl Spray—4 oz. can.
Caladryl Clear Lotion—6 fl.-oz. bottle.
Shown in Product Identification Section, page 419

GELUSIL®
[jĕl ′ū-sĭl ″]
Antacid–Anti-gas
Liquid/Tablets
Sodium Free

Each teaspoonful (5 mL) or tablet contains:
200 mg aluminum hydroxide
200 mg magnesium hydroxide
25 mg simethicone
Also contains: Liquid: Ammonia Solution Strong; Citric Acid; Flavors; Hydroxypropyl Methylcellulose; Menthol; Sodium Saccharin; Sorbitol Solution; Water; Xanthan Gum.
Tablets: Flavors; Magnesium Stearate; Mannitol; Sorbitol; Sugar.

Advantages:
● High acid-neutralizing capacity
● Sodium free
● Simethicone for antiflatulent activity
● Good taste for better patient compliance
● Fast dissolution of chewed tablets for prompt relief

Indications: For the relief of heartburn, sour stomach, acid indigestion and to relieve symptoms of gas.

Dosage and Administration: Two or more teaspoonfuls or tablets one hour after meals and at bedtime, or as directed by a physician.
Tablets should be chewed.

Warnings: Do not take more than 12 tablets or teaspoonfuls in a 24-hour period, or use this maximum dosage for more than two weeks, or use this product if you have kidney disease, except under the advice and supervision of a physician.
Keep this and all drugs out of the reach of children.

Professional Warnings: Prolonged use of aluminum-containing antacids in pa-

tients with renal failure may result in or worsen dialysis osteomalacia. Elevated tissue aluminum levels contribute to the development of the dialysis encephalopathy and osteomalacia syndromes. Small amounts of aluminum are absorbed from the gastrointestinal tract and renal excretion of aluminum is impaired in renal failure. Aluminum is not well removed by dialysis because it is bound to albumin and transferrin, which do not cross dialysis membranes. As a result, aluminum is deposited in bone, and dialysis osteomalacia may develop when large amounts of aluminum are ingested orally by patients with impaired renal function. Aluminum forms insoluble complexes with phosphate in the gastrointestinal tract, thus decreasing phosphate absorption. Prolonged use of aluminum-containing antacids by normophosphatemic patients may result in hypophosphatemia if phosphate intake is not adequate. In its more severe forms, hypophosphatemia can lead to anorexia, malaise, muscle weakness, and osteomalacia.

Drug Interaction Precaution: Do not take this product if you are presently taking a prescription antibiotic drug containing any form of tetracycline.

How Supplied:
Liquid—In plastic bottles of 12 fl oz.
Tablets—White, embossed Gelusil P-D 034—individual strips of 10 in boxes of 100.
Store at 59°–86°F (15°–30°C).
Shown in Product Identification Section, page 419

GERIPLEX-FS® KAPSEALS®
[jĕ ′rĭ-plĕx ″]

Composition: Each Kapseal represents:
Vitamin A .... (1.5 mg) 5,000 IU*
(acetate)
Vitamin C .... 50 mg
(ascorbic acid)†
Vitamin B$_1$ .... 5 mg
(thiamine mononitrate)
Vitamin B$_2$ .... 5 mg
(riboflavin)
Vitamin B$_{12}$, crystalline
(cyanocobalamin) .... 2 mcg
Choline dihydrogen
citrate .... 20 mg
Nicotinamide .... 15 mg
(niacinamide)
Vitamin E (*dl* -alpha-tocopheryl acetate) .... (5 mg) 5 IU*
Iron‡ .... 6 mg
Copper sulfate .... 4 mg
Manganese sulfate
(monohydrate) .... 4 mg
Zinc sulfate .... 2 mg

---

*International Units
†Supplied as sodium ascorbate
‡Supplied as dried ferrous sulfate equivalent to the labeled amount of elemental iron

Calcium phosphate, dibasic
(anhydrous) .... 200 mg
Taka-Diastase® (*Aspergillus oryzae* enzymes) ....2½ gr
Docusate sodium .... 100 mg
Also contains magnesium stearate, NF.

The capsule shell contains FD&C Blue No. 1, FD&C Red No. 3 and Gelatin.
Action and Uses: A preparation containing vitamins, minerals, and a fecal softener for middle-aged and older individuals. The fecal softening agent, docusate sodium, acts to soften stools and make bowel movements easier.

Administration and Dosage: USUAL DOSAGE —One capsule daily, with or immediately after a meal.

How Supplied: Bottles of 100.
Store at controlled room temperature 15°–30°C (59° to 86°F). Protect from light and moisture.

GERIPLEX-FS®
[jĕ ′rĭ-plĕx ″]
LIQUID
Geriatric Vitamin Formula with Iron and a Fecal Softener

Composition: Each 30 ml represents vitamin B$_1$ (thiamine hydrochloride), 1.2 mg; vitamin B$_2$ (as riboflavin-5′-phosphate sodium), 1.7 mg; vitamin B$_6$ (pyridoxine hydrochloride), 1 mg; vitamin B$_{12}$ (cyanocobalamin) crystalline, 5 mcg; niacinamide, 15 mg; iron (as ferric ammonium citrate, green), 15 mg; Pluronic® F-68,* 200 mg; alcohol, 18%.
Also contains: Brandy, Caramel NF, Citric Acid Anhydrous NF, D&C Red No. 33, Flavors, FD&C Red No. 40, Glucono Delta Lactone, Glucose Liquid USP, Glycerin USP, Sodium Citrate USP, Sodium Saccharin NF, Sorbitol Solution USP, Sugar, Water Purified.

Administration and Dosage: USUAL ADULT DOSAGE — Two tablespoonfuls (30 ml) daily or as recommended by the physician.

How Supplied: 16-oz bottles.
Store below 30° (86°F). Protect from light and freezing.

---

*Pluronic is a registered trademark of BASF Wyandotte Corporation for polymers of ethylene oxide and propylene oxide.

MEDI–FLU™ Caplet, Liquid

Composition:
Each Caplet contains: **Active Ingredients**—Pseudoephedrine Hydrochloride 30mg., Chlorpheniramine Maleate 2mg., Dextromethorphan Hydrobromide 15mg., Acetaminophen 500mg.
Inactive Ingredients—Cellulose derivatives, croscarmellose sodium, magnesium stearate, mauba wax, polyethylene glycol, starch, stearic acid.
Each fluid ounce contains: **Active Ingredients**—Acetaminophen 1000mg., Chlorpheniramine Maleate 4mg., Dex-

tromethorphan Hydrobromide 30mg., and Pseudoephedrine Hydrochloride 60mg. **Inactive Ingredients**—Alcohol (19%), Citric Acid, D&C Red No. 33, FD&C Red No. 40, Flavors, Glycerin, Propylene Glycol, Sodium Citrate, Sodium Chloride, Sodium Saccharin, Sorbitol Solution, Sugar and Water.

Actions: Medi-Flu provides temporary relief of these flu symptoms: Fever, body aches & pains, nasal congestion, runny nose, minor sore throat pain, coughing, sneezing, headache and watery eyes.

Warnings: Do not exceed recommended dosage because at higher doses nervousness, dizziness or sleeplessness may occur. Do not take this product for more than 7 days. If symptoms do not improve or are accompanied by fever for more than 3 days or if fever recurs after 3 days consult a doctor. Do not take this product if you have high blood pressure, heart disease, diabetes, thyroid disease, asthma, glaucoma, emphysema, chronic pulmonary disease, shortness of breath, difficulty in breathing, or difficulty in urination due to an enlargement of the prostate gland unless directed by a doctor. Do not take this product for persistent or chronic cough such as occurs with smoking, or if cough is accompanied by excessive phlegm (mucus) unless directed by a doctor. A persistent cough may be a sign of a serious condition. If cough persists for more than one week, tends to recur, or is accompanied or followed by fever, headache, rash, nausea, or vomiting consult a doctor promptly. May cause drowsiness: alcohol, sedatives, and tranquilizers may increase drowsiness effect. Avoid alcoholic beverages while taking this product. May cause excitability. Do not take this product if you are taking sedatives or tranquilizers without first consulting your doctor. Use caution when driving a motor vehicle or operating machinery. As with any drug if you are pregnant or nursing a baby, seek the advise of a health professional before using this product. KEEP THIS AND ALL DRUGS OUT OF THE REACH OF CHILDREN. In case of accidental overdose, seek professional assistance or contact a Poison Control Center immediately. Do not give this product to children under 12 years of age except under the advice and supervision of a doctor.

Drug Interaction Precaution: Do not take this product if you are presently taking a prescription drug for high blood pressure or depression without first consulting your doctor.

Dosage and Administration:
Caplets: Adults—two caplets every 6 hours, as needed, not to exceed 8 caplets in 24 hours. Under 12 consult a physician.
Liquid: 1 fluid ounce (2 tablespoonfuls) every 6 hours as needed, not to exceed 4 fluid ounces in 24 hours. Under 12 consult a physician.

How Supplied: 16 caplets or 6 fl. oz. liquid
Shown in Product Identification Section, page 419

MEDI–FLU WITHOUT DROWSINESS™

Composition: Each caplet contains:
Active Ingredients: Pseudoephedrine Hydrochloride 30mg, Dextromethorphan Hydrobromide 15mg, Acetaminophen 500mg.

Inactive Ingredients: Candelilla Wax, Corn Starch, Croscarmellose Sodium, D&C Red No. 33 Aluminum Lake, FD&C Red No. 40 Aluminum Lake, Hydroxypropyl Methylcellulose, Microcrystalline Cellulose, Polyethylene Glycol, Polysorbate 80, Titanium Dioxide, Zinc Stearate.

Indications: Medi-Flu provides temporary relief of these flu symptoms: fever, body aches and pains, nasal and sinus congestion, minor sore throat pain, coughing and headache.

Warnings: Do not exceed recommended dosage because at higher doses nervousness, dizziness or sleeplessness may occur. Do not take this product for more than 7 days. If symptoms do not improve or are accompanied by fever for more than 3 days or if fever recurs after 3 days consult a doctor. Do not take this product if you have high blood pressure, heart disease, diabetes, thyroid disease, or difficulty in urination due to an enlargement of the prostate gland unless directed by a doctor. Do not take this product for persistent or chronic cough or chronic cough such as occurs with smoking, or if cough is accompanied by phlegm (mucus) unless directed by a doctor. A persistent cough may be a sign of a serious condition. If cough persists for more than one week, tends to recur, or is accompanied or followed by fever, headache, rash, nausea, or vomiting consult a doctor promptly. As with any drug if you are pregnant or nursing a baby, seek the advise of a health professional before using this product. KEEP THIS AND ALL DRUGS OUT OF THE REACH OF CHILDREN. In case of accidental overdose, seek professional assistance or contact a Poison Control Center immediately. Do not give this product to children under 12 years of age except under the advice and supervision of a doctor.

Drug Interaction Precaution: Do not take this product if you are presently taking a prescription drug for high blood pressure or depression without first consulting your doctor.

Dosage and Administration: Adults: 2 caplets every 6 hours, as needed, not to exceed 8 caplets in 24 hours. Under 12: consult a physician.

How Supplied: 16 caplet box
Shown in Product Identification Section, page 419

MYADEC®
High Potency Multivitamin Multimineral Formula

Each Tablet Represents:
[See table top of next column]

		% of US Recommended Daily Allowances (US RDA)
Vitamins		
Vitamin A	9,000 IU*	180%
Vitamin D	400 IU	100%
Vitamin E	30 IU	100%
Vitamin C (ascorbic acid)	90 mg	150%
Folic Acid	0.4 mg	100%
Thiamine (vitamin B₁)	10 mg	667%
Riboflavin (vitamin B₂)	10 mg	588%
Niacin**	20 mg	100%
Vitamin B₆	5 mg	250%
Vitamin B₁₂	10 mcg	167%
Pantothenic Acid	20 mg	200%
Vitamin K	25 mcg	***
Biotin	45 mcg	15%
Minerals		
Iodine	150 mcg	100%
Iron	30 mg	167%
Magnesium	100 mg	25%
Copper	3 mg	150%
Zinc	15 mg	100%
Manganese	7.5 mg	***
Calcium	70 mg	7%
Phosphorus	54 mg	5%
Potassium	8 mg	***
Selenium	15 mcg	***
Molybdenum	15 mcg	***
Chromium	15 mcg	***

  * International Units
 ** Supplied as niacinamide
*** No US Recommended Daily Allowance (US RDA) has been established for this nutrient.

Ingredients: Dibasic calcium phosphate, cellulose derivatives, magnesium oxide, calcium sulfate, ascorbic acid, ferrous fumarate, *dl*-alpha tocopheryl acetate, zinc sulfate, *d*-calcium pantothenate, vitamin A acetate, magnesium sulfate, niacinamide, potassium chloride, riboflavin, thiamine mononitrate, croscarmellose sodium, stearic acid, cupric sulfate, pyridoxine hydrochloride, magnesium stearate, polyethylene glycol, biotin, phytonadione, silicon dioxide, povidone, cyanocobalamin, modified food starch, methylparaben (preservative), vitamin D₃ beadlets, folic acid, candelilla wax, vanillin, potassium iodide, propylparaben (preservative), chromium chloride, sodium molybdate, sodium selenate, FD&C Yellow #6, FD&C Red #40, titanium dioxide (color) and FD&C Blue #2.

Actions and Uses: High potency vitamin supplement with minerals for adults.

Dosage: One tablet daily with a full meal.

Continued on next page

This product information was prepared in November 1991. On these and other Parke-Davis Products, detailed information may be obtained by addressing PARKE-DAVIS, Consumer Health Products Group, Division of Warner-Lambert Company, Morris Plains, NJ 07950.

Parke-Davis—Cont.

How Supplied: In bottles of 130. Store below 30°C (86°F). Protect from moisture.

Shown in Product Identification Section, page 419

NATABEC® KAPSEALS®

Each capsule represents:

Vitamins	
Vitamin A	4,000 IU*
Vitamin D	400 IU
Vitamin C	50 mg
Vitamin B₁	3 mg
Vitamin B₂	2.0 mg
Nicotinamide†	10 mg
Vitamin B₆	3 mg
Vitamin B₁₂	5 mcg
Minerals	
Precipitated Calcium carbonate	600 mg
Iron	30 mg

*IU = International Units
†Supplied as niacinamide

Action and Uses: A multivitamin and mineral supplement for use during pregnancy and lactation.

Dosage: One capsule daily, or as directed by physician.

How Supplied: In bottles of 100. The color combination of the banded capsule is a Warner-Lambert trademark.

SINUTAB® Sinus Medication, Regular Strength Without Drowsiness Formula, Tablets

Indications: Specially formulated to provide fast, temporary relief of sinus pain and congestion due to colds, flu, allergy and hay fever without drowsiness.

Active Ingredients: Each tablet contains: Acetaminophen 325 mg., pseudoephedrine hydrochloride 30 mg.

Inactive Ingredients: Cellulose microcrystalline, croscarmellose sodium, D&C red No. 33, FD&C red No. 40, hydroxypropyl cellulose, hydroxypropyl methylcellulose, magnesium stearate, propylene glycol, simethicone, starch pregelatinized, titanium dioxide, zinc stearate.

Actions: Sinutab® Sinus Medication, Regular Strength Without Drowsiness Formula, Tablets contain an analgesic (acetaminophen) to relieve pain and a decongestant (pseudoephedrine hydrochloride) to reduce congestion of the nasopharyngeal mucosa.
Acetaminophen is both analgesic and antipyretic. Because acetaminophen is not a salicylate, Sinutab® Sinus Medication, Regular Strength Without Drowsiness Formula, Tablets can be used by patients who are allergic to aspirin.
Pseudoephedrine hydrochloride, a sympathomimetic drug, provides vasoconstriction of the nasopharyngeal mucosa resulting in a nasal decongestant effect.

The absence of antihistamine in the formula provides the added benefit of reduced likelihood of drowsiness side effects.

Warnings: Do not exceed recommended dosage. If symptoms persist, do not improve within 7 days, or are accompanied by high fever, or if new symptoms occur, see your doctor before continuing use. Do not take this product if you have high blood pressure, heart disease, diabetes, thyroid disease, or difficulty in urination due to an enlarged prostate except under doctor's supervision. Do not take this product for more than 10 days. As with any drug, if you are pregnant or nursing a baby, seek the advice of a health professional before using this product.

Drug Interaction: Do not take this product if you are presently taking a prescription drug for high blood pressure or depression without first consulting your doctor.

Precaution: Keep this and all drugs out of the reach of children.

Symptoms and Treatment of Oral Overdosage: In case of accidental overdose, seek professional help or contact a Poison Control Center immediately.

Dosage and Administration: Adults 2 tablets every 4 hours, not to exceed 8 tablets in 24 hours, or as directed by physician. Children under 12 should use only as directed by physician.

How Supplied: Sinutab® Sinus Medication, Regular Strength Without Drowsiness Formula, Tablets are pink, coated and scored so that tablets may be split in half. They are supplied in easy-to-open (exempt) blister packs of 24 tablets.

Shown in Product Identification Section, page 419

SINUTAB® Sinus Allergy Medication, Maximum Strength Formula, Tablets and Caplets

Indications: Specially formulated to provide fast, maximum strength relief of sinus pain and congestion. Sinutab Sinus Allergy Medication is a complete allergy and hay fever medication relieving runny nose, itchy watery eyes and sneezing.

Active Ingredients: Each tablet/caplet contains: Acetaminophen 500 mg., chlorpheniramine maleate 2 mg., pseudoephedrine hydrochloride 30 mg.

Inactive Ingredients:
Tablets contain: Carboxymethyl starch, cellulose, corn starch, croscarmellose sodium, hydroxypropyl cellulose, stearic acid, zinc stearate, D&C yellow No. 10 aluminum lake and FD&C yellow No. 6 aluminum lake.
Caplets contain: Microcrystalline cellulose, corn starch, croscarmellose sodium, hydroxypropyl cellulose, hydroxypropyl methylcellulose, magnesium stearate,

polyethylene glycol, sodium starch glycolate, stearic acid, titanium dioxide, zinc stearate, D&C yellow No. 10 aluminum lake, and FD&C yellow No. 6 aluminum lake.

Actions: Sinutab® Sinus Allergy Medication, Maximum Strength Formula, Tablets and Caplets contain an analgesic (acetaminophen) to relieve pain, a decongestant (pseudoephedrine hydrochloride) to reduce congestion of the nasopharyngeal mucosa, and an antihistamine (chlorpheniramine maleate) to help control allergic symptoms.
Acetaminophen is both analgesic and antipyretic. Because acetaminophen is not a salicylate, Sinutab® Sinus Allergy Medication, Maximum Strength Formula, Tablets and Caplets can be used by patients who are allergic to aspirin.
Pseudoephedrine hydrochloride, a sympathomimetic drug, provides vasoconstriction of the nasopharyngeal mucosa resulting in a nasal decongestant effect.
Chlorpheniramine maleate is an antihistamine incorporated to provide relief of running nose, sneezing, itching of the nose or throat, and itchy and watery eyes as may occur in allergic rhinitis.

Warnings: Do not exceed recommended dosage. If symptoms persist, do not improve within 7 days, or are accompanied by high fever, or if new symptoms occur, see your doctor before continuing use. Do not take this product if you have high blood pressure, heart disease, diabetes, thyroid disease, glaucoma, or difficulty in urination due to an enlarged prostate except under doctor's supervision. Do not take this product for more than 10 days. As with any drug, if you are pregnant or nursing a baby, seek the advice of a health professional before using this product. This product may cause drowsiness. Alcohol, sedatives and tranquilizers may increase the drowsiness effect. Avoid alcoholic beverages while taking this product. Do not take this product if you are taking sedatives or tranquilizers, without first consulting your doctor. Use caution when driving a motor vehicle or operating machinery.

Drug Interaction: Do not take this product if you are presently taking a prescription drug for high blood pressure or depression without first consulting your doctor.

Precaution: Keep this and all drugs out of the reach of children.

Symptoms and Treatment of Oral Overdosage: In case of accidental overdose, seek professional help or contact a Poison Control Center immediately.

Dosage and Administration: Adults 2 tablets or caplets every 6 hours, not to exceed 8 tablets or caplets in 24 hours, or as directed by physician. Children under 12 should use only as directed by physician.

How Supplied: Sinutab® Sinus Allergy Medication, Maximum Strength Formula, Caplets are yellow and coated. The Tablets are yellow and uncoated.

They are supplied in child-resistant blister packs in boxes of 24 tablets or caplets.
Shown in Product Identification Section, page 419

SINUTAB® Sinus Medication, Maximum Strength Without Drowsiness Formula, Tablets and Caplets

Indications: Specially formulated to provide fast, maximum strength relief of sinus pain and congestion due to colds, flu and allergies. Sinutab relieves sinus headache and pressure without drowsiness.

Active Ingredients: Each tablet/caplet contains: Acetaminophen 500 mg., pseudoephedrine hydrochloride 30 mg.

Inactive Ingredients:
Tablets contain: Carboxymethyl starch, cellulose, corn starch, croscarmellose sodium, hydroxypropyl cellulose, stearic acid, zinc stearate, D&C yellow No. 10 aluminum lake and FD&C yellow No. 6 aluminum lake.
Caplets contain: Cellulose, corn starch, croscarmellose sodium, hydroxypropyl cellulose, hydroxypropyl methylcellulose, magnesium stearate, polyethylene glycol, sodium starch glycolate, stearic acid, titanium dioxide, zinc stearate, D&C yellow No. 10 aluminum lake and FD&C yellow No. 6 aluminum lake.

Actions: Sinutab® Sinus Medication, Maximum Strength Without Drowsiness Formula, Tablets and Caplets contain an analgesic (acetaminophen) to relieve pain, and a decongestant (pseudoephedrine hydrochloride) to reduce congestion of the nasopharyngeal mucosa.
Acetaminophen is both analgesic and antipyretic. Because acetaminophen is not a salicylate, Sinutab® Sinus Medication, Maximum Strength Without Drowsiness Formula, can be used by patients who are allergic to aspirin.
Pseudoephedrine hydrochloride, a sympathomimetic drug, provides vasoconstriction of the nasopharyngeal mucosa resulting in a nasal decongestant effect. The absence of antihistamine in the formula provides the added benefit of reduced likelihood of drowsiness side effects.

Warnings: Do not exceed recommended dosage. If symptoms persist, do not improve within seven days, or are accompanied by high fever, or if new symptoms occur, see your doctor before continuing use. Do not take this product if you have high blood pressure, heart disease, diabetes, thyroid disease, or difficulty in urination due to an enlarged prostate except under doctor's supervision. Do not take this product for more than 10 days. As with any drug, if you are pregnant or nursing a baby, seek the advice of a health professional before using this product.

Drug Interaction: Do not take this product if you are presently taking a prescription drug for high blood pressure or depression without first consulting your doctor.

Precaution: Keep this and all drugs out of the reach of children.

Symptoms and Treatment of Oral Overdosage: In case of accidental overdose, seek professional help or contact a Poison Control Center immediately.

Dosage and Administration: Adults 2 tablets or caplets every 6 hours, not to exceed 8 tablets or caplets in 24 hours or as directed by physician. Children under 12 should use only as directed by physician.

How Supplied: Sinutab® Sinus Medication, Maximum Strength Without Drowsiness Formula, Caplets are orange and coated. The Tablets are orange and uncoated. They are supplied in child-resistant blister packs in boxes of 24 tablets or caplets and in bottles of 50 caplets with child-resistant caps.
Shown in Product Identification Section, page 419

THERA-COMBEX H-P®
High-Potency Vitamin B Complex with 500 mg Vitamin C

Composition: Each Kapseal contains:
Ascorbic acid
(vitamin C)................................. 500 mg
Thiamine (vitamin B_1)
mononitrate................................ 25 mg
Riboflavin
(vitamin B_2)................................. 15 mg
Pyridoxine hydrochloride
(vitamin B_6)................................. 10 mg
Vitamin B_{12}
(cyanocobalamin)........................ 5 mcg
Niacinamide.................................. 100 mg
dl-Panthenol .... 20 mg

Uses: For the prevention or treatment of vitamin B complex and vitamin C deficiencies.

Dosage: One or two Kapseals daily

How Supplied: Bottles of 100.

TUCKS®
Pre-moistened Hemorrhoidal/Vaginal Pads

Indications: For prompt, temporary relief of minor external itching, burning and irritation associated with hemorrhoids, rectal or vaginal surgical stitches and other minor rectal or vaginal irritation.
—Soothe, cool, and comfort itching, burning, and irritation of sensitive rectal and outer vaginal areas.
—As a compress, to help relieve discomfort from rectal/vaginal surgical stitches.
—Effective hygienic wipe to cleanse rectal area of irritation-causing residue.

Directions: For external use only. *As a hemorrhoidal treatment* —Adults: When practical, cleanse the affected area with soap and warm water, and rinse thoroughly. Gently dry by patting or blotting with toilet tissue or soft cloth before each application of this product. Gently apply to affected area by patting and then discard. Can be used up to six times daily or after each bowel movement. Children under 12 years of age: consult a physician.
As a hygienic wipe —Use as a wipe instead of toilet tissue after bowel movement or after napkin or tampon change.
As a moist compress —For soothing relief, fold pad and place in contact with irritated tissue. Leave in place for 5 to 15 minutes. Repeat as needed.

Warnings: If condition worsens or does not improve within 7 days, consult a physician. Do not exceed recommended daily dosage unless directed by a physician. In case of bleeding, consult a physician promptly. Do not put this product in the rectum by using fingers or any mechanical device or applicator. Keep this and all drugs out of the reach of children. In case of accidental ingestion, seek professional assistance or contact a Poison Control Center immediately.

Contains: Soft pads pre-moistened with a solution containing 50% Witch Hazel; also contains: Water, Glycerin, Alcohol 7%, Sodium Citrate, Citric Acid, Methylparaben, and Benzalkonium Citrate.

How Supplied: Jars of 40 and 100. Also available as Tucks Take-Alongs®, individual, foil-wrapped, nonwoven wipes, 12 per box.
Shown in Product Identification Section, page 420

TUCKS® CREAM

Active Ingredient: Witch Hazel (Hamamelis Water) 50%
Also contains: Alcohol 7%, White Petrolatum, Sorbitol Solution, Cetyl Alcohol, Polysorbate 60, Polyethylene Stearate, Anhydrous Lanolin, Glyceryl Oleate, Propylene Glycol and Benzethonium Chloride

Indications: For prompt, temporary relief of minor external ITCHING, BURNING and IRRITATION associated with Hemorrhoids.

Warnings: If condition worsens or does not improve within 7 days, consult a physician. Do not exceed the recommended daily dosage unless directed by a physician. In case of rectal bleeding, consult a physician promptly. Do not put this product into the rectum by using fingers or any other mechanical device or applicator. KEEP THIS AND ALL DRUGS OUT

Continued on next page

This product information was prepared in November 1991. On these and other Parke-Davis Products, detailed information may be obtained by addressing PARKE-DAVIS, Consumer Health Products Group, Division of Warner-Lambert Company, Morris Plains, NJ 07950.

Parke-Davis—Cont.

OF THE REACH OF CHILDREN. In case of accidental ingestion, seek professional assistance or contact a Poison Contol Center immediately.

Directions: Adults: When practical, cleanse the affected area with Tucks Hemorrhoidal Pads or mild soap and warm water and rinse thoroughly. Gently dry by patting or blotting with toilet tissue or soft cloth before each application. Remove cap and apply externally to affected area up to 6 times daily or after each bowel movement. Children under 12 years of age: Consult a physician.

How Supplied: Tucks Cream (water-washable) in 1.4 oz. tube with dispensing cap.

The Parthenon Co., Inc.
3311 W. 2400 SOUTH
SALT LAKE CITY, UTAH 84119

DEVROM® CHEWABLE TABLETS

Active Ingredients: Bismuth Subgallate 200 mg/tablet

Indications: Devrom Chewable Tablets are used as an aid to reduce odor from colostomies or ileostomies.

Warnings: This product cannot be expected to be effective in the reduction of odor due to faulty personal hygiene. Keep this and all medication out of the reach of children.
Note: The beneficial ingredient in these tablets may coat the tongue which may also darken in color. This condition is harmless and temporary. Darkening of the stool is also possible and is equally harmless.

Dosage and Administration: Take one to two tablets three times a day with meals or as directed by physician. Chew or swallow whole if desired. Keep bottle tightly closed in cool, dry place. Protect from light.

How Supplied: 100 tablets per bottle.

Pfizer Consumer Health Care Division
Division of Pfizer Inc.
100 JEFFERSON ROAD
PARSIPPANY, NJ 07054

BEN–GAY® External Analgesic Products

Description: Ben-Gay products contain menthol in an alcohol base gel, combinations of methyl salicylate and menthol in cream and ointment bases, as well as a combination of methyl salicylate, menthol and camphor in a non-greasy cream base; all suitable for topical application.
In addition to the Original Formula Pain Relieving Rub (methyl salicylate, 18.3%; menthol, 16%), Ben-Gay is offered as Regular Strength Pain Relieving Rub [formerly Ben-Gay Greaseless/Stainless] (methyl salicylate, 15%; menthol, 10%), an Extra Strength Arthritis Rub (methyl salicylate, 30%; menthol, 8%), a Sports Formula Sports and Exercise Rub [formerly Extra Strength Sports Balm] (methyl salicylate 28%; menthol 10%), an Ultra Strength Pain Relieving Rub (methyl salicylate 30%; menthol 10%; camphor 4%), a Vanishing Scent Sports and Exercise Rub [formerly Ben-Gay SportsGel] (menthol 3%), and Ben-Gay Warming Ice Vanishing Scent Formula (2.5% menthol in an alcohol base gel).

Action and Uses: Methyl salicylate, menthol and camphor are external analgesics which stimulate sensory receptors of warmth and/or cold. This produces a counter-irritant response which provides temporary relief of minor aches and pains of muscles and joints associated with simple backache, arthritis, strains, bruises and sprains.
Several double-blind clinical studies of Ben-Gay products containing menthol-methyl salicylate have shown the effectiveness of this combination in counteracting minor pain of skeletal muscle stress and arthritis.
Three studies involving a total of 102 normal subjects in which muscle soreness was experimentally induced showed statistically significant beneficial results from use of the active product vs. placebo for lowered Muscle Action Potential (spasms), greater rise in threshold of muscular pain and greater reduction in perceived muscular pain.
Six clinical studies of a total of 207 subjects suffering from minor pain due to osteoarthritis and rheumatoid arthritis showed the active product to give statistically significant beneficial results vs. placebo for greater relief of perceived pain, increased range of motion of the affected joints and increased digital dexterity. In two studies designed to measure the effect of topically applied Ben-Gay vs. Placebo on muscular endurance, discomfort, onset of exercise pain and fatigue, 30 subjects performed a submaximal three-hour run and another 30 subjects performed a maximal treadmill run. Ben-Gay was found to significantly decrease the discomfort during the submaximal and maximal runs, and increase the time before onset of fatigue during the maximal run.
Applied before workouts, Ben-Gay exercise rubs relax tight muscles and increase circulation to make exercising more comfortable, longer.
To help reduce muscle ache and soreness after exercise, a Ben-Gay exercise rub can be applied and allowed to work before taking a shower.

Directions: Apply generously and gently massage into painful area until Ben-Gay disappears. Repeat 3 to 4 times daily.

Warning: Use only as directed. Do not use with a heating pad (may blister skin). Keep away from children to avoid accidental poisoning. Do not swallow. In case of accidental ingestion, seek professional assistance or contact a Poison Control Center immediately. Keep away from eyes, mucous membrane, broken or irritated skin. If skin irritation develops, pain lasts 10 days or more, redness is present, or with arthritis-like conditions in children under 12, call a physician.

BONINE®
(meclizine hydrochloride)
Chewable Tablets

Action: BONINE (meclizine) is an H_1 histamine receptor blocker of the piperazine side chain group. It exhibits its action by an effect on the Central Nervous System (CNS), possibly by its ability to block muscarinic receptors in the brain.

Indications: BONINE is effective in the management of nausea, vomiting and dizziness associated with motion sickness.

Contraindications: Asthma, glaucoma, emphysema, chronic pulmonary disease, shortness of breath, difficulty in breathing, or difficulty in urination due to enlargement of the prostate gland unless directed by a doctor.

Warnings: May cause drowsiness; alcohol, sedatives and tranquilizers may increase the drowsiness effect. Avoid alcoholic beverages while taking this product. Do not take this product if you are taking sedatives or tranquilizers without first consulting your doctor. Do not drive or operate dangerous machinery while taking this medication.
Usage in Children: Clinical studies establishing safety and effectiveness in children have not been done; therefore, usage is not recommended in children under 12 years of age.
Usage in Pregnancy: As with any drug, if you are pregnant or nursing a baby, seek advice of a health care professional before taking this product.

Adverse Reactions: Drowsiness, dry mouth, and on rare occasions, blurred vision have been reported.

Dosage and Administration: For motion sickness, take one or two tablets of Bonine once daily, one hour before travel starts, for up to 24 hours of protection against motion sickness. The tablet can be chewed with or without water or swallowed whole with water. Thereafter, the dose may be repeated every 24 hours for the duration of the travel.

How Supplied: BONINE (meclizine hydrochloride) is available in convenient packets of 8 chewable tablets of 25 mg. meclizine hydrochloride.

Inactive Ingredients: FD&C Red #40, Lactose, Magnesium Stearate, Purified Siliceous Earth, Raspberry Flavor, Saccharin Sodium, Starch, Talc.

DESITIN® OINTMENT

Description: Desitin Ointment combines Zinc Oxide (40%) with Cod Liver

Oil (high in Vitamins A & D), in a petrolatum-lanolin base suitable for topical application.

Actions and Uses: Desitin Ointment is designed to provide relief of diaper rash, superficial wounds and burns, and other minor skin irritations. It helps prevent incidence of diaper rash, protects against urine and other irritants, soothes chafed skin and promotes healing.

Relief and protection is afforded by Zinc Oxide, Cod Liver Oil, Lanolin and Petrolatum. They provide a physical barrier by forming a protective coating over skin or mucous membrane which serves to reduce further effects of irritants on the affected area and relieves burning, pain or itch produced by them. In addition to its protective properties, Zinc Oxide acts as an astringent that helps heal local irritation and inflammation by lessening the flow of mucus and other secretions. Several studies have shown the effectiveness of Desitin Ointment in the relief and prevention of diaper rash.

Two clinical studies involving 90 infants demonstrated the effectiveness of Desitin Ointment in curing diaper rash. The diaper rash area was treated with Desitin Ointment at each diaper change for a period of 24 hours, while the untreated site served as controls. A significant reduction was noted in the severity and area of diaper dermatitis on the treated area.

Ninety-seven (97) babies participated in a 12-week study to show that Desitin Ointment helps prevent diaper rash. Approximately half of the infants (49) were treated with Desitin Ointment on a regular daily basis. The other half (48) received the ointment as necessary to treat any diaper rash which occurred. The incidence as well as the severity of diaper rash was significantly less among the babies using the ointment on a regular daily basis.

In a comparative study of the efficacy of Desitin Ointment vs. a baby powder, forty-five babies were observed for a total of eight weeks. Results support the conclusion that Desitin Ointment is a better prophylactic against diaper rash than the baby powder.

In another study, Desitin was found to be dramatically more effective in reducing the severity of medically diagnosed diaper rash than a commercially available diaper rash product in which only anhydrous lanolin and petrolatum are listed as ingredients. Fifty infants participated in the study, half of whom were treated with Desitin and half with the other product. In the group (25) treated with Desitin, seventeen infants showed significant improvement within 10 hours which increased to twenty-three improved infants within 24 hours. Of the group (25) treated with the other product, only three showed improvement at ten hours with a total of four improved within twenty-four hours. These results are statistically valid to conclude that Desitin Ointment reduces severity of diaper rash within ten hours.

Several other studies show that Desitin Ointment helps relieve other skin disorders, such as contact dermatitis.

Directions: Prevention: To prevent diaper rash, apply Desitin Ointment to the diaper area—especially at bedtime when exposure to wet diapers may be prolonged.

Treatment: If diaper rash is present, or at the first sign of redness, minor skin irritation or chafing, simply apply Desitin Ointment three or four times daily as needed. In superficial noninfected surface wounds and minor burns, apply a thin layer of Desitin Ointment, using a gauze dressing, if necessary. For external use only.

How Supplied: Desitin Ointment is available in 1 ounce (28g), 2 ounce (57g), and 4 ounce (114g) tubes, and 9 ounce (255g) and 1 lb. (454g) jars.

Shown in Product Identification Section, page 420

RHEABAN® Maximum Strength TABLETS
[rē ′ăban]
(attapulgite)

Description: Maximum Strength Rheaban is an anti-diarrheal medication containing activated attapulgite and is offered in tablet form.

Each white Rheaban tablet contains 750 mg. of colloidal activated attapulgite. Rheaban provides the maximum level of medication when taken as directed.

Rheaban contains no narcotics, opiates or other habit-forming drugs.

Actions and Uses: Rheaban is indicated for relief of diarrhea and the cramps and pains associated with it. Attapulgite, which has been activated by thermal treatment, is a highly sorptive substance which absorbs nutrients and digestive enzymes as well as noxious gases, irritants, toxins and some bacteria and viruses that are common causes of diarrhea.

In clinical studies to show the effectiveness in relieving diarrhea and its symptoms, 100 subjects suffering from acute gastroenteritis with diarrhea participated in a double-blind comparison of Rheaban to a placebo. Patients treated with the attapulgite product showed significantly improved relief of diarrhea and its symptoms vs. the placebo.

Dosage and Administration: TABLETS
Adults—2 tablets after initial bowel movement, 2 tablets after each subsequent bowel movement. For a maximum of 12 tablets in 24 hours.
Children 6 to 12 years—1 tablet after initial bowel movement, 1 tablet after each subsequent bowel movement. For a maximum of 6 tablets in 24 hours, or as directed by a physician.

Warnings: Do not exceed 12 tablets in 24 hours. Swallow tablets with water, do not chew. Do not use for more than two days, or in the presence of high fever. Tablets should not be used for infants or

children under 6 years of age unless directed by physician. If diarrhea persists consult a physician.

How Supplied:
Tablets—Boxes of 12 tablets.

Inactive Ingredients: Colloidal Silicon Dioxide, Croscarmellose Sodium, Ethylcellulose, Hydroxypropyl Methylcellulose 2910, Pectin, Pharmaceutical Glaze, Sucrose, Talc, Titanium Dioxide, Zinc Stearate.

RID® Spray
Lice Control Spray

THIS PRODUCT IS NOT FOR USE ON HUMANS OR ANIMALS

Active Ingredient:
*Permethrin 0.50%
INERT INGREDIENTS 99.50%
                                         100.00%
*(3-phenoxyphenyl) methyl (±) cis,trans 3-(2,2-dichloroethenyl) 2,2-dimethylcyclopropanecarboxylate. Cis, trans ratio: min. 35% (±) cis and max. 65% (±) trans

Actions: A highly active synthetic pyrethroid for the control of lice and louse eggs on garments, bedding, furniture and other inanimate objects.

Warnings: Harmful if swallowed. May be absorbed through skin. Avoid inhalation of spray mist. Avoid contact with skin, eyes or clothing. Wash thoroughly after handling and before smoking or eating. Avoid contamination of feed and foodstuffs. Remove pets and birds and cover fish aquaria before space spraying or surface applications. **This product is not for use on humans or animals.** If lice infestation should occur on humans, use Rid Lice Killing Shampoo. Vacate room after treatment and ventilate before reoccupying. Do not allow children or pets to contact treated areas until surfaces are dry. Do not overspray.

Physical and Chemical Hazards: Contents under pressure. Do not use or store near heat or open flame. Do not puncture or incinerate container. Exposure to temperatures above 130° F may cause bursting.
CAUTION: Avoid spraying in eyes. Avoid breathing spray mist. Use only in well ventilated areas. Avoid contact with skin. In case of contact wash immediately with soap and water. Vacate room after treatment and ventilate before reoccupying.
Statement of Practical Treatment: If inhaled: Remove affected person to fresh air. Apply artificial respiration if indicated.
If in eyes: Flush with plenty of water. Contact physician if irritation persists. If on skin: Wash affected areas immediately with soap and water.

Direction For Use: It is a violation of Federal law to use this product in a manner inconsistent with its labeling.

Continued on next page

Pfizer Consumer—Cont.

Shake well before each use. Remove protective cap. Aim spray opening away from person. Push button to spray.

To kill lice and louse eggs: Spray in an inconspicuous area to test for possible staining or discoloration. Inspect again after drying, then proceed to spray entire area to be treated.

Hold container upright with nozzle away from you. Depress valve and spray from a distance of 8 to 10 inches.

Spray each square foot for 3 seconds. Spray only those garments, parts of bedding, including mattresses and furniture that cannot be either laundered or dry cleaned. Do not overspray.

Allow all sprayed articles to dry thoroughly before use. Repeat treatment as necessary.

Buyer assumes all risks of use, storage or handling of this material not in strict accordance with direction given herewith.

STORAGE AND DISPOSAL
Store in cool, dry area. Do not store below 32°F.

Wrap container in several layers of newspaper and dispose of in trash. Do not incinerate or puncture.

How Supplied: 5 oz. aerosol can.

Also available in combination with RID® Lice Treatment Kit as the RID® Lice Elimination System.

RID®
Lice Killing Shampoo

Description: Rid contains a liquid pediculicide whose active ingredients are: pyrethrins 0.3% and piperonyl butoxide, technical 3.00%, equivalent to 2.4% (butylcarbityl) (6-propylpiperonyl) ether and to 0.6% related compounds. Also contains petroleum distillate 1.20% and benzyl alcohol 2.4%. Inert ingredients 93.1%.

Actions: RID kills head lice (*Pediculus humanus capitis*), body lice (*Pediculus humanus humanus*), and pubic or crab lice (*Phthirus pubis*).

The pyrethrins act as a contact poison and affect the parasite's nervous system, resulting in paralysis and death. The efficacy of the pyrethrins is enhanced by the synergist, piperonyl butoxide. Rid rinses out completely after treatment.

The active ingredients in RID are poorly absorbed through the skin. Of the relatively minor amounts that are absorbed, they are rapidly metabolized to water-soluble compounds and eliminated from the body without ill-effects.

Indications: RID is indicated for the treatment of infestations of head lice, body lice and pubic (crab) lice, and their eggs.

Warning: RID should be used with caution by ragweed sensitized persons.

Precautions: This product is for external use only. It is harmful if swallowed. If accidentally swallowed, call a physician

or Poison Control Center immediately. It should not be inhaled. It should be kept out of the eyes and contact with mucous membranes should be avoided. If accidental contact with eyes occur, flush eyes immediately with plenty of water and call a physician. In the case of infection or skin irritation, discontinue use immediately and consult a physician. Consult a physician before use if infestation of eyebrows or eyelashes occurs. Avoid contamination of feed or foodstuffs.

Storage and Disposal: Do not store below 32°F (0°C). Do not reuse empty container. Wrap in several layers of newspaper and discard in trash.

Dosage and Administration: (1) Shake well. Apply undiluted RID to dry hair and scalp or to any other infested area until entirely wet. Do not use on eyelashes or eyebrows. (2) Allow RID to remain on area for 10 minutes but no longer. (3) Wash thoroughly with warm water and soap or shampoo. (4) Dead lice and eggs should be removed with the special nit comb provided. (5) Repeat treatment in 7 to 10 days to kill any newly hatched lice. Do not exceed two consecutive applications within 24 hours.

Since lice infestations are spread by contact, each family member should be examined carefully. If infested, he or she should be treated promptly to avoid spread or reinfestation of previously treated individuals. Contaminated clothing and other articles, such as hats, etc. should be dry cleaned, boiled or otherwise treated until decontaminated to prevent reinfestation or spread.

How Supplied: In 2, 4 and 8 fl. oz. plastic bottles. Exclusive nit removal comb that removes nits and patient instruction booklet (English and Spanish) are included in each package of RID.

Also available in combination with RID Lice Control Spray as the RID Lice Elimination System.

UNISOM® NIGHTTIME SLEEP AID
[yu 'na-som]
(doxylamine succinate)

Description: Pale blue oval scored tablets containing 25 mg. of doxylamine succinate, 2-[α-(2-dimethylaminoethoxy)α-methylbenzyl] pyridine succinate.

Action and Uses: Doxylamine succinate is an antihistamine of the ethanolamine class, which characteristically shows a high incidence of sedation. In a comparative clinical study of over 20 antihistamines on more than 3000 subjects, doxylamine succinate 25 mg. was one of the three most sedating antihistamines, producing a significantly reduced latency to end of wakefulness and comparing favorably with established hypnotic drugs such as secobarbital and pentobarbital in sedation activity. It was chosen as the antihistamine, based on dosage, causing the earliest onset of sleep. In another clinical study, doxylamine succinate 25 mg. scored better than secobarbital 100 mg. as a nighttime hypnotic. Two addi-

tional, identical clinical studies involving a total of 121 subjects demonstrated that doxylamine succinate 25 mg. reduced the sleep latency period by a third, compared to placebo. Duration of sleep was 26.6% longer with doxylamine succinate, and the quality of sleep was rated higher with the drug than with placebo. An EEG study of 6 subjects confirmed the results of these studies. In yet another study, no statistically significant difference was found between doxylamine succinate and flurazepam in the average time required for 200 patients with mild to moderate insomnia to fall asleep over 5 nights following a nightly dose of doxylamine succinate 25 mg. or flurazepam 30 mg., nor was any statistically significant difference found in the total time the 200 patients slept. Patients on doxylamine succinate awoke an average of 1.2 times per night while those on flurazepam awoke an average of 0.9 times per night. In either case the patients awoke rested the following morning. On a rating scale of 1 to 5, doxylamine succinate was given a 3.0, flurazepam a 3.4 by patients rating the degree of restfulness provided by their medication (5 represents "very well rested"). Although statistically significant, the difference between doxylamine succinate 25 mg. and flurazepam 30 mg. in the number of awakenings and degree of restfulness is clinically insignificant.

Administration and Dosage: One tablet 30 minutes before retiring. Not for children under 12 years of age.

Side Effects: Occasional anticholinergic effects may be seen.

Precautions: Unisom® should be taken only at bedtime.

Contraindications: This product should not be taken by pregnant women, or those who are nursing a baby. This product is also contraindicated for asthma, glaucoma, enlargement of the prostate gland.

Warnings: Should be taken with caution if alcohol is being consumed. Product should not be taken if patient is concurrently on any other drug, without prior consultation with physician. Should not be taken for longer than two weeks unless approved by physician.

How Supplied: Boxes of 8, 32 or 48 tablets in child resistant blisters, and in boxes of 16 with non–child resistant packaging.

Inactive Ingredients: Dibasic Calcium Phosphate, FD&C Blue #1 Aluminum Lake, Magnesium Stearate, Microcrystalline Cellulose, Sodium Starch Glycolate.

UNISOM® WITH PAIN RELIEF
(formerly Unisom Dual Relief)
Nighttime Sleep Aid and
Pain Reliever

Description: Unisom ® With Pain Relief is a pale blue, capsule-shaped, coated tablet.

Active Ingredients: 650 mg. acetaminophen and 50 mg. diphenhydramine HCl per tablet.

Inactive Ingredients: Corn starch, FD&C Blue #1 Aluminum Lake, FD&C Blue #2 Aluminum Lake, hydroxypropyl methylcellulose, magnesium stearate, polyethylene glycol, polysorbate 80, povidone, stearic acid, titanium dioxide.

Indications: Unisom With Pain Relief (diphenhydramine sleep aid formula) is indicated to help reduce difficulty in falling asleep while relieving accompanying minor aches and pains such as headache, muscle ache or menstrual discomfort. If there is difficulty in falling asleep, but pain is not being experienced at the same time, regular Unisom sleep aid is indicated which contains doxylamine succinate as its active ingredient.

Administration and Dosage: One tablet 30 minutes before retiring. Take once daily or as directed by a physician.

Warnings: DO NOT TAKE THIS PRODUCT IF YOU HAVE ASTHMA, GLAUCOMA OR ENLARGEMENT OF THE PROSTATE GLAND EXCEPT UNDER THE ADVICE AND SUPERVISION OF A PHYSICIAN.
Do not take this product for treatment of arthritis except under the advice and supervision of a physician. Do not exceed recommended dosage because severe liver damage may occur. If symptoms persist continuously for more than ten days, consult your physician. Insomnia may be a symptom of serious underlying medical illness. Take this product with caution if alcohol is being consumed. Do not take this product if pregnant or nursing a baby. For adults only. Do not give to children under 12 years of age. Keep this and all medications out of reach of children. IN CASE OF ACCIDENTAL OVERDOSE SEEK PROFESSIONAL ADVICE OR CONTACT A POISON CONTROL CENTER IMMEDIATELY.

Caution: This product contains an antihistamine and will cause drowsiness. It should be used only at bedtime.

Drug Interaction: Monoamine oxidase (MAO) inhibitors prolong and intensify the anticholinergic effects of antihistamines. The CNS depressant effect is heightened by alcohol and other CNS depressant drugs.

Attention: Use only if tablet blister seals are unbroken. Child resistant packaging.

How Supplied: Boxes of 8 and 16 tablets in child resistant blisters.

VISINE®
Tetrahydrozoline Hydrochloride
Redness Reliever Eye Drops

Description: Visine is a sterile, isotonic, buffered ophthalmic solution containing tetrahydrozoline hydrochloride 0.05%, boric acid, sodium borate, sodium chloride and water. It is preserved with benzalkonium chloride 0.01% and ede-tate disodium 0.1%. Visine is a decongestant ophthalmic solution designed to provide symptomatic relief of conjunctival edema and hyperemia secondary to minor irritations, due to conditions such as smoke, dust, other airborne pollutants, swimming etc. and so-called nonspecific or catarrhal conjunctivitis. Relief is afforded by tetrahydrozoline hydrochloride, a sympathomimetic agent, which brings about decongestion by vasoconstriction. Reddened eyes are rapidly whitened by this effective vasoconstrictor, which limits the local vascular response by constricting the small blood vessels. The onset of vasoconstriction becomes apparent within minutes.
The effectiveness of Visine in relieving conjunctival hyperemia has been demonstrated by numerous clinicals, including several double-blind studies, involving more than 2,000 subjects suffering from acute or chronic hyperemia induced by a variety of conditions. Visine was found to be efficacious in providing relief from conjunctival hyperemia.

Indications: Relieves redness of the eye due to minor eye irritations.

Directions: Instill 1 to 2 drops in the affected eye(s) up to four times daily.

Warning: To avoid contamination, do not touch tip of container to any surface. Replace cap after using. If you experience eye pain, changes in vision, continued redness or irritation of the eye, or if the condition worsens or persists for more than 72 hours, discontinue use and consult a doctor. If you have glaucoma, do not use this product except under the advice and supervision of a doctor. Overuse of this product may produce increased redness of the eye. If solution changes color or becomes cloudy, do not use. Remove contact lenses before using.
Parents: Before using with children under 6 years of age, consult your physician. Keep this and all other drugs out of the reach of children. In case of accidental ingestion, seek professional assistance or contact a poison control center immediately.

How Supplied: In 0.5 fl. oz., 0.75 fl. oz., and 1.0 fl. oz. plastic dispenser bottle and 0.5 fl. oz. plastic bottle with dropper.
Shown in Product Identification Section, page 420

VISINE A.C.®
Astringent/Redness Reliever Eye Drops

Description: Visine A.C. is a sterile, isotonic, buffered ophthalmic solution containing tetrahydrozoline hydrochloride 0.05%, zinc sulfate 0.25%, boric acid, sodium chloride, sodium citrate and purified water. It is preserved with benzalkonium chloride 0.01% and edetate disodium 0.1%. Visine A.C. is an ophthalmic solution combining the effects of the vasoconstrictor tetrahydrozoline hydrochloride with the astringent effects of zinc sulfate. The vasoconstrictor provides symptomatic relief of conjunctival edema and hyperemia secondary to minor irritation due to conditions such as dust and airborne pollutants as well as so-called nonspecific or catarrhal conjunctivitis, while zinc sulfate provides relief from burning and itching, symptoms often associated with hay fever, allergies, etc. Beneficial effects include amelioration of burning, irritation, pruritis, and removal of mucus from the eye. Relief is afforded by both ingredients, tetrahydrozoline hydrochloride and zinc sulfate.
Tetrahydrozoline hydrochloride is a sympathomimetic agent, which brings about decongestion by vasoconstriction. Reddened eyes are rapidly whitened by this effective vasoconstrictor, which limits the local vascular response by constricting the small blood vessels. The onset of vasoconstriction becomes apparent within minutes. Zinc sulfate is an ocular astringent which, by precipitating protein, helps to clear mucus from the outer surface of the eye.
The effectiveness of Visine A.C. in relieving conjunctival hyperemia and associated symptoms induced by allergies has been clinically demonstrated. In one double-blind study allergy sufferers experienced acute episodes of minor eye irritation. Visine A.C. produced statistically significant beneficial results versus a placebo of normal saline solution in relieving irritation of bulbar conjunctiva, irritation of palpebral conjunctiva, and mucous build-up. Treatment with Visine A.C. containing zinc sulfate also significantly improved burning and itching symptoms.

Indications: For temporary relief of discomfort and redness due to minor eye irritations.

Directions: Instill 1 to 2 drops in the affected eye(s) up to 4 times daily.

Warning: To avoid contamination, do not touch tip of container to any surface. Replace cap after using. If you experience eye pain, changes in vision, continued redness or irritation of the eye, or if the condition worsens or persists for more than 72 hours, discontinue use and consult a doctor. If you have glaucoma, do not use this product except under the advice and supervision of a doctor. Overuse of this product may produce increased redness of the eye. If solution changes color or becomes cloudy, do not use. Remove contact lenses before using.
Parents: Before using with children under 6 years of age, consult your physician. Keep this and all other drugs out of the reach of children. In case of accidental ingestion, seek professional assistance or contact a poison control center immediately.

How Supplied: In 0.5 fl. oz. and 1.0 fl. oz. plastic dispenser bottle.
Shown in Product Identification Section, page 420

Continued on next page

Pfizer Consumer—Cont.

VISINE EXTRA®
Redness Reliever/Lubricant Eye Drops

Description: Visine Extra is a sterile, isotonic, buffered ophthalmic solution containing tetrahydrozoline hydrochloride 0.05%, polyethylene glycol 400 1.0%, boric acid, sodium borate, sodium chloride and water. It is preserved with benzalkonium chloride 0.013% and edetate disodium 0.1%.

Visine Extra is an ophthalmic solution combining the effects of the decongestant tetrahydrozoline hydrochloride with the demulcent effects of polyethylene glycol. It provides symptomatic relief of conjunctival edema and hyperemia secondary to ocular allergies, minor irritations and so-called nonspecific or catarrhal conjunctivitis. Tetrahydrozoline hydrochloride is a sympathomimetic agent, which brings about decongestion by vasoconstriction. Reddened eyes are rapidly whitened by this effective vasoconstrictor, which limits the local vascular response by constricting the small blood vessels. The onset of vasoconstriction becomes apparent within minutes. Additional effects include amelioration of burning, irritation, pruritus, soreness, and excessive lacrimation. Relief is afforded by polyethylene glycol.

Polyethylene glycol is an ophthalmic demulcent which has been shown to be effective for the temporary relief of discomfort of minor irritations of the eye due to exposure to wind or sun. It is effective as a protectant and lubricant against further irritation or to relieve dryness of the eye.

The effectiveness of tetrahydrozoline hydrochloride in relieving conjunctival hyperemia and associated symptoms has been demonstrated by numerous clinicals, including several double-blind studies, involving more than 2000 subjects suffering from acute or chronic hyperemia induced by a variety of conditions. Visine Extra is a product that combines the redness relieving effects of a vasoconstrictor and the soothing moisturizing and protective effects of a demulcent.

Indications: Relieves redness of the eye due to minor eye irritations. For use as a protectant against further irritation or to relieve dryness.

Directions: Instill 1 to 2 drops in the affected eye(s) up to 4 times daily.

Warning: To avoid contamination, do not touch tip of container to any surface. Replace cap after using. If you experience eye pain, changes in vision, continued redness or irritation of the eye, or if the condition worsens or persists for more than 72 hours, discontinue use and consult a doctor. If you have glaucoma, do not use this product except under the advice and supervision of a doctor. Overuse of this product may produce increased redness of the eye. If solution changes color or becomes cloudy, do not use. Remove contact lenses before using.

Parents: Before using with children under 6 years of age, consult your physician. Keep this and all other drugs out of the reach of children. In case of accidental ingestion, seek professional assistance or contact a poison control center immediately.

How Supplied: In 0.5 fl. oz. and 1.0 fl. oz. plastic dispenser bottle.

Shown in Product Identification Section, page 420

VISINE L. R.™ EYE DROPS
(oxymetazoline hydrochloride)

Description: Visine L. R. is a sterile, isotonic, buffered ophthalmic solution containing oxymetazoline hydrochloride 0.025%, boric acid, sodium borate, sodium chloride and water. It is preserved with benzalkonium chloride 0.01% and edetate disodium 0.1%.

Visine L. R. is produced by a process that assures sterility.

Indications: Visine L. R. is a decongestant ophthalmic solution designed for the relief of redness of the eye due to minor eye irritations. Visine L. R. is specially formulated to relieve redness of the eye in minutes with effective relief that lasts up to 6 hours.

Directions: *Adults and children 6 years of age and older*—Place 1 or 2 drops in the affected eye(s). This may be repeated as needed every 6 hours or as directed by a physician.

Warning: If you experience eye pain, changes in vision, continued redness or irritation of the eye, or if the condition worsens or persists for more than 72 hours, discontinue use and consult a physician. If you have glaucoma, do not use this product except under the advice and supervision of a physician. As with any medication, if you are pregnant seek the advice of a physician before using this product. Overuse of this product may produce increased redness of the eye. If solution changes color or becomes cloudy, do not use. To avoid contamination of this product, do not touch tip of container to any surface. Replace cap after using. Remove contact lenses before using this product.

Parents: Before using with children under 6 years of age, consult your physician. Keep this and all other medications out of the reach of children. In case of accidental ingestion, seek professional assistance or contact a poison control center immediately.

Caution: Should not be used if Visine-imprinted neckband on bottle is broken or missing.

Storage: Store between 2° and 30°C (36° and 86°F).

How Supplied: In 0.5 fl. oz. and 1 fl. oz. plastic dispenser bottle.

Shown in Product Identification Section, page 420

WART-OFF®
Liquid

Active Ingredient: Salicylic Acid 17% w/w.

Inactive Ingredients: Alcohol, 26.35% w/w, Flexible Collodion, Propylene Glycol Dipelargonate.

Indications: For the removal of common warts and plantar warts on the bottom of the foot. The common wart is easily recognized by the rough "cauliflower-like" appearance of the surface. The plantar wart is recognized by its location only on the bottom of the foot, its tenderness, and the interruption of the footprint pattern.

Warnings: For external use only. Keep this and all medications out of the reach of children to avoid accidental poisoning. In case of accidental ingestion, contact a physician or a Poison Control Center immediately. Do not use this product on irritated skin, on any area that is infected or reddened, if you are a diabetic, or if you have poor blood circulation. Do not use on moles, birthmarks, warts with hair growing from them, genital warts, or warts on the face or mucous membranes. If product gets into the eye, flush with water for 15 minutes. Avoid inhaling vapors. If discomfort persists, see your doctor.

Extremely Flammable—Keep away from fire or flame. Cap bottle tightly and store at room temperature away from heat (59°–86°F).

Instructions For Use: Read warnings and enclosed instructional brochure. Wash affected area. Dry area thoroughly. Using the special pinpoint applicator, apply one drop at a time to sufficiently cover each wart. Apply Wart-Off to warts only—not to surrounding skin. Let dry. Repeat this procedure once or twice daily as needed (until wart is removed) for up to 12 weeks. Replace cap tightly to prevent evaporation.

How Supplied: 0.5 fluid ounce bottle with special pinpoint plastic applicator and instructional brochure.

Procter & Gamble
P. O. BOX 5516
CINCINNATI, OH 45201

DENQUEL® Sensitive Teeth Toothpaste
Desensitizing Dentifrice

Description: Each tube contains potassium nitrate (5%) in a low-abrasion, pleasant mint-flavored dentifrice.

Dentinal hypersensitivity is a condition in which pain or discomfort arises when various stimuli, such as hot, cold, sweet, sour or touch contact exposed dentin. Exposure of dentin often occurs as a result of either gingival recession or periodontal surgery.

Daily use of Denquel can provide, within the first 2 weeks of regular brushing, a significant decrease in hypersensitivity.

See a dentist if tooth sensitivity is not reduced after 4 weeks of regular use, as this may indicate a dental condition other than hypersensitivity. The Council on Dental Therapeutics of the American Dental Association has given Denquel the ADA Seal of Acceptance as an effective desensitizing dentifrice for teeth sensitive to hot, cold or pressure (tactile) in otherwise normal teeth.

Dosage: Use twice a day or as directed by a dentist.

How Supplied: Denquel Sensitive Teeth Toothpaste is supplied in tubes containing 1.6, 3.0, or 4.5 ounces.

HEAD & SHOULDERS®
Antidandruff Shampoo

Head & Shoulders Shampoo offers effective dandruff control and beautiful hair in a formula that is pleasant to use. Independently conducted clinical testing (double-blind and dermatologist-graded) has proved that Head & Shoulders reduces dandruff flaking. Head & Shoulders is also gentle enough to use every day for clean, manageable hair.

Active Ingredient: 1.0% pyrithione zinc suspended in an anionic detergent system. Cosmetic ingredients are also included.

Indications: For effective control of typical dandruff and seborrheic dermatitis of the scalp.

Actions: Pyrithione zinc is substantive to the scalp and remains after rinsing. Its mechanism of action has not been fully established, but it is believed to control the microorganisms associated with dandruff flaking and itching.

Precautions: Not to be taken internally. Keep out of children's reach. Avoid getting shampoo in eyes—if this happens, rinse eyes with water.

Dosage and Administration: For best results in controlling dandruff, Head & Shoulders should be used regularly. It is gentle enough to use for every shampoo. In treating seborrheic dermatitis, a minimum of four shampooings are needed to achieve full effectiveness.

Composition:
Lotion—Normal to Oily Formula: Pyrithione zinc in a shampoo base of water, ammonium laureth sulfate, ammonium lauryl sulfate, cocamide MEA, glycol distearate, ammonium xylenesulfonate, fragrance, citric acid, methylchloroisothiazolinone, methylisothiazolinone, and FD&C Blue No. 1.
Lotion—Normal to Dry Formula: Pyrithione zinc in a shampoo base of water, ammonium laureth sulfate, ammonium lauryl sulfate, cocamide MEA, glycol distearate, ammonium xylenesulfonate, propylene glycol, fragrance, citric acid, methylchloroisothiazolinone, methylisothiazolinone, and FD&C Blue No. 1.
Lotion 2-in-1 (Complete Dandruff Shampoo plus Conditioner in One) Formula: Pyrithione zinc in a shampoo base of water, ammonium lauryl sulfate,

ammonium laureth sulfate, dimethicone, glycol distearate, cocamide MEA, ammonium xylenesulfonate, fragrance, tricetylmonium chloride, cetyl alcohol, stearyl alcohol, sodium chloride, DMDM hydantoin, sodium phosphate, disodium phosphate and FD&C Blue No. 1.
Cream—Normal to Oily Formula: Pyrithione zinc in a shampoo base of water, sodium cocoglyceryl ether sulfonate, sodium chloride, sodium lauroyl sarcosinate, lauramide DEA, cocoyl sarcosine, fragrance, and FD&C Blue No. 1.
Cream—Normal to Dry Formula: Pyrithione zinc in a shampoo base of water, sodium cocoglyceryl ether sulfonate, sodium chloride, sodium lauroyl sarcosinate, lauramide DEA, propylene glycol, cocoyl sarcosine, fragrance, and FD&C Blue No. 1.

How Supplied: Normal to Oily and Normal to Dry Lotion available in 4.0, 7.0, 11.0, and 15.0 fl. oz. unbreakable plastic bottles. 2-in-1 Lotion available in 9.0 and 12.5 fl. oz. unbreakable plastic bottle. Concentrate cream available in 5.5 oz. tube. Both lotion and concentrate are available in formulas for "Normal to Oily" and "Normal to Dry" hair.

HEAD & SHOULDERS® DRY SCALP SHAMPOO

Head & Shoulders Dry Scalp Shampoo offers effective control of irritating itching and flaking due to dry scalp. Dry Scalp Shampoo is gentle enough to use every day for clean, manageable hair.

Active Ingredient: 1.0% pyrithione zinc suspended in a mild surfactant base. Shampoo also includes mild conditioning agents.

Indications: For effective control of dry scalp and dry scalp symptoms.

Actions: Mild surfactants' gentle action reduces insult to the scalp, allowing the scalp to maintain its natural moisture balance. Pyrithione zinc is substantive to the scalp, and remains after rinsing.

Precautions: Not to be taken internally. Keep out of children's reach. Avoid getting shampoo in eyes—if this happens, rinse eyes with water.

Dosage and Administration: For best results in controlling dry scalp and dry scalp symptoms, Head & Shoulders Dry Scalp Shampoo should be used regularly. It is gentle enough to use for every shampoo.

Composition:
Lotion — Dry Scalp Regular Formula: Pyrithione zinc in a shampoo base of water, ammonium laureth sulfate, ammonium lauryl sulfate, cocamide MEA, glycol distearate, dimethicone, ammonium xylenesulfonate, fragrance, tricetylmonium chloride, cetyl alcohol, stearyl alcohol, DMDM hydantoin, sodium chloride, FD&C blue no. 1.
Lotion — Dry Scalp Conditioning Formula: Pyrithione zinc in a shampoo base of water, ammonium laureth sulfate, am-

monium lauryl sulfate, cocamide MEA, glycol distearate, dimethicone, ammonium xylenesulfonate, fragrance, tricetylmonium chloride, cetyl alcohol, stearyl alcohol, DMDM hydantoin, sodium chloride, FD&C blue no. 1.
Lotion — Dry Scalp 2-in-1 (Dry Scalp Shampoo Plus Conditioner in One) Formula: Pyrithione zinc in a shampoo base of water, ammonium laureth sulfate, ammonium lauryl sulfate, cocamide MEA, glycol distearate, dimethicone, ammonium xylenesulfonate, fragrance, tricetylmonium chloride, cetyl alcohol, stearyl alcohol, DMDM hydantoin, sodium chloride, and FD&C blue no. 1.

How Supplied: Dry Scalp Regular and Conditioning lotions are avilable in 7.0, 11.0, and 15.0 fl. oz. unbreakable plastic bottles. Dry Scalp 2-in-1 is available in 9.0 and 12.5 fl. oz. unbreakable plastic bottles.

HEAD & SHOULDERS® INTENSIVE TREATMENT DANDRUFF SHAMPOO

Head & Shoulders Intensive Treatment Dandruff Shampoo offers effective control of persistent dandruff, and beautiful hair from a pleasant-to-use formula. Double-blind and expert-graded testing have proven that Intensive Treatment Dandruff Shampoo reduces persistent dandruff. It is also gentle enough to use every day for clean, manageable hair.

Active Ingredient: 1% selenium sulfide suspended in a mild surfactant base. Shampoo also includes mild conditioning agents.

Indications: For effective control of seborrheic dermatitis and persistent dandruff of the scalp.

Actions: Selenium sulfide is substantive to the scalp and remains after rinsing. Its mechanism is believed to be an antihyperproliferative, and to also control the microorganisms associated with persistent dandruff flaking and itching.

Warnings: For external use only. Avoid contact with eyes—if this happens, rinse thoroughly with water. If condition worsens, or does not improve, consult a doctor. Keep out of reach of children.

Caution: If used on light, gray, or chemically treated hair, rinse (VIGOROUSLY) for 5 minutes.

Dosage and Administration: For best results in controlling persistent dandruff, Head & Shoulders Intensive Treatment Dandruff Shampoo should be used regularly. It is gentle enough to use for every shampoo.

Composition:
Lotion — Intensive Treatment Regular Formula: Ingredients: Selenium sulfide in a shampoo base of water, ammonium laureth sulfate, ammonium lauryl sulfate, cocamide MEA, glycol distearate, ammonium xylenesulfonate, dimethicone, fragrance, tricetylmonium chlo-

Continued on next page

Procter & Gamble—Cont.

ride, cetyl alcohol, DMDM hydantoin, sodium chloride, stearyl alcohol, hydroxypropyl methylcellulose, FD&C Red no. 4.

Lotion—Intensive Treatment Conditioning Formula: Ingredients: Selenium sulfide in a shampoo base of water, ammonium laureth sulfate, ammonium lauryl sulfate, cocamide MEA, glycol distearate, ammonium xylenesulfonate, dimethicone, fragrance, tricetylmonium chloride, cetyl alcohol, DMDM hydantoin, sodium chloride, stearyl alcohol, hydroxypropyl methylcellulose, FD&C Red no. 4.

Lotion — Intensive Treatment 2-in-1 (Persistent Dandruff Shampoo plus Conditioner in One) Formula: Selenium sulfide in a shampoo base of water, ammonium laureth sulfate, ammonium lauryl sulfate, cocamide MEA, glycol distearate, dimethicone, ammonium xylenesulfonate, fragrance, tricetylmonium chloride, cetyl alcohol, DMDM hydantoin, sodium chloride, stearyl alcohol, hydroxypropyl methylcellulose, FD&C Red no. 4.

How Supplied: Intensive Treatment Regular and Conditioning Lotion is available in 4.0, 7.0, and 11.0 fl. oz. unbreakable plastic bottles. Intensive Treatment 2-in-1 is available in 6.0 and 8.9 fl. oz. unbreakable plastic bottles.

PEPTO-BISMOL® ORIGINAL LIQUID
AND ORIGINAL AND CHERRY TABLETS
For diarrhea, heartburn, indigestion, upset stomach and nausea.

Description: Each Pepto-Bismol Tablet contains 262 mg bismuth subsalicylate and each tablespoonful (15 ml) of Pepto-Bismol Liquid contains 262 mg bismuth subsalicylate. Each tablet contains 102 mg salicylate (99 mg salicylate for Cherry) and each tablespoonful of liquid contains 130 mg salicylate. Liquid and tablets contain no sugar. Tablets are very low in sodium (less than 2 mg/tablet) and Liquid is low in sodium (less than 3 mg/tablespoonful). Inactive ingredients include (Tablets): adipic acid (in Cherry only), calcium carbonate, D&C Red No. 27, D&C Red No. 40 (in Cherry only), flavors, magnesium stearate, mannitol, povidone, saccharin sodium and talc; (Liquid): benzoic acid, D&C Red No. 22, D&C Red no. 28, flavor, magnesium aluminum silicate, methylcellulose, saccharin sodium, salicylic acid, sodium salicylate, sorbic acid and water.

Indications: Pepto-Bismol controls diarrhea within 24 hours, relieving associated abdominal cramps; soothes heartburn and indigestion without constipating; and relieves nausea and upset stomach.

Caution: This product contains salicylates. If taken with aspirin and ringing of the ears occurs, discontinue use. This product does not contain aspirin, but should not be administered to those patients who have a known allergy to aspirin or salicylates. Caution is advised in the administration to patients taking medication for anticoagulation, diabetes and gout.

Warning: Children and teenagers who have or are recovering from chicken pox or flu should NOT use this medicine to treat nausea or vomiting. If nausea or vomiting is present, consult a doctor because this could be an early sign of Reye Syndrome, a rare but serious illness. As with any drug, caution is advised in the administration to pregnant or nursing women.

Note: This medication may cause a temporary and harmless darkening of the tongue and/or stool. Stool darkening should not be confused with melena.

Dosage and Administration:
Tablets:
Adults—Two tablets
Children (according to age)—
9–12 yr   1 tablet
6–9 yr   ⅔ tablet
3–6 yr   ⅓ tablet
Chew or dissolve in mouth. Repeat every ½ to 1 hour as needed, to a maximum of 8 doses in a 24-hour period.
Liquid: Shake well before using.
Adults—2 tablespoonfuls
Children (according to age)—
9–12 yr   1 tablespoonful
6–9 yr   2 teaspoonfuls
3–6 yr   1 teaspoonful
Repeat dosage every ½ to 1 hour, if needed, to a maximum of 8 doses in a 24-hour period.
For children under 3 years, dose according to weight.
18–28 lb 1 teaspoonful
14–18 lb ½ teaspoonful
Repeat every 4 hours, if needed, to a maximum of 6 doses in a 24-hour period.

How Supplied:
Pepto-Bismol Liquid is available in: 4 fl oz bottle, 8 fl oz bottle, 12 fl oz bottle, 16 fl oz bottle.
Pepto-Bismol Tablets are pink, round, chewable, tablets imprinted with "Pepto-Bismol" on one side. Tablets are available in: box of 30, box of 48, and roll pack of 12 (cherry only).

PEPTO-BISMOL®
MAXIMUM STRENGTH LIQUID
For diarrhea, heartburn, indigestion, upset stomach and nausea.

Description: Each tablespoonful (15 ml) of Maximum Strength Pepto-Bismol Liquid contains 525 mg bismuth subsalicylate (236 mg salicylate). Maximum Strength Pepto-Bismol Liquid contains no sugar and is low in sodium (less than 3 mg/tablespoonful). Inactive ingredients include: benzoic acid, D&C Red No. 22, D&C Red No. 28, flavor, magnesium aluminum silicate, methylcellulose, saccharin sodium, salicylic acid, sodium salicylate, sorbic acid, and water.

Indications: Maximum Strength Pepto-Bismol controls diarrhea within 24 hours, relieving associated abdominal cramps; soothes heartburn and indigestion without constipating; and relieves nausea and upset stomach.

Caution: This product contains salicylates. If taken with aspirin and ringing of the ears occurs, discontinue use. This product does not contain aspirin, but should not be administered to those patients who have a known allergy to aspirin or salicylates. Caution is advised in the administration to patients taking medication for anticoagulation, diabetes, and gout.

Warning: Children and teenagers who have or are recovering from chicken pox or flu should NOT use this medicine to treat nausea or vomiting. If nausea or vomiting is present, consult a doctor because this could be an early sign of Reye Syndrome, a rare but serious illness. As with any drug, caution is advised in the administration to pregnant or nursing women.

Note: This medication may cause a temporary and harmless darkening of the tongue and/or stool. Stool darkening should not be confused with melena.

Dosage and Administration: Shake well before using.
Adults—2 tablespoonfuls
Children (according to age)—
9–12 yr   1 tablespoonful
6–9 yr   2 teaspoonfuls
3–6 yr   1 teaspoonful
Repeat dosage every hour, if needed, to a maximum of 4 doses in a 24-hour period.

How Supplied:
Maximum Strength Pepto-Bismol is available in:
4 fl oz bottle
8 fl oz bottle
12 fl oz bottle

EDUCATIONAL MATERIAL

Journal Reprints for Physicians
Reprints of published journal articles illustrating the effectiveness of bismuth subsalicylate (Pepto-Bismol) for the treatment of diarrhea.

IDENTIFICATION PROBLEM?
Consult the
Product Identification Section
where you'll find
products pictured
in full color.

Reed & Carnrick
Division of Block Drug Company, Inc.
JERSEY CITY, NJ 07302-9988

PHAZYME® and PHAZYME®-95
[fay-zime]
Tablets

Description: Contains simethicone, an antiflatulent to alleviate or relieve the symptoms of gas. It has no known side effects or drug interactions.

Actions: Simethicone minimizes gas formation and relieves gas entrapment in both the stomach and the lower G.I. tract. This action combats the painful sensation due to gastrointestinal gas. Also, for relief of gas distress associated with other functional or organic conditions such as: diverticulitis, spastic colitis, hyperacidity, postcholecystectomy syndrome and chronic cholecystitis.

Indication: To alleviate or relieve the symptoms of gas.

Warnings: Keep this and all drugs out of the reach of children. If condition persists, consult your physician.
Store at controlled room temperature 59–86°F (15–30°C).

PHAZYME®

Active Ingredient: Each tablet contains simethicone 60 mg.

Inactive Ingredients: acacia, calcium sulfate, carnauba wax, crospovidone, D&C red No. 7 calcium lake, FD&C blue No. 1 aluminum lake, gelatin, lactose, methylparaben, microcrystalline cellulose, polyoxyl-40 stearate, povidone, pregelatinized starch, propylparaben, rice starch, sodium benzoate, sucrose, talc, titanium dioxide, white wax.

Dosage: One tablet four times a day after meals and at bedtime. Do not exceed 8 tablets a day unless directed by a physician.

How Supplied: Pink coated tablet in bottles of 100, NDC #0021-1400-01

PHAZYME® 95

Active Ingredient: Each tablet contains simethicone 95 mg.

Inactive Ingredients: acacia, calcium sulfate, carnauba wax, crospovidone, FD&C yellow No. 6 aluminum lake, FD&C red No. 40 aluminum lake, gelatin, lactose, microcrystalline cellulose, polyoxyl-40 stearate, povidone, pregelatinized starch, rice starch, sodium benzoate, sucrose, talc, titanium dioxide, white wax.

Dosage: One tablet four times a day after meals and at bedtime. Do not exceed 5 tablets per day unless directed by a physician.

How Supplied: Red coated tablet in
10 pack,   NDC #0021-1420-02
50's   NDC #0021-1420-50
100's,   NDC #0021-1420-01
Shown in Product Identification Section, page 420

PHAZYME® DROPS
[fay-zime]

Description:
Active Ingredients: Each 0.6 mL contains simethicone 40 mg.
Inactive Ingredients: carbomer 934 P, citric acid, flavor (natural orange), hydroxypropylmethylcellulose, PEG-8 stearate, potassium sorbate, sodium citrate, sodium saccharin, water.

Actions: Simethicone minimizes gas formation and relieves gas entrapment in both the stomach and the lower G.I. tract. This action combats the painful sensation due to gastrointestinal gas. Also, for relief of gas distress associated with other functional or organic conditions such as diverticulitis, spastic colitis, hyperacidity, post-cholecystectomy syndrome and chronic cholecystitis.

Indication: To alleviate or relieve symptoms of gas.

Warnings: Keep this and all drugs out of the reach of children. If condition persists, consult your physician.

Dosage/Administration: Shake well before using.
Infants (under 2 years):
0.3 ml four times daily after meals and at bedtime or as directed by your physician. Can also be mixed with liquids for easier administration.
Children (2 to 12 years):
0.6 ml four times daily after meals and at bedtime or as directed by your physician.
Adults: 1.2 ml (take two 0.6 ml doses) four times daily after meals and at bedtime. Do not take more than six times per day unless directed by a physician.

How Supplied: Dropper bottles of 30 mL (1 fl oz)
NDC-0021-4300-17
Shown in Product Identification Section, page 420

Maximum Strength
PHAZYME®-125 Capsules

Description: A red softgel containing the highest dose of simethicone available in a single capsule.
Active Ingredient: Each capsule contains simethicone 125 mg.
Inactive Ingredients: FD&C red No. 40, gelatin, glycerin, hydrogenated soybean oil, lecithin, methylparaben, polysorbate 80, propylparaben, soybean oil, titanium dioxide, vegetable shortening, yellow wax.

Actions: Simethicone minimizes gas formation and relieves gas entrapment in both the stomach and the lower G.I. tract. This action combats the painful sensation due to gastrointestinal gas. Also, for relief of gas distress associated with other functional or organic conditions such as diverticulitis, spastic colitis, hyperacidity, post-cholecystectomy syndrome and chronic cholecystitis.

Indication: To alleviate or relieve symptoms of gas.

Warnings: Keep this and all drugs out of the reach of children. If condition persists, consult your physician.
Store at controlled room temperature 59–86°F (15–30°C).

Dosage: One softgel capsule four times a day after meals and at bedtime. Do not exceed 4 softgel capsules per day unless directed by a physician.

How Supplied: Red capsule in bottles of 50, NDC #0021-0450-50 and 10 pack, NDC #0021-0450-02
Shown in Product Identification Section, page 420

---

proctoFoam®/non-steroid
(pramoxine HCl 1%)

Composition: Active Ingredient: pramoxine hydrochloride 1%.
Inactive Ingredients: butane, cetyl alcohol, emulsifying wax, methylparaben, mineral oil, polysorbate 60, propane, propylparaben, sorbitan sesquioleate, trolamine, water.

Indication: For the temporary relief of pain and itching associated with hemorrhoids.

Warnings: Do not exceed the recommended daily dosage unless directed by a physician. If condition worsens or does not improve within 7 days, consult a physician. In case of rectal bleeding, consult a physician promptly. Do not put this product into the rectum by using fingers or any mechanical device or applicator. Certain persons can develop allergic reactions to ingredients in this product. If the symptom being treated does not subside or if redness, irritation, swelling, pain or other symptoms develop or increase, discontinue use and consult a physician.

Caution: Do not insert any part of the aerosol container into the rectum. Contents of the container are under pressure, but not flammable. Do not burn or puncture the aerosol container. Store upright at controlled room temperature, 59°–86°F (15–30°C).
SHAKE WELL BEFORE USE. DO NOT REFRIGERATE.
The contents of this can are under pressure, but not flammable. Do not burn or puncture the aerosol container. Keep this and all drugs out of the reach of children.

Directions: Adults: When practical, cleanse the affected area with mild soap and warm water and rinse thoroughly. Gently dry by patting or blotting with toilet tissue or a soft cloth before application of proctoFoam.
Children under 12 years of age: consult a physician.
Shake cannister well before each use. Dispense proctoFoam onto a clean tissue or pad and apply externally to the affected area up to 5 times daily.

How Supplied: Available in 15 g aerosol container.

Continued on next page

Reed & Carnrick—Cont.

R&C® SHAMPOO
Shampoo Pediculicide

Description: R&C SHAMPOO is a one-step pediculicide shampoo available without a prescription. Includes conditioning rinse and special comb for easy removal of lice and eggs.

Active Ingredients:
Pyrethrins 0.30%
Piperonyl Butoxide Technical* 3.00%

Inert Ingredients 96.70%
C-13-14 Isoparaffin, Fragrance, Isocetyl Alcohol, Isopropyl Alcohol, Lauramine Oxide, Laureth-4, Laureth-23, Petroleum Distillate, TEA-Lauryl Sulfate, Water.
TOTAL 100.00%

Action: R&C SHAMPOO kills head lice (pediculus capitis), crab lice (phthirus pubis) and body lice (pediculus corporis) and their eggs.

Indications: R&C SHAMPOO is indicated for the treatment of infestations with head lice, pubic (crab) lice and body lice.

Precautionary Statements: Hazard to Humans and Domestic Animals.
Caution: For external use only. In case of infection or skin irritation, discontinue use and consult a physician. Consult a physician if infestation of eyebrows and eyelashes occurs. Avoid contamination of feed or foodstuffs.
NOTE: Should not be used by ragweed-sensitized persons.
STATEMENT OF PRACTICAL TREATMENT
IF SWALLOWED: Call a physician or Poison Control Center immediately. Drink one to two glasses of water and induce vomiting by touching the back of the throat with finger.
Repeat until vomit is clear. Do not induce vomiting or give anything by mouth to an unconscious person.
IF INHALED: Remove victim to fresh air. Apply respiration if indicated.
IF IN EYES: Flush eyes with plenty of water. Call a physician if irritation persists.

Storage and Disposal:
Storage: Store below 120°F.
Disposal: Do not reuse container. Rinse thoroughly before discarding in trash.

KEEP OUT OF REACH OF CHILDREN.
CAUTION: FOR EXTERNAL USE ONLY.

Directions for Use: It is a violation of Federal law to use this product in a manner inconsistent with its label.
(Package also has Spanish instructions)
Do not use on eyelashes or eyebrows.
1. Begin with DRY hair—do not wet hair prior to using R&C Shampoo.

*Equivalent to 2.40% (butylcarbityl) (6-propylpiperonyl) ether and 0.60% related compounds.

2. SHAKE WELL. Apply enough R&C Shampoo to saturate the hair, paying particular attention to the infested and adjacent hairy areas.
3. Allow undiluted shampoo to remain on the area for ten minutes.
4. Then add small amounts of water, working the R&C Shampoo into the hair until a lather forms. Rinse thoroughly.
5. Treatment should be repeated in 7–10 days if needed. Do not apply R&C Shampoo more than twice within 24 hours.
Conditioning Rinse and Special Comb
To help remove dead lice and eggs apply enclosed conditioning rinse, leaving on the area for one minute. Rinse thoroughly.
Remove dead lice and eggs with the specially designed fine-tooth comb. Illustrated combing instructions are enclosed.
NOTE: TO AVOID REINFESTATION, wash or dry clean all clothing and linens of the infested person at time of treatment. Items that cannot be cleaned in this way, such as bedding, furniture and carpeting, should be treated with R&C Spray Lice Control Insecticide.

How Supplied: In 2 and 4 fl oz. plastic bottles with pourable cap. Fine-tooth comb, a special conditioning rinse to aid in removal of dead lice and nits, and patient booklet are included in each package of R&C SHAMPOO.

Literature Available: For free patient information brochures and film-strips, please call 1-800-KIL-LICE. A Reed & Carnrick health consultant will be glad to assist you.
Shown in Product Identification Section, page 420

R&C® SPRAY Lice Control Insecticide

Description: Insecticide: Not for use on humans or animals.
Active Ingredient: 3-Phenoxybenzyl-(1RS;3RS;1RS,3SR)-2,2-dimethyl-3-(2-methylprop-1-enyl)cyclopropane carboxylate   0.400%
Inert Ingredients: 99.600%
           100.000%

Actions: R&C SPRAY is specially formulated to kill lice and their eggs in the environment.

Indications: R&C SPRAY is recommended for use only on bedding, mattresses, furniture and other objects infested or possibly infested with lice which cannot be laundered or dry cleaned.
KEEP OUT OF REACH OF CHILDREN. Not for use on the skin or hair. Consult your physician for the treatment of lice infestations on humans.

Precautionary Statements: HAZARDS TO HUMANS AND DOMESTIC ANIMALS.
Caution: Vacate room after treatment and ventilate before reoccupying. Avoid contamination of feed and foodstuffs.

Remove pets, birds and cover fish aquariums before spraying.
Statement of Practical Treatment:
IF IN EYES: Immediately flush with large amounts of water. Get medical attention if irritation persists.
IF ON SKIN: Wash with soap and water. Get medical attention if irritation persists.
IF INHALED: Move victim to fresh air. Give artificial respiration if indicated.
IF SWALLOWED: Do not induce vomiting. Call a physician or Poison Control Center immediately.
Physical Hazard: Contents under pressure. Do not use or store near heat or open flame.
Do not puncture or incinerate container. Exposure to temperatures above 130° F may cause bursting.

Directions for Use: It is a violation of Federal law to use this product in a manner inconsistent with its labeling.
SHAKE WELL BEFORE AND OCCASIONALLY DURING USE. Spray on an inconspicuous area to test for possible staining or discoloration. Inspect after drying, then proceed to spray entire area to be treated.
Hold container upright with nozzle away from you. Depress valve and spray from a distance of 8 to 10 inches.
Spray each square foot for about three seconds. For mattresses, furniture, or similar objects (that cannot be laundered or dry cleaned): Spray thoroughly. Do not use article until spray is dry. Repeat treatment as necessary. Do not use in commercial food processing, preparation, storage or serving areas.

Storage and Disposal:
Storage: Store in a cool area away from heat or open flame.
Disposal: Replace cap and securely wrap container in several layers of newspaper and discard in trash.

How Supplied: In 5 oz. and 10 oz. aerosol container.

Literature Available: For free patient information brochures and film-strips, please call 1-800-KIL-LICE. A Reed & Carnrick health consultant will be glad to assist you.
Shown in Product Identification Section, page 420

EDUCATIONAL MATERIAL

Brochures
Questions and Answers About Head Lice
Available in English and Spanish to physicians, pharmacists and patients.

Products are indexed by generic and chemical names in the **YELLOW SECTION.**

The Reese Chemical Co.
10617 FRANK AVENUE
CLEVELAND, OHIO 44106

COLD CONTROL +
INTENSE COLD MEDICINE

Active Ingredients: Each caplet contains:
Acetaminophen 500 mg., Diphenhydramine Hydrochloride 25 mg., Pseudoephedrine Hydrochloride 60 mg.

Indications: Cold Control + provides effective temporary relief of symptoms associated with the common colds and upper respiratory infections including runny nose, sneezing, sniffles, itchy watery eyes that accompany colds or hay fever. Relieves sinus congestion due to head colds or hay fever.

Warning: Do not exceed recommended dosage or administer to children under 12 years of age. May cause marked drowsiness. Do not drive or operate machinery while taking this medication. Do not take if you have high fever, high blood pressure, diabetes, heart disease, asthma, glaucoma, thyroid disease, enlargement of the prostate gland or if you are taking a prescription drug for high blood pressure or emotional disorders. If symptoms do not improve within seven days, consult a physician before continuing use. In case of accidental over-dosage, contact a physician or a Poison Control Center immediately.

Warning: Keep this and all medication out of the reach of children. As with any drug, if you are pregnant or nursing a baby, seek the advice of a health professional before using this product.

Directions: Adults: One caplet every 4 to 6 hours. Do not exceed 4 doses in 24 hours.
CHILDREN 12 YEARS AND OLDER: Same as adult dose. Do not administer to children under 12 years.

How Supplied: Cold Control + is available in packs of 20's and 50 caplets.

COLICON® DROPS

Active Ingredient: Simethicone.

Inactive Ingredients: Citric Acid, Carbomer 934P, Hydroxypropyl methylcellulose, Sodium Benzoate, Sodium Saccharin, deionized water and flavor.

Indications: For relief of the painful symptoms of excess gas in the digestive tract.
The defoaming action of Colicon relieves flatulence by dispersing and preventing the formation of mucus-surrounded gas pockets in the gastrointestintal tract. Infants: Colicon drops are also useful for relief of the painful symptoms of excess gas associated with such conditions as colic, lactose intolerance or air swallowing.

Warnings: Keep this and all drugs out of the reach of children. In case of ac-

cidental overdose consult a physician immediately.

Dosage and Administration: Adults and children 0.6cc four times a day after meals and at bedtime or as directed by a physician. Infants (under two years) 0.3cc four times a day after meals and at bedtime, or as directed by a physician.

How Supplied: 1 Fl. oz. (30cc) plastic dropper enclosed.
NDC 10956-639-01

DENTAPAINE
Oral pain reliever and demulcent

Active Ingredients: Benzocaine 20%, Oil of Cloves and Glycerine in a soothing, nonhardening, water-soluble base.

Indications: For temporary relief of occasional minor irritation, pain, and sore mouth.

Warnings: Do not use this product for more than (7) seven days unless directed by a dentist or doctor. If sore mouth symptoms do not improve in (7) seven days; if irritation, pain or redness persists or worsens; or if swelling, rash, or fever develops, see your dentist or doctor promptly.

Warnings: Keep this and all drugs out of the reach of children. In case of accidental ingestion, seek professional assistance or contact a Posion Control immediately.

Dosage and Administration: Adults and children 12 years of age and older. Apply to affected area. Allow to remain in place at least (1) one minute and then spit out. Use up to (4) four times daily or as directed by a dentist or doctor.
Children under 12 years of age; consult a dentist or doctor.

How Supplied: Available in 11 gm. tubes

REESE'S PINWORM MEDICINE
Pyrantel Pamoate

Active Ingredient: Pyrantel pamoate, 144 mg/cc (the equivalent of 50 mg pyrantel base per cc).

Indications: For the treatment of enterobiasis (pinworm infection).

Warnings: Keep this and all drugs out of the reach of children. In case of accidental overdose, seek professional assistance or contact a poison control center immediately.

Precaution: If you are pregnant or have liver disease, do not take this product unless directed by a doctor.

Dosage and Administration: Adults, children 12 years of age and over, and children 2 years to under 12 years of age —Oral dosage is a single dose of 5 mg of pyrantel pamoate base per pound of body weight, not to exceed 1 gram.
Read package insert before taking this medicine. Do not administer to children under 2 years of age.

How Supplied: Reese's Pinworm Medicine is available in one-ounce bottles as a pleasant-tasting suspension which contains the equivalent of 50 mg pyrantel base per cc. It is supplied with English and Spanish label copy and directions.
Shown in Product Identification Section, page 420

SLEEP–ETTES–D

Active Ingredient: Diphenhydramine HCl USP 50mg.

Indications: For relief of occasional sleeplessness.

Warnings: Do not give to children under 12 years of age. If sleeplessness persists continuously for more than 2 weeks, consult your doctor. Insomnia may be a symptom of serious underlying medical illness. Do not take this product if you have asthma, glaucoma, emphysema, chronic pulmonary disease, shortness of breath, difficulty in breathing, or difficulty in urination due to enlargement of the prostate gland unless directed by a doctor. Avoid alcoholic beverages while taking this product. Do not take this product if you are taking sedatives or tranquilizers, without first consulting your doctor. As with any drug, if you are nursing a baby, seek the advice of a health professional before using this product. Keep this and all drugs out of the reach of children. In case of accidental overdose, seek professional assistance or contact a poison control center immediately.

Dosage and Administration: Adults and children 12 years of age and over: one tablet at bedtime if needed or as directed by a doctor.

How Supplied: Sleep-ettes-D is strip packed in cartons or sealed in bottles of 24 and 48 tablets.

Requa, Inc.
BOX 4008
1 SENECA PLACE
GREENWICH, CT 06830

CHARCOAID
Poison Adsorbent, liquid has sweet, pleasant taste and feel; especially good for young patients.

Active Ingredient: Activated vegetable charcoal U.S.P., 30g per bottle, suspended in 70% sorbitol solution U.S.P., 110 g.

Indication: For the emergency treatment of acute poisoning.

Action: Adsorbent

Warnings: Before using call a poison control center, emergency room, or a physician for advice. If the patient has been given Ipecac Syrup, do not give activated charcoal until after patient has

Continued on next page

Requa—Cont.

vomited. Do not use in a semi-conscious or unconscious person.

Precaution: May cause laxation. Careful attention to fluids and electrolytes is important, especially with young children and multiple dose therapy.

Dosage and Administration: Adults: Shake well and drink entire contents (add water if too sweet). To insure a full dose, rinse bottle with water and drink. For children, refer to Poison Control Center.

Professional Labeling: Some dilution may be necessary for administration via lavage tube. Add a small amount of water to bottle and shake.

How Supplied: 5 fl. oz. unit dose bottle, 30g activated charcoal U.S.P., suspended in 70% sorbitol solution U.S.P., 110 g.
U.S. Patent #4,122,169

CHARCOCAPS®
Activated Charcoal Capsules

Active Ingredient: Activated vegetable charcoal U.S.P., 260 mg per capsule.

Indications: Relief of intestinal gas, diarrhea, gastrointestinal distress associated with indigestion. Also to aid in the prevention of non-specific pruritus associated with kidney dialysis treatment.

Actions: Adsorbent, detoxicant, soothing agent. Reduces the volume of intestinal gas and allays related discomfort.

Warnings: As with all anti-diarrheals—not for children under 3 unless directed by physician. If diarrhea persists more than two days or is accompanied by high fever, consult physician.

Drug Interaction: Activated Charcoal USP can adsorb medication while they are in the digestive tract.

Precaution: General Guidelines— Take two hours before or one hour after medication including oral contraceptives.

Symptoms and Treatment of Oral Overdosage: Overdosage has not been encountered. Medical evidence indicates that high dosage or prolonged use does not cause side effect or harm the nutritional state of the patient.

Dosage and Administration: Two capsules after meals or at first sign of discomfort. Repeat as needed up to eight doses (16 capsules) per day.

Professional Labeling: None.

How Supplied: Bottles of 8, 36, 100 capsules

EDUCATIONAL MATERIAL

Questions & Answers
Brochure with questions and answers about the use of activated charcoal.

Trial Size
Free professional samples of Charcocaps, which includes coupon for regular size for the patient.

Rhône-Poulenc Rorer Pharmaceuticals Inc.
Consumer Pharmaceutical Products
**500 ARCOLA ROAD
P.O. BOX 1200
COLLEGEVILLE, PA 19426-0107**

Regular Strength
ASCRIPTIN®
[ă″skrĭp′tĭn]
Analgesic
Aspirin buffered with Maalox®

Active Ingredients: Each tablet contains Aspirin (325 mg), buffered with Maalox (Alumina-Magnesia) and Calcium Carbonate.

Inactive Ingredients: Hydroxypropyl Methylcellulose, Magnesium Stearate, Microcrystalline Cellulose, Starch, Talc, Titanium Dioxide, and other ingredients.

Description: Ascriptin is an excellent analgesic, antipyretic, and anti-inflammatory agent for general use, particularly where there is concern over aspirin-induced gastric distress. Coated tablets make swallowing easy.

Indications: As an analgesic for the relief of pain in such conditions as headache, neuralgia, minor injuries, and dysmenorrhea. As an analgesic and antipyretic in colds and influenza. As an analgesic and anti-inflammatory agent in arthritis and other rheumatic diseases. As an inhibitor of platelet aggregation, see MI's and TIA's indications.

Usual Adult Dose: Two or three tablets, four times daily. Do not exceed 12 tablets in a 24-hour period. For children under twelve, consult a doctor.

WARNINGS: Children and teenagers should not use this medicine for chicken pox or flu symptoms before a doctor is consulted about Reye syndrome, a rare but serious illness reported to be associated with aspirin. Keep this and all medicines out of children's reach. If pain persists more than 10 days, redness or swelling is present, fever persists more than 3 days, or symptoms worsen, consult a doctor immediately. If you are under medical care or have a history of stomach, kidney, or bleeding disorders or asthma, consult a doctor before using. Do not use if allergic to aspirin. As with any drug, if you are pregnant or nursing a baby, consult a doctor before using. **IT IS ESPECIALLY IMPORTANT NOT TO USE ASPIRIN DURING THE LAST 3 MONTHS OF PREGNANCY UNLESS SPECIFICALLY DIRECTED TO DO SO BY A DOCTOR BECAUSE IT MAY CAUSE PROBLEMS IN THE UNBORN CHILD OR COMPLICA-TIONS DURING DELIVERY.** If ringing in the ears or loss of hearing occurs, consult a doctor before taking any more of this product. In case of accidental overdose, contact a doctor immediately. *Drug Interaction Precaution:* Do not use if taking a prescription drug for anticoagulation (blood thinning), diabetes, gout or arthritis, or a tetracycline antibiotic unless directed by a doctor.

**Professional Labeling:
Aspirin for Myocardial Infarction**

Indication: Aspirin is indicated to reduce the risk of death and/or non-fatal myocardial infarction in patients with a previous infarction or unstable angina pectoris.

Dosage and Administration: Although most of the studies used dosages exceeding 300 mg, two trials used only 300 mg, and pharmacologic data indicate that this dose inhibits platelet function fully. Therefore, 300 mg or a conventional 325-mg aspirin dose is a reasonable, routine dose that would minimize gastrointestinal adverse reactions. This use of aspirin applies to both solid, oral dosage forms (buffered and plain aspirin), and buffered aspirin in solution. *Note:* Complete information and references available.

ASCRIPTIN FOR RECURRENT TIA's IN MEN
Clinical Trials: The indication is supported by the results of a Canadian study (1) in which 585 patients with threatened stroke were followed in a randomized clinical trial for an average of 26 months to determine whether aspirin or sulfinpyrazone, singly or in combination was superior to placebo in preventing transient ischemic attacks, stroke, or death. The study showed that, although sulfinpyrazone had no statistically significant effect, aspirin reduced the risk of continuing transient ischemic attacks, stroke, or death by 19 percent and reduced the risk of stroke or death by 31 percent. Another aspirin study carried out in the United States with 178 patients, showed a statistically significant number of "favorable outcomes" including reduced transient ischemic attacks, stroke, and death (2).

Indications: For reducing the risk of recurrent transient ischemic attacks (TIA's) or stroke in men who have had transient ischemia of the brain due to fibrin platelet emboli. There is inadequate evidence that aspirin or buffered aspirin is effective in reducing TIA's in women at the recommended dosage. There is no evidence that aspirin or buffered aspirin is of benefit in the treatment of completed strokes in men or women.

Precautions: (1) Patients presenting with signs and symptoms of TIA's should have a complete medical and neurologic evaluation. Consideration should be given to other disorders which resemble TIA's. **(2)** Attention should be given to risk factors; it is important to evaluate and treat, if appropriate, other diseases associated with TIA's and stroke such as hypertension and diabetes. **(3)** Concurrent administration of absorbable antacids at therapeutic doses may increase the clearance of salicylates in some individuals. The concurrent administration of nonabsorbable antacids may alter the rate of absorption of aspirin, thereby resulting in a decreased acetylsalicylic acid/salicylate ratio in plasma. The clinical significance on TIA's of these decreases in available aspirin is unknown.

Aspirin at dosages of 1,000 milligrams per day has been associated with small increases in blood pressure, blood urea nitrogen, and serum uric acid levels. It is recommended that patients placed on long-term aspirin treatment be seen at regular intervals to assess changes in these measurements.

Adverse Reactions: At dosages of 1,000 milligrams or higher of aspirin per day, gastrointestinal side effects include stomach pain, heartburn, nausea and/or vomiting, as well as increased rates of gross gastrointestinal bleeding.

Dosage: Adults dosage for men is 1300 mg a day, in divided doses of 650 mg twice a day or 325 mg four times a day.

References
(1) The Canadian Cooperative Study Group. "A Randomized Trial of Aspirin and Sulfinpyrazone in Threatened Stroke," *New England Journal of Medicine,*299:53–59, 1978.
(2) Fields, W.S., et al., "Controlled Trial of Aspirin in Cerebral Ischemia," *Stroke* 8:301–316, 1977.

How Supplied: Bottles of 60 tablets (NDC 0067-0145-60), 100 tablets (NDC 0067-0145-68), 160 (NDC 0067-0145-30) and 225 tablets (NDC 0067-0145-77). Bottles of 500 tablets (NDC 0067-0145-74) without child-resistant closures (for arthritic patients). Military Stock #NSN 6505-00-135-2783 V.A. Stock #6505-00-890-1979 (bottles of 500).

Shown in Product Identification Section, page 420

ASCRIPTIN® A/D for arthritis pain
Analgesic
Aspirin buffered with extra
Maalox® for pain relief
with extra stomach comfort

Active Ingredients: Each caplet contains Aspirin (325 mg), buffered with Maalox (Alumina-Magnesia) and Calcium Carbonate.

Inactive Ingredients: Hydroxypropyl Methylcellulose, Magnesium Stearate, Microcrystalline Cellulose, Starch, Talc, Titanium Dioxide, and other ingredients.

Description: Ascriptin A/D is a highly buffered analgesic, anti-inflammatory, and antipyretic agent for use in the treatment of rheumatoid arthritis, osteoarthritis, and other arthritic conditions. It is formulated with 50% more Maalox than Regular Strength Ascriptin to provide increased neutralization of gastric acid thus reducing the likelihood of GI disturbance when large antiarthritic

doses of aspirin are used. Coated caplets make swallowing easy.

Indications: As an analgesic, anti-inflammatory, and antipyretic agent in rheumatoid arthritis, osteoarthritis, and other arthritic conditions.

Usual Adult Dose: Two or three caplets, four times daily, or as directed by the physician for arthritis therapy. For children under twelve, at the discretion of the physician.

WARNINGS: Children and teenagers should not use this medicine for chicken pox or flu symptoms before a doctor is consulted about Reye syndrome, a rare but serious illness reported to be associated with aspirin. Keep this and all medicines out of children's reach. If pain persists more than 10 days, redness or swelling is present, fever persists more than 3 days, or symptoms worsen, consult a doctor immediately. If you are under medical care or have a history of stomach, kidney, or bleeding disorders or asthma, consult a doctor before using. Do not use if allergic to aspirin. As with any drug, if you are pregnant or nursing a baby, consult a doctor before using. **IT IS ESPECIALLY IMPORTANT NOT TO USE ASPIRIN DURING THE LAST 3 MONTHS OF PREGNANCY UNLESS SPECIFICALLY DIRECTED TO DO SO BY A DOCTOR BECAUSE IT MAY CAUSE PROBLEMS IN THE UNBORN CHILD OR COMPLICATIONS DURING DELIVERY.** If ringing in the ears or loss of hearing occurs, consult a doctor before taking any more of this product. **In case of accidental overdose, contact a doctor immediately.**
Drug Interaction Precaution: Do not use if taking a prescription drug for anticoagulation (blood thinning), diabetes, gout or arthritis, or a tetracycline antibiotic unless directed by a doctor.

How Supplied: Available in bottles of 60 caplets (NDC 0067-0147-60), 100 caplets (NDC 0067-0147-68), and 225 caplets (NDC 0067-0147-77) with child-resistant caps and in special bottles of 500 caplets (without child-resistant closures) for arthritic patients (NDC 0067-0147-74).

Shown in Product Identification Section, page 420

MAALOX® HRF
Heartburn Relief Formula™
Suspension
Rhône-Poulenc Rorer

Description: Maalox HRF provides symptomatic relief of heartburn, acid indigestion and/or sour stomach. Each 10 ml (2 teaspoonfuls) contains aluminum hydroxide-magnesium carbonate codried gel 280 mg and magnesium carbonate USP 350 mg. It is formulated in a pleasant, cool mint flavor to help provide a cooling and soothing sensation as it goes down the esophagus.

Inactive Ingredients: Calcium carbonate, calcium saccharin, FD&C Blue No. 1, Yellow No. 5 (tartrazine) as a color

additive, flavors, magnesium alginate, methyl and propyl parabens, potassium bicarbonate, purified water, sorbitol and other ingredients.

Directions for Use: Maalox HRF—two to four teaspoonfuls after meals and at bedtime, or as directed by a physician.

Patient Warnings: Do not take more than 16 teaspoonfuls in a 24-hour period or use the maximum dosage for more than 2 weeks or use if you have kidney disease except under the advice and supervision of a physician.

Drug Interaction Precaution: Do not use if you are taking a prescription antibiotic drug containing any form of tetracycline. Keep this and all drugs out of the reach of children.

Professional Labeling: Warnings
Prolonged use of aluminum-containing antacids in patients with renal failure may result in or worsen dialysis osteomalacia. Elevated tissue aluminum levels contribute to the development of the dialysis encephalopathy and osteomalacia syndromes. Small amounts of aluminum are absorbed from the gastrointestinal tract and renal excretion of aluminum is impaired in renal failure. Aluminum is not well removed by dialysis because it is bound to albumin and transferrin, which do not cross dialysis membranes. As a result, aluminum is deposited in bone, and dialysis osteomalacia may develop when large amounts of aluminum are ingested orally by patients with impaired renal function.

Aluminum forms insoluble complexes with phosphate in the gastrointestinal tract, thus decreasing phosphate absorption. Prolonged use of antacids containing aluminum by normophosphatemic patients may result in hypophosphatemia if phosphate intake is not adequate. In its more severe forms, hypophosphatemia can lead to anorexia, malaise, muscle weakness, and osteomalacia.

How Supplied: Maalox HRF is available in a 12 fl oz (NDC 0067-0350-71).

Shown in Product Identification Section, page 420

MAALOX® Plus
Alumina, Magnesia and Simethicone
Oral Suspension and Tablets,
Rhône-Poulenc Rorer
Antacid/Anti-Gas

Tablets
   Lemon Swiss Creme
   Cherry Creme
   ... the flavors preferred by the physician and patient.
☐ **Physician-proven Maalox® formula for antacid effectiveness.**
☐ **Simethicone, at a recognized clinical dose, for antiflatulent action.**

Description: Maalox® Plus, a balanced combination of magnesium and aluminum hydroxides plus simethicone, is a non-constipating antacid/anti-gas which comes in pleasant tasting flavors.

Continued on next page

Rhône-Poulenc Rorer—Cont.

Composition: To provide symptomatic relief of hyperacidity plus alleviation of gas symptoms, each tablet contains:

Active Ingredients	Maalox® Plus Per Tablet
Magnesium Hydroxide	250 mg
Aluminum Hydroxide (equivalent to dried gel, USP)	200 mg
Simethicone	25 mg

Inactive Ingredients: Maalox® Plus Tablets: Citric acid, confectioners' sugar, artifical colors, dextrose, flavors, glycerin, magnesium stearate, mannitol, saccharin sodium, sorbitol, starch, talc and may also contain hydrogenated vegetable oil.

To aid in establishing proper dosage schedules, the following information is provided:

Minimum Recommended Dosage:	Per Tablet
Acid neutralizing capacity	10.65 mEq
Sodium content*	0.8 mg
Sugar content	0.55 g
Lactose content	None

*Dietetically insignificant. Each Maalox® Plus Tablet contains approximately 0.03 mEq sodium per Tablet.

Indications: As an antacid for symptomatic relief of hyperacidity associated with the diagnosis of peptic ulcer, gastritis, peptic esophagitis, gastric hyperacidity, heartburn, or hiatal hernia. As an antiflatulent to alleviate the symptoms of gas, including postoperative gas pain.

Professional Labeling

Warnings: Prolonged use of aluminum-containing antacids in patients with renal failure may result in or worsen dialysis osteomalacia. Elevated tissue aluminum levels contribute to the development of the dialysis encephalopathy and osteomalacia syndromes. Small amounts of aluminum are absorbed from the gastrointestinal tract and renal excretion of aluminum is impaired in renal failure. Aluminum is not well removed by dialysis because it is bound to albumin and transferrin, which do not cross dialysis membranes. As a result, aluminum is deposited in bone, and dialysis osteomalacia may develop when large amounts of aluminum are ingested orally by patients with impaired renal function.

Aluminum forms insoluble complexes with phosphate in the gastrointestinal tract, thus decreasing phosphate absorption. Prolonged use of aluminum-containing antacids by normophosphatemic patients may result in hypophosphatemia if phosphate intake is not adequate. In its more severe forms, hypophosphatemia can lead to anorexia, malaise, muscle weakness, and osteomalacia.

Advantages: Maalox® Plus Tablets are uniquely palatable—an important feature which encourages patients to follow your dosage directions. Maalox® Plus Tablets have the time-proven, nonconstipating, sodium-free* Maalox® formula—useful for those patients suffering from the problems associated with hyperacidity. Additionally, Maalox® Plus Tablets contain simethicone to alleviate discomfort associated with entrapped gas.

Directions for Use: One to four tablets, well chewed, four times a day, taken twenty minutes to one hour after meals and at bedtime, or as directed by a physician.

Patient Warnings: Do not take more than 16 tablets in a 24-hour period or use the maximum dosage for more than 2 weeks or use if you have kidney disease except under the advice and supervision of a physician.

Drug Interaction Precaution: Do not use with patients taking a prescription antibiotic containing any form of tetracycline. As with all aluminum-containing antacids, Maalox® Plus may prevent the proper absorption of the tetracycline. Keep this and all drugs out of the reach of children.

How Supplied: Maalox® Plus Lemon Swiss Creme Tablets are available in bottles of 50 tablets (NDC 0067-0339-50) and 100 tablets (NDC 0067-0339-67), convenience packs of 12 tablets (NDC 0067-0339-19), Roll Packs of 12 tablets (NDC 0067-0339-23).

Maalox Plus Cherry Creme Tablets are available in bottles of 50 tablets (NDC 0067-0341-50) and 100 tablets (NDC 0067-0341-68), roll packs of 12 tablets (NDC 0067-0339-23) and 3 roll packs of 36 tablets (NDC 0067-0341-33).

Shown in Product Identification Section, page 421

EXTRA STRENGTH MAALOX® Plus (Reformulated Maalox Plus)
Alumina, Magnesia and Simethicone Oral Suspension and Tablets,
Rhône-Poulenc Rorer
Antacid/Anti-Gas

Liquids	Tablets
☐ Lemon Swiss Creme	Mint Creme
Cherry Creme	
Mint Creme	

  . . . the flavors preferred by the physician and patient.

☐ Physician-proven Maalox® formula for antacid effectiveness.
☐ Simethicone, at a recognized clinical dose, for antiflatulent action.

Description: Extra Strength Maalox® Plus, a balanced combination of magnesium and aluminum hydroxides plus simethicone, is a non-constipating antacid/anti-gas product to provide symptomatic relief of hyperacidity plus alleviation of gas symptoms. Available in liquid form in Cherry Creme, Mint Creme or Lemon Swiss Creme flavors, and in tablet form in the Mint Creme flavor.

Composition: To provide symptomatic relief of hyperacidity plus alleviation of gas symptoms, each teaspoonful/tablet contains:

Active Ingredients	Extra Strength Maalox® Plus Per Tsp. (5 mL)	Extra Strength Maalox® Plus Per Tablet
Magnesium Hydroxide	450 mg	350 mg
Aluminum Hydroxide (equivalent to dried gel, USP)	500 mg	350 mg
Simethicone	40 mg	30 mg

Inactive Ingredients: Extra Strength Maalox® Plus Suspension: Citric acid, flavors, methylparaben, propylparaben, purified water, saccharin sodium, sorbitol, and other ingredients.

Extra Strength Maalox® Plus Tablets: Citric acid, confectioners' sugar, D&C yellow No. 10, dextrose, FD&C Blue No. 1, flavors, glycerin, hydrogenated vegetable oil, magnesium stearate, mannitol, saccharin sodium, sorbitol, starch, talc.

To aid in establishing proper dosage schedules, the following information is provided:

Minimum Recommended Dosage: Extra Strength Maalox Plus	Per 2 Tsp. (10 mL)	Per Tablet
Acid neutralizing capacity	58.1 mEq	18.6 mEq
Sodium content*	2.3 mg	1.6 mg
Sugar content	None	0.75 g
Lactose content	None	None

*Dietetically insignificant. Contains approximately 0.05 mEq sodium per teaspoonful of Suspension. Each Extra Strength Maalox® Plus Tablet contains approximately 0.03 mEq sodium per Tablet.

Indications: As an antacid for symptomatic relief of hyperacidity associated with the diagnosis of peptic ulcer, gastritis, peptic esophagitis, gastric hyperacidity, heartburn, or hiatal hernia. As an antiflatulent to alleviate the symptoms of gas, including postoperative gas pain.

Advantages: Among antacids, Extra Strength Maalox® Plus Suspension and Extra Strength Maalox® Plus Tablets are uniquely palatable—an important feature which encourages patients to follow your dosage directions. Extra Strength Maalox® Plus Suspension and Extra Strength Maalox® Plus Tablets have the time-proven, nonconstipating, sodium-free* Maalox® formula—useful for those patients suffering from the problems associated with hyperacidity. Additionally, Extra Strength Maalox® Plus Suspension and Extra Strength Maalox® Plus Tablets contain simethicone to alleviate discomfort associated with entrapped gas.

Professional Labeling

Warnings:
(i) Prolonged use of aluminum-containing antacids in patients with renal failure may result in or worsen dialysis osteomalacia. Elevated tissue aluminum levels contribute to the development of the dialysis encephalopathy and osteomalacia syndromes. Small amounts of aluminum are absorbed from the gastrointestinal tract and renal excretion of aluminum is impaired in renal failure. Aluminum is not well removed by dialysis because it is bound to albumin and transferrin, which do not cross dialysis membranes. As a result, aluminum is deposited in bone, and dialysis osteomalacia may develop when large amounts of aluminum are ingested orally by patients with impaired renal function.
(ii) Aluminum forms insoluble complexes with phosphate in the gastrointestinal tract, thus decreasing phosphate absorption. Prolonged use of aluminum-containing antacids by normophosphatemic patients may result in hypophosphatemia if phosphate intake is not adequate. In its more severe forms, hypophosphatemia can lead to anorexia, malaise, muscle weakness, and osteomalacia.

Extra Strength Maalox® Plus Suspension

Directions for Use: Two to four teaspoonfuls, four times a day, taken twenty minutes to one hour after meals and at bedtime, or as directed by a physician. Stomach pain and discomfort should always be evaluated by a physician for proper diagnosis.

Patient Warnings: Do not take more than 12 teaspoonfuls in a 24-hour period or use the maximum dosage for more than 2 weeks or use if you have kidney disease except under the advice and supervision of a physician.

Extra Strength Maalox® Plus Tablets

Directions for Use: Chew one to three tablets twenty minutes to one hour after meals and at bedtime, or as directed by a physician.

Patient Warnings: Do not take more than 12 tablets in a 24-hour period or use the maximum dosage for more than two weeks or use if you have kidney disease except under the advice and supervision of a physician.

Drug Interaction Precaution: Do not use with patients taking a prescription antibiotic containing any form of tetracycline. As with all aluminum-containing antacids, Extra Strength Maalox® Plus may prevent the proper absorption of the tetracycline.
Keep this and all drugs out of the reach of children.

How Supplied:
Extra Strength Maalox® Plus Suspension
Available in Lemon Swiss Creme in the following sizes: 5 fl. oz. (148 mL) (NDC 0067-0333-62), 12 fl. oz. (355 mL) (NDC 0067-0333-71), and 26 fl. oz. (769 mL) (NDC 0067-0333-44).
Cherry Creme is available in plastic bottles of 5 fl. oz. (148 mL) (NDC 0067-0336-62, 12 fl. oz. (355 mL) (NDC 0067-0336-71), and 26 fl. oz. (769 mL) (NDC 0067-0336-44).
Mint Creme is available in plastic bottles of 5 fl. oz. (148 mL) (NDC 0067-0338-62), 12 fl. oz. (355 mL) (NDC 0067-0338-71) and 26 fl. oz. (769 mL) (NDC 0067-0338-44).
Extra Strength Maalox® Plus Mint Creme Tablets are available in flip-top bottles of 38 tablets (NDC 0067-0345-38) and 75 tablets (NDC 0067-0345-75).
Shown in Product Identification Section, page 420

PERDIEM®
[pĕr ″dē ′ŭm]

Indication: For relief of constipation.

Actions: Perdiem®, with its 100% natural, gentle action provides comfortable relief from constipation. Perdiem® is a unique combination of bulk-forming fiber and natural stimulant. The vegetable mucilages of Perdiem® soften the stool and provide pain-free evacuation of the bowel with no chemical stimulants. Perdiem® is effective as an aid to elimination for the hemorrhoid or fissure patient prior to and following surgery.

Composition: Perdiem® contains as its active ingredients, 82% psyllium (Plantago Hydrocolloid) a natural grain and 18% senna (Cassia Pod Concentrate), a natural vegetable derivative. Each rounded teaspoonful (6.0 g) contains 3.25 g psyllium, 0.74 g senna, 1.8 mg of sodium, 35.5 mg of potassium, and 4 calories. Perdiem® is "Dye-Free" and contains no artificial sweeteners.

Inactive Ingredients: Acacia, iron oxides, natural flavors, paraffin, sucrose, talc.

Patient Warning: Should not be used in the presence of undiagnosed abdominal pain. Frequent or prolonged use without the direction of a physician is not recommended, as it may lead to laxative dependence. Do not use in patients with a history of psyllium allergy. Psyllium allergy is rare but can be severe. If an allergic reaction occurs, discontinue use and consult a physician immediately. Bulk-forming agents have the potential to obstruct the esophagus, particularly in the presence of esophageal narrowing or when consumed with insufficient fluid. Patients should be made aware of the symptoms of esophageal obstruction, including chest pain/pressure, regurgitation, and difficulty swallowing. Patients experiencing these symptoms should seek immediate medical attention. Patients with esophageal narrowing or dysphagia should not use Perdiem®.
As with any drug, if you are pregnant or nursing a baby, seek the advice of a health professional before using this product. Keep this and all drugs out of the reach of children. In case of accidental overdose, seek professional assistance or contact a poison control center immediately.

Directions for Use: Perdiem must be taken with at least 8 ounces of liquid.
Adults and children 12 years and older: In the evening and/or before breakfast, 1–2 rounded teaspoonfuls of Perdiem® granules (in single or partial teaspoon doses) should be placed in the mouth and swallowed with at least 8 fl oz of cool beverage after the dose. Additional liquid would be helpful. Perdiem® granules should not be chewed.
Children 7 to 11 years: One rounded teaspoon one to two times daily with at least 8 ounces of cool liquid.
Perdiem® generally takes effect within 12 hours. Subsequent doses may be adjusted after adequate laxation is obtained.

Note: It is extremely important that Perdiem® be taken with at least 8 fl oz of cool liquid.

Warning: TAKE THIS PRODUCT WITH AT LEAST 8 OUNCES [A FULL GLASS] OF WATER OR OTHER FLUID. TAKING THIS PRODUCT WITHOUT ADEQUATE FLUID MAY CAUSE IT TO SWELL AND BLOCK YOUR THROAT OR ESOPHAGUS AND MAY CAUSE CHOKING. DO NOT TAKE THIS PRODUCT IF YOU HAVE EVER HAD DIFFICULTY IN SWALLOWING OR HAVE ANY THROAT PROBLEMS. IF YOU EXPERIENCE CHEST PAIN, VOMITING, OR DIFFICULTY IN SWALLOWING OR BREATHING AFTER TAKING THIS PRODUCT, SEEK IMMEDIATE MEDICAL ATTENTION.

In Severe Cases of Constipation: Perdiem® may be taken more frequently, up to 2 rounded teaspoonfuls every 6 hours not to exceed 5 teaspoonfuls in a 24-hour period. In severe cases, 24 to 72 hours may be required for optimal relief.

Continued on next page

Rhône-Poulenc Rorer—Cont.

For Patients Habituated to Strong Purgatives: Two rounded teaspoonfuls of Perdiem® in the morning and evening may be required along with half the usual dose of the purgative being used. The purgative should be discontinued as soon as possible and the dosage of Perdiem® granules reduced when and if bowel tone shows lessened laxative dependence.

For Colostomy Patients: To ensure formed stools, give one to two rounded teaspoonfuls of Perdiem® in the evening.

For Clinical Regulation: For patients confined to bed, for those of inactive habits, and in the presence of cardiovascular disease where straining must be avoided, one rounded teaspoonful of Perdiem® taken once or twice daily will provide regular bowel habits.

How Supplied: Granules: 100-gram (3.5 oz) (NDC 0067-0690-68) and 250-gram (8.8 oz) (NDC 0067-0690-70) canisters.
Shown in Product Identification Section, page 421

PERDIEM® FIBER
[pĕr ″dē ′ŭm]

Indications: Perdiem® Fiber provides gentle relief from simple, chronic, and spastic constipation. In addition, it relieves constipation associated with convalescence, pregnancy, and advanced age. Perdiem® Fiber is also indicated for use in special diets lacking in residue fiber to aid regularity and in the management of constipation associated with irritable bowel syndrome, diverticular disease, hemorrhoids, and anal fissures.

Action: Perdiem® Fiber is a 100% natural bulk-forming fiber that gently helps maintain regularity and prevents constipation. Perdiem® Fiber's unique form is easy to swallow and requires no mixing but must be followed by at least 8 ounces of cool liquid. Perdiem® Fiber contains no chemical stimulants and may be used daily by those who may lack sufficient dietary fiber. When recommended by a doctor, Perdiem Fiber is also useful for the treatment of bowel disorders other than constipation.

Composition: Perdiem® Fiber contains as its active ingredient 100% psyllium (Plantago Hydrocolloid), a natural grain with no chemical stimulants. Each rounded teaspoonful (6.0 g) contains 4.03 g of psyllium, 1.8 mg of sodium, 36.1 mg of potassium and 4 calories. Perdiem® Fiber is "Dye-Free" and contains no artificial sweeteners.

Inactive Ingredients: Acacia, iron oxides, natural flavors, paraffin, sucrose, talc, titanium dioxide.

Directions for Use: Perdiem Fiber must be taken with at least 8 ounces of cool liquid. Additional liquid is helpful.

Adults and children 12 years and older: In the evening and/or before breakfast, 1 to 2 rounded teaspoonfuls (6.0 to 12.0 g) of Perdiem® Fiber granules (in full or partial teaspoon doses) should be placed in the mouth and swallowed with at least 8 fl oz of cool beverage after the dose. Perdiem® Fiber granules should not be chewed.

During Pregnancy: Because of its natural ingredients and bulking action, Perdiem Fiber is effective for expectant mothers—follow directions.

Children 7 to 11 years: One (1) rounded teaspoonful one to two times daily with at least 8 ounces of cool liquid.

Patient Warning: Should not be used in the presence of undiagnosed abdominal pain. Frequent or prolonged use without the direction of a physician is not recommended.
Do not use in patients with a history of psyllium allergy. Psyllium allergy is rare but can be severe. If an allergic reaction occurs, discontinue use.
Bulk-forming agents have the potential to obstruct the esophagus, particularly in the presence of esophageal narrowing or when consumed with insufficient fluid. Patients should be made aware of the symptoms of esophageal obstruction, including chest pain/pressure, regurgitation, and difficulty swallowing. Patients experiencing these symptoms should seek immediate medical attention. Patients with esophageal narrowing or dysphagia should not use Perdiem® Fiber. Keep this and all drugs out of the reach of children. In case of accidental overdose, seek professional assistance or contact a poison control center immediately.

In Severe Cases of Constipation: Perdiem® Fiber may be taken more frequently, up to 2 rounded teaspoonfuls every 6 hours depending upon need and response not to exceed 5 teaspoonfuls in a 24-hour period. Perdiem Fiber generally takes effect after 24 hours; in severe cases 48 to 72 hours may be required to provide optimal benefit.

Warning: TAKE THIS PRODUCT WITH AT LEAST 8 OUNCES [A FULL GLASS] OF WATER OR OTHER FLUID. TAKING THIS PRODUCT WITHOUT ADEQUATE FLUID MAY CAUSE IT TO SWELL AND BLOCK YOUR THROAT OR ESOPHAGUS AND MAY CAUSE CHOKING. DO NOT TAKE THIS PRODUCT IF YOU HAVE EVER HAD DIFFICULTY IN SWALLOWING OR HAVE ANY THROAT PROBLEMS. IF YOU EXPERIENCE CHEST PAIN, VOMITING, OR DIFFICULTY IN SWALLOWING OR BREATHING AFTER TAKING THIS PRODUCT, SEEK IMMEDIATE MEDICAL ATTENTION.

After Rectal Surgery: The vegetable mucilages of Perdiem® Fiber soften the stool and provide pain-free evacuation of the bowel. Perdiem® Fiber is effective as an aid to elimination for the hemorrhoid or fissure patient prior to and following surgery.

For Clinical Regulation: For patients confined to bed—after an operation for example—and for those of inactive habits, 1 rounded teaspoonful of Perdiem® Fiber taken 1–2 times daily will ensure regular bowel habits.

How Supplied: Granules: 100-gram (3.5 oz) (NDC 0067-0795-68) and 250-gram (8.8 oz) (NDC 0067-0795-70) canisters, 42-gram (1.4 oz) (NDC 0067-0795-42) and 42-gram sample (1.4 oz) (NDC 0067-0795-52).
Shown in Product Identification Section, page 421

Richardson-Vicks Inc.
**ONE FAR MILL CROSSING
SHELTON, CT 06484**

CHILDREN'S CHLORASEPTIC® LOZENGES
Benzocaine/Oral Anesthetic

Active Ingredients: Benzocaine 5 mg per lozenge.

Inactive Ingredients: Corn syrup, FD&C Blue No. 1, FD&C Red No. 40, flavor, sucrose.

Indications: For temporary relief of occasional minor mouth irritation and pain, sore mouth and sore throat. Also for temporary relief of pain associated with canker sores.

Directions: Adults and children 2 years of age and older: Allow 1 lozenge to dissolve slowly in mouth. May be repeated every 2 hours as needed or as directed by a physician or dentist. Children under 2 years of age: Consult a physician or a dentist.

Warning: If sore throat is severe, or is accompanied by difficulty in breathing, or persists for more than two days, do not use, and consult a physician promptly. If sore throat is accompanied or followed by fever, headache, rash, nausea, or vomiting, consult a physician promptly. If sore mouth symptoms do not improve in 7 days, see your physician or dentist promptly. KEEP THIS AND ALL DRUGS OUT OF THE REACH OF CHILDREN. In case of accidental overdose seek professional assistance or contact a poison control center immediately. As with any drug if you are pregnant or nursing a baby, seek the advice of a health professional before using this product.

How Supplied: Cartons of 18.

CHLORASEPTIC® LIQUID
**Phenol/oral anesthetic/antiseptic
Cherry, Menthol and Cool Mint Flavors**

Active Ingredients: Liquid—Phenol 1.4%
Aerosol Spray—Phenol and sodium phenolate (total phenol 1.4%)

Inactive Ingredients:
Original Menthol Liquid: D&C Green No. 5, D&C Yellow No. 10, FD&C Green No. 3, flavor, glycerin, purified water, saccharin sodium.
Menthol Aerosol Spray: D&C Yellow No. 10, FD&C Green No. 3, flavor, glycerin, purified water and saccharin sodium.
Cherry Liquid: FD&C Red No. 40, flavor, glycerin, purified water, saccharin sodium.
Cherry Aerosol Spray: FD&C Red No. 40, flavor, glycerin, purified water, and saccharin sodium.
Cool Mint Liquid: FD&C Blue No. 1, flavor, glycerin, purified water, saccharin sodium.

Indications: For temporary relief of occasional minor sore throat pain and irritation. For pain associated with sore mouth and canker sores. Also for the temporary relief of pain associated with tonsillitis, pharyngitis and throat infections.

Administration and Dosage:
Chloraseptic Spray (Pump): Spray 5 times directly on throat or affected area. (Children 2–12 years of age, 3 times) and swallow. Repeat every 2 hours or as directed by a physician or dentist. Children under 12 years of age should be supervised in product use. Children under 2 years: consult a physician or dentist.
Chloraseptic Gargle: Adults and children 12 years of age and older: Gargle or swish around the mouth for at least 15 seconds and then spit out. Use every 2 hours or as directed by a physician or dentist. Children 6 to under 12 years: Gargle or swish around in mouth 2 teaspoonfuls for at least 15 seconds and then spit out. Use every 2 hours or as directed by a physician or dentist. Children under 12 years should be supervised in product use. Children under 6 years: Consult a physician or dentist.
Chloraseptic Aerosol Spray: Adults— Spray for 2 seconds directly on affected area (children 2 to 12 years, spray for 1 second) and swallow. Use every 2 hours or as directed by a physician or dentist. Children under 12 years of age should be supervised in the use of this product. Children under 2 years of age: Consult a physician or dentist.

Warning: If sore throat is severe, or is accompanied by difficulty in breathing, or persists for more than two days, do not use, and consult a physician promptly. If sore throat is accompanied or followed by fever, headache, rash, nausea, or vomiting, consult a physician promptly. If sore mouth symptoms do not improve in 7 days, see your physician or dentist promptly. KEEP THIS AND ALL DRUGS OUT OF THE REACH OF CHILDREN. In case of accidental overdose, seek professional assistance or contact a poison control center immediately. As with any drug, if you are pregnant or nursing a baby, seek the advice of a health professional before using this product.

For 1.5 oz. Aerosol Spray—Avoid spraying in eyes. Contents under pressure. Do not puncture or incinerate. Do not store at temperature above 120°F.

How Supplied: Available in Original Menthol, Cherry, and Cool Mint flavors in 6 fl. oz. plastic bottles with sprayer. Menthol and Cherry Flavors also available in 12 fl. oz. gargle and 1.5 oz. nitrogen-propelled aerosol sprays.

CHLORASEPTIC® LOZENGES
Cherry, Menthol, and Cool Mint Flavor
Menthol/Benzocaine
Oral Anesthetic

Active Ingredients: Benzocaine 6 mg and Menthol 10 mg

Inactive Ingredients:
Menthol Lozenges: Corn syrup, D&C Yellow No. 10, FD&C Blue No. 1, FD&C Yellow No. 6, flavor and sucrose.
Cherry Lozenges: Corn syrup, FD&C Blue No. 1, FD&C Red No. 40, flavor, and sucrose.
Cool Mint Lozenges: Corn syrup, FD&C Blue No. 1, flavor and sucrose.

Indications: For temporary relief of occasional minor mouth irritation and pain, sore mouth and sore throat. Also, for pain associated with canker sores.

Directions:
Adults and children 2 years of age and older: Allow lozenge to dissolve slowly in mouth. May be repeated every 2 hours as needed or as directed by a physician or dentist. Children under 2 years of Age: Consult a physician or a dentist.

Warning: If sore throat is severe, or is accompanied by difficulty in breathing, or persists for more than two days, do not use, and consult a physician promptly. If sore throat is accompanied or followed by fever, headache, rash, nausea, or vomiting, consult a physician promptly. If sore mouth symptoms do not improve in 7 days, see your physician or dentist promptly. KEEP THIS AND ALL DRUGS OUT OF THE REACH OF CHILDREN. In case of accidental overdose seek professional assistance or contact a Poison Control Center immediately. As with any drug if you are pregnant or nursing a baby, seek the advice of a health professional before using this product.

How Supplied: Available in Cool Mint and Cherry flavors in packages of 18 and 36. Also available in Menthol flavor in packages of 18.

OIL OF OLAY®—Daily UV Protectant SPF 15 Beauty Fluid—Regular & Fragrance Free
(Olay Co., Inc.)

Oil of Olay Daily UV Protectant Beauty Fluid is a light, greaseless lotion that is specially formulated to provide effective moisturization and SPF protection.

Oil of Olay UV Protectant is PABA free. It is non-comedeogenic and is suitable for daily use under facial make-up.

Active Ingredients: ETHYLHEXYL P-METHOXYCINNAMATE, 2-PHENYL-BENZIMIDAZOLE-5-SULFONIC ACID.

Inactive Ingredients: WATER, ISO-HEXADECANE, BUTYLENE GLYCOL, TRIETHANOLAMINE, GLYCERIN, STEARIC ACID, CETYL ALCOHOL, CETYL PALMITATE, DEA-CETYL PHOSPHATE, ALUMINUM STARCH OCTENYLSUCCINATE, TITANIUM DIOXIDE, IMIDAZOLIDINYL UREA, METHYLPARABEN, PROPYLPARABEN, CARBOMER, ACRYLATES/C10–30 ALKYL ACRYLATE CROSS-POLYMER, PEG-10 SOYA STEROL, DISODIUM EDTA, CASTOR OIL, FRAGRANCE, FD&C RED NO. 4, FD&C YELLOW NO. 5.
Available in a both lightly scented and 100% color free and fragrance free versions.

Indications: Provides SPF 15 UV protection to help protect against skin-aging UV rays in a light, greaseless moisturizer. The liberal and regular use of this product over the years may help reduce the chance of premature aging of the skin and skin cancer.

Directions: Apply liberally as needed to face, neck and other exposed areas for protection against UV rays and for moisturization.

Warning: FOR EXTERNAL USE ONLY. NOT TO BE SWALLOWED. AVOID CONTACT WITH EYES. DISCONTINUE USE IF SIGNS OF IRRITATION OR RASH APPEAR. USE ON CHILDREN UNDER SIX MONTHS OF AGE ONLY WITH THE ADVICE OF A PHYSICIAN. KEEP OUT OF REACH OF CHILDREN.

How Supplied: Available in 3.5 fl. oz. and 5.25 fl. oz. plastic bottles.

OIL OF OLAY®—Daily UV Protectant SPF 15 Moisture Replenishing Cream—Regular & Fragrance Free
(Olay Co., Inc.)

Oil of Olay Daily UV Protectant Moisture Replenishing Cream is an extra-rich cream specially formulated to provide effective moisturization and SPF protection.

Oil of Olay UV Protectant is PABA free. It is non-comedeogenic and is suitable for daily use under facial make-up.

Active Ingredients: ETHYLHEXYL P-METHOXYCINNAMATE, 2-PHENYL-BENZIMIDAZOLE-5-SULFONIC ACID.

Inactive Ingredients: WATER, ISO-HEXADECANE, GLYCERIN, BUTYLENE GLYCOL, TRIETHANOLAMINE, STEARIC ACID, CETYL ALCOHOL, CETYL PALMITATE, DEA-CETYL PHOSPHATE, ALUMINUM STARCH

Continued on next page

Richardson-Vicks—Cont.

OCTENYLSUCCINATE, TITANIUM DIOXIDE, IMIDAZOLIDINYL UREA, METHYLPARABEN, PROPYLPARABEN, CARBOMER, ACRYLATES/C10–30 ALKYL ACRYLATE CROSS-POLYMER, PEG-10 SOYA STEROL, DISODIUM EDTA, CASTOR OIL, FRAGRANCE, FD&C RED NO. 4, FD&C YELLOW NO. 5.

Available in both lightly scented and 100% color and fragrance free versions.

Indications: Provides SPF 15 UV protection to help protect against skin-aging UV rays in a light, greaseless moisturizer. The liberal and regular use of this product over the years may help reduce the chance of premature aging of the skin and skin cancer.

Directions: Apply liberally as needed to face, neck and other exposed areas for protection against UV rays and for moisturization.

Warning: FOR EXTERNAL USE ONLY. NOT TO BE SWALLOWED. AVOID CONTACT WITH EYES. DISCONTINUE USE IF SIGNS OF IRRITATION OR RASH APPEAR. USE ON CHILDREN UNDER SIX MONTHS OF AGE ONLY WITH THE ADVICE OF A PHYSICIAN. KEEP OUT OF REACH OF CHILDREN.

How Supplied: Available in 1.7 oz. glass jar.

OIL OF OLAY®—Foaming Face Wash
(Olay Co., Inc.)

Ingredients: WATER, POTASSIUM COCOYL HYDROLYZED COLLAGEN, GLYCERIN, SODIUM LAURIMINODIPROPIONATE, SODIUM ACRYLATES/STEARETH-20, METHACRYLATE COPOLYMER, SODIUM LAUROYL SARCOSINATE, DISODIUM, COCOAMPHODIACETATE, SODIUM LAURYL SULFATE, HEXYLENE GLYCOL, POLYQUATERNIUM-10, FRAGRANCE, PHENOXYETHANOL, DMDM HYDANTOIN, TETRASODIUM EDTA, MICA, TITANIUM DIOXIDE

Action and Uses: For soap-free, oil-free cleansing, removing dirt, oil and make-up—even eye make-up—without stripping or irritating skin or eyes like soaps can.

Directions: Wet your hands and face. Squeeze Foaming Face Wash into your hand. Add water, work into a rich lather and cleanse by massaging gently on your face. Rinse thoroughly. Gentle enough to use twice a day, every day.

How Supplied: Available in a regular and fragrance-free version for sensitive skin. Supplied in a 3 oz. tube and a 7 oz. pump.

PERCOGESIC®
[pĕr′kō-jē′zĭk]
Analgesic Tablets
Pain Reliever/Fever Reducer

Description: Each tablet contains:
Acetaminophen .... 325 mg
Phenyltoloxamine citrate .... 30 mg

Inactive Ingredients: Cellulose, Flavor, FD&C Yellow No. 6, Hydroxypropyl Methylcellulose, Magnesium Stearate, Polyethylene Glycol, Povidone, Silica Gel, Starch, Stearic Acid, Sucrose.

Indications: For temporary relief of minor aches and pains associated with headache, backache, muscular aches, the premenstrual and menstrual periods, the common cold and flu, toothache, and for the minor pain from arthritis, and to reduce fever.

Dosage and Administration: *Adults* (12 years and over)—1 or 2 tablets every four hours. Maximum daily dose—8 tablets
Children (6 to under 12 years)—one tablet every 4 hours. Maximum daily dose—4 tablets.
Children under 6 years of age: consult a doctor.

Warning: May cause excitability especially in children. Do not take this product if you have asthma, glaucoma, emphysema, chronic pulmonary disease, shortness of breath, difficulty in breathing, or difficulty in urination due to enlargement of the prostate gland unless directed by a doctor. May cause drowsiness; alcohol, sedatives, and tranquilizers may increase the drowsiness effect. Avoid alcoholic beverages while taking this product. Do not take this product if you are taking sedatives or tranquilizers, without first consulting your doctor. Use caution when driving a motor vehicle or operating machinery. Do not take this product for pain for more than 10 days (adults) or 5 days (children), and do not take for fever for more than 3 days unless directed by a doctor. If pain or fever persists or gets worse, if new symptoms occur, or if redness or swelling is present, consult a doctor because these could be signs of a serious condition. Do not give this product to children for the pain of arthritis unless directed by a doctor. Keep this and all drugs out of the reach of children. In case of accidental overdose, seek professional assistance or contact a poison control center immediately. Prompt medical attention is critical for adults as well as for children even if you do not notice any signs or symptoms. As with any drug, if you are pregnant or nursing a baby, seek the advice of a health professional before using this product.

How Supplied: Each light orange tablet engraved with "Percogesic". Child-resistant bottles of 24 and 90 tablets, and bottles of 50 tablets.

VICKS CHILDREN'S CHLORASEPTIC® SPRAY
Phenol/Oral
Anesthetic/Antiseptic

Children's Chloraseptic Spray is formulated especially for kids with a "child-strength" phenol formula that provides fast, effective relief with great-tasting grape flavor.

Active Ingredient: Phenol 0.5%

Inactive Ingredients: FD&C Blue No. 1, FD&C Red No. 40, flavor, glycerin, purified water, saccharin sodium, and sorbitol.

Indications: For temporary relief of your child's occasional minor sore throat pain and irritation. Also for pain associated with sore mouth and canker sores.

Directions—Children 2 Years of Age and Older: Spray 5 times directly on throat or affected area and swallow. Repeat every two hours or as directed by a physician or dentist. Children under 12 years of age should be supervised in product use.
Children Under 2 Years of Age: Consult a physician or dentist.

Warning: If sore throat is severe, or is accompanied by difficulty in breathing, or persists for more than 2 days, do not use and consult a physician promptly. If sore throat is accompanied or followed by fever, headache, rash, nausea, or vomiting, consult a physician promptly. If sore mouth symptoms do not improve in 7 days, see your physician or dentist promptly. Keep this and all drugs out of the reach of children. In case of accidental overdose, seek professional assistance or contact a poison control center immediately. As with any drug, if you are pregnant or nursing a baby, seek the advice of a health professional before using this product.

How Supplied: Available in 6 fl. oz. plastic bottles with sprayer.

VICKS® CHILDREN'S COUGH SYRUP
Cough Suppressant • Expectorant

Active Ingredients per tsp. (5 ml.): Dextromethorphan Hydrobromide 3.5 mg., Guaifenesin 50 mg.

Inactive Ingredients: Citric Acid, FD&C Green No. 3, FD&C Red No. 40, Flavor, Methylparaben, Propylene Glycol, Purified Water, Sodium Citrate, Sodium Saccharin, Sucrose.

Indications: Temporarily reduces cough due to a cold or inhaled irritants. Helps loosen phlegm (sputum) and thin bronchial secretions to drain bronchial tubes to make coughs more productive.

Actions: VICKS Children's COUGH SYRUP is an alcohol-free antitussive and expectorant. It calms, quiets coughs of colds; loosens phlegm, promotes drainage of bronchial tubes; and coats and soothes a cough irritated throat.

Direction for Use:

12 years and over:	4 teaspoons
6 to under 12 years:	2 teaspoons
2 to under 6 years:	1 teaspoon

Repeat every 4 hours or as directed by a doctor. Do not exceed 6 doses in a 24 hour period.
Children under 2 years of age: consult a doctor.

Warnings: A persistent cough may be a sign of a serious condition. If cough persists for more than 1 week, tends to recur, or is accompanied by fever, rash, or persistent headache, consult a doctor. Do not take this product for persistent or chronic cough such as occurs with smoking, asthma, chronic bronchitis, or emphysema, or where cough is accompanied by excessive phlegm (sputum) unless directed by a doctor. KEEP THIS AND ALL DRUGS OUT OF THE REACH OF CHILDREN. In case of accidental overdose, seek professional assistance or contact a poison control center immediately. As with any drug, if you are pregnant or nursing a baby, seek the advice of a health professional before using this product.

How Supplied: Available in 4 fl. oz. shatterproof bottles.

VICKS® COUGH DROPS
Menthol Cough Suppressant/Oral Anesthetic

Flavors: Available in two popular flavors: Menthol and Cherry.

Active Ingredient: Menthol.

Inactive Ingredients:
Menthol Flavor: Benzyl Alcohol, Camphor, Caramel, Corn Syrup, Eucalyptus Oil, Flavoring, Sucrose, Tolu Balsam and Thymol.
Cherry Flavor: Citric Acid, Corn Syrup, FD&C Blue No. 1, FD&C Blue No. 40, Flavor, Sucrose.

Indications: Temporarily relieves sore throat and coughs due to colds or inhaled irritants.

Directions: Adults and children 3 to 12 years: Allow drop to dissolve slowly in mouth. Cough: may be repeated every hour as needed or as directed by a doctor. Sore Throat: may be repeated every 2 hours—as needed or as directed by a doctor. Children under 3 years of age, consult a doctor.

Warning: A persistent cough may be a sign of a serious condition. If cough persists for more than 1 week, tends to recur, or is accompanied by fever, rash, or persistent headache, consult a doctor. Do not take this product for persistent chronic cough such as occurs with smoking, asthma, emphysema, or if cough is accompanied by excessive phlegm (mucus), unless directed by a doctor. If sore throat is severe, or is accompanied by difficulty in breathing, or persists for more than two days, do not use, and consult a doctor promptly. If sore throat is accompanied or followed by fever, head-

ache, rash, nausea, or vomiting, consult a doctor promptly. Keep this and all drugs out of the reach of children. As with any drug, if you are pregnant or nursing a baby, seek the advice of a health professional before using this product.

How Supplied: Vicks Cough Drops are available in boxes of 14 drops each and bags of 30 drops.

EXTRA STRENGTH VICKS®
COUGH DROPS
Menthol Cough Suppressant/Oral Anesthetic

Flavors: Available in Cherry, Menthol and Honey Lemon flavor.

Active Ingredient: Menthol Flavor: Menthol 8.4 mg. Cherry: Menthol 10 mg Honey Lemon: Menthol 10 mg

Inactive Ingredients:
Menthol Flavor: Corn Syrup, FD&C Blue No. 1, Flavor, Sucrose, Cherry Flavor: Corn Syrup, FD&C Red No. 40, FD&C Blue No. 2, Flavor, Sucrose Honey Lemon: Citric Acid, Corn Syrup, D&C Yellow No. 10, FD&C Yellow No. 6, Flavor, Sucrose

Indications: Temporarily relieves sore throat and coughs due to colds or inhaled irritants.

Directions: Adults and children 3 to 12 years: Allow drop to dissolve slowly in mouth. Cough: may be repeated every hour as needed or as directed by a doctor. Sore Throat: may be repeated every 2 hours as needed or as directed by a doctor. Children under 3 years of age, consult a doctor.

Warning: A persistent cough may be a sign of a serious condition. If cough persists for more than 1 week, tends to recur, or is accompanied by fever, rash, or persistent headache, consult a doctor. Do not take this product for persistent or chronic cough such as occurs with smoking, asthma, emphysema, or if cough is accompanied by excessive phlegm (mucus), unless directed by a doctor. If sore throat is severe, or is accompanied by difficulty in breathing, or persists for more than two days, do not use, and consult a doctor promptly. If sore throat is accompanied or followed by fever, headache, rash, nausea, or vomiting, consult a doctor promptly. Keep this and all drugs out of the reach of children. As with any drug, if you are pregnant or nursing a baby, seek the advice of a health professional before using this product.

How Supplied: Extra Strength Vicks Cough Drops are available in single sticks of 9 drops each and bags of 30 drops.

VICKS DAYCARE® LIQUID
VICKS DAYCARE® CAPLETS
Daytime Colds/Flu Medicine
Nasal Decongestant/Pain
Reliever Fever Reducer
Cough Suppressant/Expectorant

Active Ingredients: LIQUID — per fluid ounce (2 Tbs.) or **CAPLET** — per two caplets, contains Acetaminophen 650 mg., Dextromethorphan Hydrobromide 20 mg., Pseudoephedrine Hydrochloride 60 mg., Guaifenesin 200 mg.

Inactive Ingredients:
Liquid: Citric Acid, FD&C Yellow No. 6, Flavor, Glycerin, Propylene Glycol, Purified Water, Sodium Saccharin, Sodium Benzoate, Sodium Citrate, Sucrose. Also contains Alcohol 10%.
Caplets: Cellulose, Croscarmellose Sodium, FD&C Red No. 40, FD&C Yellow No. 6, Magnesium Stearate, Povidone, Starch, Stearic acid.

Indications: For the temporary relief of minor aches, pains, headache, muscular aches, sore throat and fever associated with a cold or flu. Temporarily relieves nasal congestion and coughing due to a cold. Helps loosen phlegm (sputum) and thin secretions to drain bronchial tubes and make coughs more productive.

Directions: Take as directed. Adults 12 years and over: one fluid ounce in medicine cup (2 tablespoons), or 2 caplets.
Children 6 to under 12 years of age: one half fluid ounce in medicine cup (1 tablespoon), or 1 caplet.
Children 2 to under 6 years of age: 1½ teaspoons.
Children under 2 years of age: Consult a doctor.
Repeat every 4 hours, not to exceed 4 doses per day, or as directed by a doctor.

Warning: Do not exceed recommended dosage because at higher doses, nervousness, dizziness, or sleeplessness may occur. Do not take this product if you have heart disease, high blood pressure, thyroid disease, diabetes, or difficulty in urination due to enlargement of the prostate gland unless directed by a doctor. DRUG INTERACTION PRECAUTION: Do not take this product if you are presently taking a prescription drug for high blood pressure or depression, without first consulting your doctor. Do not take this product for persistent or chronic cough such as occurs with smoking, asthma, chronic bronchitis, or emphysema, or where a cough is accompanied by excessive phlegm (sputum) unless directed by a doctor. Do not take this product for more than 7 days (for adults) or 5 days (for children). A persistent cough may be a sign of serious condition. If cough persists for more than 7 days, tends to recur, or is accompanied by rash, or persistent headache, consult a doctor. If symptoms do not improve or are accompanied by fever that lasts for more than 3 days, or if new symptoms occur, consult a doctor. If sore throat is severe, persists for more than 2 days, is accompa-

Continued on next page

Richardson-Vicks—Cont.

nied or followed by fever, headache, rash, nausea, or vomiting, consult a doctor promptly. Keep this and all drugs out of the reach of children. In case of accidental overdose, seek professional assistance or contact a poison control center immediately. Prompt medical attention is critical for adults as well as for children even if you do not notice any signs or symptoms. As with any drug, if you are pregnant or nursing a baby, seek the advice of a health professional before using this product.
TAKE ONLY AS DIRECTED.

How Supplied: Available in: **LIQUID** with child-resistant, tamper-evident cap—6 and 10 fl. oz. plastic bottles. **CAPLET** in child-resistant packages—20.

VICKS FORMULA 44® COUGH CONTROL DISCS
Cough Suppressant/Oral Anesthetic

Active Ingredients per disc: Dextromethorphan (expressed as Dextromethorphan Hydrobromide) 5 mg, Benzocaine 1.25 mg, Menthol 4.3 mg.

Inactive Ingredients: Caramel, Corn Syrup, Flavors, Silicon Dioxide, Sodium Chloride, Sucrose.

Indications: Temporarily relieves cough due to minor throat and bronchial irritation as may occur with the common cold or inhaled irritants.
Also provides temporary relief of occasional minor irritation, pain, sore mouth, and sore throat.

Actions: VICKS FORMULA 44 COUGH CONTROL DISCS have antitussive and oral-anesthetic actions in a solid disc form.

Direction for Use:
Adults 12 years and over:
Dissolve two discs in mouth, one at a time. Repeat every 4 hours not to exceed 12 discs in 24 hours or as directed by doctor.
Children 3 to under 12 years:
Dissolve one disc in mouth. Repeat every 4 hours not to exceed 6 discs in 24 hours or as directed by doctor.
Children under 3 years, consult a doctor.

Warnings: A persistent cough may be a sign of a serious condition. If cough persists for more than 1 week, tends to recur, or is accompanied by fever, rash, or persistent headache, consult a doctor. Do not take this product for persistent or chronic cough such as occurs with smoking, asthma, emphysema, or if cough is accompanied by excessive phlegm (mucus) unless directed by a doctor. If sore throat is severe, or is accompanied by difficulty in breathing, or persists for more than 2 days, do not use, and consult a doctor promptly. If sore throat is accompanied or followed by fever, headache, rash, nausea or vomiting, consult a doctor promptly. If sore mouth symptoms do not improve in 7 days, see your

physician or dentist promptly. KEEP THIS AND ALL DRUGS OUT OF THE REACH OF CHILDREN. In case of accidental overdose, seek professional assistance or contact a poison control center immediately. As with any drug, if you are pregnant or nursing a baby, seek the advice of a health professional before using this product.

How Supplied: Available as 24 discs in invididual foil-wrapped portable packets.

VICKS FORMULA 44® COUGH MEDICINE
Dextromethorphan HBr/ Cough Suppressant

Active Ingredient per 2 tsp. (10 mL.): Dextromethorphan Hydrobromide 30 mg. Also contains Alcohol 10%.

Inactive Ingredients: Caramel, Carboxymethylcellulose Sodium, Citric Acid, FD&C Red #40, Flavor, Invert Sugar, Propylene Glycol, Purified water, Sodium Citrate.

Indications: Formula 44 provides temporary relief of coughs due to minor throat and bronchial irritation associated with a cold.

Actions: VICKS FORMULA 44 COUGH MEDICINE is a cough suppressant.

Directions:
Adults:
12 years and over—2 teaspoons
Children:
6–11 years of age—1 teaspoon
2–5 years of age—½ teaspoon
Children under 2 years of age consult a doctor.
Repeat every 6–8 hours.
No more than 4 doses per day or as directed by doctor.

Warning: A persistent cough may be a sign of a serious condition. If cough persists for more than 1 week, tends to recur, or is accompanied by fever, rash, or persistent headache, consult a doctor. Do not take this product for persistent or chronic cough such as occurs with smoking, asthma, emphysema, or if cough is accompanied by excessive phlegm (mucus) unless directed by a doctor. KEEP THIS AND ALL DRUGS OUT OF THE REACH OF CHILDREN. In case of accidental overdose, seek professional assistance or contact a poison control center immediately. As with any drug, if you are pregnant or nursing a baby, seek the advice of a health professional before using this product.

How Supplied: Available in 4 fl. oz. and 8 fl. oz. squeeze bottles with Vicks AccuTip™ Dispenser for clean, easy dosing.

VICKS FORMULA 44D®
COUGH & DECONGESTANT MEDICINE
Cough Suppressant/ Nasal Decongestant

Active Ingredients per 3 tsp. (15 ml.): Dextromethorphan Hydrobromide 30 mg., Pseudoephedrine Hydrochloride 60 mg. Also contains Alcohol 10%.

Inactive Ingredients: Citric Acid, FD&C Red No. 40, Flavor, Glycerin, Propylene Glycol, Purified Water, Sodium Citrate, Sodium Saccharin, Sucrose.

Indications: Vicks Formula 44D provides temporary relief of coughs and nasal congestion due to a common cold.

Actions: VICKS FORMULA 44D is a cough suppressant and a nasal decongestant.

Dosage:
ADULT DOSE   12 years of age
             and over—
             3 teaspoons
CHILD DOSE   6–11 years of age—
             1½ teaspoons
             2–5 years of age—
             ¾ teaspoon
Children under 2 years of age, consult a doctor.
Repeat ever 6 hours. No more than 4 doses per day or as directed by a doctor.

Warning: A persistent cough may be a sign of a serious condition. If cough persists for more than 1 week, tends to recur, or is accompanied by fever, rash, or persistent headache, consult a doctor. Do not take this product for persistent or chronic cough such as occurs with smoking, asthma, emphysema, or if cough is accompanied by excessive phlegm (mucus) unless directed by a doctor. Do not exceed recommended dosage because at higher doses nervousness, dizziness, or sleeplessness may occur. Do not take this product for more than 7 days. If symptoms do not improve or are accompanied by fever, consult a doctor. Do not take this product if you have heart disease, high blood pressure, thyroid disease, diabetes, or difficulty in urination due to enlargement of the prostate gland unless directed by a doctor. *Drug Interaction Precaution.* Do not take this product if you are presently taking a prescription drug for high blood pressure or depression, without first consulting your doctor. KEEP THIS AND ALL DRUGS OUT OF THE REACH OF CHILDREN. In case of accidental overdose, seek professional assistance or contact a poison control center immediately. As with any drug, if you are pregnant, or nursing a baby, seek the advice of a health professional before using this product.

How Supplied: Available in 4 fl. oz. and 8 fl. oz. squeeze bottles with Vicks AccuTip™ Dispenser for clean, easy dosing.

VICKS FORMULA 44E®
Cough & Expectorant Medicine
Cough Suppressant/Expectorant

Active Ingredients per 3 teaspoons (15ml) Dextromethorphan Hydrobromide 20mg, Guaifenesin 200mg Also contains Alcohol 10%

Inactive Ingredients: Citric Acid, FD&C Blue No. 1, FD&C Red No. 40, Flavor, Glycerin, Propylene Glycol, Purified Water, Sodium Citrate, Sodium Saccharin, Sucrose.

Indications: Vicks Formula 44E provides temporary relief of coughs due to the common cold and helps loosen phlegm to make coughs more productive.

Actions: VICKS FORMULA 44E is a cough suppressant and expectorant.

Directions:
Adults and Children 12 years of age and over: 3 teaspoons.
Children 6–11 years of age: 1½ teaspoons.
Children 2–5 years of age: ¾ teaspoon.
Children under 2 years of age: consult a doctor.
Repeat every 4 hours. No more than 6 doses per day, or as directed by a doctor.

Warning: A persistent cough may be a sign of a serious condition. If cough persists for more than 1 week, tends to recur, or is accompanied by fever, rash, or persistent headache, consult a doctor. Do not take this product for persistent or chronic cough such as occurs with smoking, asthma, chronic bronchitis, or emphysema, or where cough is accompanied by excessive phlegm (sputum) unless directed by a doctor. KEEP THIS AND ALL DRUGS OUT OF THE REACH OF CHILDREN. In case of accidental overdose, seek professional assistance or contact a poison control center immediately. As with any drug, if you are pregnant, or nursing a baby, seek the advice of a health professional before using this product.

How Supplied: Available in 4 fl. oz. and 8 fl. oz. squeeze bottles with Vicks AccuTip™ Dispenser for clean, easy dosing.

VICKS FORMULA 44M®
MULTI-SYMPTOM COUGH & COLD MEDICINE
Cough Suppressant/Nasal Decongestant/Antihistamine/Pain Reliever-Fever Reducer

Active Ingredients per 4 tsp. (20 ml.): Dextromethorphan Hydrobromide 30 mg., Pseudoephedrine Hydrochloride 60 mg., Chlorpheniramine Maleate 4 mg., Acetaminophen 500 mg. Also contains Alcohol 20%.

Inactive Ingredients: Citric Acid, FD&C Blue No. 1, FD&C Red No. 40, Flavor, Glycerin, Purified Water, Sodium Benzoate, Sodium Citrate, Sodium Saccharin, Sucrose.

Indications: FORMULA 44M provides temporary relief of coughing, nasal congestion, runny nose, and sneezing due to a cold. Also for temporary relief of headache, fever, muscular aches and sore throat due to a cold or flu.

Actions: VICKS FORMULA 44M is a cough suppressant, nasal decongestant, antihistamine and analgesic.

Directions: Adults and children 12 years of age and over—4 teaspoons
Children 6–11 years of age—2 teaspoons
Children under 6 years of age—consult a doctor
Repeat every 6 hours. No more than 4 doses per day or as directed by a doctor.

Warning: Do not take this product for persistent or chronic cough such as occurs with smoking, asthma, or emphysema, or if cough is accompanied by excessive phlegm (mucus) unless directed by a doctor. Do not exceed recommended dosage because at higher doses nervousness, dizziness, or sleeplessness may occur. Do not take this product if you have heart disease, high blood pressure, thyroid disease, diabetes, or difficulty in urination due to enlargement of the prostate gland unless directed by a doctor. *Drug Interaction Precaution.* Do not take this product if you are presently taking a prescription drug for high blood pressure or depression, without first consulting your doctor. May cause excitability especially in children. Do not take this product if you have asthma, glaucoma, emphysema, chronic pulmonary disease, shortness of breath, or difficulty in breathing unless directed by a doctor. May cause marked drowsiness; alcohol, sedatives, and tranquilizers may increase the drowsiness effect. Avoid alcoholic beverages while taking this product. Do not take this product if you are taking sedatives or tranquilizers, without first consulting your doctor. Use caution when driving a motor vehicle or operating machinery. Do not take this product for more than 7 days (for adults) or 5 days (for children). A persistent cough may be a sign of a serious condition. If cough persists for more than 7 days, tends to recur, or is accompanied by rash, persistent headache, fever that lasts for more than 3 days, or if new symptoms occur, consult a doctor. If symptoms do not improve or are accompanied by fever that lasts for more than 3 days, or if new symptoms occur, consult a doctor. If sore throat is severe, persists for more than 2 days, is accompanied or followed by fever, headache, rash, nausea or vomiting, consult a doctor. KEEP THIS AND ALL DRUGS OUT OF THE REACH OF CHILDREN. In case of accidental overdose, seek professional assistance or contact a poison control center immediately. Prompt medical attention is critical for adults as well as for children, even if you do not notice any signs or symptoms. As with any drug, if you are pregnant or nursing a baby, seek the advice of a health professional before using this product.

How Supplied: Available in 4 fl. oz. and 8 fl. oz. squeeze bottles with Vicks AccuTip™ Dispenser for clean, easy dosing. A calibrated dose cup accompanies each bottle.

VICKS PEDIATRIC FORMULA 44®
COUGH MEDICINE
Dextromethorphan HBr/Cough Suppressant

Active Ingredients per 1 Tbs. (15 ml.): Dextromethorphan Hydrobromide 15 mg.

Inactive Ingredients: Carboxymethylcellulose Sodium, Cellulose, Citric Acid, FD&C Red No. 40, Flavors, Glycerin, Polysorbate 80, Potassium Sorbate, Propylene Glycol, Purified Water, Sodium Citrate, Sorbitol, Sucrose.

Indications: For the temporary relief of coughs due to the common cold.

Actions: Vicks Pediatric Formula 44 is a cough suppressant.

Administration and Dosage:
Directions: SHAKE WELL BEFORE USING
Squeeze bottle to accurately dispense medicine into dosage cup provided. 1 Tbs. ½ Tbs.

Dosage:

Age	Weight	Dose
Under 2 yrs	Under 28 lbs.	Consult physician*
2–5 yrs	28–47 lbs.	Fill cup to ½ Tbs.
6–11 yrs	48–95 lbs.	Fill cup to 1 Tbs.
12 yrs. and over	96 lbs. and over	2 Tbs. or Try one of the Adult Formula 44® Medicines

Repeat every 6–8 hours, no more than 4 doses in 24 hours, or as directed by a doctor.

Professional Dosage:
*Physicians: Suggested doses for children under 2 years of age.

Age	Weight	Dose
* 6–11 mo.	17–21 lbs.	1 teaspoon (5 ml.)
*12–23 mo.	22–27 lbs.	1¼ teaspoon (6.25 ml.)

Repeat every 6–8 hours, no more than 4 doses in 24 hours or as directed by doctor.

*Based on extrapolation from studies on the safety and efficacy of active ingredients conducted among older children and adults. Use caution in treating children under 2 years of age who were born prematurely.

Warnings: A persistent cough may be a sign of a serious condition. If cough persists for more than 1 week, tends to recur, or is accompanied by fever, rash, or

Continued on next page

Richardson-Vicks—Cont.

persistent headache, consult a doctor. Do not take this product for persistent or chronic cough such as occurs with smoking, asthma, emphysema, or if cough is accompanied by excessive phlegm (mucus) unless directed by a doctor. KEEP THIS AND ALL DRUGS OUT OF THE REACH OF CHILDREN. In case of accidental overdose, seek professional assistance or contact a poison control center immediately. As with any drug, if you are pregnant or nursing a baby, seek the advice of a health professional before using this product.

How Supplied: 4 fl. oz. squeeze bottles with Vicks AccuTip™ Dispenser for clean, easy, accurate dosing. Calibrated dose cup accompanies each bottle.

VICKS PEDIATRIC FORMULA 44m®
Multi-Symptom COUGH & COLD MEDICINE
Cough Suppressant/Nasal Decongestant/Antihistamine

Active Ingredients: Per 1 Tbs. (15 ml.): Dextromethorphan Hydrobromide 15 mg., Pseudoephedrine Hydrochloride 30 mg., Chlorpheniramine Maleate 2 mg.

Inactive Ingredients: Carboxymethylcellulose Sodium, Cellulose, Citric Acid, FD&C Red No. 40, Flavors, Glycerin, Polysorbate 80, Potassium Sorbate, Propylene Glycol, Purified Water, Sodium Citrate, Sorbitol, Sucrose.

Indications: For the temporary relief of coughs, nasal congestion, runny nose and sneezing due to the common cold.

Actions: Vicks Pediatric Formula 44m is a cough suppppressant, nasal decongestant and antihistamine.

Administration and Dosage:
Directions for Use: SHAKE WELL BEFORE USING
Squeeze bottle to accurately dispense medicine into dosage cup provided.   1 Tbs.   ½ Tbs.

Dosage:

Age	Weight	Dose
Under 6 yrs	Under 48 lbs.	Consult physician*
6–11 yrs	48–95 lbs.	Fill cup to 1 Tbs.
12 yrs and over	96 lbs. and over	2 Tbs. or try one of the Adult Formula 44® Medicines

Repeat every 6 hours. No more than 4 doses in 24 hours, or as directed by a doctor.

Professional Dosage:
*Physicians: Suggested doses for children under 6 years of age:

Age	Weight	Dose
*6–11 mo.	17–21 lbs.	1 teaspoon (5 ml.)
*12–23 mo.	22–27 lbs.	1¼ teaspoon (6.25 ml.)
2–5 yrs.	28–47 lbs.	½ Tbs. (7.5 ml.)

Repeat every 6 hours, no more than 4 doses in 24 hours, or as directed by doctor.
*Based on extrapolation from studies on the safety and efficacy of active ingredients conducted among older children and adults. Use caution in treating children under 2 years of age who were born prematurely.

Warnings: A persistent cough may be a sign of a serious condition. If cough persists for more than 1 week, tends to recur, or is accompanied by fever, rash, or persistent headache, consult a doctor. Do not take this product for persistent or chronic cough such as occurs with smoking, asthma, emphysema, or if cough is accompanied by excessive phlegm (mucus) unless directed by a doctor. Do not exceed recommended dosage because at higher doses nervousness, dizziness, or sleeplessness may occur. Do not take this product for more than 7 days. If symptoms do not improve or are accompanied by fever, consult a doctor. Do not take this product if you have heart disease, high blood pressure, thyroid disease, diabetes, or difficulty in urination due to enlargement of the prostate gland unless directed by a doctor. *Drug Interaction Precaution.* Do not take this product if you are presently taking a prescription drug for high blood pressure or depression, without first consulting your doctor. May cause excitability especially in children. Do not take this product if you have asthma, glaucoma, emphysema, chronic pulmonary disease, shortness of breath, or difficulty in breathing unless directed by a doctor. May cause marked drowsiness; alcohol, sedatives, and tranquilizers may increase the drowsiness effect. Avoid alcoholic beverages while taking this product. Do not take this product if you are taking sedatives or tranquilizers, without first consulting your doctor. Use caution when driving a motor vehicle or operating machinery. KEEP THIS AND ALL DRUGS OUT OF THE REACH OF CHILDREN. In case of accidental overdose, seek professional assistance or contact a poison control center immediately. As with any drug, if you are pregnant or nursing a baby, seek the advice of a health professional before using this product.

How Supplied: 4 fl. oz. squeeze bottles with Vicks AccuTip™ Dispenser for clean, easy, accurate dosing. Calibrated dose cup accompanies each bottle.

VICKS PEDIATRIC FORMULA 44d®
COUGH & DECONGESTANT MEDICINE

Active Ingredients: Per 1 Tbs. (15 ml.): Dextromethorphan Hydrobromide 15 mg., Pseudoephedrine Hydrochloride 30 mg.

Inactive Ingredients: Carboxymethylcellulose Sodium, Cellulose, Citric Acid, FD&C Red No. 40, Flavor, Glycerin, Polysorbate 80, Potassium Sorbate, Propylene Glycol, Purified Water, Sodium Citrate, Sorbitol, Sucrose.

Indications: For the temporary relief of coughs and nasal congestion due to the common cold.

Actions: Vicks Pediatric Formula 44d is a cough suppressant and decongestant.

Administration and Dosage:
Directions: SHAKE WELL BEFORE USING
Squeeze bottle to accurately dispense medicine into dosage cup provided   1 Tbs.   ½ Tbs.

Dosage:

Age	Weight	Dose
Under 2 yrs	Under 28 lbs.	Consult physician*
2–5 yrs	28–47 lbs.	Fill cup to ½ Tbs.
6–11 yrs	48–95 lbs.	Fill cup to 1 Tbs.
12 yrs and over	96 lbs. and over	2 Tbs. or try one of the Adult Formula 44® medicines

Repeat every 6 hours. No more than 4 doses in 24 hours, or as directed by a doctor.

*Professional Dosage:
Physicians: Suggested doses for children under 2 years of age.

Age	Weight	Dose
*6–11 mo.	17–21 lbs.	1 teaspoon (5 ml)
*12–23 mo.	22–27 lbs.	1¼ teaspoon 6.25 ml)

Repeat every 6 hours. No more than 4 doses in 24 hours, or as directed by doctor.
*Based on extrapolation from studies on the safety and efficacy of active ingredients conducted among older children and adults. Use caution in treating children under 2 years who were born prematurely.

Warnings: A persistent cough may be a sign of a serious condition. If cough persists for more than 1 week, tends to recur, or is accompanied by fever, rash, or persistent headache, consult a doctor. Do not take this product for persistent or chronic cough such as occurs with smoking, asthma, emphysema, or if cough is accompanied by excessive phlegm (mucus) unless directed by a doctor. Do not exceed recommended dosage because at higher doses nervousness, dizziness, or sleeplessness may occur. Do not take this product for more than 7 days. If symptoms do not improve or are accompanied by fever, consult a doctor. Do not take this product if you have heart disease, high blood pressure, thyroid disease, diabetes, or difficulty in urination due to enlargement of the prostate gland unless directed by a doctor. *Drug Interaction Precaution.* Do not take this product if you are presently taking a prescription drug for high blood pressure or depression, without first consulting your doctor. KEEP THIS AND ALL DRUGS OUT OF THE REACH OF CHILDREN. In case of accidental overdose, seek professional assistance or contact a poison control center immediately. As with any drug, if you are pregnant or nursing a baby, seek the advice of a health professional before using this product.

How Supplied: 4 fl. oz. squeeze bottles with Vicks AccuTip™ Dispenser for clean, easy, accurate dosing. Calibrated dose cup accompanies each bottle.

VICKS PEDIATRIC FORMULA 44e®
Cough & Expectorant Medicine

Active Ingredients: per 1 tablespoon (15 ml.): Dextromethorphan Hydrobromide 10 mg, Guaifenesin 100 mg

Inactive Ingredients: Carboxymethylcellulose Sodium, Cellulose, Citric Acid, FD&C Red No. 40, Flavor, Glycerin, Polysorbate 80, Potassium Sorbate, Propylene Glycol, Purified Water, Sodium Citrate, Sorbitol, Sucrose.

Indications: For the temporary relief of coughs due to the common cold and helps loosen phlegm to make coughs more productive.

Actions: Vicks Formula 44e is a cough suppressant and expectorant.

Administration and Dosage: Directions:
SHAKE WELL BEFORE USING
Squeeze bottle to accurately dispense medicine into dosage cup provided.

1 Tbs.
½ Tbs.

Dosage:

Age	Weight	Dose
Under 2 yrs	Under 28 lb.	Consult Physician*
2–5 yrs	28–47 lb.	Fill cup to ½ Tbs.
6–11 yrs	48–95 lb.	Fill cup to 1 Tbs.
12 yrs. and over	96 lb. and over	2 Tbs. or Try one of the Adult Formula 44® medicines

Repeat every 4 hours. No more than 6 doses in 24 hours, or as directed by a doctor.
*Professional Dosage:
Physicians: Suggested dose for children under 2 years of age. [See table above]

Warnings: A persistent cough may be a sign of a serious condition. If cough persists for more than 1 week, tends to recur, or is accompanied by fever, rash, or persistent headache, consult a doctor. Do not take this product for persistent or chronic cough such as occurs with smoking, asthma, chronic bronchitis, emphysema, or where cough is accompanied by

Age	Weight	Dose
* 6–11 mo.	17–21 lb.	1 teaspoon (5 ml)
*12–23 mo.	22–27 lb.	1¼ teaspoon (6.25 ml)

Repeat every 4 hours. No more than 6 doses in 24 hours, or as directed by a doctor.
*Based on extrapolation from studies on the safety and efficacy of active ingredients conducted among older children and adults. Use caution in treating children under 2 years who were born prematurely.

excessive phlegm (sputum) unless directed by a doctor. **KEEP THIS AND ALL DRUGS OUT OF THE REACH OF CHILDREN.** In case of accidental overdose, seek professional assistance or contact a poison control center immediately. As with any drug, if you are pregnant or nursing a baby, seek the advice of a health professional before using this product.

How Supplied: 4 fl. oz. squeeze bottles with Vicks AccuTip™ Dispenser for clean, easy, accurate dosing. Calibrated dose cup accompanies each bottle.

VICKS® INHALER
with decongestant action
l-Desoxyephedrine/Nasal Decongestant

Active Ingredient per inhaler: l-Desoxyephedrine 50 mg.

Inactive Ingredients: Special Vicks Vapors (bornyl acetate, camphor, lavender oil, menthol).

Indications: For the temporary relief of nasal congestion due to the common cold, hay fever, upper respiratory allergies or sinusitis.

Actions: Provides fast decongestant relief.

Directions: Adults: 2 inhalations in each nostril not more often than every 2 hours. Children 6 to under 12 years of age (under adult supervision): 1 inhalation in each nostril not more often than every 2 hours. Children under 6 years of age: consult a doctor.

Warnings: Do not exceed recommended dosage because burning, stinging, sneezing, or increase of nasal discharge may occur. The use of this container by more than one person may spread infection. Do not use this product for more than 7 days. If symptoms persist, consult a doctor. Keep this and all drugs out of the reach of children. In case of accidental ingestion, seek professional assistance or contact a poison control center immediately.

VICKS INHALER is effective for a minimum of 3 months after first use. Keep tightly closed.

How Supplied: Available as a cylindrical plastic nasal inhaler (net weight: 0.007 oz.).

VICKS CHILDREN'S NYQUIL®
NIGHTTIME COLD/COUGH MEDICINE
Antihistamine/Nasal Decongestant/ Cough Suppressant

Children's NyQuil was specially formulated with the maximum allowable nonprescription levels of three effective ingredients to relieve nighttime cough, nasal congestion, and runny nose so children can rest. Children's NyQuil is alcohol free and analgesic free and has a pleasant cherry flavor.

Active Ingredients: Each ½ oz dose (1 Tbs) Chlorpheniramine Maleate 2 mg, Pseudoephedrine HCl 30 mg, Dextromethorphan Hydrobromide 15 mg.

Inactive Ingredients: Citric Acid, FD&C Red No. 40, Flavor, Potassium Sorbate, Propylene Glycol, Purified Water, Sodium Citrate, Sucrose.

Indications: For temporary relief of nasal congestion, runny nose, sneezing, and coughing due to a cold, so your child can rest.

Directions: Take at bedtime as directed. Use medicine cup provided.
If cold symptoms keep your child at home, a total of 4 doses may be given per day, each 6 hours apart, or use as directed by a doctor.

Age	Weight	Dose
Under 6 yrs	Under 48 lb.	Consult physician*
6–11 yrs	48–95 lb.	1 Tbs.
12 yrs and over	96 lb. and over	2 Tbs.

* **Professional Labeling:** Children under 6 years of age: Use only as directed by a physician. Suggested doses for children under 6 years of age:

Age	Weight	Dose
*6–11 mo.	17–21 lb.	1 tsp. (5 ml.)
*12–23 mo.	22–27 lb.	1¼ tsp. (6.25 ml.)
2–5 yrs	28–47 lb.	½ Tbs. (7.5 ml.)

Repeat every 6 hours, not to exceed 4 doses in 24 hours, or as directed by doctor.
*Based on extrapolation from studies on the safety and efficacy of active ingredients conducted among older children and adults. Use caution in treating children under 2 years of age who were born prematurely.

Warnings: Do not exceed recommended dosage, because at higher doses nervousness, dizziness or sleeplessness may occur. Do not take this product for more than 7 days. If symptoms do not improve or are accompanied by fever, consult a doctor. Do not take this product if

Continued on next page

Richardson-Vicks—Cont.

you have heart disease, high blood pressure, thyroid disease, diabetes, or difficulty in urination due to enlargement of the prostate gland unless directed by a doctor.

Drug Interaction Precaution. Do not take this product if you are presently taking a prescription drug for high blood pressure or depression, without first consulting your doctor.

May cause excitability especially in children. Do not take this product if you have asthma, glaucoma, emphysema, chronic pulmonary disease, shortness of breath, or difficulty in breathing, unless directed by a doctor. May cause marked drowsiness; alcohol, sedatives, and tranquilizers may increase the drowsiness effect. Avoid alcoholic beverages while taking this product. Do not take this product if you are taking sedatives or tranquilizers, without first consulting your doctor. Use caution when driving a motor vehicle or operating machinery. A persistent cough may be a sign of a serious condition. If cough persists for more than 1 week, tends to recur, or is accompanied by fever, rash, or persistent headache, consult a doctor. Do not take this product for persistent or chronic cough such as occurs with smoking, asthma, emphysema, or if cough is accompanied by excessive phlegm (mucus) unless directed by a doctor.

KEEP THIS AND ALL DRUGS OUT OF THE REACH OF CHILDREN. In case of accidental overdose, seek professional assistance or contact a poison control center immediately. As with any drug, if you are pregnant or nursing a baby, seek the advice of a health professional before using this product.

How Supplied: Available in 4 fl. oz. and 8 fl. oz. bottles with child-resistant, tamper-evident cap and a calibrated medicine cup.

VICKS CHILDREN'S NYQUIL®
Nighttime Head Cold/Allergy Medicine
Antihistamine/Nasal Decongestant

Children's NyQuil Head Cold/Allergy Medicine was specially formulated with the maximum allowable non-prescription levels of two effective ingredients to relieve allergy symptoms and head colds without coughs.

Active Ingredients per ½ Oz. Dose (1 Tbs): Chlorpheniramine Maleate 2mg. Pseudoephedrine HCl 30mg

Inactive Ingredients: Citric Acid, FD&C Blue No. 1, FD&C Red No. 40, Flavors, Methylparaben, Potassium Sorbate, Propylene Glycol, Purified Water, Sodium Citrate, Sucrose and Sorbitol.

Indications: For temporary relief of nasal congestion, runny nose, and sneezing due to a cold. Also relieves nasal and sinus congestion, sneezing, runny nose, and itchy, watery eyes due to hay fever or other upper respiratory allergies.

Directions: Take at bedtime as directed. Use medicine cup provided. If symptoms keep your child at home, 4 doses may be given per day, each 6 hours apart, or use as directed by a doctor.

Age	Weight	Dose
Under 6 yrs	Under 48 lb.	Consult Physician*
6–11 yrs	48–95 lb.	1 Tbs. (½ fl. oz.)
12 yrs and over	96 lb. and over	2 Tbs. (1 fl. oz.)

*Professional Labeling: Children under 6 years of age: Use only as directed by a physician. Suggested doses for children under 6 years of age:

Age	Weight	Dose
*6–11 mo.	17–21 lb.	1 tsp. (5 ml.)
*12–23 mo.	22–27 lb.	1¼ tsp. (6.25 ml.)
2–5 yrs	28–47 lb.	½ Tbs. (7.5 ml.)

Repeat every 6 hours, not to exceed 4 doses in 24 hours, or as directed by doctor.
* Based on extrapolation from studies on the safety and efficacy of active ingredients conducted among older children and adults. Use caution in treating children under 2 years of age who were born prematurely.

Warning: Do not exceed recommended dosage, because at higher doses nervousness, dizziness or sleeplessness may occur. Do not take this product for more than 7 days. If symptoms do not improve or are accompanied by fever, consult a doctor. Do not take this product if you have heart disease, high blood pressure, thyroid disease, diabetes, or difficulty in urination due to enlargement of the prostate gland unless directed by a doctor.

Drug Interaction Precaution: Do not take this product if you are presently taking a prescription drug for high blood pressure or depression, without first consulting your doctor. May cause excitability especially in children. Do not take this product if you have asthma, glaucoma, emphysema, chronic pulmonary disease, shortness of breath, or difficulty in breathing, unless directed by a doctor. May cause drowsiness: alcohol, sedatives, and tranquilizers may increase the drowsiness effect. Avoid alcoholic beverages while taking this product. Do not take this product if you are taking sedatives or tranquilizers, without first consulting your doctor. Use caution when driving a motor vehicle or operating machinery. Keep this and all drugs out of the reach of children. In case of accidental overdose, seek professional assistance or contact a poison control center immediately. As with any drug, if you are pregnant or nursing a baby, seek the advice of a

health professional before using this product.
TAKE ONLY AS DIRECTED

How Supplied: Available in 4 fl. oz. bottles with child-resistant, tamper-evident cap and a calibrated medicine cup.

VICKS NYQUIL®
[nī'quil]
Adult Nighttime Colds/Flu Medicine in oral liquid form.
Original and Cherry Flavor
Nasal Decongestant/Antihistamine/ Cough Suppressant/Pain Reliever, Fever Reducer

Active Ingredients per fluid oz. (2 Tbs.): Acetaminophen 1000 mg., Doxylamine Succinate 7.5 mg., Pseudoephedrine HCl 60 mg, and Dextromethorphan Hydrobromide 30 mg.

Inactive Ingredients: Original Flavor: Citric Acid, FD&C Blue No. 1, Flavor, Glycerin, Purified Water, Sodium Benzoate, Sodium Citrate, Sucrose.
Contains FD&C Yellow No. 5 (tartrazine) as a color additive.
Contains alcohol 25%.
Cherry Flavor: Citric Acid, FD&C Blue No. 1, FD&C Red No. 40, Flavor, Glycerin, Purified Water, Sodium Citrate, Sodium Saccharin, Sucrose.
Contains alcohol 25%.

Indications: For the temporary relief of minor aches, pains, headache, muscular aches, sore throat, and fever associated with a cold or flu. Temporarily relieves nasal congestion, cough due to minor throat and bronchial irritations, runny nose and sneezing associated with the common cold.

Actions: Decongestant, antipyretic, antihistaminic, antitussive, analgesic. By relieving symptoms, helps patient to get the rest he needs.

Directions:
ADULTS (12 and over): One fluid ounce (2 tablespoons) at bedtime in medicine cup provided.
Not recommended for children.
If your cold or flu symptoms keep you confined to bed or at home, a total of 4 doses may be taken per day, each 6 hours apart, or as directed by a doctor.

Warning: Do not exceed recommended dosage because at higher doses nervousness, dizziness or sleeplessness may occur. Do not take this product if you have heart disease, high blood pressure, thyroid disease, diabetes, or difficulty in urination due to enlargement of the prostate gland unless directed by a doctor.
Drug Interaction Precaution: Do not take this product if you are presently taking a prescription drug for high blood pressure or depression, without first consulting your doctor.
Do not take this product for persistent or chronic cough such as occurs with smoking, asthma, emphysema, or if cough is accompanied by excessive phlegm (mucus) unless directed by a doctor. Do not take this product for more than 7 days. A

persistent cough may be a sign of a serious condition. If cough persists for more than 7 days, tends to recur, or is accompanied by rash, persistent headache, fever that lasts for more than 3 days, or if new symptoms occur, consult a doctor. May cause excitability especially in children. Do not take this product if you have asthma, glaucoma, emphysema, chronic pulmonary disease, shortness of breath, or difficulty in breathing unless directed by a doctor. May cause marked drowsiness; alcohol, sedatives, and tranquilizers may increase the drowsiness effect. Avoid alcoholic beverages while taking this product. Do not take this product if you are taking sedatives or tranquilizers, without first consulting your doctor. Use caution when driving a motor vehicle or operating machinery. If symptoms do not improve or are accompanied by fever that lasts for more than 3 days, or if new symptoms occur, consult a doctor. If sore throat is severe, persists for more than 2 days, is accompanied or followed by fever, headache, rash, nausea, or vomiting, consult a doctor promptly.
Keep this and all drugs out of the reach of children. In case of accidental overdose, seek professional assistance or contact a poison control center immediately. Prompt medical attention is critical for adults as well as for children even if you do not notice any signs or symptoms. As with any drug, if you are pregnant or nursing a baby, seek the advice of a health professional before using this product.

How Supplied: Available in 6, 10, and 14 fl. oz. plastic bottles with child-resistant, tamper-evident cap.

VICKS NYQUIL® LIQUICAPS
Adult Nighttime Colds/Flu Medicine
Nasal Decongestant/Antihistamine/
Cough Suppressant/Pain
Reliever-Fever Reducer

Active Ingredients (per softgel) Acetaminophen 250 mg, Pseudoephedrine HCl 30 mg, Dextromethorphan HBr 15 mg, Diphenhydramine HCl 25 mg

Inactive Ingredients: D&C Yellow No. 10, Edible Ink, FD&C Blue No. 1, Gelatin, Glycerin, Polyethylene Glycol, Povidone, Propylene Glycol and Purified Water. Contains no alcohol.

Indications: For the temporary relief of minor aches, pains, headache, muscular aches, sore throat, and fever associated with a cold or flu. Temporarily relieves nasal congestion, cough due to minor throat and bronchial irritations, runny nose and sneezing associated with the common cold.

Directions: ADULTS (12 years and over): Swallow two softgels, once daily, at bedtime or as directed by a doctor.
NOT RECOMMENDED FOR CHILDREN.

Warnings: Do not exceed recommended dosage because at higher doses nervousness, dizziness or sleeplessness may occur. Do not take this product if

you have heart disease, high blood pressure, thyroid disease, diabetes, or difficulty in urination due to enlargement of the prostate gland unless directed by a doctor. DRUG INTERACTION PRECAUTION: Do not take this product if you are presently taking a prescription drug for high blood pressure or depression, without first consulting your doctor. Do not take this product for persistent or chronic cough such as occurs with smoking, asthma, emphysema, or if cough is accompanied by excessive phlegm (mucus) unless directed by a doctor. May cause excitability especially in children. Do not take this product if you have asthma, glaucoma, emphysema, chronic pulmonary disease, shortness of breath, or difficulty in breathing unless directed by a doctor. May cause marked drowsiness; alcohol, sedatives, and tranquilizers may increase the drowsiness effect. Avoid alcoholic beverages while taking this product. Do not take this product if you are taking sedatives or tranquilizers, without first consulting your doctor. Use caution when driving a motor vehicle or operating machinery. Do not take this product for more than 7 days. A persistent cough may be a sign of a serious condition. If cough persists for more than 7 days, tends to recur, or is accompanied by rash, persistent headache, consult a doctor. If symptoms do not improve or are accompanied by fever that lasts for more than 3 days, or if new symptoms occur, consult a doctor. If sore throat is severe, persists for more than 2 days, is accompanied or followed by fever, headache, rash, nausea, or vomiting, consult a doctor promptly. Keep this and all drugs out of the reach of children. In case of accidental overdose, seek professional assistance or contact a poison control center immediately. Prompt medical attention is critical for adults as well as for children even if you do not notice any signs or symptoms. As with any drug, if you are pregnant or nursing a baby, seek the advice of a health professional before using this product.

How Supplied: Available in 12 and 20 softgel blister packs. Green, clear liquid filled, one piece softgel imprinted "NyQuil".

VICKS SINEX®
[sĭ 'nĕx]
Decongestant Nasal Spray and
Ultra Fine Mist

Active Ingredient: Phenylephrine Hydrochloride 0.5%.

Inactive Ingredients: Aromatic Vapors (Camphor, Eucalyptol, Menthol), Cetylpyridinium Chloride, Potassium Phosphate, Purified Water, Sodium Chloride, Sodium Phosphate, Tyloxapol. Preservative: Thimerosal 0.001%.

Indications: For temporary relief of nasal congestion due to colds, hay fever, upper respiratory allergies or sinusitis.

Actions: *Provides fast decongestant relief.*

Dosage and Administration: Keep head and dispenser upright. May be used every 4 hours as needed.
Ultra Fine Mist: Remove protective cap. Before using for the first time, prime the pump by firmly depressing its rim several times. Hold container with thumb at base and nozzle between first and second fingers. Without tilting head, insert nozzle into nostril. Fully depress rim with a firm even stroke and sniff deeply. *Adults:* 2 or 3 sprays in each nostril not more often than every 4 hours. Do not give to children under 12 years of age unless directed by a doctor.
Squeeze Bottle: *Adults:* 2 or 3 sprays in each nostril not more often than every 4 hours. Do not give to children under 12 years of age unless directed by a doctor.

Warning: Do not exceed recommended dosage because burning, stinging, sneezing, or increase of nasal discharge may occur. The use of this container by more than one person may spread infection. Do not use this product for more than 3 days. If symptoms persist, consult a doctor. Do not use this product if you have heart disease, high blood pressure, thyroid disease, diabetes, or difficulty in urination due to enlargment of the prostate gland unless directed by a doctor.
KEEP THIS AND ALL DRUGS OUT OF THE REACH OF CHILDREN. In case of accidental ingestion, seek professional assistance or contact a poison control center immediately.

How Supplied: Available in ½ fl. oz. and 1 fl. oz. plastic squeeze bottles and ½ fl. oz. measured dose atomizer.

VICKS SINEX® LONG-ACTING
[sĭ 'nĕx]
12-hour Formula Decongestant
Nasal Spray and Ultra Fine Mist

Active Ingredient: Oxymetazoline Hydrochloride 0.05%.

Inactive Ingredients: Aromatic Vapors (Camphor, Eucalyptol, Menthol), Potassium Phosphate, Purified Water, Sodium Chloride, Sodium Phosphate, Tyloxapol. Preservative: Thimerosal 0.001%.

Indications: For temporary relief of nasal congestion due to colds, hay fever, upper respiratory allergies or sinusitis.

Actions: Provides fast decongestant relief and lasts up to 12 hours.

Dosage and Administration: Keep head and dispenser upright. May be used twice daily (morning and evening) or as directed by a physician.
Ultra Fine Mist: Remove protective cap. Before using for the first time, prime the pump by firmly depressing its rim several times. Hold container with thumb at base and nozzle between first and second fingers. Without tilting head, insert nozzle into nostril. Fully depress rim with a firm even stroke and sniff deeply. *Adults and children 6 years of age*

Continued on next page

Richardson-Vicks—Cont.

and over (under adult supervision): 2 or 3 sprays in each nostril not more often than every 10 to 12 hours. Do not exceed 2 applications in any 24-hour period. Children under 6 years of age: consult a doctor.

Squeeze Bottle: *Adults and children 6 years of age and over (under adult supervision):* 2 or 3 sprays in each nostril not more often than every 10 to 12 hours. Do not exceed 2 applications in any 24-hour period. Children under 6 years of age: consult a doctor.

Warnings: Do not exceed recommended dosage because burning, stinging, sneezing or increase of nasal discharge may occur. The use of this container by more than one person may spread infection. Do not use this product for more than 3 days. If symptoms persist, consult a doctor. Do not use this product if you have heart disease, high blood pressure, thyroid disease, diabetes, or difficulty in urination due to enlargement of the prostate gland unless directed by a doctor. **KEEP THIS AND ALL MEDICINES OUT OF THE REACH OF CHILDREN.** In case of accidental ingestion, seek professional assistance or contact a poison control center immediately.

How Supplied: Available in ½ fl. oz. and 1 fl. oz. plastic squeeze bottles and ½ fl. oz. measured-dose container.

VICKS VAPORUB®
[va̅ 'pō-rub]
Nasal Decongestant/Cough Suppressant

Active Ingredients: Menthol 2.6%, Camphor 4.7%, Eucalyptus Oil 1.2%.

Inactive Ingredients: Cedarleaf Oil, Mineral Oil, Nutmeg Oil, Petrolatum, Thymol, Spirits of Turpentine.

Indications: For the temporary relief of nasal congestion and coughs associated with a cold.

Actions: The inhaled vapors of VICKS VAPORUB have a decongestant and antitussive effect.

Directions: Adults and children 2 years of age and older: Rub a thick layer of Vicks VapoRub on chest and throat. If desired, cover with a dry, warm cloth, but keep clothing loose to let vapors rise to the nose and mouth. Repeat up to three times daily, especially at bedtime, or as directed by a doctor. Children under two years of age, consult a doctor.

Warnings: For external use only. Do not take by mouth or place in nostrils. Avoid excessive heat. Never expose VapoRub to flame or place in any container in which are you heating water. Do not reheat. Never place VapoRub in a microwave oven. A persistent cough may be a sign of a serious condition. If cough persists for more than 1 week, tends to recur, or is accompanied by fever, rash,

or persistent headache, consult a doctor. Do not use this product for persistent or chronic cough such as occurs with smoking, asthma, emphysema, or if cough is accompanied by excessive phlegm (mucus) unless directed by a doctor. **KEEP THIS AND ALL DRUGS OUT OF THE REACH OF CHILDREN.** In case of accidental ingestion, seek professional assistance or contact a poison control center immediately.

How Supplied: Available in 1.5 oz., 3.0 oz. and 6.0 oz. plastic jars and 2.0 oz. tubes.

VICKS VAPOSTEAM®
[va̅ 'pō "stēm]
Liquid Medication for Hot Steam Vaporizers.
Nasal Decongestant/Cough Suppressant

Active Ingredients: Menthol 3.2%, Camphor 6.2%, Eucalyptus Oil 1.5%.

Inactive Ingredients: Cedarleaf Oil, Nutmeg Oil, Poloxamer 124, Polyoxyethylene Dodecanol, Silicone. Alcohol 74%.

Indications: For temporary relief of nasal congestion due to colds, hay fever or other upper respiratory allergies. Temporarily relieves cough occurring with a cold.

Actions: VAPOSTEAM increases the action of steam to help relieve colds symptoms in the following ways: relieves coughs of colds, eases nasal congestion, and moistens dry, irritated breathing passages.

Directions:
Adults and children 2 years of age and older: Use VAPOSTEAM in Hot/Warm Steam Vaporizers, Wash Basin or Bowl as described below. Follow directions for use carefully. Breathe in medicated vapors. May be repeated up to 3 times daily or as directed by a doctor. **Children under 2 years of age:** consult a doctor.
In Hot/Warm Steam Vaporizers: Add VAPOSTEAM directly to the water in your electric vaporizer. Add one tablespoon of VAPOSTEAM with each quart of water added to the vaporizer. For best performance, vaporizer should be thoroughly cleaned after each use according to manufacturer's instructions. In soft water areas, it may be necessary to add salt or other steaming aid to promote steaming. Follow directions of vaporizer manufacturer for best results.
In Bowl or Washbasin: Pour steaming hot water into bowl or washbasin. Then add 1½ teaspoons of VAPOSTEAM for each pint of water used. Beathe in medicated vapors.

Warning: For hot/warm steam vaporizers only. Do not use in cold steam vaporizers or humidifiers. **Not to be taken by mouth.** A persistent cough may be sign of a serious condition. If cough persists for more than one week, tends to recur or is accompanied by fever, rash, or

persistent headache, consult a doctor. Do not use this product for persistent or chronic cough such as occurs with smoking, asthma, emphysema, or if cough is accompanied by excessive phlegm (mucus) unless directed by a doctor. Store at room temperature and always keep VAPOSTEAM away from open flame or excessive heat. Do not direct steam from vaporizer towards face. Use caution in handling any container of hot water. Do not heat water containing VAPOSTEAM or use in microwave oven. **KEEP THIS AND ALL DRUGS OUT OF THE REACH OF CHILDREN.**

ACCIDENTAL INGESTION: In case of accidental ingestion, seek professional assistance or contact a poison control center immediately.

How Supplied: Available in 4 fl. oz. and 6 fl. oz. bottles.

VICKS VATRONOL®
[va̅trōnŏl]
Ephedrine Sulfate/Nasal Decongestant Nose Drops

Active Ingredient: Ephedrine Sulfate 0.5%.

Inactive Ingredients: Camphor, Cedarleaf Oil, Eucalyptol, Menthol, Nutmeg Oil, Potassium Phosphate, Purified Water, Sodium Chloride, Sodium Phosphate, Tyloxapol.
Preservative: Thimerosal 0.001%.

Indications: For temporary relief of nasal congestion due to a cold, hay fever, upper respiratory allergies or associated with sinusitis.

Actions: VICKS VATRONOL helps restore freer breathing by relieving nasal stuffiness. Relieves sinus pressure.

Dosage: *Adults:* Fill dropper to upper mark. *Children 6 to under 12 years of age (under adult supervision):* Fill dropper to lower mark. *Children under 6 years of age:* consult a doctor.
Apply in each nostril, not more often than every four hours.

Warning: Do not exceed recommended dosage because burning, stinging, sneezing, or increase of nasal discharge may occur. The use of this container by more than one person may spread infection. Do not use this product for more than 3 days. If symptoms persist, consult a doctor. Do not use this product if you have heart disease, high blood pressure, thyroid disease, diabetes, or difficulty in urination due to enlargement of the prostate gland unless directed by a doctor. Keep this and all drugs out of the reach of children. In case of accidental ingestion, seek professional assistance or contact a poison control center immediately.

How Supplied: Available in 1 fl. oz. dropper bottles.

Roberts Pharmaceutical Corporation
6 INDUSTRIAL WAY WEST
EATONTOWN, NJ 07724

CHERACOL® Nasal Spray Pump Cherry Scented

Description: CHERACOL® NASAL SPRAY PUMP is a cherry scented long acting topical nasal decongestant. One application lasts up to 12 hours.

Indications: For the temporary relief of a nasal congestion associated with colds ("flu"), hay fever, and sinusitis.

Active Ingredients: Oxymetazoline hydrochloride USP 0.05% (0.5 mg/ml).

Inactive Ingredients: Benzalkonium chloride, glycine, phenylmercuric acetate (0.02 mg/ml), sorbitol, cherry flavor, and purified water.

Dosage and Administration: CHERACOL Nasal Spray has a long duration of action lasting up to 12 hours with each topical application. One application mornings and at bedtime is usually sufficient for round-the-clock action. For adults and children 6 years of age and over: Two or three sprays in each nostril twice daily—morning and bedtime. Remove protective cap. Hold bottle with thumb at base and nozzle between first and second fingers. With head upright, insert metered pump spray nozzle in nostril. Depress pump 2 or 3 times all the way down with a firm even stroke and sniff deeply. Repeat in other nostril. Do not tilt head backward while spraying. Wipe tip clean after each use. Before using the first time, remove the protective cap from the tip and prime the metered pump by depressing pump firmly several times.

Warning: Do not give this product to children under 6 years of age except under the advice and supervision of a physician. Do not exceed recommended dosage because symptoms may occur such as burning, stinging, sneezing or increase of nasal discharge. Do not use this product for more than 3 days. If symptoms persist, consult a physician. The use of this dispenser by more than one person may spread infection. Store at room temperature. Keep this and all medicines out of children's reach. In case of accidental ingestion contact a physician or poison control center immediately.

Overdosage: For overdose treatment, contact a regional poison control center.

How Supplied: Available in 1 fluid ounce bottles fitted with a metered pump (NDC 54092-880-30).

CHERACOL® Sore Throat Spray Anesthetic/Antiseptic Liquid

Description: A pleasant tasting cherry flavored liquid spray with anesthetic and antiseptic properties.

Indications: For the temporary relief of occasional minor sore throat pain and irritation. Also for temporary relief of pain associated with sore mouth, canker sores, tonsillitis, pharnyngitis and throat infections.

Active Ingredients: Phenol 1.4%.

Inactive Ingredients: Alcohol 12.5%, citric acid, FD&C Red No. 40, flavor, glycerin, propylene glycol, sodium citrate, sodium saccharin, sorbitol and purified water.

Directions For Use: Mouthwash and gargle: Irritated throat: Spray 5 times (children 2–12 years of age, 3 times) and swallow. May be used as a gargle. Repeat every 2 hours or as directed by physician or dentist. Children under 12 years of age should be supervised in the use of this product.

Warning: If sore throat is severe, persists for more than 2 days, is accompanied or followed by fever, headache, rash, nausea or vomiting, consult a doctor promptly. If sore mouth symptoms do not improve in 7 days, see your doctor or dentist promptly. In case of accidental overdosage, seek professional assistance or contact poison control center immediately. As with any drug, if you are pregnant or nursing a baby, seek the advice of a health professional before using this product. Do not administer to children under 2 years unless directed by a physician or dentist. Keep this and all medicines out of the reach of children.

How Supplied: Available in 6 fluid ounce spray pump bottle (NDC 54092-340-06).

CHERACOL-D® Cough Formula Maximum Strength Cough Formula

Description: CHERACOL-D® is a non-narcotic cough formula which combines two important medicines in one safe, fast-acting pleasant tasting liquid:
- The highest level of cough suppressant available without prescription.
- A clinically proven expectorant to help loosen phlegm and drain bronchial tubes.

Indications: CHERACOL-D® cough formula helps quiet dry, hacking coughs, and helps loosen phlegm and mucus. Recommended for adults and children 2 years of age and older.

Active Ingredients: Each teaspoonful (5 ml) contains dextromethorphan hydrobromide, 10 mg; guaifenesin, 100 mg; alcohol, 4.75%. Also contains benzoic acid, FD&C Red #40, flavors, fragrances, fructose, glycerin, propylene glycol, sodium chloride, sucrose, and purified water.

Dosage and Administration: Adults and children 12 years of age and over: 2 teaspoonfuls. Children 6 to 12 years: 1 teaspoonful. Children 2 to 6 years: ½ teaspoonful. May be repeated every 4 hours if necessary. Children under 2 years, consult a physician.

Warnings: Keep this and all drugs out of the reach of children. In case of acci-dental overdose, seek professional assistance or contact a poison control center immediately. Do not give this product to children under 2 years of age except under the advice and supervision of a physician. Do not use this product for persistent or chronic cough such as occurs with smoking, asthma, or emphysema or where cough is accompanied by excessive secretions except under the advice and supervision of a physician. As with any drug, if you are pregnant or nursing a baby, seek the advice of a health professional before using this product.

Caution: A persistent cough may be a sign of a serious condition. If cough persists for more than 1 week, tends to recur or is accompanied by high fever, rash or persistent headache, consult a physician.

How Supplied: Available in 2 oz bottle (NDC 54092-400-60), 4 oz bottle (NDC 54092-400-04), and 6 oz bottle (NDC 54092-400-06).

Shown in Product Identification Section, page 421

CHERACOL PLUS® Cough Syrup Multisymptom cough/cold formula

Description: CHERACOL PLUS® Cough Syrup is a pleasant tasting 3-ingredient non-narcotic liquid formulation.

Indications: Cheracol Plus syrup is an effective 3-ingredient, maximum strength formula for the temporary relief of head cold symptoms and cough (without narcotic side effects).

Active Ingredients: Each tablespoonful (15ml) contains phenylpropanolamine, 25 mg; dextromethorphan hydrobromide, 20 mg; chlorpheniramine maleate, 4 mg; and alcohol, 8%.

Inactive Ingredients: Flavors, glycerin, methylparaben, propylene glycol, propylparaben, FD&C Red No. 40, sodium chloride, sorbitol solution, and purified water.

Dosage and Administration: Adults and children over 12 years of age: 1 tablespoonful (15ml) every 4 hours or as directed by a physician. Do not take more than 6 tablespoonfuls in a 24 hour period. Do not administer to children under 12 years of age.

Uses: Cheracol Plus® multisymptom head cold/cough formula provides cough suppressant and decongestant activity and controls runny nose associated with the common cold ("flu").

Warnings: Do not take this product for persistent or chronic cough such as occurs with smoking, asthma, or emphysema or where cough is accompanied by excessive secretions or if you have high blood pressure, heart or thyroid disease, diabetes, asthma, glaucoma, or difficulty in urination due to enlargement of the prostate gland except under the advice and supervision of a physician. If symptoms do not improve within 7 days or are

Continued on next page

Roberts—Cont.

accompanied by high fever, consult a physician before continuing use. May cause excitability, especially in children. Do not give this product to children under 12 years except under the advice and supervision of a physician. As with any drug, if you are pregnant or nursing a baby consult a health professional before using this product.

Drug Interaction Precaution: Do not take this product if you are presently taking antihypertensive or antidepressant medication containing a monoamine oxidase inhibitor except under the advice and supervision of a physician.

How Supplied: Available in 4 oz bottle (NDC 54092-401-04), 6 oz bottle (54092-401-06).

Shown in Product Identification Section, page 421

CITROCARBONATE® Antacid

Active Ingredients: When dissolved, each 3.9 grams (1 teaspoonful) contains approximately: sodium bicarbonate, 0.78 gram and sodium citrate, 1.82 grams. **As derived from (per teaspoonful):** sodium bicarbonate 2.34 gram; citric acid anhydrous, 1.19 gram; sodium citrate hydrous, 254 mg; calcium lactate pentahydrate, 151 mg; sodium chloride, 79 mg; monobasic sodium phosphate anhydrous, 44 mg; and, magnesium sulfate dried, 42 mg. Each 3.9 grams (teaspoonful) contains 30.46 mEq (700.6 mg) of sodium.

Indications: For the relief of heartburn, acid indigestion, and sour stomach; and upset stomach associated with these symptoms.

Dosage and Administration: Adults: 1 to 2 teaspoonfuls (not to exceed 5 level teaspoonfuls per day) in a glass of cold water after meals. Persons 60 years or older: ½ to 1 teaspoonful after meals. Children 6 to 12 years: ¼ to ½ teaspoonful. For children under 6 years: Consult physician.

How Supplied: Available in 5 oz (NDC 54092-900-05) and 10 oz (NDC 54092-900-10) bottles.

CLOCREAM®
Skin Protectant Cream

Description: CLOCREAM® skin protectant cream contains Vitamins A and D in a greaseless vanishing cream base that leaves no residue. Also contains cetylpalmitate, cottonseed oil, glyceryl monostearate, fragrance, methylparaben, mineral oil, potassium stearate, propylparaben, sodium citrate, and purified oil. Each ounce of CLOCREAM® contains Vitamins A and D equivalent to 1 ounce of cod liver oil.

Indications: CLOCREAM® is indicated for the temporary relief of chapped skin, diaper rash, wind burn and sunburn; and minor non-infected skin irrita-

tions. CLOCREAM® promotes epithelization.

Uses: CLOCREAM® may be particularly useful for health care personnel or others who frequently wash their hands and for general patient care to reduce dermal excoriation and breakdown from prolonged bed rest, bedwetting and abrasions. The vanishing action of CLOCREAM skin protectant cream makes it cosmetically acceptable when the skin treated is on an exposed part of the body such as the hands or arms.

Warnings: CLOCREAM® skin protectant cream is for external use only. Avoid contact with the eyes. If condition worsens or if symptoms persist for more than 7 days, discontinue use of this product and consult a physician. Keep this and all medications out of the reach of children. In case of accidental ingestion seek professional assistance or contact a poison control center immediately.

Dosage and Administration: Gently massage or apply liberally to unbroken skin or abraded skin where promotion of epitheliazation is denied. Use as often as desired.

How Supplied: Available in 1 ounce tubes (NDC 54092-300-30).

HALTRAN® Tablets
Ibuprofen/Analgesic
MENSTRUAL CRAMP RELIEVER

WARNING: ASPIRIN SENSITIVE PATIENTS. Do not take this product if you have had a severe allergic reaction to aspirin, eg—asthma, swelling, shock or hives, because even though this product contains no aspirin or salicylates cross-reactions may occur in patients allergic to aspirin.

Indications: For the pain of menstrual cramps and also the temporary relief of minor aches and pains associated with the common cold, headache, toothache, muscular aches, backache, for the minor pain of arthritis and for reduction of fever.

Directions: *Adults:* Take 1 tablet every 4 to 6 hours while symptoms persist. If pain or fever does not respond to 1 tablet, 2 tablets may be used, but do not exceed 6 tablets in 24 hours, unless directed by a doctor. The smallest effective dose should be used. Take with food or milk if occasional and mild heartburn, upset stomach, or stomach pain occurs with use. Consult a doctor if these symptoms are more than mild or if they persist. *Children:* Do not give this product to children under 12 except under the advice and supervision of a doctor.

Warnings: Do not take for pain for more than 10 days or for fever for more than 3 days unless directed by a doctor. If pain or fever persists or gets worse, if new symptoms occur, or if the painful area is red or swollen, consult a doctor. These could be signs of serious illness. If you are under a doctor's care for any serious condition, consult a doctor before

taking this product. As with aspirin and acetaminophen, if you have any condition which requires you to take prescription drugs or if you have had any problems or serious side effects from taking any non-prescription pain reliever, do not take HALTRAN Tablets (ibuprofen) without first discussing it with your doctor. If you experience any symptoms which are unusual or seem unrelated to the condition for which you took ibuprofen, consult a doctor before taking any more of it. Although ibuprofen is indicated for the same conditions as aspirin and acetaminophen, it should not be taken with them except under a doctor's direction. Before using any drug, including HALTRAN, you should seek the advice of a health professional if you are pregnant or nursing a baby. IT IS ESPECIALLY IMPORTANT NOT TO USE IBUPROFEN DURING THE LAST 3 MONTHS OF PREGNANCY UNLESS SPECIFICALLY DIRECTED TO DO SO BY A DOCTOR BECAUSE IT MAY CAUSE PROBLEMS IN THE UNBORN CHILD OR COMPLICATIONS DURING DELIVERY. Keep this and all drugs out of the reach of children. In case of accidental overdose, seek professional assistance or contact a poison control center immediately.

Active Ingredient: Each tablet contains ibuprofen USP 200 mg.

Other Ingredients: Carnauba wax, cornstarch, hydroxypropyl methylcellulose, propylene glycol, silicon dioxide, pregelatinized starch, stearic acid, and titanium dioxide.
Store at room temperature. Avoid excessive heat 40°C (104°F).

How Supplied: Available in bottles of 30 (NDC 54092-020-30).

Shown in Product Identification Section, page 421

KASOF® Capsules
[*kay'sof*]
High Strength Stool Softener
Laxative

Ingredients: Each capsule contains: Active: docusate potassium, 240 mg. Inactive: Blue 1, gelatin, glycerin, methylparaben, polyethylene glycol, propylparaben, purified water, Red 40, sorbitol, Yellow 10.

Indications: KASOF provides a highly efficient wetting action to restore moisture to the bowel, thus softening the stool to prevent straining. The action of KASOF does not interfere with normal peristalsis and generally does not cause griping or extreme sensation of urgency. KASOF is sodium-free, containing a unique potassium formulation, without the problems associated with sodium intake. KASOF is especially valuable for the severely constipated, as well as patients with anorectal disorders, such as hemorrhoids and anal fissures. KASOF is ideal for patients with any condition that can be complicated by straining at stool, for example, cardiac patients. The simple, one-a-day dosage helps assure patient compliance in maintaining normal bowel function.

Directions: Adults: One KASOF capsule daily for several days, or until bowel movements are normal and gentle. It is helpful to increase the daily intake of fluids by drinking a glass of water with each dose.

Store in a closed container, protect from freezing and avoid excessive heat (104°F).

Warnings: As with any drug, if you are pregnant or nursing a baby, seek the advice of a health professional before using this product. Keep out of the reach of children.

How Supplied: KASOF is available in bottles of 30, (NDC 54092-380-30) and 60 (NDC 54092-380-60) brown gelatin capsules identified "KASOF".

ORTHOXICOL® Cough Syrup
Multisymptom cough/cold formula

Description: ORTHOXICOL® Cough Syrup is a pleasant tasting 3-ingredient non-narcotic liquid formulation.

Indications: Orthoxicol syrup is an effective 3-ingredient, maximum strength formula for the temporary relief of head cold symptoms and cough (without narcotic side effects).

Active Ingredients: Each tablespoonful (15 ml) contains phenylpropanolamine, 25 mg; dextromethorphan hydrobromide, 20 mg; chlorpheniramine, 4 mg; and alcohol, 8%.

Inactive Ingredients: Flavors, glycerin, methylparaben, propylene glycol, propylparaben, FD&C Red No. 40, sodium chloride, sorbitol solution, and purified water.

Dosage and Administration: Adults and children over 12 years of age: 1 tablespoonful (15 ml) every 4 hours or as directed by a physician. Do not take more than 6 tablespoonfuls in a 24 hour period. Do not administer to children under 12 years of age.

Uses: Orthoxicol multisymptom head cold/cough formula provides cough suppressant and decongestant activity and controls runny nose associated with the common cold ("flu").

Warnings: Do not take this product for persistent or chronic cough such as occurs with smoking, asthma, or emphysema or where cough is accompanied by excessive secretions or if you have high blood pressure, heart or thyroid disease, diabetes, asthma, glaucoma, or difficulty in urination due to enlargement of the prostate gland except under the advice and supervision of a physician. If symptoms do not improve within 7 days or are accompanied by high fever, consult a physician before continuing use. May cause excitability, especially in children. Do not give this product to children under 12 years except under the advice and supervision of a physician. As with any drug, if you are pregnant or nursing a

baby consult a health professional before using this product.

Drug Interaction Precaution: Do not take this product if you are presently taking antihypertensive or antidepressant medication containing a monoamine oxidase inhibitor except under the advice and supervision of a physician.

How Supplied: Available in 2 oz bottle (NDC 54092-410-60), 4 oz bottle (NDC 54092-410-04), 16 oz bottle (NDC 54092-410-16).

P-A-C® Analgesic Tablets

Description: A combination tablet formulation providing more pain-relieving ingredients per tablet than conventional tablets.

Indications: P-A-C® tablets are indicated for the temporary relief of occasional minor aches, pains, headache and the reduction of fever.

Active Ingredients: Each tablet contains: aspirin; caffeine anhydrous, 32 mg. Contains non-standard strength of 400 mg (6.17 gr) aspirin per tablet compared to the established standard of 325 mg (5 gr) aspirin per tablet.

Inactive Ingredients: Cellulose, corn starch, croscarmellose sodium, FD&C Blue No. 2, FD&C Yellow No. 5 (tartrazine), sucrose.

Directions For Use: (except under the advice and supervision of a physician): Adults—1 or 2 tablets every 4 hours while symptoms persist not to exceed 10 tablets in 24 hours for not more than 10 days, or in the presence of fever for more than 3 days (72 hours). Children (see warnings)—9 to 12 years: 1 tablet every 4 hours while symptoms persist not to exceed 5 single doses in 24 hours for not more than 5 days, or in the presence of fever for not more than 3 days (72 hours). Do not use in children under 9 years.

Warnings: Children and teenagers should not use this product for chickenpox or flu symptoms before a physician is consulted about Reye Syndrome, a rare but serious illness reported to be associated with aspirin. Do not take this product if you are allergic to aspirin or if you have asthma. As with any drug, if you are pregnant or nursing a baby seek the advice of a health professional before you use this product. Do not exceed recommended dosage.

Cautions: (except under the advice and supervision of a physician): Do not take this product if you have stomach distress, ulcers, bleeding problems, are presently taking a prescription drug for anticoagulation (thinning of the blood), diabetes, gout, arthritis, or for the treatment of arthritis. Stop taking this product if ringing of the ears or other symptoms occur. In case of accidental overdose seek professional assistance or contact a poison control center immediately.

How Supplied: Available in bottles of 100 (NDC 54092-010-01), and 1000 (NDC 54092-010-10) tablets.

Shown in Product Identification Shown, page 421

PYRROXATE® Capsules
Extra Strength
Decongestant/Antihistamine/Analgesic Capsules

Description: *Pyrroxate®* provides single-capsule, multisymptom relief for colds, allergies, nasal/sinus congestion, runny nose, sneezing, and watery eyes. Because it contains the non-aspirin analgesic **acetaminophen**, *Pyrroxate* gives temporary relief of occasional minor aches, pains, headache, and helps in the reduction of fever. *Pyrroxate* is caffeine and aspirin-free.

Ingredients: Each *Pyrroxate* Capsule contains: chlorpheniramine maleate, 4 mg; phenylpropanolamine HCl, 25 mg; acetaminophen, 500 mg. The 500 mg (7.69 gr) strength of acetaminophen per capsule is non-standard, as compared to the established standard of 325 mg (5 gr) acetaminophen per capsule. Also contains benzyl alcohol, butylparaben, D&C yellow No. 10, erythrosine sodium, FD&C blue No. 1, FD&C yellow No. 6 (sunset yellow) as a color additive, gelatin, glycerin, magnesium stearate, methylparaben, propylparaben, sodium lauryl sulfate, sodium propionate, starch, and talc.

Indications: *Pyrroxate* Capsules are for the temporary relief of runny nose, sneezing, itching of the nose or throat; for the temporary relief of nasal congestion due to the common cold, allergies (hay fever), and sinus congestion; for the temporary relief of occasional minor aches, pains, headache, and for the reduction of fever.

Actions: Chlorpheniramine maleate is an antihistamine effective in controlling runny nose, sneezing, watery eyes, and itching of the nose and throat. Phenylpropanolamine HCl is an oral nasal decongestant effective in relieving nasal/sinus congestion due to the common cold or allergies (hay fever). Acetaminophen is a clinically effective analgesic and antipyretic without aspirin side effects.

Warnings: Do not take this product for more than 7 days. If symptoms persist, do not improve, or new ones occur, or if fever persists for more than 3 days, discontinue use and consult your physician. Do not take this product if you have asthma, glaucoma, difficulty in urination due to the enlargement of the prostate gland, high blood pressure, diabetes, thyroid disease, or if you are presently taking a prescription antihypertensive or antidepressant drug containing a monamine oxidase inhibitor, except under the advice and supervision of a physician. As with any drug, if you are pregnant or nursing a baby, seek the advice of a

Continued on next page

Roberts—Cont.

health professional before using this product. Do not exceed recommended dosage because severe liver damage may occur and at higher doses, nervousness, dizziness or sleeplessness may occur. Do not take this product for the treatment of arthritis except under the advice and supervision of a physician.

Cautions: Avoid alcoholic beverages, driving a motor vehicle, or operating heavy machinery while taking this product. This product may cause drowsiness or excitability, especially in children. Keep this and all drugs out of the reach of children. In case of accidental overdose, seek professional assistance or contact a poison control center immediately.

Dosage and Administration: Take 1 capsule every 4 hours or as directed by a physician. Do not take more than 6 capsules in a 24-hour period. Do not administer to children under 12 years of age.

How Supplied: Black/yellow capsules available in bottles of 24 (NDC 54092-040-24) and 500 (NDC 54092-040-05).

Shown in Product Identification Section, page 421

SIGTAB® Tablets
High Potency Vitamin Supplement

Each tablet contains:		% U.S. RDA*
Vitamin A	5000 IU	100
Vitamin D	400 IU	100
Vitamin E	15 IU	50
Vitamin C	333 mg	555
Folic Acid	0.4 mg	100
Thiamine	10.3 mg	686
Riboflavin	10 mg	588
Niacin	100 mg	500
Vitamin B_6	6 mg	300
Vitamin B_{12}	18 mcg	300
Pantothenic Acid	20 mg	200

*Percentage of U.S. Recommended Daily Allowance.

Recommended Dosage: 1 tablet daily

Ingredient List: Sucrose, Sodium Ascorbate (Vit. C), Calcium Sulfate, Niacinamide, Vitamin E Acetate, Calcium Pantothenate, Vitamin A Acetate, Thiamine Mononitrate (B-1), Riboflavin (B-2), Gelatin, Pyridoxine HCl (B-6), Povidone, Lacca, Magnesium Stearate, Silica, Artificial Color, Sodium Benzoate, Folic Acid, Polyethylene Glycol, Cholecalciferol (Vit. D), Carnauba Wax, Cyanocobalamin (B-12), Medical Antifoam.

How Supplied: Available in bottles of 90 (NDC 54092-033-90) and 500 (NDC 54092-033-05).

Shown in Product Identification Section, page 421

ZYMACAP® Capsules
High Potency Vitamin Supplement

Description: Dietary multivitamin supplement providing 150% of the RDA

for Vitamin B and Vitamin C plus 100% of the RDA for Vitamins A and D.

Each Capsule Contains:		% US RDA*
Vitamin A	5,000 IU	100
Vitamin D	400 IU	100
Vitamin E	15 IU	50
Vitamin C	90 mg	150
Folic Acid	400 mcg	100
Thiamine	2.25 mg	150
Riboflavin	2.6 mg	150
Niacin	30 mg	150
Vitamin B-6	3 mg	150
Vitamin B-12	9 mcg	150
Pantothenic Acid	15 mg	150

*Percentage of U.S. recommended daily allowance.

Recommended Dosage: 1 Capsule daily.

Ingredient List: Soybean oil, ascorbic acid (Vitamin C), gelatin, glycerin, niacinamide, calcium pantothenate, Vitamin E acetate, lecithin, pyridoxine hydrochloride (Vitamin B-6), yellow wax, thiamine mononitrate (Vitamin B-1), riboflavin (Vitamin B-2), Vitamin A palmitate, corn oil, FD&C Red No. 40, folic acid, titanium dioxide, ethyl vanillin, vanilla enhancer, cholecalciferol (Vitamin D), cyanocobalamin (Vitamin B-12).

How Supplied: Available in bottles of 90 capsules (NDC 54092-030-90).

A. H. Robins Company, Inc.
Subsidiary of American Home Products Corporation
CONSUMER PRODUCTS DIVISION
1405 CUMMINGS DRIVE
RICHMOND, VIRGINIA 23220

ALLBEE® C–800 TABLETS
[all 'bē]
ALLBEE® C–800 plus IRON TABLETS

Allbee C-800

One tablet daily provides:	Percentage of U.S. Recommended Daily Allowances (U.S. RDA)	
Vitamin E	150	45 I.U.
Vitamin C	1333	800 mg
Thiamine (Vitamin B_1)	1000	15 mg
Riboflavin (Vitamin B_2)	1000	17 mg
Niacin	500	100 mg
Vitamin B_6	1250	25 mg
Vitamin B_{12}	200	12 mcg
Pantothenic Acid	250	25 mg

Ingredients: Ascorbic Acid, Niacinamide Ascorbate, Modified Starch, Vitamin E Acetate, Hydrolyzed Protein, Calcium Pantothenate, Hydroxypropyl Methylcellulose, Pyridoxine Hydrochloride, Riboflavin, Stearic Acid, Thiamine Mononitrate, Artificial Color, Silicon Dioxide, Lactose, Magnesium Stearate, Povidone, Polyethylene Glycol 400 or 4000, Vanillin, Gelatin, Polysorbate 20 or 80, Sorbic Acid, Sodium Benzoate, Cyanoco-

balamin. May also contain: Hydroxypropylcellulose and Propylene Glycol.

Allbee C-800 plus Iron

One tablet daily provides: Vitamin Composition	Percentage of U.S. Recommended Daily Allowances (U.S. RDA)	
Vitamin E	150	45.0 I.U.
Vitamin C	1333	800.0 mg
Folic Acid	100	0.4 mg
Thiamine (Vitamin B_1)	1000	15.0 mg
Riboflavin (Vitamin B_2)	1000	17.0 mg
Niacin	500	100.0 mg
Vitamin B_6	1250	25.0 mg
Vitamin B_{12}	200	12.0 mcg
Pantothenic Acid	250	25.0 mg
Mineral Composition		
Iron	150	27.0 mg

Ingredients: Ascorbic Acid, Niacinamide Ascorbate, Ferrous Fumarate, Modified Starch, Vitamin E Acetate, Hydrolyzed Protein, Calcium Pantothenate, Hydroxypropyl Methylcellulose, Pyridoxine Hydrochloride, Riboflavin, Stearic Acid, Thiamine Mononitrate, Povidone, Silicon Dioxide, Artificial Color, Lactose, Magnesium Stearate, Polyethylene Glycol 400 or 4000, Vanillin, Gelatin, Folic Acid, Polysorbate 20 or 80, Sorbic Acid, Sodium Benzoate, Cyanocobalamin. May also contain: Hydroxypropylcellulose and Propylene Glycol.

Actions and Uses: The components of Allbee C-800 have important roles in general nutrition, healing of wounds, and prevention of hemorrhage. Allbee C-800 is recommended for nutritional supplementation of these components in conditions such as febrile diseases, chronic or acute infections, burns, fractures, surgery, physiologic stress, alcoholism, prolonged exposure to high temperature, geriatrics, gastritis, peptic ulcer, and colitis; and in weight-reduction and other special diets.
In dentistry, Allbee C-800 is recommended for nutritional supplementation of its components in conditions such as herpetic stomatitis, aphthous stomatitis, cheilosis, herpangina and gingivitis.
In addition, Allbee C-800 Plus Iron is recommended as a nutritional source of iron. The iron is present as ferrous fumarate, a well-tolerated salt. The ascorbic acid in the formulation enhances the absorption of iron.

Precautions: Do not take Allbee C-800 Plus Iron within two hours of oral tetracycline antibiotics, since oral iron products interfere with absorption of tetracycline. Not intended for treatment of iron-deficiency anemia.

Adverse Reactions: Iron-containing medications may occasionally cause gastrointestinal discomfort, nausea, constipation or diarrhea.

Dosage: The recommended OTC dosage for adults and children twelve or more years of age is one tablet daily. Under the direction and supervision of a physician, the dose and frequency of administration may be increased in accordance with the patient's requirements.

How Supplied: Allbee C-800—orange, film-coated, elliptically-shaped tablets engraved AHR on one side and 0677 on the other in bottles of 60 (NDC 0031-0677-62). Allbee C-800 Plus Iron—red, film-coated, elliptically-shaped tablets engraved AHR on one side and 0678 on the other in bottles of 60 (NDC 0031-0678-62).

ALLBEE® WITH C CAPLETS
[all 'bē]

One caplet daily provides:	Percentage of U.S. Recommended Daily Allowance (U.S. RDA)	
Vitamin C	500	300.0 mg
Thiamine (Vitamin B₁)	1000	15.0 mg
Riboflavin (Vitamin B₂)	600	10.2 mg
Niacin	250	50.0 mg
Vitamin B₆	250	5.0 mg
Pantothenic Acid	100	10.0 mg

Ingredients: Niacinamide Ascorbate; Ascorbic Acid; Microcrystalline Cellulose; Corn Starch; Thiamine Mononitrate; Calcium Pantothenate; Riboflavin; Hydroxypropyl Methylcellulose; Pyridoxine Hydrochloride; Magnesium Stearate; Silicon Dioxide; Propylene Glycol; Lactose; Methacrylic Acid Copolymer; Triethyl Citrate; Titanium Dioxide; Polysorbate 20; Artificial Flavor; Saccharin Sodium; Sodium Sorbate.

Action and Uses: Allbee with C is a high-potency formulation of B and C vitamins. Its components have important roles in general nutrition, healing of wounds, and prevention of hemorrhage. It is recommended for deficiencies of B-vitamins and ascorbic acid in conditions such as febrile diseases, chronic or acute infections, burns, fractures, surgery, toxic conditions, physiologic stress, alcoholism, prolonged exposure to high temperature, geriatrics, gastritis, peptic ulcer, and colitis; and in conditions involving special diets and weight-reduction diets.

In dentistry, Allbee with C is recommended for deficiencies of B-vitamins and ascorbic acid in conditions such as herpetic stomatitis, aphthous stomatitis, cheilosis, herpangina, gingivitis.

Dosage: The recommended OTC dosage for adults and children twelve or more years of age, is one caplet daily. Under the direction and supervision of a physician, the dose and frequency of administration may be increased in accordance with the patient's requirements.

How Supplied: Yellow, capsule-shaped, film-coated tablets engraved AHR on one side and Allbee C on the other in bottles of 130 (NDC 0031-0673-66) and in Dis-Co® Unit Dose Packs of 100 (NDC 0031-0673-64).

CHAP STICK® Lip Balm

Active Ingredients: 44% Petrolatums, 1.5% Padimate O.

Inactive Ingredients:
Regular: Contains FD&C Yellow 5 Aluminum Lake (Tartrazine). Also contains: Wax Paraffin, Mineral Oil, 2-Octyl Dodecanol, Arachidyl Propionate, Polyphenylmethylsiloxane 556, Oleyl Alcohol, White Wax, Isopropyl Lanolate, Lanolin, Carnauba Wax, Isopropyl Myristate, Camphor, Cetyl Alcohol, Fragrance, Methylparaben, Propylparaben, Titanium Dioxide, D&C Red 6 Barium Lake.
Cherry: Wax Paraffin, Mineral Oil, 2-Octyl Dodecanol, Arachidyl Propionate, Polyphenylmethylsiloxane 556, Flavors, White Wax, Isopropyl Lanolate, Lanolin, Isopropyl Myristate, Camphor, Carnauba Wax, Cetyl Alcohol, Methylparaben, D&C Red Barium Lake, Propylparaben, Saccharin.
Mint: Contains FD&C Yellow 5 Aluminum Lake (Tartrazine). Also contains: Wax Paraffin, Mineral Oil, 2-Octyl Dodecanol, Arachidyl Propionate, Polyphenylmethylsiloxane 556, Flavors, White Wax, Isopropyl Lanolate, Lanolin, Carnauba Wax, Isopropyl Myristate, Cetyl Alcohol, Methylparaben, Saccharin, Propylparaben, FD&C Blue 1 Aluminum Lake.
Orange: Wax Paraffin, Mineral Oil, 2-Octyl Dodecanol, Arachidyl Propionate, Polyphenylmethylsiloxane 556, Flavors, White Wax, Isopropyl Lanolate, Lanolin, Carnauba Wax, Isopropyl Myristate, Cetyl Alcohol, FD&C Yellow 6 Aluminum Lake, Methylparaben, Propylparaben, Saccharin.
Strawberry: Wax Paraffin, Mineral Oil, 2-Octyl Dodecanol, Arachidyl Propionate, Polyphenylmethylsiloxane 556, Flavors, White Wax, Isopropyl Lanolate, Lanolin, Isopropyl Myristate, Carnauba Wax, Camphor, Cetyl Alcohol, Methylparaben, Saccharin, Propylparaben, D&C Red 6 Barium Lake.

Indications: Helps prevention and healing of dry, chapped, sun and windburned lips.

Actions: A specially designed lipid complex hydrophobic base containing Padimate O which forms a barrier to prevent moisture loss and protect lips from the drying effects of cold weather, wind and sun which cause chapping. The special emollients soften the skin by forming an occlusive film thus inducing hydration, restoring suppleness to the lips, and preventing drying from evaporation of water that diffuses to the surface from the underlying layers of tissue. Chap Stick also protects the skin from the external environment and its sunscreen offers protection from exposure to the sun.

Warning: Patients should consult a physician if condition worsens or does not improve within 7 days.

Symptoms and Treatment of Oral Ingestion: The oral LD₅₀ in rats is greater than 5 gm/kg. There have been

no reported overdoses in humans. There are no known symptoms of overdosage.

Dosage and Treatment: For dry, chapped lips apply as needed. To help prevent dry, chapped sun or windburned lips, apply to lips as needed before, during and following exposure to sun, wind, water and cold weather.

How Supplied: Available in 4.25 gm tubes in Regular, Mint, Cherry, Orange, and Strawberry flavors.
Shown in Product Identification Section, page 421

CHAP STICK® SUNBLOCK 15 Lip Balm

Active Ingredients: 44% Petrolatums, 7% Padimate O, 3% Oxybenzone.

Inactive Ingredients: Contains FD&C Yellow 5 Aluminum Lake (Tartrazine). Also contains: Wax Paraffin, Mineral Oil, White Wax, Isopropyl Lanolate, Camphor, Lanolin, Isopropyl Myristate, Cetyl Alcohol, Carnauba Wax, Fragrance, Methylparaben, Propylparaben, Titanium Dioxide, D&C Red 6 Barium Lake.

Indications: Ultra Sunscreen Protection (SPF-15). Helps prevention and healing of dry, chapped, sun and windburned lips. Overexposure to sun may lead to premature aging of skin and lip cancer. Liberal and regular use may help reduce the sun's harmful effects.

Actions: Ultra sunscreen protection for the lips, plus the attributes of Chap Stick® Lip Balm. The emollients in the specially designed lipid complex hydrophobic base soften the lips by forming an occlusive film while the two sunscreens have specific ultraviolet absorption ranges which overlap to offer ultra sunscreen protection (SPF-15).

Warning: Patients should consult a physician if condition worsens or does not improve within 7 days.

Symptoms and Treatment of Oral Ingestion: Toxicity studies indicate this product to be extremely safe. The oral LD₅₀ in rats is greater than 5 gm./kg. There are no known symptoms of overdosage.

Dosage and Treatment: For ultra sunscreen protection, apply evenly and liberally to lips before exposure to sun. Reapply as needed. For dry, chapped lips, apply as needed. To help prevent dry, chapped, sun, and windburned lips, apply to lips as needed before, during, following exposure to sun, wind, water, and cold weather.

Continued on next page

Prescribing information on A.H. Robins products listed here is based on official labeling in effect November 1, 1991, with Indications, Contraindications, Warnings, Precautions, Adverse Reactions, and Dosage stated in full.

Robins—Cont.

How Supplied: 4.25 gm. tube.
*Shown in Product Identification
Section, page 421*

CHAP STICK® PETROLEUM JELLY PLUS

REGULAR:

Active Ingredients: 99% White Petrolatum, USP .

Inactive Ingredients: Aloe, Lanolin, Phenonip®, Butylated Hydroxytoluene, Fragrance.

CHERRY:

Active Ingredients: 98.85% White Petrolatum, USP.

Inactive Ingredients: Lanolin, Aloe, Phenonip®, Flavors, Butylated Hydroxytoluene, Saccharin, D&C Red 6 Barium Lake.

Indications: Helps prevent and protect against dry, chapped, sun and windburned lips.

Actions: White Petrolatum, USP forms a barrier to prevent moisture loss and protect lips from the drying effects of cold weather, wind and sun which cause chapping. White Petrolatum, USP helps soften the skin by forming an occlusive film for inducing hydration, restoring suppleness to the lips and preventing drying from evaporation of water that diffuses to the surface from the underlying layers of tissue.

Warning: Patients should consult a physician if condition worsens or does not improve within 7 days.

Dosage and Treatment: To help prevent dry, chapped, sun or wind-burned lips, apply to lips as needed before, during and following exposure to sun, wind, water and cold weather.

How Supplied: Regular and Cherry flavored available in 0.35 oz. (10 grams) polyethylene tube.
*Shown in Product Identification
Section page 421*

CHAP STICK® PETROLEUM JELLY PLUS WITH SUNBLOCK 15

Active Ingredients: 89% White Petrolatum, USP, 7% Padimate O, 3% Oxybenzone.

Inactive Ingredients: Aloe, Lanolin, Phenonip®, Butylated Hydroxytoluene, Fragrance.

Indications: Ultra Sunscreen Protection (SPF-15). Helps prevent and protect against dry, chapped, sun and windburned lips. Overexposure to sun may lead to premature aging of skin and skin cancer. Liberal and regular use may help reduce the sun's harmful effects.

Actions: Ultra sunscreen protection for the lips, plus the attributes of Chap Stick® Petroleum Jelly Plus. White Pet-

rolatum, USP forms a barrier to prevent moisture loss and protect lips from the drying effects of wind and sun while two sunscreens, which have specific ultra violet absorption ranges, overlap to provide ultra sunscreen protection (SPF-15).

Warning: Patients should consult a physician if condition worsens or does not improve within 7 days.

Dosage and Treatment: For ultra sunscreen protection, apply evenly and liberally to lips before exposure to sun. Reapply as needed. For dry chapped lips, apply as needed. To help prevent dry, chapped, sun and windburned lips, apply to lips as needed before, during and following exposure to sun, wind, water and cold weather.

How Supplied: Available in 0.35 oz (10 grams) polyethylene tube.
*Shown in Product Identification
Section, page 421*

DIMACOL® Caplets
[di 'mă-col]

Description: Each caplet contains:
Guaifenesin, USP .... 100 mg
Pseudoephedrine
   Hydrochloride, USP .... 30 mg
Dextromethorphan
   Hydrobromide, USP .... 10 mg

Inactive Ingredients: D&C Yellow 10 Aluminum Lake, FD&C Yellow 6 Aluminum Lake, Flavor, Hydroxypropyl Methylcellulose, Magnesium Stearate, Methacrylic Acid Copolymer, Methylparaben, Microcrystalline Cellulose, Polysorbate 20, Potassium Sorbate, Povidone, Propylene Glycol, Propylparaben, Saccharin Sodium, Silicon Dioxide, Titanium Dioxide, Triethyl Citrate, Xanthan Gum.

Indications: Temporarily relieves cough due to minor throat and bronchial irritation and nasal congestion as may occur with a cold. Expectorant action to help loosen phlegm and thin bronchial secretions to make coughs more productive.

Warnings: Patients with the following conditions are warned not to take this product, unless directed by a physician: persistent or chronic cough such as occurs with smoking, asthma, chronic bronchitis, emphysema, or if cough is accompanied by excessive phlegm (mucus). Likewise, patients with heart disease, high blood pressure, thyroid disease, diabetes, or difficulty in urination due to enlargement of the prostate gland are warned not to take this product unless directed by a physician.
Patients are warned not to exceed the recommended dosage because at higher doses, nervousness, dizziness or sleeplessness may occur. They also are told not to take the product for more than 7 days. A persistent cough may be a sign of a serious condition. If cough or symptoms persist for more than one week, tend to recur, or are accompanied by fever, rash, or persistent headache, patients should consult a physician.

Patients should not take this product if they are hypersensitive to any of the ingredients. As with any drug, women who are pregnant or nursing a baby should seek the advice of a health professional before using this product.

Contraindications: Hypersensitivity to any of the ingredients; marked hypertension, hyperthyroidism or in patients who are receiving monoamine oxidase inhibitors (MAOIs).

Adverse Reactions: The following adverse reactions may possibly occur: nausea, vomiting, dry mouth, nervousness, insomnia and rash (including urticaria).
NOTE: Guaifenesin has been shown to produce a color interference with certain clinical laboratory determinations of 5-hydroxyindoleacetic acid (5-HIAA) and vanillylmandelic acid (VMA).

Drug Interaction Precautions: Concomitant administration of pseudoephedrine with other sympathomimetic agents may produce additive effects and increased toxicity; with MAOIs may produce a hypertensive crisis; with certain antihypertensive agents may diminish their antihypertensive effect. Serious toxicity may result if dextromethorphan is used with MAOIs.

Directions: Adults and children 12 years and over, 2 caplets every 4 hours; children 6 to under 12 years of age, 1 caplet every 4 hours; children under 6 years—consult a doctor. DO NOT EXCEED 4 DOSES IN A 24-HOUR PERIOD.

How Supplied: Orange, film-coated caplets engraved AHR on one side and DIMACOL on the other in bottles of 100 (NDC 0031-1653-63), and 500 (NDC 0031-1653-70) and consumer packages of 12 (NDC 0031-1653-46), and 24 (NDC 0031-1653-54) (individually packaged).
Store at Controlled Room Temperature, between 15°C and 30°C (59°F and 86°F).

DIMETANE®
[dī' mě-tāne]
brand of Brompheniramine Maleate, USP
Tablets—4 mg
Elixir—2 mg/5 mL
Extentabs®—8 mg and 12 mg

Family Description: Dimetane® is Robins brand name for Brompheniramine Maleate, USP, an antihistamine. It comes in several oral dosage forms (tablets, elixir and Extentabs®) and can be used when an antihistamine is indicated.

Inactive Ingredients:
Tablets: Corn Starch, D&C Yellow 10 Aluminum Lake, Dibasic Calcium Phosphate, FD&C Yellow 6 Aluminum Lake, Lactose, Magnesium Stearate, Polyethylene Glycol.
Elixir: Alcohol 3%, Citric Acid, FD&C Yellow 6, Flavors, Glucose, Saccharin Sodium, Sodium Benzoate, Water.
Extentabs® 8 mg: Acacia, Acetylated Monoglycerides, Calcium Carbonate,

Calcium Sulfate, Carnauba Wax, Cellulose Acetate Phthalate, Corn Starch, Diethyl Phthalate, Edible Ink, FD&C Blue 2 Aluminum Lake, FD&C Red 3, Gelatin, Guar Gum, Magnesium Stearate, Pharmaceutical Glaze, Polysorbates, Stearic Acid, Sucrose, Titanium Dioxide, Wheat Flour, White Wax and other ingredients, one of which is a corn derivative. May contain FD&C Red 40 and FD&C Yellow 6 Aluminum Lakes.

Extentabs® 12 mg: Acacia, Acetylated Monoglycerides, Calcium Carbonate, Calcium Sulfate, Carnauba Wax, Cellulose Acetate Phthalate, Corn Starch, Diethyl Phthalate, Edible Ink, FD&C Blue 2 Aluminum Lake, FD&C Red 3, FD&C Yellow 6, Gelatin, Guar Gum, Magnesium Stearate, Pharmaceutical Glaze, Polysorbates, Stearic Acid, Sucrose, Titanium Dioxide, Wheat Flour, White Wax and other ingredients, one of which is a corn derivative. May contain FD&C Red 40 and FD&C Yellow 6 Aluminum Lakes.

Indications: For temporary relief of running nose, sneezing, itching of the nose or throat; and itchy, watery eyes as may occur in allergic rhinitis (such as hay fever).

Warnings: Patients with the following conditions are warned not to take any of these products, unless directed by a physician: asthma, emphysema, chronic pulmonary disease, shortness of breath, difficulty in breathing, glaucoma, or difficulty in urination due to enlargement of the prostate gland.
These products may cause drowsiness; alcohol, sedatives and tranquilizers may increase the drowsiness effect. Patients are told to avoid alcoholic beverages while taking these products and not to take them if they are taking sedatives or tranquilizers without first consulting their physician. Caution should be used when driving a motor vehicle or operating machinery. May cause excitability, especially in children.

Dimetane Extentabs should not be given to children under 12 years of age, except under the advice and supervision of a physician. Patients should not take these products if they are hypersensitive to any of the ingredients. As with any drug, women who are pregnant or nursing a baby should seek the advice of a health professional before using these products.

Directions: Tablets and Liquid—The recommended OTC dosage is: Adults and children 12 years of age and over: 1 tablet or 2 teaspoonfuls every four to six hours, not to exceed 6 tablets or 12 teaspoonfuls in 24 hours. Children 6 to under 12 years: ½ tablet or 1 teaspoonful every four to six hours, not to exceed 3 whole tablets or 6 teaspoonfuls in 24 hours.

Professional Labeling: Children under 6 years: Use only as directed by a physician. The suggested dosage for children age 2 to under 6 years, only when the child is under the care of a physician, is ½ teaspoonful every 4 to 6 hours, not to exceed 6 doses in a 24-hour period. The dosage for a child under 2 years should be determined by the physician on the basis of the patient's weight, physical condition, or other appropriate consideration. Dimetane Elixir is contraindicated in neonates (children under the age of one month).

Extentabs®—The recommended OTC dosage is: Adults and children 12 years of age and over:
8 mg Extentab: One tablet every eight to twelve hours, NOT TO EXCEED 1 TABLET EVERY 8 HOURS OR 3 TABLETS IN A 24-HOUR PERIOD.
12 mg Extentab: One tablet every twelve hours, NOT TO EXCEED 1 TABLET EVERY 12 HOURS OR 2 TABLETS IN A 24-HOUR PERIOD.
Children under 12 years of age should use only as directed by a physician.

How Supplied:
[See table below.]
Store at Controlled Room Temperature, between 15°C and 30°C (59°F and 86°F).

DIMETANE® DECONGESTANT ELIXIR
[dī' mĕ-tāne]
DIMETANE® DECONGESTANT CAPLETS

Elixir:
Each 5 mL (1 teaspoonful) contains:
Phenylephrine
  Hydrochloride, USP .... 5 mg
Brompheniramine
  Maleate, USP .... 2 mg

Inactive Ingredients: Alcohol 2.3%, Citric Acid, FD&C Blue 1, FD&C Red 40, Flavors, Sodium Benzoate, Sorbitol, Water.

Caplets:
Each caplet contains:
Phenylephrine
  Hydrochloride, USP .... 10 mg
Brompheniramine
  Maleate, USP .... 4 mg

Inactive Ingredients: Corn Starch, FD&C Blue 1 Aluminum Lake, Magnesium Stearate, Microcrystalline Cellulose.

Indications: For temporary relief of nasal congestion due to the common cold, hay fever or other upper respiratory allergies or associated with sinusitis; temporarily relieves runny nose, sneezing, itching of the nose or throat and itchy and watery eyes as may occur in allergic rhinitis (such as hay fever). Temporarily restores freer breathing through the nose.

Warnings: Patients with the following conditions are warned not to take either of these products, unless directed by a physician: asthma, emphysema, chronic pulmonary disease, shortness of breath, difficulty in breathing, high blood pressure, heart disease, diabetes, thyroid disease, glaucoma, or difficulty in urination due to enlargement of the prostate gland. These products may cause drowsiness; alcohol, sedatives, and tranquilizers may increase the drowsiness effect. Patients are told to avoid alcoholic beverages while taking these products and not to take them if they are taking sedatives or tranquilizers without first consulting their physician. Caution should be used when driving a motor vehicle or operating machinery. May cause excitability, especially in children.
Patients are warned not to exceed the recommended dosage because at higher doses, nervousness, dizziness or sleeplessness may occur. They also are told not to take the products for more than 7 days. If symptoms do not improve or are accompanied by fever, patients should consult a physician.
Patients should not take these products if they are hypersensitive to any of the

Continued on next page

Prescribing information on A.H. Robins products listed here is based on official labeling in effect November 1, 1991, with Indications, Contraindications, Warnings, Precautions, Adverse Reactions, and Dosage stated in full.

Product Name	Form	Strength	Package Size	Package Type	NDC 0031-
Dimetane Tablets	Peach-colored, compressed scored tablet	4 mg tablet	24	Blister Unit	1857-54
			100	Bottles	1857-63
Dimetane Elixir	Peach-colored liquid	2 mg/ 5 mL	4 fl. oz.	Bottles	1807-12
			1 Pint	Bottles	1807-25
Dimetane Extentabs 8 mg	Persian rose-colored, coated tablets	8 mg tablet	12	Blister Unit	1868-46
			100	Bottles	1868-63
Dimetane Extentabs 12 mg	Peach-colored, coated tablets	12 mg tablet	12	Blister Unit	1843-46
			100	Bottles	1843-63

Robins—Cont.

ingredients. As with any drug, women who are pregnant or nursing a baby should seek the advice of a health professional before using these products.

Drug Interaction Precautions: Concomitant administration of phenylephrine with other sympathomimetic agents may produce additive effects and increased toxicity: with monoamine oxidase inhibitors (MAOIs) may produce a hypertensive crisis; with certain antihypertensive agents may diminish their antihypertensive effect.

Directions: *Caplets:* Adults and children 12 years of age and over: 1 caplet every 4 hours, not to exceed 6 caplets in a 24-hour period; children 6 to under 12 years: ½ caplet every 4 hours, not to exceed 3 caplets in a 24-hour period; children under 6 years: use only as directed by a physician.
Elixir: Adults and children 12 years of age and over: 2 teaspoonfuls every 4 hours, not to exceed 12 teaspoonfuls in a 24-hour period; children 6 to under 12 years: 1 teaspoonful every 4 hours, not to exceed 6 teaspoonfuls in a 24-hour period. Children under 6 years: use only as directed by a physician.

Professional Labeling: The suggested dosage for children age 2 to under 6 years, only when the child is under the care of a physician, is ½ teaspoonful every 4 hours, not to exceed 6 doses in a 24-hour period. The dosage for a child under 2 years should be determined by the physician on the basis of the patient's weight, physical condition, or other appropriate consideration. Dimetane Decongestant is contraindicated in neonates (children under the age of one month).

How Supplied: *Caplets* —light blue, capsule-shaped, compressed tablets engraved AHR on one side and scored and engraved 2117 on the other, in cartons of 24 (NDC 0031-2117-54) and 48 (NDC 0031-2117-59) individually packaged blister units.
Elixir —red-colored, grape-flavored liquid in 4 fl oz bottle (NDC 0031-2127-12). Store at Controlled Room Temperature, between 15°C and 30°C (59°F and 86°F).

DIMETAPP® COLD AND FLU CAPLETS

[dī' mĕ-tap]

Description: Each **Dimetapp® Cold & Flu Caplet** contains:
Acetaminophen, USP .... 500 mg
Phenylpropanolamine
  Hydrochloride, USP .... 12.5 mg
Brompheniramine
  Maleate, USP .... 2 mg

Inactive Ingredients: Corn Starch, FD&C Blue 2 Aluminum Lake, Hydroxypropyl Methylcellulose, Magnesium Stearate, Microcrystalline Cellulose, Polysorbate 20, Povidone, Propylene Glycol, Stearic Acid, Titanium Dioxide. May also contain Calcium Phosphate, Hy-

droxypropyl Cellulose, Methylparaben, Propylparaben.

Indications: For the temporary relief of minor aches, pains, and headache; for the reduction of fever; for the relief of nasal congestion due to the common cold or associated with sinusitis; and for the relief of runny nose, sneezing, itching of the nose or throat and itchy and watery eyes as may occur in allergic rhinitis (such as hay fever). Temporarily restores freer breathing through the nose.

Warnings: Patients with the following conditions are warned not to take this product, unless directed by a physician: asthma, emphysema, chronic pulmonary disease, shortness of breath, difficulty in breathing, high blood pressure, heart disease, diabetes, thyroid disease, glaucoma, or difficulty in urination due to enlargement of the prostate gland.
This product may cause drowsiness; alcohol, sedatives and tranquilizers may increase the drowsiness effect. Patients are told to avoid alcoholic beverages while taking this product and not to take it if they are taking sedatives or tranquilizers without first consulting their physician. Caution should be used when driving a motor vehicle or operating machinery. May cause excitability, especially in children.
Patients are warned not to exceed the recommended dosage because at higher doses, nervousness, dizziness or sleeplessness may occur. They also are told not to take this product for more than 10 days. If symptoms do not improve or are accompanied by fever that lasts for more than 3 days, or if new symptoms occur, patients should consult a physician.
Patients should not take this product if they are hypersensitive to any of the ingredients. As with any drug, women who are pregnant or nursing a baby should seek the advice of a health professional before using this product.
NOTE: Patients are also warned that IN CASE OF ACCIDENTAL OVERDOSE, they should SEEK PROFESSIONAL ASSISTANCE OR CONTACT A POISON CONTROL CENTER IMMEDIATELY. Because of the acetaminophen content, they are told that PROMPT MEDICAL ATTENTION IS CRITICAL FOR ADULTS AS WELL AS FOR CHILDREN, EVEN IF NO SIGNS OR SYMPTOMS ARE NOTED.

Drug Interaction Precaution: Concomitant administration of phenylpropanolamine with other sympathomimetic agents may produce additive effects and increased toxicity; with monoamine oxidase inhibitors (MAOIs) may produce a hypertensive crisis; with certain antihypertensive agents may diminish their antihypertensive effect.

Directions: Adults and children (12 years and over): Two caplets every 6 hours. DO NOT EXCEED 8 CAPLETS IN A 24-HOUR PERIOD.
Not recommended for children under 12 years of age.

How Supplied: Dimetapp® Cold & Flu Caplets are supplied as blue capsule-

shaped film-coated tablets, engraved AHR on one side and 2280 on the other, in consumer packages of 24 (NDC 0031-2280-54) (individually packaged), and 48 (NDC 0031-2280-59) (bottle).
Store at Controlled Room Temperature, between 15°C and 30°C (59°F and 86°F).
Shown in Product Identification Section, page 421

DIMETAPP® Elixir

[dī' mĕ-tap]

Description: Each 5 mL (1 teaspoonful) contains:
Brompheniramine
  Maleate, USP ....2 mg
Phenylpropanolamine
  Hydrochloride, USP .... 12.5 mg

Inactive Ingredients: Alcohol 2.3%, Citric Acid, FD&C Blue 1, FD&C Red 40, Flavor, Saccharin Sodium, Sodium Benzoate, Sorbitol, Water.

Indications: For temporary relief of nasal congestion due to the common cold, hay fever or other upper respiratory allergies or associated with sinusitis; temporarily relieves runny nose, sneezing, and itchy and watery eyes as may occur in allergic rhinitis (such as hay fever). Temporarily restores freer breathing through the nose.

Warnings: Patients with the following conditions are warned not to take this product, unless directed by a physician: asthma, emphysema, chronic pulmonary disease, shortness of breath, difficulty in breathing, high blood pressure, heart disease, diabetes, thyroid disease, glaucoma, or difficulty in urination due to enlargement of the prostate gland.
This product may cause drowsiness; alcohol, sedatives and tranquilizers may increase the drowsiness effect. Patients are told to avoid alcoholic beverages while taking this product and not to take it if they are taking sedatives or tranquilizers without first consulting their physician. Caution should be used when driving a motor vehicle or operating machinery. May cause excitability, especially in children.
Patients are warned not to exceed the recommended dosage because at higher doses, nervousness, dizziness or sleeplessness may occur. They also are told not to take this product for more than 7 days. If symptoms do not improve, or are accompanied by fever, patients should consult a physician.
Patients should not take this product if they are hypersensitive to any of the ingredients. As with any drug, women who are pregnant or nursing a baby should seek the advice of a health professional before using this product.

Drug Interaction Precaution: Concomitant administration of phenylpropanolamine with other sympathomimetic agents may produce additive effects and increased toxicity; with monamine oxidase inhibitors (MAOIs) may produce a hypertensive crisis; with certain antihypertensive agents may diminish their antihypertensive effect.

Directions: Adults and children 12 years of age and over: 2 teaspoonfuls every 4 hours; children 6 to under 12 years: 1 teaspoonful every 4 hours; DO NOT EXCEED 6 DOSES IN A 24-HOUR PERIOD. Children under 6 years: use only as directed by a physician.

Professional Labeling: The suggested dosage for children age 2 to under 6 years, only when the child is under the care of a physician, is ½ teaspoonful every 4 hours, not to exceed 6 doses in a 24-hour period. The dosage for children under 2 years should be determined by the physician on the basis of the patients' weight, physical condition, or other appropriate consideration. Dimetapp Elixir is contraindicated in neonates (children under the age of one month).

How Supplied: Purple, grape-flavored liquid in bottles of 4 fl. oz. (NDC 0031-2230-12), 8 fl. oz. (NDC 0031-2230-18), 12 fl. oz. (NDC 0031-2230-22), pints (NDC 0031-2230-25), gallons (NDC 0031-2230-29), and 5 mL Dis-Co® Unit Dose Packs (10 × 10s) (NDC 0031-2230-23). Store at Controlled Room Temperature, between 15°C and 30°C (59°F and 86°F).

Shown in Product Identification Section, page 421

DIMETAPP® DM ELIXIR
[dĭ'mĕ-tap]

Description: Each 5 mL (1 teaspoonful) contains:
Brompheniramine
  Maleate, USP .... 2 mg
Phenylpropanolamine
  Hydrochloride, USP .... 12.5 mg
Dextromethorphan
  Hydrobromide, USP .... 10.0 mg

Inactive Ingredients: Alcohol 2.3%, Citric Acid, FD&C Blue 1, FD&C Red 40, Flavors, Glycerin, Propylene Glycol, Saccharin Sodium, Sodium Benzoate, Sorbitol, Water.

Indications: Temporarily relieves cough due to minor throat and bronchial irritation as may occur with a cold. For temporary relief of nasal congestion due to the common cold, hay fever or other upper respiratory allergies and associated with sinusitis; temporarily relieves runny nose, sneezing, and itchy and watery eyes as may occur in allergic rhinitis (such as hay fever). Temporarily restores freer breathing through the nose.

Warnings: Patients with the following conditions are warned not to take this product, unless directed by a physician: asthma, emphysema, chronic pulmonary disease, shortness of breath, difficulty in breathing, or other persistent or chronic cough such as occurs with smoking, or cough that is accompanied by excessive phlegm (mucus). Likewise, patients with high blood pressure, heart disease, diabetes, thyroid disease, glaucoma, or difficulty in urination due to enlargement of the prostate gland are warned not to take

this product unless directed by a physician.
This product may cause marked drowsiness; alcohol, sedatives and tranquilizers may increase the drowsiness effect. Patients are instructed to avoid alcoholic beverages while taking this product and not to take it if they are taking sedatives or tranquilizers without first consulting their physician. Caution should be used when driving a motor vehicle or operating machinery. May cause excitability, especially in children.
Patients are warned not to exceed the recommended dosage because at higher doses, nervousness, dizziness or sleeplessness may occur. They also are told not to take the product for more than 7 days. A persistent cough may be a sign of a serious condition. If cough or other symptoms persist for more than one week, tend to recur, or are accompanied by fever, rash or persistent headache, patients should consult a physician.
Patients should not take this product if they are hypersensitive to any of the ingredients. As with any drug, women who are pregnant or nursing a baby should seek the advice of a health professional before using this product.

Drug Interaction Precautions: Concomitant administration of phenylpropanolamine with other sympathomimetic agents may produce additive effects and increased toxicity; with monamine oxidase inhibitors (MAOIs) may produce a hypertensive crisis; with certain antihypertensive agents may diminish their antihypertensive effect. Serious toxicity may result if dextromethorphan is used with MAOIs.

Directions: Adults and children 12 years of age and over: Two teaspoonfuls every 4 hours; children 6 to under 12 years: one teaspoonful every 4 hours. **DO NOT EXCEED 6 DOSES IN A 24-HOUR PERIOD.** Children under 6 years: use only as directed by a physician.

Professional Labeling: The suggested dosage for children age 2 to under 6 years, only when the child is under the care of a physician, is ½ teaspoonful every 4 hours, not to exceed 6 doses in a 24-hour period. The dosage for children under 2 years should be determined by the physician on the basis of the patients' weight, physical condition, or other appropriate consideration. Dimetapp DM Elixir is contraindicated in neonates (children under the age of one month).

How Supplied: Red, grape-flavored liquid in bottles of 4 fl. oz. (NDC 0031-2240-12), 8 fl. oz. (NDC 0031-2240-18), and 12 fl. oz. (NDC 0031-2240-22). Store at Room Temperature.

Shown in Product Identification Section, page 421

DIMETAPP® Extentabs®
[dĭ' mĕ-tap]

Description: Each **Dimetapp Extentabs®** Tablet contains:

Brompheniramine Maleate,
  USP .... 12 mg
Phenylpropanolamine
  Hydrochloride, USP .... 75 mg

Inactive Ingredients: Acacia, Acetylated Monoglycerides, Calcium Sulfate, Carnauba Wax, Castor Wax or Oil, Citric Acid, Edible Ink, FD&C Blue 1 and FD&C Blue 2 Aluminum Lake, Gelatin, Magnesium Stearate, Magnesium Trisilicate, Pharmaceutical Glaze, Polysorbates, Povidone, Silicon Dioxide, Stearyl Alcohol, Sucrose, Titanium Dioxide, Wheat Flour, White Wax. May contain FD&C Red 40 and FD&C Yellow 6 Aluminum Lakes.

Indications: For temporary relief of nasal congestion due to the common cold, hay fever or other upper respiratory allergies and associated with sinusitis; temporarily relieves runny nose, sneezing, and itchy and watery eyes as may occur in allergic rhinitis (such as hay fever). Temporarily restores freer breathing through the nose.

Warnings: Patients with the following conditions are warned not to take this product, unless directed by a physician: asthma, emphysema, chronic pulmonary disease, shortness of breath, difficulty in breathing, high blood pressure, heart disease, diabetes, thyroid disease, glaucoma, or difficulty in urination due to enlargement of the prostate gland.
This product may cause drowsiness; alcohol, sedatives and tranquilizers may increase the drowsiness effect. Patients are told to avoid alcoholic beverages while taking this product and not to take it if they are taking sedatives or tranquilizers without first consulting their physician. Caution should be used when driving a motor vehicle or operating machinery. May cause excitability, especially in children.
Patients are warned not to exceed the recommended dosage because at higher doses, nervousness, dizziness or sleeplessness may occur. They also are told not to take this product for more than 7 days. If symptoms do not improve, or are accompanied by fever, patients should consult a physician.
Dimetapp Extentabs should not be given to children under 12 years, except under the advice and supervision of a physician. Patients should not take this product if they are hypersensitive to any of the ingredients. As with any drug, women who are pregnant or nursing a baby should seek the advice of a health professional before using this product.

Drug Interaction Precaution: Concomitant administration of phenylpropanolamine with other sympathomimetic

Continued on next page

Prescribing information on A.H. Robins products listed here is based on official labeling in effect November 1, 1991, with Indications, Contraindications, Warnings, Precautions, Adverse Reactions, and Dosage stated in full.

Robins—Cont.

agents may produce additive effects and increased toxicity; with monoamine oxidase inhibitors (MAOIs) may produce a hypertensive crisis; with certain antihypertensive agents may diminish their antihypertensive effect.

Directions: Adults and children 12 years of age and over: one tablet every 12 hours. DO NOT EXCEED 1 TABLET EVERY 12 HOURS OR 2 TABLETS IN A 24-HOUR PERIOD.

How Supplied: Pale blue sugar-coated tablets monogrammed DIMETAPP AHR in bottles of 100 (NDC 0031-2277-63), 500 (NDC 0031-2277-70); Dis-Co® Unit Dose Packs of 100 (NDC 0031-2277-64); and consumer packages of 12 tablets (NDC 0031-2277-46), 24 tablets (NDC 0031-2277-54) and 48 tablets (NDC 0031-2277-59) (individually packaged).

Store at Controlled Room Temperature, between 15°C and 30°C (59°F and 86°F). Dimetapp Extentabs® Tablets are the A. H. Robins Company's uniquely constructed extended action tablets.

Shown in Product Identification Section, page 421

DIMETAPP® Tablets
[dĭ' mĕ-tap]

Description: Each **Dimetapp** Tablet contains:
Brompheniramine
  Maleate, USP .... 4 mg
Phenylpropanolamine
  Hydrochloride, USP .... 25 mg

Inactive Ingredients: Corn Starch, FD&C Blue 1 Aluminum Lake, Magnesium Stearate, Microcrystalline Cellulose.

Indications: For temporary relief of nasal congestion due to the common cold, hay fever or other upper respiratory allergies or associated with sinusitis; temporarily relieves runny nose, sneezing, and itchy and watery eyes as may occur in allergic rhinitis (such as hay fever). Temporarily restores freer breathing through the nose.

Warnings: Patients with the following conditions are warned not to take this product, unless directed by a physician: asthma, emphysema, chronic pulmonary disease, shortness of breath, difficulty in breathing, high blood pressure, heart disease, diabetes, thyroid disease, glaucoma, or difficulty in urination due to enlargement of the prostate gland.

This product may cause drowsiness; alcohol, sedatives and tranquilizers may increase the drowsiness effect. Patients are told to avoid alcoholic beverages while taking this product and not to take it if they are taking sedatives or tranquilizers without first consulting their physician. Caution should be used when driving a motor vehicle or operating machinery. May cause excitability, especially in children. Patients are warned not to exceed

the recommended dosage because at higher doses, nervousness, dizziness or sleeplessness may occur. They also are told not to take this product for more than 7 days. If symptoms do not improve, or are accompanied by fever, patients should consult a physician.

Patients should not take this product if they are hypersensitive to any of the ingredients. As with any drug, women who are pregnant or nursing a baby should seek the advice of a health professional before using this product.

Drug Interaction Precaution: Concomitant administration of phenylpropanolamine with other sympathomimetic agents may produce additive effects and increased toxicity; with monoamine oxidase inhibitors (MAOIs) may produce a hypertensive crisis; with certain antihypertensive agents may diminish their antihypertensive effect.

Directions: Adults and children 12 years of age and over: one tablet every 4 hours. Children 6 to under 12 years: one-half tablet every 4 hours. DO NOT EXCEED 6 DOSES IN A 24-HOUR PERIOD. Children under 6 years: Use only as directed by a physician.

How Supplied: Blue, scored compressed tablets engraved AHR and 2254 in consumer packages of 24 (NDC 0031-2254-54) (individually packaged). Store at Controlled Room Temperature, between 15°C and 30°C (59°F and 86°F).

Shown in Product Identification Section, page 421

DONNAGEL®
[don 'nă-jel]
Liquid and Chewable Tablets

Each tablespoon (15 mL) of **Donnagel Liquid** contains: 600 mg Attapulgite, USP.

Inactive Ingredients: Alcohol 1.4%, Benzyl Alcohol, Carboxymethylcellulose Sodium, Citric Acid, FD&C Blue 1, Flavors, Magnesium Aluminum Silicate, Methylparaben, Phosphoric Acid, Propylene Glycol, Propylparaben, Saccharin Sodium, Sorbitol, Titanium Dioxide, Water, Xanthan Gum.

Each **Donnagel Chewable** Tablet contains: 600 mg Attapulgite, USP.

Inactive Ingredients: D&C Yellow 10 Aluminum Lake, FD&C Blue 1 Aluminum Lake, Flavors, Magnesium Stearate, Mannitol, Saccharin Sodium, Sorbitol, Water.

Indications: Donnagel is indicated for the symptomatic relief of diarrhea. It reduces the number of bowel movements, improves consistency of loose, watery bowel movements and relieves cramping.

Warnings: Patients are told that diarrhea may be serious. They are warned not to use this product for more than 2 days, or in the presence of fever, or in children under 3 years of age unless directed by a physician.

This product should not be taken by patients who are hypersensitive to any of the ingredients. As with any drug, women who are pregnant or nursing a baby should seek the advice of a health professional before using this product.

Dosage and Administration: Full recommended dose should be administered at the first sign of diarrhea and after each subsequent bowel movement, NOT TO EXCEED 7 DOSES IN A 24-HOUR PERIOD. [See table below.]

How Supplied: Donnagel Liquid (green suspension) in 4 fl. oz. (NDC 0031-3017-12) and 8 fl. oz. (NDC 0031-3017-18). Donnagel Chewable Tablets (light-green, flat-faced, beveled-edged, round tablets with darker green flecks; one side engraved AHR, obverse engraved Donnagel) in consumer blister packages of 18 (NDC 0031-3018-51). Store at Controlled Room Temperature, between 15°C and 30°C (59°F and 86°F).

Shown in Product Identification Section, page 422

ROBITUSSIN®
(Guaifenesin Syrup, USP)
[ro "bĭ-tuss 'ĭn]

Active Ingredients per teaspoonful (5 mL)—Guaifenesin, USP 100 mg in pleasant tasting syrup.

Inactive Ingredients: Alcohol 3.5%, Caramel, Citric Acid, FD&C Red 40, Flavors, Glucose, Glycerin, High Fructose Corn Syrup, Saccharin Sodium, Sodium Benzoate, Water.

Indications: Expectorant action to help loosen phlegm and thin bronchial secretions to make coughs more productive.

Professional Labeling: Helps loosen phlegm and thin bronchial secretions in patients with stable chronic bronchitis.

Warnings: Patients with the following conditions are warned not to take this product, unless directed by a physician: persistent or chronic cough such as occurs with smoking, asthma, chronic bronchitis, emphysema or where cough

	Liquid	Chewable Tablets
Adults	2 Tablespoons	2 Tablets
Children		
12 years and over	2 Tablespoons	2 Tablets
6 through 11 years	1 Tablespoon	1 Tablet
3 through 5 years	½ Tablespoon	½ Tablet
Under 3 years	Consult Physician	

Liquid should be shaken well. Tablets should be chewed thoroughly and swallowed.

is accompanied by excessive phlegm (sputum).

A persistent cough may be a sign of a serious condition. If cough persists for more than one week, tends to recur, or is accompanied by fever, rash, or persistent headache, patients should consult a physician.

Patients should not take this product if they are hypersensitive to any of the ingredients. As with any drug, women who are pregnant or nursing a baby should seek the advice of a health professional before using this product.

Contraindications: Hypersensitivity to any of the ingredients.

Adverse Reactions: Guaifenesin is well tolerated and has a wide margin of safety. Nausea and vomiting are the side effects that occur most commonly, and other reported adverse reactions have included dizziness, headache, and rash (including urticaria).

Note: Guaifenesin has been shown to produce a color interference with certain clinical laboratory determinations of 5-hydroxyindoleacetic acid (5-HIAA) and vanillylmandelic acid (VMA).

Directions: Adults and children 12 years and over: 2–4 teaspoonfuls every 4 hours; children 6 years to under 12 years: 1–2 teaspoonfuls every 4 hours. Children 2 years to under 6 years: ½–1 teaspoonful every 4 hours; children under 2 years—consult your doctor. DO NOT EXCEED RECOMMENDED DOSAGE.

How Supplied: Robitussin (wine-colored) in bottles of 4 fl. oz. (NDC 0031-8624-12), 8 fl. oz. (NDC 0031-8624-18), pint (NDC 0031-8624-25) and gallon (NDC 0031-8624-29).

Robitussin also available in 1 fl. oz. bottles (4 × 25's) (NDC 0031-8624-02) and Dis-Co® Unit Dose Packs of 10 × 10's in 5 mL (NDC 0031-8624-23), 10 mL (NDC 0031-8624-26) and 15 mL (NDC 0031-8624-28).

Store at Controlled Room Temperature, between 15°C and 30°C (59°F and 86°F).

Shown in Product Identification Section, page 422

ROBITUSSIN®-CF
[ro "bĭ-tuss 'ĭn]

Active Ingredients per teaspoonful (5 mL)—Guaifenesin, USP 100 mg; Phenylpropanolamine Hydrochloride, USP 12.5 mg and Dextromethorphan Hydrobromide, USP 10 mg in pleasant-tasting syrup.

Inactive Ingredients: Alcohol 4.75%, Citric Acid, FD&C Red 40, Flavors, Glycerin, Propylene Glycol, Saccharin Sodium, Sodium Benzoate, Sorbitol, Water.

Indications: Temporarily relieves coughs due to minor throat and bronchial irritation and nasal congestion as may occur with a cold. Expectorant action to help loosen phlegm and thin bronchial secretions to make coughs more productive.

Warnings: Patients with the following conditions are warned not to take this product, unless directed by a physician: persistent or chronic cough such as occurs with smoking, asthma, chronic bronchitis, emphysema, or if cough is accompanied by excessive phlegm (mucus). Likewise, patients with heart disease, high blood pressure, thyroid disease, diabetes, or difficulty in urination due to enlargement of the prostate gland are warned not to take this product unless directed by a physician.

Patients are warned not to exceed the recommended dosage because at higher doses, nervousness, dizziness or sleeplessness may occur. They also are told not to take this product for more than 7 days. A persistent cough may be a sign of a serious condition. If cough or other symptoms persist for more than one week, tend to recur, or are accompanied by fever, rash, or persistent headache, patients should consult a physician.

Patients should not take this product if they are hypersensitive to any of the ingredients. As with any drug, women who are pregnant or nursing a baby should seek the advice of a health professional before using this product.

Contraindications: Hypersensitivity to any of the ingredients; marked hypertension; hyperthyroidism; patients who are receiving monoamine oxidase inhibitors (MAOIs).

Adverse Reactions: The following adverse reactions may occur: nausea, vomiting, dizziness, nervousness, insomnia, or rash (including urticaria).

Note: Guaifenesin has been shown to produce a color interference with certain clinical laboratory determinations of 5-hydroxyindoleacetic acid (5-HIAA) and vanillylmandelic acid (VMA).

Drug Interaction Precautions: Concomitant administration of phenylpropanolamine with other sympathomimetic agents may produce additive effects and increased toxicity; with MAOIs may produce a hypertensive crisis; with certain antihypertensive agents may diminish their antihypertensive effect. Serious toxicity may result if dextromethorphan is used with MAOIs.

Directions: Adults and children 12 years and over, 2 teaspoonfuls every 4 hours; children 6 years to under 12 years, 1 teaspoonful every 4 hours; children 2 years to under 6 years, ½ teaspoonful every 4 hours; children under 2 years —as directed by a physician. DO NOT EXCEED 6 DOSES IN A 24-HOUR PERIOD.

How Supplied: Robitussin-CF (red-colored) in bottles of 4 fl. oz. (NDC 0031-8677-12), 8 fl. oz. (NDC 0031-8677-18), 12 fl. oz. (NDC 0031-8677-22), and one pint (NDC 0031-8677-25).

Store at Controlled Room Temperature, between 15°C and 30°C (59°F and 86°F).

Shown in Product Identification Section, page 422

ROBITUSSIN®-DM
[ro "bĭ-tuss 'ĭn]

Active Ingredients per teaspoonful (5 mL)—Guaifenesin, USP 100 mg and Dextromethorphan Hydrobromide, USP 10 mg in pleasant-tasting syrup.

Inactive Ingredients: Citric Acid, FD&C Red 40, Flavors, Glucose, Glycerin, High Fructose Corn Syrup, Saccharin Sodium, Sodium Benzoate, Water.

Indications: Temporarily relieves coughs due to minor throat and bronchial irritation as may occur with a cold. Expectorant action to help loosen phlegm and thin bronchial secretions to make coughs more productive.

Warnings: Patients with the following conditions are warned not to take this product, unless directed by a physician: persistent or chronic cough such as occurs with smoking, asthma, chronic bronchitis, emphysema, or if cough is accompanied by excessive phlegm (mucus).

A persistent cough may be a sign of a serious condition. If cough persists for more than one week, tends to recur, or is accompanied by a fever, rash, or persistent headache, patients should consult a physician.

Patients should not take this product if they are hypersensitive to any of the ingredients. As with any drug, women who are pregnant or nursing a baby should seek the advice of a health professional before using this product.

Contraindications: Hypersensitivity to any of the ingredients, or in patients who are receiving monoamine oxidase inhibitors (MAOIs).

Adverse Reactions: The incidence of side effects is low. Reported side effects include nausea and vomiting, dizziness, and rash (including urticaria).

Overdose: Symptoms may include ataxia, respiratory depression and convulsions in children, whereas adults may exhibit altered sensory perception, ataxia, slurred speech and dysphoria.

Note: Guaifenesin has been shown to produce a color interference with certain clinical laboratory determinations of 5-hydroxyindoleacetic acid (5-HIAA) and vanillylmandelic acid (VMA).

Drug Interaction Precaution: Serious toxicity may result if dextromethorphan is used with MAOIs.

Directions: Adults and children 12 years and over, 2 teaspoonfuls every 4 hours; children 6 years to under 12 years, 1 teaspoonful every 4 hours; children 2 years to under 6 years, ½ teaspoonful every 4 hours; children under 2 years—

Continued on next page

Prescribing information on A.H. Robins products listed here is based on official labeling in effect November 1, 1991, with Indications, Contraindications, Warnings, Precautions, Adverse Reactions, and Dosage stated in full.

Robins—Cont.

consult your doctor. DO NOT EXCEED 6 DOSES IN A 24-HOUR PERIOD.

How Supplied: Robitussin-DM (cherry-colored) in bottles of 4 fl. oz. (NDC 0031-8685-12), 8 fl. oz. (NDC 0031-8685-18), 12 fl. oz. (NDC 0031-8685-22), single doses: 6 premeasured doses—⅓ fl. oz. each (NDC 0031-8685-06), pint (NDC 0031-8685-25), and gallon (NDC 0031-8685-29).
Robitussin-DM also available in Dis-Co® Unit Dose Packs of 10 × 10's in 5 mL (NDC 0031-8685-23) and 10 mL (NDC 0031-8685-26).
Store at Controlled Room Temperature, between 15°C and 30°C (59°F and 86°F).

Shown in Product Identification Section, page 422

ROBITUSSIN®-PE
[ro"bĭ-tuss'ĭn]

Active Ingredients per teaspoonful (5 mL)—Guaifenesin, USP 100 mg and Pseudoephedrine Hydrochloride, USP 30 mg in pleasant tasting syrup.

Inactive Ingredients: Alcohol 1.4%, Citric Acid, FD&C Red 40, Flavors, Glucose, Glycerin, High Fructose Corn Syrup, Saccharin Sodium, Sodium Benzoate, Water.

Indications: Temporarily relieves nasal congestion as may occur with a cold. Expectorant action to help loosen phlegm and thin bronchial secretions to make coughs more productive.

Warnings: Patients with the following conditions are warned not to take this product, unless directed by a physician: persistent or chronic cough such as occurs with smoking, asthma, chronic bronchitis, emphysema, or if cough is accompanied by excessive phlegm (mucus). Likewise, patients with heart disease, high blood pressure, thyroid disease, diabetes, or difficulty in urination due to enlargement of the prostate gland are warned not to take this product unless directed by a physician.
Patients are warned not to exceed the recommended dosage because at higher doses, nervousness, dizziness or sleeplessness may occur. They also are told not to take this product for more than 7 days. A persistent cough may be a sign of a serious condition. If cough or other symptoms persist for more than one week, tend to recur, or are accompanied by fever, rash, or persistent headache, patients should consult a physician.
Patients should not take this product if they are hypersensitive to any of the ingredients. As with any drug, women who are pregnant or nursing a baby should seek the advice of a health professional before using this product.

Contraindications: Hypersensitivity to any of the ingredients; marked hypertension; hyperthyroidism; or in patients who are receiving monoamine oxidase inhibitors (MAOIs).

Adverse Reactions: Possible side effects include nausea, vomiting, nervousness, insomnia, or rash (including urticaria).
Note: Guaifenesin has been shown to produce a color interference with certain clinical laboratory determinations of 5-hydroxyindoleacetic acid (5-HIAA) and vanillylmandelic acid (VMA).

Drug Interaction Precautions: Concomitant administration of pseudoephedrine with other sympathomimetic agents may produce additive effects and increased toxicity; with MAOIs may produce a hypertensive crisis; with certain antihypertensive agents may diminish their antihypertensive effect.

Directions: Adults and children 12 years and over, 2 teaspoonfuls every 4 hours; children 6 years to under 12 years, 1 teaspoonful every 4 hours; children 2 years to under 6 years, ½ teaspoonful every 4 hours; children under 2 years —as directed by physician. DO NOT EXCEED 4 DOSES IN A 24-HOUR PERIOD.

How Supplied: Robitussin-PE (orange-red) in bottles of 4 fl. oz. (NDC 0031-8695-12), 8 fl. oz. (NDC 0031-8695-18) and pint (NDC 0031-8695-25).
Store at Controlled Room Temperature, between 15°C and 30°C (59°F and 86°F).

Shown in Product Identification Section, page 422

ROBITUSSIN® COUGH CALMERS
[ro"bi-tuss'in]

Description: Each lozenge contains: Dextromethorphan Hydrobromide, USP .... 5 mg

Inactive Ingredients: Corn Syrup, FD&C Red 40, flavors, glycerin, gum acacia, sucrose.

Indications: Temporarily relieves coughs due to minor throat and bronchial irritation as may occur with a cold.

Warnings: Patients with the following conditions are warned not to take this product unless directed by a physician: persistent or chronic cough such as occurs with smoking, asthma, or emphysema, or if cough is accompanied by excessive phlegm (mucus).
A persistent cough may be a sign of a serious condition. If cough persists for more than one week, tends to recur, or is accompanied by fever, rash, or persistent headache, patients should consult a physician.
Patients should not take this product if they are hypersensitive to any of the ingredients. As with any drug, women who are pregnant or nursing a baby should seek the advice of a health professional before using this product.

Contraindications: Hypersensitivity to any of the ingredients, or in patients who are receiving monoamine oxidase inhibitors (MAOIs).

Adverse Reactions: Side effects may include nausea.

Overdose: Symptoms may include ataxia, respiratory depression and convulsions in children; whereas, adults may exhibit altered sensory perception, ataxia, slurred speech and dysphoria.

Drug Interaction Precaution: Serious toxicity may result if dextromethorphan is used with MAOIs.

Directions: Adults and children 12 years and over: Dissolve 2–4 lozenges in mouth every 4 hours as needed.
Children 6 to under 12 years: Dissolve 1–2 lozenges in mouth every 4 hours or as directed by a doctor.
Children 4 to under 6 years: Dissolve one lozenge in mouth every 4 hours or as directed by a doctor.
Do not exceed recommended dosage.

How Supplied: Square, red cherry-flavored lozenge engraved AHR on both sides. Each consumer carton contains 8 tandem-joined pouches containing 2 lozenges each (16 lozenges total).
Store at Controlled Room Temperature, between 15°C and 30°C (59°F and 86°F).

ROBITUSSIN® COUGH DROPS
[ro"bĭ-tuss'in]
Menthol Eucalyptus, Cherry, and Honey-Lemon Flavors

Active Ingredients:
Menthol Eucalyptus and *Cherry:* Menthol 7.4 mg per cough drop.
Honey-Lemon: Menthol 10 mg per cough drop.

Inactive Ingredients:
Menthol Eucalyptus: Corn Syrup, Eucalyptus Oil, Sucrose, Titanium Dioxide (coloring). May contain Starch.
Cherry: Corn Syrup, Eucalyptus Oil, FD&C Red 40, Flavors, Sucrose. May contain Starch.
Honey-Lemon: Corn Syrup, D&C Yellow 10, Eucalyptus Oil, FD&C Yellow 6, Flavors, Sucrose. May contain Starch.

Indications: Temporarily relieves coughs and minor throat irritations due to colds or inhaled irritants.

Warnings: Patients with the following conditions are warned not to use these products unless directed by a physician: sore throat that lasts more than 2 days, or persistent or chronic cough such as occurs with smoking, asthma, or emphysema, or if cough is accompanied by excessive phlegm (mucus).
A persistent cough or sore throat may be a sign of a serious condition. Patients are warned to consult a physician if cough persists for more than one week, tends to recur, or is accompanied by fever, rash, or persistent headache, or if sore throat is severe, persistent or accompanied by high fever, headache, nausea, or vomiting.
These products should not be taken by patients who are hypersensitive to any of the ingredients. As with any drug, women who are pregnant or nursing a baby should seek the advice of a health professional before using these products.

Directions: Adults and children 4 years and over: allow cough drop to dissolve slowly in the mouth. May be repeated every hour, as needed, or as directed by a physician. Children under 4 years: as directed by physician.

How Supplied: All 3 flavors of Robitussin Cough Drops are available in bags of 25 drops and sticks of 9 drops: *Menthol Eucalyptus:* Bags (NDC 0031-8622-55); Sticks (NDC 0031-8622-44). *Cherry:* Bags (NDC 0031-8623-55); Sticks (NDC 0031-8623-44). *Honey-Lemon:* Bags (NDC 0031-8621-55); Sticks (NDC 0031-8621-44).
Shown in Product Identification Section, page 422

ROBITUSSIN® MAXIMUM STRENGTH COUGH SUPPRESSANT
[ro "bĭ-tuss 'ĭn]

Description: Each 5 mL (1 teaspoonful) contains:
Dextromethorphan
Hydrobromide, USP .... 15 mg
in a pleasant tasting liquid.

Inactive Ingredients: Citric Acid, FD&C Red 40, Flavors, Glucose, Glycerin, High Fructose Corn Syrup, Saccharin Sodium, Sodium Benzoate, Water.

Indications: Temporarily relieves coughs due to minor throat and bronchial irritation as may occur with a cold.

Warnings: Patients with the following conditions are warned not to take this product unless directed by a physician: persistent or chronic cough such as occurs with smoking, asthma, emphysema, or if cough is accompanied by excessive phlegm (mucus).
A persistent cough may be a sign of a serious condition. If cough persists for more than one week, tends to recur, or is accompanied by fever, rash, or persistent headache, patients should consult a physician.
Patients should not take this product if they are hypersensitive to any of the ingredients. As with any drug, women who are pregnant or nursing a baby should seek the advice of a health professional before using this product.

Contraindications: Hypersensitivity to any of the ingredients, or in patients who are receiving monoamine oxidase inhibitors (MAOIs).

Adverse Reactions: Side effects may include nausea.

Overdose: Symptoms may include ataxia, respiratory depression and convulsions in children, whereas adults may exhibit altered sensory perception, ataxia, slurred speech and dysphoria.

Drug Interaction Precaution: Serious toxicity may result if dextromethorphan is used with MAOIs.

Directions: Adults and children 12 years and over: 2 teaspoonfuls every 6–8 hours in medicine cup. Do not exceed 4 doses in a 24-hour period.

Professional Labeling: Children 6 years to under 12 years, 1 teaspoonful every 6–8 hours; children 2 years to under 6 years, ½ teaspoonful every 6–8 hours. Do not exceed 4 doses in a 24-hour period.

How Supplied: Robitussin Maximum Strength (dark red-colored) in bottles of 4 fl. oz. (NDC 0031-8670-12) and 8 fl. oz. (NDC 0031-8670-18).
Store at Controlled Room Temperature, between 15°C and 30°C (59°F and 86°F).
Shown in Product Identification Section, page 422

ROBITUSSIN® NIGHT RELIEF
[ro "bĭ-tuss 'ĭn]
COUGH/COLD/FLU FORMULA

Description:
Each fluid ounce contains:
Acetaminophen, USP .... 650 mg
Phenylephrine HCl, USP .... 10 mg
Pyrilamine Maleate, USP .... 50 mg
Dextromethorphan
Hydrobromide, USP .... 30 mg

Inactive Ingredients: Citric Acid, FD&C Blue 1, FD&C Red 40, Flavors, Glycerin, Propylene Glycol, Saccharin Sodium, Sodium Benzoate, Sorbitol, Water.

Indications: Temporarily relieves cough, runny nose, sneezing and nasal congestion as may occur with a cold. Also relieves fever, headache, minor sore throat pain, and body aches and pains as may occur with a cold.

Warnings: Patients with any of the following conditions are warned not to take this product, unless directed by a physician: asthma, emphysema, chronic pulmonary disease, shortness of breath, difficulty in breathing, or other persistent or chronic cough such as occurs with smoking, or cough that is accompanied by excessive phlegm (mucus). Likewise, patients with high blood pressure, heart disease, diabetes, thyroid disease, glaucoma, or difficulty in urination due to enlargement of the prostate gland, are warned not to take this product unless directed by a physician.
This product may cause marked drowsiness; alcohol, sedatives and tranquilizers may increase the drowsiness effect. Patients are warned to avoid alcoholic beverages while taking this product and not to take it if they are taking sedatives or tranquilizers without first consulting their physician. Caution should be used when driving a motor vehicle or operating machinery. This product may cause excitability, especially in children.
Patients are told not to exceed the recommended dosage because at higher doses, nervousness, dizziness or sleeplessness may occur. They also are told not to take the product for more than 10 days (for adults) or 5 days (for children). A persistent cough may be a sign of a serious condition. If cough or other symptoms persist for more than one week, tend to recur, or are accompanied by rash, persistent headache, fever that lasts more than

3 days, or if new symptoms occur, patients should consult a physician.
Patients should not take this product if they are hypersensitive to any of the ingredients. As with any drug, women who are pregnant or nursing a baby should seek the advice of a health professional before using this product.
NOTE: Patients are also warned that IN CASE OF ACCIDENTAL OVERDOSE, they should SEEK PROFESSIONAL ASSISTANCE OR CONTACT A POISON CONTROL CENTER IMMEDIATELY. Because of the acetaminophen content, they are told that PROMPT MEDICAL ATTENTION IS CRITICAL FOR ADULTS AS WELL AS FOR CHILDREN, EVEN IF NO SIGNS OR SYMPTOMS ARE NOTED.

Contraindications: Hypersensitivity to any of the ingredients; marked hypertension; hyperthyroidism; patients who are receiving monoamine oxidase inhibitors (MAOIs).

Adverse Effects: The following adverse reactions may possibly occur: nausea, vomiting, diarrhea, or insomnia.

Drug Interaction Precautions: Concomitant administration of phenylephrine with other sympathomimetic agents may produce additive effects and increased toxicity; with MAOIs may produce a hypertensive crisis; with certain antihypertensive agents may diminish their antihypertensive effect. Serious toxicity may result if dextromethorphan is used with MAOIs.

Dosage: If cold keeps the patient confined to bed or at home, one dose should be taken every 6 hours, not to exceed 4 doses in a 24-hour period.
Adults (and children 12 years and over): one fluid ounce in medicine cup at bedtime (2 tablespoons). Children (6 years to under 12 years): ½ fluid ounce in medicine cup at bedtime (1 tablespoon). Under 6 years—consult your physician.

How Supplied: Bottles of 4 fl. oz. (NDC 0031-8641-12) and 8 fl. oz. (NDC 0031-8641-18).
Store at Controlled Room Temperature, between 15°C and 30°C (59°F and 86°F).
Shown in Product Identification Section, page 422

ROBITUSSIN® PEDIATRIC COUGH & COLD FORMULA
[ro "bĭ-tuss 'ĭn]

Description: Each 5 mL (1 teaspoonful) contains:

Continued on next page

Prescribing information on A.H. Robins products listed here is based on official labeling in effect November 1, 1991, with Indications, Contraindications, Warnings, Precautions, Adverse Reactions, and Dosage stated in full.

Robins—Cont.

Dextromethorphan

Hydrobromide, USP .... 7.5 mg
Pseudoephedrine

Hydrochloride .... 15 mg
in a pleasant tasting nonalcoholic liquid.

Inactive Ingredients: Citric Acid, FD&C Red 40, Flavors, Glycerin, Propylene Glycol, Saccharin Sodium, Sodium Benzoate, Sorbitol, Water.

Indications: Temporarily relieves coughs due to minor throat and bronchial irritation and nasal congestion as may occur with a cold.

Warnings: Patients with the following conditions are warned not to take this product unless directed by a physician: persistent or chronic cough such as occurs with smoking, asthma, or emphysema, or if cough is accompanied by excessive phlegm (mucus). Likewise, patients with heart disease, high blood pressure, thyroid disease, diabetes, or difficulty in urination due to enlargement of the prostate gland are warned not to take this product unless directed by a physician.
Patients are warned not to exceed the recommended dosage because at higher doses, nervousness, dizziness or sleeplessness may occur. They also are told not to take this product for more than 7 days. A persistent cough may be a sign of a serious condition. If cough or other symptoms persist for more than one week, tend to recur, or are accompanied by fever, rash, or persistent headache, patients should consult a physician.
Patients should not take this product if they are hypersensitive to any of the ingredients. As with any drug, women who are pregnant or nursing a baby should seek the advice of a health professional before using this product.

Contraindications: Hypersensitivity to any of the ingredients, or in patients who are receiving monoamine oxidase inhibitors (MAOIs).

Adverse Reactions: Side effects may include nausea and restlessness.

Directions: Patients are instructed to follow recommendations on the bottle or carton (see below) or to use as directed by a physician. Doses may be repeated every 6–8 hours, not to exceed 4 doses in a 24-hour period. Dosage should be chosen by weight, if known; if weight is not known, choose by age.

[See table above.]

How Supplied: Robitussin Pediatric Cough & Cold formula (bright red) in bottles of 4 fl. oz. (NDC 0031-8609-12) and 8 fl. oz. (NDC 0031-8609-18).
Store at Controlled Room Temperature, between 15°C and 30°C (59°F and 86°F).

Shown in Product Identification Section, page 422

Age	Weight	Dose
Under 2 yrs.	Under 24 lbs.	As directed by physician.
2 to under 6 yrs.	24–27 lbs.	1 Teaspoonful
6 to under 12 yrs.	48–95 lbs.	2 Teaspoonfuls
12 yrs. and older	96 lbs. and over	4 Teaspoonfuls

ROBITUSSIN® PEDIATRIC
[ro″bi-tuss′in]
COUGH SUPPRESSANT

Description: Each 5 mL (1 teaspoonful) contains:
Dextromethorphan

Hydrobromide, USP .... 7.5 mg
in a pleasant tasting nonalcoholic liquid.

Inactive Ingredients: Citric Acid, FD&C Red 40, Flavors, Glycerin, Propylene Glycol, Saccharin Sodium, Sodium Benzoate, Sorbitol, Water.

Indications: Temporarily relieves coughs due to minor throat and bronchial irritation as may occur with a cold.

Warnings: Patients with the following conditions are warned not to take this product unless directed by a physician: persistent or chronic cough such as occurs with smoking, asthma, or emphysema, or if cough is accompanied by excessive phlegm (mucus).
A persistent cough may be a sign of a serious condition. If cough persists for more than one week, tends to recur, or is accompanied by fever, rash, or persistent headache, patients should consult a physician.
Patients should not take this product if they are hypersensitive to any of the ingredients. As with any drug, women who are pregnant or nursing a baby should seek the advice of a health professional before using this product.

Contraindications: Hypersensitivity to any of the ingredients, or in patients who are receiving monoamine oxidase inhibitors (MAOIs).

Adverse Reactions: Side effects may include nausea.

Overdose: Symptoms may include ataxia, respiratory depression and convulsions in children, whereas adults may exhibit altered sensory perception, ataxia, slurred speech and dysphoria.

Drug Interaction Precaution: Serious toxicity may result if dextromethorphan is used with MAOIs.

Directions: Patients are instructed to follow recommendations on the bottle or carton (see below) or to use as directed by a physician. Doses may be repeated every 6–8 hours, not to exceed 4 doses in a 24-hour period. Dosage should be chosen by weight, if known; if weight is not known, choose by age. [See table below.]

How Supplied: Robitussin Pediatric (cherry-colored) in bottles of 4 fl. oz.

Age	Weight	Dose
Under 2 yrs.	Under 24 lbs.	As directed by physician.
2 to under 6 yrs.	24–27 lbs.	1 Teaspoonful
6 to under 12 yrs.	48–95 lbs.	2 Teaspoonfuls
12 yrs. and older	96 lbs. and over	4 Teaspoonfuls

(NDC 0031-8610-12) and 8 fl. oz. (NDC 0031-8610-18).
Store at Controlled Room Temperature, between 15°C and 30°C (59°F and 86°F).
Shown in Product Identification Section, page 422

Z-BEC® Tablets
[zē′bĕk]
One tablet daily provides:

Vitamin Composition		Percentage of U.S. Recommended Daily Allowance (U.S. RDA)
Vitamin E	150	45.0 I.U.
Vitamin C	1000	600.0 mg
Thiamine (Vitamin B$_1$)	1000	15.0 mg
Riboflavin (Vitamin B$_2$)	600	10.2 mg
Niacin	500	100.0 mg
Vitamin B$_6$	500	10.0 mg
Vitamin B$_{12}$	100	6.0 mcg
Pantothenic Acid	250	25.0 mg

Mineral Composition
Zinc	150	22.5 mg*

*22.5 mg zinc (equivalent to zinc content in 100 mg zinc sulfate, USP)

Ingredients: Niacinamide Ascorbate, Ascorbic Acid, Microcrystalline Cellulose, Vitamin E Acetate, Zinc Sulfate, Calcium Pantothenate, Hydroxypropyl Methylcellulose, Thiamine Mononitrate, Stearic Acid, Pyridoxine Hydrochloride, Riboflavin, Propylene Glycol, Titanium Dioxide, FD&C Blue 1 Aluminum Lake, Methylparaben, Propylparaben, Xanthan Gum, Sodium Citrate, Potassium Sorbate, Silicon Dioxide, Polysorbate 20, Magnesium Stearate, Polyvinylpyrrolidone, Vanillin, Cyanocobalamin.

Actions and Uses: Z-BEC is a high potency formulation. Its components have important roles in general nutrition, healing of wounds, and prevention of hemorrhage. It is recommended for deficiencies of these components in conditions such as febrile diseases, chronic or acute infections, burns, fractures, surgery, leg ulcers, toxic conditions, physiologic stress, alcoholism, prolonged exposure to high temperature, geriatrics, gastritis, peptic ulcer, and colitis; and in conditions involving special diets and weight-reduction diets.
In dentistry, Z-BEC is recommended for deficiencies of its components in conditions such as herpetic stomatitis, aphthous stomatitis, cheilosis, herpangina and gingivitis.

Precaution: Not intended for the treatment of pernicious anemia.

Dosage: The recommended OTC dosage for adults and children 12 or more years of age is one tablet daily with food or after meals. Under the direction and supervision of a physician, the dose and frequency of administration may be increased in accordance with the patient's requirements.

How Supplied: Green film-coated, capsule-shaped tablets engraved AHR on one side and Z-BEC on the other in bottles of 60 (NDC 0031-0689-62), 500 (NDC 0031-0689-70), and Dis-Co® Unit Dose Packs of 100 (NDC 0031-0689-64).

Ross Laboratories
COLUMBUS, OH 43216

PEDIATRIC NUTRITIONAL PRODUCTS

Alimentum® Protein Hydrolysate Formula With Iron

Isomil® Soy Protein Formula With Iron

Isomil® SF Sucrose-Free Soy Protein Formula With Iron

PediaSure® Liquid Nutrition for Children

RCF® Ross Carbohydrate Free Low-Iron Soy Protein Formula Base

Similac® Low-Iron Infant Formula

Similac® PM 60/40 Low-Iron Infant Formula

Similac® Special Care® With Iron 24 Premature Infant Formula

Similac® With Iron Infant Formula

For most current information, refer to product labels.

CLEAR® EYES
[klēr īz]
Lubricating Eye Redness Reliever

Description: Clear Eyes is a sterile, isotonic, buffered solution containing the active ingredients naphazoline hydrochloride (0.012%) and glycerin (0.2%). It also contains boric acid, purified water and sodium borate. Edetate disodium (0.1%) and benzalkonium chloride (0.01%) are added as preservatives. Clear Eyes is a lubricating, decongestant ophthalmic solution specially designed for temporary relief of redness and drying due to minor eye irritation caused by dust, smoke, smog, sun glare, wearing contact lenses, colds, allergies, swimming, reading, driving, TV or close work. Clear Eyes contains laboratory-tested and scientifically blended ingredients, including an effective vasoconstrictor which narrows swollen blood vessels and rapidly whitens reddened eyes in a formulation which also contains a lubricant and produces a refreshing, soothing effect. Clear Eyes is a sterile, isotonic solution compatible with the natural fluids of the eye.

Indications: For the temporary relief of redness due to minor eye irritation AND for protection against further irritation or dryness of the eye.

Warnings: To avoid contamination, do not touch tip of container to any surface. Replace cap after using. If you experience eye pain, changes in vision, continued redness or irritation of the eye, or if the condition worsens or persists for more than 72 hours, discontinue use and consult a doctor. If you have glaucoma, do not use this product except under the advice and supervision of a doctor. Overuse of this product may produce increased redness of the eye. If solution changes color or becomes cloudy, do not use. Keep this and all drugs out of the reach of children.

Directions: Instill 1 or 2 drops in the affected eye(s), up to four times daily.

How Supplied: In 0.5-fl-oz and 1.0-fl-oz plastic dropper bottles.
(FAN 2323)
Shown in Product Identification Section, page 422

CLEAR EYES® ACR
[klēr īz]
Astringent/Lubricating Eye Redness Reliever Drops

Description: Clear Eyes ACR is a sterile, isotonic, buffered solution containing the active ingredients naphazoline hydrochloride (0.012%), zinc sulfate (0.25%) and glycerin (0.2%). It also contains boric acid, purified water and sodium borate. Edetate disodium (0.1%) and benzalkonium chloride (0.01%) are added as preservatives. Clear Eyes ACR is a lubricating, decongestant, astringent ophthalmic solution specially designed for temporary relief of redness and drying due to minor eye irritation caused by dust, smoke, smog, sun glare, wearing contact lenses, colds, allergies, swimming, reading, driving, TV or close work. Clear Eyes ACR contains laboratory-tested and scientifically blended ingredients, including an effective vasoconstrictor which narrows swollen blood vessels and rapidly whitens reddened eyes in a formulation which also contains a lubricant and produces a refreshing, soothing effect. Clear Eyes ACR also contains an ocular astringent (zinc sulfate) that precipitates the sticky mucus buildup on the eye often associated with hay fever, allergies and colds and this helps clear the mucus from the outer surface of the eye. Clear Eyes ACR is a sterile, isotonic solution compatible with the natural fluids of the eye.

Indications: For the temporary relief of redness due to minor eye irritation AND for protection against further irritation or dryness of the eye.

Warnings: To avoid contamination, do not touch tip of container to any surface. Replace cap after using. If you experience eye pain, changes in vision, continued redness or irritation of the eye, or if the condition worsens or persists for more than 72 hours, discontinue use and consult a doctor. If you have glaucoma, do not use this product except under the advice and supervision of a doctor. Overuse of this product may produce increased redness of the eye. If solution changes color or becomes cloudy, do not use. Keep this and all drugs out of the reach of children.

Directions: Instill 1 or 2 drops in the affected eye(s), up to four times daily.

How Supplied: In 0.5-fl-oz and 1.0-fl-oz plastic dropper bottles.
(FAN 2318)
Shown in Product Identification Section, page 422

EAR DROPS BY MURINE®
[myūr'ēn]
See Murine Ear Wax Removal System/Murine Ear Drops.

Shown in Product Identification Section, page 422

MURINE® EAR WAX REMOVAL SYSTEM/MURINE® EAR DROPS
[myūr'ēn]
Carbamide Peroxide
Ear Wax Removal Aid

Description: MURINE EAR DROPS contains the active ingredient carbamide peroxide, 6.5%. It also contains alcohol (6.3%), glycerin, polysorbate 20 and other ingredients. The MURINE EAR WAX REMOVAL SYSTEM includes a 1.0-fl-oz soft bulb ear syringe. This system is a complete medically approved system to safely remove ear wax. Application of carbamide peroxide drops followed by warm-water irrigation is an effective, medically recommended way to help loosen excessive and/or hardened ear wax.

Actions: The carbamide peroxide formula in MURINE EAR DROPS is an aid in the removal of wax from the ear canal. Anhydrous glycerin penetrates and softens wax while the release of oxygen from carbamide peroxide provides a mechanical action resulting in the loosening of the softened wax accumulation. It is usually necessary to remove the loosened wax by gently flushing the ear with warm water, using the soft bulb ear syringe provided.

Indications: The MURINE EAR WAX REMOVAL SYSTEM is indicated for occasional use as an aid to soften, loosen and remove excessive ear wax.

Warnings: DO NOT USE if you have ear drainage or discharge, ear pain, irritation, or rash in the ear or are dizzy; consult a doctor. DO NOT USE if you have an injury or perforation (hole) of the eardrum or after ear surgery, unless directed by a doctor.

Continued on next page

If desired, additional information on any Ross Product will be provided upon request to Ross Laboratories.

Ross—Cont.

DO NOT USE for more than 4 days; if excessive ear wax remains after use of this product, consult a doctor. Avoid contact with the eyes. KEEP THIS AND ALL MEDICINES OUT OF THE REACH OF CHILDREN.

Directions: FOR USE IN THE EAR ONLY. Adults and children over 12 years of age: Tilt head sideways and place 5 to 10 drops in ear. Tip of applicator should not enter ear canal. Keep drops in ear for several minutes by keeping head tilted or placing cotton in the ear. Use twice daily for up to 4 days if needed, or as directed by a doctor. Any wax remaining after treatment may be removed by gently flushing the ear with warm water, using a soft bulb ear syringe. Children under 12 years, consult a doctor.

Note: When the ear canal is irrigated, the tip of the ear syringe should not obstruct the flow of water leaving the ear canal.

How Supplied: The MURINE EAR WAX REMOVAL SYSTEM contains 0.5-fl-oz drops and a 1.0-fl-oz soft bulb ear syringe.

Also available in 0.5-fl-oz drops only, MURINE EAR DROPS.
(FAN 2273)

Shown in Product Identification Section, page 422

MURINE®
[*myūr'ēn*]
Eye Lubricant

Description: Murine eye lubricant is a sterile buffered solution containing the active ingredients 1.4% polyvinyl alcohol and 0.6% povidone. Also contains benzalkonium chloride, dextrose, disodium edetate, potassium chloride, purified water, sodium bicarbonate, sodium chloride, sodium citrate and sodium phosphate (mono- and dibasic). Murine is a clear solution formulated to more closely match the natural tear fluid of the eye for gentle, soothing relief from minor eye irritation while moisturizing and relieving dryness. Use as desired to temporarily relieve minor eye irritation, dryness and burning due to dust, smoke, smog, sun glare, wearing contact lenses, colds, allergies, swimming, reading, driving, TV or close work.

Indications: For the temporary relief or prevention of further discomfort due to minor eye irritations and symptoms related to dry eyes.

Warnings: To avoid contamination, do not touch tip of container to any surface. Replace cap after using. If you experience eye pain, changes in vision, continued redness or irritation of the eye, or if the condition worsens or persists for more than 72 hours, discontinue use and consult a doctor. If solution changes color or becomes cloudy, do not use. Keep this and all drugs out of the reach of children.

Directions: Instill 1 or 2 drops in the affected eye(s) as needed.

How Supplied: In 0.5-fl-oz and 1.0-fl-oz plastic dropper bottles.
(FAN 2321)

Shown in Product Identification Section, page 422

MURINE® PLUS
[*myūr'ēn*]
Lubricating Eye Redness Reliever

Description: Murine Plus is a sterile, non-staining, buffered solution containing the active ingredients 1.4% polyvinyl alcohol, 0.6% povidone and 0.05% tetrahydrozoline hydrochloride. Also contains benzalkonium chloride, dextrose, disodium edetate, potassium chloride, purified water, sodium bicarbonate, sodium chloride, sodium citrate and sodium phosphate (mono- and dibasic). Murine Plus is an isotonic, sterile ophthalmic solution, formulated to more closely match the natural tear fluid of the eye. It contains demulcents for gentle, soothing relief from minor eye irritation as well as the sympathomimetic agent, tetrahydrozoline hydrochloride, which produces local vasoconstriction in the eye. Thus, the drug effectively narrows swollen blood vessels locally and provides symptomatic relief of edema and hyperemia of conjunctival tissues due to eye allergies, minor local irritations and conjunctivitis. Use up to four times daily, to remove redness due to minor eye irritation caused by dust, smoke, smog, sun glare, wearing contact lenses, colds, allergies, swimming, reading, driving, TV or close work. The effect of Murine Plus is prompt (apparent within minutes) and sustained.

Indications: For the temporary relief or prevention of further discomfort due to minor eye irritations and symptoms related to dry eyes PLUS removal of redness.

Warnings: To avoid contamination, do not touch tip of container to any surface. Replace cap after using. If you experience eye pain, changes in vision, continued redness or irritation of the eye, or if the condition worsens or persists for more than 72 hours, discontinue use and consult a doctor. If you have glaucoma, do not use this product except under the advice and supervision of a doctor. Overuse of this product may produce increased redness of the eye. If solution changes color or becomes cloudy, do not use. Keep this and all drugs out of the reach of children.

Directions: Instill 1 or 2 drops in the affected eye(s), up to four times daily.

How Supplied: In 0.5-fl-oz and 1.0-fl-oz plastic dropper bottles.
(FAN 2321)

Shown in Product Identification Section, page 422

PEDIALYTE®
[*pē'dē-ah-līt"*]
Oral Electrolyte Maintenance Solution

Usage: To restore fluid and minerals lost in diarrhea and vomiting by infants and children; to maintain water and electrolytes following corrective parenteral therapy for severe diarrhea.

Features:
* Ready To Use—no mixing or dilution necessary.
* Balanced electrolytes to replace usual stool losses and provide maintenance requirements.
* Provides glucose to promote sodium and water absorption.
* Fruit-flavored form available to enhance compliance in older infants and children. Unflavored form available for younger infants.
* Plastic quart bottles are resealable, easy to pour and easy to measure.
* No coloring added.
* Widely available in grocery, drug and convenience stores.

Availability:
32-fl-oz plastic bottles; 8 per case; Unflavored, No. 336—NDC 0074-6470-32; Fruit-flavored, No. 365—NDC 0074-6471-32.
8-fl-oz bottles; 4 six-packs per case; Unflavored, No. 160—NDC 0074-6470-08. For hospital use, Pedialyte is available in the Ross Hospital Formula System.

Dosage: See Administration Guide to restore fluid and minerals lost in diarrhea and vomiting (Pedialyte Unflavored or Fruit-flavored) and to manage mild to moderate dehydration secondary to moderate to severe diarrhea (Rehydralyte® Oral Electrolyte Rehydration Solution). Pedialyte (Unflavored or Fruit-flavored) or Rehydralyte should be offered frequently in amounts tolerated. Total daily intake should be adjusted to meet individual needs, based on thirst and response to therapy. The suggested intakes for maintenance are based on water requirements for ordinary energy expenditure.[1] The suggested intakes for replacement are based on fluid losses of 5% or 10% of body weight, including maintenance requirement.
[See table on next page.]

Composition: Unflavored Pedialyte (Fruit-flavored Pedialyte has similar composition and nutrient value. For specific information, see product label.)

Ingredients: (Pareve, Ⓤ) Water, dextrose, potassium citrate, sodium chloride and sodium citrate.

Provides:	Per 8 Fl Oz	Per Liter	Per 32 Fl Oz
Sodium (mEq)	10.6	45	42.4
Potassium (mEq)	4.7	20	18.8
Chloride (mEq)	8.3	35	33.2
Citrate (mEq)	7.1	30	28.4
Dextrose (g)	5.9	25	23.6
Calories	24	100	96

(FAN 718-01)

Pedialyte, Rehydralyte Administration Guide

For Infants and Young Children

Age	2 Weeks	3 Months	6 Months	9 Months	1 Years	1½ Years	2 Years	2½ Years	3 Years	3½ Years	4 Years
Approximate Weight[2]											
(lb)	7	13	17	20	23	25	28	30	32	35	38
(kg)	3.2	6.0	7.8	9.2	10.2	11.4	12.6	13.6	14.6	16.0	17.0
PEDIALYTE UNFLAVORED or FRUIT-FLAVORED fl oz/day for maintenance*	13 to 16	28 to 32	34 to 40	38 to 44	41 to 46	45 to 50	48 to 53	51 to 56	54 to 58	56 to 60	57 to 62
REHYDRALYTE fl oz/day for Replacement for 5% Dehydration (including maintenance)*	18 to 21	38 to 42	47 to 53	53 to 59	58 to 63	64 to 69	69 to 74	74 to 79	78 to 82	83 to 87	85 to 90
REHYDRALYTE fl oz/day for Replacement for 10% Dehydration (including maintenance)*	23 to 26	48 to 52	60 to 66	68 to 74	75 to 80	83 to 88	90 to 95	97 to 102	102 to 106	110 to 114	113 to 118

Administration Guide does not apply to infants less than 1 week of age. For children over 4 years, maintenance intakes may exceed 2 qt daily.

1. Extrapolated from Barness L: Nutrition and nutritional disorders, in Behrman RE, Vaughan VC III: *Nelson Textbook of Pediatrics*, ed 12. Philadelphia: WB Saunders Co, 1983, pp 136-138.
2. Weight based on the 50th percentile of weight for age of the National Center for Health Statistics (NCHS) reference data. Hamill PVV, Drizd TA, Johnson CL, et al: Physical growth: National Center for Health Statistics percentiles. *Am J Clin Nutr* 1979; 32:607-629.
* Fluid intakes do not take into account ongoing stool losses. Fluid loss in the stool should be replaced by consumption of an extra amount of Pedialyte or Rehydralyte equal to stool losses in addition to the amounts given in this Administration Guide.

REHYDRALYTE®

[rē-hī 'drə-līt ″]

Oral Electrolyte Rehydration Solution

Usage: For replacement of water and electrolytes lost during moderate to severe diarrhea.

Features:
- Ready To Use—no mixing or dilution necessary.
- Safe, economical alternative to IV therapy.
- 75 mEq of sodium per liter for effective replacement of fluid deficits.
- 2½% glucose solution to promote sodium and water absorption and provide energy.
- Available in pharmacies.

Availability: 8-fl-oz bottles; 4 six-packs per case; No. 162; NDC 0074-0162-01.

Dosage: (See Administration Guide under Pedialyte®.)

Ingredients: (Pareve, Ⓤ) Water, dextrose, sodium chloride, potassium citrate and sodium citrate.

Provides:	Per 8 Fl Oz	Per Liter
Sodium (mEq)	17.7	75
Potassium (mEq)	4.7	20
Chloride (mEq)	15.4	65
Citrate (mEq)	7.1	30
Dextrose (g)	5.9	25
Calories	24	100

(FAN 564-01)

SELSUN BLUE®

[sel 'sun blü]

Dandruff Shampoo

(selenium sulfide lotion, 1%)

Selsun Blue is a non-prescription anti-dandruff shampoo containing the active ingredient selenium sulfide, 1%, in a freshly scented, pH-balanced formula to leave hair clean and manageable. Available in Dry, Oily, Regular, Extra Conditioning and Extra Medicated (also contains 0.5% menthol) formulas.

Inactive ingredients:

Dry formula —Acetylated lanolin alcohol, ammonium laureth sulfate, ammonium lauryl sulfate, cetyl acetate, citric acid, cocamide DEA, cocamidopropyl betaine, DMDM hydantoin, FD&C blue No. 1, fragrance, hydroxypropyl methylcellulose, magnesium aluminum sili-cate, polysorbate 80, sodium chloride, titanium dioxide, water and other ingredients.

Regular formula —Ammonium laureth sulfate, ammonium lauryl sulfate, citric acid, cocamide DEA, cocamidopropyl betaine, DMDM hydantoin, FD&C blue No. 1, fragrance, hydroxypropyl methylcellulose, magnesium aluminum silicate, sodium chloride, titanium dioxide, water and other ingredients.

Oily formula —Ammonium laureth sulfate, ammonium lauryl sulfate, citric acid, cocamide DEA, cocamidopropyl betaine, DMDM hydantoin, FD&C blue No. 1, fragrance, hydroxypropyl methylcellulose, magnesium aluminum silicate, sodium chloride, titanium dioxide, water and other ingredients.

Extra Conditioning formula — Acetylated lanolin alcohol, aloe, ammonium laureth sulfate, ammonium lauryl sulfate, cetyl acetate, citric acid, cocamide DEA, cocamidopropyl betaine, DMDM hydantoin, FD&C blue No. 1, fragrance, glycol distearate, hydroxypropyl methylcellulose, magnesium aluminum silicate, polysorbate 80, propylene glycol, sodium chloride, TEA-lauryl sulfate, titanium dioxide, water and other ingredients.

Extra Medicated formula — Ammonium laureth sulfate, ammonium lauryl sulfate, citric acid, cocamide DEA, cocamidopropyl betaine, DMDM hydantoin, D&C red No. 33, FD&C blue No. 1, fragrance, hydroxypropyl methylcellulose, magnesium aluminum silicate, sodium chloride, TEA-lauryl sulfate, water and other ingredients.

Clinical testing has shown Selsun Blue to be as safe and effective as other leading shampoos in helping control dandruff symptoms with regular use.

Directions: Shake well. Lather, rinse, repeat. For best results, use regularly.

Warnings: For external use only. Avoid contact with eyes—if this happens, rinse thoroughly with water. If condition worsens or does not improve, consult doctor. Keep out of the reach of children. **Caution:** If used on bleached, tinted, or permanent-waved hair, rinse for 5 minutes.

How Supplied: 4-, 7- and 11-fl-oz plastic bottles.

(FAN 2301-02)

Shown in Product Identification Section, page 422

TRONOLANE®

[tron 'ə-lān]

Anesthetic Cream for Hemorrhoids

Description: The active ingredient in Tronolane cream is the topical anesthetic agent, pramoxine hydrochloride, 1% (chemically unrelated to the benzoate esters of the "caine" type), which is chemically designated as a 4-n-butox-

Continued on next page

Ross—Cont.

yphenyl gammamor-pholinopropyl-ether hydrochloride. Also contains the following inactive ingredients: A nongreasy cream base containing beeswax, cetyl alcohol, cetyl esters wax, glycerin, methylparaben, propylparaben, sodium lauryl sulfate and zinc oxide.

Tronolane cream contains a rapidly acting topical anesthetic producing analgesia that lasts up to 5 hours. Because the drug is chemically unrelated to other anesthetics, cross-sensitization is unlikely. Patients who are already sensitized to the "caine" anesthetics can generally use Tronolane cream.

The emollient/emulsion base of Tronolane cream provides soothing lubrication. Tronolane cream is in a nondrying base that is nongreasy and nonstaining to undergarments.

Indications: Tronolane cream is indicated for the temporary relief of the pain, burning, itching and discomfort that accompany hemorrhoids.

Warnings: If condition worsens or does not improve within 7 days, consult a doctor. Do not exceed the recommended daily dosage unless directed by a doctor. In case of bleeding, consult a doctor promptly. Do not put this product into the rectum by using fingers or any mechanical device or applicator. Certain persons can develop allergic reactions to ingredients in this product. If the symptom being treated does not subside, or if redness, irritation, swelling, pain or other symptoms develop or increase, discontinue use and consult a doctor. As with any drug, if you are pregnant or nursing a baby, seek the advice of a health care professional before using this product. Keep this and all drugs out of the reach of children.

Dosage and Administration (Directions): Adults—When practical, cleanse the affected area with mild soap and warm water and rinse thoroughly or cleanse by patting or blotting with an appropriate cleansing pad. Gently dry by patting or blotting with toilet tissue or a soft cloth before application of this product. Apply externally to the affected area up to five times daily. Children under 12 years of age—Consult a doctor.

How Supplied: Tronolane cream is available in 1-oz and 2-oz tubes. (FAN 2313-02)

Shown in Product Identification Section, page 422

TRONOLANE®
[tron'ə-lān]
Hemorrhoidal Suppositories

Description: The active ingredients in Tronolane suppositories are zinc oxide, 5%, and hard fat, 95%. Zinc oxide (an astringent) and hard fat (a skin protectant) afford temporary relief of hemorrhoidal itching and burning and protect irritated hemorrhoidal areas.

Indications: Tronolane suppositories are indicated for the temporary relief of the itching and burning associated with hemorrhoids and the protection of irritated hemorrhoidal areas.

Warnings: If condition worsens or does not improve within 7 days, consult a doctor. Do not exceed the recommended daily dosage unless directed by a doctor. In case of bleeding, consult a doctor promptly. As with any drug, if you are pregnant or nursing a baby, seek the advice of a health care professional before using this product. Keep this and all drugs out of the reach of children.

Dosage and Administration (Directions): Adults—When practical, cleanse the affected area with mild soap and warm water and rinse thoroughly or cleanse by patting or blotting with an appropriate cleansing pad. Gently dry by patting or blotting with toilet tissue or a soft cloth before application of this product. Remove foil wrapper before inserting into the rectum. Use up to six times daily or after each bowel movement. Children under 12 years of age—Consult a doctor.

How Supplied: Tronolane suppositories are available in 10- and 20-count boxes. (FAN 2313-02)

Shown in Product Identification Section, page 422

If desired, additional information on any Ross Product will be provided upon request to Ross Laboratories.

Rydelle Laboratories
Division of S. C. Johnson & Son, Inc.
**1525 HOWE STREET
RACINE, WI 53403**

AVEENO® ANTI-ITCH
[ah-ve'no]
**CREAM AND LOTION
(External analgesic/Skin protectant)**

AVEENO® Anti-Itch Cream provides fast temporary relief of the itching and pain associated with many minor skin irritations such as chicken pox rash, poison ivy/oak/sumac, and insect bites. Unlike hydrocortisone products, AVEENO® Anti-Itch Cream contains calamine to dry up weepy rashes, help control further spreading and promote healing. Aveeno's soothing oatmeal-enriched formula is non-greasy and invisible when rubbed into the skin.

Directions: Adults and children 2 years and older: Apply no more than 4 times daily. Children under 2: Consult a physician.

Warnings: For external use only. Avoid contact with eyes. If condition does not improve or recurs within 7 days, discontinue use and consult a physician. Keep out of children's reach. If ingested, contact a physician or poison control center. Store at 59°–86°F.

Active Ingredients: CALAMINE 3.0%, PRAMOXINE HCl 1.0%, CAMPHOR 0.3% IN A BASE OF WATER, GLYCERIN, DISTEARYLDIMONIUM CHLORIDE, PETROLATUM, OATMEAL FLOUR, ISOPROPYL PALMITATE, CETYL ALCOHOL, DIMETHICONE, SODIUM CHLORIDE.

How Supplied: 1 oz. tube of cream and 4 oz. bottle of lotion.
Shown in Product Identification Section, page 423

AVEENO® BATH TREATMENTS
[ah-ve'no]
REGULAR FORMULA AND OILATED FOR DRY SKIN

AVEENO® BATH TREATMENTS contain colloidal oatmeal, a natural oat derivative developed especially for soothing and cleaning itchy, sore, sensitive skin.
AVEENO® BATH TREATMENTS contain no soaps or synthetic detergents that may be harmful to the skin. They cleanse naturally because of their unique adsorptive properties.
AVEENO® BATH TREATMENTS can be used in the care of itch due to dry skin, rashes, psoriasis, hemorrhoidal and genital irritations, poison ivy/oak, and sunburn. They are safe for use on children and can be used in the treatment of chicken pox, diaper rash, prickly heat and hives.

Ingredients: AVEENO® Bath Regular: 100% colloidal oatmeal; AVEENO® Bath Oilated: 43% colloidal oatmeal, mineral oil.
Shown in Product Identification Section, page 423

AVEENO® CLEANSING BAR
[ah-ve'no]
FOR COMBINATION SKIN

AVEENO® Cleansing Bar For Normal To Oily Skin is made especially for itchy, sensitive skin that is irritated by ordinary soaps.
More than 50% of this mild skin cleanser is colloidal oatmeal, noted for its soothing and protective qualities.
AVEENO® Cleansing Bar is completely soap-free. It leaves no harsh alkaline film to irritate delicate skin, and it leaves skin feeling soft and comfortable.

Ingredients: AVEENO® Colloidal Oatmeal, 51%; in a sudsing soap-free base containing a mild surfactant.
Shown in Product Identification Section, page 423

AVEENO® CLEANSING BAR
[ah-ve'no]
FOR ACNE

AVEENO® Cleansing Bar For Acne is a unique soap-free cleanser. It combines colloidal oatmeal, a long recognized, natural anti-itch treatment and gentle adsorbing cleanser, with special medication to eliminate most blackheads or acne pimples.

Ingredients: AVEENO® Colloidal Oatmeal, 51%; salicylic acid 2%; in a sudsing soap-free base containing a mild surfactant.
Shown in Product Identification Section, page 423

AVEENO® CLEANSING BAR
[ah-ve 'no]
FOR DRY SKIN

AVEENO® Cleansing Bar For Dry Skin is a unique, soap-free cleanser for itchy, dry, sensitive skin that is irritated by ordinary soaps. It contains over 15% skin-softening emollients to help replace natural skin oils and 51% colloidal oatmeal, recommended for its soothing and protective qualities.

Ingredients: AVEENO® Colloidal Oatmeal, 51%, in a sudsing soap-free base containing vegetable oils, glycerine, and a mild surfactant.
Shown in Product Identification Section, page 423

AVEENO® MOISTURIZING CREAM
Soothing Therapy for Dry, Itchy Skin

Aveeno® Moisturizing Cream has been clinically proven to relieve dry skin. The natural colloidal oatmeal in Aveeno Cream allows it to go beyond soothing and moisturizing dry skin to provide prompt relief from persistent itch. Aveeno Cream is noncomedogenic and contains no fragrance, parabens, or lanolin which could cause allergic reactions. Cream formula is especially effective for extra-dry hands, feet and elbows.

Active Ingredient: Colloidal oatmeal 1% in a base of water, glycerin, distearyldimonium chloride, petrolatum, isopropyl palmitate, 1-hexadecanol, dimethicone, sodium chloride, phenylcarbinol. For External Use Only.

How Supplied: 4 oz. jar.
Distributed by:
RYDELLE LABORATORIES
Division of S.C. Johnson & Son, Inc., Racine, WI 53403
ⓒ1991 S.C. Johnson & Son, Inc.
Questions? Call (800) 558-5252 weekdays, 9-5 EST.
See bottom for lot code.
All rights reserved   400740
Made in Canada
Shown in Product Identification Section, page 423

AVEENO® MOISTURIZING LOTION
[ah-ve 'no]
FOR RELIEF OF DRY, ITCHY SKIN

AVEENO® Moisturizing Lotion has been clinically proven to relieve dry skin. It contains natural colloidal oatmeal to relieve the itch often associated with dry skin. It is noncomedogenic and contains no fragrance, parabens, or lanolin which can cause allergic reactions.

Active Ingredient: Colloidal oatmeal 1%.

Also Contains: Water, glycerin, distearyldimonium chloride, petrolatum, isopropyl palmitate, cetyl alcohol, dimethicone, sodium chloride, benzyl alcohol.
Shown in Product Identification Section, page 423

AVEENO® SHOWER AND BATH OIL
[ah-ve 'no]
FOR RELIEF OF DRY, ITCHY SKIN

AVEENO® Shower and Bath Oil combines the lubricating properties of mineral oil with the natural anti-itch benefits of colloidal oatmeal for the relief of dry, itchy skin. It contains no fragrance, parabens or lanolin which can cause allergic reactions.

Active Ingredient: Colloidal oatmeal 5%.
Also contains: Mineral oil, glyceryl stearate and PEG 100 stearate, laureth-4, benzyl alcohol, silica, benzaldehyde.
Shown in Product Identification Section, page 423

RHULICREAM®
(External analgesic/Skin protectant)

Rhulicream® works on contact to provide fast, soothing, temporary relief of the itching and pain associated with many minor skin irritations. Apply this non-greasy calamine formula after exposure to poison ivy/oak/sumac to dry oozing and weeping, help to control further spreading and promote healing.

Directions: Adults and children 2 years and older: Apply to affected area no more than 4 times daily. Children under 2: Consult a physician.

Warnings: For external use only. Avoid contact with eyes. If condition does not improve or recurs within 7 days, discontinue use and consult a physician. Keep out of children's reach. If ingested contact a physician or poison control center. Store at 59°–86°F.

Active Ingredients: CALAMINE 3.0%, PRAMOXINE HCl 1.0%, CAMPHOR 0.3% IN A BASE OF WATER, GLYCERIN, DISTEARYLDIMONIUM CHLORIDE, PETROLATUM, ISOPROPYL PALMITATE, CETYL ALCOHOL, DIMETHICONE, SODIUM CHLORIDE.

How Supplied: 2 oz. tube.
Shown in Product Identification Section, page 423

RHULIGEL®
(External analgesic)

Rhuligel® provides fast, cooling, temporary relief of the itching and pain associated with many minor skin irritations, including poison ivy/oak/sumac, insect bites, and sunburn. Clear Rhuligel® is non-greasy and invisible on the skin. Won't stain clothing.

Directions: Adults and children 2 years and older: Apply to affected area

no more than 4 times daily. Children under 2: Consult a physician.

Warnings: For external use only. Avoid contact with eyes. If condition does not improve or recurs within 7 days, discontinue use and consult a physician. Keep out of children's reach. If ingested contact a physician or poison control center. Store at 59°–86°F.

Active Ingredients: Benzyl Alcohol 2%, Menthol 0.3%, Camphor 0.3% in a base of SD Alcohol 23A 31% w/w, Purified Water, Propylene Glycol, Carbomer 940, Triethanolamine, Benzophenone-4, EDTA.

How Supplied: 2 oz. tube.
Shown in Product Identification Section, page 423

RHULISPRAY®
(External analgesic/Skin protectant)

Rhulispray® works on contact to provide fast, cooling, temporary relief of the itching and pain associated with many minor skin irritations. Calamine-based formula dries the oozing and weeping of poison ivy/oak/sumac. Convenient spray action eliminates the need to touch delicate inflamed skin.

Directions: Shake well before use. Adults and children 2 years and older: Apply to affected area no more than 4 times daily. Children under 2: Consult a physician.

Warnings: For external use only. Avoid contact with eyes. If condition does not improve or recurs within 7 days, discontinue use and consult a physician. Keep out of children's reach. If ingested contact a physician or poison control center. Store at 59°–86°F.

Caution: Flammable. Contents under pressure. Do not puncture or incinerate. Intentional misuse by deliberately concentrating and inhaling the contents can be harmful or fatal. Do not use near an open flame. May burst at temperatures above 120°F.

Active Ingredients (in concentrate): Calamine 13.8%, Benzocaine 5.0%, Camphor 0.7% in a base of Benzyl Alcohol, Hydrated Silica, Isobutane, Isopropyl Alcohol 70% w/w (concentrate), Oleyl Alcohol, Sorbitan Trioleate.

How Supplied: 4 oz. aerosol.
Shown in Product Identification Section, page 423

Products are indexed
by product category
in the
BLUE SECTION.

Sandoz Pharmaceuticals/ Consumer Division
59 ROUTE 10
EAST HANOVER, NJ 07936

ACID MANTLE® CREME
[ă'sĭd-mănt'l]
Acid pH

Description: A greaseless, water-miscible preparation containing buffered aluminum acetate. Other ingredients: aluminum sulfate, calcium acetate, cetearyl alcohol, glycerin, light mineral oil, methylparaben, purified water, sodium lauryl sulfate, synthetic beeswax, white petrolatum, white potato dextrin. May also contain: ammonium hydroxide, citric acid.

Indications: A vehicle for compatible topical drugs. Restores and maintains protective acidity of the skin. Provides relief of mildly irritated skin due to exposure to soaps, detergents, chemicals, alkalis. Aids in the treatment of bath dermatitis, athlete's foot, anogenital pruritis, acne, winter eczema and dry, rough, scaly skin of varied causes.

Caution: Limited compatibility and stability with Vitamin A, neomycin and other water-sensitive antibiotics. For external use only. Not for ophthalmic use.

Warnings: Keep this and all drugs out of the reach of children. In case of accidental ingestion, seek professional assistance or contact a Poison Control Center immediately.

Directions: Apply several times daily, especially after wet work.

How Supplied: 1 oz tubes; 4 oz and 1 lb jars.

BiCOZENE® Creme External Analgesic
[bī-cō-zēn]

Active Ingredients: Benzocaine 6%, resorcinol 1.67% in a specially prepared cream base.

Inactive Ingredients: Castor Oil, Chlorothymol, Ethanolamine Stearates, Glycerin, Glyceryl Borate, Glyceryl Stearates, Parachlorometaxylenol, Polysorbate 80, Sodium Stearate, Triglycerol Diisostearate, Perfume.

Indications: For the temporary relief of pain and itching associated with minor burns, sunburn, minor cuts, scrapes, insect bites or minor skin irritations.

Actions: Benzocaine is a topical anesthetic and resorcinol is a topical antipruritic, at the concentrations used in BiCozene Creme. Both exert their actions by depressing cutaneous sensory receptors.

Warnings: Do not apply over large areas of the body. Caution: Use only as directed. Keep away from the eyes. Not for prolonged use. If the symptoms persist for more than seven days or clear up and reoccur within a few days, or if a rash or irritation develops, discontinue use and consult a physician. For external use only. **KEEP THIS AND ALL DRUGS OUT OF THE REACH OF CHILDREN.** In case of accidental ingestion, seek professional assistance or contact a Poison Control Center immediately.

Drug Interaction Precautions: No known drug interaction.

Dosage and Administration: Adults and children 2 years of age and older: apply to affected area not more than 3 to 4 times daily. Children under 2 years of age: consult a physician. Apply liberally to affected area as needed, several times a day.

How Supplied: BiCozene Creme is available in 1-ounce tubes.
Shown in Product Identification Section, page 423

CAMA® ARTHRITIS PAIN RELIEVER
[kă'măh]

Description: Each CAMA Inlay-Tab contains: aspirin USP, 500 mg (7.7 grains); magnesium oxide, USP, 150 mg; dried aluminum hydroxide gel, USP, equivalent to 125 mg aluminum hydroxide. Other ingredients: colloidal silicon dioxide, croscarmellose sodium, hydrogenated vegetable oil, methylcellulose, methylparaben, microcrystalline cellulose, polyethylene glycol, povidone, pregelatinized starch, starch, Yellow 6, Yellow 10.

Indications: For the temporary relief of minor arthritic pain.

Warnings: Children and teenagers should not use this medicine for chicken pox or flu symptoms before a doctor is consulted about Reye syndrome, a rare but serious illness reported to be associated with aspirin. If redness or swelling is present, consult a doctor because these could be signs of a serious condition. Do not take this drug if you have asthma unless directed by a doctor. Do not take this product if you have stomach problems (such as heartburn, upset stomach, or stomach pain) that persists or recurs, or if you have ulcers or bleeding problems, unless directed by a doctor. If pain persists for more than 10 days, consult a physician immediately. As with any drug, if you are pregnant or nursing a baby, seek the advice of a health professional before using this product. **IT IS ESPECIALLY IMPORTANT NOT TO USE ASPIRIN DURING THE LAST 3 MONTHS OF PREGNANCY UNLESS SPECIFICALLY DIRECTED TO DO SO BY A DOCTOR BECAUSE IT MAY CAUSE PROBLEMS IN THE UNBORN CHILD OR COMPLICATIONS DURING DELIVERY.** Stop taking this product if ringing in the ears, loss of hearing, or dizziness occur. Do not take this product if you are presently taking a prescription drug for anticoagulation (thinning the blood), diabetes, arthritis, gout or if you have an aspirin allergy unless directed by a doctor. Keep this and all medicines out of the reach of children. In case of accidental overdose, contact a physician immediately.

Directions For Use: Adults: 2 tablets with a full glass of water every 6 hours. Not to exceed 8 tablets in 24 hours unless directed by a physician. Do not use in children under 12 years of age except under the advice and supervision of a physician.

How Supplied: CAMA Arthritis Pain Reliever Tablets (white with salmon inlay), imprinted "Cama 500" on one side, "Dorsey" on the other, in bottles of 100.

DORCOL® CHILDREN'S COUGH SYRUP
[door'call]

Description: Each teaspoonful (5 ml) of DORCOL Children's Cough Syrup contains pseudoephedrine hydrochloride 15 mg, guaifenesin 50 mg, dextromethorphan hydrobromide 5 mg. Other ingredients: benzoic acid, Blue 1, edetate disodium, flavors, glycerin, propylene glycol, purified water, Red 40, sodium hydroxide, sucrose, tartaric acid.

Indications: Temporarily relieves your child's cough due to minor throat and bronchial irritation as may occur with the common cold. Helps loosen phlegm (mucus) and thin bronchial secretions to rid the bronchial passageways of bothersome mucus. Helps drain bronchial tubes and makes coughs more productive. Temporarily relieves nasal stuffiness due to the common cold and promotes nasal and/or sinus drainage.

Warnings: Do Not give your child more than the recommended dosage because at higher doses nervousness, dizziness or sleeplessness may occur. Do Not give this preparation if your child has high blood pressure, heart disease, diabetes or thyroid disease. Do Not give this product for persistent or chronic cough such as occurs with asthma or where cough is accompanied by excessive secretions. Keep this and all drugs out of the reach of children. In case of accidental overdose, seek professional assistance or contact a Poison Control Center immediately. A persistent cough may be a sign of a serious condition. If cough or other symptoms persist for more than one week, tend to recur or are accompanied by high fever, rash or persistent headache, consult a physician before continuing use. *Drug Interaction Precaution:* Do not give this product if your child is presently taking a prescription antihypertensive or antidepressant drug containing a monoamine oxidase inhibitor except under the advice and supervision of a physician.

Directions For Use: Children under 2 years—consult physician.
By age:
Children 2 to under 6 years: 1 teaspoonful every 4 hours.
Children 6 to under 12 years: 2 teaspoonfuls every 4 hours.

By weight:

Children 25 to 45 pounds: 1 teaspoonful every 4 hours.

Children 46 to 85 pounds: 2 teaspoonfuls every 4 hours.

Unless directed by a physician, do not exceed 4 doses in 24 hours.

Professional Labeling: The suggested dosage for pediatric patients is:

3–12 months	3 drops/Kg of body weight every 4 hours
12–24 months	7 drops (0.2 ml)/Kg of body weight every 4 hours

Maximum 4 doses in 24 hours.

How Supplied: DORCOL Children's Cough Syrup (grape colored), in 4 fl oz and 8 fl oz plastic bottles with tamper-evident band around child-resistant cap.

Shown in Product Identification Section, page 423

DORCOL® CHILDREN'S DECONGESTANT LIQUID
[door 'call]

Description: Each teaspoonful (5 ml) of DORCOL Children's Decongestant Liquid contains pseudoephedrine hydrochloride 15 mg. Other ingredients: benzoic acid, edetate disodium, flavors, purified water, sodium hydroxide, sorbitol, sucrose, Yellow 6, Yellow 10.

Indications: Provides temporary relief of nasal congestion due to the common cold, hay fever or other upper respiratory allergies, or associated with sinusitis. Reduces swelling of nasal passages to restore freer breathing through the nose. Promotes nasal and sinus drainage; relieves sinus pressure.

Directions For Use: Children under 2 years—consult physician.

By age:

Children 2 to under 6 years: 1 teaspoonful every 4 to 6 hours.

Children 6 years and older: 2 teaspoonfuls every 4 to 6 hours.

By weight:

Children 25 to 45 pounds: 1 teaspoonful every 4 to 6 hours.

Children 46 to 85 pounds: 2 teaspoonfuls every 4 to 6 hours.

Unless directed by a physician, do not exceed 4 doses in 24 hours.

Professional Labeling: The suggested dosage for pediatric patients is:

3–12 Months	3 drops/Kg of body weight every 4–6 hours
12–24 months	7 drops (0.2 ml)/Kg of body weight every 4–6 hours

Maximum of 4 doses in 24 hours.

Warnings: Do not give your child more than the recommended dosage because at higher doses nervousness, dizziness, or sleeplessness may occur. If symptoms do not improve within seven days or are accompanied by high fever, consult a physician before continuing use. Do not give this preparation if your child has high blood pressure, heart disease, diabetes, or thyroid disease except under the advice and supervision of a physician. Keep this and all drugs out of the reach of children. In case of accidental overdose, seek professional assistance or contact a Poison Control Center immediately. *Drug Interaction Precaution:* Do not give this product if your child is presently taking a prescription antihypertensive or antidepressant drug containing a monoamine oxidase inhibitor except under the advice and supervision of a physician.

How Supplied: DORCOL Children's Decongestant Liquid (pale orange), in 4 fl oz bottles with tamper-evident band around child-resistant cap.

Shown in Product Identification Section, page 423

DORCOL® CHILDREN'S LIQUID COLD FORMULA
[door 'call]

Description: Each teaspoonful (5 ml) of DORCOL Children's Liquid Cold Formula contains: pseudoephedrine hydrochloride 15 mg and chlorpheniramine maleate 1 mg. Other ingredients: benzoic acid, Blue 1, flavors, purified water, Red 40, sorbitol, sucrose, Yellow 10. May also contain sodium hydroxide.

Indications: Provides temporary relief of nasal congestion, sneezing and rhinorrhea due to the common cold, hay fever or other upper respiratory allergies or associated with sinusitis. Reduces swelling of nasal passages and restores freer breathing. Promotes nasal and sinus drainage; relieves sinus pressure.

Directions For Use: Children under 6 years—consult physician.

By age:

Children 6 to under 12 years: 2 teaspoonfuls every 4 to 6 hours.

By weight:

Children 45 to 85 pounds: 2 teaspoonfuls every 4 to 6 hours.

Unless directed by a physician, do not exceed 4 doses in 24 hours.

Professional Labeling: The suggested dosage for pediatric patients is:

3–12 months	2 drops/Kg of body weight every 4–6 hours
12–24 months	5 drops (0.2 ml)/Kg of body weight every 4–6 hours
2–6 years	1 teaspoonful every 4–6 hours

Maximum of 4 doses in 24 hours.

Warnings: Do not give your child more than the recommended dosage because at higher doses nervousness, dizziness, or sleeplessness may occur. Do not give this preparation if your child has high blood pressure, heart disease, diabetes, thyroid disease, asthma, or glaucoma, except under the advice and supervision of a physician. If symptoms do not improve within 7 days or are accompanied by high fever, consult a physician before continuing use. May cause drowsiness. May cause excitability especially in children. Keep this and all drugs out of the reach of children. In case of accidental overdose, seek professional assistance or contact a Poison Control Center immediately. *Drug Interaction Precaution:* Do not give this product if your child is presently taking a prescription antihypertensive, sedatives, tranquilizers, or antidepressant drug containing a monoamine oxidase inhibitor except under the advice and supervision of a physician.

Caution: Avoid alcoholic beverages or operating a motor vehicle or heavy machinery while taking this product.

How Supplied: DORCOL Children's Liquid Cold Formula (light brown), in 4 fl oz bottles with tamper-evident band around child-resistant cap.

Shown in Product Identification Section, page 423

EX–LAX® Chocolated Laxative Tablets

Active Ingredient: Yellow phenolphthalein, 90 mg. phenolphthalein per tablet.

Inactive Ingredients: Cocoa, Confectioners' Sugar, Hydrogenated Palm Kernel Oil, Lecithin, Nonfat Dry Milk, Vanillin.

Indication: For relief of occasional constipation (irregularity).

Caution: Do not take any laxative when abdominal pain, nausea, or vomiting are present. Frequent or prolonged use of this or any other laxative may result in dependence on laxatives. If skin rash appears, do not use this or any other preparation containing phenolphthalein.

Warnings: Keep this and all drugs out of the reach of children. In case of accidental overdose, seek professional assistance or contact a poison control center immediately. As with any drug, if you are pregnant or nursing a baby, seek the advice of a health care professional before using this product.

Drug Interaction Precautions: No known drug interaction.

Dosage and Administration: Adults: Chew 1 to 2 tablets, preferably at bedtime. Children over 6 years: Chew ½ to 1 tablet.

How Supplied: Available in boxes of 6, 18, 48, and 72 chewable chocolate-flavored tablets.

Shown in Product Identification Section, page 423

EX–LAX® Laxative Pills

**Regular Strength Ex-Lax®
Laxative Pills
Extra Gentle Ex-Lax® Laxative Pills
Maximum Relief Formula Ex-Lax®
Laxative Pills**

Active Ingredients: Regular Strength Ex-Lax Laxative Pills—Yellow phe-

Continued on next page

Sandoz Pharm.—Cont.

nolphthalein, 90 mg. phenolphthalein per pill. **Extra Gentle Ex-Lax Laxative Pills**—Docusate sodium, 75 mg. and yellow phenolphthalein, 65 mg. per pill. **Maximum Relief Formula Ex-Lax Laxative Pills**—Yellow phenolphthalein, 135 mg. phenolphthalein per pill.

Inactive Ingredients: Regular Strength Ex-Lax Laxative Pills—Acacia, Alginic Acid, Carnauba Wax, Colloidal Silicon Dioxide, Dibasic Calcium Phosphate, Iron Oxides, Magnesium Stearate, Microcrystalline Cellulose, Sodium Benzoate, Sodium Lauryl Sulfate, Starch, Stearic Acid, Sucrose, Talc, Titanium Dioxide. **Extra Gentle Ex-Lax Laxative Pills**—Acacia, Croscarmellose Sodium, Dibasic Calcium Phosphate, Colloidal Silicon Dioxide, Magnesium Stearate, Microcrystalline Cellulose, Red 7, Stearic Acid, Sucrose, Talc, Titanium Dioxide. **Maximum Relief Formula Ex-Lax Laxative Pills**—Acacia, Alginic Acid, Blue No. 1, Carnauba Wax, Colloidal Silicon Dioxide, Dibasic Calcium Phosphate, Magnesium Stearate, Microcrystalline Cellulose, Povidone, Sodium Benzoate, Sodium Lauryl Sulfate, Starch, Stearic Acid, Sucrose, Talc, Titanium Dioxide.

Indication: For relief of occasional constipation (irregularity).

Caution: Do not take any laxative when abdominal pain, nausea, or vomiting are present. Frequent or prolonged use of this or any other laxative may result in dependence on laxatives. If skin rash appears, do not use this or any other preparation containing phenolphthalein.

Warnings: Keep this and all drugs out of the reach of children. In case of accidental overdose, seek professional assistance or contact a Poison Control Center immediately. As with any drug, if you are pregnant or nursing a baby, seek the advice of a health care professional before using this product.

Drug Interaction Precautions: No known drug interaction.

Dosage and Administration: Regular Strength Ex-Lax Laxative Pills and Extra Gentle Ex-Lax Laxative Pills—Adults take 1 to 2 pills with a glass of water, preferably at bedtime. Children over 6 years: 1 pill, as needed. **Maximum Relief Formula Ex-Lax Laxative Pills**—Adults and children over 12 years of age, take 1 to 2 pills with a glass of water, preferably at bedtime. Consult with a physician for children under 12 years of age.

How Supplied: Extra Strength Ex-Lax Laxative Pills—Available in boxes of 8, 30, and 60 pills. **Extra Gentle Ex-Lax Laxative Pills and Maximum Relief Formula Ex-Lax Laxative Pills**—Available in boxes of 24 pills.
Shown in Product Identification Section, page 423

GAS-X® AND EXTRA STRENGTH GAS-X®
High–Capacity Antiflatulent Tablets

Active Ingredients: GAS-X®—Each tablet contains 80 mg. simethicone. EXTRA STRENGTH GAS-X®—Each tablet contains 125 mg. simethicone.

Inactive Ingredients: calcium phosphates dibasic and tribasic, colloidal silicon dioxide, calcium silicate, microcrystalline cellulose, flavors, compressible sugar and talc. Extra strength Gas-X also contains Red 30 and Yellow 10.

Indications: For relief of the pain and pressure symptoms of excess gas in the digestive tract, which is often accompanied by complaints of bloating, distention, fullness, pressure, pain, cramps or excess anal flatus.

Actions: GAS-X acts in the stomach and intestines to disperse and reduce the formation of mucus-trapped gas bubbles. The GAS-X defoaming action reduces the surface tension of gas bubbles so that they are more easily eliminated.

Warning: Keep this and all medicines out of the reach of children.

Drug Interaction Precautions: No known drug interaction.

Dosage and Administration: Adults: Chew thoroughly and swallow one or two tablets as needed after meals and at bedtime. Do not exceed six GAS-X tablets or four EXTRA STRENGTH GAS-X tablets in 24 hours, except under the advice and supervision of a physician.

Professional Labeling: GAS-X may be useful in the alleviation of postoperative gas pain, and for use in endoscopic examination.

How Supplied: GAS-X is available in white, chewable, scored tablets in boxes of 36 tablets and convenience packages of 12 tablets.
EXTRA STRENGTH GAS-X is available in yellow, chewable, scored tablets in boxes of 18 tablets and 48 tablets.
Shown in Product Identification Section, page 423

GENTLE NATURE®
Natural Vegetable Laxative Tablets

Active Ingredients: 20 mg. Sennosides per tablet.

Inactive Ingredients: Alginic Acid, Calcium Phosphate Dibasic, Magnesium Stearate, Microcrystalline Cellulose, Silicon Dioxide, Sodium Lauryl Sulfate, Starch, Stearic Acid.

Indications: For short-term relief of constipation.

Actions: Sennosides is a highly purified form of senna. The purification process removes components found in senna concentrate which may cause griping and cramps.
Sennosides has no laxative effect until they are carried to the lower part of the

alimentary system by the regular working of the digestive process. In the bowel, the active glycosides are freed by the natural bowel micro-organisms. The freed laxative agent then gently encourages the muscle wave action of elimination. The gentle, predictable working of the laxative in the bowel, usually in 8–10 hours, or overnight if taken at bedtime, is apt to produce a well-formed stool in a natural-feeling way.

Caution: Not to be used when abdominal pain, nausea, or vomiting are present. Take only as needed. Frequent or prolonged use may result in dependence on laxatives. Keep this and all medications out of reach of children. In case of accidental overdose, seek professional assistance or contact a Poison Control Center immediately.

Drug Interaction Precautions: No known drug interaction.

Warning: As with any drug, if you are pregnant or nursing a baby, seek the advice of a health professional before using this product.

Dosage and Administration: Adults—Take 1 or 2 tablets daily with water, preferably at bedtime, or as directed by your physician. Children over 6 years—1 tablet daily as required.

How Supplied: Available in boxes of 16 blister packed uncoated pills.
Shown in Product Identification Section, page 423

THERAFLU®
Flu and Cold Medicine
Flu, Cold & Cough Medicine

Description: Each packet of TheraFlu Flu and Cold Medicine contains: acetaminophen 650 mg, pseudoephedrine hydrochloride 60 mg, and chlorpheniramine maleate 4 mg. Each packet of TheraFlu Flu, Cold & Cough Medicine also contains dextromethorphan hydrobromide 20 mg. Other ingredients: ascorbic acid, citric acid, natural lemon flavors, sodium citrate, sucrose, titanium dioxide, tribasic calcium phosphate, pregelatinized starch, Yellow 6, and Yellow 10.

Indications: Provides temporary relief of the symptoms associated with flu, common cold and other upper respiratory infections including: headache, body-aches, fever, minor sore throat pain, nasal and sinus congestion, runny nose and sneezing. TheraFlu Flu, Cold & Cough Medicine also suppresses coughs due to minor throat and bronchial irritation.

Warnings: Keep this and all drugs out of the reach of children. In case of accidental overdose, seek professional assistance or contact a Poison Control Center immediately. Prompt medical attention is critical for adults as well as children even if you do not notice any signs or symptoms. Unless directed by a doctor, do not take this product if you have heart disease, high blood pressure, thyroid disease, diabetes, asthma, glaucoma, difficulty in breathing, or difficulty in urination due to enlargement of the prostate gland or are taking a prescription drug for high blood pressure or depression or are taking sedatives or tranquilizers without first consulting your doctor. Do not exceed recommended dosage or take for more than 7 days. If symptoms persist or new ones occur, or if fever persists for more than 3 days or recurs, consult a doctor. May cause excitability, especially in children. May cause marked drowsiness. Avoid drinking alcohol since alcohol may increase the drowsiness effect. Do not drive or operate machinery while taking this product. As with any drug, if you are pregnant or nursing a baby, seek the advice of a health professional before using this product. Do not take the cough formula if cough is accompanied by excessive secretions, for persistent cough such as occurs with smoking, asthma, or emphysema. A persistent cough may be sign of a serious condition. If cough recurs, or is accompanied by fever, rash or persistent headache, consult a doctor.

Dosage and Administration: Adults and children 12 years and over—dissolve one packet in 6 oz. cup of hot water. Sip while hot. If using microwave, add contents of packet and 6 oz. of cool water to a microwave-safe cup and stir briskly. Microwave on high 1½ minutes or until water is hot. Do not boil water or overheat and remember to stir liquid between reheatings. May repeat every 4 hours, but not to exceed 4 doses in 24 hours.

How Supplied: TheraFlu Flu and Cold Medicine powder in foil packets, 6 or 12 packets per carton. TheraFlu Flu, Cold & Cough Medicine powder in foil packets, 6 or 12 packets per carton.
Shown in Product Identification Section, page 423

TRIAMINIC® ALLERGY TABLETS
[trī"ah-mĭn'ĭc]

Description: Each tablet contains: phenylpropanolamine hydrochloride 25 mg and chlorpheniramine maleate 4 mg. Other ingredients: calcium stearate, calcium sulfate, colloidal silicon dioxide, methylcellulose, methylparaben, microcrystalline cellulose, polyethylene glycol, povidone, pregelatinized starch, titanium dioxide, Yellow 10.

Indications: For the temporary relief of runny nose, nasal congestion, sneezing, itching of the eyes, nose or throat and watery eyes as may occur in hay fever or other upper respiratory allergies (allergic rhinitis).

Warnings: Do not take this product if you have high blood pressure, heart disease, diabetes, thyroid disease, asthma, glaucoma, emphysema, chronic pulmonary disease, shortness of breath, difficulty in breathing or difficulty in urination due to enlargement of the prostate gland or are taking a prescription drug for high blood pressure or depression unless directed by a doctor. Do not exceed the recommended dosage because at

higher doses nervousness, dizziness or sleeplessness may occur or take for more than 7 days. This preparation may cause drowsiness; alcohol, sedatives and tranquilizers may increase the drowsiness effect; avoid alcoholic beverages; do not operate machinery or drive a motor vehicle while taking this product; this preparation may cause excitability, especially in children. If symptoms do not improve within seven days or are accompanied by high fever, consult a doctor. As with any drug, if you are pregnant or nursing a baby, seek the advice of a health professional before using this product. Keep this and all drugs out of the reach of children. In case of accidental overdose, seek professional assistance or contact a Poison Control Center immediately.

Directions: Adults and children over 12 years of age—1 tablet every 4 hours. Children 6 to under 12 years, ½ tablet every 4 hours. Unless directed by physician, do not exceed 6 doses in 24 hours or give to children under 6 years.

How Supplied: Triaminic Allergy Tablets (yellow), scored, in blister packs of 24.

TRIAMINIC® CHEWABLES
[trī"ah-mĭn'ĭc]

Description: Each TRIAMINIC Chewable contains: phenylpropanolamine hydrochloride 6.25 mg, chlorpheniramine maleate 0.5 mg. Other ingredients: calcium stearate, citric acid, flavors, magnesium trisilicate, mannitol, microcrystalline cellulose, saccharin sodium, sucrose, Yellow 6, Yellow 10.

Indications: For the temporary relief of children's nasal congestion, runny nose, and sneezing due to the common cold or hay fever.

Warnings: Do not exceed recommended dosage because at higher doses nervousness, dizziness, or sleeplessness may occur. Do not give this product to children for more than 7 days. If symptoms do not improve or are accompanied by fever, consult a doctor. Do not give this product to children who have heart disease, high blood pressure, thyroid disease, diabetes, asthma, emphysema, shortness of breath, chronic pulmonary disease or glaucoma unless directed by a doctor. May cause drowsiness. Sedatives and tranquilizers may increase the drowsiness effect. May cause excitability.
Drug Interaction Precaution: Do not give this product to a child who is taking a prescription drug for high blood pressure or depression, without first consulting the child's doctor. Keep this and all drugs out of the reach of children. In case of accidental overdose, seek professional assistance or contact a Poison Control Center immediately.

Dosage: Children 6 to 12 years—2 tablets every 4 hours. Children under 6, consult your physician.

Professional Labeling: The suggested dosage for children 2 to 6 years is 1 tablet every 4 hours.

How Supplied: TRIAMINIC Chewables (hexagonal, yellow), in blister packs of 24. Orange flavor.

TRIAMINIC® COLD TABLETS
[trī"ah-mĭn'ĭc]

Description: Each tablet contains: phenylpropanolamine hydrochloride 12.5 mg and chlorpheniramine maleate 2 mg. Other ingredients: calcium stearate, colloidal silicon dioxide, flavor, lactose, methylcellulose, methylparaben, microcrystalline cellulose, polyethylene glycol, povidone, pregelatinized starch, Red 40, titanium dioxide, Yellow 6.

Indications: For the temporary relief of nasal congestion due to the common cold, hay fever or other upper respiratory allergies and associated with sinusitis. Helps decongest sinus openings, sinus passages, promotes nasal and/or sinus drainage, temporarily restores freer breathing through the nose. For temporary relief of runny nose, sneezing, itching of the nose or throat and itchy and watery eyes as may occur in allergic rhinitis (such as hay fever).

Warnings: Do not take this product if you have high blood pressure, heart disease, diabetes, thyroid disease, asthma, glaucoma, emphysema, chronic pulmonary disease, shortness of breath, difficulty in breathing or difficulty in urination due to enlargement of the prostate gland or are taking a prescription drug for high blood pressure or depression unless directed by a doctor. Do not exceed the recommended dosage because at higher doses nervousness, dizziness or sleeplessness may occur or take for more than 7 days. This preparation may cause drowsiness; alcohol, sedatives and tranquilizers may increase the drowsiness effect; avoid alcoholic beverages; do not operate machinery or drive a motor vehicle while taking this product; this preparation may cause excitability, especially in children. If symptoms do not improve within seven days or are accompanied by high fever, consult a doctor. As with any drug, if you are pregnant or nursing a baby, seek the advice of a health professional before using this product. Keep this and all drugs out of the reach of children. In case of accidental overdose, seek professional assistance or contact a Poison Control Center immediately.

Directions: Adults and children 12 years of age and older: 2 tablets every 4 hours. Children 6 to under 12 years, 1 tablet every 4 hours. Unless directed by physician, do not exceed 6 doses in 24 hours or give to children under 6 years.

How Supplied: Triaminic Cold Tablets (orange) imprinted "DORSEY" on one side, "TRIAMINIC" on the other, in blister packs of 24.

Shown in Product Identification Section, page 424

Continued on next page

Sandoz Pharm.—Cont.

TRIAMINIC® EXPECTORANT
[trī"ah-mĭn'ĭc]

Description: Each teaspoonful (5 ml) of TRIAMINIC Expectorant contains: phenylpropanolamine hydrochloride 12.5 mg and guaifenesin 100 mg in a palatable, citrus-flavored alcohol-free liquid. Other ingredients: benzoic acid, edetate disodium, flavors, purified water, saccharin, saccharin sodium, sodium hydroxide, sorbitol, sucrose, Yellow 6, Yellow 10.

Indications: Provides prompt relief of nasal congestion due to the common cold. The expectorant component helps loosen bronchial secretions and rid the bronchial passageways of bothersome mucus. The decongestant and expectorant are provided in an antihistamine-free formula.

Warnings: Do not take this product: 1) if cough is accompanied by excessive secretions, 2) for persistent cough such as occurs with smoking, asthma or emphysema, or 3) if you have heart disease, high blood pressure, thyroid disease, diabetes, difficulty in urination due to enlargement of the prostate gland, or are taking a prescription drug for high blood pressure or depression, unless directed by a doctor. Do not: 1) give this product to children under two years of age, 2) exceed recommended dosage, or 3) take for more than 7 days, unless directed by a doctor. If symptoms persist, are accompanied by a fever, rash or persistent headache or if cough recurs, consult a doctor. As with any drug, if you are pregnant or nursing a baby, seek advice from a health professional before using this product. Keep this and all drugs out of the reach of children. In case of accidental overdose, seek professional assistance or contact a Poison Control Center immediately.

Dosage and Administration: Adults and children 12 and over (96+ lbs)— 2 teaspoonfuls every 4 hours. Children 6 to under 12 years (48–95 lbs)—1 teaspoonful every 4 hours. Children 2 to under 6 years (24–47 lbs)—½ teaspoonful every 4 hours. Unless directed by physician, do not exceed 6 doses in 24 hours or give to children under 2 years of age.

Professional Labeling: The suggested dosage for pediatric patients is:

3–12 months	.75 ml (⅛ tsp)*	
(12–17 lbs)	every 4 hours	
12–24 months	1.25 ml (¼ tsp)	
(18–23 lbs)	every 4 hours	

*(⅛ tsp is appproximately .75 ml)

How Supplied: TRIAMINIC Expectorant (yellow), in 4 fl oz and 8 fl oz plastic bottles with tamper-evident band around child-resistant cap. Citrus flavored, Alcohol free.

Shown in Product Identification Section, page 424

TRIAMINIC® NITE LIGHT®
Nighttime Cough and Cold Medicine for Children
[trī"ah-mĭn'ĭc]

Description: Each teaspoonful (5 ml) of Triaminic® Nite Light® contains: Pseudoephedrine hydrochloride 15 mg, chlorpheniramine maleate 1 mg, dextromethorphan hydrobromide 7.5 mg in a palatable, grape-flavored, alcohol-free liquid. Other ingredients: benzoic acid, Blue 1, citric acid, flavors, propylene glycol, purified water, Red 33, dibasic sodium phosphate, sorbitol, sucrose.

Indications: Temporarily quiets your child's cough associated with the common cold. Also, provides temporary relief of nasal stuffiness, sneezing, runny nose, and itchy watery eyes caused by the common cold, hay fever or other upper respiratory allergies.

Warnings: Do not exceed recommended dosage or take for more than 7 days. A persistent cough may be a sign of a serious condition. If symptoms persist for more than one week, tend to recur, or are accompanied by fever, rash, or persistent headache, consult a physician. May cause excitability especially in children. Unless directed by a physician, do not take this product: 1) if cough is accompanied by excessive phlegm (mucus), 2) for persistent or chronic cough such as occurs with smoking, asthma or emphysema, or 3) if you or your child has heart disease, high blood pressure, thyroid disease, diabetes, asthma, glaucoma, difficulty in breathing, or difficulty in urination due to enlargement of the prostate gland. May cause marked drowsiness. Alcohol, sedatives, and tranquilizers may increase the drowsiness effect. Avoid alcoholic beverages while taking this product. Avoid driving a motor vehicle or operating machinery. As with any drug, if you are pregnant or nursing a baby, seek the advice of a health professional before using this product. Keep this and all drugs out of the reach of children. In case of accidental overdose, seek professional assistance, or call a Poison Control Center immediately.

Drug Interaction Precaution: Do not take this product if you are taking a prescription drug for high blood pressure or depression, or if you are taking sedatives or tranquilizers, without first consulting your physician.

Dosage and Administration: Children 12 and over (96+ lbs.)—4 teaspoonfuls every 6–8 hours. Children 6 to under 12 years (48–95 lbs.)—2 teaspoonfuls every 6–8 hours. Unless directed by physician, do not exceed 4 doses in 24 hours. For convenience, a True-Dose™ dosage cup is provided with each 4 fl. oz. and 8 fl. oz. bottle.

Professional Labeling: The suggested dosage for pediatric patients is:

3 to under 12 months (12–17 lbs.)	¼ teaspoon or 1.25 ml	
12 months to under 2 years (18–23 lbs.)	½ teaspoon or 2.5 ml	
2 to under 6 years	1 teaspoonful or 5 ml	

How Supplied: Triaminic® Nite Light™ Nighttime Cough and Cold Medicine for Children (purple), in 4 fl. oz. and 8 fl. oz. plastic bottles packaged in cartons with tamper-evident band around child-resistant cap. Grape flavored. Alcohol free.

Shown in Product Identification Section, page 424

TRIAMINIC® SYRUP
[trī"ah-mĭn'ĭc]

Description: Each teaspoonful (5 ml) of TRIAMINIC Syrup contains: phenylpropanolamine hydrochloride 12.5 mg and chlorpheniramine maleate 2 mg in a palatable, orange-flavored, alcohol-free liquid. Other ingredients: benzoic acid, edetate disodium, flavors, purified water, sodium hydroxide, sorbitol, sucrose. Contains FD&C Yellow No. 6 as a color additive.

Indications: Provides temporary relief of nasal congestion, runny nose and sneezing that may occur with the common cold or with hay fever or other upper respiratory allergies. Relieves itching of the nose or throat and itchy, watery eyes.

Warnings: Do not take this product: 1) if you have heart disease, high blood pressure, thyroid disease, diabetes, asthma, glaucoma, emphysema, shortness of breath, chronic pulmonary disease, difficulty in breathing, difficulty in urination due to enlargement of the prostate gland, or 2) if you are taking a prescription drug for high blood pressure or depression, or 3) if you are taking sedatives or tranquilizers, unless directed by a doctor. Do not exceed recommended dosage because at higher doses nervousness, dizziness, or sleeplessness may occur. Do not take for more than 7 days. If symptoms persist or are accompanied by fever, consult a doctor. May cause excitability especially in children. May cause drowsiness. Alcohol, sedatives, or tranquilizers may increase drowsiness. Avoid driving a motor vehicle or operating machinery while taking this product. As with any drug, if you are pregnant or nursing a baby, seek the advice of a health professional before using this product. Keep this and all drugs out of the reach of children. In case of accidental overdose, seek professional assistance or contact a Poison Control Center immediately.

Dosage and Administration: Adults and children 12 and over (96+ lbs)— 2 teaspoonfuls every 4 hours. Children 6 to under 12 years (48–95 lbs)—1 teaspoonful every 4 hours. Unless directed by physician, do not exceed 6 doses in 24 hours. Consult physician for dosage under 6 years of age.

Professional Labeling: The suggested dosage for pediatric patients is:

3–12 months	.75 ml (⅛ tsp)*
(12–17 lbs)	every 4 hours
12–24 months	1.25 ml (¼ tsp)
(18–23 lbs)	every 4 hours
2–6 years	2.5 ml (½ tsp)
(24–47 lbs)	every 4 hours

*(⅛ tsp is approximately .75 ml)

How Supplied: TRIAMINIC Syrup (orange), in 4 fl oz and 8 fl oz plastic bottles with tamper-evident band around child-resistant cap. Orange flavored. Alcohol-free.

Shown in Product Identification Section, page 423

TRIAMINIC–DM® SYRUP
[trī "ah-mĭn 'ĭc]

Description: Each teaspoonful (5 ml) of TRIAMINIC-DM Syrup contains: phenylpropanolamine hydrochloride 12.5 mg and dextromethorphan hydrobromide 10 mg in a palatable, berry-flavored alcohol-free liquid. Other ingredients: benzoic acid, Blue 1, flavors, propylene glycol, purified water, Red 40, sodium chloride, sorbitol, sucrose.

Indications: Provides relief of cough due to minor throat and bronchial irritation as may occur with the common cold or inhaled irritants. Promotes nasal and sinus drainage. The decongestant and antitussive are provided in an alcohol-free and antihistamine-free formula.

Warnings: Do not take this product: 1) if cough is accompanied by excessive secretions, 2) for persistent cough such as occurs with smoking, asthma or emphysema, or 3) if you have heart disease, high blood pressure, thyroid disease, diabetes, difficulty in urination due to enlargement of the prostate gland, or are taking a prescription drug for high blood pressure or depression, unless directed by a doctor. Do not exceed recommended dosage because at higher doses nervousness, dizziness or sleeplessness may occur. Do not take for more than 7 days. If symptoms persist, are accompanied by a fever, rash or persistent headache or if cough recurs, consult a doctor. As with any drug, if you are pregnant or nursing a baby, seek the advice of a health professional before using this product. Keep this and all drugs out of the reach of children. In case of accidental overdose, seek professional assistance or contact a Poison Control Center immediately.

Dosage and Administration: Adults and children 12 and over (96+ lbs)—2 teaspoonfuls every 4 hours. Children 6 to under 12 years (48–95 lbs)—1 teaspoonful every 4 hours. Children 2 to under 6 years (24–47 lbs)—½ teaspoonful every 4 hours. Unless directed by physician, do not exceed 6 doses in 24 hours or give to children under 2 years of age.

Professional Labeling: The suggested dosage for pediatric patients is:

3–12 months	.75 ml (⅛ tsp)*
(12–17 lbs)	every 4 hours
12–24 months	1.25 ml (¼ tsp)
(18–23 lbs)	every 4 hours

---

*(⅛ tsp is approximately .75 ml)

How Supplied: TRIAMINIC-DM Syrup (dark red), in 4 fl oz and 8 fl oz plastic bottles with tamper-evident band around child-resistant cap. Berry flavored. Alcohol-free.

Shown in Product Identification Section, page 423

TRIAMINIC–12® TABLETS
[trī "ah-mĭn 'ĭc]

Description: Each tablet contains: phenylpropanolamine hydrochloride 75 mg and chlorpheniramine maleate 12 mg. Other ingredients: carnauba wax, colloidal silicon dioxide, lactose, methylcellulose, polyethylene glycol, povidone, Red 30, stearic acid, titanium dioxide, Yellow 6. Triaminic-12 Tablets contain the nasal decongestant phenylpropanolamine, and the antihistamine chlorpheniramine, in a formulation providing 12 hours of symptomatic relief.

Indications: For the temporary relief of nasal congestion due to the common cold, hay fever or other upper respiratory allergies and associated with sinusitis. Helps decongest sinus openings, sinus passages; promotes nasal and/or sinus drainage; temporarily restores freer breathing through the nose. For temporary relief of running nose, sneezing, itching of the nose or throat and itchy and watery eyes as may occur in allergic rhinitis (such as hay fever).

Warnings: Do not give this product to children under 12 years except under the advice and supervision of a physician. Do not take this product if you are taking another medication containing phenylpropanolamine. Do not take this preparation if you have high blood pressure, heart disease, diabetes, thyroid disease, asthma, glaucoma, emphysema, chronic pulmonary disease, shortness of breath, difficulty in breathing or difficulty in urination due to enlargement of the prostate gland except under the advice and supervision of a physician. Do not exceed the recommended dosage because at higher doses nervousness, dizziness or sleeplessness may occur. This preparation may cause drowsiness; alcohol may increase the drowsing effect; this preparation may cause excitability, especially in children. If symptoms do not improve within seven days or are accompanied by high fever, consult a physician before continuing use. As with any drug, if you are pregnant or nursing a baby, seek the advice of a health professional before using this product. Keep this and all drugs out of the reach of children. In case of accidental overdose, seek professional assistance or contact a Poison Control Center immediately.

Caution: Avoid driving a motor vehicle or operating heavy machinery. Avoid alcoholic beverages while taking this product.

Drug Interaction Precaution: Do not take this product if you are presently taking a prescription antihypertensive or antidepressant drug containing a monoamine oxidase inhibitor except under the advice and supervision of a physician.

Directions: Adults and children over 12 years of age—1 tablet swallowed whole every 12 hours. Unless directed by physician, do not exceed 2 tablets in 24 hours.

Note: The nonactive portion of the tablet that supplies the active ingredients may occasionally appear in your stool as a soft mass.

How Supplied: Triaminic-12 Tablets (orange) imprinted "DORSEY" on one side, "TRIAMINIC-12" on the other, in blister packs of 10 and 20.

Shown in Product Identification Section, page 424

TRIAMINICIN® TABLETS
[trī "ah-mĭn 'ĭ-sĭn]

Description: Each tablet contains: phenylpropanolamine hydrochloride 25 mg and chlorpheniramine maleate 4 mg and acetaminophen 650 mg. Other ingredients: colloidal silicon dioxide, croscarmellose sodium, hydroxypropyl cellulose, lactose, magnesium stearate, methylcellulose, methylparaben, polyethylene glycol, povidone, pregelatinized starch, Red 40, titanium dioxide, Yellow 10.

Indications: Temporarily relieves runny nose, sneezing, itching of the nose or throat, and itchy, watery eyes due to hay fever or other upper respiratory allergies (allergic rhinitis). Temporarily relieves nasal congestion due to hay fever or other upper respiratory allergies or associated with sinusitis. Temporarily relieves nasal congestion, runny nose and sneezing associated with the common cold. For the temporary relief of occasional minor aches, pains, headache and for the reduction of fever associated with the common cold.

Warnings: Do not take this product if you have high blood pressure, heart disease, diabetes, thyroid disease, asthma, glaucoma, emphysema, chronic pulmonary disease, shortness of breath, difficulty in breathing or difficulty in urination due to enlargement of the prostate gland or are taking a prescription drug for high blood pressure or depression unless directed by a doctor. Do not exceed recommended dosage because at higher doses nervousness, dizziness, or sleeplessness may occur. This preparation may cause drowsiness; alcohol, sedatives and tranquilizers may increase the drowsiness effect; avoid alcoholic beverages; do not operate machinery or drive a motor

Continued on next page

Sandoz Pharm.—Cont.

vehicle while taking this product; this preparation may cause excitability, especially in children. Do not take this product for more than 7 days. If symptoms do not improve, new ones occur, or if fever persists for more than 3 days (72 hours) or recurs, consult a doctor. As with any drug, if you are pregnant or nursing a baby, seek the advice of a health professional before using this product. Keep this and all drugs out of the reach of children. In case of accidental overdose, seek professional assistance or contact a Poison Control Center immediately. Prompt medical attention is critical for adults as well as for children even if you do not notice any signs or symptoms.

Directions: Adults and children 12 years and older: Take 1 tablet every 4 hours. Unless directed by a doctor, do not exceed 6 doses in 24 hours or give to children under 12 years.

How Supplied: TRIAMINICIN Tablets (yellow) imprinted "DORSEY" on one side, "TRIAMINICIN" on the other, in blister packs of 12, 24 and 48, and bottles of 100 tablets.
Shown in Product Identification Section, page 424

TRIAMINICOL® MULTI-SYMPTOM COLD TABLETS
[trī″ah-mĭn′ĭ-call]

Description: Each tablet contains: phenylpropanolamine hydrochloride 12.5 mg, chlorpheniramine maleate 2 mg and dextromethorphan hydrobromide 10 mg. Other ingredients: calcium stearate, colloidal silicon dioxide, lactose, methylcellulose, methylparaben, microcrystalline cellulose, polyethylene glycol, povidone, pregelatinized starch, Red 40, titanium dioxide.

Indications: For the temporary relief of nasal congestion due to the common cold, hay fever or other upper respiratory allergies and associated with sinusitis. Helps decongest sinus openings, sinus passages, promotes nasal and/or sinus drainage, temporarily restores freer breathing through the nose. For temporary relief of runny nose, sneezing, itching of the nose or throat and itchy and watery eyes as may occur in allergic rhinitis (such as hay fever). For temporary relief of cough due to minor throat and bronchial irritation as may occur with the common cold or with inhaled irritants.

Warnings: Do not take this product: 1) if cough is accompanied by excessive secretions, 2) for persistent cough such as occurs with smoking, asthma or emphysema, or 3) if you have high blood pressure, heart disease, diabetes, thyroid disease, asthma, glaucoma, chronic pulmonary disease, shortness of breath, difficulty in breathing or difficulty in urination due to enlargement of the prostate gland or are taking a prescription drug for high blood pressure or depression un-

less directed by a doctor. Do not exceed recommended dosage because at higher doses nervousness, dizziness, or sleeplessness may occur or take for more than 7 days. This preparation may cause drowsiness; alcohol, sedatives, and tranquilizers may increase the drowsiness effect; avoid alcoholic beverages; do not operate machinery or drive a motor vehicle while taking this product; this preparation may cause excitability, especially in children. If symptoms do not improve within seven days or are accompanied by fever, rash or persistant headache or if cough recurs, consult a doctor. As with any drug, if you are pregnant or nursing a baby, seek the advice of a health professional before using this product. Keep this and all drugs out of the reach of children. In case of accidental overdose, seek professional assistance or contact a Poison Control Center immediately.

Directions: Adults and children 12 years of age and older: 2 tablets every 4 hours. Children 6 to under 12 years, 1 tablet every 4 hours. Unless directed by physician, do not exceed 6 doses in 24 hours or give to children under 6 years.

How Supplied: Triaminicol Tablets (cherry red) imprinted "DORSEY" on one side, "TRIAMINICOL" on the other, in blister packs of 24.
Shown in Product Identification Section, page 424

TRIAMINICOL® MULTI-SYMPTOM RELIEF
[trī″ah-mĭn′ĭ-call]

Description: Each teaspoonful (5 ml) of TRIAMINICOL Multi-Symptom Relief contains: phenylpropanolamine hydrochloride 12.5 mg, chlorpheniramine maleate 2 mg, dextromethorphan hydrobromide 10 mg in a palatable, cherry flavored alcohol-free liquid. Other ingredients: benzoic acid, flavors, propylene glycol, purified water, Red 40, saccharin sodium, sodium chloride, sorbitol, sucrose.

Indications: Provides relief of runny nose, nasal congestion and sneezing that may occur with the common cold. Suppresses cough due to minor throat and bronchial irritation. Promotes nasal and sinus drainage.

Warnings: Do not take this product: 1) if cough is accompanied by excessive secretions, 2) for persistent cough such as occurs with smoking, asthma or emphysema, or 3) if you have heart disease, high blood pressure, thyroid disease, diabetes, asthma, glaucoma, emphysema, shortness of breath, chronic pulmonary disease, difficulty in breathing, difficulty in urination due to enlargement of the prostate gland, or 4) if you are taking a prescription drug for high blood pressure or depression, or are taking sedatives or tranquilizers, unless directed by a doctor. Do not exceed recommended dosage because at higher doses nervousness, dizziness or sleeplessness may occur, or take for more than 7 days. If symptoms persist, are accompanied by a fever, rash or

persistent headache, or if cough recurs, consult a doctor. May cause excitability especially in children. May cause marked drowsiness. Alcohol, sedatives or tranquilizers may increase drowsiness. Avoid alcoholic beverages. Do not operate machinery or drive a motor vehicle while taking this product. As with any drug, if you are pregnant or nursing a baby, seek the advice of a health professional before using this product. Keep this and all drugs out of the reach of children. In case of accidental overdose, seek professional assistance or contact a Poison Control Center immediately.

Dosage and Administration: Adults and children 12 and over (96+ lbs)—2 teaspoonfuls every 4 hours. Children 6 to under 12 years (48–95 lbs)—1 teaspoonful every 4 hours. Unless directed by physician, do not exceed 6 doses in 24 hours or give to children under 6 years of age.

Professional Labeling: The suggested dosage for pediatric patients is:

3–12 months	.75 ml (⅛ tsp)*	
(12–17 lbs)		every 4 hours
12–24 months	1.25 ml (¼ tsp)	
(18–23 lbs)		every 4 hours
2–6 years	2.5 ml (½ tsp)	
(24–47 lbs)		every 4 hours

*(⅛ tsp is approximately .75 ml)

How Supplied: TRIAMINICOL Multi-Symptom Relief (red), in 4 fl oz and 8 fl oz plastic bottles with tamper-evident band around child-resistant cap. Cherry flavored. Alcohol-free.
Shown in Product Identification Section, page 424

URSINUS® INLAY-TABS®
[yur″sīgn′us]

Description: Each URSINUS Inlay-Tab contains: pseudoephedrine hydrochloride 30 mg and aspirin (USP) 325 mg. Other ingredients: calcium stearate, lactose, microcrystalline cellulose, pregelatinized starch, sodium starch, Yellow 6, Yellow 10.

Indications: For the temporary relief of nasal congestion due to the common cold, hay fever or associated with sinusitis. For the temporary relief of occasional minor aches, pains and headache and for the reduction of fever associated with the common cold.

Warnings: Children and teenagers should not use this medicine for chicken pox or flu symptoms before a doctor is consulted about Reye syndrome, a rare but serious illness reported to be associated with aspirin. Unless directed by a doctor: 1) Do not take this product if you are allergic to aspirin or if you have asthma, or if you have stomach distress, ulcers or bleeding problems; 2) Do not take this product if you have heart disease, thyroid disease, or difficulty in urination due to enlargement of the prostate gland, and 3) Do not exceed recommended dosage because at higher doses nervousness, dizziness, or sleeplessness may occur. Do not take this product for more than 7 days. If symptoms do not improve, are accompanied by fever, or new symptoms occur, consult a doctor. Stop taking this product if ringing in the ears or other symptoms occur. As with any drug, if you are pregnant or nursing a baby, seek the advice of a health professional before using this product. **IT IS ESPECIALLY IMPORTANT NOT TO USE ASPIRIN DURING THE LAST 3 MONTHS OF PREGNANCY UNLESS SPECIFICALLY DIRECTED TO DO SO BY A DOCTOR BECAUSE IT MAY CAUSE PROBLEMS IN THE UNBORN CHILD OR COMPLICATIONS DURING DELIVERY.**

Drug Interaction Precaution: Do not take this product if you are presently taking a prescription drug for high blood pressure or depression without first consulting your doctor. Do not take this product if you are presently taking a prescription drug for anticoagulation (thinning the blood), diabetes, arthritis or gout unless directed by a doctor. **Keep this and all medicines out of the reach of children. In case of accidental overdose, contact a physician immediately.**

Directions for Use: Adults and children 12 years and older: 2 tablets with a full glass of water every 4 hours while symptoms persist or as directed by a physician. Do not take more than 4 doses in 24 hours. For chicken pox or flu see Warnings.

How Supplied: URSINUS INLAYTABS (white with yellow inlay), in bottles of 24.

Sanofi Winthrop Pharmaceuticals
90 PARK AVENUE
NEW YORK, NY 10016

BRONKOLIXIR®
Bronchodilator • Decongestant

Description: Each 5 mL teaspoonful contains:
Ephedrine sulfate, USP .... 12 mg
Guaifenesin, USP .... 50 mg
Theophylline, USP .... 15 mg
Phenobarbital, USP .... 4 mg
 (Warning: May be habit forming.)
Also contains: Alcohol 19% (v/v), FD&C Red #40, Flavors, Glycerin, Purified Water, Saccharin Sodium, Sodium Chloride, Sodium Citrate, Sucrose.

Indications: For symptomatic control of bronchial asthma. BRONKOLIXIR is also helpful in overcoming the nonproductive cough often associated with bronchitis or colds.

Warnings: Frequent or prolonged use may cause nervousness, restlessness, or sleeplessness. Phenobarbital may cause drowsiness. Do not use if high blood pressure, heart disease, diabetes, or thyroid disease is present, unless directed by a physician. Ephedrine may cause urinary retention, especially in the presence of

partial obstruction, as in prostatism. Keep this and all drugs out of the reach of children. In case of accidental overdose, seek professional assistance or contact a poison control center immediately. As with any drug, if you are pregnant or nursing a baby, seek the advice of a health professional before using this product.

Dosage: *Adults*—2 teaspoons every three or four hours, not to exceed four times daily. *Children*—**over six**—one half the adult dose; **under six**—as directed by physician.

How Supplied: Bottle of 16 fl oz (NDC 0024-1004-16)

BRONKOTABS®
Bronchodilator • Decongestant

Description: Each tablet contains ephedrine sulfate, USP, 24 mg; guaifenesin, USP, 100 mg; theophylline, USP, 100 mg; phenobarbital, USP, 8 mg. (Warning: May be habit forming.)
Also contains: Magnesium Stearate, Magnesium Trisilicate, Microcrystalline Cellulose, Starch.

Indications: For symptomatic control of bronchial asthma.

Warnings: Frequent or prolonged use may cause nervousness, restlessness, or sleeplessness. Phenobarbital may cause drowsiness. Do not use if high blood pressure, heart disease, diabetes, or thyroid disease is present unless directed by a physician. Ephedrine may cause urinary retention, especially in the presence of partial obstruction, as in prostatism. Keep this and all drugs out of the reach of children. In case of accidental overdose, seek professional assistance or contact a poison control center immediately. As with any drug, if you are pregnant or nursing a baby, seek the advice of a health professional before using this product.

Dosage: *Adults* — 1 tablet every three or four hours, four to five times daily. *Children:* **over six** — one half the adult dose; **under six** — as directed by physician.

How Supplied: Bottle of 100 (NDC 0024-1006-10)

DRISDOL®
brand of ergocalciferol oral solution, USP (in propylene glycol)
Vitamin D Supplement

Description: 200 International Units (5 µg) per drop. The dropper supplied delivers 40 drops per mL.

Indication: For the prevention of vitamin D deficiency in infants, children, and adults.

Warnings: Keep this and all drugs out of the reach of children. In case of accidental overdose, seek professional assistance or contact a poison control center immediately.

Dosage: 2 drops daily. This dose provides the US Recommended Daily Allowance for vitamin D for infants, children, and adults.

How Supplied: Bottles of 2 fl oz (NDC 0024-0391-02)

---

pHisoDerm
(See Sterling Health.)

ZEPHIRAN® CHLORIDE
brand of benzalkonium chloride
ANTISEPTIC
AQUEOUS SOLUTION 1:750
TINTED TINCTURE 1:750
SPRAY—TINTED TINCTURE 1:750

Description: ZEPHIRAN Chloride, brand of benzalkonium chloride, NF, a mixture of alkylbenzyldimethylammonium chlorides, is a cationic quaternary ammonium surface-acting agent. It is very soluble in water, alcohol, and acetone. Aqueous solutions of ZEPHIRAN Chloride are neutral to slightly alkaline, generally colorless, and nonstaining. They have a bitter taste, aromatic odor, and foam when shaken. ZEPHIRAN Chloride Tinted Tincture 1:750 contains alcohol 50 percent and acetone 10 percent by volume. ZEPHIRAN Chloride Spray—Tinted Tincture 1:750 contains alcohol 92 percent. The Tinted Tincture and Spray also contain an orange-red coloring agent.

Clinical Pharmacology: ZEPHIRAN Chloride solutions are rapidly acting anti-infective agents with a moderately long duration of action. They are active against bacteria and some viruses, fungi, and protozoa. Bacterial spores are considered to be resistant. Solutions are bacteriostatic or bactericidal according to their concentration. The exact mechanism of bactericidal action is unknown but is thought to be due to enzyme inactivation. Activity generally increases with increasing temperature and pH. Gram-positive bacteria are more susceptible than gram-negative bacteria (TABLE 1).

TABLE 1
Highest Dilution of ZEPHIRAN Chloride Aqueous Solution Destroying the Organism in 10 but not in 5 Minutes

Organisms	20°C
Streptococcus pyogenes	1:75,000
Staphylococcus aureus	1:52,500
Salmonella typhosa	1:37,500
Escherichia coli	1:10,500

Continued on next page

This product information was effective as of October 31, 1991. Current detailed information may be obtained directly from Sanofi Winthrop Pharmaceuticals by writing to 90 Park Avenue, New York, NY 10016.

Sanofi Winthrop—Cont.

Pseudomonas is the most resistant gram-negative genus. Using the AOAC Use-Dilution Confirmation Method, no growth was obtained when *Staphylococcus aureus*, *Salmonella choleraesuis*, and *Pseudomonas aeruginosa* (strain PRD-10) were exposed for ten minutes at 20°C to ZEPHIRAN Chloride Aqueous Solution 1:750 and Tinted Tincture 1:750.

ZEPHIRAN Chloride Aqueous Solution 1:750 has been shown to retain its bactericidal activity following autoclaving for 30 minutes at 15 lb pressure, freezing, and then thawing.

The tubercle bacillus may be resistant to aqueous ZEPHIRAN Chloride solutions but is susceptible to the 1:750 tincture (AOAC Method, 10 minutes at 20°C).

ZEPHIRAN Chloride solutions also demonstrate deodorant, wetting, detergent, keratolytic, and emulsifying activity.

Indications and Usage: ZEPHIRAN Chloride aqueous solutions in appropriate dilutions (see Recommended Dilutions) are indicated for the antisepsis of skin, mucous membranes, and wounds. They are used for preoperative preparation of the skin, surgeons' hand and arm soaks, treatment of wounds, preservation of ophthalmic solutions, irrigations of the eye, body cavities, bladder, urethra, and vaginal douching.

ZEPHIRAN Chloride Tinted Tincture 1:750 and Spray are indicated for preoperative preparation of the skin and for treatment of minor skin wounds and abrasions.

Contraindication: The use of ZEPHIRAN Chloride solutions in occlusive dressings, casts, and anal or vaginal packs is inadvisable, as they may produce irritation or chemical burns.

Warnings: Sterile Water for Injection, USP, should be used as diluent in preparing diluted aqueous solutions intended for use on deep wounds or for irrigation of body cavities. Otherwise, freshly distilled water should be used. Tap water, containing metallic ions and organic matter, may reduce antibacterial potency. Resin deionized water should not be used since it may contain pathogenic bacteria.

Organic, inorganic, and synthetic materials and surfaces may adsorb sufficient quantities of ZEPHIRAN Chloride to significantly reduce its antibacterial potency in solutions. This has resulted in serious contamination of solutions of ZEPHIRAN Chloride with viable pathogenic bacteria. Solutions should not be stored in bottles stoppered with cork closures, but rather in those equipped with appropriate screw-caps. Cotton, wool, rayon, and other materials should not be stored in ZEPHIRAN Chloride solutions. Gauze sponges and fiber pledgets used to apply solutions of ZEPHIRAN Chloride to the skin should be sterilized and stored in separate containers. Only immediately prior to application should they be immersed in ZEPHIRAN Chloride solutions.

Since ZEPHIRAN Chloride solutions are inactivated by soaps and anionic detergents, thorough rinsing is necessary if these agents are employed prior to their use.

Antiseptics such as ZEPHIRAN Chloride solutions must not be relied upon to achieve complete sterilization, because they do not destroy bacterial spores and certain viruses, including the etiologic agent of infectious hepatitis, and may not destroy *Mycobacterium tuberculosis* and other rare bacterial strains.

ZEPHIRAN Chloride Tinted Tincture 1:750 and Spray contain flammable organic solvents and should not be used near an open flame or cautery.

If solutions stronger than 1:3000 enter the eyes, irrigate immediately and repeatedly with water. Prompt medical attention should then be obtained. Concentrations greater than 1:5000 should not be used on mucous membranes, with the exception of the vaginal mucosa (see Recommended Dilutions).

Precautions: In preoperative antisepsis of the skin, ZEPHIRAN Chloride solutions should not be permitted to remain in prolonged contact with the patient's skin. Avoid pooling of the solution on the operating table.

ZEPHIRAN Chloride solutions that are used on inflamed or irritated tissues must be more dilute than those used on normal tissues (see Recommended Dilutions). ZEPHIRAN Chloride Tinted Tincture 1:750 and Spray, which contain irritating organic solvents, should be kept away from the eyes or other mucous membranes.

Preoperative periorbital skin or head prep should be performed only before the patient, or eye, is anesthetized.

Adverse Reactions: ZEPHIRAN Chloride solutions in normally used concentrations have low systemic and local toxicity and are generally well tolerated, although a rare individual may exhibit hypersensitivity.

Directions for Use:

General: For most surgical applications, the recommended concentration of ZEPHIRAN Chloride Aqueous Solution or ZEPHIRAN Chloride Tinted Tincture is 1:750 (0.13 percent). Liberal use of the solution is recommended to compensate for any adsorption of ZEPHIRAN Chloride by cotton or other materials.

To use ZEPHIRAN Chloride Spray—Tinted Tincture 1:750, remove protective cap, hold in an UPRIGHT position several inches away from the surgical field or injured area, and apply by spraying freely.

Preoperative preparation of skin: ZEPHIRAN Chloride solutions 1:750 are recommended as an antiseptic for use on unbroken skin in the preoperative preparation of the surgical field. Detergents and soaps should be thoroughly rinsed from the skin before applying ZEPHIRAN Chloride solutions. The detergent action of ZEPHIRAN Chloride solutions, particularly when used alternately with alcohol, leaves the skin smooth and clean. When ZEPHIRAN

Chloride solutions are applied by friction (using several changes of sponges), dirt, skin fats, desquamating epithelium, and superficial bacteria are effectively removed, thus exposing the underlying skin to the antiseptic activity of the solutions.

The following procedure has been found satisfactory for preparation of the surgical field. On the day prior to surgery, the operative site is shaved and then scrubbed thoroughly with ZEPHIRAN Chloride Aqueous Solution 1:750. Immediately before surgery, ZEPHIRAN Chloride Tinted Tincture 1:750 or Spray is applied to the site in the usual manner (see Precautions). If the red tinted solution turns yellow during the preparation of patient's skin for surgery, it usually indicates the presence of soap (alkali) residue which is incompatible with ZEPHIRAN solutions. Therefore, rinse thoroughly and reapply the antiseptic. Because ZEPHIRAN Chloride Tinted Tincture 1:750 contains alcohol and acetone, its cleansing action on the skin is particularly effective and it dries more rapidly than the aqueous solution. The Tinted Tincture is recommended when it is desirable to outline the operative site.

Recommended Dilutions: For specific directions, see TABLES 2 and 3.

Surgery

Preoperative preparation of skin: Aqueous solution 1:750 and Tinted Tincture 1:750 or Spray

Surgeons' hand and arm soaks: Aqueous solution 1:750

Treatment of minor wounds and lacerations: Tinted Tincture 1:750 or Spray

Irrigation of deep infected wounds: Aqueous solution 1:3000 to 1:20,000

Denuded skin and mucous membranes: Aqueous solution 1:5000 to 1:10,000

Obstetrics and Gynecology

Preoperative preparation of skin: Aqueous solution 1:750 and Tinted Tincture 1:750 or Spray

Vaginal douche and irrigation: Aqueous solution 1:2000 to 1:5000

Postepisiotomy care: Aqueous solution 1:5000 to 1:10,000

Breast and nipple hygiene: Aqueous solution 1:1000 to 1:2000

Urology

Bladder and urethral irrigation: Aqueous solution 1:5000 to 1:20,000

Bladder retention lavage: Aqueous solution 1:20,000 to 1:40,000

Dermatology

Oozing and open infections: Aqueous solution 1:2000 to 1:5000

Wet dressings by irrigation or open dressing (Use in occlusive dressings is inadvisable.): Aqueous solution 1:5000 or less

Ophthalmology

Eye irrigation: Aqueous solution 1:5000 to 1:10,000

TABLE 2
Correct Use of ZEPHIRAN Chloride

ZEPHIRAN Chloride solutions must be prepared, stored, and used correctly to achieve and maintain their antiseptic action. Serious inactivation and contamination of ZEPHIRAN Chloride solutions may occur with misuse.

CORRECT DILUENTS	INCOMPATIBILITIES	PREFERRED FORM

Sterile Water for Injection is recommended for irrigation of body cavities.

Sterile distilled water is recommended for irrigating traumatized tissue and in the eye.

Freshly distilled water is recommended for skin antisepsis.

Resin deionized water should not be used because the deionizing resins can carry pathogens (especially gram-negative bacteria); they also inactivate quaternary ammonium compounds.

Stored water is not recommended since it may contain many organisms.

Saline should not be used since it may decrease the antibacterial potency of ZEPHIRAN Chloride solutions.

Anionic detergents and soaps should be thoroughly rinsed from the skin or other areas prior to use of ZEPHIRAN Chloride solutions because they reduce the antibacterial activity of the solutions.

Serum and protein material also decrease the activity of ZEPHIRAN Chloride solutions.

Corks should not be used to stopper bottles containing ZEPHIRAN Chloride solutions.

Fibers or fabrics when stored in ZEPHIRAN Chloride solutions adsorb ZEPHIRAN from the surrounding liquid. Examples are:

Cotton	Gauze sponges
Wool	Rayon
	Rubber materials

Applicators or sponges, intended for a skin prep, should be stored separately and dipped in ZEPHIRAN Chloride solutions immediately before use.

Under certain circumstances the following commonly encountered substances are incompatible with ZEPHIRAN Chloride solutions:

Iodine	Aluminum
Silver nitrate	Caramel
Fluorescein	Kaolin
Nitrates	Pine oil
Peroxide	Zinc sulfate
Lanolin	Zinc oxide
Potassium permanganate	Yellow oxide of mercury

ZEPHIRAN Chloride Tinted Tincture 1:750 is recommended for preoperative skin preparation because it contains alcohol and acetone which enhance its cleansing action and promote rapid drying.

ZEPHIRAN Chloride Tinted Tincture 1:750, containing acetone, is recommended when it is desirable to outline the operative site. (Aqueous solutions of ZEPHIRAN Chloride used in skin preparation have a tendency to "run off" the skin.)

Caution: Because of the flammable organic solvents in ZEPHIRAN Chloride Tinted Tincture 1:750 and Spray, these products should be kept away from open flame or cautery.

TABLE 3
Dilutions of ZEPHIRAN Chloride
Aqueous Solution 1:750

Final Dilution	ZEPHIRAN Chloride Aqueous Solution 1:750 (parts)	Distilled Water (parts)
1:1000	3	1
1:2000	3	5
1:2500	3	7
1:3000	3	9
1:4000	3	13
1:5000	3	17
1:10,000	3	37
1:20,000	3	77
1:40,000	3	157

Preservation of ophthalmic solutions: Aqueous solution 1:5000 to 1:7500

Accidental Ingestion: If ZEPHIRAN Chloride solution, particularly a concentrated solution, is ingested, marked local irritation of the gastrointestinal tract, manifested by nausea and vomiting, may occur. Signs of systemic toxicity include

restlessness, apprehension, weakness, confusion, dyspnea, cyanosis, collapse, convulsions, and coma. Death occurs as a result of paralysis of the respiratory muscles.

Treatment: Immediate administration of several glasses of a mild soap solution, milk, or egg whites beaten in water is recommended. This may be followed by gastric lavage with a mild soap solution. Alcohol should be avoided as it promotes absorption.

To support respiration, the airway should be clear and oxygen should be administered, employing artificial respiration if necessary. If convulsions occur, a short-acting barbiturate may be given parenterally with caution.

How Supplied:

ZEPHIRAN Chloride Aqueous Solution 1:750
    Bottles of 8 fl oz (NDC 0024-2521-04) and 1 gallon (NDC 0024-2521-08)
ZEPHIRAN Chloride Tinted Tincture 1:750 (*flammable*)
    Bottles of 1 gallon (NDC 0024-2523-08)

ZEPHIRAN Chloride Spray—Tinted Tincture 1:750 (*flammable*)
    Bottles of 1 fl oz (NDC 0024-2527-01) and 6 fl oz (NDC 0024-2527-03)

ZW-83-H

This product information was effective as of October 31, 1991. Current detailed information may be obtained directly from Sanofi Winthrop Pharmaceuticals by writing to 90 Park Avenue, New York, NY 10016.

IDENTIFICATION PROBLEM?
Consult the
Product Identification Section
where you'll find products pictured in full color.

Schering-Plough HealthCare Products
LIBERTY CORNER, NJ 07938

A and D Ointment
REG. T.M.

Description: An ointment containing the emollients, anhydrous lanolin and petrolatum. Also contains: Cholecalciferol, Fish Liver Oil, Fragrance, Mineral Oil, Paraffin.

Indications: *Diaper rash*—**A and D Ointment** provides prompt, soothing relief for diaper rash and helps heal baby's tender skin; forms a moisture-proof shield that helps protect against urine and detergent irritants; comforts baby's skin and helps prevent chafing.
Chafed Skin—**A and D Ointment** helps skin retain its vital natural moisture; quickly soothes chafed skin in adults and children and helps prevent abnormal dryness.
Abrasions and Minor Burns—**A and D Ointment** soothes and helps relieve the smarting and pain of abrasions and minor burns, encourages healing and prevents dressings from sticking to the injured area.

Warning: Keep this and all drugs out of the reach of children.

Overdosage: In case of accidental ingestion, seek professional assistance or contact a poison control center immediately.

Dosage and Administration: *Diaper Rash*—Simply apply a thin coating of **A and D Ointment** at each diaper change. A modest amount is all that is needed to provide protective and healing action.
Chafed Skin—Gently smooth a small quantity of **A and D Ointment** over the area to be treated.
Abrasions, Minor Burns—Wash with lukewarm water and mild soap. When dry, apply **A and D Ointment** liberally. When a sterile dressing is used, change the dressing daily and apply fresh **A and D Ointment**. If no improvement occurs after 48 to 72 hours or if condition worsens, consult your physician.

How Supplied: A and D Ointment is available in 1½-ounce (42.5 g) and 4-ounce (113 g) tubes and 1-pound (454 g) jars and 2.5 oz. pumps.
Store away from heat.
Shown in Product Identification Section, page 424

AFRIN®
[a 'frin]
Nasal Spray 0.05%
Nasal Spray Pump 0.05%
Cherry Scented Nasal Spray 0.05%
Menthol Nasal Spray 0.05%
Nose Drops 0.05%
Children's Strength Nose Drops 0.025%

Description: AFRIN products contain oxymetazoline hydrochloride, the longest acting topical nasal decongestant available. Each ml of AFRIN Nasal Spray, Nasal Spray Pump, and Nose Drops contains Oxymetazoline Hydrochloride, USP 0.5 mg (0.05%); Benzalkonium Chloride, Glycine, Phenylmercuric Acetate, Sorbitol, and Water.
Each ml of AFRIN Children's Strength Nose Drops contains Oxymetazoline Hydrochloride, USP 0.25 mg (0.025%); Benzalkonium Chloride, Glycine, Phenylmercuric Acetate, Sorbitol, and Water.
AFRIN Menthol Nasal Spray contains cooling aromatic vapors of menthol, eucalyptol and camphor and polysorbate, in addition to the ingredients of AFRIN Nasal Spray.
AFRIN Cherry Scented Nasal Spray contains artificial cherry flavor in addition to the ingredients in regular AFRIN.

Indications: For temporary relief of nasal congestion associated with colds, hay fever and sinusitis.

Actions: The sympathomimetic action of AFRIN products constricts the smaller arterioles of the nasal passages, producing a prolonged, gentle and predictable decongesting effect. In just a few minutes a single dose, as directed, provides prompt, temporary relief of nasal congestion that lasts up to 12 hours. AFRIN products last up to 3 or 4 times longer than most ordinary nasal sprays.
AFRIN products used at bedtime help restore freer nasal breathing through the night.

Warnings: Do not exceed recommended dosage because burning, stinging, sneezing or increase of nasal discharge may occur. Do not use these products for more than 3 days. If nasal congestion persists, consult a physician. As with any drug, if you are pregnant or nursing a baby, seek the advice of a health professional before using this product. The use of the dispensers by more than one person may spread infection. Keep these and all medicines out of the reach of children.

Overdosage: In case of accidental ingestion, seek professional assistance or contact a Poison Control Center immediately.

Dosage and Administration: Because AFRIN has a long duration of action, twice-a-day administration—in the morning and at bedtime—is usually adequate.
AFRIN Nasal Spray, Cherry Scented Nasal Spray and Menthol Nasal Spray, 0.05%—For adults and children 6 years of age and over: With head upright, spray 2 or 3 times into each nostril twice daily—morning and evening. To spray, squeeze bottle quickly and firmly. Do not tilt head backward while spraying. Wipe nozzle clean after use. Not recommended for children under six.
Afrin Nasal Spray Pump, 0.05%—For adults and children 6 years of age and over: Two or three sprays in each nostril twice daily—morning and bedtime. Remove protective cap. Hold bottle with thumb at base and nozzle between first and second fingers. With head upright, insert metered pump spray nozzle in nos-tril. Depress pump 2 or 3 times, all the way down, with a firm even stroke and sniff deeply. Repeat in other nostril. Do not tilt head backward while spraying. Wipe tip clean after each use. Before using the first time, remove the protective cap from the tip and prime the metered pump by depressing pump firmly several times.
AFRIN Nose Drops—For adults and children 6 years of age and over: Tilt head back, apply 2 or 3 drops into each nostril twice daily—morning and evening. Immediately bend head forward toward knees. Hold a few seconds, then return to upright position. Wipe dropper clean after each use. Not recommended for children under six.
AFRIN Children's Strength Nose Drops—Children 2 through 5 years of age: Tilt head back, apply 2 or 3 drops into each nostril twice daily—morning and evening. Promptly move head forward toward knees. Hold a few seconds, then return child to upright position. Wipe dropper clean after each use. For children under 2 years, use only as directed by a physician.

How Supplied: AFRIN Nasal Spray 0.05% (1:2000), 15 ml and 30 ml plastic squeeze bottles.
AFRIN Nasal Spray Pump 0.05% (1:2000), 15 ml spray pump bottles.
AFRIN Cherry Scented Nasal Spray 0.05% (1:2000), 15 ml plastic squeeze bottle.
AFRIN Menthol Nasal Spray 0.05% (1:2000), 15 ml plastic squeeze bottle.
AFRIN Nose Drops, 0.05% (1:2000), 20 ml dropper bottle.
AFRIN Children's Strength Nose Drops, 0.025% (1:4000), 20 ml dropper bottle.
Store all nasal sprays and nose drops between 2° and 30°C (36° and 86°F).
Shown in Product Identification Section, page 424

AFRIN™
[a 'frin]
Saline Mist

Ingredients: Water, Sodium Chloride, Disodium Phosphate, Sodium Phosphate, Benzalkonium Chloride, Phenyl Mercuric Acetate.

Indications: Provides soothing moisture to dry, inflamed nasal membranes due to colds, allergies, low humidity, and other minor nasal irritations. Afrin Saline Mist loosens and thins mucus secretions to aid removal of mucus from nose and sinuses. Afrin Saline Mist can be used as often as needed, and is safe to use with cold, allergy, and sinus medications.

Directions: For infants, children, and adults, 2 to 6 sprays/drops in each nostril as often as needed or as directed by a physician. For a fine mist, keep bottle upright; for nose drops, keep bottle upside down; for a stream, keep bottle horizontal. Wipe nozzle clean after use.

Keep out of the reach of children. As with any drug, if you are pregnant or nursing a baby, seek the advice of a health professional before using this product.

The use of this dispenser by more than one person may spread infection.

CONTAINS NO ALCOHOL
Shown in Product Identification Section, page 424

AFRIN Tablets
[*a'frin*]

Active Ingredients: Each Extended Release Tablet contains: 120 mg pseudoephedrine sulfate. Each tablet also contains: Acacia, Butylparaben, Calcium Sulfate, Carnauba Wax, Corn Starch, FD&C Blue No. 1, Gelatin, Lactose, Magnesium Stearate, Neutral Soap, Oleic Acid, Povidone, Rosin, Sugar, Talc, White Wax, Zein. Half the dose (60 mg) is released after the tablet is swallowed and the other half is released hours later; continuous relief is provided for up to 12 hours . . . without drowsiness.

Indications: For temporary relief of nasal congestion due to the common cold, hay fever or other upper respiratory allergies, and nasal congestion associated with sinusitis.

Actions: Promotes nasal and/or sinus drainage, helps decongest sinus openings, sinus passages.

Warnings: Do not exceed recommended dosage because at higher doses nervousness, dizziness or sleeplessness may occur. Do not take this preparation if you have high blood pressure, heart disease, diabetes, or thyroid disease, except under the advice and supervision of a physician. If symptoms do not improve within 7 days or are accompanied by fever, consult a physician before continuing use. Keep this and all drugs out of the reach of children.

As with any drug, if you are pregnant or nursing a baby, seek the advice of a health professional before using this product.

Drug Interactions: Do not take this product if you are presently taking a prescription drug for high blood pressure or depression, without first consulting your physician.

Overdosage: In case of accidental overdose, seek professional assistance or contact a poison control center immediately.

Dosage and Administration: Adults and children 12 years and over—One tablet every 12 hours. AFRIN Tablets is not recommended for children under 12 years of age.

How Supplied: AFRIN Extended Release Tablets—Boxes of 12 and 24 and bottles of 100.
Store between 2° and 30°C (36° and 86° F). Protect from excessive moisture.
Shown in Product Identification Section, page 424

AFTATE® Antifungal
Aerosol Liquid
Aerosol Powder
Gel
Powder

Active Ingredient: Tolnaftate 1% (Also contains: Aerosol Spray Liquid-36% alcohol; Aerosol Spray Powder-14% alcohol.)

How Supplied:
AFTATE for Athlete's Foot
Sprinkle Powder—2.25 oz. bottle
Aerosol Spray Powder—3.5 oz can
Gel—.5 oz. tube
Aerosol Spray Liquid—4 oz. can
AFTATE for Jock Itch
Aerosol Spray Powder—3.5 oz. can
Sprinkle Powder—1.5 oz. bottle
Gel—.5 oz. tube
Shown in Product Identification Section, page 424

CHLOR–TRIMETON®
[*klor-tri'mĕ-ton*]
Allergy Syrup
Allergy Tablets 4 mg
Long Acting Allergy REPETABS®
  Tablets 8 mg and 12 mg

Active Ingredients: Each Allergy Tablet contains: 4 mg chlorpheniramine maleate, USP; also contains: Corn Starch, D&C Yellow No. 10 Al Lake, Lactose, Magnesium Stearate. Each REPETABS® Tablet contains: 8 mg or 12 mg chlorpheniramine maleate; 8 mg Repetabs also contains: Acacia, Butylparaben, Calcium Phosphate, Calcium Sulfate, Carnauba Wax, Corn Starch, D&C Yellow No. 10 Al Lake, FD&C Yellow No.6 Al Lake, Lactose, Magnesium Stearate, Neutral Soap, Oleic Acid, Povidone, Rosin, Sugar, Talc, White Wax, Zein.
12 mg Repetabs also contains: Acacia, Butylparaben, Calcium Phosphate, Calcium Sulfate, Carnauba Wax, Corn Starch, D&C Yellow No. 10 Al Lake, FD&C Blue No. 2 Al Lake, FD&C Yellow No. 6, FD&C Yellow No. 6 Al Lake, Lactose, Magnesium Stearate, Neutral Soap, Oleic Acid, Potato Starch, Rosin, Sugar, Talc, White Wax, Zein. Half the dose is released after the tablet is swallowed, and the other half is released hours later; continuous relief is provided for up to 12 hours.
Each teaspoonful (5 ml) of Allergy Syrup contains: 2 mg CHLOR-TRIMETON (brand of chlorpheniramine maleate) in a pleasant-tasting syrup containing approximately 7% alcohol. Also contains: Benzaldehyde, FD&C Green No. 3, FD&C Yellow No. 6, Flavor, Glycerin, Menthol, Methylparaben, Propylene Glycol, Propylparaben, Sugar, Vanillin, Water.

Indications: For temporary relief of hay fever symptoms: sneezing; runny nose; watery, itchy eyes, itching of the nose or throat.

Actions: The active ingredient in CHLOR-TRIMETON is an antihistamine with anticholinergic (drying) and sedative side effects. Antihistamines appear to compete with histamine for cell receptor sites on effector cells.

Warnings: May cause excitability especially in children. Do not give the REPETABS Tablets to children under 12 years, or the Allergy Syrup and Tablets to children under 6 years except under the advice and supervision of a physician. Do not take this product if you have asthma, glaucoma, emphysema, chronic pulmonary disease, shortness of breath, difficulty in breathing, or difficulty in urination due to enlargement of the prostate gland unless directed by a physician. May cause drowsiness; alcohol may increase the drowsiness effect. Avoid alcoholic beverages while taking this product. Use caution when driving a motor vehicle or operating machinery. As with any drug, if you are pregnant or nursing a baby, seek the advice of a health professional before using this product. Keep this and all drugs out of the reach of children. In case of accidental overdose, seek professional assistance or contact a Poison Control Center immediately.

Dosage and Administration: Allergy Syrup—Adults and Children 12 years and over: Two teaspoonfuls (4 mg) every 4 to 6 hours, not to exceed 12 teaspoonfuls in 24 hours. Children 6 through 11 years: one teaspoonful (2 mg) every 4 to 6 hours, not to exceed 6 teaspoonfuls in 24 hours. For children under 6 years, consult a physician.
Allergy Tablets—Adults and Children 12 years and over: One tablet (4 mg) every 4 to 6 hours, not to exceed 6 tablets in 24 hours. Children 6 through 11 years: One half the adult dose (break tablet in half) every 4 to 6 hours, not to exceed 3 whole tablets in 24 hours. For children under 6 years, consult a physician.
Allergy REPETABS Tablets—Adults and Children 12 years and over: One tablet in the morning and one tablet in the evening, not to exceed 24 mg (3 tablets of 8 mg; 2 tablets of 12 mg) in 24 hours. For children under 12 years, consult a physician.

Professional Labeling: Dosage—Allergy Syrup: Children 2 through 5 years: ½ teaspoonful (1 mg) every 4 to 6 hours; Allergy Tablets: Children 2 through 5 years: one-quarter tablet (1 mg) every 4 to 6 hours.
Allergy REPETABS Tablets—Children 6 to 12 years: One tablet (8 mg) at bedtime or during the day, as indicated.

How Supplied: CHLOR-TRIMETON Allergy Tablets, 4 mg, yellow compressed, scored tablets impressed with the Schering trademark and product identification letters, TW or numbers, 080; box of 24, bottles of 100.
CHLOR-TRIMETON Allergy Syrup: 2 mg per 5 ml, blue-green-colored liquid; 4-fluid ounce (118 ml). Protect from light;

Continued on next page

Information on Schering-Plough HealthCare Products appearing on these pages is effective as of November 1991.

Schering-Plough—Cont.

however, if color fades potency will not be affected.

CHLOR-TRIMETON Allergy REPE-TABS Tablets, 8 mg, sugar-coated, yellow tablets branded in red with the Schering trademark and product identification letters, CC or numbers, 374; boxes of 24, 48, bottles of 100.

CHLOR-TRIMETON REPETABS Tablets, 12 mg, sugar coated orange tablets branded in black with Schering trademark and product identification letters AAE or numbers 009; boxes of 12 and 24, bottles of 100.

Store the tablets and syrup between 2° and 30°C (36° and 86°F).

Shown in Product Identification Section, pages 424 and 425

CHLOR–TRIMETON®
[*klor 'tri 'mĕ-ton*]
Antihistamine and Decongestant Tablets
Long Acting CHLOR–TRIMETON®
Antihistamine and Decongestant REPETABS® Tablets

Active Ingredients: Each tablet contains: 4 mg chlorpheniramine maleate, USP and 60 mg pseudoephedrine sulfate. Each tablet also contains: Corn Starch, FD&C Blue No. 1, Lactose, Magnesium Stearate, Povidone.

Each REPETABS Tablet contains: 8 mg chlorpheniramine maleate and 120 mg pseudoephedrine sulfate. Each repetab also contains: Acacia, Butylparaben, Calcium Sulfate, Carnauba Wax, Corn Starch, D&C Yellow No. 10 Al Lake, FD&C Blue No. 1 Al Lake, FD&C Yellow No. 6 Al Lake, Gelatin, Lactose, Magnesium Stearate, Neutral Soap, Oleic Acid, Povidone, Rosin, Sugar, Talc, White Wax, Zein. Half the dose of each ingredient is released after the tablet is swallowed and the other half is released hours later providing continuous long-lasting relief up to 12 hours.

Indications: For temporary relief of hay fever symptoms (sneezing; running nose; watery, itchy eyes, itching of the nose or throat) and nasal congestion due to hay fever and associated with sinusitis.

Actions: The antihistamine, chlorpheniramine maleate, provides temporary relief of running nose, sneezing, itching of the nose or throat, and itchy and watery eyes as may occur in allergic rhinitis (such as hayfever). The decongestant, pseudoephedrine sulfate reduces swelling of nasal passages; shrinks swollen membranes; and temporarily restores freer breathing through the nose.

Warnings: If symptoms do not improve within 7 days or are accompanied by fever, consult a physician before continuing use. May cause excitability especially in children. Do not exceed recommended dosage because at higher doses nervousness, dizziness or sleeplessness may oc-

cur. Do not take this product if you have asthma, glaucoma, emphysema, chronic pulmonary disease, shortness of breath, difficulty in breathing, heart disease, high blood pressure, thyroid disease, diabetes, or difficulty in urination due to enlargement of the prostate gland. Do not give the Decongestant Tablets to children under 6 years or the REPETABS Tablets to children under 12 years unless directed by a physician. May cause drowsiness; alcohol may increase the drowsiness effect. Avoid alcoholic beverages while taking this product. Use caution when driving a motor vehicle or operating machinery. Keep this and all drugs out of the reach of children. In case of accidental overdose, seek professional assistance or contact a Poison Control Center immediately. As with any drug, if you are pregnant or nursing a baby, seek the advice of a health professional before using this product.

Drug Interaction Precaution: Do not take this product if you are presently taking a prescription drug for high blood pressure or depression, without first consulting your doctor.

Dosage and Administration: Tablets —ADULTS AND CHILDREN 12 YEARS AND OVER: One tablet every 4 to 6 hours, not to exceed 4 tablets in 24 hours. CHILDREN 6 THROUGH 11 YEARS —One half the adult dose (break tablet in half) every 4 to 6 hours not to exceed 2 whole tablets in 24 hours. For children under 6 years, consult a physician. REPETABS Tablets—ADULTS AND CHILDREN 12 YEARS AND OVER: one tablet every 12 hours.

Professional Labeling: Tablets— Children 2-5 years—one quarter the adult dose every 4 hours, not to exceed 1 tablet in 24 hours.

How Supplied: CHLOR-TRIMETON Decongestant Tablets—boxes of 24 and 48. Long Acting CHLOR-TRIMETON Decongestant REPETABS Tablets boxes of 12 and 36.
Store these CHLOR-TRIMETON Products between 2° and 30°C (36°and 86°F); and protect from excessive moisture.

Shown in Product Identification Section, page 425

CHOOZ® ANTACID GUM

Active Ingredients: 500 mg. of calcium carbonate per tablet.

Inactive Ingredients: Sucrose, gum base, glucose, cornstarch, peppermint oil, hydrated silica, gelatin, glycerin, acacia, carnauba, beeswax, sodium benzoate.

Indications: For relief from acid indigestion, sour stomach, heartburn, and upset stomach associated with these symptoms. Five tablets provide 100% of the adult U.S. Recommended Daily Allowance for calcium. Chooz Anatcid Gum is dietically sodium-free, an important benefit for those watching their sodium and salt consumption.

Warnings: Adults—Do not take more than 14 tablets in a 24-hour period. Do not use the maximum dosage of this product for more than 2 weeks except under the advice and supervision of a physician. Children 6 to 12 years—Do not take more than 8 tablets in a 24-hour period. Keep this and all drugs out of reach of children.

Dosage and Administration: Adults chew 1 to 2 tablets every 2 to 4 hours. Children 6 to 12 years of age chew 1 tablet every 2 to 4 hours. Or take as directed by physician.

How Supplied: Tablets—individually foil-backed safety sealed blister packaging in boxes of 16 tablets.
Shown in Product Identification Section, page 425

COMPLEX 15®
Phospholipid Hand & Body Moisturizing Cream
Formulated For Mild To Severe Dry Skin

Ingredients: Water, Mineral Oil, Glycerin, Squalane, Caprylic/Capric Triglyceride, Dimethicone, Glyceryl Stearate, Glycol Stearate, PEG-50 Stearate, Stearic Acid, Cetyl Alcohol, Myristyl Myristate, Lecithin, Diazolidinyl Urea, Carbomer 934, Magnesium Aluminum Silicate, C10–30 Carboxylic Acid Sterol Ester, Sodium Hydroxide, Tetrasodium EDTA, BHT

COMPLEX 15® Hand and Body Cream is formulated for mild to severe dry skin with a system modeled from nature. It contains lecithin, a phospholipid water-binding agent found naturally in the skin. Each phospholipid molecule holds 15 molecules of water, restoring the natural moisture balance. COMPLEX 15 Hand and Body Cream is nongreasy and absorbs quickly into the skin. COMPLEX 15 Hand and Body Cream is unscented, contains no parabens or lanolin. COMPLEX 15 Hand and Body Cream is proven to be hypoallergenic and non-comedogenic.

Directions: Apply to the hands and body as needed or as directed by a physician. Avoid contact with eyes.
FOR EXTERNAL USE ONLY

How Supplied: COMPLEX 15® Hand & Body Moisturizing Cream is available in 4 ounce jars (0085-4151-04).
Shown in Product Identification Section, page 425

COMPLEX 15®
Phospholipid Hand & Body Moisturizing Lotion
Formulated For Mild To Severe Dry Skin

Ingredients: Water, Caprylic/Capric Triglyceride, Glycerin, Glyceryl Stearate, Dimethicone, PEG-50 Stearate, Squalane, Cetyl Alcohol, Glycol Stearate, Myristyl Myristate, Stearic Acid, Lecithin, C10–30 Carboxylic Acid Sterol Ester, Diazolidinyl Urea, Carbomer 934, Magnesium Aluminum Silicate, Sodium Hydroxide, BHT, Tetrasodium EDTA

COMPLEX 15® Hand and Body Lotion is formulated for mild to severe dry skin with a system modeled from nature. It contains lecithin, a phospholipid water-binding agent found naturally in the skin. Each phospholipid molecule holds 15 molecules of water, restoring the natural moisture balance. COMPLEX 15 Hand and Body Lotion is nongreasy and absorbs quickly into the skin. COMPLEX 15 Hand and Body Lotion is unscented, contains no parabens, lanolin, or mineral oil. COMPLEX 15 Hand and Body Lotion is proven to be hypoallergenic and non-comedogenic.

Directions: Apply to the hands and body as needed, or as directed by a physician. Avoid contact with eyes.
FOR EXTERNAL USE ONLY

How Supplied: COMPLEX 15® Hand and Body Moisturizing Lotion is available in 8 fluid ounce and 4 fluid ounce bottles (0085-4115-08).
Shown in Product Identification Section, page 425

COMPLEX 15®
Phospholipid Moisturizing Face Cream

Ingredients: Water, Caprylic/Capric Triglyceride, Glycerin, Squalane, Glyceryl Stearate, Propylene Glycol, PEG-50 Stearate, Cetyl Alcohol, Dimethicone, Glycol Stearate, Myristyl Myristate, Stearic Acid, Carbomer 934, Magnesium Aluminum Silicate, Diazolidinyl Urea, Lecithin, Sodium Hydroxide, C10–30 Carboxylic Acid Sterol Ester, BHT, Tetrasodium EDTA

COMPLEX 15® Face Cream is formulated for mild to severe dry skin with a system modeled from nature. It contains lecithin, a phospholipid water-binding agent found naturally in the skin. Each phospholipid molecule holds 15 molecules of water, restoring the natural moisture balance. COMPLEX 15 Face Cream is nongreasy and absorbs quickly into the skin. COMPLEX 15 Face Cream is unscented, contains no parabens, lanolin or mineral oil. COMPLEX 15 Face Cream is proven to be hypoallergenic and noncomedogenic.

Directions: Apply to the face as needed or as directed by a physician. Avoid contact with eyes.
FOR EXTERNAL USE ONLY

How Supplied: COMPLEX 15® Moisturizing Face Cream is available in 2.5 oz. tubes (0085-4100-25).
Shown in Product Identification Section, page 425

CORICIDIN® Tablets
[*kor-a-see 'din*]
CORICIDIN 'D'® Decongestant Tablets

Active Ingredients: CORICIDIN Tablets—2 mg chlorpheniramine maleate, USP; 325 mg (5 gr) acetaminophen.
CORICIDIN 'D' Decongestant Tablets—2 mg chlorpheniramine maleate, USP; 12.5 mg phenylpropanolamine hydrochloride, USP; 325 mg (5 gr) acetaminophen.

Inactive Ingredients: CORICIDIN Tablets—Acacia, Butylparaben, Calcium Sulfate, Carnauba Wax, Cellulose, Corn Starch, FD&C Red No. 40, FD&C Yellow No. 6 Aluminum Lake, Lactose, Magnesium Stearate, Povidone, Sugar, Titanium Dioxide, and White Wax. May also contain Talc.
CORICIDIN 'D' Decongestant Tablets—Acacia, Butylparaben, Calcium Sulfate, Carnauba Wax, Cellulose, Corn Starch, Magnesium Stearate, Povidone, Sugar, Titanium Dioxide, and White Wax. May also contain Talc.

Indications: CORICIDIN Tablets—For effective, temporary relief of cold and flu symptoms.
CORICIDIN 'D' Decongestant Tablets—For effective, temporary relief of congested cold, flu and sinus symptoms.

Actions: CORICIDIN Tablets relieve annoying cold and flu symptoms such as minor aches and pains, fever, sneezing, running nose and watery/itchy eyes.
CORICIDIN 'D' Tablets relieve the same annoying cold and flu symptoms as well as stuffy nose, nasal membrane swelling and sinus headache.

Warnings: CORICIDIN Tablets: Do not take this product for pain for more than 10 days (for adults) or 5 days (for children 6 years through 11 years), and do not take for fever for more than 3 days unless directed by a physician. If pain or fever persists or gets worse, if new symptoms occur, or if redness or swelling is present, consult a physician because these could be signs of a serious condition. May cause excitability especially in children. Do not take this product if you have asthma, glaucoma, emphysema, chronic pulmonary disease, shortness of breath, difficulty in breathing, difficulty in urination due to enlargement of the prostate gland, or give this product to children under 6 years, unless directed by a physician. May cause drowsiness; alcohol, sedatives, and tranquilizers may increase the drowsiness effect. Avoid alcoholic beverages while taking this product. Do not take this product if you are taking sedatives or tranquilizers, without first consulting your physician. Use caution when driving a motor vehicle or operating machinery. Keep this and all drugs out of the reach of children. In case of accidental overdose, seek professional assistance or contact a Poison Control Center immediately. Prompt medical attention is critical for adults as well as for children even if you do not notice any signs or symptoms. As with any drug, if you are preg-

nant or nursing a baby, seek the advice of a health professional before using this product.
CORICIDIN 'D' Decongestant Tablets: Do not take this product for pain or congestion for more than 7 days (adults) or 5 days (children 6 through 11 years), and do not take for fever for more than 3 days unless directed by a physician. If pain or fever persists or gets worse, if new symptoms occur, or if redness or swelling is present, consult your physician because these could be signs of a serious condition. May cause excitability, especially in children. Do not exceed recommended dosage because at higher doses nervousness, dizziness, or sleeplessness may occur. Do not take this product if you have asthma, glaucoma, emphysema, chronic pulmonary disease, shortness of breath, difficulty in breathing, heart disease, high blood pressure, thyroid disease, diabetes, difficulty in urination due to enlargement of the prostate gland, or give this product to children under 6 years unless directed by a physician. May cause drowsiness; alcohol, sedatives, and tranquilizers may increase the drowsiness effect. Avoid alcoholic beverages while taking this product. Use caution when driving a motor vehicle or operating machinery. Keep this and all drugs out of the reach of children. In case of accidental overdose, seek professional assistance or contact a Poison Control Center immediately. Proper medical attention is critical for adults and children even if you do not notice any signs or symptoms. As with any drug, if you are pregnant or nursing a baby, seek the advice of a health care professional before using this product. *Drug Interaction Precaution:* Do not take this product if you are presently taking a prescription drug for high blood pressure or depression, sedatives, tranquilizers or appetite-controlling medication containing phenylpropanolamine without first consulting your physician.

Dosage and Administration: CORICIDIN Tablets—Adults and children 12 years and over—2 tablets every 4 hours not to exceed 12 tablets in 24 hours. Children 6 through 11 years: 1 tablet every 4 hours not to exceed 5 tablets in 24 hours.
CORICIDIN 'D' Decongestant Tablets—Adults and children 12 years and over: 2 tablets every 4 hours not to exceed 12 tablets in 24 hours. Children 6 through 11 years: 1 tablet every 4 hours not to exceed 5 tablets in 24 hours.

How Supplied: CORICIDIN Tablets—bottles of 12, 24, 48, and 100.
CORICIDIN 'D' Decongestant Tablets—bottles of 12, 24, 48, and 100.
Store the tablets between 2° and 30°C (36° and 86°F).
Shown in Product Identification Section, page 425

Continued on next page

Information on Schering-Plough HealthCare Products appearing on these pages is effective as of November 1991.

Schering-Plough—Cont.

CORICIDIN® DEMILETS®
[kor-a-see'din dem'ē-lets]
Tablets for Children

CORICIDIN DEMILETS Tablets—1.0 mg chlorpheniramine maleate, USP; 80 mg acetaminophen, USP; 6.25 mg phenylpropanolamine hydrochloride, USP.

Inactive Ingredients: Corn Starch, D&C Yellow No. 10 Al Lake, FD&C Yellow No. 6 Al Lake, Flavor, Lactose, Magnesium Stearate, Mannitol, Saccharin, Stearic Acid.

Indications: CORICIDIN DEMILETS Tablets—For temporary relief of children's congested cold, flu and sinus symptoms.

Actions: CORICIDIN DEMILETS Tablets provide relief of annoying cold, flu and sinus symptoms: running nose, stuffy nose, sneezing, watery/itchy eyes, minor aches, pains and fever.

Warnings: CORICIDIN DEMILETS Tablets—Give water with each dose. Do not give this product for more than 5 days, but if fever is present, persists or recurs, limit dosage to 3 days; if symptoms persist or new ones occur, consult a physician. This product may cause drowsiness, therefore, driving a motor vehicle or operating heavy machinery must be avoided while taking it. Alcoholic beverages must also be avoided while taking this product. It may cause excitability, especially in children. Do not exceed recommended dosage because at higher doses severe liver damage, nervousness, dizziness, elevation of blood pressure or sleeplessness is more likely to occur. Do not administer this product to persons who have asthma, glaucoma, difficulty in urination due to enlargement of the prostate gland, high blood pressure, heart disease, diabetes or thyroid disease, or give this product to children less than 6 years old, except under the advice and supervision of a physician. Keep this and all drugs out of the reach of children. As with any drug, if you are pregnant or nursing a baby, seek the advice of a health professional before using this product.

Drug Interactions: CORICIDIN DEMILETS Tablets—Do not give this product to persons who are presently taking a prescription antihypertensive or antidepressant medication containing a monoamine oxidase inhibitor or an appetite-controlling medication containing phenylpropanolamine except under the advice and supervision of a physician.

Overdosage: In case of accidental overdose, seek professional assistance or contact a Poison Control Center immediately.

Dosage and Administration:
CORICIDIN DEMILETS Tablets—Under 6 years: As directed by a physician. 6 through 11 years: Two DEMILETS Tablets every 4 hours not to exceed 12 tablets in a 24-hour period, or as directed by a physician.

How Supplied: CORICIDIN DEMILETS Tablets—boxes of 36, individually wrapped in a child's protective pack. Store the tablets between 2° and 30°C (36° and 86°F). Protect from excessive moisture.

CORRECTOL®
Laxative
Tablets

Active Ingredients: Tablets—Yellow phenolphthalein, 65 mg. and docusate sodium, 100 mg. per tablet.

Inactive Ingredients: Butylparaben, calcium gluconate, calcium sulfate, carnauba wax, D&C No. 7 calcium lake, gelatin, magnesium stearate, sugar, talc, titanium dioxide, wheat flour, white wax, and other ingredients.

Indications: For relief of occasional constipation or irregularity. CORRECTOL generally produces bowel movement in 6 to 8 hours.

Actions: Yellow phenolphthalein—stimulant laxative; docusate sodium—fecal softener.

Warnings: Not to be taken in case of nausea, vomiting, abdominal pain, or signs of appendicitis. Take only as needed —as frequent or continued use of laxatives may result in dependence on them. If skin rash appears, do not use this or any other preparation containing phenolphthalein. As with any drug, if you are pregnant or nursing a baby, seek the advice of a health professional before using this product.

Dosage and Administration
Dosage: Adults—1 or 2 tablets daily as needed, at bedtime or on arising.
Children over 6 years—1 tablet daily as needed.

How Supplied: Tablets—Individual foil-backed safety sealed blister packaging in boxes of 15, 30, 60 and 90 tablets.
Shown in Product Identification Section, page 425

DI–GEL®
Antacid · Anti-Gas
Tablets/Liquid

DI-GEL Tablets: Active Ingredients: (Per Tablet)—Simethicone 20 mg., Calcium Carbonate 280 mg., Magnesium Hydroxide 128 mg. **Inactive Ingredients:** D & C yellow No. 10 aluminum lake, dextrin, FD&C yellow No. 6 aluminum lake, flavor, magnesium stearate, mannitol, povidone, stearic acid, sucrose, talc.
Dietetically sodium free, calcium rich.

DI-GEL Liquid: Active Ingredients—per teaspoonful (5 ml): Simethicone 20 mg., aluminum hydroxide (equivalent to aluminum hydroxide dried gel USP) 200 mg., magnesium hydroxide 200 mg. **Also contains:** Flavor, methylcellu-

lose, methylparaben, propylparaben, sodium saccharin, sorbitol, water.
Dietetically sodium free.

Indications: For fast, temporary relief of acid indigestion, heartburn, sour stomach and accompanying painful gas symptoms.

Actions: The antacid system in DI-GEL relieves and soothes acid indigestion, heartburn and sour stomach. At the same time, the simethicone "defoamers" eliminate gas.
When air becomes entrapped in the stomach, heartburn and acid indigestion can result, along with sensations of fullness, pressure and bloating.

Warnings: Do not take more than 20 teaspoonfuls or 24 tablets in a 24 hour period, or use the maximum dosage of this product for more than 2 weeks, except under the advice and supervision of a physician. If you have kidney disease do not use this product except under the advice and supervision of a physician. May cause constipation or have a laxative effect.

Drug Interaction: (Liquid Only) This product should not be taken if patient is presently taking a prescription antibiotic drug containing any form of tetracycline.

Dosage and Administration: Two teaspoonfuls or tablets every 2 hours, or after or between meals and at bedtime, not to exceed 20 teaspoonfuls or 24 tablets per day, or as directed by a physician.

How Supplied:
DI-GEL Liquid in Mint Flavor - 6 and 12 fl. oz. bottles, safety sealed and Lemon/Orange Flavors - 6 and 12 fl. oz. bottles, safety sealed.
DI-GEL Tablets in Mint and Lemon/Orange Flavors - In boxes of 30 and 90 in handy portable safety sealed blister packaging. Also available in Mint 60-tablet bottles.
Shown in Product Identification Section, page 425

DRIXORAL®
[dricks-or'al]
Antihistamine/Nasal Decongestant
Syrup

Description: Each 5 ml (1 teaspoonful) of DRIXORAL Syrup contains 2 mg brompheniramine maleate and 30 mg pseudoephedrine sulfate; also contains Citric Acid, D&C Red No. 33, FD&C Yellow No. 6, Flavor, Propylene Glycol, Sodium Benzoate, Sodium Citrate, Sorbitol, Sugar, Water. Drixoral Syrup is alcohol-free.

Indications: DRIXORAL Syrup contains a nasal decongestant with an antihistamine in a pleasant-tasting wild cherry flavor to provide temporary relief of nasal congestion due to the common cold, hay fever or other upper respiratory allergies. Helps decongest sinus openings, sinus passages. Alleviates running nose, sneezing, itching of the nose or throat, and itchy and watery eyes due to hay fever. DRIXORAL Syrup is ideal for adults and children who prefer a syrup instead of tablets or capsules.

Warnings: If symptoms do not improve within 7 days or are accompanied by fever, consult a physician before continuing use. May cause drowsiness. May cause excitability especially in children. Do not exceed recommended dosage because at higher doses nervousness, dizziness, or sleeplessness may occur. Do not give this product to children under 6 years except under the advice and supervision of a physician. Do not take this product if you have asthma, glaucoma, emphysema, chronic pulmonary disease, shortness of breath, difficulty in breathing, difficulty in urination due to enlargement of the prostate gland, high blood pressure, heart disease, diabetes, or thyroid disease except under the advice and supervision of a physician. As with any drug, if you are pregnant or nursing a baby, seek the advice of a health professional before using this product. CAUTION: Avoid driving a motor vehicle or operating heavy machinery. Avoid alcoholic beverages while taking this product. Keep this and all drugs out of the reach of children. In case of accidental overdose, seek professional assistance or contact a Poison Control Center immediately.

Drug Interaction Precaution: Do not take this product if you are presently taking a prescription drug for high blood pressure or depression, without first consulting your doctor.

Directions: Adults and children 12 years of age and over: two teaspoonfuls every 4–6 hours. Children 6 to under 12 years of age: 1 teaspoonful every 4–6 hours. Do not exceed 4 doses in 24 hours. Children under 6 years of age, consult a physician.
Store between 2° and 30°C (36° and 86°F).

Overdosage: In case of accidental overdose, seek professional assistance or contact a Poison Control Center immediately.

How Supplied: DRIXORAL Syrup is available in 4 fl. oz. (118 ml) bottles.

DRIXORAL®
[dricks-or 'al]
Sustained-Action Tablets

Description: EACH DRIXORAL SUSTAINED-ACTION TABLET CONTAINS: 120 mg of pseudoephedrine sulfate and 6 mg of dexbrompheniramine maleate. Half of the medication is released after the tablet is swallowed and the remaining amount of medication is released hours later providing continuous long-lasting relief for 12 hours. Also contains: Acacia, Butylparaben, Calcium Sulfate, Carnauba Wax, Corn Starch, D&C Yellow No. 10 Al Lake, FD&C Blue No. 1 Al Lake, FD&C Yellow No. 6 Al Lake, Gelatin, Lactose, Magnesium Stea-

rate, Neutral Soap, Oleic Acid, Povidone, Rosin, Sugar, Talc, White Wax, Zein.

Indications: For temporary relief of nasal congestion due to the common cold, hay fever, or other upper respiratory allergies, and associated with sinusitis. Helps decongest sinus openings, sinus passages. Reduces swelling of nasal passages; shrinks swollen membranes; and temporarily restores freer breathing through the nose. Alleviates running nose, sneezing, itching of the nose or throat, and itchy and watery eyes as may occur in allergic rhinitis (such as hay fever).

Actions: The antihistamine, dexbrompheniramine maleate, provides temporary relief of sneezing; watery, itchy eyes; running nose due to hay fever and other upper respiratory allergies. The decongestant, pseudoephedrine sulfate, temporarily restores freer breathing through the nose and promotes sinus drainage.

Warnings: If symptoms do not improve within 7 days or are accompanied by fever, consult a physician before continuing use. May cause excitability especially in children. Do not exceed recommended dosage because at higher doses nervousness, dizziness, or sleeplessness may occur. Do not take this product if you have asthma, glaucoma, emphysema, chronic pulmonary disease, high blood pressure, thyroid disease, diabetes, or difficulty in urination due to enlargement of the prostate gland or give this product to children under 12 years, unless directed by a physician. May cause drowsiness; alcohol may increase the drowsiness effect. Avoid alcoholic beverages while taking this product. Use caution when driving a motor vehicle or operating machinery. Keep this and all drugs out of the reach of children. In case of accidental overdose, seek professional assistance or contact a Poison Control Center immediately. As with any drug, if you are pregnant or nursing a baby, seek the advice of a health professional before using this product.

Drug Interaction Precaution: Do not take this product if you are presently taking a prescription drug for high blood pressure or depression, without first consulting your physician.

Dosage and Administration: ADULTS AND CHILDREN 12 YEARS AND OVER—one tablet every 12 hours. Do not exceed two tablets in 24 hours.

How Supplied: DRIXORAL Sustained-Action Tablets, green, sugar-coated tablets branded in black with the product name, boxes of 10, 20, and 40, bottle of 100.
Store between 2° and 30°C (36° and 86°F).

Shown in Product Identification Section, page 425

DRIXORAL® NON-DROWSY FORMULA
[dricks-or 'al]
Long-Acting Nasal Decongestant

DRIXORAL NON-DROWSY FORMULA Long-Acting Nasal Decongestant Tablets contain pseudoephedrine sulfate, a nasal decongestant, in a special timed-release tablet providing up to 12 hours of continuous relief . . . without drowsiness.

Indications: For temporary relief of nasal congestion due to the common cold, hay fever or other upper respiratory allergies, and nasal congestion associated with sinusitis. Helps decongest sinus openings and sinus passages.

Directions: Adults and Children 12 Years and Over—One tablet every 12 hours. DRIXORAL NON-DROWSY FORMULA is not recommended for children under 12 years of age.

Each Extended-Release Tablet Contains: 120 mg pseudoephedrine sulfate. Half the dose is released after the tablet is swallowed and the other half is released hours later, providing continuous relief for up to 12 hours.

Warnings: Do not exceed recommended dosage because at higher doses, nervousness, dizziness, or sleeplessness may occur. Do not take this product if you have heart disease, high blood pressure, thyroid disease, diabetes, difficulty in urination due to enlargement of the prostate gland, or give this product to children under 12 years unless directed by a physician. If symptoms do not improve within 7 days or are accompanied by fever, consult your physician before continuing use. Keep this and all drugs out of the reach of children. In case of accidental overdose, seek professional assistance or contact a Poison Control Center immediately. As with any drug, if you are pregnant or nursing a baby, seek the advice of a health professional before using this product.

Drug Interaction Precautions: Do not take this product if you are presently taking a prescription drug for high blood pressure or depression, without first consulting your physician.

Active Ingredients: Pseudoephedrine Sulfate

Also Contains: Acacia, Butylparaben, Calcium Sulfate, Carnauba Wax, Corn Starch, FD&C Blue No. 1, Gelatin, Lactose, Magnesium Stearate, Neutral Soap, Oleic Acid, Povidone, Rosin, Sugar, Talc, White Wax, Zein.
Store between 2° and 30°C (36° and 86°F).

Continued on next page

Information on Schering-Plough HealthCare Products appearing on these pages is effective as of November 1991.

Schering-Plough—Cont.

Protect from excessive moisture.
Shown in Product Identification Section, page 425

DRIXORAL® PLUS
[*dricks-or 'al*]
Extended-Release Tablets

Active Ingredients: Acetaminophen, Dexbrompheniramine Maleate, Pseudoephedrine Sulfate.

Also Contains: Calcium Phosphate, Carnauba Wax, D&C Yellow No. 10 Al Lake, FD&C Blue No. 1 Al Lake, FD&C Yellow No. 6 Al Lake, Hydroxypropyl Methylcellulose, Magnesium Stearate, Methylparaben, PEG, Propylparaben, Stearic Acid.
DRIXORAL® *PLUS* Extended-Release Tablets combine a nasal decongestant and an antihistamine with a nonaspirin analgesic in a special 12-hour continuous-acting timed-release tablet.

Indications: The *decongestant* temporarily relieves nasal congestion due to the common cold, hay fever or other upper respiratory allergies, and associated with sinusitis. Reduces swelling of nasal passages; shrinks swollen membranes; and temporarily restores freer breathing through the nose. Also helps decongest sinus openings, sinus passages. The *nonaspirin analgesic* temporarily relieves occasional minor aches, pains, and headache and reduces fever due to the common cold. The *antihistamine* alleviates running nose, sneezing, itching of the nose or throat, and itchy and watery eyes as may occur in allergic rhinitis (such as hay fever).
EACH DRIXORAL PLUS EXTENDED-RELEASE TABLET CONTAINS: 60 mg of pseudoephedrine sulfate, 3 mg of dexbrompheniramine maleate and 500 mg of acetaminophen. These ingredients are released continuously, providing long-lasting relief for 12 hours.

Directions: ADULTS AND CHILDREN 12 YEARS AND OVER—two tablets every 12 hours. Do not exceed four tablets in 24 hours. Children under 12 years of age: consult a doctor.

Warnings: Do not take this product for more than 7 days. If symptoms do not improve, or are accompanied by fever that lasts for more than three days (72 hours) or recurs, or if new symptoms occur, consult a physician before continuing use. If pain or fever persists or gets worse, or if redness or swelling is present, consult a physician because these could be signs of a serious condition. May cause excitability especially in children. Do not exceed recommended dosage because at higher doses nervousness, dizziness, or sleeplessness may occur. Do not take this product if you have asthma, glaucoma, emphysema, chronic pulmonary disease, shortness of breath, difficulty in breathing, heart disease, high blood pressure, thyroid disease, difficulty in urination due to enlargement of the prostate gland, or

give this product to children under 12 years unless directed by a physician. May cause drowsiness; alcohol, sedatives, and tranquilizers may increase the drowsiness effect. Avoid alcoholic beverages while taking this product. Use caution when driving a motor vehicle or operating machinery. Keep this and all drugs out of the reach of children. In case of accidental overdose, seek professional assistance or contact a Poison Control Center immediately. Prompt medical attention is critical for adults as well as for children even if you do not notice any signs or symptoms. As with any drug, if you are pregnant or nursing a baby, seek the advice of a health professional before using this product.

Drug Interaction Precaution: Do not take this product if you are presently taking a prescription drug for high blood pressure or depression, sedatives or tranquilizers, without first consulting your physician.

How Supplied: DRIXORAL PLUS Extended-Release Tablets are available in boxes of 12's and 24's and bottles of 48. **Store between 2° and 30°C (36° and 86°F).**
Protect from excessive moisture.
Shown in Product Identification Section, page 425

DRIXORAL® SINUS
[*dricks-or 'al*]
Nasal decongestant/Pain reliever/Antihistamine
DRIXORAL® SINUS Extended-Release Tablets combine a nasal decongestant, and a non-aspirin analgesic, with an antihistamine in a special 12-hour continuous-acting timed-release tablet.

Indications: The *decongestant* temporarily relieves nasal congestion due to sinusitis, the common cold, and hay fever or other upper respiratory allergies. Helps decongest sinus openings, sinus passages; relieves sinus pressure. Reduces swelling of nasal passages; shrinks swollen membranes; and temporarily restores freer breathing through the nose. The *non-aspirin analgesic* temporarily relieves occasional headaches, minor aches and pains, and reduces fever due to the common cold. The *antihistamine* alleviates runny nose, sneezing, itching of the nose or throat, and itchy and watery eyes as may occur in allergic rhinitis (such as hay fever).

Each Drixoral Sinus Extended-Release Tablet Contains: 60 mg of pseudoephedrine sulfate, 3 mg of dexbrompheniramine maleate, and 500 mg of acetaminophen. These ingredients are released continuously, providing long-lasting relief for 12 hours.

Directions: ADULTS AND CHILDREN 12 YEARS AND OVER—two tablets every 12 hours. Do not exceed four tablets in 24 hours. Children under 12 years of age: consult a physician.

Store between 2° and 26°C (36° and 77°F).
Protect from excessive moisture.

Warnings: Do not take this product for more than 7 days. If symptoms do not improve, or are accompanied by fever that lasts for more than three days (72 hours) or recurs, or if new symptoms occur, consult a physician before continuing use. If pain or fever persists or gets worse, or if redness or swelling is present, consult a physician because these could be signs of a serious condition. May cause excitability especially in children. Do not exceed recommended dosage because at higher doses nervousness, dizziness, or sleeplessness may occur. Do not take this product if you have asthma, glaucoma, emphysema, chronic pulmonary disease, shortness of breath, difficulty in breathing, heart disease, high blood pressure, thyroid disease, diabetes, difficulty in urination due to enlargement of the prostate gland, or give this product to children under 12 years unless directed by a physician. May cause drowsiness; alcohol, sedatives, and tranquilizers may increase the drowsiness effect. Avoid alcoholic beverages while taking this product. Use caution when driving a motor vehicle or operating machinery. Keep this and all drugs out of the reach of children. In case of accidental overdose, seek professional assistance or contact a Poison Control Center immediately. Prompt medical attention is critical for adults as well as for children even if you do not notice any signs or symptoms. As with any drug, if you are pregnant or nursing a baby, seek the advice of a health care professional before using this product.

Drug Interaction Precaution: Do not take this product if you are presently taking a prescription drug for high blood pressure or depression, sedatives, or tranquilizers, without first consulting your physician.
Shown in Product Identification, Section, page 426

DUOFILM® LIQUID

Active Ingredient: Salicylic Acid 17% (w/w).

Inactive Ingredients: Alcohol 15.8% w/w, castor oil, ether 42.6% w/w, ethyl lactate, and polybutene in flexible collodion.

Indications: For the removal of common and plantar warts. Common warts can be easily recognized by the rough, cauliflower-like appearance of the surface. Plantar warts are found on the bottom of the foot.

Warnings: For external use only. Do not use this product on irritated skin, on any area that is infected or reddened, if you are a diabetic, or if you have poor blood circulation. If discomfort persists, see your doctor. Do not use on moles, birthmarks, warts with hair growing from them, genital warts, or warts on the face or mucous membranes. Keep out of reach of children. If DuoFilm Liquid gets in eyes, flush with water for 15 minutes. Avoid inhaling vapors. DuoFilm Liquid is extremely flammable. Keep away from fire or flame. Cap bottle tightly when not in use. Store at room temperature away from heat.

Dosage and Administration: Wash affected area. Soak wart in warm water for five minutes. Dry area thoroughly with a clean towel. Apply a thin layer of Duo-Film Liquid directly to wart with the brush applicator. Repeat procedure once or twice daily as needed (until wart is removed) for up to 12 weeks.

How Supplied: DuoFilm Liquid is available in ½ fluid oz. spill-resistant bottles with brush applicator for pinpoint application.
Shown in Product Identification Section, page 426

DUOPLANT® GEL

Active Ingredient: Salicylic Acid 17% (w/w).

Inactive Ingredients: Alcohol 57.6% w/w, ether 16.42% w/w, ethyl lactate, hydroxypropyl cellulose, and polybutene in flexible collodion, USP.

Indications: For the removal of plantar and common warts. Plantar warts are found on the bottom of the foot. Common warts can be easily recognized by the rough, cauliflower-like appearance of the surface.

Warnings: For external use only. Do not use this product on irritated skin, on any area that is infected or reddened, if you are a diabetic, or if you have poor blood circulation. If discomfort persists, see your doctor. Do not use on moles, birthmarks, warts with hair growing from them, genital warts, or warts on the face or mucous membranes. Keep out of reach of children. If DuoPlant Gel gets in eyes, flush with water for 15 minutes. Avoid inhaling vapors. DuoPlant Gel is extremely flammable. Keep away from fire or flame. Keep tube tightly capped when not in use. Store at room temperature away from heat.

Dosage and Administration: Wash affected area. Soak wart in warm water for five minutes. Dry area thoroughly with a clean towel. Apply a thin layer of Duo-Plant Gel directly to wart. Cover treated area with adhesive tape. Repeat procedure once or twice daily as needed (until wart is removed) for up to 12 weeks.

How Supplied: DuoPlant Gel is available in ½ oz. tubes with applicator tip for pinpoint application.
Shown in Product Identification Section, page 426

DURATION®
12 Hour Nasal Spray
Topical Nasal Decongestant

Active Ingredient:
12 Hour Nasal Spray:
Oxymetazoline HCl 0.05%

Other Ingredients:
12 Hour Nasal Spray: Preservative Phenylmercuric Acetate

Indications: Immediate relief for up to 12 hours of nasal congestion due to colds, hay fever and sinusitis.

Actions: The sympathomimetic action of DURATION constricts the smaller arterioles of the nasal passages, producing a gentle and predictable decongesting effect.

Warnings: Do not exceed recommended dosage because symptoms may occur such as burning, stinging, sneezing, or increase of nasal discharge. Do not use this product for more than 3 days. If symptoms persist, consult a physician. As with any drug, if you are pregnant or nursing a baby, seek the advice of a health professional before using this product. The use of dispenser by more than one person may spread infection. Keep this and all medication out of the reach of children. In case of accidental ingestion, seek professional assistance or contact a Poison Control Center immediately.

Dosage and Administration:
DURATION 12 Hour Nasal Spray— With head upright, spray 2 or 3 times in each nostril twice daily—morning and evening. To spray, squeeze bottle quickly and firmly. Not recommended for children under 6.

How Supplied:
DURATION 12 Hour Nasal Spray—½ and 1 fl. oz. plastic squeeze bottle. All bottles in safety sealed cartons.
Shown in Product Identification Section, page 426

DURATION®
12 Hour Nasal Spray Pump

Active Ingredients: Oxymetazoline Hydrochloride 0.05%

Inactive Ingredients: Aminoacetic Acid, Benzalkonium Chloride, Phenylmercuric Acetate (Preservative), Sorbitol, Water.

Indications: Delivers a measured dosage every time. Immediate relief of nasal congestion for up to 12 hours due to common cold, hay fever and sinusitis.

Warnings: Do not exceed recommended dosage because symptoms may occur such as burning, stinging, sneezing, or increase of nasal discharge. Do not use this product for more than 3 days. If symptoms persist, consult a physician. As with any drug, if you are pregnant or nursing a baby, seek the advice of a health professional before using this product. The use of dispenser by more than one person may spread infection.

Keep this and all medications out of the reach of children.

Symptoms and Treatment of Oral Overdosage: In case of accidental ingestion, seek professional assistance or contact a Poison Control Center immediately.

Dosage and Administration: Before using first time, remove protective cap. Prime the metered pump by depressing several times. Hold bottle with thumb at base and nozzle between first and second fingers. With head upright (do not tilt backward), insert pump-spray nozzle in nostril. Depress pump completely 2 or 3 times. Sniff deeply. Repeat in other nostil. Wipe tip clean after each use.

How Supplied: Available in ½ fl. oz. pump spray.
Shown in Product Identification Section, page 426

FEEN-A-MINT®
Laxative Gum/Pills

Active Ingredients: Gum—yellow phenolphthalein 97.2 mg. per tablet. Pills—yellow phenolphthalein 65 mg., and docusate sodium 100 mg. per pill.

Indications: For relief of occasional constipation or irregularity. FEEN-A-MINT generally produces bowel movement in 6 to 8 hours.

Inactive Ingredients: Gum—Acacia, butylated hydroxyanisole, gelatin, glycerin, glucose, gum base, peppermint oil, sodium benzoate, starch, sugar, talc, water.
Pills—Butylparaben, calcium gluconate, calcium slufate, carnauba wax, gelatin, magnesium stearate, sugar, talc, titanium dioxide, wheat flour, white wax and other ingredients.

How Supplied: Gum—Individual foil-backed safety sealed blister packaging in boxes of 5 and 16 tablets.
Pills—Safety sealed boxes of 15, 30, and 60 tablets.
Shown in Product Identification Section, page 426

GYNE–LOTRIMIN®
Clotrimazole
Vaginal Cream
Antifungal

Active Ingredient: Clotrimazole 1%

Inactive Ingredients: Benzyl alcohol, cetearyl alcohol, cetyl esters wax, octyldodecanol, polysorbate 60, purified water, sorbitan monostearate.

Indications: Gyne-Lotrimin® will cure most recurrent vaginal yeast (Candida)

Continued on next page

Information on Schering-Plough HealthCare Products appearing on these pages is effective as of November 1991.

Schering-Plough—Cont.

infections. Gyne-Lotrimin® usually starts to relieve the itching and other symptoms of vaginal yeast infection within 3 days. If the patient does not improve in 3 days or if the patient does not get well in 7 days, a condition other than yeast infection may exist. The patient should discontinue use of the product and consult a doctor. Also, if symptoms recur within a 2-month period, patient should consult a doctor.

Important: In order to kill the yeast completely, GYNE-LOTRIMIN must be used the full seven days, even if symptoms are relieved sooner.

WARNINGS:
• Do not use if you have abdominal pain, fever, or a foul-smelling vaginal discharge. You may have a condition which is more serious than a yeast infection. Contact your doctor immediately.
• Do not use if this is your first experience with vaginal itch and discomfort. See your doctor.
• If there is no improvement within 3 days, you may have a condition other than a yeast infection. Stop using this product and see your doctor.
• If symptoms recur within a 2-month period, contact your doctor.
• Do not use during pregnancy except under the advice and supervision of a doctor.
• This medication is for vaginal use only. It is not for use in the mouth or the eyes. In case accidentally swallowed, seek professional assistance or contact a Poison Control Center immediately.
• Keep this and all drugs out of reach of children. This product is not to be used on children less than 12 years of age.

Dosage: Fill the applicator with the cream and then insert one applicatorful of cream into the vagina every day, preferably at bedtime. Repeat this procedure for seven consecutive days.
Shown in Product Identification Section, page 426

GYNE–LOTRIMIN®
Clotrimazole
Vaginal Inserts
Antifungal

Active Ingredient: Each insert contains Clotrimazole 100 mg.

Inactive Ingredients: Corn starch, lactose, magnesium stearate, povidone.

Indications: Gyne-Lotrimin® will cure most vaginal yeast (Candida) infections. Gyne-Lotrimin® usually starts to relieve the itching and other symptoms of vaginal yeast infection within 3 days. If the patient does not improve in 3 days or if the patient does not get well in 7 days, a condition other than yeast infection may exist. The patient should discontinue use of the product and consult a doctor. Also, if symptoms recur within a 2-month period, patient should consult a doctor.

Important: In order to kill the yeast completely, GYNE-LOTRIMIN must be used the full seven days, even if symptoms are relieved sooner.

WARNINGS:
• Do not use if you have abdominal pain, fever, or a foul-smelling vaginal discharge. You may have a condition which is more serious than a yeast infection. Contact your doctor immediately.
• Do not use if this is your first experience with vaginal itch and discomfort. See your doctor.
• If there is no improvement within 3 days, you may have a condition other than a yeast infection. Stop using this product and see your doctor.
• If symptoms recur within a 2-month period, contact your doctor.
• Do not use during pregnancy except under the advice and supervision of a doctor.
• This medication is for vaginal use only. It is not for use in the mouth or the eyes. In case accidentally swallowed, seek professional assistance or contact a Poison Control Center immediately.
• Keep this and all drugs out of reach of children. This product is not to be used on children less than 12 years of age.

Dosage: Using the applicator, place one insert into the vagina, preferably at bedtime. Repeat this procedure for seven consecutive days.
Shown in Product Identification Section, page 426

GYNE–MOISTRIN™
Vaginal Moisturizing Gel

Description: Gyne-Moistrin Vaginal Moisturizing Gel was specially developed to soothe and relieve vaginal dryness. Gyne-Moistrin provides natural feeling moisture and lubrication. It is clear, colorless, odorless and proven to be non-irritating. Gyne-Moistrin is water-based, greaseless and non-staining; and it contains no hormones or medication, so it can be used as often as needed.

Actions: When used as directed, Gyne-Moistrin will relieve vaginal dryness. Gyne-Moistrin forms a non-occlusive layer of moisture over the vaginal epithelium, gradually hydrating a dry irritated area. Gyne-Moistrin can be used as often as needed.
Externally, in the vulvar area, Gyne-Moistrin will also moisturize tissues.

Ingredients: Polyglycerylmethacrylate, water, propylene glycol, methylparaben, propylparaben.

Warnings: Gyne-Moistrin is not a contraceptive.

Directions: Gyne-Moistrin may be applied externally and internally according to personal preference using fingertip application or the reusable applicator.
FOR FINGERTIP APPLICATION: Squeeze out small amount of gel to cover fingertip and apply to the vaginal opening and external area as needed. Actual amount applied may be increased or decreased according to personal preference.

FOR INTERNAL USE: Remove reusable applicator from sealed wrapper. Fill with gel to line on applicator. Gently insert front end well into vagina; push end of applicator to fully release gel; remove applicator. Actual amount used may be increased or decreased according to personal preference. Wash applicator in warm soapy water then thoroughly rinse and dry before and after each use.

How Supplied: Gyne-Moistrin is available in 1.5 oz. and 2.5 oz. tubes.
Shown in Product Identification Section, page 426

LOTRIMIN® AF ANTIFUNGAL
[lo-tre-min]
Cream 1%
Solution 1%
Lotion 1%

Description: Lotrimin® AF Cream 1% is a white fully vanishing homogeneous cream containing 1% clotrimazole. The cream contains no sensitizing parabens and is totally grease free and non-staining.
Lotrimin® AF Solution 1% is a nonaqueous liquid, containing polyethylene glycol.
Lotrimin® AF Lotion 1% is light penetrating buffered emulsion also containing no common sensitizing agents and is greaseless and nonstaining.

Indications: Lotrimin® AF Cream, Solution and Lotion contain 1% clotrimazole, a synthetic broad-spectrum antifungal agent. Clotrimazole is used for the treatment of dermal infections caused by a variety of pathogenic dermatophytes, yeasts and *Malassezia furfur*. The primary action of clotrimazole is against dividing and growing organisms. Lotrimin® AF was first made available as an over-the-counter drug in 1990 and is indicated for superficial dermatophyte infections: athlete's foot (tinea pedis), jock itch (tinea cruris) and ringworm (tinea corporis). Lotrimin® remains on prescription for topical candidiasis due to *Candida albicans* and tinea versicolor due to *Malassezia furfur*.

Directions: Cleanse skin with soap and water and dry thoroughly. Apply a thin layer over affected area morning and evening or as directed by a physician. For athlete's foot, pay special attention to the spaces between the toes. It is also helpful to wear well-fitting, ventilated shoes and to change shoes and socks at least once daily. Best results in athlete's foot and ringworm are usually obtained with 4 weeks' use of this product, and in jock itch, with 2 weeks' use. If satisfactory results have not occurred within these times, consult a physician or pharmacist. Children under 12 years of age should be supervised in the use of this product. This product is not effective on the scalp or nails.

How Supplied: Lotrimin® AF Antifungal Cream is available in a 0.42 oz. tube (12 grams) and a 0.84 oz. tube (24 grams).

Inactive ingredients include: benzyl alcohol, cetearyl alcohol, cetyl esters wax, octyldodecanol, polysorbate, sorbitan monostearate and water.

Lotrimin® AF Antifungal Solution is available in a 0.33 fl. oz. (10 milliliters) bottle. Inactive ingredients include polyethylene glycol.

Lotrimin® AF Antifungal Lotion is available in a 0.66 fl. oz. (20 milliliters) bottle. Inactive ingredients include benzyl alcohol, cetearyl alcohol, cetyl esters wax, octyldodecanol, polysorbate, sodium phosphate, sorbitan monostearate and water.

Storage: Keep Lotrimin® AF products between 2° and 30°C (36° and 86°F).

Shown in Product Identification Section, page 426

ST. JOSEPH®
ADULT CHEWABLE ASPIRIN
Low Strength Caplets (81 mg. each)

Active Ingredient: Each St. Joseph Adult Chewable Aspirin caplet contains 81 mg. (1.25 grains) aspirin in a chewable, pleasant citrus-flavored form.

Inactive Ingredients: D&C yellow No. 10 aluminum lake, FD&C yellow No. 6 aluminum lake, flavor, hydrogenated vegetable oil, maltodextrin, mannitol, saccharin, starch.

Indications: For safe, effective, temporary relief from: headache, muscular aches, minor aches and pain associated with overexertion, sprains, menstrual cramps, neuralgia, bursitis, and discomforts of fever due to colds.

Actions: Analgesic/Antipyretic.

Warnings: Children and teenagers should not use this medicine for chicken pox or flu symptoms before a doctor is consulted about Reye syndrome, a rare but serious illness reported to be associated with aspirin. As with any drug, if you are pregnant or nursing a baby, seek the advice of a health professional before using this product. **IT IS ESPECIALLY IMPORTANT NOT TO USE ASPIRIN DURING THE LAST 3 MONTHS OF PREGNANCY UNLESS SPECIFICALLY DIRECTED TO DO SO BY A DOCTOR BECAUSE IT MAY CAUSE PROBLEMS IN THE UNBORN CHILD OR COMPLICATIONS DURING DELIVERY.** Keep out of reach of children. In case of an accidental overdose, seek professional assistance or contact a poison control center immediately.

Dosage and Administration: Adult Dose—Analgesic/Antipyretic Indication: Take from 4 to 8 caplets (325 mg. to 650 mg.) every 4 hours as needed. Do not exceed 48 caplets in 24 hours. For professional dosage see below.

IN MYOCARDIAL INFARCTION PROPHYLAXIS

Indication: Aspirin is indicated to reduce the risk of death and/or nonfatal myocardial infarction in patients with a previous infarction or unstable angina pectoris.

Advantages of Product Form: Four St. Joseph Adult Chewable Aspirin caplets give patients the appropriate dosage (325 mg.) of aspirin to help prevent secondary MI. Because they're chewable, they can be taken anytime and anyplace. And they have a pleasant-tasting citrus flavor.

Clinical Trials: The indication is supported by the results of six, large, randomized, multicenter, placebo-controlled studies[1-7] involving 10,816, predominantly male, post–myocardial infarction (MI) patients and one randomized placebo-controlled study of 1,266 men with unstable angina. Therapy with aspirin was begun at intervals after the onset of acute MI varying from less than 3 days to more than 5 years and continued for periods of from less than 1 year to 4 years. In the unstable angina study, treatment was started within 1 month after the onset of unstable angina and continued for 12 weeks; complicating conditions, such as congestive heart failure were not included in the study.

Aspirin therapy in MI patients was associated with about a 20% reduction in the risk of subsequent death and/or nonfatal reinfarction, a median absolute decrease of 3% from the 12 to 22% event rates in the placebo groups. In aspirin-treated unstable angina patients the reduction in risk was about 50%, a reduction in event rate of 5% from the 10% rate in the placebo group over the 12 weeks of the study.

Daily dosage of aspirin in the post–myocardial infarction studies was 300 mg. in one study and 900 to 1500 mg. in five studies. A dose of 325 mg. was used in the study of unstable angina.

Adverse Reactions: Gastrointestinal Reactions—Doses of 1000 mg. per day of aspirin caused gastrointestinal symptoms and bleeding that in some cases were clinically significant. In the largest postinfarction study, the Aspirin Myocardial Infarction Study (AMIS) trial with 4,500 people, the percentage incidences of gastrointestinal symptoms for the aspirin (1000 mg. of a standard, solid-tablet formulation) and placebo-treated subjects, respectively, were: stomach pain (14.3%; 4.4%); heartburn (11.9%; 4.3%); nausea and/or vomiting (7.3%; 2.1%); hospitalization for GI disorder (4.9%; 3.3%). In the AMIS and other trials, aspirin-treated patients had increased rates of gross gastrointestinal bleeding.

Cardiovascular and Biochemical: In the AMIS trial, the dosage of 1000 mg. per day of aspirin was associated with small increases in systolic blood pressure (BP) (average 1.5 to 2.1 mm) and diastolic BP (0.5 to 0.6 mm), depending upon whether maximal or last available readings were used. Blood urea nitrogen and

uric acid levels were also increased, but by less than 1.0 mg.%. Subjects with marked hypertension or renal insufficiency had been excluded from the trial so that the clinical importance of these observations for such subjects or for any subjects treated over more prolonged periods is not known. It is recommended that patients placed on long-term aspirin treatment, even at doses of 300 mg. per day, be seen at regular intervals to assess changes in these measurements.

Dosage and Administration: Although most of the studies used dosages exceeding 300 mg., two trials used only 300 mg. daily, and pharmacologic data indicate that this dose inhibits platelet function fully. Therefore, 300 mg. or a conventional 325 mg. aspirin dose daily is a reasonable routine dose that would minimize gastrointestinal adverse reactions.

How Supplied: Chewable citrus-flavored caplets in plastic bottles of 36 caplets each.

References: (1) Elwood, P.C., et al.: A Randomized Controlled Trial of Acetylsalicylic Acid in the Secondary Prevention of Mortality from Myocardial Infarction, *British Medical Journal*, 1:436–440, 1974. (2) The Coronary Drug Project Research Group: "Aspirin in Coronary Heart Disease," *Journal of Chronic Disease*, 29:625–642, 1976. (3) Breddin, K., et al.: "Secondary Prevention of Myocardial Infarction: A Comparison of Acetylsalicylic Acid, Placebo and Phenprocoumon, *Homeostasis*, 9:325–344, 1980. (4) Aspirin Myocardial Infarction Study Research Group, "A Randomized, Controlled Trial of Aspirin in Persons Recovered from Myocardial Infarction," *Journal American Medical Association*, 245:661–669, 1980. (5) Elwood, P.C., and Sweetnam, P.M., "Aspirin and Secondary Mortality After Myocardial Infarction," *Lancet*, pp. 1313–1315, December 22–29, 1979. (6) The Persantine-Aspirin Reinfarction Study Research Group, "Persantine and Aspirin in Coronary Heart Disease," *Circulation*, 62: 449–460, 1980. (7) Lewis, H.D., et al., "Protective Effects of Aspirin Against Acute Myocardial Infarction and Death in Men with Unstable Angina. Results of a Veterans Administration Cooperative Study," *New England Journal of Medicine*, 309:396–403, 1983.

ST. JOSEPH® Aspirin–Free Fever Reducer
for Children
Chewable Tablets

Active Ingredient: Each Children's St. Joseph Aspirin-Free Chewable Tablet contains 80 mg. acetaminophen in a fruit-flavored tablet.

Continued on next page

Information on Schering-Plough HealthCare Products appearing on these pages is effective as of November 1991.

Schering-Plough—Cont.

ST. JOSEPH CHILDREN'S DOSAGE CHART

Age	0–3 (months)	4–11 (months)	12–23 (months)	2–3 (years)	4–5 (years)	6–8 (years)	9–10 (years)	11 (years)	12+ (years)
Weight (lbs.)	7–12	13–21	22–26	27–35	36–45	46–65	66–76	77–83	84+
Chewable Tablets Acetaminophen (80 mg. each)	—	—	1½	2	3	4	5	6	8

All dosages may be repeated every 4 hours, but do not exceed 5 dosages daily.
Note: Since St. Joseph pediatric products are available without prescription, parents are advised on the package label to consult a physician for use in children under two years.

Inactive Ingredients: Tablets: Cellulose, D&C red No. 7 calcium lake, D&C red No. 30 aluminum lake, flavor, mannitol, silicon dioxide, sodium saccharin, zinc stearate.

Indications: For temporary reduction of fever, relief of minor aches and pains of colds and flu.

Actions: Analgesic/Antipyretic

Warnings: Do not administer this product for more than 5 days. If symptoms persist or new ones occur, consult physician. If fever persists for more than three days, or recurs, consult physician. When using St. Joseph Aspirin-Free products do not give other medications containing acetaminophen unless directed by your physician. NOTE: SEVERE OR PERSISTENT SORE THROAT, HIGH FEVER, HEADACHES, NAUSEA OR VOMITING MAY BE SERIOUS. DISCONTINUE USE AND CONSULT PHYSICIAN IF NOT RELIEVED IN 24 HOURS. Do not exceed recommended dosage because severe liver damage may occur. As with any drug, if you are pregnant or nursing a baby, seek the advice of a health professional before using this product.

Dosage and Administration: [See table above.]
ST. JOSEPH Aspirin-Free Fever Reducer Tablets for Children may be given one of three ways. Always follow with ½ glass of water, milk or fruit juice.
1. Chewed, followed by liquid.
2. Crushed or dissolved in a teaspoon of liquid (for younger children).
3. Powdered for infant use, when so directed by physician.

How Supplied: Chewable fruit flavored tablets in plastic bottles of 30 tablets.
All packages have child resistant safety caps and safety sealed packaging.

ST. JOSEPH® Cold Tablets for Children

Active Ingredients: Per tablet: Acetaminophen 80 mg and phenylpropanolamine hydrochloride 3.125 mg.

Inactive Ingredients: Cellulose, FD&C Yellow No. 6 aluminum lake, flavor, mannitol, silica, sodium saccharin, zinc stearate.

Indications: ST. JOSEPH Cold Tablets combine acetaminophen with a gentle nasal decongestant to relieve congestion, runny nose, difficult breathing, and fever which accompany colds in children. (1) Acetaminophen is widely recommended by pediatricians to reduce fever fast and relieve the aches and pains of cold and flu without causing stomach upset or irritation. (2) The gentle nasal decongestant quickly relieves a stuffy nose and helps restore easier breathing without causing drowsiness. ST. JOSEPH Cold Tablets are sugar-free and fruit-flavored.

DOSAGE BY AGE AND WEIGHT
To be administered under adult supervision

Age (Years)	Weight (lbs.)	Dosage
Under 2	below 27	As directed by physician.
2–3	27–35	2 tablets
4–5	36–45	3 tablets
6–8	46–65	4 tablets
9–10	66–76	5 tablets
11	77–83	6 tablets
12+	84 & over	8 tablets

May be repeated every 4 hours, but do not exceed 4 doses daily, unless prescribed by your doctor.
ST. JOSEPH Cold Tablets for Children may be dissolved on the child's tongue, chewed or swallowed whole. Always follow immediately with liquid. For younger children crush and dissolve in spoon of liquid.
Each tablet contains: Acetaminophen 80 mg. and phenylpropanolamine hydrochloride 3.125 mg.

Warning: Do not take this product for more than five days. If symptoms persist, or new ones occur, consult your physician. If fever persists for more than three days, or recurs, consult your physician.
Do not exceed recommended dosage because severe liver damage may occur.
When using ST. JOSEPH Cold Tablets do not give other medications containing acetaminophen unless directed by your physician. NOTE: SEVERE OR PERSISTENT SORE THROAT, HIGH FEVER, HEADACHE, NAUSEA OR VOMITING MAY BE SERIOUS. DISCONTINUE USE AND CONSULT PHYSICIAN IF NOT RELIEVED IN 24 HOURS. As with any drug, if you are pregnant or nursing a baby, seek the advice of a health professional before using this product. Keep this and all drugs out of the reach of children. In case of accidental overdose, seek professional assistance or contact a Poison Control center immediately.

How Supplied: In bottle with 30 fruit flavored chewable tablets.

ST. JOSEPH® Cough Suppressant for Children
Pediatric
Antitussive Suppressant

Active Ingredient: Dextromethorphan hydrobromide 7.5 mg. per 5 cc. (teaspoonful)

Inactive Ingredients: Caramel, citric acid, flavor, glycerin, methylparaben, propylparaben, sodium benzoate, sodium citrate, sucrose, water.

Indications: Temporarily relieves cough associated with a common cold or inhaled irritants. Quiets coughing to help you and your child get needed sleep. The non-narcotic SUPPRESSIN® formula gives advantages of codeine without its side effects.

Dose

Age (yrs.)	WT. (lbs.)	Dosage
Under 2	Below 27	As directed by physician.
2–6	27–45	1 teaspoon every 6 to 8 hours (not to exceed 4 tsp. daily)
6–12	46–83	2 teaspoons every 6 to 8 hours (not to exceed 8 tsp. daily)
12+	84+	4 teaspoons every 6 to 8 hours (not to exceed 16 tsp. daily)

Do not exceed 4 doses per day.

Warnings: Do not give this product to children under 2 years except under the advice and supervision of a physician. Do not take this product for persistent or chronic cough such as occurs with smoking, asthma, or emphysema, or where cough is accompanied by excessive mucus unless directed by a doctor. As with any drug, if you are pregnant or nursing a baby, seek the advice of a health professional before using this product.

Caution: A persistent cough may be a sign of serious condition. If cough persists for more than 1 week, tends to recur or is accompanied by high fever, rash or persistent headache, consult a physician. Keep this and all drugs out of the reach of children. In case of accidental overdose, seek professional assistance or contact a Poison Control Center immediately.

How Supplied: Alcohol-Free Cherry tasting suppressant in plastic bottle of 2 and 4 fl. ozs. In safety sealed packaging.

TINACTIN® Antifungal
[tin-ak'tin]
Cream 1%
Solution 1%
Powder 1%
Powder (1%) Aerosol
Liquid (1%) Aerosol
Deodorant Powder Aerosol 1%
Jock Itch Cream 1%
Jock Itch Spray Powder 1%

Description: TINACTIN Cream 1% is a white homogeneous, nonaqueous preparation containing the highly active synthetic fungicidal agent, tolnaftate. Each gram contains 10 mg tolnaftate solubilized in BHT, Carbomer 934 P, Monoamylamine, PEG, Propylene Glycol, and Titanium Dioxide.

TINACTIN Jock Itch Cream 1% is a smooth white homogeneous cream containing the highly active synthetic fungicidal agent, tolnaftate. Each gram contains 10 mg tolnaftate finely dispersed in a water-washable emulsion containing: Cetearyl Alcohol, Ceteareth-30, Chlorocresol, Mineral Oil, Petrolatum, Propylene Glycol, Sodium Phosphate and Water. Phosphoric acid and sodium hydroxide used to adjust pH.

TINACTIN Solution 1% contains in each ml tolnaftate 10 mg, BHT, and PEG. The solution solidifies at low temperatures but liquefies readily when warmed, retaining its potency.

TINACTIN Liquid Aerosol contains 91 mg tolnaftate in a vehicle of Alcohol SD-40-2 (36% w/w), BHT and PPG-12 Buteth-16. The spray deposits solution containing a concentration of 1% tolnaftate.
Each gram of **TINACTIN Powder 1%** contains tolnaftate 10 mg in a vehicle of corn starch and talc.

TINACTIN Powder Aerosol contains 91 mg tolnaftate in a vehicle of Alcohol SD-40-2 (14% w/w), BHT, Hydrocarbon Propellant, PPG-12 Buteth-16 and Talc.

The spray deposits a white clinging powder containing a concentration of 1% tolnaftate.

TINACTIN Deodorant Powder Aerosol contains tolnaftate in a vehicle of SD Alcohol 40 (14% w/w), talc, PPG-12-Buteth-16, starch/acrylates/acrylamide copolymer, fragrance, BHT. The spray deposits a white clinging powder containing a concentration of 1% tolnaftate.

TINACTIN Jock Itch Spray Powder contains 91 mg tolnaftate in a vehicle of Alcohol SD-40-2 (14% w/w), BHT, Hydrocarbon Propellant, PPG-12 Buteth-16, Talc. The spray deposits a white clinging powder containing a concentration of 1% tolnaftate.

Indications: TINACTIN Cream, Solution, Liquid Aerosol and **TINACTIN Jock Itch Cream** are highly active antifungal agents that are effective in killing superficial fungi of the skin which cause tinea pedis (athlete's foot), tinea cruris (jock itch) and tinea corporis (body ringworm).

TINACTIN Powder, Powder Aerosol, Deodorant Powder Aerosol and **TINACTIN Jock Itch Spray Powder** are effective in killing superficial fungi of the skin which cause tinea cruris (jock itch) and tinea pedis (athlete's foot). All forms begin to relieve burning, itching and soreness within 24 hours. The powder and powder aerosol forms aid the drying of naturally moist areas. The deodorant powder aerosol provides additional protection against odor and wetness.

Actions: The active ingredient in TINACTIN, tolnaftate, is a highly active synthetic fungicidal agent that is effective in the treatment of superficial fungous infections of the skin. It is inactive systemically, virtually nonsensitizing, and does not ordinarily sting or irritate intact or broken skin, even in the presence of acute inflammatory reactions. TINACTIN products are odorless, greaseless, and do not stain or discolor the skin, hair, or nails.

Warnings: Keep these and all drugs out of the reach of children. Do not use in children under 2 years of age except under the advice and supervision of a physician.

TINACTIN Powder Aerosol, Deodorant Powder Aerosol and **Liquid Aerosol:** Avoid spraying in eyes. Contents under pressure. Do not puncture or incinerate. Flammable mixture, do not use or store near heat or open flame. Exposure to temperatures above 120°F may cause bursting. Never throw container into fire or incinerator. Use only as directed. Intentional misuse by deliberately concentrating and inhaling the contents can be harmful or fatal.

Precautions: If irritation occurs or symptoms do not improve within 10 days, discontinue use and consult your physician or podiatrist.

TINACTIN products are for external use only. Keep out of eyes.

TINACTIN is not effective on nail or scalp infections.

Overdosage: In case of accidental ingestion, seek professional assistance or contact a Poison Control Center immediately.

Dosage and Administration: Children under 12 years of age should be supervised in the use of TINACTIN.

TINACTIN Cream and **TINACTIN Jock Itch Cream**—Wash and dry infected area. Then apply one-half inch ribbon of cream and rub gently on infected area morning and evening or as directed by a doctor. Spread evenly. Best results in athlete's foot and body ringworm are usually obtained with 4 weeks' use of this product and in jock itch, with 2 weeks' use. To help prevent recurrence of athlete's foot, continue treatment for two weeks after disappearance of all symptoms.

TINACTIN Solution—Wash and dry infected area. Then apply two or three drops morning and evening or as directed by a doctor, and massage gently to cover the infected area. Best results in athlete's foot and body ringworm are usually obtained with 4 weeks' use of this product and in jock itch, with 2 weeks' use. To help prevent recurrence of athlete's foot, continue treatment for two weeks after disappearance of all symptoms.

TINACTIN Liquid Aerosol—Wash and dry infected area. Spray from a distance of 6 to 10 inches morning and evening or as directed by a doctor. For athlete's foot, spray between toes and on feet. For jock itch, spray infected area. Best results in athlete's foot are usually obtained with 4 weeks' use of this product and in jock itch, with 2 weeks' use. Continue treatment for two weeks after symptoms disappear. To help prevent reinfection of athlete's foot, bathe daily, dry carefully and apply **TINACTIN Powder** daily.

TINACTIN Powder—Wash and dry infected area. Sprinkle powder liberally on all areas of infection and in shoes or socks morning and evening or as directed by a doctor. Best results in athlete's foot are usually obtained with 4 weeks' use of this product and in jock itch, with 2 weeks' use. Continue treatment for two weeks after symptoms disappear. To prevent recurrence of athlete's foot, bathe daily, dry carefully and apply **TINACTIN Powder.**

TINACTIN Powder Aerosol, Deodorant Powder Aerosol and **TINACTIN Jock Itch Spray Powder**—Wash and dry infected area. Shake container well before using. Spray liberally from a distance of 6 to 10 inches onto affected area morning and night or as directed by a doctor. Best results in athlete's foot are

Continued on next page

Information on Schering-Plough HealthCare Products appearing on these pages is effective as of November 1991.

Schering-Plough—Cont.

usually obtained with 4 weeks' use of this product and in jock itch, with 2 weeks' use. To help prevent recurrence of athlete's foot, bathe daily, dry carefully and apply **TINACTIN Powder Aerosol or TINACTIN Deodorant Powder Aerosol.**

How Supplied: TINACTIN Antifungal Cream 1%, 15 g (½ oz) and 30 g (1 oz) collapsible tube with dispensing tip. **TINACTIN Antifungal Solution 1%,** 10 ml (⅓ oz) plastic squeeze bottle. **TINACTIN Antifungal Liquid (1%) Aerosol,** 113 g (4 oz) spray can. **TINACTIN Antifungal Powder 1%,** 45 g (1.5 oz) and 90 g (3.0 oz) plastic containers. **TINACTIN Antifungal Powder (1%) Aerosol,** 100 g (3.5 oz) and 150 g (5.0 oz) spray containers. TINACTIN Antifungal Deodorant Powder Aerosol 100 g (3.5 oz.) spray container. **TINACTIN Antifungal Jock Itch Cream 1%,** 15 g (½ oz) collapsible tube with dispensing tip. **TINACTIN Antifungal Jock Itch Spray Powder (1%),** 100 g (3.5 oz) spray can.
Store TINACTIN products between 36° and 86°F (2° and 30°C).
Shown in Product Identification Section, page 426

SmithKline Beecham Consumer Brands
Unit of SmithKline Beecham Inc.
POST OFFICE BOX 1467
PITTSBURGH, PA 15230

A–200® Pediculicide Shampoo Concentrate
A–200® Pediculicide Gel Concentrate

Description: Active ingredients: Pyrethrins 0.33%, Piperonyl butoxide technical 4.00% – Equivalent to 3.2% (butylcarbityl) (6-propylpiperonyl) ether and 0.8% related compounds. **Inactive Ingredients:** Shampoo—Benzyl alcohol, Butyl Stearate, Fragrance, Mineral Spirits, Octoxynol 9, Oleic Acid, Oleoresin Parsley Seed and Water. Gel—Benzyl alcohol, Butyl Stearate, Carbomer 940, Fragrance, Mineral Spirits, Octoxynol 9, Oleic Acid, Oleoresin Parsley Seed, Triisopropanolamine, and Water.

Inert ingredients: 95.67%.

Indications: A-200 is indicated for the treatment of human pediculosis—head lice, body lice and pubic lice, and their eggs. A-200 Gel is specially formulated for pubic lice and head lice in children, where control of application is desirable.

Actions: A-200 is an effective pediculicide for control of head lice (*Pediculus humanus capitis*), pubic lice (*Phthirus pubis*) and body lice (*Pediculus humanus corporis*), and their nits.

Precautionary Statements: Hazards to Humans and Domestic Animals

Warnings: KEEP OUT OF THE REACH OF CHILDREN. FOR EXTERNAL USE ONLY. May cause eye injury. Do not get in eyes or permit contact with mucous membranes. Harmful if swallowed. Wash thoroughly after handling. Do not leave children unattended with product on their heads.

Precaution: If in Eyes: Flush with plenty of water. Get medical attention.

Drug Interaction: NOT TO BE USED BY PERSONS ALLERGIC TO RAGWEED. If skin irritation or infection is present or develops, discontinue use and consult a physician.

Symptoms and Treatment of Oral Overdosage: If swallowed: Call a physician, local Poison Control Center, or the Rocky Mountain Poison Control Center at 303-592-1710 (Collect) 24 hours a day. Drink 1 or 2 glasses of water and induce vomiting by touching the back of throat with finger. Do not induce vomiting or give anything by mouth to an unconscious person.

Dosage and Administration: It is a violation of Federal law to use this product in a manner inconsistent with its labeling.

Directions for Use: 1. Apply A-200 Shampoo to **dry** hair and scalp or other infested areas. Use enough to completely wet area being treated. Massage in. (For head lice, avoid getting product into eyes. Helpful hint: When shampooing a child's head, place towel across forehead.) 2. Allow product to remain for 10 minutes, but no longer. 3. Add small quantities of water, and work rich lather into hair and scalp. 4. Rinse thoroughly with warm water. Towel dry. 5. Comb hair with special A-200 precision comb to remove dead lice and eggs. (See left side panel for combing suggestions.) Repeat treatment in 7–10 days or earlier if reinfestation has occurred. Do not use more than 2 applications of A-200 Shampoo in 24 hours. When used on children, adult supervision is recommended.

Additional Control Measures: At time of shampoo treatment, all infested clothing, bed linen and other articles should be laundered in hot water or dry cleaned. Carpets, upholstery and mattresses should be vacuumed thoroughly. Combs and brushes should be soaked in hot water (above 130°) for 5 to 10 minutes.

Storage and Disposal: Store at room temperature. Do not reuse empty bottle. Wrap and put in trash.

How Supplied: A-200 Shampoo Concentrate in 2 and 4 fl. oz. unbreakable plastic bottles and A-200 Gel Concentrate in 1 oz. tubes, all with special comb and bilingual patient insert.

Literature Available: Additional patient literature available upon request.
Shown in Product Identification Section, page 426

CLEAR BY DESIGN®
Medicated Acne Gel for Sensitive Skin

Product Information: CLEAR BY DESIGN contains benzoyl peroxide, an effective anti-acne agent available without a prescription in a lower 2.5% strength. CLEAR BY DESIGN is as effective as 10% benzoyl peroxide but with less of the irritation and redness that you may get with the higher strengths. Greaseless, colorless CLEAR BY DESIGN is invisible while it works fast. Helps prevent new acne pimples and blackheads from forming.

Directions: Wash problem areas thoroughly but gently and dry well. Using fingertips, apply CLEAR BY DESIGN to all affected and surrounding areas of face, neck, and body. Apply one or two times a day or as directed by a physician.

Warnings: Persons with a known allergy to benzoyl peroxide should not use this medication. To test for an allergy, apply CLEAR BY DESIGN on a small affected area once a day for two days. If discomforting irritation or undue dryness occurs during treatment, reduce frequency of use or amount. If excessive itching, redness, burning, swelling, irritation or dryness occurs, discontinue use and consult a physician. Avoid contact with eyes, lips and mouth. May bleach hair or dyed fabrics. Keep tightly closed. Keep this and all drugs out of reach of children. Store at controlled room temperature (59°–86°F.); avoid excessive heat.
FOR EXTERNAL USE ONLY

Formula: Active Ingredient: Benzoyl Peroxide, 2.5% in a gel base. Inactive ingredients: Purified water, carbomer 940, dioctyl sodium sulfosuccinate, sodium hydroxide, and edetate disodium.

How Supplied: Available in 1.5 oz. tubes.
Shown in Product Identification Section, page 426

CONTAC®
MAXIMUM STRENGTH
Continuous Action Nasal Decongestant/Antihistamine Caplets

Composition: [See table on page 706.]

Product Information: Each CONTAC Maximum Strength continuous action caplet provides up to 12 hours of relief. Part of the caplet goes to work right away for fast relief; the rest is released gradually to provide up to 12 hours of prolonged relief. With just *one* caplet in the morning and *one* at bedtime, you feel better all day, sleep better at night, breathing freely without congestion. CONTAC Maximum Strength provides:
- A NASAL DECONGESTANT which helps clear nasal passages, shrinks swollen membranes and helps decongest sinus openings.

• AN ANTIHISTAMINE at the maximum level to help relieve itchy, watery eyes, sneezing, and runny nose.

Indications: For temporary relief of nasal congestion due to the common cold, hay fever or other upper respiratory allergies, and nasal congestion associated with sinusitis.

Directions: One caplet every 12 hours. Do not exceed 2 caplets in 24 hours.

NOTE: The nonactive portion of the caplet that supplies the active ingredients may occasionally appear in your stool as a soft mass.

This carton is protected by a clear overwrap printed with "safety-sealed"; do not use if overwrap is missing or broken.

TAMPER-RESISTANT PACKAGING FEATURES FOR YOUR PROTECTION:

• Each caplet is encased in a plastic cell with a foil back; do not use if cell or foil is broken.
• The name CONTAC appears on each caplet; do not use this product if the CONTAC name is missing.

Warnings: Do not give this product to children under 12 years except under the advice and supervision of a physician. Do not exceed recommended dosage because at higher doses nervousness, dizziness, or sleeplessness may occur. Do not take this product if you have high blood pressure, heart disease, diabetes or thyroid disease except under the advice and supervision of a physician. If symptoms do not improve within 7 days or are accompanied by high fever, consult a physician before continuing use. Do not take this product if you have asthma, glaucoma or difficulty in urination due to enlargement of the prostate gland except under the advice and supervision of a physician. Do not take this product if you are taking another medication containing phenylpropanolamine. Avoid alcoholic beverages while taking this product. Do not drive or operate heavy machinery. May cause drowsiness. May cause excitability, especially in children. Keep this and all drugs out of reach of children. In case of accidental overdose, seek professional assistance or contact a poison control center immediately. As with any drug, if you are pregnant or nursing a baby, seek the advice of a health professional before using this product. Store at controlled room temperature (59°–86°F.).

Drug Interaction Precaution: Do not take this product if you are presently taking a prescription antihypertensive or antidepressant drug containing monoamine oxidase inhibitor except under the advice and supervision of a physician.

Formula: Active Ingredients: Each Maximum Strength caplet contains Phenylpropanolamine Hydrochloride 75 mg.; Chlorpheniramine Maleate 12 mg. (which is a higher dose of antihistamine than CONTAC capsules). **Inactive Ingredients (listed for individuals with specific allergies):** Acetylated Monoglycerides, Carnauba Wax, Colloidal Silicon

Dioxide, Ethylcellulose, Hydroxypropyl Methylcellulose, Lactose, Stearic Acid, Titanium Dioxide.

How Supplied: Consumer packages of 10, 20 and 40 caplets.
Note: There are other CONTAC products. Make sure this is the one you are interested in.
Shown in Product Identification Section, page 426

CONTAC®
MAXIMUM STRENGTH SINUS
Caplets/Tablets
Non-Drowsy Formula
Decongestant • Analgesic

Indications: Provides temporary relief from sinus pressure, nasal congestion, headache and pain.

Directions: Adults (12 years and older): Take two caplets every 6 hours not to exceed 8 caplets in any 24 hour period.

Product Benefits: CONTAC SINUS contains a decongestant and a non-aspirin analgesic. These safe and effective ingredients provide temporary relief from these major sinusitis symptoms: sinus pressure, nasal congestion, headache and pain.

NO ANTIHISTAMINE DROWSINESS

This carton is protected by a clear overwrap printed with "safety-sealed"; do not use if overwrap is missing or broken.

TAMPER-RESISTANT PACKAGING FEATURES FOR YOUR PROTECTION:

• Two caplets/tablets (one dose) are encased in a clear plastic cell with a foil back; do not use if cell or foil is broken.
• The name CONTAC-S appears on each caplet; do not use this product if the CONTAC-S name is missing.
The letters C-S appear on each tablet; do not use the product if these letters are missing.

Warnings: Do not take this product for more than 10 days. If symptoms do not improve or are accompanied by fever that lasts for more than 3 days, or if new symptoms occur, consult a physician. Do not take this product if you have heart disease, high blood pressure, thyroid disease, diabetes, or difficulty in urination due to enlargement of the prostate gland unless directed by a physician. Do not exceed recommended dosage. At higher doses nervousness, dizziness, or sleeplessness may occur. Keep this and all drugs out of the reach of children. In case of accidental overdose, seek professional assistance or contact a poison control center immediately. Prompt medical attention is critical for adults as well as for children even if you do not notice any signs or symptoms. As with any drug, if you are pregnant or nursing a baby, seek the advice of a health professional before using this product. Store at controlled room temperature (59°–86°F).

Formula: Active Ingredients: Each caplet/tablet contains Decongestant—Pseudoephedrine Hydrochloride 30 mg., Analgesic and Fever Reducer—

Acetaminophen 500 mg. (500 mg. is a non-standard dosage of acetaminophen, as compared to the standard of 325 mg.). **Inactive Ingredients (listed for individuals with specific allergies):** Cellulose, Crospovidone, D&C Red 30, Hydroxypropyl Methylcellulose, Magnesium Stearate, Polyethylene Glycol, Polysorbate 80, Povidone, Starch, Titanium Dioxide and trace amounts of other inactive ingredients.

Drug Interaction Precaution: Do not take this product if you are presently taking a prescription drug for high blood pressure or depression without first consulting your physician.

How Supplied: Consumer packages of 24 caplets or 24 tablets.

Note: There are other CONTAC products. Make sure this is the one you are interested in.
Shown in Product Identification Section, page 427

CONTAC®
Continuous Action Nasal Decongestant/Antihistamine Capsules

Composition: [See table on next page.]

Product Information: Each CONTAC continuous action capsule contains over 600 "tiny time pills." Some go to work right away. The rest are scientifically timed to dissolve slowly to give up to 12 hours of relief. With just *one* capsule in the morning and *one* at bedtime, you feel better all day, sleep better at night, breathing freely without congestion. CONTAC provides:

• A NASAL DECONGESTANT which helps clear nasal passages, shrinks swollen membranes and helps decongest sinus openings.
• AN ANTIHISTAMINE to help relieve itchy, watery eyes, sneezing, and runny nose.

Indications: For temporary relief of nasal congestion due to the common cold, hay fever or other upper respiratory allergies, and nasal congestion associated with sinusitis.

Directions: One capsule every 12 hours. Do not exceed 2 capsules in 24 hours.

This carton is protected by a clear overwrap printed with "safety-sealed"; do not use if overwrap is missing or broken.

TAMPER-RESISTANT PACKAGING FEATURES FOR YOUR PROTECTION:

• Each capsule is encased in a plastic cell with a foil back; do not use if cell or foil is broken.
• Each CONTAC capsule is protected by a red Perma-Seal™ band which bonds the two capsule halves together; do not use if capsule or band is broken.

Warnings: Do not give this product to children under 12 years except under the advice and supervision of a physician. Do not exceed recommended dosage because

Continued on next page

SmithKline Beecham—Cont.

at higher doses nervousness, dizziness, or sleeplessness may occur. Do not take this product if you have high blood pressure, heart disease, diabetes or thyroid disease except under the advice and supervision of a physician. If symptoms do not improve within 7 days or are accompanied by a high fever, consult a physician before continuing use. Do not take this product if you have asthma, glaucoma or difficulty in urination due to enlargement of the prostate gland except under the advice and supervision of a physician. Do not take this product if you are taking another medication containing phenylpropanolamine. Avoid alcoholic beverages while taking this product. Do not drive or operate heavy machinery. May cause drowsiness. May cause excitability, especially in children. Keep this and all drugs out of reach of children. In case of accidental overdose, seek professional assistance or contact a poison control center immediately. As with any drug, if you are pregnant or nursing a baby, seek the advice of a health professional before using this product. Store at controlled room temperature (59°–86°F.).

Drug Interaction Precaution: Do not take this product if you are presently taking a prescription antihypertensive or antidepressant drug containing monoamine oxidase inhibitor except under the advice and supervision of a physician.

Each Capsule Contains: Phenylpropanolamine Hydrochloride 75 mg. and Chlorpheniramine Maleate 8 mg. Also Contains: Benzyl Alcohol, Butylparaben, Carboxymethylcellulose Sodium, D&C Red No. 33, D&C Yellow No. 10, Edetate Calcium Disodium, FD&C Red No. 3, FD&C Yellow No. 6, Gelatin, Methylparaben, Pharmaceutical Glaze, Polysorbate 80, Propylparaben, Sodium Lauryl Sulfate, Sodium Propionate, Starch, Sucrose and other ingredients.

How Supplied: Consumer packages of 10, 20 and 40 capsules.

Note: There are other CONTAC products. Make sure this is the one you are interested in.

Shown in Product Identification Section, page 426

CONTAC®
Severe Cold and Flu Formula Caplets
Analgesic • Decongestant
Antihistamine • Cough Suppressant

Composition:
[See table below.]

Product Information: Two caplets every 6 hours to help relieve the discomforts of severe colds with flu-like symptoms.

Product Benefits: CONTAC Severe Cold and Flu Formula contains a non-aspirin analgesic, a decongestant, an antihistamine and a cough suppressant. These safe and effective ingredients provide temporary relief from these major cold symptoms: fever, body aches and pains, minor sore throat pain, headache, runny nose, postnasal drip, sneezing, itchy, watery eyes, nasal and sinus congestion, and temporarily relieves cough due to the common cold.

Directions: Adults (12 years and over): Two caplets every 6 hours, not to exceed 8 caplets in any 24 hour period.

This carton is protected by a clear overwrap printed with "safety-sealed". Do not use if overwrap is missing or broken.

TAMPER-RESISTANT PACKAGING FEATURES FOR YOUR PROTECTION:
• Caplets are encased in a plastic cell with a foil back; do not use if cell or foil is broken.
• The letters SCF appear on each caplet; do not use this product if these letters are missing.

Warnings: Do not administer to children under 12. Do not take this product for more than 7 days or for fever for more than 3 days unless directed by a doctor. If symptoms do not improve or are accompanied by fever, consult a doctor. A persistent cough may be a sign of a serious condition. If cough persists for more than one week, tends to recur or is accompanied by fever, rash, or persistent headache, consult a doctor. Do not take this product for persistent or chronic coughs such as occurs with smoking, asthma, emphysema, or if cough is accompanied by excessive phlegm (mucus), unless directed by a doctor. Do not exceed recommended dosage because at higher doses nervousness, dizziness, or sleeplessness may occur. May cause excitability, especially in children. Do not take this product if you have asthma, glaucoma, heart

disease, high blood pressure, emphysema, chronic pulmonary disease, shortness of breath, difficulty in breathing, diabetes, thyroid disease, or difficulty in urination due to enlargement of the prostate gland unless directed by a doctor. Do not take this product if you are taking another medication containing phenylpropanolamine. May cause marked drowsiness. Alcohol may increase the drowsiness effect. Avoid alcoholic beverages while taking this product. Use caution when driving a motor vehicle or operating machinery. Keep this and all medication out of the reach of children. As with any drug, if you are pregnant or nursing a baby, seek the advice of a health professional before using this product. In case of accidental overdose, contact a physician or poison control center immediately. Prompt medical attention is critical for adults as well as for children even if you do not notice any signs or symptoms.

Drug Interaction Precaution: Do not take this product if you are presently taking a prescription drug for high blood pressure or depression without first consulting your doctor.

Formula: Active Ingredients: Each caplet contains Acetaminophen, 500 mg., Dextromethorphan Hydrobromide, 15 mg.; Phenylpropanolamine Hydrochloride, 12.5 mg.; Chlorpheniramine Maleate, 2 mg. **Inactive Ingredients (listed for individuals with specific allergies):** Cellulose, FD&C Blue 1, Hydroxypropyl Methylcellulose, Polyethylene Glycol, Polysorbate 80, Povidone, Sodium Starch Glycolate, Starch, Stearic Acid, Titanium Dioxide.

How Supplied: Consumer packages of 10, 20 and 40 caplets.

Note: There are other CONTAC products. Make sure this is the one you are interested in.

Shown in Product Identification Section, page 427

CONTAC® Cough & Chest Cold

Composition: [See table on next page.]

Indications: Temporarily relieves cough, nasal and chest congestion, and minor aches and pains as may occur with chest colds, the common cold or respiratory allergies.

CONTAC	CONTAC Maximum Strength Continuous Action Decongestant Caplets	CONTAC Continuous Action Decongestant Capsules	CONTAC Severe Cold and Flu Formula Caplets (each 2 caplet dose)	CONTAC Severe Cold and Flu Hot Medicine Drink (each Packet dose)	CONTAC Severe Cold and Flu Nighttime Liquid (each fluid dose)
Phenylpropanolamine HCl	75.0 mg	75.0 mg	25.0 mg	—	—
Chlorpheniramine Maleate	12.0 mg	8.0 mg	4.0 mg	4.0 mg	4.0 mg
Pseudoephedrine HCl				60.0 mg	60.0 mg
Acetaminophen	—	—	1000.0 mg	650.0 mg	1000.0 mg
Dextromethorphan Hydrobromide	—	—	30.0 mg	20.0 mg	30.0 mg
Alcohol					18.5% by volume

CONTAC Liquid	CONTAC Cough & Chest Cold (each adult dose)	CONTAC Cough & Sore Throat Formula (each adult dose)	CONTAC JR. (each 5cc)
Pseudoephedrine Hydrochloride	60.0 mg	—	15.0 mg
Acetaminophen	500.0 mg	500.0 mg	160.0 mg
Dextromethorphan Hydrobromide	20.0 mg	20.0 mg	5.0 mg
Guaifenesin	200.0 mg	—	—
Alcohol	10%	10%	—

Directions: Adults and children 12 and older: take 4 tsps. every 4–6 hours, as needed. Do not exceed 4 doses in 24 hours.

Warning: Do not exceed recommended dosage, as at higher doses, dizziness, sleeplessness, or nervousness may occur. A persistent cough may be a sign of a serious condition. Do not use this product if: cough or other symptoms do not improve within 7 days, worsen, recur, or are accompanied by fever, rash, redness, swelling, or persistent headache; fever lasts for more than three days; you have high blood pressure, heart disease, diabetes, thyroid disease, or difficulty in urination due to an enlarged prostate gland; you have persistent or chronic cough such as occurs with smoking, asthma, emphysema or if cough is accompanied by excessive phlegm (mucus), unless directed by a doctor. As with any drug, if you are pregnant or nursing a baby, seek the advice of a health professional before using this product. Keep this and all drugs out of reach of children. In case of accidental overdose, seek professional assistance or contact a poison control center immediately. Prompt medical attention is critical for adults as well as for children even if you do not notice any signs or symptoms.

TAMPER RESISTANT PACKAGE FEATURE. DO NOT USE IF PRINTED SEAL AROUND BOTTLE CAP IS MISSING OR BROKEN.

Drug Interaction Precaution: Do not take if you are presently taking a prescription drug for high blood pressure or depression, without first consulting a doctor.

Active Ingredients: Per dose (4 tsps.): Acetaminophen 500 mg., Dextromethorphan Hydrobromide 20 mg., Pseudoephedrine Hydrochloride 60 mg., Guaifenesin 200 mg. Alcohol content: 10% by volume. Contains no sugar or aspirin.

Inactive Ingredients: Alcohol, Flavor, Glycerin, Maltitol Solution, Monobasic Sodium Phosphate, Phosphoric Acid, Polyethylene Glycol, Potassium Sorbate, Povidone, Red 33, Red 40, Saccharin Sodium, Sorbitol, Water.

How Supplied: In 4 fl. oz. bottles.
Note: There are other CONTAC products. Make sure this is the one you are interested in.

CONTAC® Cough & Sore Throat Formula
Cough Suppressant • Expectorant and Non-Aspirin Analgesic

Composition:
[See table above.]

Indications: Temporarily relieves both coughs and sore throats which often accompany coughs. Also temporarily relieves minor aches and pains and fever as may occur with the common cold or respiratory allergies.

Directions: Adults and children 12 and older: take 4 tsps. every 4–6 hours, as needed. Not to exceed 4 doses in 24 hours.

Warning: A persistent cough may be a sign of a serious condition. Do not use this product if: cough or other symptoms do not improve within 7 days, worsen, recur, or are accompanied by fever, rash, redness, swelling, or persistent headache; fever lasts for more than three days; you have persistent or chronic cough such as occurs with smoking, asthma, emphysema or if cough is accompanied by excessive phlegm (mucus), unless directed by a doctor. As with any drug, if you are pregnant or nursing a baby, seek the advice of a health professional before using this product. Keep this and all drugs out of reach of children. In case of accidental overdose, seek professional assistance or contact a poison control center immediately. Prompt medical attention is critical for adults as well as for children even if you do not notice any signs or symptoms.

TAMPER RESISTANT PACKAGE FEATURE. DO NOT USE IF PRINTED SEAL AROUND BOTTLE CAP IS MISSING OR BROKEN.

Active Ingredients: Per dose (4 tsps.): Acetaminophen 500 mg., Dextromethorphan Hydrobromide 20 mg. Alcohol content: 10% by volume. Contains no sugar or aspirin.

Inactive Ingredients: Alcohol, Flavor, Glycerin, Maltitol Solution, Monobasic Sodium Phosphate, Phosphoric Acid, Polyethylene Glycol, Potassium Sorbate, Povidone, Red 33, Red 40, Saccharin Sodium, Sorbitol, Water.

How Supplied: In 4 fl. oz. bottles.
Note: There are other CONTAC products. Make sure this is the one you are interested in.
Shown in Product Identification Section, page 427

CONTAC JR.®
Non-Drowsy Cold Liquid
Analgesic • Decongestant
Cough Suppressant

Composition:
[See table above.]
PRODUCT INFORMATION

Indications: Temporarily relieves cough and occasional sore throat pain, aches, pains, headache, fever, and nasal congestion as may occur with the common cold, hay fever, or other upper respiratory allergies.

PRODUCT BENEFITS
The good medicines in Contac Jr. were specially chosen to help gently relieve your child's nasal and sinus congestion, coughing, body aches and pains due to colds.
DOES NOT CONTAIN ANTIHISTAMINES WHICH MAY CAUSE DROWSINESS.
Medical authorities know that for children, dose by weight—not age—means the dose you give is right for consistent, controlled relief. Use the enclosed dosage cup to measure the right dose for your child's body weight.
SHAKE WELL BEFORE USING

Directions: Give one dose every 4 to 6 hours as needed by weight as detailed below:

Child's Weight	Dosage (teaspoonfuls)
Over 85 lbs.	2 tsps.
66–85 lbs.	1½ tsps.
48–65 lbs.	1 tsp.
31–47 lbs.	½ tsp.

Do not administer to children under 31 lbs. or under 3 years of age, unless directed by a doctor.

TAMPER-RESISTANT PACKAGING FEATURES FOR YOUR PROTECTION:
• Imprinted seal around bottle cap.
• DO NOT USE THIS PRODUCT IF THIS TAMPER-RESISTANT FEATURE IS MISSING OR BROKEN.

Warnings: Do not exceed recommended dosage for your child's body weight. Do not exceed recommended dosage because at higher doses nervousness, dizziness, or sleeplessness may occur. A persistent cough or sore throat may be a sign of a serious condition. Do not give this product to children who have heart disease, high blood pressure, thyroid disease or diabetes, unless directed by a doctor. If symptoms persist for more than 1 week, recur, or are accompanied by fever, rash, headache, nausea or vomiting,

Continued on next page

SmithKline Beecham—Cont.

consult a doctor. If symptoms get worse, if new symptoms occur, or if redness or swelling are present, consult a doctor because these could be signs of a serious condition. Do not give this product for persistent or chronic cough such as occurs with asthma, or where cough is accompanied by excessive phlegm (mucus) unless directed by a doctor. As with any drug, if you are pregnant or nursing a baby, seek the advice of a health professional before using this product. In case of accidental overdose, seek professional assistance or contact a poison control center immediately. Prompt medical attention is critical for adults as well as for children even if you do not notice any signs or symptoms.

Drug Interaction Precaution: Do not give this product to a child who is taking a prescription drug for high blood pressure or depression without first consulting the child's doctor.

Store at controlled room temperature (59°–86°).

KEEP THIS AND ALL DRUGS OUT OF REACH OF CHILDREN.

Active Ingredients: Each teaspoon contains: Acetaminophen 160 mg., Pseudoephedrine Hydrochloride 15 mg., Dextromethorphan Hydrobromide 5 mg.

Inactive Ingredients: Citric Acid, Flavors, Methylparaben, Polyethylene Glycol, Propylene Glycol, Propylparaben, D&C Red 33, Saccharin Sodium, Sodium Benzoate, Sodium Citrate, Sorbitol, Water and FD&C Yellow 6.

Comments or Questions? Call toll-free 1-800-245-1040 Weekdays.

How Supplied: A clear red liquid in 4 oz. size bottle.

Note: There are other CONTAC products. Make sure this is the one you are interested in.

Shown in Product Identification Section, page 427

CONTAC®
SEVERE COLD & FLU NIGHTTIME
Antihistamine • Analgesic
Cough Suppressant • Nasal
Decongestant

Composition: See table on page 706.]

Product Information: CONTAC Severe Cold & Flu Nighttime:
• Provides temporary relief from nasal and sinus congestion, runny nose, coughing, postnasal drip, sneezing, itchy, watery eyes and minor aches and pains associated with the common cold, sore throat, and flu, so you can get the rest you need.
• Contains a non-aspirin analgesic and fever reducer, a cough suppressant, a nasal decongestant and an antihistamine.

Directions: Adults and children 12 years and older: Take 2 Tbsps. every 6 hours in dosage cup provided. May be repeated every 6 hours as needed, not to exceed 8 Tbsps. in 24 hours.

TAMPER RESISTANT PACKAGE FEATURE: DO NOT USE IF PRINTED SEAL AROUND BOTTLE CAP IS MISSING OR BROKEN.

Warnings: Do not administer to children under 12. Do not take this product for more than 7 days or for fever for more than 3 days unless directed by a doctor. If symptoms do not improve or are accompanied by fever, consult a doctor. A persistent cough may be a sign of a serious condition. If cough persists for more than one week, tends to recur or is accompanied by fever, rash, or persistent headache, consult a doctor. Do not take this product for persistent or chronic coughs such as occurs with smoking, asthma, emphysema, or if cough is accompanied by excessive phlegm (mucus) unless directed by a doctor. Do not exceed recommended dosage because at higher doses nervousness, dizziness, or sleeplessness may occur. May cause excitability, especially in children. Do not take this product if you have asthma, glaucoma, heart disease, high blood pressure, emphysema, chronic pulmonary disease, shortness of breath, difficulty in breathing, diabetes, thyroid disease, or difficulty in urination due to enlargement of the prostate gland unless directed by a doctor. May cause drowsiness. Alcohol may increase the drowsiness effect. Avoid alcoholic beverages while taking this product. Use caution when driving a motor vehicle or operating machinery.

Keep this and all medication out of the reach of children. As with any drug, if you are pregnant or nursing a baby, seek the advice of a health professional before using this product. In case of accidental overdose, contact a physician or poison control center immediately. Prompt medical attention is critical for adults as well as children even if you do not notice any signs or symptoms.

Drug Interaction Precaution: Do not take this product if you are presently taking a prescription drug for high blood pressure or depression without first consulting your doctor.

Active Ingredients: Per dose (2 Tbsps.):
Acetaminophen 1000 mg
Pseudoephedrine Hydrochloride 60 mg
Dextromethorphan Hydrobromide 30 mg
Chlorpheniramine Maleate 4 mg
Alcohol content: 18.5% by volume.
Contains no sugar or aspirin.

Inactive Ingredients: Alcohol, Blue 1, Dibasic Sodium Phosphate, Flavors, Glycerin, Hydrogenated Glucose Syrup, Phosphoric Acid, Potassium Sorbate, Povidone, Red 33, Red 40, Saccharin Sodium, Sorbitol, Water.

How Supplied: In 6 fl. oz. bottles.
Note: There are other CONTAC products. Make sure this is the one you are interested in.

ECOTRIN®
Enteric-Coated Aspirin
Antiarthritic, Antiplatelet

Description: 'Ecotrin' is enteric-coated aspirin (acetylsalicylic acid, ASA) available in tablet and caplet forms in 325 mg and 500 mg dosage units.

The enteric coating covers a core of aspirin and is designed to resist disintegration in the stomach, dissolving in the more neutral-to-alkaline environment of the duodenum. Such action helps to protect the stomach from injury that may result from ingestion of plain, buffered or highly buffered aspirin (see SAFETY).

Indications: 'Ecotrin' is indicated for:
• conditions requiring chronic or long-term aspirin therapy for pain and/or inflammation, e.g., rheumatoid arthritis, juvenile rheumatoid arthritis, systemic lupus erythematosus, osteoarthritis (degenerative joint disease), ankylosing spondylitis, psoriatic arthritis, Reiter's syndrome and fibrositis,
• antiplatelet indications of aspirin (see the ANTIPLATELET-EFFECT section) and
• situations in which compliance with aspirin therapy may be affected because of the gastrointestinal side effects of plain, i.e., non-enteric-coated, or buffered aspirin.

Dosage: For analgesic or anti-inflammatory indications, the OTC maximum dosage for aspirin is 4000 mg per day in divided doses, i.e., two-325 mg tablets or caplets every 4 hours, or three-325 mg tablets or caplets every 6 hours, or two-500 mg tablets or caplets every 6 hours.

For antiplatelet effect dosage: see the ANTIPLATELET EFFECT section.

Under a physician's direction, the dosage can be increased or otherwise modified as appropriate to the clinical situation. When 'Ecotrin' is used for anti-inflammatory effect, the physician should be attentive to plasma salicylate levels, and may also caution the patient to be alert to the development of tinnitus as an indicator of elevated salicylate levels. It should be noted that patients with a high frequency hearing loss (such as may occur in older individuals) may have difficulty perceiving the tinnitus. Tinnitus would then not be a reliable indicator in such individuals.

Inactive Ingredients: Cellulose, Cellulose Acetate Phthalate, D&C Yellow 10, Diethyl Phthalate, FD&C Yellow 6, Silicon Dioxide, Sodium Starch Glycolate, Starch, Stearic Acid, Titanium Dioxide, and trace amounts of other inactive ingredients.

Bioavailability: The bioavailability of aspirin from 'Ecotrin' has been demonstrated in a number of salicylate excretion studies. The studies show levels of salicylate (and metabolites) in urine excreted over 48 hours for 'Ecotrin' do not differ statistically from plain, i.e., non-enteric-coated, aspirin.

Plasma studies, in which 'Ecotrin' has been compared with plain aspirin in steady-state studies over eight days, also demonstrate that 'Ecotrin' provides plasma salicylate levels not statistically different from plain aspirin.

Information regarding salicylate levels over a range of doses was generated in a study in which 24 healthy volunteers (12 male and 12 female) took daily (divided) doses of either 2600 mg, 3900 mg, or 5200 mg of 'Ecotrin'. Plasma salicylate levels generally acknowledged to be anti-inflammatory (15 mg/dL.) were attained at daily doses of 5200 mg, on Day 2 by females and Day 3 by males. At 3900 mg, anti-inflammatory levels were attained at Day 3 by females and Day 4 by males. Dissolution of the enteric coating occurs at a neutral-to-basic pH and is therefore dependent on gastric emptying into the duodenum. With continued dosing, appropriate plasma levels are maintained.

Safety: The safety of 'Ecotrin' has been demonstrated in a number of endoscopic studies comparing 'Ecotrin', plain aspirin, buffered aspirin and highly buffered aspirin preparations. In these studies, all forms of aspirin were dosed to the OTC maximum (3900–4000 mg per day) for up to 14 days. The normal healthy volunteers participating in these studies were gastroscoped before and after the courses of treatment and 14-day drug-free periods followed active drug. Compared to all the other preparations, there was less gastric damage at a statistically significant level during the 'Ecotrin' courses. There was also statistically less duodenal damage when compared with the plain, i.e., non-enteric-coated, aspirin.

Details of studies demonstrating the safety and bioavailability of 'Ecotrin' are available to health care professionals. Write: Professional Services Department, SmithKline Beecham Consumer Brands, P.O. Box 1467, Pittsburgh, Pa. 15230.

Warning:
Consumer Warning: Children and teenagers should not use this medicine for chicken pox or flu symptoms before a doctor is consulted about Reye syndrome, a rare but serious illness. Do not take this product for pain for more than 10 days unless directed by a physician. If pain persists or gets worse, if new symptoms occur, or if redness or swelling is present, consult a physician because these could be signs of a serious condition. Also, consult a physician before using this medicine to treat arthritic or rheumatic conditions affecting children under 12. Discontinue use if dizziness occurs. Do not take this product if you are allergic to aspirin, have asthma, or if you have ulcers or bleeding problems unless directed by a physician. If ringing in the ears or a loss of hearing occurs, consult a physician before taking any more of this product. If you experience persistent or unexplained stomach upset, consult a physician. Keep this and all drugs out of children's reach. In case of accidental overdose, seek professional assistance or contact a poison control center immediately. As with any medicine, if you are pregnant or nursing a baby, seek the advice of a health professional before using this

product. IT IS ESPECIALLY IMPORTANT NOT TO USE ASPIRIN DURING THE LAST 3 MONTHS OF PREGNANCY UNLESS SPECIFICALLY DIRECTED TO DO SO BY A DOCTOR, BECAUSE IT MAY CAUSE PROBLEMS IN THE UNBORN CHILD OR COMPLICATIONS DURING DELIVERY. Store at controlled room temperature (59°–86°F.).

Drug Interaction Precaution: Do not take this product if you are taking a prescription drug for anticoagulation (thinning of the blood), diabetes, gout, or arthritis unless directed by a physician.

Professional Warning: There have been occasional reports in the literature concerning individuals with impaired gastric emptying in whom there may be retention of one or more 'Ecotrin' tablets over time. This unusual phenomenon may occur as a result of outlet obstruction from ulcer disease alone or combined with hypotonic gastric peristalsis. Because of the integrity of the enteric coating in an acidic environment, these tablets may accumulate and form a bezoar in the stomach. Individuals with this condition may present with complaints of early satiety or of vague upper abdominal distress. Diagnosis may be made by endoscopy or by abdominal films which show opacities suggestive of a mass of small tablets (*Ref.: Bogacz, K. and Caldron, P.: Enteric-coated Aspirin Bezoar: Elevation of Serum Salicylate Level by Barium Study. Amer. J. Med. 1987:83, 783–6.*). Management may vary according to the condition of the patient. Options include: gastrotomy and alternating slightly basic and neutral lavage (*Ref.: Baum, J.: Enteric-Coated Aspirin and the Problem of Gastric Retention. J. Rheum., 1984:11, 250–1.*). While there have been no clinical reports, it has been suggested that such individuals may also be treated with parenteral cimetidine (to reduce acid secretion) and then given sips of slightly basic liquids to effect gradual dissolution of the enteric coating. Progress may be followed with plasma salicylate levels or via recognition of tinnitus by the patient.

It should be kept in mind that individuals with a history of partial or complete gastrectomy may produce reduced amounts of acid and therefore have less acidic gastric pH. Under these circumstances, the benefits offered by the acid-resistant enteric coating may not exist.

Antiplatelet Effect FDA approved professional labeling permits the use of aspirin to reduce the risk of death and/or nonfatal myocardial infarction (MI) in patients with a previous infarction or unstable angina pectoris and its use in reducing the risk of transient ischemic attacks in men.

Labeling for both indications follows:
ASPIRIN FOR MYOCARDIAL INFARCTION
Indication: Aspirin is indicated to reduce the risk of death and/or nonfatal myocardial infarction in patients with a previous infarction or unstable angina pectoris.

Clinical Trials: The indication is supported by the results of six, large, randomized multicenter, placebo-controlled studies involving 10,816 predominantly male, post-myocardial infarction (MI) patients and one randomized placebo-controlled study of 1,266 men with unstable angina.[1-7] Therapy with aspirin was begun at intervals after the onset of acute MI varying from less than three days to more than five years and continued for periods of from less than one year to four years. In the unstable angina study, treatment was started within one month after the onset of unstable angina and continued for 12 weeks, and patients with complicating conditions such as congestive heart failure were not included in the study.

Aspirin therapy in MI patients was associated with about a 20 percent reduction in the risk of subsequent death and/or nonfatal reinfarction, a median absolute decrease of 3 percent from the 12 to 22 percent event rates in the placebo groups. In aspirin-treated unstable angina patients, the reduction in risk was about 50 percent, a reduction in event rate to 5% from the 10% in the placebo group over the 12 weeks of the study. Daily dosage of aspirin in the post-myocardial infarction studies was 300 mg in one study and 900 to 1500 mg in five studies. A dose of 325 mg was used in the study of unstable angina.

Adverse Reactions
Gastrointestinal Reactions: Doses of 1000 mg per day of plain aspirin caused gastrointestinal symptoms and bleeding that in some cases were clinically significant. In the largest postinfarction study (the Aspirin Myocardial Infarction Study [AMIS] with 4,500 people), the percentage incidences of gastrointestinal symptoms of a standard, solid-tablet formulation and placebo-treated subjects, respectively, were: stomach pain (14.5%; 4.4%); heartburn (11.9%; 4.8%); nausea and/or vomiting (7.6%; 2.1%); hospitalization for gastrointestinal disorder (4.9%; 3.5%). In the AMIS and other trials, plain aspirin-treated patients had increased rates of gross gastrointestinal bleeding. Symptoms and signs of gastrointestinal irritation were not significantly increased in subjects treated for unstable angina with buffered aspirin in solution.

Cardiovascular and Biochemical: In the AMIS trial, the dosage of 1000 mg per day of plain aspirin was associated with small increases in systolic blood pressure (BP) (average 1.5 to 2.1 mmHg) and diastolic BP (0.5 to 0.6 mmHg), depending upon whether maximal or last available readings were used. Blood urea nitrogen and uric acid levels were also increased, but by less than 1.0 mg%. Subjects with marked hypertension or renal insufficiency had been excluded from the trial so that the clinical importance of these observations for such subjects or for any subjects treated over more prolonged periods is not known. It is recommended that patients placed on long-term aspirin

Continued on next page

SmithKline Beecham—Cont.

treatment, even at doses of 300 mg per day, be seen at regular intervals to assess changes in these measurements.

Sodium in Buffered Aspirin for Solution Formulations: One tablet daily of buffered aspirin in solution adds 553 mg of sodium to that in the diet and may not be tolerated by patients with active sodium-retaining states such as congestive heart or renal failure. This amount of sodium adds about 30 percent to the 70 to 90 meq intake suggested as appropriate for dietary hypertension in the 1984 Report of the Joint National Committee on Detection, Evaluation, and Treatment of High Blood Pressure.[8]

Dosage and Administration: Although most of the studies used dosages exceeding 300 mg daily, two trials used only 300 mg and pharmacologic data indicate that this dose inhibits platelet function fully. Therefore, 300 mg or a conventional 325 mg aspirin dose daily is a reasonable, routine dose that would minimize gastrointestinal adverse reactions for both solid oral dosage forms (buffered and plain aspirin) and buffered aspirin in solution.

References:
1. Elwood, P.C., et al.: A Randomized Controlled Trial of Acetylsalicylic Acid in the Secondary Prevention of Mortality from Myocardial Infarction, *Br. Med. J.* 1:436–440, 1974.
2. The Coronary Drug Project Research Group: Aspirin in Coronary Heart Disease, *J. Chronic Dis.* 29:625–642, 1976.
3. Breddin, K., et al.: Secondary Prevention of Myocardial Infarction: A Comparison of Acetylsalicylic Acid, Phenprocoumon or Placebo, *Homeostasis* 470:263–268, 1979.
4. Aspirin Myocardial Infarction Study Research Group: A Randomized Controlled Trial of Aspirin in Persons Recovered from Myocardial Infarction, *J.A.M.A.* 243:661–669, 1980.
5. Elwood, P.C., and Sweetnam, P.M.: Aspirin and Secondary Mortality After Myocardial Infarction, *Lancet* pp. 1313–1315, Dec. 22–29, 1979.
6. The Persantine-Aspirin Reinfarction Study Research Group, Persantine and Aspirin in Coronary Heart Disease, *Circulation* 62: 449–469, 1980.
7. Lewis, H.D., et al.: Protective Effects of Aspirin Against Acute Myocardial Infarction and Death in Men with Unstable Angina, Results of a Veterans Administration Cooperative Study, *N. Engl. J. Med.* 309:396–403, 1983.
8. 1984 Report of the Joint National Committee on Detection, Evaluation, and Treatment of High Blood Pressure, U.S. Department of Health and Human Services and U.S. Public Health Service, National Institutes of Health. NIH Pub. No. 84–1088.

Aspirin for Transient Ischemic Attacks

Indication For reducing the risk of recurrent transient ischemic attacks (TIAs) or stroke in men who have had transient ischemia of the brain due to fibrin platelet emboli. There is inadequate evidence that aspirin or buffered aspirin is effective in reducing TIAs in women at the recommended dosage. There is no evidence that aspirin or buffered aspirin is of benefit in the treatment of completed strokes in men or women.

Clinical Trials The indication is supported by the results of a Canadian study[1] in which 585 patients with threatened stroke were followed in a randomized clinical trial for an average of 26 months to determine whether aspirin or sulfinpyrazone, singly or in combination, was superior to placebo in preventing transient ischemic attacks, stroke or death. The study showed that, although sulfinpyrazone had no statistically significant effect, aspirin reduced the risk of continuing transient ischemic attacks, stroke or death by 19 percent and reduced the risk of stroke or death by 31 percent. Another aspirin study carried out in the United States with 178 patients showed a statistically significant number of "favorable outcomes," including reduced transient ischemic attacks, stroke and death.[2]

Precautions Patients presenting with signs and/or symptoms of TIAs should have a complete medical and neurologic evaluation. Consideration should be given to other disorders that resemble TIAs. Attention should be given to risk factors: it is important to evaluate and treat, if appropriate, other diseases associated with TIAs and stroke, such as hypertension and diabetes.

Concurrent administration of absorbable antacids at therapeutic doses may increase the clearance of salicylates in some individuals. The concurrent administration of nonabsorbable antacids may alter the rate of absorption of aspirin, thereby resulting in a decreased acetylsalicylic acid/salicylate ratio in plasma. The clinical significance of these decreases in available aspirin is unknown. Aspirin at dosages of 1,000 mg per day has been associated with small increases in blood pressure, blood urea nitrogen, and serum uric acid levels. It is recommended that patients placed on long-term aspirin treatment be seen at regular intervals to assess changes in these measurements.

Adverse Reactions: At dosages of 1,000 mg or higher of aspirin per day, gastrointestinal side effects include stomach pain, heartburn, nausea and/or vomiting, as well as increased rates of gross gastrointestinal bleeding.

Dosage and Administration Adult dosage for men is 1,300 mg a day, in divided doses of 650 mg twice a day or 325 mg four times a day.

References:
1. The Canadian Cooperative Study Group: Randomized Trial of Aspirin and Sulfinpyrazone in Threatened Stroke, *N. Engl. J. Med.* 299:53, 1978.
2. Fields, W. S., et al.: Controlled Trial of Aspirin in Cerebral Ischemia, *Stroke* 8:301–316, 1980.

Supplied:
'Ecotrin' Tablets
  325 mg in bottles of 100*, 250 and 1000.
  500 mg in bottles of 60* and 150.
'Ecotrin' Caplets
  325 mg in bottles of 100.
  500 mg in bottles of 60.

TAMPER-RESISTANT PACKAGE FEATURES FOR YOUR PROTECTION:
- Bottle has imprinted seal under cap.
- The words ECOTRIN REG or ECOTRIN MAX appear on each tablet or caplet (see product illustration printed on carton).
- **DO NOT USE THIS PRODUCT IF ANY OF THESE TAMPER-RESISTANT FEATURES ARE MISSING OR BROKEN.**

Comments or Questions? Call Toll-Free 800-245-1040 weekdays.

* Without child-resistant caps.

Shown in Product Identification Section, page 427

FEOSOL® CAPSULES
Hematinic

Product Information: FEOSOL capsules provide the body with ferrous sulfate, iron in its most efficient form, for iron deficiency and iron-deficiency anemia when the need for such therapy has been determined by a physician.
The special targeted-release capsule is formulated to reduce stomach upset, a common problem with iron.

Directions: *Adults:* 1 or 2 capsules daily or as directed by a physician. *Children:* As directed by a physician.
- The carton is protected by a clear overwrap printed with "safety sealed"; do not use if overwrap is missing or broken.

TAMPER-RESISTANT PACKAGING FEATURES FOR YOUR PROTECTION:
- Each capsule is encased in a plastic cell with a foil back; do not use if cell or foil is broken.
- Each FEOSOL capsule is protected by a red Perma-Seal™ band which bonds the two capsule halves together; do not use if capsule is broken or band is missing or broken.

Warnings: Do not exceed recommended dosage. The treatment of any anemic condition should be under the advice and supervision of a physician. Iron-containing medication may occasionally cause constipation or diarrhea. Since oral iron products interfere with absorption of oral tetracycline antibiotics, these products should not be taken within two hours of each other. Keep this and all drugs out of reach of children. In case of accidental overdose, seek professional assistance or contact a poison control center immediately. As with any drug, if you are pregnant or nursing a baby, seek the advice of a health professional before using this product. Store at controlled room temperature (59°–86°F.).

Formula: Active Ingredients: Each capsule contains 159 mg. of dried ferrous sulfate USP (50 mg. of elemental iron), equivalent to 250 mg. of ferrous sulfate USP. **Inactive Ingredients (listed for individuals with specific allergies):** Benzyl Alcohol, Cetylpyridinium Chloride, D&C Red 33, Yellow 10, FD&C Blue 1, D&C Red #7, Red 40, Gelatin, Glyceryl Stearates, Iron Oxide, Polyethylene Glycol, Povidone, Sodium Lauryl Sulfate, Starch, Sucrose, White Wax and trace amounts of other inactive ingredients.

How Supplied: Packages of 30 and 60 capsules, bottles of 500; in Single Unit Packages of 100 capsules (intended for institutional use only).
Also available in Tablets and Elixir.
Note: There are other FEOSOL products. Make sure this is the one you are interested in.
Shown in Product Identification Section, page 427

FEOSOL® ELIXIR
Hematinic

Product Information: FEOSOL Elixir, an unusually palatable iron elixir, provides the body with ferrous sulfate—iron in its most efficient form. The standard elixir for simple iron deficiency and iron-deficiency anemia when the need for such therapy has been determined by a physician.

Directions: Adults: 1 to 2 teaspoonfuls three times daily. Children: ½ to 1 teaspoonful three times daily preferably between meals. Infants: as directed by physician. Mix with water or fruit juice to avoid temporary staining of teeth; do not mix with milk or wine-based vehicles.

TAMPER-RESISTANT PACKAGE FEATURE: Imprinted seal around top of bottle; do not use if seal is missing.

Warnings: The treatment of any anemic condition should be under the advice and supervision of a physician. Since oral iron products interfere with absorption of oral tetracycline antibiotics, these products should not be taken within two hours of each other. Occasional gastrointestinal discomfort (such as nausea) may be minimized by taking with meals and by beginning with one teaspoonful the first day, two the second, etc. until the recommended dosage is reached. Iron-containing medication may occasionally cause constipation or diarrhea, and liquids may cause temporary staining of the teeth (this is less likely when diluted). Keep this and all drugs out of reach of children. In case of accidental overdose, seek professional assistance or contact a poison control center immediately.
As with any drug, if you are pregnant or nursing a baby, seek the advice of a health professional before using this product.
Store at controlled room temperature (59°–86°F.).

Formula: Each 5 ml. (1 teaspoonful) contains ferrous sulfate USP, 220 mg.

(44 mg. of elemental iron); alcohol, 5%.
Inactive Ingredients (listed for individuals with specific allergies): Citric Acid, FD&C Yellow 6 (Sunset Yellow) as a color additive, Flavors, Glucose, Saccharin Sodium, Sucrose, Purified Water.

How Supplied: A clear orange liquid in 16 fl. oz. bottles.
Also available in Tablets and Capsules.

Note: There are other FEOSOL products. Make sure this is the one you are interested in.
Shown in Product Identification Section, page 427

FEOSOL® TABLETS
Hematinic

Product Information: FEOSOL Tablets provide the body with ferrous sulfate, iron in its most efficient form, for iron deficiency and iron-deficiency anemia when the need for such therapy has been determined by a physician. The distinctive triangular-shaped tablet has a coating to prevent oxidation and improve palatability.

Directions: *Adults*—one tablet 3 to 4 times daily after meals and upon retiring or as directed by a physician. *Children 6 to 12 years*—one tablet three times a day after meals. *Children under 6 and infants*—use Feosol® Elixir.
• The carton has been sealed at the factory with a clear overwrap printed with "safety sealed."

TAMPER-RESISTANT PACKAGE FEATURES FOR YOUR PROTECTION:
• Bottle has imprinted "SKCP" seal under cap.
• FEOSOL Tablets are triangular shaped (see product illustration printed on carton).
• **DO NOT USE THIS PRODUCT IF ANY OF THESE TAMPER-RESISTANT FEATURES ARE MISSING OR BROKEN.**

Comments or Questions? Call Toll-Free 800-245-1040 Weekdays.

Warnings: Do not exceed recommended dosage. The treatment of any anemic condition should be under the advice and supervision of a physician. Since oral iron products interfere with absorption of oral tetracycline antibiotics, these products should not be taken within two hours of each other.
Occasional gastrointestinal discomfort (such as nausea) may be minimized by taking with meals and by beginning with one tablet the first day, two the second, etc. until the recommended dosage is reached. Iron-containing medication may occasionally cause constipation or diarrhea.
Keep this and all drugs out of reach of children. In case of accidental overdose, seek professional assistance or contact a poison control center immediately.
As with any drug, if you are pregnant or nursing a baby, seek the advice of a health professional before using this product.

Store at controlled room temperature (59°–86°F.).

Formula: Active Ingredients: Each tablet contains 200 mg. of dried ferrous sulfate USP (65 mg. of elemental iron), equivalent to 325 mg. (5 grains) of ferrous sulfate USP. **Inactive Ingredients (listed for individuals with specific allergies):** Calcium Sulfate, D&C Yellow 10, FD&C Blue 2, Glucose, Hydroxypropyl Methylcellulose, Mineral Oil, Polyethylene Glycol, Sodium Lauryl Sulfate, Starch, Stearic Acid, Talc, Titanium Dioxide, and trace amounts of other inactive ingredients.

How Supplied: Bottles of 100 and 1000 tablets; in Single Unit Packages of 100 tablets (intended for institutional use only).
Also available in Capsules and Elixir.

Note: There are other FEOSOL products. Make sure this is the one you are interested in.
Shown in Product Identification Section, page 427

GERITOL COMPLETE™ Tablets
[*jer ′e-tol*]
The High Iron Multi-Vitamin/Mineral

Active Ingredients (Per Tablet): Vitamin A (6000 IU as Beta Carotene); Vitamin E (30 IU); Vitamin C (60 mg.); Folic Acid (400 mcg.); Vitamin B_1 (1.5 mg.); Vitamin B_2 (1.7 mg.); Niacin (20 mg.); Vitamin B_6 (2 mg.); Vitamin B_{12} (6 mcg.); Vitamin D (400 IU); Biotin (45 mcg.); Pantothenic Acid (10 mg.); Vitamin K (25 mcg.); Calcium (162 mg.); Phosphorus (125 mg.); Iodine (150 mcg.); Iron (50 mg.); Magnesium (100 mg.); Copper (2 mg.); Manganese (2.5 mg.); Potassium (37.5 mg.); Chloride (34 mg.); Chromium (15 mcg.); Molybdenum (15 mcg.); Selenium (15 mcg.); Zinc (15 mg.); Nickel (5 mcg.); Silicon (80 mcg.); Tin (10 mcg); Vanadium (10 mcg).

Inactive Ingredients: Carnauba wax, Crospovidone, Flavors, Gelatin, Glycerides of Stearic and Palmitic acids, Hydroxypropyl cellulose, Hydroxypropyl methylcellulose, Magnesium stearate, Microcrystalline cellulose, Polyethylene glycol, Silicon dioxide, Stearic acid, White wax, FD&C Red #40, FD&C Blue #2, FD&C Yellow #6, Titanium dioxide.

Indications: For use as a dietary supplement.

Actions: Help treat and prevent iron deficiency.

Warnings: Keep out of reach of children.

Precaution: Alcoholics and individuals with chronic liver or pancreatic disease may have enhanced iron absorption with the potential for iron overload.
NOTE: Unabsorbed iron may cause some darkening of the stool.

Symptoms and Treatment of Oral Overdose: Toxicity and symptoms are

Continued on next page

SmithKline Beecham—Cont.

primarily due to iron overdose. Abdominal pain, nausea, vomiting and diarrhea may occur, with possible subsequent acidosis and cardiovascular collapse with severe poisoning. If an overdose is suspected, immediately seek professional assistance by contacting your physician, the local poison control center, or the Rocky Mt. Poison Control Center at 303-592-1710 (Collect), 24 hours a day.

Dosage and Administration (Adults): One (1) tablet daily after mealtime.

How Supplied: Bottles of 14, 40, 100, and 180 tablets.

GERITOL EXTEND™ Tablets or Caplets
Nutritional Supplement

Active Ingredients (per tablet): Vitamin A (3333 IU, including 1250 IU from Beta Carotene); Vitamin D (200 IU); Vitamin E (15 IU); Vitamin C (60 mg); Folic Acid (0.2 mg); Vitamin B_1 (1.2 mg); Vitamin B_2 (1.4 mg); Niacin (15 mg); Vitamin B_6 (2.0 mg); Vitamin B_{12} (2 mcg); Vitamin K (80 mcg); Calcium (130 mg); Phosphorus (100 mg); Magnesium (35 mg); Zinc (15 mg); Iodine (150 mcg); Iron (10 mg); Selenium (70 mcg)

Inactive Ingredients: Carnauba Wax, Croscarmelose Sodium, Flavors, Gelatin, Glycerides of Stearic and Palmitic Acids, Hydroxypropyl Methylcellulose, Magnesium Stearate, Microcrystalline Cellulose, Polyethylene Glycol, Silicon Dioxide, Stearic Acid, White Wax, FD&C Red #40, FD&C Blue #2, Titanium Dioxide.

Indications: For use as a dietary supplement. Recommended for active adults over 50.

Actions: Help treat and prevent iron deficiency.

Warnings: Keep out of reach of children.

Precaution: Alcoholics and individuals with chronic liver or pancreatic disease may have enhanced iron absorption with the potential for iron overload.
NOTE: Unabsorbed iron may cause some darkening of the stool.
Symptoms and Treatment of Oral Overdose: Toxicity and symptoms are primarily due to iron overdose. Abdominal pain, nausea, vomiting, and diarrhea may occur with possible subsequent acidosis and cardiovascular collapse with severe poisoning. If an overdose is suspected, immediately seek professional assistance by contacting your physician, the local poison control center, or the Rocky Mountain Poison Control Center at 303-592-1710 (collect), 24 hours a day.

Dosage and Administration (Adults 50+): One (1) tablet/caplet daily after mealtime.

How Supplied: Bottles of 40 and 100 tablets or caplets in blister-pack cartons.

GERITOL® Liquid
[jer 'e-tol]
High Potency Iron &
Vitamin Tonic

Active Ingredients Per Dose (½ fluid ounce): Iron (as ferric ammonium citrate) 50 mg; Thiamine (B_1) 2.5 mg; Riboflavin (B_2) 2.5 mg; Niacinamide 50 mg; Panthenol 2 mg; Pyridoxine (B_6) 0.5 mg; Cyanocobalamin (B_{12}) 0.75 mcg; Methionine 25 mg; Choline Bitartrate 50 mg.

Inactive Ingredients: Alcohol, Benzoic acid, Caramel color, Citric acid, Invert sugar, Sucrose, Water, Flavors.

Indications: For use as a dietary supplement.

Actions: Help treat and prevent iron deficiency.

Warnings: Keep out of reach of children.

Precaution: Alcohol accelerates absorption of ferric iron. Alcoholics and individuals with chronic liver or pancreatic disease may have enhanced iron absorption with the potential for iron overload.
NOTE: Unabsorbed iron may cause some darkening of the stool.

Symptoms and Treatment of Oral Overdose: Toxicity and symptoms are primarily due to iron overdose. Abdominal pain, nausea, vomiting and diarrhea may occur, with possible subsequent acidosis and cardiovascular collapse with severe poisoning. If an overdose is suspected, immediately seek professional assistance by contacting your physician, the local poison control center, or the Rocky Mt. Poison Control Center at 303-592-1710 (Collect), 24 hours a day.

Dosage and Administration (Adults): As an iron supplement and for normal menstrual needs: One (1) tablespoonful (0.5 fl. oz.) daily at mealtime. For iron deficiency: One (1) tablespoonful (0.5 fl. oz.) three times daily at mealtime or as directed by a physician.

How Supplied: Bottles of 4 oz., and 12 oz.

7001M
11/14/83

MASSENGILL® Douches
[mas 'sen-gil]

PRODUCT OVERVIEW

Key Facts
Massengill is the brand name for a line of douches which are recommended for routine cleansing and for temporary relief of vaginal itching and irritation. Massengill Disposable douches are available in two Vinegar & Water formulas (Extra Mild and Extra Cleansing), a Baking Soda formula, three Cosmetic solutions (Country Flowers, Belle-Mai Powder (Fresh Baby Powder Scent), and Mountain Breeze) a Fragrance-Free solution, and a Medicated formula (with povidone-iodine). Massengill also is available in a

Medicated liquid concentrate (povidone-iodine) and a Non-Medicated liquid concentrate and powder form.

Major Uses: Massengill's Vinegar & Water, Baking Soda & Water, Fragrance-Free, and Cosmetic douches are recommended for routine douching, or for cleansing following menstruation, prescribed use of vaginal medication or use of contraceptives. Massengill Medicated is recommended in a seven day regimen for the symptomatic relief of minor itching and irritation associated with vaginitis due to Candida albicans, Trichomonas vaginalis, and Gardnerella vaginalis.

Safety Information: Do not douche during pregnancy unless directed by a physician. Douching does not prevent pregnancy. Do not use this product and consult your physician if you are experiencing any of the following symptoms: unusual vaginal discharge, painful and/or frequent urination, lower abdominal pain, or you or your sex partner has genital sores or ulcers.
Massengill Vinegar & Water, Baking Soda & Water, Fragrance-Free, and Cosmetic Douches—If irritation occurs, discontinue use.
Massengill Medicated — Women with iodine-sensitivity should not use this product. If symptoms persist after seven days, or if redness, swelling or pain develop, consult a physician. Do not use while nursing unless directed by a physician.

PRODUCT INFORMATION

MASSENGILL®
[mas 'sen-gil]
Disposable Douches
MASSENGILL®
Liquid Concentrate
MASSENGILL® Powder

Ingredients:
DISPOSABLES: Extra Mild Vinegar and Water—Water and Vinegar.
Extra Cleansing Vinegar and Water—Water, Vinegar, Puraclean™ (Cetylpyridinium Chloride), Diazolidinyl Urea, Disodium EDTA.
Baking Soda and Water—Sanitized Water, Sodium Bicarbonate (Baking Soda).
Belle-Mai Powder (Fresh Baby Powder Scent)—Water, SD Alcohol 40, Lactic Acid, Sodium Lactate, Octoxynol-9, Cetylpyridinium Chloride, Propylene Glycol (and) Diazolidinyl Urea (and) Methyl Paraben (and) Propyl Paraben, Disodium EDTA, Fragrance, FD&C Blue #1.
Country Flowers—Water, SD Alcohol 40, Lactic Acid, Sodium Lactate, Octoxynol-9, Cetylpyridinium Chloride, Propylene Glycol (and) Diazolidinyl Urea (and), Methyl Paraben (and) Propyl Paraben, Disodium EDTA, Fragrance, D&C Red #28, FD&C Blue #1.
Mountain Breeze—Water, SD Alcohol 40, Lactic Acid, Sodium Lactate, Octoxynol-9, Cetylpyridinium Chloride, Propylene Glycol (and) Diazolidinyl Urea (and) Methyl Paraben (and) Propyl Paraben, Disodium EDTA, Fragrance, D&C Yellow #10, FD&C Blue #1.
Fragrance-Free—Water, SD Alcohol 40, Lactic Acid, Sodium Lactate, Octoxynol-

9, Cetylpyridinium Chloride, Propylene Glycol (and) Diazolidinyl Urea (and) Methyl Paraben (and) Propyl Paraben, Disodium EDTA.
LIQUID CONCENTRATE: Water, SD Alcohol 40, Lactic Acid, Sodium Bicarbonate, Octoxynol-9, Methyl Salicylate, Liquid Menthol, Eucalyptol, Thymol, D&C Yellow #10, FD&C Yellow #6 (Sunset Yellow).
POWDER: Sodium Chloride, Ammonium alum, PEG-8, Phenol, Methyl Salicylate, Eucalyptus Oil, Menthol, Thymol, D&C Yellow #10, FD&C Yellow #6 (Sunset Yellow).
FLORAL POWDER: Sodium Chloride, Ammonium alum, Octoxynol-9, SD Alcohol 23-A, Fragrance, and FD&C Yellow #6 (Sunset Yellow).

Indications: Recommended for routine cleansing at the end of menstruation, after use of contraceptive creams or jellies (check the contraceptive package instructions first) or to rinse out the residue of prescribed vaginal medication (as directed by physician).

Actions: The buffered acid solutions of Massengill Douches are valuable adjuncts to specific vaginal therapy following the prescribed use of vaginal medication or contraceptives and in feminine hygiene.

Directions:
DISPOSABLES: Twist off flat, wing-shaped tab from bottle containing premixed solution, attach nozzle supplied and use. The unit is completely disposable.
LIQUID CONCENTRATE: Fill cap ¾ full, to measuring line, and pour contents into douche bag containing 1 quart of warm water. Mix thoroughly.
POWDER: Dissolve two rounded teaspoonfuls in a douche bag containing 1 quart of warm water. Mix thoroughly.

Warning: Douching does not prevent pregnancy. If vaginal dryness or irritation occurs discontinue use. Do not use during pregnancy except under the advice and supervision of your physician. If you are experiencing vaginal discharge of an unusual amount, color, or odor, or painful and/or frequent urination, lower abdominal pain or genital sores or ulcers, or have had sex with a partner who has genital symptoms, you may have a serious condition. Do not use this product and contact your doctor immediately.
Use this product only as directed for routine cleansing. You should douche no more than twice a week except on the advice of your doctor.
An association has been reported between frequent douching and pelvic inflammatory disease (PID), a serious infection of the reproductive system. Douches should not be used for self-treatment of sexually transmitted diseases or PID. If you suspect you have one of these infections, stop using this product and see your doctor immediately.
Keep out of reach of children. In case of accidental ingestion, seek professional assistance by contacting your physician,

the local poison control center, or the Rocky Mt. Poison Control Center at 303-592-1710 (collect), 24 hours a day.

How Supplied:
Disposable—6 oz. disposable plastic bottle.
Liquid Concentrate—4 oz., 8 oz., plastic bottles.
Powder—4 oz., 8 oz., 16 oz., Packettes—10's, 12's.

MASSENGILL® Medicated
[mas 'sen-gil]
Disposable Douche
MASSENGILL® Medicated
Liquid Concentrate

Active Ingredient:
DISPOSABLE: Cepticin™ (povidone-iodine)
LIQUID CONCENTRATE: Cepticin™ (povidone-iodine)

Indications: For symptomatic relief of minor vaginal irritation or itching associated with vaginitis due to Candida albicans, Trichomonas vaginalis, and Gardnerella vaginalis.

Action: Povidone-iodine is widely recognized as an effective broad spectrum microbicide against both gram negative and gram positive bacteria, fungi, yeasts and protozoa. While remaining active in the presence of blood, serum or bodily secretions, it possesses virtually none of the irritating properties of iodine.

Warnings: Douching does not prevent pregnancy. Do not use during pregnancy or while nursing except under the advice and supervision of your physician. If vaginal dryness or irritation occurs discontinue use. If you are experiencing vaginal discharge of an unusual amount, color, or odor or painful and/ or frequent urination, lower abdominal pain or genital sores or ulcers, or have had sex with a partner who has genital symptoms, you may have a serious condition. Do not use this product and contact your doctor immediately.
Use this product only as directed. Do not use this product for routine cleansing.
An association has been reported between frequent douching and pelvic inflammatory disease (PID), a serious infection of the reproductive system. Douches should not be used for self-treatment of sexually transmitted diseases or PID. If you suspect you have one of these infections, stop using this product and see your doctor immediately. Women with iodine sensitivity should not use this product. Keep out of the reach of children. In case of accidental ingestion, seek professional assistance by contacting your physician, the local poison control center, or the Rocky Mt. Poison Control Center at 303-592-1710 (Collect), 24 hours a day.

Dosage and Administration:
DISPOSABLE: Dosage is provided as a single unit concentrate to be added to 6 oz. of sanitized water supplied in a disposable bottle. A specially designed nozzle is

provided. After use, the unit is discarded. Use one bottle a day. Although symptoms may be relieved earlier, for maximum relief, use for seven days.
LIQUID CONCENTRATE: Pour one capful into douche bag containing one quart of water. Mix thoroughly. Use once daily. Although symptoms may be relieved earlier, for maximum relief, use for seven days.

How Supplied:
Disposable—6 oz. bottle of sanitized water with 0.17 oz. vial of povidone-iodine and nozzle.
Liquid Concentrate—4 oz., 8 oz. plastic bottles.
Shown in Product Identification Section, page 427

MASSENGILL®
[mas 'sen-gil]
Fragrance-Free Soft Cloth Towelette

Inactive Ingredients: Water, Octoxynol-9, Lactic Acid, Sodium Lactate, Potassium Sorbate, Disodium EDTA, and Cetylpyridinium Chloride.

Indications: For cleansing and refreshing the external vaginal area.

Actions: Massengill Fragrance-Free Soft Cloth Towelettes safely cleanse the external vaginal area and do not contain fragrance. The towelette delivery system makes the application soft and gentle.

Warnings: For external use only. Avoid contact with eyes.

Directions: Remove towelette from foil packet, unfold, and gently wipe. Throw away towelette after it has been used once.

How Supplied: Sixteen individually wrapped, disposable towelettes per carton.

MASSENGILL® Medicated
[mas 'sen-gil]
Soft Cloth Towelette

Active Ingredient: Hydrocortisone (0.5%).
Inactive Ingredients: Diazolidinyl Urea, DMDM Hydantoin, Isopropyl Myristate, Methylparaben, Polysorbate 60, Propylene Glycol, Propylparaben, Sorbitan Stearate, Steareth-2, Steareth-21, Water.
Also available in non-medicated Baby Powder Scent and Unscented formulas to freshen and cleanse the external vaginal area.

Indications: For soothing relief of minor external feminine itching or other itching associated with minor skin irritations, inflammation and rashes. Other uses of this product should be only under the advice and supervision of a physician.

Action: Massengill Medicated Soft Cloth Towelettes contain hydrocortisone, a proven anti-inflammatory, anti-pruritic

Continued on next page

SmithKline Beecham—Cont.

ingredient. The towelette delivery system makes the application soothing, soft, and gentle.

Warnings: For external use only. Avoid contact with eyes. if condition worsens, symptoms persist for more than seven days, or symptoms recur within a few days, do not use this or any other hydrocortisone product unless you have consulted a physician. If experiencing a vaginal discharge, see a physician. Do not use this product for the treatment of diaper rash.

Keep this and all drugs out of the reach of children. As with any drug, if pregnant or nursing a baby, seek the advice of a health professional before using this product. In case of accidental ingestion, seek professional assistance or contact a Poison Control Center immediately.

Directions: Adults and Children two years of age and older—apply to the affected area not more than three to four times daily. Remove towelette from foil packet, gently wipe, and discard. Throw away towelette after it has been used once. Children under 2 years of age: DO NOT USE.

How Supplied: Ten individually wrapped, disposable towelettes per carton.

NATURE'S REMEDY®
Natural Vegetable Laxative

Active Ingredients: Cascara Sagrada 150 mg, Aloe 100 mg.

Inactive Ingredients: Calcium Stearate, Cellulose, Lactose, Coating, Colors (contains FD&C Yellow No. 6).

Indications: For gentle, overnight relief of constipation.

Actions: Nature's Remedy has two natural active ingredients that give gentle, overnight relief of constipation. These ingredients, Cascara Sagrada and Aloe, gently stimulate the body's natural function.

Dosage and Administration: Adults, swallow two tablets daily along with a full glass of water; children (8–15 yrs.), one tablet daily; or as directed by a physician.

Warnings: Do not take any laxative when nausea, vomiting, abdominal pain, or other symptoms of appendicitis are present. Frequent or prolonged use of laxatives may result in dependence on them. As with any drug, if you are pregnant or nursing a baby, seek the advice of a health professional before using this product.
KEEP OUT OF THE REACH OF CHILDREN.

Symptoms and Treatment of Oral Overdosage: If an overdose is suspected, immediately seek professional assistance by contacting your physician, local poison control center, or the Rocky Moun-

tain Poison Control Center at 303-592-1710 (Collect) 24 hours a day.

How Supplied: Beige, film-coated tablets with foil-backed blister packaging in boxes of 12s, 30s and 60s.

*Shown in Product Identification
Section, page 427*

NATURE'S REMEDY Regular Enema and Mineral Oil Enema

Product Information: Nature's Remedy Regular Enema and Mineral Oil Enema are packaged in a unique flex-neck bottle for easy, comfortable insertion. The safety-sealed bottle assures purity and freshness. The soft enema applicator tip is lubricated and wrapped for patient comfort and protection.

REGULAR ENEMA

Indications: For the relief of constipation and for cleansing the bowel before rectal examinations.

Active Ingredients: Each 118 ml (delivered dose) contains 19g Sodium Biphosphate and 7g Sodium Phosphate. Sodium content 4.4g per delivered dose.

Dosage: Adult: One bottle (118 ml, delivered dose) or as directed by physician. Children over 2 years: One-half adult dose or as directed by physician. Do not administer to children under 2 years of age. If you administer the enema solution and do not pass the liquid, contact a physician immediately as a more serious condition could occur.

MINERAL OIL ENEMA

Indications: For the relief of fecal impaction or constipation without straining or irritating the mucosa of the bowel. For cleansing and removal of residue after barium enema administration.

Active Ingredients: Each 118 ml (delivered dose) contains Mineral Oil, USP.

Dosage: Adult: One bottle (118 ml delivered dose), or as directed by physician. Children over 2 years: One-half adult dose or as directed by physician. Do not administer to children under 2 years of age.

Directions for Both: Twist-off flat, wing-shaped tab. Carefully line up applicator tip with bottle threads and screw onto the bottle until it is firmly attached. Do not overtighten. If applicator tip slips or comes off, repeat process. Hold bottle upright until ready to use. Grasp protective cap and pull gently to remove. With steady pressure, gently insert enema into the rectum with applicator tip pointing toward navel. Squeeze bottle until nearly all liquid is dispensed. Bottle contains more than the amount of liquid needed for effective use. A small amount of liquid will remain in bottle after squeezing. Remove applicator tip from rectum. Retain enema in solution internally for the length of time directed by physician. After administering, simply throw away used enema. Open carton along perforation for more complete directions (administration position, etc).

Warnings for Both: Do not use laxative products when nausea, vomiting, or abdominal pain is present. If you notice a sudden change in bowel habits that persists over a period of 2 weeks, consult a physician. Rectal bleeding or failure to have a bowel movement after use of a laxative may indicate a serious condition. Discontinue use and consult a physician. Laxative products should not be used longer than 1 week unless directed by a physician. Frequent or prolonged use of a laxative may result in dependence. As with any drug, if you are pregnant or nursing a baby, seek the advice of a health care professional before using this product. Keep this and all drugs out of the reach of children. In case of accidental ingestion or overdose, seek professional assistance or contact a Poison Control Center immediately.

How Supplied: Available in 4.5 fl. oz. flex-neck bottle.

*Shown in Product Identification
Section, page 427*

N'ICE® Sugarless Vitamin C Drops
[nis]

Description: Lemon, Orange—One drop provides: Vitamin C 60 mg. (100% U.S. Recommended Daily Allowance). Grape —One drop provides: Vitamin C 45 mg. (100% Children's U.S. Recommended Dietary Allowance).

Ingredients: Lemon—Sorbitol, Ascorbic Acid, Citric Acid, Natural and Artificial Flavoring, Menthol, and Artificial Color (including Yellow 5). Orange—Sorbitol, Ascorbic Acid, Natural and Artificial Flavoring, Citric Acid, Sodium Citrate, Menthol, and Artificial Color (including Yellow 6). Grape—Sorbitol, Ascorbic Acid, Natural and Artificial Flavoring, Tartaric Acid, Propylene Glycol, Menthol, and Artificial Color.

Indication: Dietary Supplementation.

How Supplied: Available in packages of 2 and 16 drops.

*Shown in Product Identification
Section, page 427*

N'ICE® Medicated Sugarless Sore Throat and Cough Lozenges
[nis]

Active Ingredient: Cherry—Each lozenge contains 5.0 mg. menthol in a sorbitol base. Citrus—Each lozenge contains 5.0 mg. menthol in a sorbitol base. Menthol Eucalyptus—Each lozenge contains 5.0 mg. menthol in a sorbitol base. Menthol Mint—Each lozenge contains 5.0 mg. menthol in a sorbitol base. Children's Berry—Each lozenge contains 3.0 mg. menthol in a sorbitol base.

Inactive Ingredients: Cherry—Flavors, Red 33, Sorbitol, Tartaric Acid, Yellow 6, Citrus—Citric Acid, Flavors, Saccharin Sodium, Sodium Citrate, Sorbitol, Yellow 10. Menthol Eucalyptus—Citric Acid, Flavors, Sorbitol. Menthol

Mint—Blue 1, Flavor, Hydrogenated Glucose Syrup, Sorbitol, Yellow 10. Children's Berry—Citric Acid, Flavors, Red 33, Sodium Citrate, Sorbitol.

Indications: Temporarily suppresses cough due to minor throat and bronchial irritation associated with a cold or inhaled irritants. Temporarily relieves minor sore throat pain.

Warnings: Do not administer to children under six years of age unless directed by a physician. Severe or persistent sore throat or sore throat accompanied by high fever, headache, nausea, and vomiting may be serious. Consult a physician in such case, or if sore throat persists for more than two days. A persistent cough may be a sign of a serious condition. If cough persists for more than one week, tends to recur, or is accompanied by fever, rash, or persistent headache, consult a physician. Do not take this product for persistent or chronic cough such as occurs with smoking, asthma, emphysema, or if cough is accompanied by excessive phlegm, unless directed by a physician.
Keep this and all medicines out of the reach of children.

Drug Interaction: No known drug interaction.

Dosage and Administration: Cherry, Citrus, Menthol Eucalyptus, Menthol Mint—Let lozenge dissolve slowly in the mouth. Repeat as needed, up to 10 lozenges per day. Children's Berry—Take two lozenges. Let lozenges dissolve slowly in the mouth. Repeat as needed, up to 10 lozenges per day.

Professional Labeling: For the temporary relief of pain associated with tonsillitis, pharyngitis, throat infections or stomatitis.

How Supplied: Available in packages of 2, 8 and 16 lozenges.
Shown in Product Identification Section, page 427

OXY ACNE MEDICATIONS
**OXY-5® and OXY-10®
with SORBOXYL®
Benzoyl peroxide lotion 5% and 10%
with silica oil absorber
Vanishing and Tinted Formulas**

Description: Active Ingredient: Oxy-5: Benzoyl peroxide 5%. Oxy-10: Benzoyl peroxide 10%.

Inactive Ingredients: Oxy-5 Vanishing: Cetyl alcohol, citric acid, methylparaben, propylene glycol, propylparaben, silica (Sorboxyl®), sodium lauryl sulfate, sodium PCA, and water.
Oxy-5 Tinted: Cetyl alcohol, citric acid, iron oxides, methylparaben, propylene glycol, propylparaben, silica (Sorboxyl®), sodium lauryl sulfate, stearyl alcohol, sodium PCA, titanium dioxide and water.
Oxy-10 Vanishing: Cetyl alcohol, citric acid, methylparaben, propylene glycol, propylparaben, silica (Sorboxyl®), so-

dium citrate, sodium lauryl sulfate, and water.
Oxy-10 Tinted: Cetyl alcohol, citric acid, glyceryl stearate, iron oxides, methylparaben, propylene glycol, propylparaben, silica (Sorboxyl®), sodium citrate, sodium lauryl sulfate, stearic acid, titanium dioxide and water.

Indications: Topical medications for the treatment of acne vulgaris.

Action: Provides antibacterial activity against Propionibacterium acnes.

Additional Benefits: Absorbs excess skin oil up to 12 hours. Vanishing formulas are colorless, odorless, greaseless lotions that vanish upon application. Tinted formulas are flesh tone, odorless, greaseless lotions that cover up acne pimples while they treat them.

Directions: Wash skin thoroughly and dry well. Shake well before using. Dab on Oxy 5 or Oxy 10, smoothing it into acne pimple areas of face, neck, and body (see Warnings). Apply once a day initially, then two or three times a day, or as directed by a physician.

Warnings: FOR EXTERNAL USE ONLY. Using other topical acne medications at the same time or immediately following use of this product may increase dryness or irritation of the skin. If this occurs only one medication should be used unless directed by a doctor. Do not use this medication if you have very sensitive skin or if you are sensitive to benzoyl peroxide. To test for sensitivity, apply to a small affected area once a day for two days. Follow label instructions and continue use if no discomfort or burning occurs. This product may cause irritation, characterized by redness, burning, itching, peeling, or possibly swelling. More frequent use or higher concentrations may aggrevate such irritation. Mild irritation may be reduced by using the product less frequently or in lower concentration. If irritation becomes severe, discontinue use. If irritation still continues, consult a doctor. Keep away from eyes, lips, and mouth. Keep this and all drugs out of reach of children. This product may bleach hair or dyed fabrics, including clothing and carpeting. Keep tightly closed. Store at room temperature, avoid excessive heat.

Symptoms and Treatment of Ingestion: These symptoms are based upon medical judgment, not on actual experience. Theoretically, ingestion of very large amounts may cause nausea, vomiting, abdominal discomfort, and diarrhea. If an oral overdose is suspected, contact a physician, the local poison control center, or the Rocky Mountain Poison Control Center at 303-592-1710 (Collect) 24 hours a day.

How Supplied: 1 fl. oz. plastic bottles.
Shown in Product Identification Section, page 427

OXY®
Medicated Cleanser, Medicated Soap, and Lathering Facial Scrub

Active Ingredient: Oxy® Medicated Cleanser: Salicylic Acid* 0.5%.
Oxy® Medicated Soap: Triclosan 1.0%.
Oxy® Lathering Facial Scrub: None.

Inactive Ingredients:
Oxy® Medicated Cleanser: Citric acid, menthol, propylene glycol, sodium lauryl sulfate, and water. Also contains Alcohol 40%.
Oxy® Lathering Facial Scrub: Sodium borate, sodium methyl cocoyl taurate, sodium laureth sulfate, sodium lauryl sulfoacetate, glyceryl stearate, PEG-100 stearate, potassium undecylenoyl, hydrolyzed animal protein, fragrance, oleth-20, potassium sorbate, and triclosan.
Oxy® Medicated Soap: Bentonite, cocoamphodipropionate, fragrance, glycerin, iron oxides, magnesium silicate, sodium borohydride, sodium chloride, sodium cocoate, sodium tallowate, talc, tetrasodium EDTA, titanium dioxide, trisodium HEDTA, water.

Indications: These skin care products are useful for opening plugged pores and for removing excess dirt and oil. Also helps remove and prevent blackheads.

Additional Benefits: When used regularly cleanses acne-prone skin and removes dirt, grime and excess skin oil. For a complete anti-acne program, after using Oxy® Cleansing Products follow use with Oxy-5® Tinted and Vanishing, or Oxy-10® Tinted and Vanishing acne pimple medications.

Warning (Oxy® Medicated Cleanser and Soap): FOR EXTERNAL USE ONLY. Using other topical acne medications at the same time or immediately following use of this product may increase dryness or irritation of the skin. If this occurs, only one medication should be used unless directed by a doctor. Do not leave pad on skin for an extended period of time. May be irritating to eyes or mucous membranes. If contact occurs, flush thoroughly with water. Keep this and all drugs out of reach of children. Store at room temperature. Flammable. Keep away from flame, fire and heat.

Warning (Oxy Medicated Soap): Do not use this product on infants under six months of age.

Warning (Oxy Lathering Facial Scrub): Avoid contact with eyes. If particles get into eyes, flush thoroughly with water and avoid rubbing eyes. Discontinue use if skin irritation or excessive dryness develops and consult your physician. FOR EXTERNAL USE ONLY. Not to be used on infants or children under 3 years of age. Do not use on inflamed skin. Keep out of reach of children.

Symptoms and Treatment of Ingestion: If large amounts are ingested, nausea, vomiting, or gastrointestinal irritation may develop. If an oral overdose

*Salicylic Acid (2-Hydroxybenzoic Acid).

Continued on next page

SmithKline Beecham—Cont.

is suspected, contact a physician, the local poison control center, or the Rocky Mountain Poison Control Center at 303-592-1710 (Collect) 24 hours a day.

Dosage and Administration: See labeling instructions for use.

How Supplied:
Medicated Liquid Cleanser—4 fl. oz.
Medicated Soap—3.25 oz. soap bar.
Lathering Facial Scrub—2.65 oz. Plastic Tube.

Shown in Product Identification Section, page 428

OXY® MEDICATED PADS
Regular, Sensitive Skin, and Maximum Strength

Active Ingredient:
Oxy® Medicated Pads Regular Strength: Salicylic Acid* 0.5%.
Oxy® Medicated Pads Sensitive Skin: Salicylic Acid* 0.5%.
Oxy® Medicated Pads Maximum Strength: Salicylic Acid* 2.0%.

Inactive Ingredients:
Oxy® Medicated Pads Regular Strength: Citric acid, fragrance, menthol, propylene glycol, sodium lauryl sulfate, water. Also contains Alcohol 40%.
Oxy® Medicated Pads Sensitive Skin: Disodium lauryl sulfosuccinate, fragrance, menthol, PEG-4, sodium lauroyl sarcosinate, sodium PCA, trisodium EDTA, water. Also contains Alcohol 22%.
Oxy® Medicated Pads Maximum Strength: Citric acid, fragrance, menthol, PEG-8, propylene glycol, sodium lauryl sulfate, water. Also contains Alcohol 50%.

Indications: These medicated pad products are useful for opening plugged pores and for removing excess dirt and oil. Also helps remove and prevent blackheads.

Additional Benefits: When used regularly cleanses acne-prone skin and removes dirt, grime and excess skin oil.

Warnings: FOR EXTERNAL USE ONLY. Using other topical acne medications at the same time or immediately following use of this product may increase dryness or irritation of the skin. If this occurs, only one medication should be used unless directed by a doctor. Do not leave pad on skin for an extended period of time. May be irritating to eyes or mucous membranes. If contact occurs, flush thoroughly with water. Keep this and all drugs out of reach of children. Store at room temperature. Flammable. Keep away from flame, fire and heat.

Symptoms and Treatment of Ingestion: If large amounts are ingested, nausea, vomiting, or gastrointestinal irritation may develop. If an oral overdose is suspected, contact a physician, the local poison control center, or the Rocky

*Salicylic Acid (2-Hydroxybenzoic Acid).

Mountain Poison Control Center at 303-592-1710 (Collect) 24 hours a day.

Dosage and Administration: See labeling instructions for use.

How Supplied:
Medicated Pads Regular Strength—Plastic Jar/50 pads or 90 pads
Medicated Pads Sensitive Skin—Plastic Jar/50 pads or 90 pads
Medicated Pads Maximum Strength—Plastic Jar/50 pads or 90 pads

Shown in Product Identification Section, page 427

OXY NIGHT WATCH™
Maximum Strength and Sensitive Skin Formulas

Active Ingredient:
Oxy Night Watch™ Maximum Strength: Salicylic Acid (2-Hydroxybenzoic Acid) 2.0%.
Oxy Night Watch™ Sensitive Skin: Salicylic Acid (2-Hydroxybenzoic Acid) 1.0%.

Inactive Ingredients: Cetyl alcohol, disodium EDTA, methylparaben, propylene glycol, propylparaben, silica (Sorboxyl®), sodium lauryl sulfate, stearyl alcohol, and water.

Indications: These medicated skin products help unplug clogged pores and penetrate pores to treat pimples and blackheads before they form.

Additional Benefits: Absorbs excess skin oil up to 12 hours. Stays on all night to treat and prevent pimples and blackheads.

Directions:
Before Using: At bedtime, wash your face gently using a non-abrasive soap. Rinse thoroughly and pat dry.
Usage: Squeeze out a small amount of lotion. Smooth a thin layer evenly over your entire face, avoiding eyes, lips, and mouth. Do not wash off. OXY NIGHT WATCH works best when left on overnight. The next morning, wash your face and pat dry.

Warnings: FOR EXTERNAL USE ONLY. Some skin types may experience sensitivity to this medication. To test sensitivity, apply to a small facial area once a night for two nights. If skin irritation, excessive drying, or discomfort develops, use less frequently or discontinue use. Using other topical acne medications at the same time or immediately following use of this product may increase dryness or irritation of the skin. If this occurs, only one medication should be used unless directed by a doctor. May be irritating to eyes or mucous membranes. If contact occurs, flush thoroughly with water. Keep this and all drugs out of reach of children. Store at room temperature. Flammable. Keep away from flame, fire and heat.

How Supplied: 2.0 oz. plastic tubes.
Shown in Product Identification Section, page 428

OXY 10® DAILY FACE WASH

Active Ingredient: Benzoyl peroxide 10%.

Inactive Ingredients: Citric acid, cocamidopropyl betaine, diazolidinyl urea, methylparaben, propylparaben, sodium citrate, sodium cocoyl isethionate, sodium lauroyl sarcosinate, water, and xanthan gum.

Indications: Antibacterial skin wash used as an aid in the treatment of acne vulgaris.

Actions: Promotes antibacterial activity against Propionibacterium acnes.

Additional Benefits: When used instead of regular soap, cleanses acne-prone skin and removes dirt, grime and excess skin oil.

Directions: Shake well. Wet area to be washed. Apply Oxy 10 Daily Face Wash and work into lather, massaging gently for 1 to 2 minutes. Rinse thoroughly. Use 2 to 3 times daily or as directed by a physician.

Warnings: FOR EXTERNAL USE ONLY. Using other topical acne medications at the same time or immediately following use of this product may increase dryness or irritation of the skin. If this occurs, only one medication should be used unless directed by a doctor. Do not use this medication if you have very sensitive skin or if you are sensitive to benzoyl peroxide. To test for sensitivity, apply to a small affected area once a day for two days. Follow label instructions and continue use if no discomfort or burning occurs. This product may cause irritation, characterized by redness, burning, itching, peeling, or possibly swelling. More frequent use or higher concentrations may aggravate such irritation. Mild irritation may be reduced by using the product less frequently or in a lower concentration. If irritation becomes severe, discontinue use; if irritation still continues, consult a doctor. Keep away from eyes, lips, and mouth. Keep this and all drugs out of reach of children. This product may bleach hair or dyed fabrics, including clothing and carpeting. Keep tightly closed. Store at room temperature; avoid excessive heat.

Symptoms and Treatment of Ingestion: These symptoms are based upon medical judgment, not on actual experience. Theoretically, ingestion of very large amounts may cause nausea, vomiting, abdominal discomfort, and diarrhea. If an oral overdose is suspected, contact a physician, the local poison control center, or the Rocky Mountain Poison Control Center at 303-592-1710 (Collect) 24 hours a day.

How supplied: 4 fl. oz. plastic bottles.
Shown in Product Identification Section, page 427

SINE-OFF Each tablet/ caplet contains:	SINE-OFF Tablets-Aspirin Formula	SINE-OFF Maximum Strength Allergy/Sinus Formula Caplets	SINE-OFF Maximum Strength No Drowsiness Formula Caplets
Chlorpheniramine maleate	2.0 mg	2.0 mg	—
Phenylpropanolamine HCl	12.5 mg	—	—
Aspirin	325.0 mg	—	—
Acetaminophen	—	500.0 mg	500.0 mg
Pseudoephedrine HCl	—	30.0 mg	30.0 mg

SINE–OFF® Maximum Strength Allergy/Sinus Formula Caplets

Composition:
[See table above.]

Product Information: SINE-OFF Maximum Strength Allergy/Sinus Formula provides maximum strength relief from upper respiratory allergy, hay fever and sinusitis symptoms. This formula contains acetaminophen, a non-aspirin pain reliever.

Product Benefits: Relieves itchy, watery eyes, sneezing, runny nose and postnasal drip • Eases headache pain and pressure • Promotes sinus drainage • Shrinks swollen membranes to relieve congestion.

Directions: Adults and children over 12 years of age: 2 caplets every 6 hours, not to exceed 8 caplets in any 24-hour period. Children under 12 should use only as directed by a physician.

TAMPER-RESISTANT PACKAGING FEATURES FOR YOUR PROTECTION:
• Each caplet is encased in a clear plastic cell with a foil back.
• The name SINE-OFF appears on each caplet (see product illustration on front of carton).
• **DO NOT USE THIS PRODUCT IF ANY OF THESE TAMPER-RESISTANT FEATURES ARE MISSING OR BROKEN.**
Comments or Questions? Call Toll-Free 800-245-1040 Weekdays.

Warnings: Do not exceed recommended dosage. If symptoms do not improve within 7 days, consult a physician before continuing use. Individuals being treated for depression, high blood pressure, asthma, heart disease, diabetes, thyroid disease, glaucoma or difficulty urinating due to an enlarged prostate gland should use only as directed by a physician. Do not take this product if you are taking sedatives or tranquilizers. Avoid alcoholic beverages while taking this product. Do not drive or operate heavy machinery. May cause drowsiness. Stop use if dizziness, sleeplessness or nervousness occurs. May cause excitability, especially in children. **This package is child-safe;** however, keep this and all drugs out of reach of children. In case of accidental overdose, seek professional assistance or contact a poison control center immediately. As with any drug, if you are pregnant or nursing a baby, seek the advice of a health professional before using this product.

Store at controlled room temperature (59°–86°F.).

Formula: Active Ingredients: Each caplet contains Chlorpheniramine Maleate 2 mg., Pseudoephedrine Hydrochloride 30 mg., Acetaminophen 500 mg. *(500 mg. is a non-standard dosage of acetaminophen as compared to the standard of 325 mg.).* **Inactive Ingredients (listed for individuals with specific allergies):** Blue 2, Cellulose, Crospovidone, Hydroxypropyl Methylcellulose, Magnesium Stearate, Polyethylene Glycol, Povidone, Red 30, Starch, Titanium Dioxide, Yellow 10, and trace amounts of other inactive ingredients.
How Supplied: Consumer packages of 24 caplets.

Note: There are other SINE-OFF products. Make sure this is the one you are interested in.

Also Available: SINE-OFF® Sinus Medicine Tablets with Aspirin in 24's, 48's, 100's. SINE-OFF® Maximum Strength No Drowsiness Formula Caplets 24's.
Shown in Product Identification Section, page 428

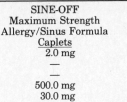

SINE–OFF® Maximum Strength No Drowsiness Formula Caplets

Composition: [See table above.]

Product Information: SINE-OFF Maximum Strength No Drowsiness Formula provides maximum strength relief from headache and sinus pain. Relieves pressure and congestion due to sinusitis, allergic sinusitis or the common cold. This formula contains acetaminophen, a non-aspirin pain reliever.

NO ANTIHISTAMINE DROWSINESS

Product Benefits: Eases headache, pain and pressure • Promotes sinus drainage • Shrinks swollen membranes to relieve congestion.

Directions: Adults and children over 12 years of age: 2 caplets every 6 hours, not to exceed 8 caplets in any 24-hour period. Children under 12 should use only as directed by physician.

TAMPER-RESISTANT PACKAGE FEATURES FOR YOUR PROTECTION:
• Each caplet is encased in a clear plastic cell with a foil back.
• The name SINE-OFF appears on each caplet (see product illustration on front of carton).
• **DO NOT USE THIS PRODUCT IF ANY OF THESE TAMPER-RESISTANT FEATURES ARE MISSING OR BROKEN.**
Comments or Questions? Call Toll-Free 800-245-1040 Weekdays.
For maximum strength relief of headache and sinus pain, without antihistamine drowsiness. Relieves pressure and congestion due to sinusitis, or the common cold. This formula contains acetaminophen, a non-aspirin pain reliever.

Directions: Adults and children over 12 years of age: 2 caplets every 6 hours, not to exceed 8 caplets in 24 hours. Children under 12 should use only as directed by physician.

Warnings: Do not exceed recommended dosage because dizziness, sleeplessness, or nervousness may occur. Do not take this product for more than 10 days. If symptoms do not improve or are accompanied by fever that lasts more than 3 days, or if new symptoms occur, consult a physician. Do not take this product if you have heart disease, high blood pressure, diabetes, thyroid disease, or difficulty in urination due to enlargement of the prostate gland unless directed by a physician. Keep this and all drugs out of reach of children. In case of accidental overdose, seek professional assistance or contact a poison control center immediately. Prompt medical attention is critical for adults as well as children even if you do not notice any signs or symptoms. As with any drug, if you are pregnant or nursing a baby, seek the advice of a health professional before using this product.

Drug Interaction Precaution: Do not take this product if you are presently taking a prescription drug for high blood pressure or depression, without first consulting your physician.
Avoid storing at high temperatures (greater than 100°F).

Active Ingredients: Each caplet contains: 30 mg. Pseudoephedrine Hydrochloride, 500 mg. Acetaminophen (500 mg. is a non-standard dosage of acetaminophen, as compared to the standard of 325 mg.).

Inactive Ingredients: Crospovidone, Hydroxypropyl Methylcellulose, Magnesium Stearate, Microcrystalline Cellulose, Polyethylene Glycol, Polysorbate 80, Povidone, FD&C Red 40, Starch, Titanium Dioxide.

How Supplied: Consumer packages of 24 caplets.

Continued on next page

SmithKline Beecham—Cont.

Note: There are other SINE-OFF products. Make sure this is the one you are interested in.

Also Available:
SINE-OFF® Tablets with Aspirin
SINE-OFF® Maximum Strength Allergy/Sinus Formula Caplets
Shown in Product Identification Section, page 428

SINE–OFF® Sinus Medicine Tablets–Aspirin Formula
Relieves sinus headache and congestion.

Composition: [See table on page 717.]

Product Information: SINE-OFF relieves headache, pain, pressure and congestion due to sinusitis, allergic sinusitis, or the common cold.

Product Benefits: Eases headache, pain and pressure • Promotes sinus drainage • Shrinks swollen membranes to relieve congestion • Relieves postnasal drip.

Directions: Adults: 2 tablets every 4 hours, not to exceed 8 tablets in any 24-hour period. Children (6–12) one-half the adult dosage. Children under 6 years should use only as directed by a physician.

TAMPER-RESISTANT PACKAGE FEATURES FOR YOUR PROTECTION:
• Each tablet is encased in a clear plastic cell with a foil back.
• The name SINE-OFF appears on each tablet (see product illustration on front of carton).
• **DO NOT USE THIS PRODUCT IF ANY OF THESE TAMPER-RESISTANT FEATURES ARE MISSING OR BROKEN.**

Comments or Questions? Call Toll-Free 800-245-1040 Weekdays.

Warnings: Children and teenagers should not use this medicine for chicken pox or flu symptoms before a doctor is consulted about Reye Syndrome, a rare but serious illness. Do not take this product for more than 10 days. If symptoms do not improve or are accompanied by fever that lasts for more than 3 days, or if new symptoms occur, consult a doctor. Do not take this product if you have asthma, glaucoma, heart disease, high blood pressure, thyroid disease, diabetes, emphysema, chronic pulmonary disease, shortness of breath, difficulty in breathing or difficulty in urination due to enlargement of the prostate gland unless directed by a doctor. Do not take this product if you are allergic to aspirin, have stomach problems, ulcers or bleeding problems unless directed by a doctor. Do not exceed recommended dosage. At higher doses nervousness, dizziness or sleeplessness may occur. May cause excitability, especially in children. May cause drowsiness. Avoid alcoholic beverages while taking this product. Do not drive or operate heavy machinery. Keep this and all drugs out of reach of children. In case of accidental overdose, seek professional assistance or contact a poison control center immediately. As with any drug, if you are pregnant or nursing a baby, seek the advice of a health professional before using this product. IT IS ESPECIALLY IMPORTANT NOT TO USE ASPIRIN DURING THE LAST 3 MONTHS OF PREGNANCY UNLESS SPECIFICALLY DIRECTED TO DO SO BY A DOCTOR BECAUSE IT MAY CAUSE PROBLEMS IN THE UNBORN CHILD OR COMPLICATIONS DURING DELIVERY.

Drug Interaction Precaution: Do not take this product if you are taking a prescription drug for anticoagulation (thinning the blood), high blood pressure, depression, diabetes, gout or arthritis unless directed by a doctor.
Store at controlled room temperature (59°–86°F.).

Each tablet contains: Active Ingredients: Aspirin, 325 mg.; Chlorpheniramine Maleate, 2 mg.; Phenylpropanolamine Hydrochloride, 12.5 mg.

Inactive Ingredients: Acacia, Calcium Sulfate, Carnauba Wax, D&C Yellow 10, Ethylcellulose, FD&C Yellow 6, Gelatin, Guar Gum, Polysorbate 80, Silicon Dioxide, Starch, Sucrose, Titanium Dioxide, and trace amounts of other inactive ingredients.

How Supplied: Consumer packages of 24, 48 and 100 tablets.

Note: There are other SINE-OFF products. Make sure this is the one you are interested in.

Also Available: SINE-OFF® Maximum Strength Allergy/Sinus Formula Caplets 24's. SINE-OFF® Maximum Strength No Drowsiness Formula Caplets 24's.
Shown in Product Identification Section, page 428

SOMINEX®
[*som 'in-ex*]
Tablets and Caplets

Active Ingredients: Each tablet contains Diphenhydramine HCl, 25 mg. Each caplet contains Diphenhydramine HCl, 50 mg.

Inactive Ingredients Tablets: Dibasic Calcium Phosphate, Magnesium Stearate, Microcrystalline Cellulose, Silicon Dioxide, Starch, FD&C Blue #1.

Inactive Ingredients Caplets: Carnauba Wax, Crospovidone, Dibasic Calcium Phosphate, Hydroxypropyl Methylcellulose, Magnesium Stearate, Microcrystalline Cellulose, Polyethylene Glycol, Polysorbate 80, Silicon Dioxide, Starch, Titanium Dioxide, White Wax, FD&C Blue #1.

Indications: Helps to reduce difficulty falling asleep.

Action: An antihistamine with anticholinergic and sedative effects.

Directions: Take 50 mg. (2 tablets or 1 caplet) at bedtime if needed, or as directed by a doctor.

Warnings: Do not give to children under 12 years of age. If sleeplessness persists continuously for more than two weeks, consult your doctor. Insomnia may be a symptom of serious underlying medical illness. Avoid alcoholic beverages while taking this product. Do not take this product if you are taking sedatives or tranquilizers, without first consulting your doctor. Do not take this product if you have asthma, glaucoma, emphysema, chronic pulmonary disease, shortness of breath, difficulty in breathing, or difficulty in urination due to enlargement of the prostate gland unless directed by a doctor. As with any drug, if you are pregnant or nursing a baby, seek the advice of a health professional before using this product. Keep this and all drugs out of the reach of children. In case of accidental overdose, seek professional assistance or contact a poison control center immediately or the Rocky Mountain Poison Control Center at 303-592-1710 (Collect) 24 hours a day.

Drug Interaction: Monoamine oxidase (MAO) inhibitors prolong and intensify the anticholinergic effects of antihistamines. The CNS depressant effect is heightened by alcohol and other CNS depressant drugs.

Symptoms and Treatment of Oral Overdosage: Antihistamine overdosage reactions may vary from central nervous system depression to stimulation. Stimulation is particularly likely in children. Atropine-like signs and symptoms, such as dry mouth, fixed and dilated pupils, flushing, and gastrointestinal symptoms, may also occur.

How Supplied Tablets: Available in blister packs of 16, 32, and 72.

How Supplied Caplets: Available in blister packs of 8, 16, and 32.
Shown in Product Identification Section, page 428

SOMINEX® Pain Relief Formula
[*som 'in-ex*]

Active Ingredients: Each tablet contains 500 mg. Acetaminophen and 25 mg. Diphenhydramine HCl.

Inactive Ingredients: Crospovidone, Povidone, Silicon Dioxide, Starch, Stearic Acid, FD&C Blue #1.

Indications: For sleeplessness with accompanying occasional minor aches, pains, or headache.

Action: An antihistamine with sedative effects combined with an internal analgesic.

Directions: Take two tablets thirty minutes before bedtime, or as directed by a physician.

Warnings: Do not give to children under 12 years of age. If symptoms persist continuously for more than 10 days, or if new ones occur, consult your physician. Do not exceed recommended dosage because severe liver damage may occur. Insomnia may be a symptom of serious underlying medical illness. Take this product with caution if alcohol is being consumed. Do not take this product for the treatment of arthritis, except under the advice and supervision of a physician. As with any drug, if you are pregnant or nursing a baby, seek the advice of a health professional before using this product. Keep this and all drugs out of the reach of children. In case of accidental overdose, seek professional assistance by contacting your physician, the local poison control center, or the Rocky Mountain Poison Control Center at 303-592-1710 (Collect), 24 hours a day. DO NOT TAKE THIS PRODUCT IF YOU HAVE ASTHMA, GLAUCOMA OR ENLARGEMENT OF THE PROSTATE GLAND, EXCEPT UNDER THE ADVICE AND SUPERVISION OF A PHYSICIAN.

Drug Interaction: Monoamine oxidase (MAO) inhibitors prolong and intensify the anticholinergic effects of antihistamines. The CNS depressant effect is heightened by alcohol and other CNS depressant drugs.

Symptoms and Treatment of Oral Overdosage: Antihistamine overdosage reactions may vary from central nervous system depression to stimulation. Stimulation is particularly likely in children. Atropine-like signs and symptoms, such as dry mouth, fixed and dilated pupils, flushing, and gastrointestinal symptoms, may also occur.

How Supplied: Available in blister packs of 16 tablets and bottles of 32 tablets.
Shown in Product Identification Section, page 428

SUCRETS® (Original Mint) Sore Throat Lozenges
[su'krets]

Active Ingredient: Hexylresorcinol, 2.4 mg. per lozenge.

Inactive Ingredients: Blue 1, Corn Syrup, Flavors, Sucrose, Yellow 10.

Indications: For temporary relief of occasional minor sore throat pain and mouth irritations.

Actions: Hexylresorcinol's soothing anesthetic action quickly relieves minor throat irritations.

Warnings: If sore throat is severe, persists more than 2 days, is accompanied or followed by fever, rash, nausea or vomiting, see a doctor promptly. If sore mouth symptoms do not improve in 7 days, see a doctor or dentist promptly. KEEP THIS AND ALL MEDICINES OUT OF THE REACH OF CHILDREN.

Drug Interaction: No known drug interaction.

Symptoms and Treatment of Oral Overdosage: Should a large overdose of Sucrets Original Mint be suspected,

with symptoms of profuse sweating, nausea, vomiting and diarrhea, seek professional assistance. Call your physician, local poison control center or the Rocky Mountain Poison Control Center at 303-592-1710 (Collect) 24 hours a day.

Dosage and Administration: Adults and children 2 years of age and older: Dissolve slowly in the mouth. Repeat as needed.

Professional Labeling: For the temporary relief of pain associated with tonsillitis, pharyngitis, throat infections or stomatitis.

How Supplied: Available in tins of 24 individually wrapped lozenges.
Shown in Product Identification Section, page 428

SUCRETS® Cold Formula
[su'krets]
Lozenges

Active Ingredients: Each lozenge contains Hexylresorcinol 2.4 mg., Menthol 10 mg.

Inactive Ingredients: Blue 1, Corn Syrup, Flavors, Silicon Dioxide, Sucrose.

Indications: For temporary relief of occasional minor sore throat pain, cough, and nasal congestion associated with a cold.

Warnings: A persistent cough may be a sign of a serious condition. If sore throat, cough or congestion is severe, lasts more than 2 days, is accompanied or followed by fever, rash, nausea, vomiting or persistent headache, see a doctor promptly. Do not take this product for chronic cough such as occurs with smoking, asthma, emphysema, or if cough is accompanied by excessive phlegm, unless directed by a doctor. KEEP THIS AND ALL MEDICINES OUT OF THE REACH OF CHILDREN.

Drug Interaction: No known drug interaction.

Symptoms and Treatment of Oral Overdosage: Should a large overdose of Sucrets Cold Formula be suspected, with symptoms of profuse sweating, nausea, vomiting and diarrhea, seek professional assistance. Call your doctor, local poison control center, or the Rocky Mountain Poison Control Center at 303-592-1710 (collect) 24 hours a day.

Dosage and Administration: Adults and children 2 years of age and older: Dissolve slowly in the mouth. Repeat every two hours as needed. Do not administer to children under 2 years of age, unless directed by a doctor.

Professional Labeling: For the temporary relief of pain associated with tonsillitis, pharyngitis, throat infections or stomatitis.

How Supplied: Available in tins of 24 individually wrapped lozenges.
Shown in Product Identification Section, page 428

SUCRETS® Maximum Strength Wintergreen
SUCRETS® Wild Cherry Regular Strength
SUCRETS® Children's Cherry Flavored
Sore Throat Lozenges
[su'krets]

Active Ingredient: Maximum Strength Wintergreen: Dyclonine Hydrochloride 3.0 mg. per lozenge. Wild Cherry, Regular Strength: Dyclonine Hydrochloride 2.0 mg. per lozenge. Children's Cherry: Dyclonine Hydrochloride 1.2 mg. per lozenge.

Inactive Ingredients: Maximum Strength Wintergreen: Citric Acid, Corn Syrup, Silicon Dioxide, Sucrose, Yellow 10. Wild Cherry Regular Strength: Blue 1, Corn Syrup, Flavor, Red 40, Silicon Dioxide, Sucrose, Tartaric Acid. Children's Cherry: Blue 1, Citric Acid, Corn Syrup, Red 40, Silicon Dioxide, Sucrose.

Indications: For temporary relief of occasional minor sore throat pain and mouth irritations.

Actions: Dyclonine Hydrochloride's soothing anesthetic action relieves minor throat irritations.

Warnings: If sore throat is severe, persists more than 2 days, is accompanied or followed by fever, headache, rash, nausea, or vomiting, consult a doctor promptly. If sore mouth symptoms do not improve in 7 days, see your dentist or doctor promptly. KEEP THIS AND ALL MEDICINES OUT OF THE REACH OF CHILDREN.

Drug Interaction: No known drug interaction.

Symptoms and Treatment of Oral Overdosage: Reactions due to large overdosage are systemic and involve the central nervous system and cardiovascular system. Central nervous system reactions are characterized by excitation and/or depression. Nervousness, dizziness, blurred vision or tremors may occur. Reactions involving the cardiovascular system include depression of the myocardium, hypotension or bradycardia. Should a large overdose be suspected seek professional assistance. Call your physician, local poison control center or the Rocky Mountain Poison Control Center at 303-592-1710 (Collect), 24 hours a day.

Dosage and Administration: Adults and children 2 years of age or older: Allow to dissolve slowly in the mouth. Repeat every two hours as needed. Do not administer to children under 2 years of age unless directed by a doctor.

Professional Labeling: For the temporary relief of pain associated with tonsillitis, pharyngitis, throat infections or stomatitis.

How Supplied: Available in tins of 24 lozenges.
Shown in Product Identification Section, page 428

Continued on next page

SmithKline Beecham—Cont.

SUCRETS MAXIMUM STRENGTH SPRAYS
[su'krets]

Active Ingredient: Dyclonine Hydrochloride 0.1%.

Inactive Ingredients: Cherry: Alcohol (10%), Dibasic Sodium Phosphate, Flavor, Glycerin, Monobasic Sodium Phosphate, Phosphoric Acid, Potassium Sorbate, Red 33, Sorbitol, Water, Yellow 6. Mint: Alcohol (8.9%), Blue 1, Flavor, Glycerin, Monobasic Sodium Phosphate, Phosphoric Acid, Sodium Benzoate, Sorbitol, Water, Yellow 10.

Indications: Temporary relief of occasional minor sore throat pain due to colds, throat irritations, and mouth and gum irritations.

Actions: Dyclonine Hydrochloride's soothing anesthetic action quickly relieves minor throat irritations.

Warnings: If sore throat is severe, persists for more than 2 days, is accompanied or followed by fever, headache, rash, nausea or vomiting, consult a doctor promptly. If sore mouth symptoms do not improve in 7 days, see your dentist or doctor promptly. KEEP THIS AND ALL MEDICINES OUT OF THE REACH OF CHILDREN.

Drug Interaction: No known drug interaction.

Symptoms and Treatment of Oral Overdosage: Reactions due to large overdosage are systemic and involve the central nervous system and cardiovascular system. Central nervous system reactions are characterized by excitation and/or depression. Nervousness, dizziness, blurred vision or tremors may occur. Reactions involving the cardiovascular system include depression of the myocardium, hypotension or bradycardia. Should a large overdose be suspected seek professional assistance. Call your physician, local poison control center or the Rocky Mountain Poison Poison Control Center at 303-592-1710 (Collect), 24 hours a day.

Dosage and Administration: Adults and children 2 years of age and older: Spray four times and swallow. Gargle/rinse affected area for 15 seconds then spit out. Repeat up to 4 times daily, as needed. Do not administer to children under 2 years of age unless directed by a doctor.

Professional Labeling: For the temporary relief of pain associated with tonsillitis, pharyngitis, throat infections or stomatitis.

How Supplied: Available in 6 fl. oz. and 3 fl. oz. plastic bottle sprayers.

Shown in Product Identification Section, page 428

TELDRIN®
Chlorpheniramine Maleate
Timed-Release Allergy Capsules
Maximum Strength 12 mg.

Product Information: Hay fever and allergies are caused by grass and tree pollen, dust and pollution. TELDRIN provides up to 12 hours of relief from hay fever/upper respiratory allergy symptoms: sneezing, runny nose, itchy, watery eyes. TELDRIN is formulated to release some medication initially and the rest gradually over a prolonged period.

Directions: Adults and children over 12: Just one capsule in the morning, and one in the evening. Do not give to children under 12 without the advice and consent of a physician. Not to exceed 24 mg. (2 capsules) in 24 hours.

- The carton is protected by a clear overwrap printed with "safety sealed"; do not use if overwrap is missing or broken.

TAMPER-RESISTANT PACKAGING FEATURES FOR YOUR PROTECTION:

- Each capsule is encased in a plastic cell with a foil back; do not use if the cell or foil is broken.
- Each TELDRIN capsule is protected by a green PERMA-SEAL™ band which bonds the two capsule halves together; do not use if capsule or band is broken.

Warnings: Do not take this product if you have asthma, glaucoma, or difficulty in urination due to enlargement of the prostate gland, except under the advice and supervision of a physician. Do not drive or operate heavy machinery. May cause drowsiness. Avoid alcoholic beverages while taking this product. May cause excitability, especially in children. Keep this and all drugs out of the reach of children. In case of accidental overdose, seek professional assistance or contact a poison control center immediately. As with any drug, if you are pregnant or nursing a baby, seek the advice of a health professional before using this product.

Formula:
Active Ingredient: Each capsule contains Chlorpheniramine Maleate, 12 mg. Inactive Ingredients (listed for individuals with specific allergies): Benzyl Alcohol, Cetylpyridinium Chloride, D&C Red 27, Red 30, Red 33, Ethylcellulose, FD&C Green 3, Red 40, Yellow 6, Gelatin, Hydrogenated Castor Oil, Silicon Dioxide, Sodium Lauryl Sulfate, Starch, Sucrose, and trace amounts of other inactive ingredients.
Store at controlled room temperature (59°–86°F.).

How Supplied: Maximum Strength 12 mg. Timed-Release capsules in packages of 12, 24 and 48 capsules.
Shown in Product Identification Section, page 428

TUMS® Antacid Tablets
TUMS E–X® Antacid Tablets

Description: Tums: Active Ingredient: Calcium Carbonate, precipitated U.S.P. 500 mg.
Tums Original Flavor: Inactive Ingredients: Flavor, mineral oil, sodium polyphosphate, starch, sucrose, talc.
Tums Assorted Flavors: Inactive Ingredients: Adipic acid, colors (contains FD&C Yellow No. 6), flavors, mineral oil, sodium polyphosphate, starch, sucrose, talc.
An antacid composition providing liquid effectiveness in a low-cost, pleasant-tasting tablet. Tums tablets are free of the chalky aftertaste usually associated with calcium carbonate therapy and remain pleasant tasting even during long-term therapy. Each TUMS tablet contains not more than 2 mg of sodium and is considered to be dietetically sodium free. Non-laxative/non-constipating.
Tums E-X: Active Ingredient: Calcium Carbonate, 750 mg.
Tums E-X Wintergreen Flavor Inactive Ingredients: Colors (contains FD&C Yellow No. 6), flavor, mineral oil, sodium polyphosphate, starch, sucrose, talc.
Tums E-X Cherry Flavor Inactive Ingredients: Adipic acid, color, flavor, mineral oil, sodium polyphosphate, starch, sucrose, talc.
Tums E-X Peppermint Flavor Inactive Ingredients: Flavor, mineral oil, sodium polyphosphate, starch, sucrose, talc.
Tums E-X Assorted Flavors Inactive Ingredients: Adipic acid, colors (contains FD&C Yellow No. 6), flavors, mineral oil, sodium polyphosphate, starch, sucrose, talc.
Each tablet contains not more than 2 mg of sodium and is considered to be dietetically sodium free. Non-laxative/non-constipating.

Indications: For fast relief of acid indigestion, heartburn, sour stomach and upset stomach associated with these symptoms.

Actions: Tums lowers the upper limit of the pH range without affecting the innate antacid efficiency of calcium carbonate. One tablet, when tested *in vitro* according to the *Federal Register* procedure (*Fed. Reg.* 39-19862, June 4, 1974), neutralizes 10 mEq of 0.1N HCl. This high neutralization capacity combined with a rapid rate of reaction makes Tums an ideal antacid for management of conditions associated with hyperacidity. It effectively neutralizes free acid yet does not cause systemic alkalosis in the presence of normal renal function. A double-blind placebo-controlled clinical study demonstrated that calcium carbonate taken at a dosage of 16 Tums tablets daily for a two-week period was non-constipating/non-laxative.

Warnings: Tums: Do not take more than 16 tablets in a 24-hour period or use the maximum dosage of this product for more than 2 weeks, except under the advice and supervision of a physician.

Tums E-X: Do not take more than 10 tablets in a 24-hour period or use the maximum dosage of this product for more than two weeks, except under the advice and supervision of a physician. Keep this and all drugs out of the reach of children.

Dosage and Administration: Chew 1 or 2 TUMS tablets as symptoms occur. Repeat hourly if symptoms return, or as directed by a physician. No water is required. Simulated Drip Method: The pleasant-tasting TUMS tablet may be kept between the gum and cheek and allowed to dissolve gradually by continuous sucking to prolong the effective relief time.

Important Dietary Information—As a Source of Extra Calcium—Chew 1 or 2 tablets after meals or as directed by a physician.

Tums Original and Assorted Flavors: The 500 mg of calcium carbonate in each tablet provide 200 mg of elemental calcium which is 20% of the adult U.S. RDA for calcium. Five tablets provide 100% of the daily calcium needs for adults.

Tums E-X: The 750 mg of calcium carbonate in each tablet provide 300 mg of elemental calcium which is 30% of the adult U.S. RDA for calcium. Four tablets provide 120% of the daily calcium needs for adults.

Professional Labeling: Indicated for the symptomatic relief of hyperacidity associated with the diagnosis of peptic ulcer, gastritis, peptic esophagitis, gastric hyperacidity, and hiatal hernia.

How Supplied: Tums: Peppermint and Assorted Flavors of Cherry, Lemon, Orange and Lime are available in 12-tablet rolls, 3-roll wraps, and bottles of 75 and 150 tablets. **Tums E-X Wintergreen, E-X Cherry, E-X Peppermint, and Assorted Flavors of Cherry, Lemon, Lime and Orange:** 8-tablet rolls, 3-roll wraps and bottles of 48 and 96 tablets.
Shown in Product Identification Section, page 428

TUMS PLUS Antacid Anti-gas Tablets

Active Ingredients: 500 mg of calcium carbonate and 20 mg of simethicone per tablet.

Tums Plus Peppermint Flavor Inactive Ingredients: Corn Syrup, FD&C Blue 1, Flavor, Microcrystalline Cellulose, Mineral Oil, Sodium Polyphosphate, Starch, Sucrose, Talc, Triglycerol Monooleate.

Tums Plus Assorted Fruit Flavor Inactive Ingredients: Adipic Acid, Corn Syrup, D&C Red 27, D&C Red 30, D&C Yellow 10, FD&C Blue 1, FD&C Yellow 6, Flavors, Microcrystalline Cellulose, Mineral Oil, Sodium Polyphosphate, Starch, Sucrose, Talc, Triglycerol Monooleate.
Each tablet contains not more than 2 mg of sodium and is considered dietetically sodium free.

The 500 mg of calcium carbonate in each tablet provide 200 mg of elemental calcium.
Non-laxative/non-constipating.

Indications: For fast relief of acid indigestion, heartburn, and sour stomach accompanied by gas and upset stomach associated with these symptoms.

Actions: Calcium carbonate in Tums Plus lowers the upper limit of the pH range without affecting the innate antacid efficiency of calcium carbonate. Calcium carbonate, when tested in vitro according to the Federal Register procedure (Fed. Reg. 39-19862, June 4, 1974), neutralizes 10 mEq of 0.1N HCl. This high neutralization capacity combined with a rapid rate of reaction makes calcium carbonate an ideal antacid for management of conditions associated with hyperacidity. It effectively neutralizes free acid yet does not cause systemic alkalosis in the presence of normal renal function.

Warnings: Do not take more than 16 tablets in a 24-hour period or use the maximum dosage of this product for more than two weeks, except under the advice and supervision of a physician. Keep this and all drugs out of the reach of children.

Dosage and Administration: Chew 1 or 2 tablets as symptoms occur. Repeat hourly if symptoms return, or as directed by a physician. No water is required. Simulated Drip Method: The pleasant-tasting Tums Plus tablet may be kept between the gum and cheek and allowed to dissolve gradually by continually sucking to prolong the effective relief time.

Professional Labeling: Indicated for the symptomatic relief of hyperacidity associated with the diagnosis of peptic ulcer, gastritis, peptic esophagitis, gastric hyperacidity, and hiatal hernia.

How Supplied: 48 tablet bottles 4770D
Shown in Product Identification Section, page 428

VIVARIN® Stimulant Tablets and Caplets
[*vi 'va-rin*]

Active Ingredient: Each tablet/caplet contains 200 mg. Caffeine Alkaloid.

Inactive Ingredients Tablets: Dextrose, Magnesium Stearate, Microcrystalline Cellulose, Powdered Cellulose, Silicon Dioxide, Starch, FD&C Yellow #6, D&C Yellow #10.

Inactive Ingredients Caplets: Carnauba Wax, Dextrose, Hydroxypropyl Methylcellulose, Magnesium Stearate, Microcrystalline Cellulose, Polyethylene Glycol, Polysorbate 80, Powdered Cellulose, Silicon Dioxide, Starch, Titanium Dioxide, White Wax, FD&C Yellow #6, D&C Yellow #10.

Indications: Helps restore mental alertness or wakefulness when experiencing fatigue or drowsiness.

Actions: Stimulates cerebrocortical areas involved with active mental processes.

Directions: Adults and children 12 years of age and over: Oral dosage is 1 tablet or caplet (200 mg) not more often than every 3 to 4 hours.

Warnings: The recommended dose of this product contains about as much caffeine as two cups of coffee. Limit the use of caffeine containing medications, foods, or beverages while taking this product because too much caffeine may cause nervousness, irritability, sleeplessness, and, occasionally, rapid heart beat. For occasional use only. Not intended for use as a substitute for sleep. If fatigue or drowsiness persists or continues to recur, consult a doctor. Do not give to children under 12 years of age. As with any drug, if you are pregnant or nursing a baby, seek the advice of a health professional before using this product. In case of accidental overdose, seek professional assistance or contact a poison control center immediately. Keep this and all drugs out of the reach of children.

Drug Interaction: Use of caffeine should be lowered or avoided if drugs are being used to treat cardiovascular ailments, psychological problems, or kidney trouble.

Precaution: Higher blood glucose levels may result from caffeine use.

Symptoms and Treatment of Oral Overdosage: Convulsions may occur if caffeine is consumed in doses larger than 10 g. Emesis should be induced to empty the stomach. In case of accidental overdose, seek professional assistance by contacting your physician, the local poison control center, or the Rocky Mt. Poison Control Center at 303-592-1710 (Collect), 24 hours a day.

How Supplied Tablets: Available in packages of 16, 40 and 80 tablets.

How Supplied Caplets: Available in packages of 24 and 48.

Booklets:
"A Personal Guide to Feminine Freshness"
A 16 page illustrated booklet on vaginal infections, feminine hygiene and douching. Free to physicians, pharmacists and patients in limited quantities by writing SmithKline Beecham Consumer Brands or calling 800-233-2426.
"Myths and Truths About STDS: An Easy Guide For Women"
A 16 page booklet on the common types of STDs and prevention. Free to physicians, pharmacists and patients in lim-

Continued on next page

SmithKline Beecham—Cont.

ited quantities by sending a SASE to: SmithKline Beecham Consumer Brands or calling 800-233-2426.

Film, Video:

"Feminine Hygiene and You"

This 14 minute color film begins with a simple explanation of how a woman's body works (reproductive system, menstrual cycle, and vaginal secretions) then explains douching. Free loan to physicians, pharmacists and clinics. Available in 16mm, and VHS by writing Smith-Kline Beecham Consumer Brands or calling 800-233-2426.

E.R. Squibb & Sons, Inc.
Apothecon
A Bristol-Myers Squibb Company
P.O. BOX 4000
PRINCETON, NJ 08540

Theragran Liquid, Theragran Stress Formula, Theragran Tablets and Theragran-M Tablets are distributed by Apothecon. For the Theragran listing, please see Apothecon.

Standard Homeopathic Company
210 WEST 131st STREET
BOX 61067
LOS ANGELES, CA 90061

HYLAND'S BED WETTING TABLETS

Active Ingredients: *Equisetum hyemale* (Scouring Rush) 2X HPUS, *Rhus aromatica* (Fragrant Sumac) 3X HPUS, *Belladonna* 3X HPUS (0.0003% Alkaloids).

Inactive Ingredients: Lactose USP.

Indications: A homeopathic combination for the temporary relief of involuntary urination (common bed wetting) in children.

Directions: Children 3 to 12 years: 2 to 3 tablets before meals and at bedtime, or as directed by a licensed health care practitioner. Children over 12 years: double the above recommended dose.

Warnings: If symptoms persist for more than seven days or worsen, consult a Health Care Professional. As with any drug, if you are pregnant or nursing a baby, seek the advice of a health professional before using this product. Keep this and all medication out of the reach of children.

How Supplied: Bottles of 125—one grain sublingual tablets (NDC 54973-7501-01). Store at room temperature.

HYLAND'S CALMS FORTÉ TABLETS

Active Ingredients: *Passiflora* (Passion Flower) 1X triple strength HPUS, *Avena sativa* (Oat) 1X triple strength HPUS, *Humulus lupulus* (Hops) 1X double strength HPUS, *Chamomilla* (Chamomile) 2X HPUS, *Calcarea Phosphorica* (Calcium Phosphate) 3X HPUS, *Ferrum Phosphorica* (Iron Phosphate) 3X HPUS, *Kali Phosphoricum* (Potassium Phosphate) 3X HPUS, *Natrum Phosphoricum* (Sodium Phosphate) 3X HPUS, *Magnesia Phosphoricum* (Magnesium Phosphate) 3X HPUS.

Inactive Ingredients: Lactose USP.

Indications: Temporary symptomatic relief of simple nervous tension and insomnia.

Directions: Adults, As a relaxant: 1 to 2 tablets as needed or 3 times daily between meals. In insomnia: 1 to 3 tablets ½ to 1 hour before retiring. Repeat as needed without danger of side effects. Children, As a relaxant: 1 tablet as needed or 3 times daily before meals. In insomnia: 1 to 2 tablets 1 hour before retiring. Non-habit-forming.

Warnings: If symptoms persist for more than seven days or worsen, consult a Health Care Professional. As with any drug, if you are pregnant or nursing a baby, seek the advice of a health professional before using this product. Keep this and all medication out of the reach of children.

How Supplied: Bottles of 100 four grain tablets (NDC 54973-1121-02). Store at room temperature. Bottles of 50 four grain tablets (NDC 54973-1121-01). Store at room temperature.

HYLAND'S COLIC TABLETS

Active Ingredients: *Disocorea* (Wild Yam) 2X HPUS, *Chamomilla* (Chamomile) 3X HPUS, *Colocynth* (Bitter Apple) 3X HPUS.

Inactive Ingredients: Lactose USP.

Indications: A homeopathic combination for the temporary relief of colic and gas pains caused by irritating food, feeding too quickly, swallowing air and similar conditions during teething, colds and other minor upset periods in children.

Directions: For children to 2 years of age: administer 2 tablets dissolved in a teaspoon of water or on the tongue every 15 minutes until relieved; then every 2 hours as required. Children over 2 years: 3 tablets dissolved on the tongue as above; or as recommended by a licensed health care practitioner.

Warnings: If symptoms persist for more than seven days or worsen, consult a Health Care Professional. Keep this and all medication out of the reach of children.

How Supplied: Bottles of 125—one grain sublingual tablets (NDC 54973-7502-01). Store at room temperature.

HYLAND'S COUGH SYRUP WITH HONEY™

Active Ingredients: Each fluid ounce contains: *Ipecacuanha* (Ipecac) 3X HPUS, *Aconitum napellus* (Aconite) 3X HPUS, *Spongia Tosta* (Sponge) 3X HPUS, *Antimonium Tartaricum* (Potassium Antimony Tartrate) 6X HPUS.

Inactive Ingredients: Simple syrup and honey.

Indications: A homeopathic combination for the temporary relief of symptoms of simple, dry, tight or tickling coughs due to colds in children.

Directions: Children 1 to 12 years: 1 to 3 teaspoonfuls as required. Children over 12 years and adults: 3 to 4 teaspoonfuls as required. May be taken with or without water. Repeat as often as necessary to relieve symptoms. For children under 1 year of age, consult a licensed health care practitioner.

Warnings: Do not use this product for persistent or chronic cough such as occurs with asthma, smoking or emphysema; or if cough is accompanied with excessive mucus, unless directed by a licensed health care practitioner. If symptoms persist for more than seven days, tend to recur, or are accompanied by a high fever, rash, or persistent headache, consult a Health Care Professional. As with any drug, if you are pregnant or nursing a baby, seek the advice of a health professional before using this product. Keep this and all medication out of the reach of children.

How Supplied: Bottles of 4 fluid ounces (120 ml) (NDC 54973-7503-02). Store at room temperature.

HYLAND'S C–PLUS™ COLD TABLETS

Active Ingredients: *Eupatorium perfoliatum* (Boneset) 2X HPUS, *Euphrasia officinalis* (Eyebright) 2X HPUS, *Gelsemium sempervirens* (Yellow Jasmine) 3X HPUS, *Kali Iodatum* (Potassium Iodide) 3X HPUS.

Inactive Ingredients: Lactose USP, Natural Raspberry Flavor.

Indications: A homeopathic combination for the temporary relief of symptoms of runny nose and sneezing due to common head colds in children.

Directions: Children 1 to 3 years: 2 tablets every 15 minutes for 4 doses, then hourly until relieved. For children 3 to 6 years: 3 tablets as above; for children 6 and older: 6 tablets as above or as directed by a licensed health care practitioner.

Warnings: If symptoms persist for more than seven days or worsen, consult a Health Care Professional. As with any drug, if you are pregnant or nursing a baby, seek the advice of a health professional before using this product. Keep this and all medication out of the reach of children.

How Supplied: Bottles of 125—one grain sublingual tablets (NDC 54973-7505-01). Store at room temperature.

HYLAND'S TEETHING TABLETS

Active Ingredients: *Calcarea Phosphorica* (Calcium Phosphate) 3X HPUS, *Chamomilla* (Chamomile) 3X HPUS, *Coffea Cruda* (Coffee) 3X HPUS, *Belladonna* 3X HPUS (Alkaloids 0.0003%).

Inactive Ingredients: Lactose USP.

Indications: A homeopathic combination for the temporary relief of symptoms of simple restlessness and wakeful irritability due to cutting of teeth.

Directions: 2 to 3 tablets in a teaspoon of water or on the tongue, 4 times per day. If the child is restless or wakeful, 2 tablets every hour for 6 doses or as directed by a licensed health care practitioner.

Warnings: If symptoms persist for more than seven days or worsen, consult a Health Care Professional. As with any drug, if you are pregnant or nursing a baby, seek the advice of a health professional before using this product. Keep this and all medication out of the reach of children.

How Supplied: Bottles of 125—one grain sublingual tablets (NDC 54973-7504-01). Store at room temperature.

HYLAND'S VITAMIN C FOR CHILDREN™

Active Ingredients: 25 mg Vitamin C as Sodium Ascorbate (30 mg).

Inactive Ingredients: Lactose USP, Natural Lemon Flavor.

Indications: Each tablet provides children with 55% of the daily recommended requirement of Vitamin C. Sodium Ascorbate is preferred to Ascorbic Acid when gastric irritation may result from free acid.

Directions: Children 2 years and older: 1 to 2 tablets on the tongue or as directed by a licensed health care practitioner.

Warning: Keep this and all medication out of the reach of children.

How Supplied: Bottles of 125—one grain sublingual tablets (NDC 54973-7506-01). Store at room temperature. Tablets may turn brown in color with exposure to light. Color change does not affect potency.

> ### EDUCATIONAL MATERIAL

Booklets—Brochures
"Homeopathy—What it is, How it Works," A Consumer's Guide to Homeopathic Medicine, Free

"Homeopathy—A Guide for Pharmacists," An ACPE (0.2 CEU) program on the basic principles of homeopathy.

Stellar Pharmacal Corp.
Div./Star Pharmaceuticals, Inc.
1990 N.W. 44TH STREET
POMPANO BEACH, FL
33064-8712

STAR–OPTIC™ EYE WASH
[*star op'tik*]
STERILE, ISOTONIC, BUFFERED SOLUTION

Description: STAR-OPTIC Eye Wash is specially formulated to soothe irritating 'Swimmers Eye'™ by bathing (washing) the eye providing cooling, refreshing relief. STAR-OPTIC Eye Wash is a sterile, isotonic buffered solution containing sodium chloride, sodium phosphate monobasic and sodium phosphate dibasic, preserved with edetate disodium and benzalkonium chloride in purified water, USP. CONTAINS NO BORIC ACID or THIMEROSAL (MERCURY).

Indications: For irrigating the eye to help relieve irritation, discomfort, burning, stinging or itching by removing loose foreign material, air pollutants (smog or pollen) or CHLORINATED WATER.

Directions: If eye cup is used, rinse cup with STAR-OPTIC Eye Wash or clean water immediately before and after each use. Avoid contamination of rim and inside surfaces of cup. Fill cup one-half full with STAR-OPTIC Eye Wash. Apply cup tightly to the affected eye to prevent leakage and tilt head backward. Open eyelids wide and rotate eyeball to ensure thorough bathing with the wash.
Note: Enclosed eye cup is sterile if package is intact. If cup is not used, flush affected eye by controlling the rate of flow of solution by pressure on the bottle.

Warnings: To avoid contamination, do not touch tip of container to any surface. Replace cap after using. If you experience eye pain, changes in vision, continued redness or irritation of the eye or if the condition worsens or persists, consult a physician. Obtain immediate medical treatment for all open wounds in or near the eyes. If solution changes color or becomes cloudy, do not use.
Keep out of the reach of children. Not for use with contact lenses. DO NOT USE IF IMPRINTED SAFETY SEAL ON CAP IS BROKEN OR MISSING AT TIME OF PURCHASE.
Store at room temperature. Use before expiration date marked on bottle and carton.

How Supplied: Bottles of 4 fl. oz. (118 ml) with eye cup.
Shown in Product Identification Section, page 428

STAR–OTIC® EAR SOLUTION
Antibacterial, Antifungal, Nonaqueous Ear Solution

Active Ingredients: Acetic acid nonaqueous, Burow's solution, Boric acid, in a propylene glycol vehicle, with an acid pH and a low surface tension.

Indications: For the prevention of otitis externa, commonly called "Swimmer's Ear".

Actions: Star-Otic Ear Solution is antibacterial, antifungal, hydrophilic, has an acid pH and a low surface tension. Acetic acid and boric acid inhibit the rapid multiplication of microorganisms and help maintain the lining mantle of the ear canal in its normal acid state. Burow's solution (aluminum acetate) is a mild astringent. Propylene glycol reduces moisture in the ear canal.

Warning: Do not use in ear if tympanic membrane (ear drum) is perforated or punctured.

Symptoms and Treatment of Overdosage: Discontinue use if undue irritation or sensitivity occurs.

Dosage and Administration: Adults and Children: To help restore normal pH to the outer ear canal. In susceptible persons, instill 3–5 drops of Star-Otic Ear Solution in each ear before and after swimming or bathing, or as directed by physician.

Professional Labeling: Same as those outlined under Indications.

How Supplied: Available in ½ oz measured drop, safety tip, plastic bottle.
Shown in Product Identification Section, page 428

> ### EDUCATIONAL MATERIAL

First Aid Prevention of Swimmer's Ear
Public health information on cause and care of preventing swimmer's ear.
Star-Otic Patient Instruction Pads
Instructions for patients on use of Star-Otic antibacterial-antifungal ear solution.

IDENTIFICATION PROBLEM?
Consult the
Product Identification Section
where you'll find
products pictured
in full color.

Sterling Health
DIVISION OF STERLING
WINTHROP INC.
90 PARK AVENUE
NEW YORK, NY 10016

Children's BAYER® Chewable Aspirin
Aspirin (Acetylsalicylic Acid)

Active Ingredients: Children's Bayer Chewable Aspirin—Aspirin 1¼ grains (81 mg) per orange flavored chewable tablet.

Inactive Ingredients: Dextrose excipient, FD&C Yellow No. 6, flavor, saccharin sodium, starch.

Actions and Uses: Analgesic, antipyretic, anti-inflammatory. For effective, gentle relief of painful discomforts, sore throat; fever of colds; headache; teething pain, toothache; and other minor aches and pains.

Warnings: Children and teenagers should not use this medicine for chicken pox or flu symptoms before a doctor is consulted about Reye syndrome, a rare but serious illness reported to be associated with aspirin. Keep this and all drugs out of the reach of children. In case of accidental overdose, seek professional assistance or contact a poison control center immediately. As with any drug, if you are pregnant or nursing a baby, seek the advice of a health professional before using this product. **IT IS ESPECIALLY IMPORTANT NOT TO USE ASPIRIN DURING THE LAST THREE MONTHS OF PREGNANCY UNLESS SPECIFICALLY DIRECTED TO DO SO BY A DOCTOR BECAUSE IT MAY CAUSE PROBLEMS IN THE UNBORN CHILD OR COMPLICATIONS DURING DELIVERY.**
IMPORTANT NOTICE: Do not take this product if you are allergic to aspirin, have asthma, stomach problems that persist or recur, gastric ulcers or bleeding, or if you are taking a prescription drug for arthritis, anticoagulation (thinning of the blood), diabetes, or gout unless directed by a doctor. If ringing in the ears or loss of hearing occurs, consult a doctor before taking any more of this product.

Administration and Dosage: The following dosages are those provided in the packaging, as appropriate for self-medication.
Children's Dose: To be administered only under adult supervision. For children under 3 consult physician.

Age (Years)	Weight (lb)	Dosage
3 up to 4	32 to 35	2 tablets
4 up to 6	36 to 45	3 tablets
6 up to 9	46 to 65	4 tablets
9 up to 11	66 to 76	5 tablets
11 up to 12	77 to 83	6 tablets
12 and over	84 and over	8 tablets

Indicated dosage may be repeated every four hours up to but not more than five times a day. Larger dosage may be prescribed by a physician.

Ways to Administer: CHEW, then follow with a half glass of water, milk or fruit juice.
SWALLOW WHOLE with a half a glass of water, milk or fruit juice.
DISSOLVE ON TONGUE, follow with a half a glass of water, milk or fruit juice.
DISSOLVE TABLET in a little water, milk or fruit juice and drink the solution.
CRUSHED in a teaspoonful of water—followed with part of a glass of water.

How Supplied: Children's Bayer Chewable Aspirin 1¼ grains (81 mg) is supplied in bottles of 36 tablets with child-resistant safety closure.

Shown in Product Identification Section, page 429

Genuine BAYER® Aspirin
Aspirin (Acetylsalicylic Acid)
Tablets and Caplets

Active Ingredients: Each Bayer-Aspirin contains aspirin 5 grains (325 mg) in a thin, inert, hydroxypropyl methylcellulose coating for easier swallowing. This is not an enteric coating and does not alter the onset of action of Genuine Bayer Aspirin.

Inactive Ingredients: Starch and Triacetin.

Actions and Uses: Analgesic, antipyretic, anti-inflammatory. For relief of headache; painful discomfort and fever of colds and flu; sore throats; muscular aches and pains; temporary relief of minor pains of arthritis, rheumatism†, bursitis, lumbago, sciatica; toothache, teething pains, and pain following dental procedures; neuralgia and neuritic pain; functional menstrual pain; minor painful discomfort; painful discomfort and fever accompanying immunizations.

†**Caution:**If pain persists for more than 10 days, or redness is present, or in conditions affecting children under 12 years of age, consult a physician immediately.

Warnings: Children and teenagers should not use this medicine for chicken pox or flu symptoms before a doctor is consulted about Reye syndrome, a rare but serious illness reported to be associated with aspirin. Keep this and all drugs out of the reach of children. In case of accidental overdose, seek professional assistance or contact a poison control center immediately. As with any drug, if you are pregnant or nursing a baby, seek the advice of a health professional before using this product. **IT IS ESPECIALLY IMPORTANT NOT TO USE ASPIRIN DURING THE LAST 3 MONTHS OF PREGNANCY UNLESS SPECIFICALLY DIRECTED TO DO SO BY A DOCTOR BECAUSE IT MAY CAUSE PROBLEMS IN THE UNBORN CHILD OR COMPLICATIONS DURING DELIVERY.**
IMPORTANT NOTICE: Do not take this product if you are allergic to aspirin, have asthma, stomach problems that persist or recur, gastric ulcers or bleeding, or if you are taking a prescription drug for arthritis, anticoagulation (thin-

ning of the blood), diabetes, or gout unless directed by a doctor. If ringing in the ears or loss of hearing occurs, consult a doctor before taking any more of this product.

Administration and Dosage: The following dosages are those provided in the packaging, as appropriate for self-medication. Larger or more frequent dosage may be necessary as appropriate to the condition or needs of the patient.
The hydroxypropyl methylcellulose coating makes Genuine Bayer Aspirin particularly appropriate for those who must take frequent doses of aspirin and for those who have difficulty in swallowing uncoated tablets and caplets.
Usual Adult Dose: One or two tablets/caplets with water. May be repeated every four hours as necessary up to 12 tablets/caplets a day.
FOR ANTIPLATELET USE: RECURRENT TIA
There is evidence that aspirin is safe and effective for reducing the risk of recurrent transient ischemic attacks or stroke in men who have had transient ischemia of the brain due to fibrin platelet emboli. There is no evidence that aspirin is effective in reducing TIAs in women, or that it is of benefit in the treatment of completed strokes in men or women. Patients presenting with signs and symptoms of TIAs should have a complete medical and neurologic evaluation. Consideration should be given to other disorders which resemble TIAs.
It is important to evaluate and treat, if appropriate, other diseases associated with TIAs and stroke, such as hypertension and diabetes.

Dosage: The recommended dosage for this new indication is 1,300 mg/day (650 mg twice a day or 325 mg four times a day).

Precautions: A complete medical and neurologic evaluation should be performed on the male patient with recurrent TIA prior to instituting antiplatelet therapy with aspirin. The differential diagnosis should include consideration of disorders that resemble TIAs. An assessment of the presence and need for treatment of other diseases associated with TIAs or stroke, such as diabetes and hypertension, should be made.
IN MI PROPHYLAXIS
Aspirin is indicated to reduce the risk of death and/or nonfatal myocardial infarction in patients with a previous infarction or unstable angina pectoris.
Clinical Trials: The indication is supported by the results of six, large, randomized multicenter, placebo-controlled studies[1-6] by the word-studies involving 10,816, predominantly male, post-myocardial infarction (MI) patients and one randomized placebo-controlled study[7] by the word study of 1,266 men with unstable angina. Therapy with aspirin was begun at intervals after the onset of acute MI varying from less than 3 days to more than 5 years and continued for periods of from less than 1 year to 4 years. In the unstable angina study, treatment was started within 1 month after the onset of unstable angina and

continued for 12 weeks and complicating conditions, such as congestive heart failure, were not included in the study.

Aspirin therapy in MI patients was associated with about a 20 percent reduction in the risk of subsequent death and/or nonfatal reinfarction, a median absolute decrease of 3 percent from the 12 to 22 percent event rates in the placebo groups. In aspirin-treated unstable angina patients the reduction in risk was about 50 percent, a reduction in event rate of 5 percent from the 10 percent rate in the placebo group over the 12 weeks of the study.

Daily dosage of aspirin in the post–myocardial infarction studies was 300 mg in one study and 900–1500 mg in five studies. A dose of 325 mg was used in the study of unstable angina.

Adverse Reactions: Gastrointestinal Reactions: Doses of 1000 mg per day of aspirin caused gastrointestinal symptoms and bleeding that in some cases were clinically significant. In the largest post-infarction study (the Aspirin Myocardial Infarction Study [AMIS] trial with 4,500 people), the percentage incidences of gastrointestinal symptoms for the aspirin (1000 mg of a standard, solid-tablet formulation) and placebo-treated subjects, respectively, were: stomach pain (14.5%; 4.4%); heartburn (11.9%; 4.8%); nausea and/or vomiting (7.6%; 2.1%) hospitalization for GI disorder (4.9%; 3.5%). In the AMIS and other trials, aspirin-treated patients had increased rates of gross gastrointestinal bleeding. Symptoms and signs of gastrointestinal irritation were not significantly increased in subjects treated for unstable angina with buffered aspirin in solution.

Cardiovascular and Biochemical: In the AMIS trial, the dosage of 1000 mg per day of aspirin was associated with small increases in systolic blood pressure (BP) (average 1.5 to 2.1 mm) and diastolic BP (0.5 to 0.6 mm), depending upon whether maximal or last available readings were used. Blood urea nitrogen and uric acid levels were also increased, but by less than 1.0 mg%. Subjects with marked hypertension or renal insufficiency had been excluded from the trial so that the clinical importance of these observations for such subjects or for any subjects treated over more prolonged periods is not known. It is recommended that patients placed on long-term aspirin treatment, even at doses of 300 mg per day, be seen at regular intervals to assess changes in these measurements.

Sodium in Buffered Aspirin for Solution Formulations: One tablet daily of buffered aspirin in solution adds 553 mg of sodium to that in the diet and may not be tolerated by patients with active sodium-retaining states such as congestive heart or renal failure. This amount of sodium adds about 30 percent to the 70 to 90 meq intake suggested as appropriate for dietary treatment of essential hypertension in the 1984 Report of the Joint National Committee on Detection, Eval-

uation, and Treatment of High Blood Pressure.[8]

Dosage and Administration: Although most of the studies used dosages exceeding 300 mg, two trials used only 300 mg, daily, and pharmacologic data indicate that this dose inhibits platelet function fully. Therefore, 300 mg or a conventional 325 mg aspirin dose daily, is a reasonable routine dose that would minimize gastrointestinal adverse reactions. This use of aspirin applies to both solid, oral dosage forms (buffered and plain aspirin) and buffered aspirin in solution.

REFERENCES

(1) Elwood, P.C., et al., A Randomized Controlled Trial of Acetylsalicylic Acid in the Secondary Prevention of Mortality from Myocardial Infarction, *British Medical Journal*, 1:436–440, 1974.
(2) The Coronary Drug Project Research Group, "Aspirin in Coronary Heart Disease," *Journal of Chronic Disease*, 29:625–642, 1976.
(3) Breddin, K., et al., "Secondary Prevention of Myocardial Infarction: A Comparison of Acetylsalicylic Acid, Phenprocoumon or Placebo," *Homeostasis*, 470:263–268, 1979.
(4) Aspirin Myocardial Infarction Study Research Group, "A Randomized, Controlled Trial of Aspirin in Persons Recovered from Myocardial Infarction," *Journal American Medical Association* 245:661–669, 1980.
(5) Elwood, P.C., and Sweetnam P.M., "Aspirin and Secondary Mortality after Myocardial Infarction," *Lancet,* pp. 1313–1315, December 22–29, 1979.
(6) The Persantine-Aspirin Reinfarction Study Research Group, "Persantine and Aspirin in Coronary Heart Disease," *Circulation,* 62: 449–460, 1980.
(7) Lewis, H.D., et al., "Protective Effects of Aspirin Against Acute Myocardial Infarction and Death in Men with Unstable Angina. Results of a Veterans Administration Cooperative Study," *New England Journal of Medicine* 309:396–403, 1983.
(8) "1984 Report of the Joint National Committee on Detection, Evaluation and Treatment of High Blood Pressure," U.S. Department of Health and Human Services and United States Public Health Service, National Institutes of Health.

How Supplied:
Genuine Bayer Aspirin 5 grains (325 mg) is supplied in packs of 12 tablets, bottles of 24, 50, 100, 200 and 300 tablets, and bottles of 50, 100 and 200 caplets.
Child-resistant safety closures on 12's, 24's, 50's, 200's, 300's tablets and 50's and 200's caplets. Bottles of 100's tablets and caplets available without safety closure for households without small children.
Shown in Product Identification Section, page 428

Maximum BAYER® Aspirin
Aspirin (Acetylsalicylic Acid)
Tablets and Caplets

Active Ingredients: Maximum Bayer Aspirin—Aspirin 500 mg (7.7 grains) contains a thin, inert, hydroxypropyl methylcellulose coating for easier swallowing. This is not an enteric coating and does not alter the onset of action of Bayer Aspirin.

Inactive Ingredients: Starch and triacetin.

Actions and Uses: Analgesic, antipyretic, anti-inflammatory. For relief of headache; painful discomfort and fever of colds and flu; sore throats; muscular aches and pains; temporary relief of minor pains of arthritis, rheumatism†, bursitis, lumbago, sciatica; toothache, teething pains, and pain following dental procedures; neuralgia and neuritic pain; functional menstrual pain; minor painful discomforts; painful discomfort and fever accompanying immunizations.

†Caution: If pain persists for more than 10 days or redness is present, or in conditions affecting children under 12 years of age, consult a physician immediately.

Warnings: Children and teenagers should not use this medicine for chicken pox or flu symptoms before a doctor is consulted about Reye syndrome, a rare but serious illness reported to be associated with aspirin. Keep this and all drugs out of the reach of children. In case of accidental overdose, seek professional assistance or contact a poison control center immediately. As with any drug, if you are pregnant or nursing a baby, seek the advice of a health professional before using this product. IT IS ESPECIALLY IMPORTANT NOT TO USE ASPIRIN DURING THE LAST 3 MONTHS OF PREGNANCY UNLESS SPECIFICALLY DIRECTED TO DO SO BY A DOCTOR BECAUSE IT MAY CAUSE PROBLEMS IN THE UNBORN CHILD OR COMPLICATIONS DURING DELIVERY.
IMPORTANT NOTICE: Do not take this product if you are allergic to aspirin, have asthma, stomach problems that persist or recur, gastric ulcers or bleeding, or if you are taking a prescription drug for arthritis, anticoagulation (thinning of the blood), diabetes, or gout unless directed by a doctor. If ringing in the ears or loss of hearing occurs, consult a doctor before taking any more of this product.

Administration and Dosage: The following dosages are those provided on the packaging, as appropriate for self-

Continued on next page

This product information was effective as of November 1, 1991. Current information may be obtained directly from Sterling Health, by writing to 90 Park Avenue, New York, NY 10016.

Sterling Health—Cont.

medication. Larger or more frequent dosage may be necessary as appropriate for the condition or needs of the patient. The hydroxypropyl methylcellulose coating makes Maximum Bayer Aspirin particularly appropriate for those who must take frequent doses of aspirin and for those who have difficulty in swallowing uncoated tablets/caplets.

Maximum Bayer Aspirin—500 mg (7.7 grains) tablets/caplets.

Usual Adult Dose: One or two tablets/caplets with water. May be repeated every four hours as necessary up to 8 tablets/caplets a day.

How Supplied:

Maximum Bayer Aspirin 500 mg (7.7 grains) is available in bottles of 30, 60 and 100 tablets, and bottles of 30 and 60 caplets.

Child-resistant safety closures on 30's bottles of tablets and caplets, 60's, bottles of caplets, and 100's bottles of tablets. Bottle of 60's tablets available without safety closure for households without young children.

Shown in Product Identification Section, page 429

8-Hour BAYER®
Timed-Release Aspirin
Aspirin (acetylsalicylic acid)

Active Ingredients: Each oblong white scored caplet contains 10 grains (650 mg) of aspirin in microencapsulated form.

Inactive Ingredients: Guar gum, microcrystalline cellulose, starch and other ingredients.

Indications: 8-Hour Bayer Timed-Release Aspirin is indicated for the temporary relief of low-grade pain amenable to relief with salicylates, such as in rheumatoid arthritis, osteoarthritis, spondylitis, bursitis and other forms of rheumatism, as well as in many common musculoskeletal disorders. It possesses the same advantages for other types of prolonged aches and pains, such as minor injuries, dental pain and dysmenorrhea. Its long-lasting effectiveness should also make it valuable as an analgesic in simple headache, colds, grippe, flu and other similar conditions in which aspirin is indicated for symptomatic relief, either by itself or as an adjunct to specific therapy.

Caution: If pain persists for more than 10 days, or redness is present, or in conditions affecting children under 12 years, consult a physician immediately.

Warnings: Children and teenagers should not use this medicine for chicken pox or flu symptoms before a doctor is consulted about Reye syndrome, a rare but serious illness reported to be associated with aspirin. Keep this and all drugs out of the reach of children. In case of accidental overdose, seek professional assistance or contact a poison control center immediately. As with any drug, if you are pregnant or nursing a baby, seek the advice of a health professional before using this product. **IT IS ESPECIALLY**

IMPORTANT NOT TO USE ASPIRIN DURING THE LAST 3 MONTHS OF PREGNANCY UNLESS SPECIFICALLY DIRECTED TO DO SO BY A DOCTOR BECAUSE IT MAY CAUSE PROBLEMS IN THE UNBORN CHILD OR COMPLICATIONS DURING DELIVERY.

Administration and Dosage: Two 8-Hour Bayer Timed-Release Aspirin caplets q. 8 h. provide effective long-lasting pain relief. This two-caplet (20 grain or 1300 mg) dose of timed-release aspirin promptly produces salicylate blood levels greater than those achieved by a 10-grain (650 mg) dose of regular aspirin, and in the second 4-hour period produces a salicylate blood level curve which approximates that of two successive 10-grain (650 mg) doses of regular aspirin at 4-hour intervals. The 10-grain (650 mg) scored 8-Hour Bayer Timed-Release Aspirin caplets permit administration of aspirin in multiples of 5 grains (325 mg) allowing individualization of dosage to meet the specific needs of the patient. For the convenience of patients on a regular aspirin dosage schedule, two 10-grain (650 mg) 8-Hour Bayer Timed-Release Aspirin caplets may be administered with water every 8 hours. Whenever necessary, two caplets (20 grains or 1300 mg) should be given before retiring to provide effective analgesic and anti-inflammatory action—for relief of pain throughout the night and lessening of stiffness upon arising. Do not exceed 6 caplets in 24 hours. 8-Hour Bayer Timed-Release Aspirin has been made in a special caplet to permit easy swallowing. However, for patients who do have difficulty, 8-Hour Bayer Timed-Release Aspirin caplets may be gently crumbled in the mouth and swallowed with water without loss of timed-release effect. There is no bitter "aspirin" taste. For children under 12, consult physician.

Side Effects: Side effects encountered with regular aspirin may be encountered with 8-Hour Bayer Timed-Release Aspirin. Tinnitus and dizziness are the ones most frequently encountered.

Contraindications and Precautions: 8-Hour Bayer Timed-Release Aspirin is contraindicated in patients with marked aspirin hypersensitivity, and should be given with extreme caution to any patient with a history of adverse reaction to salicylates. It may cautiously be tried in patients intolerant to aspirin because of gastric irritation, but the usual precautions for any form of aspirin should be observed in patients with gastric ulcers, bleeding tendencies, asthma, or hypoprothrombinemia.

How Supplied: 8-Hour Bayer Aspirin 650 mg (10 grains) is supplied in bottles of 30, 72 and 125 caplets.

All sizes packaged in child-resistant safety closure except 72's, which is a size recommended for households without young children.

Shown in Product Identification Section, page 429

BAYER® PLUS
Buffered Aspirin

Active Ingredients: Each Bayer Plus contains aspirin (325 mg), in a formulation buffered with Calcium Carbonate, Magnesium Carbonate, and Magnesium Oxide.

Inactive Ingredients: Corn Starch, Ethylcellulose, FD&C Blue #2, Hydroxypropyl Methylcellulose, Microcrystalline Cellulose, Pharmaceutical Glaze, Sodium Starch Glycolate, Talc, Zinc Stearate.

Actions and Uses: Analgesic, antipyretic, anti-inflammatory. For relief of headache; painful discomfort and fever of colds and flu; muscular aches and pains; temporary relief of minor pains of arthritis, rheumatism†, bursitis, lumbago, sciatica; toothache, teething pains, and pain following dental procedures; neuralgia and neuritic pain; functional menstrual pain; minor painful discomfort; painful discomfort and fever accompanying immunizations.

†Caution: If pain persists for more than 10 days, or redness is present, or in conditions affecting children under 12 years of age, consult a physician immediately.

Warnings: Children and teenagers should not use this medicine for chicken pox or flu symptoms before a doctor is consulted about Reye syndrome, a rare but serious illness reported to be associated with aspirin. Keep this and all drugs out of the reach of children. In case of accidental overdose, seek professional assistance or contact a poison control center immediately. As with any drug, if you are pregnant or nursing a baby, seek the advice of a health professional before using this product. **IT IS ESPECIALLY IMPORTANT NOT TO USE ASPIRIN DURING THE LAST 3 MONTHS OF PREGNANCY UNLESS SPECIFICALLY DIRECTED TO DO SO BY A DOCTOR BECAUSE IT MAY CAUSE PROBLEMS IN THE UNBORN CHILD OR COMPLICATIONS DURING DELIVERY.**

IMPORTANT NOTICE: Do not take this product if you are allergic to aspirin, have asthma, stomach problems that persist or recur, gastric ulcers or bleeding, or if you are taking a prescription drug for arthritis, anticoagulation (thinning of the blood), diabetes, or gout unless directed by a doctor. If ringing in the ears or loss of hearing occurs, consult a doctor before taking any more of this product.

Administration and Dosage: The following dosages are those provided in the packaging, as appropriate for self-medication. Larger or more frequent dosage may be necessary as appropriate to the condition or needs of the patient. The hydroxypropyl methylcellulose coating makes Bayer® Plus particularly appropriate for those who must take frequent doses of aspirin and for those who have difficulty in swallowing uncoated tablets and caplets.

Usual Adult Dose: One or two tablets with water. May be repeated every four hours as necessary up to 12 tablets a day.

FOR ANTIPLATELET USE: RECURRENT TIA

There is evidence that aspirin is safe and effective for reducing the risk of recurrent transient ischemic attacks or stroke in men who have had transient ischemia of the brain due to fibrin platelet emboli. There is no evidence that aspirin is effective in reducing TIAs in women, or that it is of benefit in the treatment of completed strokes in men or women. Patients presenting with signs and symptoms of TIAs should have a complete medical and neurologic evaluation. Consideration should be given to other disorders which resemble TIAs.

It is important to evaluate and treat, if appropriate, other diseases associated with TIAs and stroke, such as hypertension and diabetes.

Dosage: The recommended dosage for this new indication is 1,300 mg/day (650 mg twice a day or 325 mg four times a day).

Precautions: A complete medical and neurologic evaluation should be performed on the male patient with recurrent TIA prior to instituting antiplatelet therapy with aspirin. The differential diagnosis should include consideration of disorders that resemble TIAs. An assessment of the presence and need for treatment of other diseases associated with TIAs or stroke, such as diabetes and hypertension, should be made.

IN MI PROPHYLAXIS

Aspirin is indicated to reduce the risk of death and/or nonfatal myocardial infarction in patients with a previous infarction or unstable angina pectoris.

Clinical Trials: The indication is supported by the results of six, large, randomized multicenter, placebo-controlled studies[1–6] by the word-studies involving 10,816, predominantly male, post-myocardial infarction (MI) patients and one randomized placebo-controlled study[7] by the word study of 1,266 men with unstable angina. Therapy with aspirin was begun at intervals after the onset of acute MI varying from less than 3 days to more than 5 years and continued for periods of from less than 1 year to 4 years. In the unstable angina study, treatment was started within 1 month after the onset of unstable angina and continued for 12 weeks and complicating conditions, such as congestive heart failure, were not included in the study.

Aspirin therapy in MI patients was associated with about a 20 percent reduction in the risk of subsequent death and/or nonfatal reinfarction, a median absolute decrease of 3 percent from the 12 to 22 percent event rates in the placebo groups. In aspirin-treated unstable angina patients the reduction in risk was about 50 percent, a reduction in event rate of 5 percent from the 10 percent rate in the placebo group over the 12 weeks of the study.

Daily dosage of aspirin in the post–myocardial infarction studies was 300 mg in one study and 900–1500 mg in five studies. A dose of 325 mg was used in the study of unstable angina.

Adverse Reactions: Gastrointestinal Reactions: Doses of 1000 mg per day of aspirin caused gastrointestinal symptoms and bleeding that in some cases were clinically significant. In the largest post-infarction study (the Aspirin Myocardial Infarction Study [AMIS] trial with 4,500 people), the percentage incidences of gastrointestinal symptoms for the aspirin (1000 mg of a standard, solid-tablet formulation) and placebo-treated subjects, respectively, were: stomach pain (14.5%; 4.4%); heartburn (11.9%; 4.8%); nausea and/or vomiting (7.6%; 2.1%) hospitalization for GI disorder (4.9%; 3.5%). In the AMIS and other trials, aspirin-treated patients had increased rates of gross gastrointestinal bleeding. Symptoms and signs of gastrointestinal irritation were not significantly increased in subjects treated for unstable angina with buffered aspirin in solution.

Cardiovascular and Biochemical: In the AMIS trial, the dosage of 1000 mg per day of aspirin was associated with small increases in systolic blood pressure (BP) (average 1.5 to 2.1 mm) and diastolic BP (0.5 to 0.6 mm), depending upon whether maximal or last available readings were used. Blood urea nitrogen and uric acid levels were also increased, but by less than 1.0 mg%. Subjects with marked hypertension or renal insufficiency had been excluded from the trial so that the clinical importance of these observations for such subjects or for any subjects treated over more prolonged periods is not known. It is recommended that patients placed on long-term aspirin treatment, even at doses of 300 mg per day, be seen at regular intervals to assess changes in these measurements.

Sodium in Buffered Aspirin for Solution Formulations: One tablet daily of buffered aspirin in solution adds 553 mg of sodium to that in the diet and may not be tolerated by patients with active sodium-retaining states such as congestive heart or renal failure. This amount of sodium adds about 30 percent to the 70 to 90 meq intake suggested as appropriate for dietary treatment of essential hypertension in the 1984 Report of the Joint National Committee on Detection, Evaluation, and Treatment of High Blood Pressure.[8]

Dosage and Administration: Although most of the studies used dosages exceeding 300 mg, two trials used only 300 mg, daily, and pharmacologic data indicate that this dose inhibits platelet function fully. Therefore, 300 mg or a conventional 325 mg aspirin dose daily, is a reasonable routine dose that would minimize gastrointestinal adverse reactions. This use of aspirin applies to both solid, oral dosage forms (buffered and plain aspirin) and buffered aspirin in solution.

REFERENCES

(1) Elwood, P.C., et al., A Randomized Controlled Trial of Acetylsalicylic Acid in the Secondary Prevention of Mortality from Myocardial Infarction, *British Medical Journal*, 1:436–440, 1974.

(2) The Coronary Drug Project Research Group, "Aspirin in Coronary Heart Disease," *Journal of Chronic Disease*, 29:625–642, 1976.

(3) Breddin, K., et al., "Secondary Prevention of Myocardial Infarction: A Comparison of Acetylsalicylic Acid, Phenprocoumon or Placebo," *Homeostasis*, 470:263–268, 1979.

(4) Aspirin Myocardial Infarction Study Research Group, "A Randomized, Controlled Trial of Aspirin in Persons Recovered from Myocardial Infarction," *Journal American Medical Association* 245:661–669, 1980.

(5) Elwood, P.C., and Sweetnam P.M., "Aspirin and Secondary Mortality after Myocardial Infarction," *Lancet*, pp. 1313–1315, December 22–29, 1979.

(6) The Persantine-Aspirin Reinfarction Study Research Group, "Persantine and Aspirin in Coronary Heart Disease," *Circulation*, 62: 449–460, 1980.

(7) Lewis, H.D., et al., "Protective Effects of Aspirin Against Acute Myocardial Infarction and Death in Men with Unstable Angina. Results of a Veterans Administration Cooperative Study," *New England Journal of Medicine* 309:396–403, 1983.

(8) "1984 Report of the Joint National Committee on Detection, Evaluation and Treatment of High Blood Pressure," U.S. Department of Health and Human Services and United States Public Health Service, National Institutes of Health.

How Supplied: Bayer® Plus Aspirin (325 mg) is available in bottles of 8, 24, 50, and 100 tablets.

Child resistant closures on 8's, 24's and 50's tablets. Bottles of 100's tablets available without safety closure for households without young children.

Shown in Product Identification Section, page 429

Extra Strength BAYER® PLUS
Aspirin plus Stomach Guard™
Buffered Aspirin

Active Ingredients: Each Extra Strength Bayer Plus contains aspirin (500 mg), in a formulation buffered with Calcium Carbonate, Magnesium Carbonate, and Magnesium Oxide.

Inactive Ingredients: Corn Starch, FD&C Blue #2, Hydroxypropyl Methylcellulose, Methylparaben, Microcrystalline Cellulose, Propylene Glycol, Propylparaben, Sodium Starch Glycolate, Zinc Stearate.

Continued on next page

This product information was effective as of November 1, 1991. Current information may be obtained directly from Sterling Health, by writing to 90 Park Avenue, New York, NY 10016.

Sterling Health—Cont.

Actions and Uses: Analgesic, antipyretic, anti-inflammatory. For relief of headache; painful discomfort and fever of colds and flu; muscular aches and pains; temporary relief of minor pains of arthritis, rheumatism†, bursitis, lumbago, sciatica; toothache, teething pains, and pain following dental procedures; neuralgia and neuritic pain; functional menstrual pain; minor painful discomfort; painful discomfort and fever accompanying immunizations.

†Caution: If pain persists for more than 10 days, or redness is present, or in conditions affecting children under 12 years of age, consult a physician immediately.

Warnings: Children and teenagers should not use this medicine for chicken pox or flu symptoms before a doctor is consulted about Reye's Syndrome, a rare but serious illness reported to be associated with aspirin. Keep this and all drugs out of the reach of children. In case of accidental overdose, seek professional assistance or contact a poison control center immediately. As with any drug, if you are pregnant or nursing a baby, seek the advice of a health professional before using this product. **IT IS ESPECIALLY IMPORTANT NOT TO USE ASPIRIN DURING THE LAST 3 MONTHS OF PREGNANCY UNLESS SPECIFICALLY DIRECTED TO DO SO BY A DOCTOR BECAUSE IT MAY CAUSE PROBLEMS IN THE UNBORN CHILD OR COMPLICATIONS DURING DELIVERY.**
IMPORTANT NOTICE: Do not take this product if you are allergic to aspirin, have asthma, stomach problems that persist or recur, gastric ulcers or bleeding, or if you are taking a prescription drug for arthritis, anticoagulation (thinning of the blood), diabetes, or gout unless directed by a doctor. If ringing in the ears or loss of hearing occurs, consult a doctor before taking any more of this product.

Administration and Dosage: The following dosages are those provided in the packaging, as appropriate for self-medication. Larger or more frequent dosage may be necessary as appropriate to the condition or needs of the patient. The hydroxypropyl methylcellulose coating makes Extra Strength Bayer® Plus particularly appropriate for those who must take frequent doses of aspirin and for those who have difficulty in swallowing uncoated tablets and caplets.
Usual Adult Dose: One or two caplets with water. May be repeated every four hours as necessary up to 8 caplets a day.

How Supplied: Extra Strength Bayer® Plus Aspirin (500 mg) is available in bottles of 30 and 60 caplets. Child resistant closure on 30's caplets. Bottles of 60's caplets available without safety closure for households without young children.

Shown in Product Identification Section, page 429

Therapy BAYER® ENTERIC Aspirin
Delayed-Release Enteric Aspirin (Acetylsalicylic Acid) Caplets
Antiarthritic, Antiplatelet

Composition: Therapy BAYER is 325 mg enteric-coated aspirin available in caplet form. The enteric coating prevents disintegration in the stomach and promotes dissolution in the duodenum, where there is a more neutral-to-alkaline environment. This action aids in protecting the stomach against injuries that may occur as a result of ingesting non-enteric-coated aspirin (see **Safety**).

Inactive Ingredients: D&C Yellow No. 10, FD&C Yellow No. 6, hydroxypropyl methylcellulose, methacrylic acid, copolymer, starch, titanium dioxide, triacetin, polysorbate 80, and sodium lauryl sulfate.

Indications: Therapy BAYER ENTERIC is an anti-inflammatory, analgesic, and antiplatelet agent indicated for the relief of painful discomfort and muscular aches and pains associated with conditions requiring long-term aspirin therapy, e.g., arthritis or rheumatism and for situations where compliance with aspirin is hindered by the gastrointestinal side effects of non-enteric-coated or buffered aspirin.

Dosage: For analgesic or anti-inflammatory indications, the OTC maximum dosage for aspirin is 4,000 mg per day in divided doses, i.e., two 325 mg caplets every 4 hours or three 325 mg caplets every six hours. For antiplatelet effect dosage, see the **Antiplatelet Effect** section.

Caution: If pain persists for more than 10 days or redness is present, or in conditions affecting children under 12 years of age, consult a physician immediately.

Consumer Warning: Children and teenagers should not use this medicine for chicken pox or flu symptoms before a doctor is consulted about Reye syndrome, a rare but serious illness reported to be associated with aspirin. Keep this and all drugs out of the reach of children. In case of accidental overdose, seek professional assistance or contact a poison control center immediately. As with any drug, if you are pregnant or nursing a baby, seek the advice of a health professional before using this product. **IT IS ESPECIALLY IMPORTANT NOT TO USE ASPIRIN DURING THE LAST 3 MONTHS OF PREGNANCY UNLESS SPECIFICALLY DIRECTED TO DO SO BY A DOCTOR BECAUSE IT MAY CAUSE PROBLEMS IN THE UNBORN CHILD OR COMPLICATIONS DURING DELIVERY.**

IMPORTANT NOTICE: Do not take this product if you are allergic to aspirin, have asthma, stomach problems that persist or recur, gastric ulcers or bleeding, or if you are taking a prescription drug for arthritis, anticoagulation (thin-

ning of the blood), diabetes, or gout unless directed by a doctor. If ringing in the ears or loss of hearing occurs, consult a doctor before taking any more of this product.

Professional Warning: Occasional reports have documented individuals with impaired gastric emptying in whom there may be retention of one or more enteric-coated aspirin caplets over time. This phenomenon may occur as a result of outlet obstruction from ulcer disease alone or combined with hypotonic gastric peristalsis. Because of the integrity of the enteric coating in an acidic environment, these caplets may accumulate and form a bezoar in the stomach. Individuals with this condition may present with complaints of early satiety or of vague upper abdominal distress. Diagnosis may be made by endoscopy or by abdominal films, which show opacities suggestive of a mass of small caplets.[1] Management may vary according to the condition of the patient. Options include gastrotomy and alternating slightly basic and neutral lavage.[2] While there have been no clinical reports, it has been suggested that such individuals may also be treated with parenteral cimetidine (to reduce acid secretion) and then given sips of slightly basic liquids to effect gradual dissolution of the enteric coating. Progress may be followed with plasma salicylate levels or via recognition of tinnitus by the patient.
It should be kept in mind that individuals with a history of partial or complete gastrectomy may produce reduced amounts of acid and therefore have less acidic gastric pH. Under these circumstances, the benefits offered by the acid-resistant enteric coating may not exist.

Safety: The safety of enteric-coated aspirin has been demonstrated in a number of endoscopic studies comparing enteric-coated aspirin and plain aspirin, as well as plain buffered and "arthritis-strength" preparations. In these studies, endoscopies were performed in healthy volunteers before and after either two-day or 14-day administration of aspirin doses of 3,900 or 4,000 mg/day. Compared to all the other preparations, the enteric-coated aspirin produced significantly less damage to the gastric mucosa. There was also statistically less duodenal damage when compared with the plain, i.e., non-enteric-coated, aspirin.

Bioavailability: A single-dose bioavailability study[3] has demonstrated that plasma acetylsalicylic acid and salicylic acid concentrations resulting from Therapy BAYER ENTERIC are equivalent to those from plain aspirin, i.e., non-enteric-coated aspirin. As expected, enteric coating on Therapy BAYER ENTERIC results in delayed absorption (peak achieved at approximately five hours postdosing) relative to plain aspirin. Dissolution of the enteric coating occurs at a neutral-to-basic pH and is therefore dependent on gastric emptying into the duodenum. With continued dosing, appropriate therapeutic plasma levels are maintained.

Antiplatelet Effect:
IN MI PROPHYLAXIS

Indication: Aspirin is indicated to reduce the risk of death and/or nonfatal myocardial infarction in patients with a previous infarction or unstable angina pectoris.

Clinical Trials: The indication is supported by the results of six large randomized, multicenter, placebo-controlled studies[4-10] involving 10,816, predominantly male, post–myocardial infarction (MI) patients and one randomized placebo-controlled study of 1,266 men with unstable angina. Therapy with aspirin was begun at intervals after the onset of acute MI varying from less than three days to more than five years and continuing for periods of from less than 1 year to 4 years. In the unstable angina study, treatment was started within 1 month after the onset of unstable angina and continued for 12 weeks, and complicating conditions, such as congestive heart failure, were not included in the study. Aspirin therapy in MI patients was associated with about a 20% reduction in the risk of subsequent death and/or nonfatal reinfarction, a median absolute decrease of 3% from the 12% to 22% event rates in the placebo groups. In the aspirin-treated unstable angina patients the reduction in risk was about 50%, a reduction in event rate of 5% from the 10% rate in the placebo group over the 12 weeks of the study.

Daily dosage of aspirin in the post–myocardial infarction studies was 300 mg in one study and 900–1,500 mg in five studies. A dose of 325 mg was used in the study of unstable angina.

Adverse Reactions: Gastrointestinal reactions: Doses of 1,000 mg per day of aspirin caused gastrointestinal symptoms and bleeding that, in some cases were clinically significant. In the largest postinfarction study (the Aspirin Myocardial Infarction Study [AMIS] with 4,500 people), the percentage of incidences of gastrointestinal symptoms for the aspirin (1,000 mg of a standard, solid-tablet formulation) and placebo-treated subjects, respectively, were: stomach pain (14.5%; 4.4%); heartburn (11.9%; 4.8%); nausea and/or vomiting (7.6%; 2.1%), hospitalization for GI disorder (4.9%; 3.5%). In the AMIS and other trials, aspirin-treated patients had increased rates of gross gastrointestinal bleeding. Symptoms and signs of gastrointestinal irritation were not significantly increased in subjects treated for unstable angina with buffered aspirin in solution.

Cardiovascular and Biochemical: In the AMIS trial, the dosage of 1,000 mg per day of aspirin was associated with small increases in systolic blood pressure (BP) (average 1.5 to 2.1 mm) and diastolic BP (0.5 to 0.6 mm), depending upon whether maximal or last available readings were used. Blood urea nitrogen and uric acid levels were also increased but by less than 1.0 mg percent. Subjects with marked hypertension or renal insufficiency had been excluded from the trial so that the clinical importance of these observations for such subjects or for any subjects treated over more prolonged periods is not known. It is recommended that patients placed on long-term aspirin treatment, even at doses of 300 mg per day, be seen at regular intervals to assess changes in these measurements.

Sodium in Buffered Aspirin for Solution Formulations: One tablet daily of buffered aspirin in solution adds 553 mg of sodium to that in the diet and may not be tolerated by patients with active sodium-retaining states, such as congestive heart or renal failure. This amount of sodium adds about 30% to the 70 to 90 meq intake suggested as appropriate for dietary treatment of essential hypertension in the 1984 Report of the Joint National Committee on Detection, Evaluation, and Treatment of High Blood Pressure.[11]

Dosage and Administration: Although most of the studies used dosages exceeding 300 mg, two trials used only 300 mg daily, and pharmacologic data indicate that this dose inhibits platelet function fully. Therefore, 300 mg or a conventional 325 mg aspirin dose daily, is a reasonable routine dose that would minimize gastrointestinal adverse reactions. This use of aspirin applies to both solid oral dosage forms (buffered and plain aspirin) and buffered aspirin in solution.

For Recurrent TIAs in Men: There is evidence that aspirin is safe and effective for reducing the risk of recurrent transient ischemic attacks (TIAs) or stroke in men who have had transient ischemia of the brain due to fibrin platelet emboli. There is no evidence that aspirin is effective in reducing TIAs in women or is of benefit in the treatment of completed strokes in men or women.

Patients presenting with signs and/or symptoms of TIAs should have a complete medical and neurologic evaluation. Consideration should be given to other disorders that may resemble TIAs. It is important to evaluate and treat, if appropriate, other diseases associated with TIAs and stroke, such as hypertension and diabetes.

Dosage: The recommended dosage for this new indication is 1300 mg/day (650 mg b.i.d. or 325 mg q.i.d.). Store at controlled room temperature (59°–86°F).

References: 1. Bogacz, K, Caldron, P: Enteric-coated aspirin bezoar: Elevation of serum salicylate level by barium study. *Am J Med* 1987;83:783–786. 2. Baum, J: Enteric-coated aspirin and the problem of gastric retention. *J Rheumatol* 1984; 11:250–251. 3. Data on file, Glenbrook Laboratories. 4. Elwood, PC, et al: A randomized controlled trial of acetylsalicylic acid in the secondary prevention of mortality from myocardial infarction. *Br Med J* 1974;1:436–440. 5. The Coronary Drug Project Research Group: Aspirin in coronary heart disease. *J Chronic Dis* 1976;29:625–642. 6. Breddin, K, et al: Secondary prevention of myocardial infarction: A comparison of acetylsalicylic acid, phenprocoumon or placebo. *Homeostasis* 1979; 470:263–268. 7. Aspirin Myocardial Infarction Study Research Group: A randomized, controlled trial of aspirin in persons recovered from myocardial infarction. *JAMA* 1980;245:661–669. 8. Elwood, PC, Sweetnam, PM: Aspirin and secondary mortality after myocardial infarction. *Lancet*, December 22–29, 1979, pp 1313–1315. 9. The Persantine-Aspirin Reinfarction Study Research Group: Persantine and aspirin in coronary heart disease. *Circulation* 1980;62:449–460. 10. Lewis, HD, et al: Protective effects of aspirin against acute myocardial infarction and death in men with unstable angina: Results of a Veterans Administration Cooperative Study. *N Eng J Med* 1983;309:396–403. 11. *1984 Report of the Joint National Committee on Detection, Evaluation and Treatment of High Blood Pressure*, U.S. Dept of Health and Human Services and US Public Health Service, National Institutes of Health.

How Supplied: Therapy BAYER ENTERIC 325 mg caplets in bottles of 50, 100. Child-resistant safety closure on 50's caplets. Bottles of 100's caplets available without safety closure for households without small children.

Shown in Product Identification Section, page 429

BRONKAID® Mist
(Epinephrine)

Description: BRONKAID Mist, brand of epinephrine inhalation aerosol. Contains: Epinephrine, USP, 0.5% (w/w) (as nitrate and hydrochloric salts). Also contains: Alcohol 33% (w/w), ascorbic acid dichlorodifluoromethane, dichlorotetrafluoroethane, purified water. Each spray delivers 0.25 mg epinephrine. Contains no sulfites.

Indication: For temporary relief of shortness of breath, tightness of chest and wheezing due to bronchial asthma.

Warnings: FOR ORAL INHALATION ONLY. Do not use this product unless a diagnosis of asthma has been made by a doctor, or if you have heart disease, high blood pressure, thyroid disease, diabetes, or difficulty in urination due to enlargement of the prostate gland, if you have ever been hospitalized for asthma or if you are taking any prescription drug for asthma. **Do not use this product more frequently or at higher doses than recommended, unless directed by a doctor.** Keep this and all drugs out of the

Continued on next page

This product information was effective as of November 1, 1991. Current information may be obtained directly from Sterling Health, by writing to 90 Park Avenue, New York, NY 10016.

Sterling Health—Cont.

reach of children. In case of accidental overdose, seek professional assistance or contact a poison control center immediately. As with any drug, if you are pregnant or nursing a baby, seek the advice of a health professional before using this product.

Excessive use may cause nervousness and rapid heart beat, and, possibly, adverse effects on the heart. **Do not continue to use this product, but seek medical assistance immediately if symptoms are not relieved within 20 minutes or become worse.**

Drug Interaction Precaution: Do not use this product if you are presently taking a prescription drug for high blood pressure or depression, without first consulting your doctor.

Warnings: Avoid spraying in eyes. Contents under pressure. Do not break or incinerate. Using or storing near open flame or heating above 120°F may cause bursting.

Dosage: Inhalation dosage for adults and children 4 years of age and older. Start with one inhalation, then wait at least one (1) minute. If not relieved, use once more. Do not use again for at least 3 hours. The use of this product by children should be supervised by an adult. Children under 4 years of age, consult a doctor.

Directions for Use:
1. Remove cap and mouthpiece from bottle.
2. Remove cap from mouthpiece.
3. Turn mouthpiece sideways and fit metal stem of nebulizer into hole in flattened end of mouthpiece.
4. Exhale, as completely as possible. Now, hold bottle **upside down** between thumb and forefinger and close lips loosely around end of mouthpiece.
5. Inhale deeply while pressing down firmly on bottle, once only.
6. Remove mouthpiece and hold your breath a moment to allow for maximum absorption of medication. Then exhale slowly through nearly closed lips.

After use, remove mouthpiece from bottle and replace cap. Slide mouthpiece over bottle for protection. When possible rinse mouthpiece with tap water immediately after use. Soap and water will not hurt it. A clean mouthpiece always works better.

How Supplied: Bottles of ½ fl oz (15 mL) with actuator. Also available— refills (no mouthpiece) in 15 mL (½ fl oz) and 22.5 mL (¾ fl oz).

Shown in Product Identification Section, page 429

BRONKAID® Mist Suspension (Epinephrine Bitartrate)

Active Ingredients: Each spray delivers 0.3 mg epinephrine bitartrate equivalent to 0.16 mg epinephrine base. Contains epinephrine bitartrate 7.0 mg per cc. Also contains: Cetylpyridinium chloride, dichlorodifluoromethane, dichlorotetrafluoroethane, sorbitan trioleate, trichloromonofluoromethane. Contains no sulfites.

Indication: Provides temporary relief of shortness of breath, tightness of chest, and wheezing due to bronchial asthma.

Warnings: FOR ORAL INHALATION ONLY. Do not use this product unless a diagnosis of asthma has been made by a doctor, or if you have heart disease, high blood pressure, thyroid disease, diabetes, or difficulty in urination due to enlargement of the prostate gland, if you have ever been hospitalized for asthma or if you are taking any prescription drug for asthma. **Do not use this product more frequently or at higher doses than recommended, unless directed by a doctor.** Keep this and all drugs out of the reach of children. In case of accidental overdose, seek professional assistance or contact a poison control center immediately. As with any drug, if you are pregnant or nursing a baby, seek the advice of a health professional before using this product.

Excessive use may cause nervousness and rapid heart beat, and, possibly, adverse effects on the heart. **Do not continue to use this product, but seek medical assistance immediately if symptoms are not relieved within 20 minutes or become worse.**

Drug Interaction Precaution: Do not use this product if you are presently taking a prescription drug for high blood pressure or depression, without first consulting your doctor.

Warning: Avoid spraying in eyes. Contents under pressure. Do not break or incinerate. Using or storing near open flame or heating above 120°F may cause bursting.

Administration:
1. SHAKE WELL.
2. HOLD INHALER WITH NOZZLE DOWN WHILE USING. Empty the lungs as completely as possible by exhaling.
3. Purse the lips as in saying the letter "O" and hold the nozzle up to the lips, keeping the tongue flat. As you start to take a deep breath, squeeze nozzle and can together, releasing one full application. Complete taking deep breath, drawing medication into your lungs.
4. Hold breath for as long as comfortable. This distributes the medication in the lungs. Then exhale slowly keeping the lips nearly closed.
5. Rinse nozzle daily with soap and hot water after removing from vial. Dry with clean cloth.

Before each use, remove dust cap and inspect mouthpiece for foreign objects. Replace dust cap after each use.

Dosage: Inhalation dosage for adults and children 4 years of age and older. Start with one inhalation, then wait at least one (1) minute. If not relieved, use once more. Do not use again for at least 3 hours. The use of this product by children should be supervised by an adult. Children under 4 years of age; consult a doctor.

Professional Labeling: Same as stated under Indication.

How Supplied:
⅓ fl oz (10 cc) pocketsize aerosol inhaler, with actuator.
Shown in Product Identification Section, page 429

BRONKAID® Tablets

Description: Each tablet contains ephedrine sulfate 24 mg, guaifenesin (glyceryl guaiacolate) 100 mg, and theophylline 100 mg. Also contains: magnesium stearate, magnesium trisilicate, microcrystalline cellulose, starch.

Indication: For symptomatic control of bronchial congestion and bronchial asthma. Clears bronchial passages. Helps relieve shortness of breath, plus helps loosen phlegm.

Warnings: Do not use this product unless a diagnosis of asthma has been made by a doctor, or if you have heart disease, diabetes, difficulty in urination due to enlargement of the prostate gland, if you have ever been hospitalized for asthma or if you are taking any prescription drug for asthma unless directed by a doctor. Do not continue to use this product, but seek medical assistance immediately if symptoms are not relieved within an hour or become worse. Some users of this product may experience nervousness, tremor, sleeplessness, nausea, and loss of appetite. If these symptoms persist or become worse, consult your doctor.

Drug Interaction Precaution: Do not use this product if you are presently taking a prescription drug for high blood pressure or depression. Do not exceed recommended dosage unless directed by a physician.

Warnings: As with any drug, if you are pregnant or nursing a baby, seek the advice of a health professional before using this product. Keep this and all drugs out of the reach of children. In case of accidental overdose, seek professional assistance or contact a poison control center immediately.

Dosage and Administration: *Adult Dosage:* 1 tablet every four hours. Do not take more than 5 tablets in a 24-hour period. Swallow tablets whole with water. *Children under 12 years of age:* Consult a doctor. *Morning Dose:* An early dose of 1 tablet (for adults) can relieve the coughing and wheezing caused by the night's accumulation of mucus, and can help you start the day with better breathing capacity. *Before an Attack:* Many persons feel an attack of asthma coming on. One BRONKAID tablet beforehand may stop the attack before it starts. *During the Day:* The precise dose of BRONKAID tablets can be varied to meet your individual needs as you gain experience with this product. It is advisable to take 1 tablet before going to bed, for nighttime relief. However, be sure not to exceed recommended daily dosage.

How Supplied:
Boxes of 24 and 60.
*Shown in Product Identification
Section, page 429*

CAMPHO-PHENIQUE®
[*kam 'fo-finēk*]
COLD SORE GEL

Description: Contains phenol 4.7% (w/w) and camphor 10.8% (w/w). Also contains: colloidal silicon dioxide, eucalyptus oil, glycerin, light mineral oil.
Use at the first sign of cold sore, fever blister and sun blister. Symptoms (tingling, pain, itching).

Indications: For relief of pain and itching due to cold sores and fever blisters. To combat infection from minor injuries and skin lesions.
Also effective for:
Minor skin injuries: abrasions, cuts, scrapes, burns, razor nicks and chafed or irritated skin.
Insect bites: mosquitoes, black flies, sandfleas, chiggers.

Warnings: Not for prolonged use. Not to be used on large areas. In case of deep or puncture wounds, serious burns, or persisting redness, swelling or pain, or if rash or infection develops, discontinue use and consult physician. Do not bandage if applied to fingers or toes.
Avoid using near eyes. If product gets into the eye, flush thoroughly with water and obtain medical attention. Keep this and all drugs out of the reach of children. In case of accidental ingestion, seek professional assistance or contact a poison control center immediately.

Directions for Use: For external use. Apply directly to cold sore, fever blister or injury three or four times a day.

How Supplied: Tubes of 0.23 oz (6.5 g) and 0.50 oz (14 g).
*Shown in Product Identification
Section, page 429*

CAMPHO-PHENIQUE® Liquid
[*kam 'fo-finēk*]

Description: Contains phenol 4.7% (w/w) and camphor 10.8% (w/w). Also contains: Eucalyptus oil, light mineral oil.

Actions: Pain-relieving antiseptic for scrapes, cuts, burns, insect bites, fever blisters, and cold sores.

Indications: For relief of pain and to combat infection from minor injuries and skin lesions.

Warnings: Not for prolonged use. Not to be used on large areas or in or near the eyes. In case of deep or puncture wounds, serious burns, or persisting redness, swelling or pain, or if rash or infection develops, discontinue use and consult

physician. Do not bandage if applied to fingers or toes.
Keep this and all drugs out of the reach of children. In case of accidental ingestion, seek professional assistance or contact a poison control center immediately.

Directions for Use: For external use. Apply with cotton three or four times daily.
4 oz size only: Do not use more than ½ the contents of the 4 fl oz bottle in any 24-hour period.

How Supplied:
Bottles of ¾, 1½ and 4 fl oz.
*Shown in Product Identification
Section, page 429*

CAMPHO-PHENIQUE™
[*kam 'fo-finēk*]
TRIPLE ANTIBIOTIC OINTMENT PLUS PAIN RELIEVER

Description: Contains bacitracin 500 units, neomycin sulfate 5 mg (equiv to 3.5 mg neomycin base), polymyxin B sulfate 5000 units, lidocaine HCl 40 mg (or diperodon HCl 10 mg) (Pain Reliever). Also contains white petrolatum.

Actions: Pain-relieving triple antibiotic with anesthetic to help prevent infection in minor cuts, scrapes, burns and other minor wounds.

Indications: Helps prevent infections in minor cuts, burns, and other minor wounds. Provides soothing, nonstinging temporary relief of pain and itching associated with these conditions.

Warnings: For external use only. In case of deep or puncture wounds, animal bites or serious burns, consult physician. If redness, irritation, swelling or pain persists or increases, or if infection occurs, discontinue use and consult physician. Do not use in eyes or over large areas of the body. Do not use longer than 1 week unless directed by doctor. Keep this and all drugs out of the reach of children. In case of accidental ingestion seek professional assistance or contact a poison control center immediately.

Directions: Clean the affected area. Apply a small amount (an amount equal to the surface area of the tip of a finger) on the area 1 to 3 times daily. May be covered.

How Supplied: Tubes of 0.50 oz and 1.0 oz.
*Shown in Product Identification
Section, page 429*

DAIRY EASE® Tablets/Caplets
Lactase Enzyme

Ingredients: Each Tablet/Caplet contains 3000 FCC Lactase units (derived from Aspergillus Oryzae). Other ingredients are: (Tablets) Dibasic Calcium Phosphate, Mannitol, Colloidal Silicon Dioxide, Magnesium Stearate. (Caplets): Colloidal Silicon Dioxide, Dibasic Calcium Phosphate, FD&C Blue No. 2, Hydroxypropyl Methylcellulose, Magne-

sium Stearate, Microcrystalline Cellulose, Polyethylene Glycol, Potassium Sorbate, Pregelantized Starch, Titanium Dioxide and Xanthan Gum.

Indications: Lactase insufficiency, suspected from gastrointestinal disturbances after consumption of milk or milk-containing products (i.e., Gas, Bloating, Flatulence, Cramps and Diarrhea) or identified by a lactose intolerance test.

Action: Hydrolysis converts the lactose into its simple sugar components: glucose and galactose.

Product Uses: Dairy Ease is a natural lactase enzyme which supplements the natural level of lactase in the body and helps make lactose more easily digestible. The most common products where lactose can be found are Milk, Cheese, Ice Cream & Chocolate and it is also found in some vitamins and medications. Dairy Ease can also be used with other foods which contain lactose such as pizza, hot dogs, pancakes, creamed salad dressings and soups, instant cocoa mix, puddings and other foods where milk, milk solids, whey, whey protein concentrate or cheese are listed on the ingredient panel.

Dosage: Recommended dosage is 2–3 chewable tables/swallowable caplets along with or immediately following each dairy food occasion. However, since natural lactase levels vary, actual dosage may differ from person to person.

Toxicity: None.

Drug Interactions: None. Dairy Ease Tablets and Caplets are classified as food products.

Warnings: Should hypersensitivity occur, discontinue use.

Precautions: Diabetics should be aware that the milk sugar will now be metabolically available and must be taken into account (17.5 gm glucose and 17.5 gm galactose per quart at 70% hydrolysis). No reports received of any diabetics' reactions. Galactosemics may not have milk in any form, lactase enzyme modified or not.

Note: Possible adverse reactions are mainly gastrointestinal in nature, sometimes mimicking the symptoms of lactose intolerance and sometimes involving vomiting. Skin rashes possibly due to allergic reactions have been reported. Persons sensitive to penicillin and other molds may be particularly susceptible. Discontinue use of tablets/caplets immediately and consult a physician.

How Supplied: Dairy Ease Chewable Tablets are available in 12, 36, 60 and

Continued on next page

This product information was effective as of November 1, 1991. Current information may be obtained directly from Sterling Health, by writing to 90 Park Avenue, New York, NY 10016.

Sterling Health—Cont.

100 counts. Dairy Ease Swallowable Caplets are available in a 40 count bottle.

Shown in Product Identification Section, page 429

DAIRY EASE® Drops
Lactase Enzyme

Ingredients: Water, Glycerol, Lactase Enzyme (derived from Kluyveromyces Lactis). One ml contains no less than 5400 Neutral Lactase units.

Indications: Lactase insufficiency, suspected from gastrointestinal disturbances after consumption of milk or milk-containing products (i.e., Gas, Bloating, Flatulence, Cramps and Diarrhea) or identified by a lactose tolerance test.

Product Uses: Dairy Ease Drops are a natural lactase enzyme which when added to milk, make the lactose more easily digestible. Dairy Ease Drops can be used in any kind of milk including: whole, 1%, 2%, low fat, nonfat, skim, canned, powdered and chocolate. Also, cream, baby formulas containing milk and high protein diet formulas. The treated milk can be used for cooking, on cereal or directly from the carton.

Action: Hydrolysis converts the lactose into its simple sugar components: glucose and galactose.

Dosage: Add Dairy Ease Drops to a quart of milk, shake gently and refrigerate for 24 hours. Five drops will remove 70% of the lactose, 10 drops, 90% and 15 drops, 97 + %. Since the degree of natural lactase levels vary, each person may have to adjust the number of drops that work best.

Toxicity: None.

Drug Interactions: None. Dairy Ease Drops are classified as food products.

Warnings: Should hypersensitivity occur, discontinue use.

Precautions: Diabetics should be aware that the milk sugar will now be metabolically available and must be taken into account (17.5 gm glucose and 17.5 gm galactose per quart at 70% hydrolysis). No reports received of any diabetics' reactions. Galactosemics may not have milk in any form, lactose enzyme modified or not.

Adverse Reactions: No reactions of any kind have been observed from Dairy Ease liquid drops.

How Supplied: Dairy Ease Drops are available in a 7ml size which work for up to 32 quarts of milk.

Shown in Product Identification Section, page 429

DAIRY EASE® Real Milk
Lactose Reduced Milk

Dairy Ease is also available in Real Milk which is 70% lactose reduced and contains vitamins A & D. A one quart size in three varieties is available: Nonfat, 1% low fat, and 2% low fat. Dairy Ease Real Milk can be used for cooking, on cereal or directly from the carton.

Shown in Product Identification Section, page 429

FERGON® Iron Supplement
[fur-gone]
brand of ferrous gluconate
FERGON® ELIXIR

Composition: FERGON (ferrous gluconate, USP) is stabilized to maintain a minimum of ferric ions. It contains not less than 11.5 percent iron.
Each FERGON Iron Supplement tablet contains 320 mg (5 grains) ferrous gluconate equal to approximately 36 mg ferrous iron. Also contains: acacia, carnauba wax, dextrose excipient, FD&C Red No. 40, D&C Yellow No. 10, FD&C Blue No. 1, gelatin, kaolin, magnesium stearate, parabens, povidone, precipitated calcium carbonate, sodium benzoate, starch, sucrose, talc, titanium dioxide, yellow wax. Not USP for dissolution.
FERGON Elixir contains: ferrous gluconate 6%. Also contains: alcohol 7%, flavor, glycerin, liquid glucose, purified water, saccharin sodium. Each teaspoon (5 mL) contains 300 mg (5 grains) ferrous gluconate equivalent to approximately 34 mg ferrous iron.

Action and Uses: For use as a dietary supplement.

Warnings: Keep this and all drugs out of the reach of children. If you are pregnant or nursing a baby, seek the advice of a health professional before using this product. In case of accidental overdose, seek professional assistance or contact a poison control center immediately. Avoid excessive heat.

Dosage and Administration: *Adults* —One FERGON tablet or one to two teaspoonfuls of FERGON Elixir daily. *For children and infants,* as prescribed by physician.

How Supplied: FERGON Tablets of 320 mg (5 grains) bottle of 100. FERGON Elixir, 6% (5 grains per teaspoonful) bottle of 1 pint.

Shown in Product Indentification Section, page 429

HALEY'S M-O®

Active Ingredients: A suspension of magnesium hydroxide in purified water plus mineral oil. Haley's M-O contains 301 mg per teaspoon (5 mL) of magnesium hydroxide and 1.25 mL of mineral oil.

Inactive Ingredients: Purified water. For flavored Haley's M-O only, D&C Red No. 28, flavor, purified water, saccharin sodium.

Indications: For the relief of occasional constipation or irregularity accompanied by hemorrhoids.

Action at Laxative Dosage: Haley's M-O is a mild saline laxative which acts by drawing water into the gut, increasing intraluminal pressure, and increasing intestinal motility. This product generally produces bowel movement in ½ to 6 hours.

Administration and Dosage: As a laxative, especially for hemorrhoid sufferers, adults 1–2 tbsp at bedtime and upon arising. For constipation relief, adults 2 tbsp at bedtime and upon arising; children 6–12, minimum single dose; 1 tsp, maximum daily dose; 1 tbsp. For adults and children, as bowel function improves reduce dose gradually.

Caution: Do not take this product if you are presently taking a stool softener laxative unless directed by a doctor. Do not take with meals.

Warnings: Do not use laxative products when abdominal pain, nausea or vomiting are present unless directed by a doctor. If you have noticed a sudden change in bowel habits that persists over a period of 2 weeks, consult a doctor before using a laxative. Laxative products should not be used for a period longer than 1 week unless directed by a doctor. Rectal bleeding, or failure to have a bowel movement after use of a laxative may indicate a serious condition; discontinue use and consult your doctor. Do not administer to children under 6 years of age, to pregnant women, to bedridden patients, or to persons with difficulty swallowing. As with any drug, if you are nursing a baby, seek the advice of a health professional before using this product. Keep this and all drugs out of the reach of children. In case of accidental overdose, seek professional assistance or contact a poison control center immediately.

How Supplied: Haley's M-O is available in regular and flavored liquids in 12 and 26 fl oz bottles.

Shown in Product Identification Section, page 429

Regular Strength
MIDOL®
Multi-Symptom Menstrual Formula

Active Ingredients: Each caplet contains: acetaminophen 325 mg and pyrilamine maleate 12.5 mg.

Inactive Ingredients: Croscarmellose sodium, hydroxypropyl methylcellulose, magnesium stearate, microcrystalline cellulose, pregelatinized starch and triacetin.

Action and Uses: For relief of physical symptoms suffered during menstrual cycle: cramps, headaches, backaches and muscle aches.
Regular Strength Midol Multi-Symptom Menstrual Formula provides:

Relief from cramps, headaches, back-aches and muscle aches.

Caution: If pain persists for more than 10 days, consult a physician immediately. May cause drowsiness. Use caution when driving or operating machinery. Alcohol, sedatives or tranquilizers may increase drowsiness.

Warnings: Keep this and all drugs out of the reach of children. In case of accidental overdose, seek professional assistance or contact a poison control center immediately. As with any drug, if you are pregnant or nursing a baby, seek the advice of a health professional before using this product.

Dosage: Take 2 caplets with water. Repeat every four hours as needed up to a maximum of 12 caplets per day. Under age 12: Consult your physician.

How Supplied:
White, capsule-shaped caplets in bottles of 16 and 32 caplets.
Child-resistant safety closures on bottles of 32 caplets.
Shown in Product Identification Section, page 430

Maximum Strength
MIDOL®
Premenstrual Pain Formula

Active Ingredients: Each caplet contains acetaminophen 500 mg, pamabrom 25 mg, pyrilamine maleate 15 mg.

Inactive Ingredients: Croscarmellose sodium, hydroxypropyl methylcellulose, magnesium stearate, microcrystalline cellulose, pregelatinized starch, and triacetin.

Action and Uses: Relieves the physical symptoms of premenstrual pain. Contains maximum strength medication for bloating, water-weight gain, cramps, backaches, and headaches. Unlike general pain relievers, which contain only analgesics, Midol Premenstrual Pain Formula contains a combination of ingredients (an analgesic and diuretic) for the physical symptoms associated with the premenstrual period.

Dosage: Take 2 caplets with water. Repeat every 4 hours as needed, up to a maximum of 8 caplets per day. Under age 12: Consult your physician.

Caution: If pain persists for more than 10 days, consult a physician immediately. May cause drowsiness. Use caution when driving or operating machinery. Alcohol, sedatives or tranquilizers may increase drowsiness.

Warnings: Keep this and all drugs out of the reach of children. In case of accidental overdose, seek professional assistance or contact a poison control center immediately. As with any drug, if you are pregnant or nursing a baby, seek the advice of a health professional before using this product.

How Supplied: White capsule-shaped caplets available in 2-caplet packets for sample use, bottles of 8 and 32 caplets,

and in packages of 2 blisters of 8 caplets each.
Child-resistant safety closure on bottles of 8 and 32 caplets.
Shown in Product Identification Section, page 430

MIDOL® IB
CRAMP RELIEF FORMULA
Ibuprofen Tablets, USP 200 mg
Menstrual Pain/Cramp Reliever

Warning: Aspirin-Sensitive Patients —Do not take this product if you have had a severe allergic reaction to aspirin, eg, asthma, swelling, shock or hives, because even though this product contains no aspirin or salicylates, cross-reactions may occur in patients allergic to aspirin.

Indications: For the temporary relief of painful menstrual cramps (dysmenorrhea); also headaches, backaches and muscular aches and pains associated with Premenstrual Syndrome.

Directions:
Adults: Take 1 tablet every 4 to 6 hours at the onset of menstrual symptoms and while pain persists. If pain does not respond to 1 tablet, 2 tablets may be used but do not exceed 6 tablets in 24 hours, unless directed by a doctor. The smallest effective dose should be used. Take with food or milk if occasional and mild heartburn, upset stomach, or stomach pain occurs with use. Consult a doctor if these symptoms are more than mild or if they persist. *Children:* Do not give this product to children under 12 except under the advice and supervision of a doctor.

Warnings: Do not take for pain for more than 10 days unless directed by a doctor. If pain persists or gets worse, or if new symptoms occur, consult a doctor. These could be signs of serious illness. If you are under a doctor's care for any serious condition, consult a doctor before taking this product. As with aspirin and acetaminophen, if you have any condition which requires you to take prescription drugs or if you have had any problems or serious side effects from taking any nonprescription pain reliever, do not take this product without first discussing it with your doctor. If you experience any symptoms which are unusual or seem unrelated to the condition for which you took ibuprofen, consult a doctor before taking any more of it. Although ibuprofen is indicated for the same conditions as aspirin and acetaminophen, it should not be taken with them except under a doctor's direction. Do not combine this product with any other ibuprofen-containing product. As with any drug, if you are pregnant or nursing a baby, seek the advice of a health professional before using this product. **IT IS ESPECIALLY IMPORTANT NOT TO USE IBUPROFEN DURING THE LAST 3 MONTHS OF PREGNANCY UNLESS SPECIFICALLY DIRECTED TO DO SO BY A DOCTOR BECAUSE IT MAY CAUSE PROBLEMS IN THE UNBORN CHILD OR COMPLICA-**

TIONS DURING DELIVERY. Keep this and all drugs out of the reach of children. In case of accidental overdose, seek professional assistance or contact a poison control center immediately.

Action and Uses: Ibuprofen is used for the relief of painful menstrual cramps and the pain associated with Premenstrual Syndrome. Ibuprofen has been proven more effective in relieving menstrual pain and cramps than aspirin and is gentler on the stomach. Ibuprofen had been widely prescribed for years and is now available in nonprescription strength.

Active Ingredient: Each tablet contains ibuprofen USP 200 mg.

Inactive Ingredients: Calcium phosphate, cellulose, magnesium stearate, silicon dioxide, sodium lauryl sulfate, sodium starch glycolate, stearic acid, titanium dioxide.
Store at room temperature; avoid excessive heat 40℃ (104°F).

How Supplied:
White tablets in bottles of 16 and 32 tablets.
Child-resistant safety closure on bottles of 32 tablets.
Shown in Product Identification Section, page 430

Maximum Strength
MIDOL®
Multi-Symptom Menstrual Formula

Active Ingredients: Each caplet contains acetaminophen 500 mg, caffeine 60 mg and pyrilamine maleate 15 mg.

Inactive Ingredients: Croscarmellose sodium, hydroxypropyl methylcellulose, magnesium stearate, microcrystalline cellulose, pregelatinized starch and triacetin.

Action and Uses: Maximum strength medication for the relief of multiple symptoms suffered during menstrual cycle: cramps, bloating, water-weight gain, headaches, backaches, and muscle aches.
Unlike general pain relievers, which contain only analgesics, Midol Maximum Strength Multi-Symptom Menstrual Formula has a combination of ingredients (an analgesic and diuretic) specially formulated to give:
1. Maximum strength relief from cramps, headaches, backaches and muscle aches.
2. Plus maximum strength relief of bloating and water-weight gain.

Caution: If pain persists for more than 10 days, consult a physician immedi-

Continued on next page

This product information was effective as of November 1, 1991. Current information may be obtained directly from Sterling Health, by writing to 90 Park Avenue, New York, NY 10016.

Sterling Health—Cont.

ately. May cause drowsiness. Use caution when driving or operating machinery. Alcohol, sedatives or tranquilizers may increase drowsiness.

Warnings: Keep this and all drugs out of the reach of children. In case of accidental overdose, seek professional assistance or contact a poison control center immediately. As with any drug, if you are pregnant or nursing a baby, seek the advice of a health professional before using this product.

Dosage: Take 2 caplets with water. Repeat every 4 hours, as needed, up to a maximum of 8 caplets per day.
Under age 12: Consult your physician.

How Supplied: White capsule-shaped caplets available in 2-caplet packets for sample use, bottles of 8 and 32 caplets, and packages of 2 blisters of 8 caplets each.
Child-resistant safety closures on bottles of 8 and 32 caplets.

*Shown in Product Identification
Section, page 430*

**Teen Formula
MIDOL®
Multi-Symptom Menstrual Formula**

Active Ingredients: Each caplet contains Acetaminophen 400mg and Pamabrom 25mg.

Inactive Ingredients: Croscarmellose Sodium, Hydroxypropyl Methylcellulose, Magnesium Stearate, Microcrystalline Cellulose, Pregelatinized Starch, and Triacetin.

Action and Uses: Aspirin-free and Caffeine-free medication for the relief of multiple symptoms suffered by teens during menstrual cycle: cramps, bloating, water-weight gain, headaches, backaches and muscle aches. Unlike general pain relievers, which contain only analgesics, Teen Formula MIDOL contains a combination of ingredients (an analgesic and diuretic) specially formulated to give:
1. Relief from cramps, headaches and muscle aches.
2. Plus relief from bloating and water-weight gain.

Caution: If pain persists for more than 10 days, consult a physician immediately.

Warnings: Keep this and all drugs out of the reach of children. In case of accidental overdose, seek professional assistance or contact a poison control center immediately. As with any drug, if you are pregnant or nursing a baby, seek the advice of a health professional before using this product.

Dosage: Take 2 caplets with water. Repeat every 4 hours as needed, up to a maximum of 8 caplets per day. Under age 12: Consult your physician.

How Supplied: White capsule-shaped caplets available in 2-caplet packets for sample use, packages of 2 blisters of 8 caplets each, and bottles of 32 caplets. Child resistant safety closure on bottles of 32 caplets.

*Shown in Product Identification
Section, page 430*

**NaSal™Moisturizer AF
Saline (buffered)
0.65% Sodium chloride
Nasal Spray and Drops**

Description: The nasal spray, nasal spray pump and nose drops contain sodium chloride 0.65%. Also contains: benzalkonium chloride and thimerosal 0.001% as preservative, mono- and dibasic sodium phosphates as buffers, purified water.
Contains No Alcohol.

Actions: Immediate relief for dry nose. Formulated to match the pH of normal nasal secretions to help prevent stinging or burning.

Indications: Provides immediate relief for dry, inflamed nasal membranes due to colds, low humidity, allergies, minor nose bleeds, overuse of topical nasal decongestants, and other nasal irritations. As an ideal nasal moisturizer, it can be used in conjunction with oral decongestants.

Adverse Reactions: No associated side effects.

Warnings: In case of accidental ingestion seek professional assistance or contact a poison control center immediately. The use of the dispenser by more than one person may spread infection.

Dosage and Administration: *Spray* —For adults and children: with head upright, spray twice in each nostril as needed or as directed by physician. To spray, squeeze bottle quickly and firmly. *Nose Drops* —For infants and adults: 2 to 6 drops in each nostril as needed or as directed by physician.

How Supplied: Nasal Spray—plastic squeeze bottles of 15 mL (½ fl. oz.).
Nose Drops—MonoDrop® bottles of 15 mL (½ fl. oz.).

*Shown in Product Identification
Section, page 430*

**NEO-SYNEPHRINE®
Pediatric Formula, Mild Formula,
Regular Strength, and
Extra Strength.
phenylephrine hydrochloride**

Description: This line of Nasal Sprays, Drops and Spray Pumps contains phenylephrine hydrochloride in strengths ranging from 0.125% (drops only) to 1%. Also contains: benzalkonium chloride and thimerosal 0.001% as preservatives, citric acid, purified water, sodium chloride, sodium citrate.

Action: Rapid-acting nasal decongestant.

Directions: For adults: with head upright, spray 2 or 3 times, or squeeze 2 or 3 drops into each nostril. May be repeated in four hours as needed.

Indications: For temporary relief of nasal congestion due to common cold, hay fever, sinusitis, or other upper respiratory allergies.

Warnings: Do not exceed recommended dosage because symptoms may occur such as burning, stinging, sneezing or increased nasal discharge. Do not use this product for more than 3 days. If symptoms persist, consult a doctor. Frequent and continued usage of the higher concentrations (especially the 1% solution) occasionally may cause a rebound congestion of the nose. Therefore, longterm or frequent use of this solution is not recommended without the advice of a physician.
Prolonged exposure to air or strong light will cause oxidation and some loss of potency. Do not use if brown in color or contains a precipitate.
Keep these and all drugs out of the reach of children. In case of accidental ingestion seek professional assistance or contact a poison control center immediately. The use of the dispenser by more than one person may spread infection.
<u>Do</u> <u>not</u> <u>use</u> <u>this</u> <u>product</u> <u>if</u> <u>you</u> <u>have</u> <u>heart</u> <u>disease, high blood pressure, thyroid disease, diabetes, or difficulty in urination</u> <u>due to enlargement of the prostate gland</u> <u>unless</u> <u>directed</u> <u>by</u> <u>a</u> <u>doctor.</u>

Adverse Reactions: Generally very well tolerated; systemic side effects such as tremor, insomnia, or palpitation rarely occur at recommended dosages.

Dosage and Administration: *Topical* —dropper or spray. The *0.25% solution* is adequate in most cases *(0.125% for children 2 to 6 years).* In resistant cases, or if more powerful decongestion is desired, the *0.5% or 1% solution* should be used.

How Supplied: Nasal spray 0.25%—15 ml (for children and for adults who prefer a mild nasal spray); nasal spray 0.5%—15 ml (for adults); nasal spray 1%—15 ml (extra strength for adults); nasal solution 0.125% (for infants and small children), 15 ml bottles; nasal solution 0.25% (for children and adults who prefer a mild solution), 15 ml bottles; nasal solution 0.5% (for adults), 15 ml bottles; nasal solution 1% (extra strength for adults), 15 ml bottles.

*Shown in Product Identification
Section, page 430*

**NEO-SYNEPHRINE®
Maximum Strength 12 Hour
oxymetazoline hydrochloride
Nasal Spray 0.05%**

Description: *Adult Strength Nasal Spray* and *Nasal Spray Pump* contain: Oxymetazoline Hydrochloride 0.05%. Also contain: Benzalkonium Chloride and Phenylmercuric Acetate 0.002% as preservatives, Glycine, Purified Water,

Sorbitol, may also contain Sodium Chloride.

Action: 12 HOUR Nasal Decongestant.

Indications: Provides temporary relief, for up to 12 HOURS, of nasal congestion due to colds, hay fever, sinusitis, or other upper respiratory allergies. NEO-SYNEPHRINE MAXIMUM STRENGTH 12-HOUR Nasal Spray and Pump contain oxymetazoline which provides the longest-lasting relief of nasal congestion available.

Warnings: Do not exceed recommended dosage because symptoms may occur such as burning, stinging, sneezing, or increase of nasal discharge. Do not use these products for more than 3 days. If symptoms persist, consult a physician. The use of the dispenser by more than one person may spread infection. Do not use this product if you have heart disease, high blood pressure, thyroid disease, diabetes, or difficulty in urination due to enlargement of the prostate gland unless directed by a doctor. Keep this and all drugs out of the reach of children. In case of accidental ingestion, seek professional assistance or contact a poison control center immediately.

Dosage and Administration: *Adult Strength Nasal Spray*—For adults and children 6 to under 12 years of age (with adult supervision): 2 or 3 sprays in each nostril not more often than every 10 to 12 hours. Do not exceed 2 applications in any 24-hour period. Children under 6 years of age: consult a doctor. To administer, hold head upright, spray 2 or 3 times in each nostril twice daily—morning and evening. To spray, squeeze bottle quickly and firmly. *Nasal Spray Pump*—For adults and children 6 to under 12 years of age (with adult supervision): 2 or 3 sprays in each nostril not more often than every 10–12 hours. Do not exceed 2 applications in any 24 hour period. Children under 6 years of age: consult a doctor. Hold bottle with thumb at base and nozzle between first and second fingers. To administer, hold head upright and insert spray nozzle in nostril. Depress pump 2 or 3 times, all the way down, with a firm even stroke and sniff deeply. Repeat in other nostril. Do not tilt head backward while spraying.

How Supplied: *Nasal Spray Adult Strength* — plastic squeeze bottles of 15 ml (½ fl. oz.); *Nasal Spray Pump* —15 ml bottle (½ fl. oz.).

Shown in Product Identification Section, page 430

NTZ®
Long Acting
Oxymetazoline hydrochloride
Nasal Spray 0.05%
Nose Drops 0.05%

Description: Both the nasal spray and nose drops contain Oxymetazoline Hydrochloride 0.05%. Also contain: Benzalkonium Chloride and Phenylmercuric Acetate 0.002% as preservatives, Gly-

cine, Purified Water, Sorbitol, and may also contain Sodium Chloride.

Actions: 12 Hour Nasal Decongestant.

Indications: Provides temporary relief, for up to 12 hours, of nasal congestion due to colds, hay fever, sinusitis, or allergies. Oxymetazoline hydrochloride provides the longest-lasting relief of nasal congestion available. It decongests nasal passages up to 12 hours, reduces swelling of nasal passages, and temporarily restores freer breathing through the nose.

Warnings: Not recommended for children under six. Do not exceed recommended dosage because symptoms may occur such as burning, stinging, sneezing, or increase of nasal discharge. Do not use these products for more than 3 days. If symptoms persist, consult a physician. The use of the dispenser by more than one person may spread infection. Do not use this product if you have heart disease, high blood pressure, thyroid disease, diabetes, or difficulty in urination due to enlargement of the prostate gland unless directed by a doctor. Keep these and all drugs out of the reach of children. In case of accidental ingestion seek professional assistance or contact a poison control center immediately.

Dosage and Administration: Intranasally by spray and dropper. *Nasal Spray* —For adults and children 6 years of age and over: With head upright, spray 2 or 3 times in each nostril twice daily—morning and evening. To spray, squeeze bottle quickly and firmly. *Nose Drops*— For adults and children 6 years of age and over: 2 or 3 drops in each nostril twice daily—morning and evening.

How Supplied: *Nasal Spray* —plastic squeeze bottles of 15 ml (½ fl. oz.). *Nose Drops* —bottles of 15 ml (½ fl. oz.) with dropper.

Children's PANADOL®
Acetaminophen Chewable Tablets,
Liquid, Drops.

Description: Each Children's PANADOL Chewable Tablet contains 80 mg acetaminophen in a fruit-flavored sugar-free tablet. Children's PANADOL Acetaminophen Liquid is fruit-flavored, red in color, and is alcohol-free, sugar-free and aspirin-free. Each ½ teaspoonful contains 80 mg of acetaminophen. Infant's PANADOL Drops are fruit-flavored, red in color, and are alcohol-free, sugar-free and aspirin-free. Each 0.8 mL (one calibrated dropperful) contains 80 mg acetaminophen.

Actions and Indications: Acetaminophen, the active ingredient in Children's PANADOL, is the analgesic/antipyretic most widely recommended by pediatricians for fast, effective relief of children's fevers. It also relieves the aches and pains of colds and flu, earaches, headaches, teething, immunizations, tonsillectomy, and childhood illnesses.

Children's PANADOL Tablets, Liquid, and Drops are aspirin-free and contain no alcohol or sugar. The pleasant-tasting formulations are not likely to upset or irritate children's stomachs.

Usual Dosage: Dosing is based on single doses in the range of 10–15 mg/kg body weight. Doses may be repeated every four hours up to 4 or 5 times daily, but not to exceed 5 doses in 24 hours. To be administered to children under 2 years only on advice of a physician.
Children's PANADOL Chewable Tablets: 2–3 yr, 24–35 lb, 2 tablets; 4–5 yr, 36–47 lb, 3 tablets; 6–8 yr, 48–59 lb, 4 tablets; 9–10 yr, 60–71 lb, 5 tablets; 11–12 yr, 72–95 lb, 6 tablets. May be repeated every 4 hours, up to 5 times in a 24-hour period.
Children's PANADOL Liquid: (a special 3 teaspoon cup for accurate measurement is provided.) 0–4 mo, 6–11 lb, ¼ teaspoonful; 4–11 mo, 12–17 lb, ½ teaspoonful; 12–23 mo, 18–23 lb, ¾ teaspoonful; 2–3 yr, 24–35 lb, 1 teaspoonful; 4–5 yr, 36–47 lb, 1½ teaspoonfuls; 6–8 yr, 48–59 lb, 2 teaspoonfuls; 9–10 yr, 60–71 lb, 2½ teaspoonfuls; 11–12 yr, 72–95 lb, 3 teaspoonfuls. May be repeated every 4 hours up to 5 times in a 24-hour period. May be administered alone or mixed with formula, milk, juice, cereal, etc.
Infant's PANADOL Drops: 0–4 mo, 6–11 lb, ½ dropperful (0.4 mL); 4–11 mo, 12–17 lb, 1 dropperful (0.8 mL); 12–23 mo, 18–23 lb, 1½ dropperfuls (1.2 mL); 2–3 yr, 24–35 lb, 2 dropperfuls (1.6 mL); 4–5 yr, 36–47 lb, 3 dropperfuls (2.4 mL); 6–8 yr, 48–59 lb, 4 dropperfuls (3.2 mL). May be repeated every 4 hours, up to 5 times in a 24-hour period. May be administered alone or mixed with formula, milk, juice, cereal, etc.

Warnings: Since Children's PANADOL Acetaminophen Chewable Tablets, Liquid, and Drops are available without a prescription as an analgesic/antipyretic, the following appears on the package labels: "WARNINGS: Do not take this product for more than 5 days. If symptoms persist or new ones occur, consult a physician. If fever persists for more than 3 days, or recurs, consult a physician. Keep this and *all* drugs out of the reach of children. In case of accidental overdose, seek professional assistance or contact a poison control center immediately. High fever, severe or persistent sore throat, cough, headache, nausea or vomiting may be serious; consult a physician."
Tamper Resistant: Children's PANADOL Acetaminophen Chewable Tablets packaging provides tamper-resistant features on both the outer carton and bottle. The following copy appears on the end

Continued on next page

This product information was effective as of November 1, 1991. Current information may be obtained directly from Sterling Health, by writing to 90 Park Avenue, New York, NY 10016.

Sterling Health—Cont.

flaps of this carton—"Purchase only if carton end flaps are sealed." "Use only if seal under bottle cap with white G/W print is intact. The outer carton of the liquid and drops contain the following copy: "Purchase only if overwrap printed with red Panda bears is intact."

Children's PANADOL Liquid and Drops provide tamper-resistant features on the carton. The following copy appears on the carton: "Purchase only if Red Tear Tape and Plastic Overwrap are intact," and bottle—"Use only if Carton Overwrap and Red Tear Tape Are Intact."

Composition:
Tablets: Active Ingredient: Acetaminophen. Inactive Ingredients: FD&C Red No. 28, FD&C Red No. 40, flavor, mannitol, saccharin sodium, starch, stearic acid and other ingredients.

Liquid: Active Ingredient: Acetaminophen. Inactive Ingredients: Benzoic acid, FD&C Red No. 40, flavor, glycerin, polyethylene glycol, potassium sorbate, propylene glycol, purified water, saccharin sodium, sorbitol solution. May also contain sodium chloride or sodium hydroxide.

Drops: Active Ingredient: Acetaminophen. Inactive Ingredients: Citric acid, FD&C Red No. 40, flavors, glycerin, parabens, polyethylene glycol, propylene glycol, purified water, saccharin sodium, sodium chloride, sodium citrate.

How Supplied: Chewable Tablets (colored pink and scored)—bottles of 30. Liquid (colored red)—bottles of 2 fl. oz. and 4 fl. oz. Drops (colored red)—bottles of ½ oz. (15 mL).

All packages listed above have child-resistant safety caps and tamper-resistant features.

Shown in Product Identification Section, page 430

Junior Strength PANADOL®

Description: Each Junior Strength PANADOL® Caplet contains 160 mg of acetaminophen.

Actions and Indications: Acetaminophen, the active ingredient in Junior Strength PANADOL®, is the analgesic/antipyretic most widely recommended by pediatricians for fast, effective relief of children's fevers. It also relieves the aches and pains of colds and flu, earaches, headaches, teething, immunizations, tonsillectomy, menstrual discomfort, and childhood illness.

Junior Strength PANADOL® Caplets are aspirin-free, sugar-free.

Usual Dosage: Dosing is based on single doses in the range of 10–15 mg/kg body weight. Doses may be repeated every 4 hours up to 4 or 5 times daily, but not to exceed 5 doses in 24 hours. To be administered to children under 2 years only on the advice of a physician.

2–3 yr, 24–35 lb, 1 caplet; 4–5 yr, 36–47 lb, 1½ caplets; 6–8 yr, 48–59 lb, 2 caplets; 9–10 yr, 60–71 lb, 2½ caplets; 11–12 yr,

72–95 lb, 3 caplets. Over 12 yr, 96 lb and over, 4 caplets. Dosage may be repeated every 4 hours, up to 5 times in a 24-hour period.

Inactive Ingredients: Hydroxypropyl methylcellulose, potassium sorbate, povidone, pregelatinized starch, starch, stearic acid, talc, triacetin.

Warnings: If symptoms persist or new ones occur, consult physician. If fever persists for more than 3 days, or recurs, consult a physician. Do not take this product for more than 5 days. Keep this and all drugs out of the reach of children. In case of accidental overdose, seek professional assistance or contact a poison control center immediately. As with any drug, if you are pregnant, or nursing a baby, seek the advice of a health professional before using this product.

How Supplied: Swallowable caplets (white)—blister-pack of 30. Package has child-resistant and tamper-resistant features.

Shown in Product Identification Section, page 430

Maximum Strength PANADOL® Tablets and Caplets

Active Ingredients: Each Maximum Strength PANADOL micro-thin coated tablet and caplet contains acetaminophen 500 mg.

Inactive Ingredients: Hydroxypropyl methylcellulose, potassium sorbate, povidone, pregelatinized starch, starch, stearic acid, talc, triacetin.

Actions: PANADOL acetaminophen has been clinically proven as a fast, effective analgesic (pain reliever) and antipyretic (fever reducer). PANADOL acetaminophen is a nonaspirin product designed to provide relief without stomach upset. Its patented micro-thin coating makes each 500 mg tablet or caplet easy to swallow.

Indications: For the temporary relief from pain of headaches, colds or flu, sinusitis, backaches, muscle aches, and menstrual discomfort. Also to reduce fever and for temporary relief of minor arthritis pain and toothache.

Precautions: If a rare sensitivity reaction occurs, the drug should be stopped. PANADOL acetaminophen has rarely been found to produce any side effects. It is usually well tolerated by aspirin-sensitive patients.

Severe recurrent pain or high continued fever may indicate a serious condition. Under these circumstances consult a physician.

Warnings: As with other products available without prescription, the following appears on the label of PANADOL acetaminophen: Do not give to children under 12 or use for more than 10 days unless directed by a physician. Keep this and all drugs out of the reach of children. In case of accidental overdose, seek

professional assistance or contact a poison control center immediately. As with any drug, if you are pregnant or nursing a baby, seek the advice of a health professional before using this product.

Usual Dosage: *Adults:* Two tablets or caplets every 4 hours as needed. Do not exceed 8 tablets or caplets in 24 hours unless directed by a physician.

Overdosage: In massive overdosage acetaminophen may cause hepatic toxicity in some patients. Clinical and laboratory evidence of overdosage may be delayed up to 7 days. Under circumstances of suspected overdose, contact your regional poison control center immediately.

How Supplied: Tablets and caplets (white, micro-thin coated, imprinted "PANADOL" and "500"). Tablets packaged in tamper-evident bottles of 30 and 60. Caplets packaged in tamper-evident bottles of 24.

Shown in Product Identification Section, page 430

PHILLIPS'® LAXCAPS®

Active Ingredients: A combination of phenolphthalein (90 mg) and docusate sodium (83 mg) per gelatin capsule.

Inactive Ingredients: FD&C Blue No. 1, Red No. 3, Red No. 40 and Yellow No. 6, gelatin, glycerin, PEG 400 and 3350, propylene glycol, sorbitol, and titanium dioxide.

Indications: For relief of occasional constipation (irregularity).

Action: Phenolphthalein is a stimulant laxative which increases the peristaltic activity of the intestine. Docusate sodium is a stool softener which allows easier passage of the stool. This product generally produces bowel movement in 6 to 12 hours.

Administration and Dosage: Adults and children 12 and over take one (1) or two (2) capsules daily with a full glass (8 oz) of liquid, or as directed by a physician. For children under 12, consult your physician.

Warnings: Do not take any laxative if abdominal pain, nausea, vomiting, change in bowel habits persisting for over 2 weeks, rectal bleeding or kidney disease is present. Laxative products should not be used for a period longer than one week, unless directed by a physician. If there is a failure to have a bowel movement after use, discontinue and consult your doctor. If a skin rash appears do not take this or any other preparation which contains phenolphthalein. Keep this and all drugs out of the reach of children. In case of accidental overdose, seek professional assistance or contact a Poison Control Center immediately. As with any drug, if you are pregnant or nursing a baby, seek the advice of a health professional before using this product.

How Supplied: Blister packs of 24's for safety:

Shown in Product Identification Section, page 430

PHILLIPS' ® MILK OF MAGNESIA

Active Ingredients: A suspension of magnesium hydroxide in purified water meeting all USP specifications. Phillips' Milk of Magnesia contains 400 mg per teaspoon (5 mL) of magnesium hydroxide.

Inactive Ingredients: Purified water, and for Mint Flavored Phillips' Milk of Magnesia only—flavor, mineral oil and saccharin sodium.

Indications: For relief of occasional constipation (irregularity), relief of acid indigestion, sour stomach and heartburn.

Action at Laxative Dosage: Phillips' Milk of Magnesia is a mild saline laxative which acts by drawing water into the gut, increasing intraluminal pressure, and increasing intestinal motility. This product generally produces bowel movement in ½ to 6 hours.
At Antacid Dosage: Phillips' Milk of Magnesia is an effective acid neutralizer.

Administration and Dosage: As a laxative, adults and children 12 years and older, 2–4 tbsp; children 6–11, 1–2 tbsp; children 2–5, 1–3 tsp followed by a full glass (8 oz) of liquid. Children under 2, consult a physician.
As an antacid, 1–3 tsp with a little water, up to four times a day, or as directed by your physician.

Cautions: Antacids may interact with certain prescription drugs. If you are taking a prescription drug do not take this product without checking with your physician.

Laxative Warnings: Do not take any laxative if abdominal pain, nausea, vomiting, change in bowel habits persisting for over 2 weeks, rectal bleeding, or kidney disease is present. Laxative products should not be used for a period longer than 1 week, unless directed by a doctor. If there is a failure to have a bowel movement after use, discontinue and consult your doctor.

Antacid Warnings: Do not take more than the maximum recommended daily dosage in a 24-hour period (see Directions), or use the maximum dosage of this product for more than two weeks, or use this product if you have kidney disease, except under the advice and supervision of a physician. May have laxative effect.

General Warnings: As with any drug, if you are pregnant or nursing a baby, seek the advice of a health professional before using this product. Keep this and all drugs out of reach of children. In case of accidental overdose, seek professional assistance or contact a poison control center immediately.

How Supplied: Phillips' Milk of Magnesia is available in regular and mint flavor in 4, 12 and 26 fl oz bottles.
Also available in tablet form and concentrated liquid form.

Shown in Product Identification Section, page 430

Concentrated PHILLIPS'® MILK OF MAGNESIA

Active Ingredients: A suspension of magnesium hydroxide in purified water meeting all USP specifications. Concentrated Phillips' Milk of Magnesia contains 800 mg per teaspoon (5 ml) of magnesium hydroxide.

Inactive Ingredients: Carboxymethylcellulose Sodium, Citric Acid, D&C Red #28 or FD&C Yellow #6, Flavor, Glycerin, Microcrystalline Cellulose, Propylene Glycol, Purified Water, Sorbitol, Sugar, Xanthan Gum.

Indications: For relief of occasional constipation (irregularity), relief of acid indigestion, sour stomach and heartburn.

Action at Laxative Dosage: Concentrated Phillips' Milk of Magnesia is a mild saline laxative which acts by drawing water into the gut, increasing intraluminal pressure, and increasing intestinal motility. This product generally produces bowel movement in ½ hour to 6 hours.
At Antacid Dosage: Concentrated Phillips' Milk of Magnesia is an effective acid neutralizer.

Laxative Warnings: Do not take any laxative if abdominal pain, nausea, vomiting, change in bowel habits (that persists for over two weeks), rectal bleeding, or kidney disease are present. Laxative products should not be used for a period longer than 1 week, unless directed by a physician. If there is a failure to have a bowel movement after use, discontinue and consult a doctor.

Antacid Warnings: Do not take more than the maximum recommended daily dosage in a 24 hour period (see directions), or use the maximum dosage of this product for more than two weeks, or use this product if you have kidney disease, except under the advice and supervision of a physician. May have laxative effect.

General Warnings: As with any drug, if you are pregnant or nursing a baby, seek the advice of a health professional before using this product. Keep this and all drugs out of reach of children. In case of accidental overdose seek professional assistance or contact a poison control center immediately.

Drug Interaction: Antacids may interact with certain prescription drugs. If you are presently taking a prescription drug, do not take this product without checking with your physician.

Dosage and Administration: As a laxative, adults and children 12 years and older, 1–2 tbsp.; children 6–11, ½–

---

1 tbsp.; children 2–5, ½ to 1½ tsp. followed by a full glass (8 oz.) of liquid. Children under 2, consult a physician.
As an antacid, adults and children 12 years and older, ½ to 1½ tsp. with a little water, up to four times a day or as directed by a physician.

How Supplied: Concentrated Phillips' Milk of Magnesia is available in strawberry creme and orange vanilla creme flavors in bottles of 8 fl. oz.

Shown in Product Identification Section, page 430

PHILLIPS'® MILK OF MAGNESIA TABLETS

Active Ingredients: Each Tablet contains 311 mg of magnesium hydroxide.

Inactive Ingredients: Flavor, starch, sucrose. Product description not USP.

Indications: For relief of acid indigestion, sour stomach, heartburn and occasional constipation (irregularity).

Action at Laxative Dosage: Phillips' Milk of Magnesia Tablets offer the same mild saline laxative ingredient as liquid Phillips' Milk of Magnesia in a convenient, chewable tablet form. It acts by drawing water into the gut, increasing intraluminal pressure, and increasing intestinal motility. This product generally produces bowel movement in ½ to 6 hours.
At Antacid Dosage: Phillips' Milk of Magnesia Tablets are effective acid neutralizers.

Administration and Dosage:
As an Antacid—Adults chew thoroughly 2 to 4 tablets up to 4 times a day. Children 7 to 14 years, 1 tablet up to 4 times a day or as directed by a physician.
As a Laxative—Adults and children 12 years of age and older chew thoroughly 6 to 8 tablets. Children 6 to 11, 3 to 4 tablets; children 2 to 5, 1 to 2 tablets, preferably before bedtime and follow with a full glass (8 oz) of liquid. Children under 2, consult a physician.

Laxative Warnings: Do not take any laxative if abdominal pain, nausea, vomiting, change in bowel habits (that persists for over 2 weeks), rectal bleeding, or kidney disease are present. Laxative products should not be used for a period longer than 1 week, unless directed by a doctor. If there is a failure to have a bowel movement after use, discontinue and consult your doctor.

Antacid Warnings: Do not take more than the maximum recommended daily dosage in a 24-hour period (see Directions), or use the maximum dosage of this

Continued on next page

This product information was effective as of November 1, 1991. Current information may be obtained directly from Sterling Health, by writing to 90 Park Avenue, New York, NY 10016.

Sterling Health—Cont.

product for more than two weeks, or use this product if you have kidney disease, except under the advice and supervision of a physician. May have laxative effect.

General Warnings: As with any drug, if you are pregnant or nursing a baby, seek the advice of a health professional before using this product. Keep this and *all* drugs out of reach of children. In case of accidental overdose, seek professional assistance or contact a poison control center immediately.

How Supplied: Phillips' Milk of Magnesia Tablets are available in a mint flavored chewable tablet in blister packs of 24, and bottles of 100 and 200.
Also available in liquid form.
Shown in Product Identification Section, page 430

---

pHisoDerm®
[fi-zo-derm]
Skin Cleanser and Conditioner

Description: pHisoDerm, a nonsoap emollient skin cleanser, is a unique liquid emulsion containing sodium octoxynol-2 ethane sulfonate solution, water, petrolatum, octoxynol-3, mineral oil (with lanolin alcohol and oleyl alcohol), cocamide MEA, imidazolidinyl urea, sodium benzoate, tetrasodium EDTA, and methylcellulose. Adjusted to normal skin pH with hydrochloric acid. Contains no hexachlorophene. pHisoDerm contains no soap, perfumes, or irritating alkali. Its pH value, unlike that of soap, lies within the pH range of normal skin. pHisoDerm Lightly Scented contains fragrance.

Actions: pHisoDerm is well tolerated and can be used frequently by those persons whose skin may be irritated by the use of soap or other alkaline cleansers, or by those who are sensitive to the fatty acids contained in soap. pHisoDerm contains an effective detergent for removing soil and acts as an active emulsifier of all types of oil—animal, vegetable, and mineral.
pHisoDerm produces suds when used with any kind of water—hard or soft, hot or cold (even cold seawater)—at any temperature and under acid, alkaline, or neutral conditions.
pHisoDerm deposits a fine film of lanolin components and petrolatum on the skin during the washing process and, thereby, helps protect against the dryness that soap can cause.

Indications: A sudsing emollient cleanser for use on skin of infants, children, and adults.
Useful for removal of ointments and cosmetics from the skin.

Directions: For external use only.
HANDS. Squeeze a few drops of pHisoDerm into the palm, add a little water, and work up a lather. Rinse thoroughly.
FACE. After washing your hands, squeeze a small amount of pHisoDerm

into the palm or onto a small sponge or washcloth, and work up a lather by adding a little water. Massage the suds onto the face for approximately one minute. Rinse thoroughly. Avoid getting suds into the eyes.
BATHING. First wet the body. Work a small amount of pHisoDerm into a lather with hands or a soft wet sponge, gradually adding small amounts of water to make more lather. Rinse thoroughly.

Caution: pHisoDerm suds that get into the eyes accidentally during washing should be rinsed out promptly with a sufficient amount of water.
pHisoDerm is intended for external use only. pHisoDerm should not be poured into measuring cups, medicine bottles, or similar containers since it may be mistaken for baby formula or medications. If swallowed, pHisoDerm may cause gastrointestinal irritation.
pHisoDerm should not be used on persons with sensitivity to any of its components.

How Supplied: pHisoDerm is supplied in three formulations: Regular Formula Unscented, Regular Formula Lightly Scented and Oily Skin Formula Unscented. It is packaged in sanitary squeeze bottles of 5 and 16 ounces. The Regular Unscented and Lightly Scented Formulas are also supplied in squeeze bottles of 9 ounces. The Regular Unscented is also available in bottles of 1 gallon.
Shown in Product Identification Section, page 430

---

pHisoDerm®
Cleansing Bar

Description: pHisoDerm Cleansing Bar, is a unique cleansing bar containing sodium tallowate, coconut oil, water, glycerin, petrolatum, lanolin, sodium chloride, BHT, trisodium HEDTA, and titanium dioxide.

Actions: pHisoDerm Cleansing Bar is formulated to clean thoroughly, removing dirt and oil. Special emollients leave skin feeling soft and smooth, not tight and dry. pHisoDerm Cleansing Bar contains no detergents or harsh ingredients which could irritate delicate skin.

Administration: Use every time you wash. First wet area to be washed. Using hands, sponge or washcloth, mix with water and work up a creamy lather. Massage the suds onto the area to be washed for approximately one minute. Rinse thoroughly. Avoid getting suds into the eyes.

Precautions: pHisoDerm Cleansing Bar suds that get into the eyes accidentally during washing should be rinsed out promptly with a sufficient amount of water. pHisoDerm Cleansing Bar is intended for external use only. It should not be used on persons with sensitivity to any of its components.

How Supplied: pHisoDerm Cleansing Bar is supplied in an Unscented and Lightly Scented formula. It is packaged

in specially coated cardboard cartons containing a 3.3 oz. bar.
Shown in Product Identification Section, page 430

---

pHisoDerm® FOR BABY
[fi 'zo-derm]
Skin Cleanser

Description: pHisoDerm FOR BABY, a nonsoap emollient skin cleanser, is a unique liquid emulsion containing sodium octoxynol-2 ethane sulfonate solution, water, petrolatum, octoxynol-3, mineral oil (with lanolin alcohol and oleyl alcohol), cocamide MEA, fragrance, imidazolidinyl urea, sodium benzoate, tetrasodium EDTA, and methylcellulose. Adjusted to normal skin pH with hydrochloric acid. Contains no hexachlorophene or irritating alkali. Its pH value, unlike that of soap, lies within the pH range of normal skin.

Actions: pHisoDerm FOR BABY gently cleans babies' delicate skin without irritating. Petrolatum and lanolin leave skin soft and smooth and protect against dryness.
pHisoDerm FOR BABY rinses easily without leaving a soapy film. The powder fragrance leaves skin smelling fresh and clean.

Precautions: pHisoDerm FOR BABY suds that get into babies' eyes accidentally during washing should be rinsed out promptly with a sufficient amount of water.
pHisoDerm FOR BABY is intended for external use only. It should not be poured into measuring cups, medicine bottles, or similar containers since it may be mistaken for baby formula or medications. If swallowed, pHisoDerm FOR BABY may cause gastrointestinal irritation.
pHisoDerm FOR BABY should not be used on babies with sensitivity to any of its components.

Administration: First wet the baby's body. Work a small amount of pHisoDerm FOR BABY into a lather with hands or a soft wet sponge, gradually adding small amounts of water to make more lather. Spread the lather over all parts of the baby's body, including the head. Avoid getting suds into the baby's eyes. Wash the diaper area last. Be sure to carefully cleanse all folds and creases. Rinse thoroughly. Pat the baby dry with a soft towel.

How Supplied: pHisoDerm FOR BABY is packaged in soft plastic, sanitary, squeeze bottles of 5 and 9 ounces and can be opened and closed with one hand.
Shown in Product Identification Section, page 430

---

pHisoPUFF®
[fi-zo-puf]
Nonmedicated Cleansing Sponge

Description: pHisoPUFF is a nonmedicated cleansing sponge with a special dual layer construction combining a white polyester fiber side and a green sponge side.

Actions: pHisoPUFF cleanses two ways: (1) white fiber side for extra thorough cleansing to gently remove the top layer of dead skin cells, free dirt, debris, and oil trapped in this layer and reveal new, fresh skin cells and (2) green sponge side works to cleanse and rinse skin clean. Using this side will help apply your cleanser or soap more evenly. Also good for removing eye makeup.

Precautions: Do not use pHisoPUFF fiber side on skin that is irritated, sunburned, windburned, damaged, broken, or infected. Do not use on skin which is prone to rashes or itching.

Administration: For the green sponge side: Wet pHisoPUFF with warm water, apply pHisoDerm® or another skin cleanser of your choice, and develop a lather. Glide sponge over your face up and down, back and forth, or in a circle; whatever is the easiest for you. Rinse face and dry.
For the white fiber side: Wet pHisoPUFF with warm water, apply pHisoDerm or another skin cleanser of your choice, and develop a lather. Try pHisoPUFF on the back of your hand before using it on your face. Experiment by changing the pressure and speed with which you move it. Now move pHisoPUFF gently and slowly over your face. Use no more than a few seconds on each area. You can move it in any direction, whichever comes natural to you. Rinse face and dry. As you use this fiber side more often, usage and pressure may be increased to best fit your skin sensitivity. Always rinse your pHisoPUFF thoroughly each time you use it. Hold under running water, let it drain, then give it a few quick shakes.

How Supplied: Box of 1 pHisoPUFF.
*Shown in Product Identification
Section, page 430*

STRI–DEX® DUAL TEXTURED PADS
Regular Strength
STRI–DEX® DUAL TEXTURED PADS
Maximum Strength
STRI–DEX® DUAL TEXTURED PADS
Sensitive Skin
STRI–DEX® SUPER SCRUB
Oil Fighting Formula

Active Ingredients:
Stri-Dex® Regular Strength: Salicylic acid 0.5%, SD alcohol 23% (w/w).
Stri-Dex® Maximum Strength: Salicylic acid 2.0%, SD alcohol 37% (w/w).
Stri-Dex® Sensitive Skin: Salicylic acid 0.5%, SD alcohol 23% (w/w).
Stri-Dex® Super Scrub: Salicylic acid 2.0%, SD alcohol 46% (w/w).

Inactive Ingredients:
Stri-Dex® Regular Strength: Citric acid, fragrance, menthol, purified water, simethicone emulsion, sodium carbonate, sodium dodecylbenzenesulfonate, sodium xylenesulfonate.

Stri-Dex® Maximum Strength: Ammonium xylenesulfonate, citric acid, fragrance, menthol, purified water, simethicone emulsion, sodium carbonate, sodium dodecylbenzenesulfonate.
Stri-Dex® Sensitive Skin: Aloe vera, citric acid, fragrance, menthol, purified water, simethicone emulsion, sodium carbonate, sodium dodecylbenzenesulfonate, sodium xylenesulfonate.
Stri-Dex® Super Scrub: Ammonium xylenesulfonate, citric acid, fragrance, menthol, purified water, simethicone emulsion, sodium carbonate, sodium lauroyl sarcosinate.

Indications: For the treatment of acne. Reduces the number of acne pimples and blackheads, and allows the skin to heal. Helps prevent new acne pimples from forming.

Directions: Cleanse the skin thoroughly before using Stri-Dex medicated pad. Use the deep cleaning textured side first to open pores and loosen the oil and dirt that can clog them. Then use the soothing soft side to wipe away oil and dirt and leave behind a tough pimple fighting medicine that will treat your pimples and help prevent new ones from forming. Use the pad to wipe the entire affected area one to three times daily. Because excessive drying of the skin may occur, start with one application daily, then gradually increase to two or three times daily if needed or as directed by a doctor. For Stri-Dex Super Scrub Pads cleanse the skin thoroughly before using.

Warnings: FOR EXTERNAL USE ONLY: Using other topical acne medications at the same time or immediately following use of this product may increase dryness or irritation of the skin. If this occurs, only one medication should be used unless directed by a doctor. Persons with very sensitive skin or known allergy to salicylic acid should not use this medication. If irritation or excessive dryness and/or peeling occurs, reduce frequency of use or dosage. If excessive itching, dryness, redness, or swelling occurs, discontinue use. If these symptoms persist, consult a physician promptly.
Keep away from eyes, lips, and other mucous membranes. Keep this and all drugs out of reach of children. In the case of accidental ingestion, seek professional assistance or contact a Poison Control Center immediately.

Dosage and Administration: See Labeling instructions for use. Stri-Dex Pads have never contained benzoyl peroxide.

How Supplied:
Stri-Dex Regular Strength is available in packages of 32 and 50 pads.
Stri-Dex Maximum Strength is available in packages of 32 and 50 pads.
Stri-Dex Sensitive Skin is available in a package of 32 pads.
Stri-Dex Super Scrub is available in a package of 32 pads.
*Shown in Product Identification
Section, page 431*

VANQUISH® Analgesic Caplets

Active Ingredients: Each caplet contains aspirin 227 mg, acetaminophen 194 mg, caffeine 33 mg, dried aluminum hydroxide gel 25 mg, magnesium hydroxide 50 mg.

Inactive Ingredients: Acacia, colloidal silicon dioxide, hydrogenated vegetable oil, microcrystalline cellulose, powdered cellulose, sodium lauryl sulfate, starch, talc.

Action and Uses: A buffered analgesic, antipyretic for relief of headache; muscular aches and pains; neuralgia and neuritic pain; toothache; pain following dental procedures; for painful discomforts and fever of colds and flu; sinusitis; functional menstrual pain, headache and pain due to cramps; temporary relief from minor pains of arthritis†, rheumatism, bursitis, lumbago, sciatica.

†Caution: If pain persists for more than 10 days, or redness is present or in conditions affecting children under 12 years of age, consult a physician immediately.

Warnings: Children and teenagers should not use this medicine for chicken pox or flu symptoms before a doctor is consulted about Reye syndrome, a rare but serious illness reported to be associated with aspirin. Keep this and all drugs out of the reach of children. In case of accidental overdose, seek professional assistance or contact a poison control center immediately. As with any drug, if you are pregnant or nursing a baby, seek the advice of a health professional before using this product. IT IS ESPECIALLY IMPORTANT NOT TO USE ASPIRIN DURING THE LAST THREE MONTHS OF PREGNANCY UNLESS SPECIFICALLY DIRECTED TO DO SO BY A DOCTOR BECAUSE IT MAY CAUSE PROBLEMS IN THE UNBORN CHILD OR COMPLICATIONS DURING DELIVERY.
IMPORTANT NOTICE: Do not take this product if you are allergic to aspirin, have asthma, stomach problems that persist or recur, gastric ulcers or bleeding, or if you are taking a prescription drug for arthritis, anticoagulation (thinning of the blood), diabetes, or gout unless directed by a doctor. If ringing in the ears or loss of hearing occurs, consult a doctor before taking any more of this product.

Usual Adult Dosage: Two caplets with water. May be repeated every four hours if necessary up to 12 tablets per day. Larger or more frequent doses may be prescribed by physician if necessary.

Contraindications: Hypersensitivity to salicylates and acetaminophen. (To be

Continued on next page

This product information was effective as of November 1, 1991. Current information may be obtained directly from Sterling Health, by writing to 90 Park Avenue, New York, NY 10016.

Sterling Health—Cont.

used with caution during anticoagulant therapy or in asthmatic patients).

How Supplied:
White, capsule-shaped caplets in bottles of 30, 60 and 100 caplets.
Shown in Product Identification Section, page 431

WinGel®
[win 'jel]
Liquid Antacid

Description: Each teaspoon (5 mL) of liquid contains a specially processed, short polymer, hexitol-stabilized aluminum-magnesium hydroxide equivalent to 180 mg of aluminum hydroxide and 160 mg of magnesium hydroxide. Also contains: benzoic acid, flavor, methylcellulose, purified water, red ferric oxide, saccharin sodium, sodium hypochlorite solution, sorbitol solution.

Action: Antacid.

Indications: An antacid for the relief of acid indigestion, heartburn, and sour stomach. Nonconstipating. For the symptomatic relief of hyperacidity associated with the diagnosis of peptic ulcer, gastritis, peptic esophagitis, gastric hyperacidity, and hiatal hernia.

Warnings: *Adults and children over 6* —Patients should not take more than eight teaspoonfuls in a 24-hour period or use the maximum dosage of the product for more than 2 weeks, except under the advice and supervision of a physician. Keep this and all drugs out of the reach of children. In case of accidental overdose, seek professional assistance or contact a poison control center immediately.

Drug Interaction Precautions: Antacids may react with certain prescription drugs. Do not take this product if you are presently taking a prescription antibiotic drug containing any form of tetracycline. If the patient is presently taking a prescription drug, this product should not be taken without checking with the physician.

Dosage and Administration: *Adults and children over 6* —1 to 2 teaspoonfuls up to four times daily, or as directed by a physician.
Acid Neutralization: The acid neutralization capacity of WinGel liquid is not less than 10 mEq/5 ml.

How Supplied: WinGel liquid is supplied in a 12 fl oz bottle.

Products are indexed by
generic and chemical names
in the
YELLOW SECTION.

Stuart Pharmaceuticals
a business unit of
ICI Americas Inc.
WILMINGTON, DE 19897 USA

HIBICLENS® Antiseptic/
Antimicrobial
[hi 'bi-klenz]
Skin Cleanser
(chlorhexidine gluconate)

Description: HIBICLENS is an antiseptic antimicrobial skin cleanser possessing bactericidal activities. HIBICLENS contains 4% w/v HIBITANE® (chlorhexidine gluconate), a chemically unique hexamethylenebis biguanide with inactive ingredients: fragrance, isopropyl alcohol 4%, purified water, Red 40, and other ingredients, in a mild, sudsing base adjusted to pH 5.0–6.5 for optimal activity and stability as well as compatability with the normal pH of the skin.

Action: HIBICLENS is bactericidal on contact. It has antiseptic activity and a persistent antimicrobial effect with rapid bactericidal activity against a wide range of microorganisms, including gram-positive bacteria, and gram-negative bacteria such as *Pseudomonas aeruginosa*. The effectiveness of HIBICLENS is not significantly reduced by the presence of organic matter, such as blood.[1]
In a study[2] simulating surgical use, the immediate bactericidal effect of HIBICLENS after a single six-minute scrub resulted in a 99.9% reduction in resident bacterial flora, with a reduction of 99.98% after the eleventh scrub. Reductions on surgically gloved hands were maintained over the six-hour test period.
HIBICLENS displays persistent antimicrobial action. In one study,[2] 93% of a radiolabeled formulation of HIBICLENS remained present on uncovered skin after five hours.
HIBICLENS prevents skin infection thereby reducing the risk of cross-infection.

Indications: HIBICLENS is indicated for use as a surgical scrub, as a health-care personnel handwash, for patient preoperative showering and bathing, as a patient preoperative skin preparation, and as a skin wound cleanser and general skin cleanser.

Safety: The extensive use of chlorhexidine gluconate for over 20 years outside the United States has produced no evidence of absorption of the compound through intact skin. The potential for producing skin reactions is extremely low. HIBICLENS can be used many times a day without causing irritation, dryness, or discomfort. Experimental studies indicate that when used for cleaning superficial wounds, HIBICLENS will neither cause additional tissue injury nor delay healing.

WARNINGS: FOR EXTERNAL USE ONLY. KEEP OUT OF EYES, EARS AND MOUTH. HIBICLENS SHOULD NOT BE USED AS A PREOPERATIVE SKIN PREPARATION OF THE FACE OR HEAD. MISUSE OF HIBICLENS HAS BEEN REPORTED TO CAUSE SERIOUS AND PERMANENT EYE INJURY WHEN IT HAS BEEN PERMITTED TO ENTER AND REMAIN IN THE EYE DURING SURGICAL PROCEDURES. IF HIBICLENS SHOULD CONTACT THESE AREAS, RINSE OUT PROMPTLY AND THOROUGHLY WITH WATER. Avoid contact with meninges. HIBICLENS should not be used by persons who have a sensitivity to it or its components. Chlorhexidine gluconate has been reported to cause deafness when instilled in the middle ear through perforated ear drums. Irritation, sensitization and generalized allergic reactions have been reported with chlorhexidine-containing products, especially in the genital areas. If adverse reactions occur, discontinue use immediately and if severe, contact a physician. Keep this and all drugs out of the reach of children. In case of accidental ingestion, seek professional assistance or contact a Poison Control Center immediately.
Accidental ingestion: Chlorhexidine gluconate taken orally is poorly absorbed. Treat with gastric lavage using milk, egg white, gelatin or mild soap. Employ supportive measures as appropriate. Avoid excessive heat (above 104°F).

DIRECTIONS FOR USE:
Patient preoperative skin preparation:
Apply HIBICLENS liberally to surgical site and swab for at least two minutes. Dry with a sterile towel. Repeat procedure for an additional two minutes and dry with a sterile towel.
Preoperative showering and whole-body bathing
The patient should be instructed to wash the entire body, including the scalp, on two consecutive occasions immediately prior to surgery. Each procedure should consist of two consecutive thorough applications of HIBICLENS followed by thorough rinsing. If the patient's condition allows, showering is recommended for whole-body bathing. The recommended procedure is: Wet the body, including hair. Wash the hair using 25 mL of HIBICLENS and the body with another 25 mL of HIBICLENS. Rinse. Repeat. Rinse thoroughly after second application.
Skin wound and general skin cleansing:
Wounds which involve more than the superficial layers of the skin should not be routinely treated with HIBICLENS. HIBICLENS should not be used for repeated general skin cleansing of large body areas except in those patients whose underlying skin condition makes it necessary to reduce the bacterial population of the skin. To use, thoroughly rinse the area to be cleansed with water. Apply the minimum amount of HIBICLENS necessary to cover the skin or wound area and wash gently. Rinse again thoroughly.

Health-care personnel use
Surgical Hand Scrub
Directions for use of HIBICLENS Liquid: Wet hands and forearms to the elbows with warm water. (Avoid using very cold or very hot water.) Dispense about 5 mL of HIBICLENS into cupped hands. Spread over both hands. Scrub hands and forearms for 3 minutes without adding water, using a brush or sponge. (Avoid using extremely hard-bristled brushes.) While scrubbing, pay particular attention to fingernails, cuticles, and interdigital spaces. (Do not use excessive pressure to produce additional lather.) Rinse thoroughly with warm water. Dispense about 5 mL of HIBICLENS into cupped hands. Wash for an additional 3 minutes. (No need to use brush or sponge.) Then rinse thoroughly. Dry thoroughly.

Hand Wash:
Wet hands with water. (Avoid using very cold or very hot water.) Dispense about 5 mL of HIBICLENS into cupped hands. Wash for 15 seconds. (Do not use excessive pressure to produce additional lather.) Rinse thoroughly with warm water. Dry thoroughly.

Directions for use of HIBICLENS® Sponge/Brush: Open package and remove nail cleaner. Wet hands. Use nail cleaner under fingernails and to clean cuticles. Wet hands and forearms to the elbow with warm water. (Avoid using very cold or very hot water.) Wet sponge side of sponge/brush. Squeeze and pump immediately to work up adequate lather. Apply lather to hands and forearms using *sponge* side of the product. *Start 3 minute scrub* by using the brush side of the product to scrub *only* nails, cuticles, and interdigital areas. Use sponge side for scrubbing hands and forearms. (Avoid using brush on these more sensitive areas.) Rinse thoroughly with warm water. Scrub for an additional 3 minutes *using sponge side* only. To produce additional lather, add a small amount of water and pump the sponge. (While scrubbing, do not use excessive pressure to produce lather—a small amount of lather is all that is required to adequately cleanse skin with HIBICLENS.) Rinse and dry thoroughly, blotting hands and forearms with a soft sterile towel.

IMPORTANT LAUNDERING ADVICE FOR HOSPITAL STAFF AND OTHER USERS OF ANTISEPTIC PATIENT SKIN PREPARATIONS CONTAINING CHLORHEXIDINE GLUCONATE
Chlorhexidine gluconate is a unique agent that most closely fits the definition of an ideal antimicrobial agent, having (among others) one of the most important characteristics of persistent activity. This persistence is due to chlorhexidine gluconate binding to the protein of the skin and, thus, being available for residual activity over a relatively long period of time.
Chlorhexidine gluconate, however, binds not only to protein of the skin, but also to many fabrics, particularly cotton. Thus, special laundering procedures should be considered when such products contact these fabrics. As a result of such contact, chlorhexidine gluconate may become adsorbed onto the fabric and not be removed by washing. If sufficient available chlorine is present during the washing procedure, a fast brown stain may develop due to a chemical reaction between chlorhexidine gluconate and chlorine.

SUGGESTED LAUNDERING PROCEDURES TO LIMIT STAINING
1. **Not Aging.** Avoid allowing the product to age (set) on unwashed linens.
2. **Flushing and Washing.** A flush operation as the initial step in the wash process is helpful in the laundering of linen exposed to chlorhexidine gluconate. Such flushing is also important in the laundering of linen which contains organic materials such as blood or pus. For best results, warm water flushes (90°–100°F) are recommended. After a number of initial flushings followed by a washing with a low alkaline/nonchlorine detergent, most articles which come in contact with chlorhexidine gluconate should have an acceptable level of whiteness. If a rewash process using bleach is necessary to achieve a greater degree of whiteness, the bleach used should be a nonchlorine bleach.
3. **Not Using Chlorine Bleach.** Modern laundering methods often make the use of chlorine bleach unnecessary. It is worthwhile trying to wash without chlorine to ascertain if the resulting degree of whiteness is acceptable. Omission of chlorine from the laundering process can extend the useful life of cotton articles since oxidizing bleaches such as chlorine may cause some damage to cellulose even when used in low concentration.
4. **Changing to a Peroxide-Type Bleach, Such as Sodium Perborate, Sodium Percarbonate or Hydrogen Peroxide.** This should eliminate the reaction which could occur with the use of chlorine bleaches. If a chlorine bleach must be used, a concentration of less than 7 ppm available chlorine ($\frac{1}{10}$ the normal bleach level) is suggested to minimize possible staining.

A NOTE ON LAUNDERING OF PERSONAL CLOTHING
The laundering procedures set forth above using low alkaline, nonchlorinated laundry detergents are also applicable to laundering of uniforms and lab coats.

Commercially available laundry detergents which do not contain chlorine include Borax, Borateem, Dreft, Oxydol, and Ivory Snow. These products, however, will not remove stains previously set into the fabric.

RECLAMATION OF STAINED LINENS
For those linens which previously have been stained due to the chemical reaction between chlorhexidine gluconate and chlorine, the following laundering procedure may be helpful in reducing the visible stain:
[See table above.]

How Supplied: *For general handwashing locations:* pocket-size, 15 mL foil Packettes; plastic disposable bottles of 4 oz and 8 oz with dispenser caps; and 16 oz filled globes. *For surgical scrub areas:* disposable, unit-of-use 22 mL impregnated Sponge/Brushes with nail cleaner; plastic disposable bottles of 32 oz and 1 gal. The 32-oz bottle is designed for a special foot-operated wall dispenser. A hand-operated wall dispenser is available for the 16-oz globe. Hand pumps are available for 16 oz, 32 oz, and 1 gal sizes.
Liquid NDC 0038-0575.
Sponge/Brush NDC 0038-0577.

References:
1. Lowbury EJL, and Lilly HA: The effect of blood on disinfection of surgeons' hands, Brit. J. Surg. 61:19–21 (Jan.) 1974.
2. Peterson AF, Rosenberg A, Alatary SD: Comparative evaluation of surgical scrub preparations, Surg. Gynecol. Obstet. 146:63–65 (Jan.) 1978.

Stuart Pharmaceuticals
A business unit of ICI Americas Inc.
Wilmington, DE 19897 USA
Shown in Product Identification Section, page 431

HIBISTAT®
Germicidal Hand Rinse
HIBISTAT® TOWELETTE
Germicidal Hand Wipe
[*hi'bi-stat*]
(chlorhexidine gluconate)

Description: HIBISTAT is a germicidal hand rinse which provides rapid bactericidal action and has a persistent antimicrobial effect against a wide range of microorganisms. HIBISTAT is a clear,

Continued on next page

Operation	Water Level	Temperature	Time (Min)	Supplies/ 100 lb
Break	Low	180°F	20	1.5 lb oxalic acid
Flush	High	Cold	1	—
Emulsify	Low	160°F	5	18 oz emulsifier
Flush	High	Cold	1	—
Bleach	Low	180°F	20	2 lb alkali builder and 1 lb organic bleach
Rinse	High	Cold	1	
Antichlor	High	Cold	2	4 oz antichlor
Rinse	High	Cold	1	—
Rinse	High	Cold	1	—
Sour	Low	Cold	4	2 oz rust removing sour

Stuart—Cont.

colorless liquid containing 0.5% w/w HIBITANE® (chlorhexidine gluconate) with inactive ingredients: emollients, isopropanol 70%, purified water.

Indications: HIBISTAT is indicated for health-care personnel use as a germicidal hand rinse. HIBISTAT is for hand hygiene on physically clean hands. It is used in those situations where hands are physically clean, but in need of degerming, when routine handwashing is not convenient or desirable. HIBISTAT provides rapid germicidal action and has a persistent effect.
HIBISTAT should be used in-between patients and procedures where there are no sinks available or continued return to the sink area is inconvenient. HIBISTAT can be used as an alternative to detergent-based products when hands are physically clean. Also, HIBISTAT is an effective germicidal hand rinse following a soap and water handwash.

Warning: Flammable. This product is alcohol based. Alcohol is extremely flammable. It should be kept away from flame or devices which may generate an electrical spark.

FOR EXTERNAL USE ONLY. KEEP OUT OF EYES, EARS AND MOUTH. HIBISTAT SHOULD NOT BE USED AS A PREOPERATIVE SKIN PREPARATION OF THE FACE OR HEAD. MISUSE OF CHLORHEXIDINE-CONTAINING PRODUCTS HAS BEEN REPORTED TO CAUSE SERIOUS AND PERMANENT EYE INJURY WHEN IT HAS BEEN PERMITTED TO ENTER AND REMAIN IN THE EYE DURING SURGICAL PROCEDURES. IF HIBISTAT SHOULD CONTACT THESE AREAS, RINSE OUT PROMPTLY AND THOROUGHLY WITH WATER. Avoid contact with meninges. HIBISTAT should not be used by persons who have a sensitivity to it or its components. Chlorhexidine gluconate has been reported to cause deafness when instilled in the middle ear through perforated ear drums. Irritation, sensitization and generalized allergic reactions have been reported with chlorhexidine-containing products, especially in the genital areas. If adverse reactions occur, discontinue use immediately and if severe, contact a physician. Keep this and all drugs out of the reach of children. In case of accidental ingestion, seek professional assistance or contact a Poison Control Center immediately.
Avoid excessive heat (above 104°F).
Accidental ingestion: Chlorhexidine gluconate taken orally is poorly absorbed. Treat with gastric lavage using milk, egg white, gelatin or mild soap avoiding pulmonary aspiration. Do not use apomorphine. Assist respiration if necessary and keep patient warm. Intravenous levulose can accelerate alcohol metabolism. In severe cases, hemodialysis or peritoneal dialysis may be appropriate.

DIRECTIONS FOR USE: HIBISTAT Towelette: Rub hands vigorously with the HIBISTAT Towelette for approximately 15 seconds, paying particular attention to nails and interdigital spaces. HIBISTAT dries rapidly in use. No water or towel drying is necessary. The emollients contained in the HIBISTAT Towelette protect the hands from the potential drying effect of alcohol.
HIBISTAT Liquid: Dispense about 5 mL of HIBISTAT into cupped hands and rub vigorously until dry (about 15 seconds), paying particular attention to nails and interdigital spaces. HIBISTAT dries rapidly in use. No water or toweling are necessary. The emollients contained in HIBISTAT protect the hands from the potential drying effect of alcohol.
Laundering: Chlorhexidine gluconate chemically reacts with chlorine to form a brown stain on fabric. Fabric which has come in contact with chlorhexidine gluconate should be rinsed well and washed without the addition of chlorine products. If bleach is desired, only non-chlorine bleach should be used. Full laundering instructions are packed with each case of HIBISTAT. (Please see HIBICLENS® for full laundering instructions.)

How Supplied: In plastic disposable bottles of 4 oz and 8 oz with flip-top cap, and in disposable towelettes containing 5 mL, packaged 50 towelettes to a carton.
NDC 0038-0585 (bottles)
NDC 0038-0587 (towelettes)
Stuart Pharmaceuticals
A business unit of ICI Americas Inc.
Wilmington, Delaware 19897 USA

STUART PRENATAL® Tablets
Multivitamin/Multimineral
Supplement

One Tablet Daily Provides

VITAMINS	RDA*	
A	90%	4,000 IU
D	100%	400 IU
E	90%	11 mg
C	110%	100 mg
Folic Acid	200%	0.8 mg
B₁ (thiamin)	90%	1.5 mg
B₂ (riboflavin)	90%	1.7 mg
Niacin	90%	18 mg
B₆ (pyridoxine hydrochloride)	120%	2.6 mg
B₁₂ (cyanocobalamin)	150%	4 mcg

MINERALS	RDA*	
Calcium	20%	200 mg
Iron	200%**	60 mg
Zinc	130%	25 mg

*Recommended Dietary Allowances (Food and Nutrition Board, NAS/NRC-1989) for pregnant and/or lactating women.

Ingredients
Active: calcium sulfate, ferrous fumarate, ascorbic acid, dl-alpha tocopheryl acetate, zinc oxide, niacinamide, vitamin A acetate, pyridoxine hydrochloride, riboflavin, thiamin mononitrate, folic acid, cholecalciferol, cyanocobalamin. Inactive: croscarmellose sodium, hydroxypropyl methylcellulose, microcrystalline cellulose, pregelatinized starch, red iron oxide, titanium dioxide.

Indications: STUART PRENATAL is a nonprescription multivitamin/multimineral supplement for use before, during, and after pregnancy. It provides essential vitamins and minerals, including 60 mg of elemental iron as well-tolerated ferrous fumarate, and 200 mg of elemental calcium (nonalkalizing and phosphorus-free), and 25 mg zinc. STUART PRENATAL also contains 0.8 mg folic acid.

Directions: Before, during and after pregnancy, one tablet daily, or as directed by a physician.

Warning: In case of accidental overdose, seek professional assistance or contact a Poison Control Center immediately. Keep out of the reach of children.

How Supplied: Bottles of 100 light pink tablets imprinted "STUART 071". A child-resistant safety cap is standard on 100 tablet bottles as a safeguard against accidental ingestion by children. NDC 0038-0071.
Shown in Product Identification Section, page 431

Sublingual Products International, Inc.
1229 WEST CORPORATE DRIVE
ARLINGTON, TX 76006

SUBLINGUAL B–TOTAL™
[seb-lin-g(ye-)wel]

Composition: Each 1.0 mL supplies:

		% U.S. RDA
Vitamin C (ascorbic acid)	60 mg	100%
Vitamin B₁ (thiamin)	1.5 mg	100%
Vitamin B₂ (riboflavin)	1.7 mg	100%
Vitamin B₃ (niacin)	20 mg	100%
Vitamin B₆ (pyridoxine HCL)	2.0 mg	100%
Vitamin B₁₂ (cyanocobalamin)	1,000 mcg	16,666%
Vitamin B₅ (pantothenic acid)	30 mg	300%

Administration and Dosage: As a dietary supplement, drop under the tongue with calibrated dose dropper, hold for 30 seconds and then swallow. **Dose:** 1.0 mL daily or as indicated.

How Supplied: Available in a 30 mL (1 mo. supply) bottle. It is also available to doctors and pharmacists in full-size packages.
Shown in Product Identification Section, page 431

SUBLINGUAL C WITH NIACIN™
[seb-lin-g(ye-)wel]

Composition: Each 1.0 mL supplies:

		% U.S. RDA
Vitamin C .... (ascorbic acid)	180 mg	300%
Vitamin B₃ .... (niacin)	20 mg	100%

Administration and Dosage: As a dietary supplement, drop under the tongue with calibrated dose dropper, hold for 30 seconds and then swallow. **Dose:** 1.0 mL daily or as indicated.

How Supplied: Available in a 30 mL (1 mo. supply) bottle. It is also available to doctors and pharmacists in full-size packages.

SUBLINGUAL ZINC™
[seb-lin-g(ye-)wel]

Composition: Each 1.0 mL supplies:

		% U.S. RDA
Zinc .... (Complex Zinc Carbonates)	15 mg	100%

Administration and Dosage: As a dietary supplement, drop under the tongue with calibrated dose dropper, hold for 30 seconds and then swallow. **Dose:** 1.0 mL daily or as indicated.

How Supplied: Available in a 30 mL (1 mo. supply) bottle. It is also available to doctors and pharmacists in full-size packages.

EDUCATIONAL MATERIAL

Samples and clinical information are available to physicians and pharmacists on request.
Patient Brochure—"Why Liquid Sublingual?"

IDENTIFICATION PROBLEM?
Consult the
Product Identification Section
where you'll find
products pictured
in full color.

Syntex Laboratories, Inc
**3401 HILLVIEW AVENUE
PALO ALTO, CA 94304**

CARMOL® 10
10% urea lotion
for total body
dry skin care.

Active Ingredient: Urea 10% in a scented lotion of purified water, carbomer 940, cetyl alcohol, isopropyl palmitate, PEG-8 dioleate, PEG-8 distearate, propylene glycol, propylene glycol dipelargonate, stearic acid, sodium laureth sulfate, trolamine, and xanthan gum.

Indications: For total body dry skin care.

Actions: Keratolytic CARMOL 10 is non-occlusive, contains no mineral oil or petrolatum. CARMOL 10 is hypoallergenic; contains no lanolin, parabens or other preservatives.

Precautions: For external use only. Discontinue use if irritation occurs. Keep out of the reach of children. In case of accidental ingestion, seek professional assistance or contact a poison control center immediately.

Dosage and Administration: Rub in gently on hands, face or body. Repeat as necessary.

How Supplied: 6 fl. oz. bottle.

CARMOL® 20
20% Urea Cream
Extra strength for
rough, dry skin

Active Ingredients: Urea 20% in a non-lipid vanishing cream containing carbomer 940, hypoallergenic fragrance, isopropyl myristate, isopropyl palmitate, propylene glycol, purified water, sodium laureth sulfate, stearic acid, trolamine, xanthan gum.

Indications: Especially useful on rough, dry skin of hands, elbows, knees and feet.

Actions: Keratolytic. Contains no parabens, lanolin or mineral oil.

Precautions: For external use only. Keep away from eyes. Use with caution on face or broken or inflamed skin; transient stinging may occur. Discontinue use if irritation occurs. Keep out of the reach of children. In case of accidental ingestion, seek professional assistance or contact a poison control center immediately.

Dosage and Administration: Apply once or twice daily or as directed. Rub in well.

How Supplied: 3 oz. tubes, 1 lb. jars.

Thompson Medical Company, Inc.
**222 LAKEVIEW AVENUE
WEST PALM BEACH
FLORIDA 33401**

ASPERCREME®
[ăs-per-crēme]
External Analgesic Rub

Description: ASPERCREME® is available as an odor-free creme and lotion for use as a topical massage rub that temporarily relieves minor muscle aches and pains without stomach upset.
Aspercreme does not contain aspirin.

Active Ingredients: Salycin® 10% (Thompson Medical's brand of Trolamine Salicylate).

Other Ingredients: <u>Creme:</u> Cetyl Alcohol, Glycerin, Methylparaben, Mineral Oil, Potassium Phosphate, Propylparaben, Stearic Acid, Triethanolamine, Water. <u>Lotion:</u> Cetyl Alcohol, Fragrance, Glyceryl Stearate, Isopropyl Palmitate, Lanolin, Methylparaben, Potassium Phosphate, Propylene Glycol, Propylparaben, Sodium Lauryl Sulfate, Stearic Acid, Water.

Actions: External analgesic rub.

Indications: Analgesic rub for temporary relief of minor aches and pains of muscles associated with simple strains and sprains. **Aspercreme contains no aspirin.**

Warnings: Use only as directed. If prone to allergic reaction from aspirin or salicylate, consult your doctor before using. If redness is present or condition worsens, or if pain persists for more than 7 days or clears up and occurs again within a few days, discontinue use and consult a doctor. Do not use on children under 10 years of age. Do not apply if skin is irritated or if irritation develops. As with any drug, if you are pregnant or nursing a baby, seek the advice of a health professional before using this product. For external use only. Avoid contact with eyes. Keep this and all medicines out of the reach of children. In case of accidental ingestion seek professional assistance or contact a Poison Control Center immediately.

Dosage and Administration: Apply generously directly to affected area. Massage into painful area until thoroughly absorbed into skin, repeat as necessary, especially before retiring but not more than 4 times daily.

How to Store: Store at controlled room temperature 59°–86°F (15°–30°C).

How Supplied: Creme: 1¼ oz., 3 oz. and 5 oz. tubes. Lotion: 6 oz. bottle.

CORTIZONE-5®
Creme, Ointment, and Wipes
Anti-itch
(0.5% hydrocortisone)

Description: CORTIZONE-5® creme, ointment, and wipes are topical anti-itch preparations.

Continued on next page

Thompson Medical—Cont.

Active Ingredient: Hydrocortisone 0.5%.

Other Ingredients: Creme: Aluminum Sulfate, Calcium Acetate, Glycerin, Light Mineral Oil, Methylparaben, Potato Dextrin, Purified Water, Sodium Lauryl Sulfate, White Petroleum. May Also Contain: Cetearyl Alcohol, Propylparaben, Sodium C$_{12-15}$ Alcohols Sulfate, Synthetic Beeswax, White Wax. Ointment: White Petrolatum. Wipes: Methylparaben, Octoxynol 9, Propylene Glycol, Propylparaben, Purified Water.

Indications: CORTIZONE-5® is recommended for the temporary relief of itching associated with minor skin irritations, inflammations and rashes due to: eczema, insect bites, poison ivy, oak, sumac, soaps, detergents, cosmetics, jewelry, seborrheic dermatitis, psoriasis, external anal and genital itching. Other uses of this product should be only under the advice and supervision of a physician.

Warnings: For external use only. Avoid contact with the eyes. If condition worsens, or if symptoms persist for more than 7 days or clear up and occur again within a few days, stop use of this product and do not begin use of any hydrocortisone product unless you have consulted a physician. Do not use in genital area if you have a vaginal discharge. Consult a physician. Do not use for the treatment of diaper rash. Consult a physician. Warnings For External Anal Itching Users: Do not exceed the recommended daily dosage unless directed by a physician. In case of bleeding, consult a physician promptly. Do not put this product into the rectum by using fingers or any mechanical device or applicator. KEEP THIS AND ALL MEDICINES OUT OF THE REACH OF CHILDREN. In case of accidental ingestion, seek professional assistance or contact a poison control center immediately.

Dosage and Administration: Adults and children 2 years of age and older: Apply to affected area not more than 3 to 4 times daily. Children under 2 years of age: Do not use, consult a physician. Directions For External Anal Itching Users: Adults: When practical, cleanse the affected area with mild soap and warm water and rinse thoroughly. Gently dry by patting or blotting with toilet tissue or a soft cloth before application of this product. Children under 12 years of age: Consult a physician.

How to Store: Store at room temperature.

How Supplied: CORTIZONE-5 creme: 1 oz. and 2 oz. tubes. CORTIZONE-5 ointment: 1 oz. tube. CORTIZONE-5 wipes: carton containing 14 individual packets.

Shown in Product Identification Section, page 431

CORTIZONE-10™
Creme and Ointment
Anti-itch
(1.0% hydrocortisone)

Description: CORTIZONE-10™ creme and ointment are topical anti-itch preparations.

Active Ingredient: Hydrocortisone 1.0%.

Other Ingredients: Creme: Aluminum Sulfate, Calcium Acetate, Cetearyl Alcohol, Glycerin, Light Mineral Oil, Methylparaben, Potato Dextrin, Sodium Lauryl Sulfate, Water, White Petroleum, White Wax. May Also Contain: Sodium C12–15 Alcohols Sulfate, Propylparaben. Ointment: White Petrolatum.

Indications: Cortizone-10™ is recommended for the temporary relief of itching associated with minor skin irritations, inflammation and rashes due to: eczema, insect bites, poison ivy, oak, sumac, soaps, detergents, cosmetics, jewelry, seborrheic dermatitis, psoriasis, external anal and genital itching. Other uses of this product should be only under the advice and supervision of a physician.

Warnings: For external use only. Avoid contact with the eyes. If condition worsens, or if symptoms persist for more than 7 days or clear up and occur again within a few days, stop use of this product and do not begin use of any hydrocortisone product unless you have consulted a physician. Do not use in genital area if you have a vaginal discharge. Consult a physician. Do not use for the treatment of diaper rash. Consult a physician. **Warnings For External Anal Itching Users:** Do not exceed the recommended daily dosage unless directed by a physician. In case of bleeding, consult a physician promptly. Do not put this product into the rectum by using fingers or any mechanical device or applicator. KEEP THIS AND ALL MEDICINES OUT OF THE REACH OF CHILDREN. In case of accidental ingestion, seek professional assistance or contact a poison control center immediately.

Dosage and Administration: Adults and children 2 years of age and older: Apply to affected area not more than 3 to 4 times daily. Children under 2 years of age: Do not use, consult a physician.

Directions For External Anal Itching Users: Adults: When practical, cleanse the affected area with mild soap and warm water and rinse thoroughly. Gently dry by patting or blotting with toilet tissue or a soft cloth before application of this product. Children under 12 years of age: consult a physician.

How to Store: Store at room temperature.

How Supplied: CORTIZONE-10 creme: 1 oz. and 2 oz. tubes. CORTIZONE-10 ointment: 1 oz. tube.

DEXATRIM® Capsules, Caplets, and Tablets
[dĕx-a-trĭm]
Prolonged action anorectic for weight control

DEXATRIM® Maximum Strength Plus Vitamin C/Caffeine-Free Capsules and Caffeine-Free Capsules phenylpropanolamine HCl   75mg (time release) (180 mg Vitamin C, immediate release, added for nutritional supplementation)

DEXATRIM® Maximum Strength Plus Vitamin C/Caffeine-Free Caplets and Caffeine-Free Caplets phenylpropanolamine HCl   75mg (time release) (180 mg Vitamin C, immediate release, added for nutritional supplementation)

DEXATRIM® Maximum Strength Extended Duration Time Tablets phenylpropanolamine HCl   75mg (time release)

Indication: DEXATRIM® is an aid for effective appetite control to assist weight reduction. It is available in a time release dosage form.

Caution: READ BEFORE USING. FOR ADULT USE ONLY. Do not give this product to children under 12 years of age. Persons between the ages of 12 and 18 or over 60 are advised to consult their physician or pharmacist before using this or any drug. If nervousness, dizziness, headaches, rapid pulse, palpitations, sleeplessness, or other symptoms occur, stop using and consult your physician.

Warning: DO NOT EXCEED RECOMMENDED DOSAGE. Taking more of this or any drug than is recommended can cause untoward health complications. It is sensible to check your blood pressure regularly. Do not use if you have high blood pressure, diabetes, heart, thyroid, kidney, or other disease or are being treated for high blood pressure or depression except under the advice and supervision of a physician. If you are taking a cough/cold allergy medication containing any form of phenylpropanolamine, do not take this product. As with any drug if you are pregnant or nursing a baby, seek the advice of a health professional before using this product. Do not use continuously for more than 3 months. When you have reached your desired weight or are able to control your appetite by yourself, use DEXATRIM only as needed.

Drug Interaction Precaution: Do not take if you are presently taking another medication containing phenylpropanolamine, or any type of nasal decongestant, or a prescription drug for high blood pressure or depression, or any other type of prescription medication except under the advice and supervision of a physician. KEEP THIS AND ALL MEDICATION OUT OF THE REACH OF CHILDREN. In case of accidental overdose seek professional assistance or contact a Poison Control Center immediately.

Dosage and Administration:
Capsule Dosage Forms: DEXATRIM® Maximum Strength Plus Vitamin C, DEXATRIM® Maximum Strength/Caffeine-Free.
Caplet Dosage Forms: DEXATRIM® Maximum Strength Plus Vitamin C, DEXATRIM® Maximum Strength/Caffeine-Free.
Tablet Dosage Form: DEXATRIM® Maximum Strength Extended Duration Time Tablets.
Administration: One capsule or caplet at midmorning (10 am) with a full glass of water.

How Supplied: All Dexatrim products are supplied in tamper-evident blister packages. Do not use if individual seals are broken.
DEXATRIM® Maximum Strength Plus Vitamin C/Caffeine-Free Capsules: Packages of 10, 20 and 40 with 1250 calorie DEXATRIM Diet Plan.
DEXATRIM® Maximum Strength Plus Vitamin C/Caffeine-Free Caplets: Packages of 20 and 40 with 1250 calorie DEXATRIM Diet Plan.
DEXATRIM® Maximum Strength Extended Duration Time Tablets: Packages of 20 and 40 with 1250 calorie DEXATRIM Diet Plan.

References: Altschuler, S., and Frazer, D.L., Double-Blind Clinical Evaluation of the Anorectic Activity of Phenylpropanolamine Hydrochloride Drops and Placebo Drops in the Treatment of Exogenous Obesity. *Current Therapeutic Research,* 40(1), 211–217, July 1986. Altschuler, S., et. al., Three Controlled Trials of Weight Loss with Phenylpropanolamine, *Int J Obesity,* 1982;6:549–556. Blackburn, G.L., et. al., Determinants of the Pressor Effect of Phenylpropanolamine in Healthy Subjects. *JAMA,* 1989; 261:3267–3272.
Morgan, J.P., et. al., Subjective Profile of Phenylpropanolamine: Absence of Stimulant or Euphorigenic Effects at Recommended Dose Levels. *J Clin Psychopharm,* 1989;9(1):33–38.
Lasagna, L., *Phenylpropanolamine—A Review,* New York, John Wiley and Sons, 1988.
All referenced materials available on request.
Shown in Product Identification Section, page 431

ENCARE®
[en 'kar]
Vaginal Contraceptive Suppositories

Description: Encare is a safe and effective contraceptive in a convenient vaginal suppository form available without a prescription. Encare is reliable because it offers two-way protection: (1) Encare kills sperm on contact by releasing a precise dose of nonoxynol 9, the spermicide most recommended by doctors. (2) Encare gently disperses a physical barrier of protection against the cervix to help prevent pregnancy.

Encare is an effective contraceptive in vaginal suppository form.

Active Ingredient: Each Suppository contains 2.27% Nonoxynol 9.

Other Ingredients: Fragrance, Lactalbumin, Polyethylene Glycols, Potassium Coco-Hydrolyzed Animal Protein, Sodium Bicarbonate, Sodium Lauryl Sulfate, Sodium Tartrate, Tartaric Acid.

Indications: Encare is effective in the prevention of pregnancy.

Action: Encare is 100% free of hormones and free of the serious side effects associated with oral contraceptives.
Encare is convenient and easy to use. Women like Encare because each insert is individually wrapped and can be easily carried in a pocket or purse. There are other reasons why women use Encare. It is approximately as effective as vaginal foam contraceptives in actual use, yet there is no applicator, so there is nothing to fill, remove, or clean. In addition, women may find Encare convenient to use in place of a second application of jelly or cream in conjunction with a diaphragm.
Because Encare can be inserted as much as an hour before intercourse, it does not interfere with spontaneity or ruin the mood. Many men are not even aware a woman is using Encare. Encare has been used successfully by millions of women throughout Europe and America.

Special Warning: Spermicidal contraceptives should not be used during pregnancy. Some experts believe that there may be an increased risk of birth defects occurring in children whose mothers used a spermicidal contraceptive at the time of conception or during pregnancy. If you believe you may be pregnant, have a pregnancy test before using a spermicidal contraceptive. If you have used a spermicidal contraceptive after becoming pregnant, or used a spermicidal contraceptive when you became pregnant, discuss this issue with your physician.

Cautions: If your doctor has told you that you should not become pregnant, consult him as to which method, including Encare, is best for you.
If vaginal irritation occurs and continues, contact your physician.
Do not take orally. **KEEP THIS AND ALL DRUGS OUT OF THE REACH OF CHILDREN.** In case of accidental ingestion, call a Poison Control Center, emergency medical facility or a doctor immediately.
Encare should be kept away from excessive heat. Store at room temperature. Should the product inadvertently be exposed to higher temperatures, hold under cold water for two minutes before removing protective wrap.

Dosage and Administration: For best protection against pregnancy, it is essential to follow package instructions. At least 10 minutes before intercourse, place one Encare insert with your fingertip as far as possible into the vagina, towards the small of your back. Best pro-

tection will occur when Encare is placed deep into the vagina. You may feel a pleasant sensation of warmth as Encare effervesces and distributes the spermicide, nonoxynol 9, within the vagina. This is a natural attribute to the product. **IMPORTANT:** It is essential to insert Encare at least 10 minutes before intercourse. If one chooses, Encare can be inserted up to one hour before intercourse. If intercourse has not taken place within one hour after insertion, use a new Encare insert. Use a new Encare insert each time intercourse is repeated. Encare can be used safely as frequently as needed. Douching after use of Encare is not required; however, should you desire to do so, wait at least six hours after intercourse.

How Supplied: Boxes of 12.

References: Barwin, B., Encare Oval: A Clinical Study, *Contraceptive Delivery System,* 4, 331–334, 1983. Masters, W., In Vivo Evaluation of an Effervescent Intravaginal Contraceptive Inserted by Simulated Coital Activity, *Fertility and Sterility,* 32, 161–165, 1979.

LACTOGEST™ SOFTGEL CAPSULES

PRODUCT OVERVIEW

Description: Each easy to swallow softgel capsule of Lactogest™ contains Lactase 125 mg (1750 FCC Lactase Units), Refined Soybean Oil, Gelatin, Glycerin, Purified Water, Hydrogenated Vegetable Oil, Lecithin, Beeswax, Titanium Dioxide.

Indications: Lactogest™ supplies the lactase enzyme missing in people who are lactose intolerant, and suffer from gastrointestinal disturbances such as gas, cramps, bloating, or diarrhea after consuming dairy products such as cheese and milk.

Action: Adult ethnic groups such as Blacks, Orientals, American Indians, and Eastern European Jews have low lactose enzymes, therefore making it difficult to digest all but small quantities of lactose containing products. Lactogest's™ natural lactase enzyme converts the lactose in milk and dairy foods into easily digestible simple sugars. Lactogest™ softgel capsules are taken orally just before consuming food containing lactose.
When there is insufficient lactase to digest the lactose, the unabsorbed sugars remain in the small intestine for longer than usual. This causes many of the gastrointestinal disturbances. The undigested lactose is then broken down in the intestine and produces gases which contribute to flatulence.

Precautions: Recommended for adult use only. Diabetics should consult a doctor before using Lactogest™, as the milk sugar will metabolically available and may result in increased blood glucose level. For maximum effectiveness, the

Continued on next page

Thompson Medical—Cont.

softgels should not be chewed, nor their contents added directly to milk or dairy products. Should hypersensitivity occur, discontinue use.

Directions: One to four softgels is recommended dosage to be taken just before consuming foods or drinks containing lactose. More or less may be taken according to the level of intolerance and the amount of dairy foods being consumed.

How Supplied: Lactogest™ softgel capsules are an opaque beige color. They are supplied in packages of 50 and 100 softgels. Store at controlled room temperature of 15–30 C (59–86 F).

Shown in Product Identification Section, page 431

NP–27®
Cream, Solution, Spray Powder and Powder
Antifungal
(tolnaftate)

Description: NP-27 contains the maximum strength available without a prescription of tolnaftate, a clinically proven ingredient which cures athlete's foot and jock itch. It is available as a cream, solution, spray powder and powder.

Active Ingredients: Cream, Solution and Powder: Tolnaftate 1%. Spray Powder: Tolnaftate 1%.

Other Ingredients: Cream: BHT, Polyethylene Glycol 400, Propylene Glycol, Titanium Dioxide. May also contain: n-Amylamine, Carbomer 934P, Carbomer 940, Diisopropanolamine. Solution: BHT, Polyethylene Glycol 400. May also contain: Propylene Glycol. Spray Powder: Isobutane, Isopropyl Myristate, SD Alcohol 40 14.9%, Talc. Powder: Cornstarch, Talc.

Indications: An effective antifungal agent that cures athlete's foot fungus and jock itch fungus and helps prevent athlete's foot reinfection. Provides effective relief of the itching, burning, scaling and discomfort that can accompany these conditions.

Warnings: For external use only. Avoid contact with eyes. Do not use on children under 2 years of age except under the advice and supervision of a doctor. If irritation occurs or if there is no improvement within 4 weeks (for athlete's foot), or within 2 weeks (for jock itch), discontinue use and consult a doctor. Keep this and all medications out of the reach of children. In case of accidental ingestion, seek professional assistance or contact a Poison Control Center immediately.

Dosage and Administration: Cleanse skin with soap and water and dry thoroughly. Apply a thin layer over affected area morning and night or as directed by a doctor. For athlete's foot, pay special attention to the spaces between the toes. It is also helpful to wear well-fitting, ventilated shoes and to change shoes and socks at least once daily. Best results in athlete's foot are usually obtained with 4 weeks use of this product and in jock itch, with 2 weeks use. If satisfactory results have not occurred within these times, consult a doctor. Children under 12 years of age should be supervised in the use of this product. This product is not effective on the scalp or nails.

How Supplied: Available in 0.5 oz. cream; 0.5 oz. solution; 3.5 oz. spray powder; 1.5 oz. powder.

Warning: Flammable. Contents under pressure. Do not puncture or incinerate. Exposure to temperatures above 120°F may cause bursting. Use only as directed. Intentional misuse by deliberately concentrating and inhaling products can be harmful or fatal. Do not use or store near heat or open flame.

How to Store: Store at room temperature.

Shown in Product Identification Section, page 431

SLEEPINAL®
Night-time Sleep Aid Capsules
(Diphenhydramine HCl)

Description: SLEEPINAL is a night-time sleep aid. When taken prior to bedtime, it helps to relieve sleeplessness and aids in falling asleep.

Active Ingredient: Diphenhydramine HCl 50 mg.

Other Ingredients: FD&C Blue No. 1, Gelatin, Lactose, Magnesium Stearate, Povidone, Talc.

Indications: For relief of occasional sleeplessness.

Action: SLEEPINAL is an antihistamine with anticholinergic and sedative action.

Warnings: Read before using. Do not exceed recommended dosage. Do not give to children under 12 years of age. If sleeplessness persists continuously for more than 2 weeks, consult a physician. Insomnia may be a symptom of serious underlying medical illness. Do not take this product if you have asthma, glaucoma, emphysema, chronic pulmonary disease, shortness of breath, difficulty in breathing, or difficulty in urination due to enlargement of the prostate gland unless directed by a physician. Avoid alcoholic beverages while taking this product. Do not take this product if you are taking sedatives or tranquilizers, without first consulting your physician. As with any drug, if you are pregnant or nursing a baby, seek the advice of a health professional before using this product. **KEEP THIS AND ALL MEDICATIONS OUT OF THE REACH OF CHILDREN.** In the case of accidental overdose, seek professional assistance or contact a Poison Control Center immediately.

Dosage and Administration: Adults and children 12 years of age and over: Oral dosage, one capsule at bedtime if needed, or as directed by a physician.

How to Store: Store in a dry place at controlled room temperature 15° C–30° C (59° F–86° F).

How Supplied: Sleepinal is supplied in tamper-evident blister packages. Do not use if individual seals are broken. Packages of 16 and 32 capsules.

Shown in Product Identification Section, page 431

SLEEPINAL®
MEDICATED NIGHT TEA
Night-time Sleep Aid
(Diphenhydramine HCl)

Description: SLEEPINAL MEDICATED NIGHT TEA is a night-time sleep aid in a flavored powder that mixes with hot water. When taken prior to bedtime, it helps to relieve sleeplessness and aids in falling asleep.
EACH PACKET CONTAINS:
Active Ingredient: Diphenhydramine HCl 50 mg.

Other Ingredients: Aspartame, Citric Acid, Colloidal Silicon Dioxide, D&C Yellow No. 10, FD&C Blue No. 1, FD&C Red No. 40, Flavors, Lactose, Polyethylene Glycol, Povidone, Sodium Chloride, Sodium Citrate.

Indication: For relief of occasional sleeplessness.

Action: SLEEPINAL MEDICATED NIGHT TEA is an antihistamine with anticholinergic and sedative action.

Warnings: Read before using. Do not exceed recommended dosage. Do not give to children under 12 years of age. If sleeplessness persists continuously for more than 2 weeks, consult a physician. Insomnia may be a symptom of serious underlying medical illness. Do not take this product if you have asthma, glaucoma, emphysema, chronic pulmonary disease, shortness of breath, difficulty in breathing, or difficulty in urination due to enlargement of the prostate gland unless directed by a physician. Avoid alcoholic beverages while taking this product. Do not take this product if you are taking sedatives or tranquilizers, without first consulting your physician. As with any drug, if you are pregnant or nursing a baby, seek the advice of a health professional before using this product.
KEEP THIS AND ALL MEDICATIONS OUT OF THE REACH OF CHILDREN.
In the case of accidental overdose, seek professional assistance or contact a Poison Control Center immediately.
Phenylketonurics: Contains Phenylalanine 16.8 mg. per packet.

Dosage and Administration: Adults and children 12 years of age and over: To open, cut along dotted line, pour contents and dissolve one packet into 8 ounces of hot water. Sip while hot at bedtime, if needed, or as directed by a physician.

How to Store: Store at controlled room temperature 15°C–30°C (59°F–86°F).

How Supplied: SLEEPINAL MEDI-CATED NIGHT TEA is supplied in packages containing single-dose packets. Do not use if foil packet is torn or broken. Packages contain 8 or 16 packets.

Triton Consumer Products, Inc.
**561 W. GOLF ROAD
ARLINGTON HEIGHTS, IL 60005**

MG 217® PSORIASIS MEDICATION
**Skin Care: Ointment and Lotion
Scalp: Shampoo and Conditioner**

Active Ingredients: OINTMENT—Coal Tar Solution USP 2%, Salicylic Acid 1.5% and Colloidal Sulfur 1.1%. **LOTION—**Coal Tar Solution USP 5% with Jojoba. **SHAMPOO—**Coal Tar Solution USP 5%, Salicylic Acid 2% and Colloidal Sulfur 1.5%. **CONDITIONER—**Coal Tar Solution USP 2%.

Action/Uses: Relief for itching, scaling and flaking of Psoriasis or Seborrhea.

Caution: For external use only. Keep out of the reach of children. Avoid contact with eyes. If undue skin irritation occurs, discontinue use. For shampoo/conditioner, temporary discoloration of blond, bleached or tinted hair may occur.

Administration: OINTMENT or LOTION—Wash affected areas of skin with mild soap/water and dry. Rub MG 217 in well. Apply twice daily or as needed. Not for use on the scalp. **SHAMPOO—**Shake well before using. Wet hair, then massage liberal amount of MG 217 into scalp and leave on for 5–10 minutes. Use daily or as needed. **CONDITIONER**—After shampooing, massage liberal amount of MG 217 into scalp and leave on for several minutes. Rinse thoroughly. Use daily or as needed.

How Supplied: OINTMENT—3.8 oz. jars. **LOTION—**4 oz. bottles. **SHAMPOO—**4 oz. and 8 oz. bottles. **CONDITIONER—**4 oz. bottles.

UAS Laboratories
**9201 PENN AVENUE SOUTH
#10
MINNEAPOLIS, MN 55431**

DDS–ACIDOPHILUS
Capsule, Tablet & Powder free of dairy products, corn, soy, and preservatives

Description: DDS-Acidophilus is the source of a special strain of Lactobacillus acidophilus free of dairy products, corn, soy and preservatives. Each capsule or tablet contains one billion viable DDS-1 L.acidophilus at the time of manufacturing. One gram of powder contains two billion viable DDS-1 L.acidophilus.

Indications and Usages: An aid in implanting the gut with beneficial Lactobacillus acidophilus under conditions of digestive disorders, acne, yeast infections, and following antibiotic therapy.

Administration: One to two capsules or tablets twice daily before meals. One-fourth teaspoon powder can be substituted for two capsules or tablets.

How Supplied: Bottles of 100 capsules or tablets. 12 bottles per case. Powder is available in 2 oz. bottle; 12 bottles per case.

Storage: Keep refrigerated under 40°F.

EDUCATIONAL MATERIAL

DDS-Acidophilus
Booklet describing superior-strain Acidophilus without dairy products, corn, soy, or preservatives. Two billion viable DDS-L. acidophilus per gram.

The Upjohn Company
KALAMAZOO, MI 49001

Regular Strength CORTAID® Cream with Aloe, Ointment with Aloe, Spray and Lotion (hydrocortisone 0.5%)
Anti-itch products

Description: Regular Strength CORTAID provides safe, effective regular strength relief of many different types of itches and rashes and is the brand recommended most by physicians and pharmacists. It is available in 1) a greaseless, odorless vanishing cream that contains aloe and leaves no residue; 2) a soothing, lubricating ointment with aloe, 3) a quick-drying non-staining, non-aerosol spray; and 4) a greasless, odorless vanishing lotion.

Active Ingredients: Regular Strength CORTAID Cream and Regular Strength CORTAID Ointment: hydrocortisone acetate (equivalent to 0.5% hydrocortisone). Also contains soothing aloe.
Regular Strength CORTAID Spray: hydrocortisone 0.5%
Regular Strength CORTAID Lotion: hydrocortisone acetate (equivalent to hydrocortisone 0.5%)

Other Ingredients:
Cream: aloe vera, butylparaben, cetyl palmitate, glyceryl stearate, methylparaben, polyethylene glycol, stearamidoethyl diethylamine, and purified water.
Ointment: aloe vera, butylparaben, cholesterol, methylparaben, mineral oil, white petrolatum, and microcrystalline wax.
Spray: alcohol, glycerin, methylparaben, and purified water
Lotion: butylparaben, cetyl palmitate, glyceryl monostearate, methylparaben, polysorbate 80, propylene glycol, stearamidoethyl diethylamine, and purified water

Indications: Use Regular Strength CORTAID for the temporary relief of itching associated with minor skin irritations, inflammation, and rashes due to insect bites, soaps, detergents, cosmetics, jewelry, eczema, psoriasis, seborrheic dermatitis, poison ivy, poison oak, or poison sumac, and for external feminine and anal itching. Other uses of this product should be only under the advice and supervision of a physician.

Uses: The vanishing action of CORTAID Cream with Aloe makes it cosmetically acceptable when the skin itch or rash treated is on exposed parts of the body such as the hands or arms. CORTAID Ointment with Aloe is best used where protection, lubrication and soothing of dry and scaly lesions is required. CORTAID Spray is a quick-drying, nonstaining formulation suitable for covering large areas of the skin. CORTAID Lotion is a free-flowing lotion and is especially suitable for hairy body areas such as the scalp or arms.

Warnings: For external use only. Avoid contact with the eyes. If condition worsens, or if symptoms persist for more than 7 days or clear up and occur again within a few days, stop use of this product and do not begin use of any other hydrocortisone product unless you have consulted a physician. Do not use for the treatment of diaper rash. Consult a physician. For external feminine itching, do not use if you have a vaginal discharge. Consult a physician. For external anal itching, do not exceed the recommended daily dosage unless directed by a physician. In case of bleeding, consult a physician promptly. Do not put this product into the rectum by using fingers or any mechanical device or applicator.

Dosage and Administration: *Adults and children 2 years of age and older:* Apply to affected area not more than 3 to 4 times daily. *Children under 2 years of age:* Do not use, consult a physician. *Adults:* For external anal itching, when practical, cleanse the affected area with mild soap and warm water and rinse thoroughly by patting or blotting with an appropriate cleansing pad. Gently dry by patting or blotting with toilet tissue or a soft cloth before application of this product. *Children under 12 years of age:* For external anal itching, consult a physician.

How Supplied:
Cream with Aloe: ½ oz., 1 oz., and 1.5 oz. bonus pack tubes
Ointment with Aloe: ½ oz. and 1 oz. tubes and 1.5 oz. bonus pack tubes
Non-Aerosol Spray: 1.5 fluid oz.
Lotion: 1 oz. bottle
Shown in Product Identification Section, page 431

Continued on next page

Upjohn—Cont.

Maximum Strength CORTAID®
Cream, Ointment and Spray
(hydrocortisone 1%)
Anti-itch products

Description: Maximum Strength COR-
TAID is the same strength and form of
hydrocrtisone relief formerly available
only with a prescription. Maximum
Strength CORTAID provides safe, effective regular strength relief of many different types of itches and rashes and is
the brand recommended most by physicians and pharmacists. It is available in
1) a greaseless, odorless vanishing cream
that leaves no residue; 2) a soothing, lubricating ointment; 3) a quick-drying
non-staining, non-aerosol spray.

Active   Ingredients: Maximum
Strength CORTAID Cream and Maximum Strength CORTAID Ointment: hydrocortisone acetate (equivalent to 1%
hydrocortisone).
Maximum Strength CORTAID Spray:
hydrocortisone 1%

Other Ingredients:
Cream: butylparaben, cetyl alcohol, glycerin, methylparaben, sodium lauryl sulfate, stearic acid, stearyl alcohol, purified water, and white petrolatum.
Ointment: butylparaben, cholesterol,
methylparaben, microcrystalline wax,
mineral oil, and white petrolatum.
Spray: alcohol, glycerin, methylparaben,
and purified water

Indications: Use Maximum Strength
CORTAID for the temporary relief of
itching associated with minor skin irritations, inflammation, and rashes due to
eczema, psoriasis, seborrheic dermatitis,
poison ivy, poison oak, or poison sumac,
insect bites, soaps, detergents, cosmetics,
jewelry, and for external feminine and
anal itching. Other uses of this product
should be only under the advice and supervision of a physician.

Uses: The vanishing action of COR-
TAID Cream makes it cosmetically acceptable when the skin itch or rash
treated is on exposed parts of the body
such as the hands or arms. CORTAID
Ointment is best used where protection,
lubrication and soothing of dry and scaly
lesions is required. The ointment is also
recommended for treating itchy genital
and anal areas. CORTAID Spray is a
quick-drying, non-staining formulation
suitable for covering large areas of the
skin.

Warnings: For external use only.
Avoid contact with the eyes. If condition
worsens, or if symptoms persist for more
than 7 days or clear up and occur again
within a few days, stop use of this product and do not begin use of any other hydrocortisone product unless you have
consulted a physician. Do not use for the
treatment of diaper rash. Consult a physician. For external feminine itching, do
not use if you have a vaginal discharge.
Consult a physician. For external anal
itching, do not exceed the recommended

daily dosage unless directed by a physician. In case of bleeding, consult a physician promptly. Do not put this product
into the rectum by using fingers or any
mechanical device or applicator.

Dosage and Administration: *Adults
and children 2 years of age and older:* Apply to affected area not more than 3 to 4
times daily. *Children under 2 years of age:*
Do not use, consult a physician. *Adults:*
For external anal itching, when practical, cleanse the affected area with mild
soap and warm water and rinse thoroughly by patting or blotting with an appropriate cleansing pad. Gently dry by
patting or blotting with toilet tissue or a
soft cloth before application of this product. *Children under 12 years of age:* For
external anal itching, consult a physician.

How Supplied:
Cream: ½ oz. and 1 oz. tubes
Ointment: ½ oz. and 1 oz. tubes
Non-Aerosol Spray: 1.5 fluid oz.
*Shown in Product Identification
Section, page 431*

CORTEF® Feminine Itch Cream
(hydrocortisone acetate)
Anti-itch Cream

Description: CORTEF Feminine Itch
Cream contains hydrocortisone—the
only ingredient approved by the Food
and Drug Administration for safe and
effective relief of external feminine itching. CORTEF, from the makers of COR-
TAID, is an unscented vanishing cream
that relieves itching fast and quickly disappears into the skin to avoid staining of
clothing.

Active Ingredient: hydrocortisone acetate (equivalent to hydrocortisone 0.5%)

Other Ingredients: aloe vera, butylparaben, cetyl palmitate, glyceryl monostearate, methylparaben, polyethylene
glycol, stearamidoethyl diethylamine,
and purified water.

Indications: The Food and Drug Administration has approved the use of
CORTEF for the temporary relief of itching associated with minor skin irritations, inflammation and rashes due to
external feminine itching.

Warnings: For external use only.
Avoid contact with eyes. If condition
worsens, or if symptoms persist for more
than 7 days or clear up and occur again
within a few days, stop use of this product and do not begin use of any other hydrocortisone product unless you have
consulted a physician. Do not use for the
treatment of diaper rash. Consult a physician. For external feminine itching, do
not use if you have a vaginal discharge.
Consult a physician.

Dosage and Administration: *Adults
and children 2 years of age and older:* Apply to affected area not more than 3 to 4
times daily. *Children under 2 years of age:*
Do not use, consult a physician.

How Supplied: ½ oz. tube.

DOXIDAN® LIQUI-GELS®
Stimulant/Stool Softener Laxative

Active Ingredients: Each soft gelatin
capsule contains 65 mg yellow phenolphthalein and 60 mg docusate calcium.

Inactive Ingredients: Alcohol up to
1.5% (w/w), corn oil, FD&C Blue #1 and
Red #40, gelatin, glycerin, hydrogenated vegetable oil, lecithin, parabens,
sorbitol, titanium dioxide, vegetable
shortening, yellow wax, and other
ingredients.

Indications: DOXIDAN is a safe, reliable laxative for the relief of occasional
constipation. The combination of a stim-
ulant/stool softener laxative allows positive laxative action on a softened stool
for gentle evacuation without straining.
DOXIDAN generally produces a bowel
movement in 6 to 12 hours.

Dosage and Administration: Adults
and children 12 years of age and over:
one or two capsules by mouth daily.
For use in children under 12, consult a
physician.

Warnings: Do not use laxative products when abdominal pain, nausea, or
vomiting are present unless directed by a
doctor. If you have noticed a sudden
change in bowel habits that persists over
a period of 2 weeks, consult a doctor before using a laxative. Laxative products
should not be used for a period longer
than 1 week unless directed by a doctor.
Rectal bleeding or failure to have a bowel
movement after use of a laxative may
indicate a serious condition. Discontinue
use and consult your doctor. If skin rash
appears, do not use this product or any
other preparation containing phenolphthalein. Keep this and all drugs out of
the reach of children. In case of accidental overdose, seek professional assistance
or contact a poison control center immediately. As with any drug, if you are pregnant or nursing a baby, seek the advice of
a health professional before using this
product.

How Supplied: Packages of 10, 30, 100
and 1,000 maroon soft gelatin capsules,
and Unit Dose 100s (10 × 10 strips).
LIQUI-GELS® Reg TM R P Scherer
Corp
*Shown in Product Identification
Section, page 431*

DRAMAMINE® Liquid
(dimenhydrinate syrup USP)
DRAMAMINE® Tablets
(dimenhydrinate USP)
DRAMAMINE® Chewable Tablets
(dimenhydrinate USP)

Description: Dimenhydrinate is the
chlorotheophylline salt of the antihistaminic agent diphenhydramine. Dimenhydrinate contains not less than 53%
and not more than 56% of diphenhydramine, and not less than 44% and not
more than 47% of 8-chlorotheophylline,
calculated on the dried basis.

Active Ingredients:
DRAMAMINE Tablets and Chewable Tablets: Dimenhydrinate 50 mg.
DRAMAMINE Liquid: Dimenhydrinate 12.5 mg. per 5 ml, Ethyl Alcohol 5%.

Inactive Ingredients:
DRAMAMINE Tablets: Acacia, Carboxymethylcellulose Sodium, Corn Starch, Magnesium Stearate, and Sodium Sulfate.
DRAMAMINE Liquid: FD&C Red No. 40, Flavor, Glycerin, Methylparaben, Sucrose, and Water. Ethyl Alcohol 5%.
DRAMAMINE Chewable Tablets: Aspartame, Citric Acid, FD&C Yellow No. 6, Flavor, Magnesium Stearate, Methacrylic Acid Copolymer, Sorbitol. Phenylketonurics: Contains Phenylalanine 1.5 mg per tablet.
Contains FD&C Yellow No. 5 (tartrazine) as a color additive.

Actions: While the precise mode of action of dimenhydrinate is not known, it has a depressant action on hyperstimulated labyrinthine function.

Indications: For the prevention and treatment of the nausea, vomiting, or dizziness associated with motion sickness.

Directions:
DRAMAMINE Tablets and Chewable Tablets: To prevent motion sickness, the first dose should be taken one half to one hour before starting activity.
ADULTS: 1 to 2 tablets every 4 to 6 hours, not to exceed 8 tablets in 24 hours or as directed by a doctor.
CHILDREN 6 TO UNDER 12: ½ to 1 tablet every 6 to 8 hours, not to exceed 3 tablets in 24 hours or as directed by a doctor.
CHILDREN 2 to UNDER 6: ¼ to ½ tablet every 6 to 8 hours not to exceed 1½ tablets in 24 hours or as directed by a doctor.
Children may also be given DRAMAMINE Cherry Flavored Liquid in accordance with directions for use.
DRAMAMINE Liquid: To prevent motion sickness, the first dose should be taken one half to one hour before starting activity. ADULTS: 4 to 8 teaspoons (5 ml per teaspoonful) every 4 to 6 hours, not to exceed 32 teaspoonfuls in 24 hours or as directed by a doctor. CHILDREN 6 TO UNDER 12: 2 to 4 teaspoonfuls every 6 to 8 hours, not to exceed 12 teaspoonfuls in 24 hours or as directed by a doctor. CHILDREN 2 TO UNDER 6: 1 to 2 teaspoonfuls every 6 to 8 hours not to exceed 6 teaspoonfuls in 24 hours or as directed by a doctor. Use of a measuring device is recommended for all liquid medication.

Warnings: Do not take this product if you have asthma, glaucoma, emphysema, chronic pulmonary disease, shortness of breath, difficulty in breathing, or difficulty in urination due to enlargement of the prostate gland unless directed by a doctor. Do not give to children under 2 years of age unless directed by a doctor. May cause marked drowsiness; alcohol, sedatives, and tranquilizers may increase the drowsiness effect. Avoid alcoholic beverages while taking this product. Do not take this product if you are taking sedatives or tranquilizers, without first consulting your doctor. Use caution when driving a motor vehicle or operating machinery. Not for frequent or prolonged use except on advice of a doctor. Do not exceed recommended dosage. Keep this and all drugs out of the reach of children. In case of accidental overdose, seek professional assistance or contact a poison control center immediately. As with any drug, if you are pregnant or nursing a baby, seek the advice of a health professional before using this product.

How Supplied: *Tablets* —scored, white tablets available in packets of 12 and 36 and bottles of 100 (OTC); *Liquid* —Available in bottles of 3 fl oz (OTC); *Chewables* —scored, orange tablets available in packets of 8 and 24 (OTC).
Shown in Product Identification Section, page 431

KAOPECTATE®
Concentrated Anti-Diarrheal, Peppermint Flavor and Regular Flavor

Active Ingredient: Each tablespoon contains 600 mg attapulgite.

Inactive Ingredients: Flavors, glucono-delta-lactone, magnesium aluminum silicate, methylparaben, sorbic acid, sucrose, titanium dioxide, xanthan gum and purified water; Peppermint flavor contains FD&C Red #40.

Indications: For the fast relief of diarrhea and cramping.

Dosage and Administration: For best results, take full recommended dose at first sign of diarrhea and after each subsequent bowel movement. (Maximum 7 times in 24 hours.) Adults and children 12 years of age and over: 2 tablespoons. Children 6 to under 12 years of age: 1 tablespoon. Children 3 to under 6 years of age: ½ tablespoon.

Warnings: Unless directed by a physician, do not use in infants and children under 3 years of age or for more than two days or in the presence of high fever. Keep this and all drugs out of the reach of children. In case of accidental overdose, seek professional assistance or contact a poison control center immediately.

How Supplied: Regular flavor available in 8 oz, 12 oz and 16 oz bottles. Peppermint flavor available in 8 oz and 12 oz bottles.
Shown in Product Identification Section, page 431

KAOPECTATE® Children's Liquid and Chewable Tablets, Anti-Diarrheal

Active Ingredient: Each ½ tablespoon of liquid or chewable tablet contains 300 mg attapulgite.

Inactive Ingredients: Children's Liquid includes FD&C Red #40, flavors, glucono-delta-lactone, magnesium aluminum silicate, methylparaben, sorbic acid, sucrose, titanium dioxide, xanthan gum, and purified water. Children's Chewable Tablets include cornstarch, dextrins, dextrose, D&C Red #27, D&C Red #30, flavor, magnesium stearate, sucrose and titanium dioxide.

Indications: For the fast relief of diarrhea and cramping; in good-tasting, easy-to-take forms. Especially formulated to meet the needs of children age 3 and up.

Dosage and Administration: For best results, take full recommended dose at first sign of diarrhea and after each subsequent bowel movement (maximum 7 times in 24 hours). Liquid—Children 3 to under 6 years of age: ½ tablespoon; Children 6 to under 12 years of age: 1 tablespoon; children (and adults) 12 years of age and older: 2 tablespoons. Chewable Tablets—Children 3 to under 6 years of age: 1 tablet; Children 6 to under 12 years of age: 2 tablets; Children (and adults) 12 years of age and over: 4 tablets.

Warnings: Unless directed by a physician, do not use in infants and children under 3 years of age or for more than two days or in the presence of high fever. Keep this and all drugs out of the reach of children. In case of accidental overdose, seek professional assistance or contact a poison control center immediately.

How Supplied: Available in 6 oz bottles (liquid) and blister packs of 16 chewable tablets.
Shown in Product Identification Section, page 431

KAOPECTATE® Maximum Strength Caplets
Anti-Diarrheal

Active Ingredient: Each caplet contains 750 mg attapulgite.

Inactive Ingredients: Croscarmellose sodium, hydroxypropyl cellulose, hydroxypropyl methylcellulose, methylparaben, pectin, propylene glycol, propylparaben, sucrose, titanium dioxide and zinc stearate.

Indications: For the fast relief of diarrhea and cramping.

Dosage and Administration: Swallow whole caplets with water; do not chew. For best results, take full recommended dose.
Adults: Take 2 caplets after the initial bowel movement and 2 caplets after each subsequent bowel movement, not to exceed 12 caplets in 24 hours. Children 6 to 12 years of age: Take 1 caplet after the initial bowel movement and 1 caplet after each subsequent bowel movement, not to exceed 6 caplets in 24 hours.
Children 3 to under 6 years of age: Use Cherry Flavor Children's Liquid or

Continued on next page

Upjohn—Cont.

Chewable Tablets, or Advanced Formula KAOPECTATE Liquid.

Warnings: Unless directed by a physician, do not use in infants and children under 6 years of age or for more than two days or in the presence of high fever. Keep this and all drugs out of the reach of children. In case of accidental overdose, seek professional assistance or contact a poison control center immediately.

How Supplied: Available in blister packs of 12 and 20 caplets.
Shown in Product Identification Section, page 431

MOTRIN® IB
Caplets or Tablets
(ibuprofen, USP)
Pain Reliever/Fever Reducer

WARNING: ASPIRIN-SENSITIVE PATIENTS. Do not take this product if you have had a severe allergic reaction to aspirin, eg—asthma, swelling, shock or hives because even though this product contains no aspirin or salicylates, cross-reactions may occur in patients allergic to aspirin.

Indications: For the temporary relief of headache, muscular aches, minor pain of arthritis, toothache, backache, minor aches and pains associated with the common cold, pain of menstrual cramps, and for reduction of fever.

Directions: Adults: Take 1 caplet or tablet every 4 to 6 hours while symptoms persist. If pain or fever does not respond to 1 caplet or tablet, 2 caplets or tablets may be used, but do not exceed 6 caplets or tablets in 24 hours, unless directed by a doctor. The smallest effective dose should be used. Take with food or milk, if occasional and mild heartburn, upset stomach or stomach pain occurs with use. Consult a doctor if these symptoms are more than mild or if they persist. Children: Do not give this product to children under 12 except under the advice and supervision of a doctor.

Warnings: Do not take for pain for more than 10 days or for fever for more than 3 days unless directed by a doctor. If pain or fever persists or gets worse, if new symptoms occur, or if the painful area is red or swollen, consult a doctor. These could be signs of serious illness. If you are under a doctor's care for any serious condition, consult a doctor before taking this product. As with aspirin and acetaminophen, if you have any condition which requires you to take prescription drugs or if you have had any problems or serious side effects from taking any nonprescription pain reliever, do not take MOTRIN® IB without first discussing it with your doctor. If you experience any symptoms which are unusual or seem unrelated to the condition for which you took ibuprofen, consult a doctor before taking any more of it. Although ibuprofen is indicated for the same conditions as aspirin and acetami-

nophen, it should not be taken with them except under a doctor's direction. Do not combine this product with any other ibuprofen-containing product. As with any drug, if you are pregnant or nursing a baby, seek the advice of a health professional before using this product. IT IS ESPECIALLY IMPORTANT NOT TO USE IBUPROFEN DURING THE LAST 3 MONTHS OF PREGNANCY UNLESS SPECIFICALLY DIRECTED TO DO SO BY A DOCTOR BECAUSE IT MAY CAUSE PROBLEMS IN THE UNBORN CHILD OR COMPLICATIONS DURING DELIVERY. Keep this and all drugs out of the reach of children. In case of accidental overdose, seek professional assistance or contact a poison control center immediately. **Store at room temperature. Avoid excessive heat 40°C (104°F).**

Active Ingredient: Each caplet or tablet contains ibuprofen 200 mg.

Other Ingredients: Carnauba wax, cornstarch, hydroxypropyl methylcellulose, propylene glycol, silicon dioxide, pregelatinized starch, stearic acid, titanium dioxide.

How Supplied: Bottles of 24, 50, 100, and 165 Caplets or Tablets.
Shown in Product Identification Section, page 432

Maximum Strength MYCITRACIN®
Triple Antibiotic First Aid Ointment
MYCITRACIN® Plus Pain Reliever

Description: MYCITRACIN combines three topical antibiotics in a soothing, non-irritating petrolatum base that does not sting, aids healing, and helps prevent infection.

Indications: Maximum Strength MYCITRACIN and MYCITRACIN Plus Pain Reliever are first aid ointments to help prevent infection in minor burns, cuts, nicks, scrapes, scratches and abrasions. MYCITRACIN Plus Pain Reliever also temporarily relieves pain.

Directions: *For adults and children (all ages):* Clean the affected area. Apply a small amount of MYCITRACIN (an amount equal to the surface area of the tip of a finger) on the affected area 1 to 3 times daily. If desired, cover the affected area with a sterile bandage.

Warnings: For external use only. Do not use in the eyes or apply over large areas of the body. In case of deep or puncture wounds, animal bites, or serious burns, consult a physician. Stop use and consult a physician if the condition persists or gets worse. Do not use longer than 1 week unless directed by a physician. Keep this and all medications out of the reach of children. In case of accidental ingestion, seek professional assistance or contact a poison control center immediately.

Active Ingredients:
Maximum Strength MYCITRACIN: Each gram contains bacitracin, 500 units; neomycin sulfate equiv. to 3.5 mg

neomycin; polymyxin B sulfate, 5,000 units.
MYCITRACIN Plus Pain Reliever: Each gram contains bacitracin, 500 units; neomycin sulfate equiv. to 3.5 mg neomycin; polymyxin B sulfate, 5000 units; lidocaine, 40 mg.

Other Ingredients:
Maximum Strength MYCITRACIN: butylparaben, cholesterol, methylparaben, microcrystalline wax, mineral oil, and white petrolatum.
MYCITRACIN Plus Pain Reliever: butylparaben, cholesterol, methylparaben, microcrystalline wax, mineral oil, and white petrolatum.

How Supplied:
Maximum Strength MYCITRACIN: ½ oz. tubes, 1 oz. tubes and ¹⁄₃₂ oz. foil packets (144 per carton)
MYCITRACIN Plus Pain Reliever: ½ oz. and 1 oz. tubes
Shown in Product Identification Section, page 432

PROGAINE®
Shampoo for Thinning Hair

Description: PROGAINE Shampoo has been scientifically formulated to clean delicate thinning hair without damaging while adding body and manageability. PROGAINE is also an ideal shampoo for the user of thinning hair treatments. The exclusive, patented formula for PROGAINE Shampoo has been dermatologist tested on over 1000 adults in 31 medical clinics and proven safe for delicate thinning hair. PROGAINE Shampoo is different from many other shampoos in that PROGAINE contains none of the commonly used coating ingredients such as oils, waxes, silicones, proteins, quaternary ammonium salts, or cationic polymers which may leave a deposit on hair and scalp. PROGAINE is also hypoallergenic; it contains no harsh detergents or additives such as dyes, added formaldehydes, or parabens, commonly found in other shampoos, which may irritate sensitive scalps. PROGAINE Shampoo is pH balanced, ranging from 5.4 to 5.7, and will not affect the scalp's normal pH.

Ingredients:
Normal-to-Oily formula: Water, TEA lauryl sulfate, sodium laureth sulfate, cocamide DEA, cocamidopropyl betaine, propylene glycol, citric acid, disodium EDTA, fragrance, and sodium chloride.
Normal-to-Dry formula: Water, sodium laureth sulfate, TEA lauryl sulfate, cocamide DEA, cocamidopropyl betaine, acetamide MEA, citric acid, disodium EDTA, fragrance, sodium chloride.

Directions: PROGAINE Shampoo is gentle enough to use for every shampoo. For best results, wet hair and scalp, apply PROGAINE Shampoo, bring to a lather, then rinse. Repeat if desired.

How Supplied: Both the Normal-to-Oily and Normal-to-Dry formulas are available in 5 oz. and 8 oz. bottles.

SURFAK® LIQUI-GELS®
Stool Softener Laxative

Active Ingredients: Each soft gelatin capsule contains 240 mg docusate calcium.

Inactive Ingredients: Alcohol up to 3% (w/w), corn oil, FD&C Blue #1 and Red #40, gelatin, glycerin, parabens, sorbitol, and other ingredients.

Indications: SURFAK is indicated for the relief of occasional constipation. SURFAK generally produces a bowel movement in 12 to 72 hours. SURFAK is useful when only stool softening (without propulsive action) is required to relieve constipation.

Dosage and Administration: Adults and children 12 years of age and over: one capsule by mouth daily for several days or until bowel movements are normal. For use in children under 12, consult a physician.

Warnings: Do not use laxative products when abdominal pain, nausea, or vomiting are present unless directed by a doctor. If you have noticed a sudden change in bowel habits that persists over a period of 2 weeks, consult a doctor before using a laxative. Laxative products should not be used for a period longer than 1 week unless directed by a doctor. Rectal bleeding or failure to have a bowel movement after use of a laxative may indicate a serious condition. Discontinue use and consult your doctor. Keep this and all drugs out of the reach of children. In case of accidental overdose, seek professional assistance or contact a poison control center immediately. As with any drug, if you are pregnant or nursing a baby, seek the advice of a health professional before using this product.

How Supplied: Packages of 10, 30, 100 and 500 red soft gelatin capsules and Unit Dose 100s (10 × 10 strips). LIQUI-GELS® Reg TM R P Scherer Corp

Shown in Product Identification Section, page 432

UNICAP® Capsules/Tablets
Multivitamin Supplement
100% RDA of Essential Vitamins in Easy to Swallow Capsule
Sugar and Sodium Free Tablet

Indications: Dietary multivitamin supplement of ten essential vitamins for health-conscious families (adults and children 4 or more years of age).
Each capsule contains:
[See table above]

Ingredient List:
Capsules: Gelatin, Ascorbic Acid (Vit. C), Soybean Oil, Glycerin, Vitamin E Acetate, Niacinamide, Yellow Wax, Lecithin, Pyridoxine Hydrochloride (B-6), Thiamine Mononitrate (B-1), Riboflavin (B-2), Vitamin A Palmitate, Titanium Dioxide, Corn Oil, Folic Acid, FD&C Yellow No. 5, Ethyl Vanillin, Vanilla Enhancer, FD&C Yellow No. 6, Cholecalciferol (Vit. D), Cyanocobalamin (B-12).

		% U.S. RDA*
Vitamin A	5000 Int. Units	100
Vitamin D	400 Int. Units	100
Vitamin E	30 Int. Units	100
Vitamin C	60 mg	100
Folic Acid	400 mcg	100
Thiamine	1.5 mg	100
Riboflavin	1.7 mg	100
Niacin	20 mg	100
Vitamin B_6	2 mg	100
Vitamin B_{12}	6 mcg	100

Each tablet has same content except:

Vitamin E	15 Int. Units	50

*Percentage of U.S. Recommended Daily Allowance.

Tablets: Calcium Phosphate, Ascorbic Acid (Vit. C), Vitamin E Acetate, Hydroxypropyl Methylcellulose, Niacinamide, Artificial Color, Vitamin A Acetate, Magnesium Stearate, Pyridoxine Hydrochloride (B-6), Riboflavin (B-2), Silica Gel, Thiamine Mononitrate (B-1), FD&C Yellow No. 5, Folic Acid, Artificial Flavor, Cholecalciferol (Vit. D), Carnauba Wax, Cyanocobalamin (B-12).

Recommended Dosage: 1 capsule or tablet daily.

How Supplied: Available in bottles of 120 capsules or tablets.
Shown in Product Identification Section, page 432

UNICAP Jr.® Chewable Tablets
Good-tasting, Orange-flavored Chewable Tablet

Indications: Dietary multivitamin supplement providing up to 100% of the RDA of essential vitamins. For **children** 4 or more years of age.

		% U.S. RDA*
Vitamin A	5000 Int. Units	100
Vitamin D	400 Int. Units	100
Vitamin E	15 Int. Units	50
Vitamin C	60 mg	100
Folic Acid	400 mcg	100
Thiamine	1.5 mg	100
Riboflavin	1.7 mg	100
Niacin	20 mg	100
Vitamin B_6	2 mg	100
Vitamin B_{12}	6 mcg	100

*Percentage of U.S. Recommended Daily Allowance.

Ingredient List: Sucrose, Mannitol, Sodium Ascorbate (Vit C), Lactose, Cornstarch, Niacinamide, Citric Acid, Vitamin E Acetate, Povidone, Artificial Flavor, Dextrins, Silica, Calcium Stearate, Pyridoxine HCl (B-6), Artificial Color, Vitamin A Acetate, Thiamine Mononitrate (B-1), Riboflavin (B-2), Folic Acid, Cyanocobalamin (B-12), Cholecalciferol (Vit D).

Recommended Dosage: 1 tablet daily.

How Supplied: Available in bottles of 120 tablets.

UNICAP M® Tablets
Multivitamins and Minerals
Sugar Free and Sodium Free

Indications: Dietary supplement providing up to 100% of the RDA for essential vitamins and minerals, including vitamin C and B-complex vitamins your body cannot store.

Each tablet contains:		% U.S. RDA
Vitamin A	5000 Int. Units	100
Vitamin D	400 Int. Units	100
Vitamin E	30 Int. Units	100
Vitamin C	60 mg	100
Folic Acid	400 mcg	100
Thiamine	1.5 mg	100
Riboflavin	1.7 mg	100
Niacin	20 mg	100
Vitamin B_6	2 mg	100
Vitamin B_{12}	6 mcg	100
Pantothenic Acid	10 mg	100
Iodine	150 mcg	100
Iron	18 mg	100
Copper	2 mg	100
Zinc	15 mg	100
Calcium	60 mg	6
Phosphorus	45 mg	5
Manganese	1 mg	+
Potassium	5 mg	+

+Recognized as essential in human nutrition, but no U.S. Recommended Daily Allowance (U.S. RDA) has been established.

Ingredient List: Calcium Phosphate, Ascorbic Acid (Vit C), Vitamin E Acetate, Ferrous Fumarate, Cellulose, Niacinamide, Artificial Color, Zinc Oxide, Calcium Pantothenate, Vitamin A Acetate, Potassium Sulfate, Magnesium Stearate, Cupric Sulfate, Silica Gel, Manganese Sulfate, Pyridoxine Hydrochloride, Riboflavin (B-2), Thiamine Mononitrate (B-1), FD&C Yellow No. 5, Folic Acid, Artificial Flavor, Cholecalciferol (Vit D), Potassium Iodide, Carnauba Wax, Cyanocobalamin (B-12).

Recommended Dosage: 1 tablet daily.

How Supplied: Available in bottles of 120 and 500 tablets.
Shown in Product Identification Section, page 432

UNICAP® Plus Iron Tablets
Multivitamin Supplement With
100% of the U.S. RDA of Essential Vitamins Plus Calcium and Extra Iron
Sugar Free and Sodium Free

Indications: Dietary multivitamin supplement providing essential vitamins. 125% of the RDA of Iron plus Calcium for women 12 or more years of age.
Each tablet contains:
[See table top of next page]

Ingredient List: Calcium Phosphate, Cellulose, Ascorbic Acid (Vit C), Ferrous Fumarate, Vitamin E Acetate, Artificial Color, Niacinamide, Vitamin A Acetate, Calcium Pantothenate, Magnesium Stearate, Silica Gel, Pyridoxine HCl

Continued on next page

Upjohn—Cont.

Vitamins

		% U.S. RDA*
Vitamin A	5000 Int. Units	100
Vitamin D	400 Int. Units	100
Vitamin E	30 Int. Units	100
Vitamin C	60 mg	100
Folic Acid	400 mcg	100
Thiamine	1.5 mg	100
Riboflavin	1.7 mg	100
Niacin	20 mg	100
Vitamin B6	2 mg	100
Vitamin B12	6 mcg	100
Pantothenic Acid	10 mg	100

Minerals

Iron	22.5 mg	125
Calcium	100 mg	10

*Percentage of U.S. Recommended Daily Allowance.

(B-6), Riboflavin (B-2), Thiamine Mononitrate (B-1), Folic Acid, Artificial Flavor, Cholecalciferol (Vit D), Carnauba Wax, Cyanocobalamin (B-12).

Recommended Dosage: 1 tablet daily.

How Supplied: Available in bottles of 120 tablets.

UNICAP Sr.® Tablets
Vitamins and Minerals for Adults 50+ Based on the National Academy of Sciences–National Research Council Recommendations
Sugar Free and Sodium Free

Indications: Dietary supplement of essential vitamins and minerals formulated for the nutritional needs of adults 50+.

Each tablet contains:

		% RDDA*
Vitamin A	5000 Int. Units	100
(as Acetate and Beta Carotene)		
Vitamin D	200 Int. Units	100
Vitamin E	15 Int. Units	50
Vitamin C	60 mg	100
Folic Acid	400 mcg	100
Thiamine	1.2 mg	100
Riboflavin	1.4 mg	100
Niacin	16 mg	100
Vitamin B6	2.2 mg	100
Vitamin B12	3 mcg	100
Pantothenic Acid	10 mg	100
Iodine	150 mcg	100
Iron	10 mg	100
Copper	2 mg	100
Zinc	15 mg	100
Calcium	100 mg	12
Phosphorus	77 mg	10
Magnesium	30 mg	9
Manganese	1 mg	+
Potassium	5 mg	+

* Percentage of Recommended Daily Dietary Allowance for Adults 51 years and over, National Academy of Sciences–National Research Council.
+Recognized as essential in human nutrition, but no U.S. Recommended Daily Allowance (U.S. RDA) has been established.

Ingredient List: Calcium Phosphate, Cellulose, Ascorbic Acid (Vit C), Magnesium Oxide, Vitamin E Acetate, Ferrous Fumarate, Artificial Color, Zinc Oxide, Niacinamide, Calcium Pantothenate, Vitamin A Acetate, Magnesium Stearate, Potassium Sulfate, Cupric Sulfate, Silica Gel, Beta-Carotene, Manganese Sulfate, Pyridoxine Hydrochloride (B-6), Riboflavin (B-2), Thiamine Mononitrate (B-1), Folic Acid, Artificial Flavor, Cholecalciferol (Vit D), Potassium Iodide, Carnauba Wax, Cyanocobalamin (B-12).

Recommended Dosage: 1 tablet daily.

How Supplied: Available in bottles of 120 tablets.

Shown in Product Identification Section, page 432

UNICAP T® Tablets
Stress Formula
A More Complete Vitamin and Mineral Supplement
Sugar Free and Sodium Free

Indications: Dietary supplement offering higher levels of vitamin C and B-complex vitamins essential for the return to, and maintenance of good health.

Each tablet contains:

		% U.S. RDA
Vitamin A	5000 Int. Units	100
Vitamin D	400 Int. Units	100
Vitamin E	30 Int. Units	100
Vitamin C	500 mg	833
Folic Acid	400 mcg	100
Thiamine	10 mg	667
Riboflavin	10 mg	588
Niacin	100 mg	500
Vitamin B6	6 mg	300
Vitamin B12	18 mcg	300
Pantothenic Acid	25 mg	250
Iodine	150 mcg	100
Iron	18 mg	100
Copper	2 mg	100
Zinc	15 mg	100
Manganese	1 mg	+
Potassium	5 mg	+
Selenium	10 mcg	+

+Recognized as essential in human nutrition, but no U.S. Recommended Daily Allowance (U.S. RDA) has been established.

Ingredient List: Ascorbic Acid (Vit C), Niacinamide, Cellulose, Hydroxypropyl Methylcellulose, Vitamin E Acetate, Ferrous Fumarate, Artificial Color, Calcium Pantothenate, Calcium Phosphate, Zinc Oxide, Vitamin A Acetate, Magnesium Stearate, Potassium Sulfate, Thiamine Mononitrate (B-1), Riboflavin (B-2), Selenium Yeast, Pyridoxine Hydrochloride (B-6), Cupric Sulfate, Silica Gel, Manganese Sulfate, FD&C Yellow No. 5, Folic Acid, Artificial Flavor, Cholecalciferol (Vit D), Potassium Iodide, Carnauba Wax, Cyanocobalamin (B-12).

Recommended Dosage: 1 tablet daily.

How Supplied: Available in bottles of 60 tablets.

Shown in Product Identification Section, page 432

Wakunaga of America Co., Ltd.
Subsidiary of Wakunaga Pharmaceutical Co., Ltd.
23501 MADERO
MISSION VIEJO, CA 92691

KYOLIC®
Odor Modified Garlic

Active Ingredient: Aged Garlic Extract.™

Indications: Dietary Supplement.

Suggested Use: Average serving, four capsules or tablets a day during or after meals.

How Supplied: Liquid—Kyolic-Aged Garlic Extract Flavor and Odor Modified Enriched with Vitamin B1 and B12 (and empty gelatine capsules) 2 fl oz (62 capsules) and 4 fl oz (124 capsules). Kyolic-Aged Garlic Extract Flavor and Odor Modified Plain (and empty gelatine capsules) 2 fl oz (62 capsules) and 4 fl oz (124 capsules).

Tablets and Capsules—Ingredients per Tablet or Capsule:
Kyolic—Super Formula 100 Tablets: Aged Garlic Extract Powder (300 mg), Whey (168 mg) blended with natural vegetable sources: Cellulose and Algin, bottles of 100 and 200 tablets.
Kyolic—Super Formula 100 Capsules: Aged Garlic Extract Powder (300 mg), Whey (168 mg), bottles of 100 and 200 capsules.
Kyolic—Super Formula 101 Garlic Plus® Tablets: Aged Garlic Extract Powder (270 mg) blended with Brewer's Yeast (27 mg), Kelp (9 mg), bottles of 100 and 200 tablets.
Kyolic—Super Formula 101 Garlic Plus® Capsules: Aged Garlic Extract Powder (270 mg) blended with Brewer's Yeast (27 mg), Kelp (9 mg), bottles of 50, 100 and 200 capsules.
Kyolic—Super Formula 102 Tablets: Aged Garlic Extract Powder (350 mg), "Kyolic Enzyme Complex™" [Amylase, Protease, Cellulase and Lipase] (30 mg), bottles of 100 and 200 tablets.
Kyolic—Super Formula 102 Capsules: Aged Garlic Extract Powder (350 mg), "Kyolic Enzyme Complex™" [Amylase, Protease, Cellulase and Lipase] (30 mg), bottles of 100 and 200 tablets.
Kyolic—Super Formula 103 Capsules: Aged Garlic Extract Powder (220 mg), Ester C® [Calcium Ascorbate] (150 mg), Astragulus membranaceous (100 mg), Calcium citrate (80 mg), bottles of 100 and 200 capsules.
Kyolic—Super Formula 104 Capsules: Aged Garlic Extract Powder (300 mg), Lecithin (200 mg), bottles of 100 and 200 capsules.
Kyolic—Super Formula 105 Capsules: Aged Garlic Extract Powder (250 mg), Beta-Carotene (37.5 mg) d-Alpha-Tocopheryl Acid Succinate [Vitamin E] (50 mg) in a base of Alfalfa and Parsley, bottles of 100 capsules.

Kyolic—Super Formula 106 Capsules: Aged Garlic Extract Powder (300 mg), *d*-Alpha Tocopheryl Succinate [Vitamin E] (90 mg), Hawthorn Berry (50 mg), Cayenne Pepper (10 mg), bottles of 50 and 100 capsules.

Professional label "SGP" is available in Aged Garlic Extract powder forms.
Shown in Product Identification Section, page 432

EDUCATIONAL MATERIAL

From Soil to Shelf
Brochure describing our company, garlic fields, aging tanks and factory, plus our product line.

Walker, Corp & Co., Inc.
P.O. BOX 1320
EASTHAMPTON PL. &
N. COLLINGWOOD AVE.
SYRACUSE, NY 13201

EVAC–U–GEN®
[e-vak-ū-jen]

Description: Evac-U-Gen® is available as purple scored tablets, each containing 97.2 mg of yellow phenolphthalein. Also contains anise oil, corn syrup solids, D&C red 7, FD&C blue 1, lactose, magnesium stearate, saccharin sodium and sugar.

Action and Uses: For temporary relief of occasional constipation and to help restore a normal pattern of evacuation. A mild, non-griping, stimulant laxative in chewable, anise-flavored form, Evac-U-Gen provides gentle, overnight relief by softening of the feces through selective action on the intramural nerve plexus of intestinal smooth muscle, and increases the propulsive peristaltic activity of the colon. It is frequently helpful in preparing the bowel for diagnostic procedures.

Indications: Because of its gentle and non-toxic nature, Evac-U-Gen is especially recommended for persons over 55, and in the presence of hemorrhoids. It is also suitable in pregnancy and for children. Safe for nursing mothers, Evac-U-Gen does not affect the infant. It may be useful when straining at the stool is a hazard, as in hernia, cardiac or hypertensive patients.

Contraindications: Contraindicated in patients with a history of sensitivity to phenolphthalein. Evac-U-Gen should not be used when abdominal pain, nausea, vomiting, or other symptoms of appendicitis are present.

Side Effects: If skin rash appears, use of Evac-U-Gen or other preparations containing phenolphthalein should be discontinued. May cause coloration of feces or urine if such are sufficiently alkaline.

Warning: Frequent or prolonged use may result in dependence on laxatives. Keep this and all medication out of reach of children.

Administration and Dosage: Adults: chew one or two tablets night or morning. **Children:** Over 6, chew ½ tablet daily. Intensity of action is proportional to dosage, but individually effective doses vary. Evac-U-Gen is usually active 6 to 8 hours after administration, but residual action may last 3 to 4 days.

How Supplied: Evac-U-Gen is available in bottles of 35, 100, 500, 1000 and 6000 tablets.
Shown in Product Identification Section, page 432

Walker Pharmacal Company
4200 LACLEDE AVENUE
ST. LOUIS, MO 63108

PRID SALVE
(Smile's PRID Salve)
Drawing Salve and Anti-infectant

Active Ingredients: Ichthammol (Ammonium Ichthosulfonate) Phenol (Carbolic Acid) Lead Oleate, Rosin, Bees Wax, Lard.

Description: PRID has a very stiff consistency and is almost black in color.

Indication: PRID is an anti-infective salve, which also serves as a skin protective ointment. As a drawing salve, PRID softens the skin around the foreign body, and assists the natural rejection. PRID also helps to prevent the spread of infection. PRID aids in relieving the discomfort of minor skin irritations, superficial cuts, scratches and wounds. PRID is also helpful in the treatment of boils and carbuncles. PRID has been used with some success in the treatment of acne and furunculosis as well as other skin disorders.

Warning: When applied to fingers or toes, do not use a bandage; use loose gauze so as to not interfere with circulation. Apply according to directions for use and in no case to large areas of the body without a physician's direction. Keep out of eyes.

Caution: If PRID salve is not effective in 10 days, see your physician.

Directions For Use: Wash affected parts thoroughly with hot water; dry and apply PRID at least twice daily on a clean bandage or gauze. After irritation subsides, repeat application once a day for several days. DO NOT irritate by squeezing or pressing skin area.

How Supplied: PRID is packaged in a telescoping orange metal can containing 20 grams of PRID salve.

Wallace Laboratories
P.O. BOX 1001
HALF ACRE ROAD
CRANBURY, NJ 08512

MALTSUPEX®
(malt soup extract)
Powder, Liquid, Tablets

Composition: 'Maltsupex' is a nondiastatic extract from barley malt, which is available in powder, liquid, and tablet form. 'Maltsupex' has a gentle laxative action and promotes soft, easily passed stools. Each **Tablet** contains 750 mg of 'Maltsupex' and approximately 0.15 to 0.25 mEq of potassium. Tablet Ingredients: acetylated monoglycerides, FD&C Yellow #5, FD&C Yellow #6, flavor (artificial), hydroxypropyl methylcellulose, polyethylene glycol, povidone, stearic acid, talc, titanium dioxide. Each tablespoonful (½ fl oz) of **Liquid** and each heaping tablespoonful of **Powder** contains the equivalent of 16 g of Malt Soup Extract Powder and 3.1 to 5.5 mEq of potassium. Other Ingredients: none.

Indications: 'Maltsupex' is indicated for the dietary management and treatment of functional constipation in infants and children. It is also useful in treating constipation in adults, including those with laxative dependence.

Warnings: Do not use when abdominal pain, nausea or vomiting are present. If constipation persists, consult a physician. Keep this and all medications out of the reach of children.
'Maltsupex' Powder and Liquid only—Do not use these products except under the advice and supervision of a physician if you have kidney disease.
As with any drug, if you are pregnant or nursing a baby, seek the advice of a health professional before using this product.

Precautions: In patients with diabetes, allow for carbohydrate content of approximately 14 grams per tablespoonful of **Liquid** (56 calories), 13 grams per tablespoonful of **Powder** (52 calories), and 0.6 grams per Tablet (3 calories). **Tablets only:** This product contains FD&C Yellow No. 5 (tartrazine) which may cause allergic-type reactions (including bronchial asthma) in certain susceptible individuals. Although the overall incidence of FD&C Yellow No. 5 (tartrazine) sensitivity in the general population is low, it is frequently seen in patients who also have aspirin hypersensitivity.

Dosage and Administration: General—The recommended daily dosage of 'Maltsupex' may vary from 6 to 32 grams for infants (2 years or less) and 12 to 64 grams for children and adults, accompanied by adequate fluid intake with each dose. Use the smallest dose that is effective and lower dosage as improvement occurs. Use heaping measures of the **Powder**. 'Maltsupex' **Liquid** mixes more

Continued on next page

Wallace—Cont.

easily if stirred first in one or two ounces of warm water.

Powder and Liquid (Usual Dosage)—
Adults: 2 tablespoonfuls (32 g) twice daily for 3 or 4 days, or until relief is noted, then 1 to 2 tablespoonfuls at bedtime for maintenance, as needed. Drink a full glass (8 oz) of liquid with each dose. **Children:** 1 or 2 tablespoonfuls in 8 ounces of liquid once or twice daily (with cereal, milk or preferred beverage). **Bottle-Fed Infants (over 1 month):** ½ to 2 tablespoonfuls in the day's total formula, or 1 to 2 teaspoonfuls in a single feeding to correct constipation. To prevent constipation (as when switching to whole milk) add 1 to 2 teaspoonfuls to the day's formula or 1 teaspoonful to every second feeding. **Breast-Fed Infants (over one month):** 1 to 2 teaspoonfuls in 2 to 4 ounces of water or fruit juice once or twice daily.

Tablets—**Adults:** Start with 4 tablets (3 g) four times daily (with meals and bedtime) and adjust dosage according to response. Drink a full glass (8 oz) of liquid with each dose.

How Supplied: 'Maltsupex' is supplied in 8 ounce (NDC 0037-9101-12) and 16 ounce (NDC 0037-9101-08) jars of 'Maltsupex' Powder; 8 fluid ounce (NDC 0037-9001-12) and 1 pint (NDC 0037-9001-08) bottles of 'Maltsupex' Liquid; and in bottles of 100 'Maltsupex' Tablets (NDC 0037-9201-01).

'Maltsupex' **Powder** and **Liquid** are Distributed by

WALLACE LABORATORIES
Division of
CARTER-WALLACE, INC.
Cranbury, New Jersey 08512

'Maltsupex' **Tablets** are Manufactured by

WALLACE LABORATORIES
Division of
CARTER-WALLACE, INC.
Cranbury, New Jersey 08512
Rev. 10/85

Shown in Product Identification Section, page 432

RYNA®
(Liquid)
RYNA–C®   ℭ
(Liquid)
RYNA–CX®   ℭ
(Liquid)

Description:
RYNA Liquid—Each 5 mL (one teaspoonful) contains:
Chlorpheniramine maleate .... 2 mg
Pseudoephedrine hydrochloride....30 mg
Other ingredients: flavor (artificial), glycerin, malic acid, sodium benzoate, sorbitol, purified water, in a clear, slightly yellow colored, lemon-vanilla flavored demulcent base containing no sugar, dyes, or alcohol.
RYNA-C Liquid—Each 5 mL (one teaspoonful) contains, in addition:

Codeine phosphate ....10 mg
(WARNING: May be habit-forming)
Other ingredients: flavor (artificial), glycerin, malic acid, purified water, saccharin sodium, sodium benzoate, sorbitol, in a clear, colorless to slightly yellow, cinnamon-flavored, demulcent base containing no sugar, dyes, or alcohol.
RYNA-CX Liquid—Each 5 mL (one teaspoonful) contains:
Codeine phosphate ....10 mg
(WARNING: May be habit-forming)
Pseudoephedrine hydrochloride....30 mg
Guaifenesin ....100 mg
Other ingredients: flavors (artificial), glycerin, glycine, malic acid, povidone, propylene glycol, purified water, saccharin sodium, sorbitol, in a clear, colorless, cherry-vanilla-menthol flavored demulcent base containing no sugar, dyes, or alcohol.

Actions:
Chlorpheniramine maleate in RYNA and RYNA-C is an antihistamine that antagonizes the effects of histamine.
Codeine phosphate in RYNA-C and RYNA-CX is a centrally-acting antitussive that relieves cough.
Pseudoephedrine hydrochloride in RYNA, RYNA-C and RYNA-CX is a sympathomimetic nasal decongestant that acts to shrink swollen mucosa of the respiratory tract.
Guaifenesin in RYNA-CX is an expectorant that increases mucus flow to help prevent dryness and relieve irritated respiratory tract membranes.

Indications:
RYNA: For the temporary relief of nasal congestion due to the common cold, hay fever or other upper respiratory allergies. Temporarily relieves runny nose, sneezing, itching of the nose or throat, and itchy, watery eyes due to hay fever or other respiratory allergies such as allergic rhinitis.
RYNA-C: Temporarily relieves cough, nasal congestion, runny nose and sneezing as may occur with the common cold.
RYNA-CX: Temporarily relieves cough and nasal congestion as may occur with the common cold. Relieves irritated membranes in the respiratory passageways by preventing dryness through increased mucus flow.

Warnings:
For RYNA:
Do not give this product to children taking other medication or to children under 6 years except under the advice and supervision of a physician. Do not exceed recommended dosage because nervousness, dizziness or sleeplessness may occur. Do not take this product for more than 7 days. If symptoms do not improve or are accompanied by fever, consult a doctor. Do not take this product except under the advice and supervision of a physician if you have any of the following symptoms or conditions: high blood pressure; heart disease; thyroid disease; diabetes; asthma; glaucoma; emphysema; chronic pulmonary disease; shortness of breath; difficulty in breathing; or difficulty in urination due to enlargement of the prostate.

For RYNA-C and RYNA-CX:
Adults and children who have a chronic pulmonary disease or shortness of breath, or children who are taking other drugs, should not take these products unless directed by a physician. Do not give these products to children under 6 years of age except under the advice and supervision of a physician. A persistent cough may be a sign of a serious condition. If cough persists for more than one week, tends to recur, or is accompanied by fever, rash or persistent headache, consult a physician. Do not take these products for persistent or chronic cough such as occurs with smoking, asthma, emphysema, or if cough is accompanied by excessive phlegm (mucus) unless directed by a physician. Do not take these products if you have glaucoma, asthma, emphysema, difficulty in breathing, difficulty in urination due to enlargement of the prostate gland, heart disease, high blood pressure, thyroid disease, or diabetes unless directed by a physician. May cause or aggravate constipation.

Do not take these products or give to children for more than 7 days. If symptoms do not improve or are accompanied by fever, consult a physician. Unless directed by a physician, do not exceed recommended dosage because nervousness, dizziness or sleeplessness may occur at higher doses.
For RYNA and RYNA-C:
These products contain an antihistamine which may cause excitability, especially in children, or may cause drowsiness. Alcohol may increase the drowsiness effect. Do not drive motor vehicles, operate machinery, or drink alcoholic beverages while taking these products.
As with any drug, if you are pregnant or nursing a baby, seek the advice of a health professional before using these products.

Drug Interaction Precaution: Do not use these products if you are presently taking a prescription drug for high blood pressure or depression without first consulting your doctor.

Dosage and Administration:
Adults: 2 teaspoonfuls every 6 hours
Children 6 to under 12 years: 1 teaspoonful every 6 hours.
Children under 6 years: Do not take except under the advice and supervision of a physician.
DO NOT EXCEED 4 DOSES IN 24 HOURS.
Ryna-C and Ryna-CX:
A special measuring device should be used to give an accurate dose of these products to children under 6 years of age. Giving a higher dose than recommended by a physician could result in serious side effects for the child.

How Supplied:
RYNA: bottles of 4 fl oz (NDC 0037-0638-66) and one pint (NDC 0037-0638-68).
RYNA-C: bottles of 4 fl oz (NDC 0037-0522-66) and one pint (NDC 0037-0522-68).

RYNA-CX: bottles of 4 fl oz (NDC 0037-0801-66) and one pint (NDC 0037-0801-68).

TAMPER-RESISTANT BAND ON CAP, PRINTED "WALLACE LABORATORIES". DO NOT USE IF BAND IS MISSING OR BROKEN.

Storage:
RYNA: Store below 30°C (86°F).
RYNA-C and RYNA-CX: Store at controlled room temperature. Protect from excessive heat and freezing.
KEEP THESE AND ALL DRUGS OUT OF THE REACH OF CHILDREN. IN CASE OF ACCIDENTAL OVERDOSE, SEEK PROFESSIONAL ASSISTANCE OR CONTACT A POISON CONTROL CENTER IMMEDIATELY.

WALLACE LABORATORIES
Division of
CARTER-WALLACE, Inc.
Cranbury, New Jersey 08512
Rev. 4/91
*Shown in Product Identification
Section, page 432*

SYLLACT®
(Psyllium Hydrophilic Mucilloid for Oral Suspension, U.S.P.)
(Powdered Psyllium Seed Husks)

Description: Each rounded teaspoonful of fruit-flavored **'Syllact'** contains approximately 3.3 g of powdered psyllium seed husks and an equal amount of dextrose as a dispersing agent, and provides about 14 calories. Potassium sorbate, methyl and propylparaben are added as preservatives. Other ingredients: citric acid, dextrose, FD&C Red #40, flavor (artificial), and saccharin sodium.

Actions: The active ingredient in 'Syllact' is hydrophilic mucilloid, non-absorbable dietary fiber derived from the powdered husks of natural psyllium seed, which acts by increasing the water content and bulk volume of stools. It gives 'Syllact' a bland, non-irritating, laxative action and promotes physiologic evacuation of the bowel.

Indications: 'Syllact' is indicated for the relief of occasional constipation. This product generally produces bowel movement in 12 to 72 hours.

Warnings: Do not use laxative products when abdominal pain, nausea or vomiting are present unless directed by a physician. If you have noticed a sudden change in bowel habits that persists over a period of 2 weeks, consult a physician before using a laxative. Laxative products should not be used for a period longer than 1 week unless directed by a physician. Rectal bleeding or failure to have a bowel movement after use of a laxative may indicate a serious condition. Discontinue use and consult a physician. Bulk-forming agents should not be swallowed dry. They should not be used if impaction or gross intestinal pathology is present.
WARNING: MIX THIS PRODUCT WITH AT LEAST 8 OUNCES (A FULL GLASS) OF WATER OR OTHER FLUID. TAKING THIS PRODUCT WITHOUT ADEQUATE FLUID MAY CAUSE IT TO SWELL AND TO BLOCK YOUR THROAT OR ESOPHAGUS AND MAY CAUSE CHOKING. DO NOT TAKE THIS PRODUCT IF YOU HAVE EVER HAD DIFFICULTY IN SWALLOWING OR HAVE ANY THROAT PROBLEMS.
IF YOU EXPERIENCE CHEST PAIN, VOMITING, OR DIFFICULTY IN SWALLOWING OR BREATHING AFTER TAKING THIS PRODUCT, SEEK IMMEDIATE MEDICAL ATTENTION. Keep this and all medications out of the reach of children. This product may cause allergic reactions in people sensitive to inhaled or ingested psyllium powder. As with any drug, if you are pregnant or nursing a baby, seek the advice of a health professional before using this product.

Dosage and Administration: The actual daily dosage depends on the need and response of the patient. Adults may take up to 9 teaspoonfuls daily, in divided doses, for several days to provide optimum benefit when constipation is chronic or severe. Lower the dosage as improvement occurs. Use a dry spoon to measure powder. Tighten lid to keep out moisture.
Drink a full glass (8 ounces) of liquid with each dose.
Adults and children 12 years of age and over: Oral dosage is 1 rounded teaspoonful in a full glass of liquid, one to three times daily, before or after meals.
Children 6 to under 12 years of age: ½ to 1 rounded teaspoonful in a full glass of liquid, one to three times daily.
Children under 6 years of age: Consult a physician.
For best results, place powder in a dry glass, add about ½ inch of liquid and stir briskly. Add remainder of liquid, stir and drink immediately. Follow with an additional glass of water if desired.

How Supplied: 'Syllact' Powder—in 10 oz jars (NDC 0037-9501-13).
Rev. 2/91
WALLACE LABORATORIES
Division of
CARTER-WALLACE, INC.
Cranbury, New Jersey 08512
*Shown in Product Identification
Section, page 432*

IDENTIFICATION PROBLEM?
Consult the
Product Identification Section
where you'll find
products pictured
in full color.

Warner-Lambert Company
Consumer Health Products Group
201 TABOR ROAD
MORRIS PLAINS, NJ 07950

PROFESSIONAL STRENGTH EFFERDENT
Denture Cleanser

Cleansing Ingredients: Potassium monopersulfate, sodium perborate, sodium carbonate, sodium tripolyphosphate, EDTA and surfactants.

Other Ingredients: Sodium bicarbonate, citric acid, colors and flavors.

Indications: For effective and convenient daily denture cleaning to remove plaque and stains and to inhibit bacterial growth on dentures and removable orthodontic appliances.

Actions: Efferdent's effervescent cleansing action removes stubborn stains between teeth, whitens and brightens, fights plaque and leaves dentures and removable orthodontic appliances fresh tasting and odor free.

Warnings: Keep out of the reach of children. DO NOT PUT TABLETS IN MOUTH.

Dosage and Administration: For best results, use at least once daily. Dentures may be soaked safely in Efferdent overnight.

How Supplied: Available in boxes of 20, 40, 60, 90, and 120 tablets.
*Shown in Product Identification
Section, page 432*

HALLS® MENTHO–LYPTUS®
Cough Suppressant Tablets

Active Ingredients: Each tablet contains eucalyptus oil and menthol.

Inactive Ingredients: Corn Syrup, Flavoring, Sugar and Artificial Colors.

Indications: For temporary relief of minor throat irritation and coughs due to colds or inhaled irritants. Makes nasal passages feel clearer.

Warning: A persistent cough or sore throat may be a sign of a serious condition. If cough persists for more than 1 week, tends to recur, or is accompanied by fever, rash or persistent headache, or if sore throat is severe, persistent or accompanied by high fever, headache, nausea, and vomiting, consult a doctor. Do not take this product for sore throat lasting more than 2 days or persistent or chronic cough such as occurs with smoking, asthma, emphysema, or if cough is accompanied by excessive phlegm (mucus) unless directed by a doctor. Keep this and all drugs out of the reach of children.

Dosage and Administration: Adults and children 5 years and over: dissolve one tablet slowly in mouth. Repeat every

Continued on next page

Warner-Lambert—Cont.

hour as needed or as directed by a doctor. Children under 5 years: consult a doctor.

How Supplied: Halls Mentho-Lyptus Cough Suppressant Tablets are available in single sticks of 9 tablets each, in 5-stick packs, and in bags of 30 tablets. They are available in five flavors: Regular, Cherry, Honey-Lemon, Ice Blue–Peppermint, and Spearmint.
Shown in Product Identification Section, page 432

HALLS® PLUS
Cough Suppressant Tablets

Active Ingredients: Each centerfilled tablet contains eucalyptus oil and menthol.

Inactive Ingredients: Corn Syrup, Flavoring, Glycerin, High Fructose Corn Syrup, Sugar and Artificial Colors

Indications: For temporary relief of minor throat irritation and coughs due to colds or inhaled irritants. Makes nasal passages feel clearer.

Warnings: A persistent cough or sore throat may be a sign of a serious condition. If cough persists for more than 1 week, tends to recur, or is accompanied by fever, rash or persistent headache or if sore throat is severe, persistent or accompanied by high fever, headache, nausea, and vomiting, consult a doctor. Do not take this product for sore throat lasting more than 2 days or persistent or chronic cough such as occurs with smoking, asthma, emphysema, or if cough is accompanied by excessive phlegm (mucus) unless directed by a doctor. Keep this and all drugs out of the reach of children.

Dosage and Administration: Adults and children 5 years and over dissolve one centerfilled tablet slowly in mouth. Repeat every hour as needed or as directed by a doctor. Children under 5 years: consult a doctor.

How Supplied: Halls Plus Cough Suppressant Tablets are available in single sticks of 10 tablets each and in bags of 25 tablets. They are available in three flavors: Regular, Cherry and Honey-Lemon.
Shown in Product Identification Section, page 432

HALLS® Vitamin C Drops

Description: Halls Vitamin C Drops are a delicious way to get 100% of the U.S. Recommended Daily Allowance of Vitamin C. Each drop provides 60 mg. of Vitamin C (100% U.S. RDA).

Ingredients: Sugar, Glucose Syrup, Sodium Ascorbate, Citric Acid, Ascorbic Acid, Natural Flavoring and Artificial Color (Including Yellow 5 and Yellow 6).

Indication: Dietary Supplementation.

How Supplied: Halls Vitamin C Drops are available in single sticks of 9 drops

each and in bags of 30 drops. They are available in 2 great-tasting assortments: All-natural citrus flavors (tangerine, lemon, sweet grapefruit, lime and orange) and berry flavors (grape, cherry, strawberry and raspberry).
Shown in Product Identification Section, page 433

LISTERINE® Antiseptic

Active Ingredients: Thymol .06%, Eucalyptol .09%, Methyl Salicylate .06% and Menthol .04%. Also contains: Water, Alcohol 26.9%, Benzoic Acid, Poloxamer 407 and Caramel.

Indications: To help prevent and reduce supragingival plaque and gingivitis; for general oral hygiene and bad breath.

Actions: Listerine Antiseptic has been shown to help prevent and reduce supragingival plaque and gingivitis when used in a conscientiously applied program of daily oral hygiene and regular professional care. Its effect on periodontitis has not been determined. Listerine is the only leading nonprescription mouthrinse that has received the American Dental Association's Council on Dental Therapeutics Seal of Acceptance for helping to prevent and reduce plaque above the gumline and gingivitis.

Directions: Rinse full strength for 30 seconds with ⅔ ounce (4 teaspoonfuls) morning and night. If bad breath persists, see your dentist.

How Supplied: Listerine Antiseptic is supplied in 3, 6, 12, 18, 24, 32, 48, 58 fl. oz. bottles, and professional gallons.
Shown in Product Identification Section, page 433

LISTERMINT®
Mouthwash with Fluoride

Active Ingredient: Sodium Fluoride (0.02%). Also contains: Water, SD alcohol 38-B (6.65%), glycerin, poloxamer 407, sodium lauryl sulfate, sodium citrate, flavoring, sodium saccharin, zinc chloride, citric acid, D&C Yellow No. 10, FD&C Green No. 3.

Indications: Aids in prevention of dental cavities and freshens breath.

Directions: Adults and children 6 years of age and older: Use twice a day after brushing teeth with toothpaste. Vigorously swish 10 ml. (2 teaspoonfuls) of rinse between teeth for 1 minute and spit out. Do not swallow the rinse. Do not eat or drink for 30 minutes after rinsing.

Warnings: Children under 12 years of age should be supervised in the use of this product. Consult a dentist or physician for use in children under 6 years of age. Developing teeth of children under 6 years of age may become permanently discolored if excessive amounts of fluoride are repeatedly swallowed. This is not a dentifrice and should not be used as a substitute for regular toothbrushing.

Keep this and all drugs out of reach of children.

How Supplied: Listermint with Fluoride is supplied to consumers in 6, 12, 18, 24 and 32 fl. oz. bottles.
Shown in Product Identification Section, page 433

LUBRIDERM BODY BAR®
Extremely Mild Lathering Cleanser Unscented

Ingredients: Sodium Cocoyl Isethionate, Stearic Acid, Sodium Tallowate, Water, Sodium Dodecylbenzene Sulfonate, Sodium Palm Kernelate, Coconut Fatty Acid, Masking Fragrance, Pentasodium Pentetate, Tetrasodium Etidronate. May also contain Sodium Cocoate.

Actions and Uses: Lubriderm Moisturizing Body Bar contains essential moisturizing ingredients in a formula that provides a balance between cleansing and mildness. Luibriderm Moisturizing Bar contains no harsh detergents that might dry or irritate the skin and is non-comedogenic to promote clear skin.

Administration and Dosage: Wash daily with Lubriderm Moisturizing Body Bar and warm water.

How Supplied: Unscented 4oz (Net Wt.)
Shown in Product Identification Section, page 433

LUBRIDERM® LOTION
Skin Lubricant Moisturizer

Composition:
Scented—Contains Water, Mineral Oil, Petrolatum, Sorbitol, Lanolin, Lanolin Alcohol, Stearic Acid, Triethanolamine, Cetyl Alcohol, Fragrance, Butylparaben, Methylparaben, Propylparaben, Sodium Chloride.
Fragrance Free—Contains Water, Mineral Oil, Petrolatum, Sorbitol, Lanolin, Lanolin Alcohol, Stearic Acid, Triethanolamine, Cetyl Alcohol, Butylparaben, Methylparaben, Propylparaben, Sodium Chloride.

Actions and Uses: Lubriderm Lotion is an oil-in-water emulsion indicated for use in softening, soothing and moisturizing dry chapped skin. Lubriderm relieves the roughness, tightness and discomfort associated with dry or chapped skin and helps protect the skin from further drying.
Lubriderm's formula smoothes easily into skin without leaving a greasy feeling.

Administration and Dosage: Apply as often as needed to hands and body to restore and maintain the skin's natural suppleness.

Precautions: For external use only.

How Supplied:
Scented: Available in 1, 4, 8, 12 and 16 fl. oz. plastic bottles, and a 2.5 ounce tube.

Fragrance Free: Available in 1, 8, 12 and 16 fl. oz. plastic bottles, and a 2.5 ounce tube.

Shown in Product Identification Section, page 433

LUBRIDERM® BATH OIL
Skin Conditioning Oil

Composition: Contains Mineral Oil, PPG-15 Stearyl Ether, Oleth-2, Nonoxynol-5, Fragrance, D&C Green No. 6.

Actions and Uses: Lubriderm Skin Conditioning Oil is a lanolin-free, mineral oil–based, bath oil designed for softening and soothing dry skin during the bath. The formula disperses into countless droplets of oil that coat the skin and help lubricate and soften. It is equally effective in hard or soft water and provides an excellent way to moisturize the skin and help counterbalance the drying effects of harsh soaps and hot water.

Administration and Dosage: One to two capfuls in bath, or apply with hand or moistened cloth in shower and rinse. For use as a skin cleanser, rub into wet skin and rinse.

Precautions: Avoid getting in eyes; if this occurs, flush with clear water. When using any bath oil, take precautions against slipping. For external use only.

How Supplied: Available in 8 fl. oz. plastic bottles.

Shown in Product Identification Section, page 433

REPLENS® Vaginal Moisturizer
[ree 'plenz]

Description: Replens relieves the discomfort of vaginal dryness for days with a single application. Replens non-hormonal vaginal moisturizer provides natural moisture to continuously hydrate vaginal tissue. Replens is non-staining, fragrance free, unflavored, non-greasy and non-irritating.

Actions: When used as directed, Replens provides long-lasting relief from the discomfort of vaginal dryness by providing continuous hydration to the vaginal tissue.

Ingredients: Purified water, glycerin, mineral oil, polycarbophil, Carbomer 934P, hydrogenated palm oil glyceride, and sorbic acid.

Warnings: Keep out of the reach of children. Replens is not a contraceptive. Does not contain spermicide.

Usage: Use as needed. One application 2 to 3 times a week is recommended.

How Supplied: Replens is available in boxes containing 3, 8, or 12 pre-filled disposable applicators. Each applicator delivers 2.5 grams.

Shown in Product Identification Section, page 433

ROLAIDS®

Active Ingredient: Dihydroxyaluminum Sodium Carbonate 300 mg.

Inactive Ingredients: Corn Starch, Corn Syrup, Flavoring, Magnesium Stearate and Sugar. May also contain pregelatinized starch. Contains 50 mg. sodium per tablet.

Indications: For the relief of heartburn, sour stomach or acid indigestion and upset stomach associated with these symptoms.

Actions: Rolaids® provides rapid neutralization of stomach acid. Each tablet has acid-neutralizing capacity of 75–80 ml. of 0.1N hydrochloric acid and the ability to maintain the pH of the stomach contents close to 3.5 for a significant period of time.
Due to the relatively low solubility and other physical and chemical properties of dihydroxyaluminum sodium carbonate (DASC), it is for the most part non-absorbed.
Although sodium is present in DASC, the sodium is available for absorption only when the antacid reacts with stomach acid. When Rolaids are consumed in excess of the amount of acid present in the stomach, this sodium is unavailable for absorption and the active ingredient is passed through the digestive system unchanged, with no sodium released.

Warnings: Keep this and all drugs out of the reach of children. Do not take more than 24 tablets in a 24-hour period, nor use the maximum dosage of this product for more than two weeks, nor use this product if you are on a sodium-restricted diet, except under the advice and supervision of a physician.

Professional Warnings: Prolonged use of aluminum-containing antacids in patients with renal failure may result in or worsen dialysis osteomalacia. Elevated tissue aluminum levels contribute to the development of the dialysis encephalopathy and osteomalacia syndromes. Small amounts of aluminum are absorbed from the gastrointestinal tract and renal excretion of aluminum is impaired in renal failure. Aluminum is not well removed by dialysis because it is bound to albumin and transferrin, which do not cross dialysis membranes. As a result, aluminum is deposited in bone, and dialysis osteomalacia may develop when large amounts of aluminum are ingested orally by patients with impaired renal function. Aluminum forms insoluble complexes with phosphate in the gastrointestinal tract, thus decreasing phosphate absorption. Prolonged use of aluminum-containing antacids by normophosphatemic patients may result in hypophosphatemia if phosphate intake is not adequate. In its more severe forms, hypophosphatemia can lead to anorexia, malaise, muscle weakness, and osteomalacia.

Drug Interaction Precaution: Do not take this product if you are presently taking a prescription antibiotic drug containing any form of tetracycline.

Dosage and Administration: Chew 1 or 2 tablets as symptoms occur. Repeat hourly if symptoms return or as directed by a physician.

How Supplied: Rolaids is available in Regular (Peppermint), Spearmint and Wintergreen Flavors. One roll contains 12 tablets; 3-pack contains three 12-tablet rolls; one bottle contains 75 tablets; one bottle contains 150 tablets.

Shown in Product Identification Section, page 433

CALCIUM RICH/SODIUM FREE ROLAIDS®

Active Ingredient: Calcium Carbonate 550 mg. per tablet.

Inactive Ingredients:
Cherry Flavor: Corn Starch, D&C Red No. 27, Flavoring, Magnesium Stearate, Mannitol, Polyethylene Glycol, Sugar and Titanium Dioxide.
Assorted Fruit Flavors: Colors (D&C Red No. 27, FD&C Blue No. 1, Red 40, Yellow 5 [Tartrazine] and Yellow 6), Corn Starch, Flavoring, Magnesium Stearate, Mannitol, Pregelatinized Starch and Sugar.
Peppermint Flavor: Corn Starch, Flavoring, Magnesium Stearate, Mannitol, Pregelatinized Starch, Sugar and Titanium Dioxide.

Indications: For the relief of heartburn, sour stomach or acid indigestion and upset stomach associated with these symptoms.

Actions: Calcium Rich/Sodium Free Rolaids provides rapid neutralization of stomach acid. Each tablet has an acid neutralizing capacity of 110 ml of 0.1N hydrochloric acid and the ability to maintain the pH of the stomach contents at 3.5 or greater for a significant period of time. Each tablet contains less than 0.4 mg of sodium and provides 22% of the Adult U.S. RDA for calcium.

Warnings: Do not take more than 14 tablets in a 24-hour period or use the maximum dosage of this product for more than 2 weeks except under the advice and supervision of a physician. Keep this and all drugs out of the reach of children.

Dosage and Administration: Chew 1 or 2 tablets as symptoms occur. Repeat hourly if symptoms return or as directed by a physician.

How Supplied: Calcium Rich/Sodium Free Rolaids is available in Peppermint, Cherry and Assorted Fruit Flavors. One roll contains 12 tablets: 3-pack contains three 12-tablet rolls; one bottle contains 75 tablets; one bottle contains 150 tablets.

Shown in Product Identification Section, page 433

Continued on next page

Warner-Lambert—Cont.

EXTRA STRENGTH ROLAIDS®

Active Ingredient: Calcium Carbonate 1000 mg. per tablet.

Inactive Ingredients: Acesulfame Potassium, Colors (FD&C Blue No. 1, FD&C Yellow No. 5 [Tartrazine] and Titanium Dioxide), Corn Syrup, Flavoring, Magnesium Stearate, Pregelatinized Starch and Sugar.

Indications: For the relief of heartburn, sour stomach or acid indigestion and upset stomach associated with these symptoms.

Actions: Extra Strength Rolaids provides rapid neutralization of stomach acid. Each tablet has an acid-neutralizing capacity of 200 ml. of 0.1N hydrochloric acid and the ability to maintain the pH of the stomach contents at 3.5 or greater for a significant period of time. Each tablet contains less than 0.4 mg. of sodium.

Warnings: Do not take more than 8 tablets in a 24-hour period or use the maximum dosage of this product for more than 2 weeks except under the advice and supervision of a physician. Keep this and all drugs out of the reach of children.

Dosage and Administration: Chew 1 or 2 tablets as symptoms occur. Repeat hourly if symptoms return or as directed by a physician.

How Supplied: Extra Strength Rolaids is available in Assorted Mint Flavors. One roll contains 10 tablets: 3-pack contains three 10-tablet rolls; one bottle contains 55 tablets; one bottle contains 110 tablets.
Shown in Product Identification Section, page 433

SOOTHERS® Throat Drops
From the makers of Halls

Active Ingredients: Each centerfilled tablet contains menthol 2 mg.

Inactive Ingredients: Colors (Including Yellow 6), Corn Syrup, Flavoring, Glycerin, High Fructose Corn Syrup, Honey and Sugar.

Indications: For temporary relief of occasional minor irritation, pain, sore mouth, sore throat or pain associated with canker sores.

Warnings: If sore throat is severe, persists for more than 2 days, is accompanied or followed by fever, headache, rash, nausea, or vomiting, consult a doctor promptly. If sore mouth symptoms do not improve in 7 days, see your dentist or doctor promptly. Keep this and all drugs out of the reach of children.

Dosage and Administration: Adults and children 5 years of age and older: dissolve 1 drop slowly in mouth. May be repeated every 2 hours as needed or as di-

rected by a dentist or doctor. Children under 5 years of age: consult a dentist or doctor.

How Supplied: Soothers Throat Drops are available in packages of 10 tablets each and in bags of 25 tablets. They are available in cherry and orange flavors.
Shown in Product Identification Section, page 433

Water-Jel Technologies, Inc.
**243 VETERANS BLVD.
CARLSTADT, NJ 07072**

WATER–JEL® Sterile Burn Dressings
One-Step Emergency Burn Care Product for all types of burns

Key Facts: Water-Jel is a unique, patented one-step product ideal for emergency first aid burn care, to extinguish flame on a victim, and protect from heat. The scientifically formulated gel combines with a special carrier material to: Ease pain, prevent burn progression, cool the skin and stabilize skin temperature, protect the covered wound from contamination, facilitate removal of burnt clothing or jewelry; Won't harm skin or eyes, does not require a water source to continue cooling, and is non-allergenic.

Major Uses: Burns of all types—Fire, steam, heat, electrical, boiling water. Emergency First Aid for all burns.

Safety Information: Chemical burns must be thoroughly flushed before applying Water-Jel. Consult a physician if the burn is severe, covers an area larger than your palm, or involves your face.

Description: Each packet contains a gel-soaked polyester fabric.
The gel is an off-white translucent color. It has a characteristic odor. It is sterile. A freezing point of $-15°C$ and a boiling point of $+92°C$. The gel is a proprietary formulation of natural gums and oils in a preserved, sterile, easily washed-off aqueous base.

Indications: Emergency First Aid for all burns. Water-Jel provides fast relief of pain due to burns. It soothes and cools the burned area and protects the covered wound from contamination. It stops burn progress and is easily removed without re-injuring the wound. It is non-allergenic.

Application: Simply open the package and apply the dressing to the burned area. Pour the excess gel from the package onto the dressing. Keep in place for approximately 15 to 20 minutes.

Warning: In the case of chemical burns, the wound must be thoroughly flushed before applying Water-Jel. Consult a physician if the burn is severe, covers an area larger than your palm, or involves the face.

How Supplied: Water-Jel Sterile Burn Dressings are available in several sizes for use on different size burns—$2''\times6''$;

$4''\times4''$; $4''\times16''$; and $8''\times18''$. Water-Jel is contained in heat-sealed foil packets.

EDUCATIONAL MATERIAL

"Since the Dawn of Civilization..."
4-page, full color brochure.
Descriptive use and application of all Water-Jel® Fire Rescue, Heat Shield and Emergency Burn care products.
"Technical Specifications"
2-page, in-depth specifications of all Water-Jel® products.
"Presentation Video"
11-minute video on the use of Water-Jel® products.

Westwood-Squibb Pharmaceuticals Inc.
**100 FOREST AVENUE
BUFFALO, NY 14213**

MOISTUREL® CREAM
Skin Protectant—Moisturizer

Description: A highly effective, concentrated formula clinically proven to relieve dry skin and designed not to cause acne or blemishes. Ideal for sensitive skin. Free of lanolins, fragrances, and parabens that can sensitize or irritate skin.

Directions: Apply liberally as often as needed. If used for diaper rash, change wet diapers promptly, cleanse the diaper area and allow to dry. Apply cream liberally with each changing.

Indications: Helps prevent and temporarily protects chafed, chapped, cracked or windburned skin. For temporary protection of minor cuts, scrapes, burns and sunburn. Helps treat and prevent minor skin irritation due to diaper rash and helps seal out wetness.

Active Ingredients: Dimethicone 1%, petrolatum 30%. Also contains: Water, glycerin, PG dioctanoate, cetyl alcohol, steareth-2, PVP/hexadecene copolymer, laureth-23, magnesium aluminum silicate, diazolidinyl urea, carbomer-934, sodium hydroxide, methylchloroisothiazolinone and methylisothiazolinone.

Warnings: For external use only. Avoid contact with the eyes. Not to be applied over puncture wounds or infections.

How Supplied: 4 oz. (NDC 0072-9500-04) and 16 oz. (NDC 0072-9500-16) plastic jars.
Shown in Product Identification Section, page 433

MOISTUREL® LOTION
Skin Protectant—Moisturizer

Directions: Apply liberally as often as needed to soothe and soften sensitive skin. If used for diaper rash, change wet diapers promptly, cleanse the diaper area and allow to dry. Apply lotion liberally with each changing.

Indications: Generalized dry skin. Helps prevent and temporarily protects chafed, chapped, cracked or windburned skin. Helps treat and prevent minor skin irritation due to diaper rash and helps seal out wetness.

Warnings: For external use only. Avoid contact with the eyes. Not to be applied over puncture wounds or infections.

Active Ingredient: Dimethicone 3%. Also contains: Water, petrolatum, glycerin, steareth-2, cetyl alcohol, benzyl alcohol, laureth-23, magnesium aluminum silicate, carbomer-934, sodium hydroxide, quaternium-15.

How Supplied: 8 oz. (NDC 0072-9100-08) and 12 oz. (NDC 0072-9100-12) plastic bottles.
Shown in Product Identification Section, page 433

MOISTUREL®
SENSITIVE SKIN CLEANSER
Pure, Clear and Soap-Free

Composition: Sodium laureth sulfate and laureth-6 carboxylic acid and disodium laureth sulfosuccinate, methyl gluceth-20, cocamidopropyl betaine, water, diazolidinyl urea, and methylchloroisothiazolinone and methylisothiazolinone.

Actions and Uses: Moisturel Sensitive Skin Cleanser is a crystal clear, lathering, soap-free cleanser. It cleans thoroughly without stinging, irritating, or drying. Unlike soaps, Moisturel Sensitive Skin Cleanser rinses refreshingly clean without leaving a film or residue. Its pure and gentle formula makes it ideal for facial use. Its nondrying, noncomedogenic, and fragrance-free formula makes it ideal for cleansing:
● Sensitive skin—even a baby's
● Dry, itchy skin caused by cold and wind, or overexposure to sun
● Skin robbed of moisture by use and removal of cosmetics
● Irritated, allergic skin
● Skin dried by harsh acne medications

Administration and Dosage: With skin wet, gently work Moisturel Sensitive Skin Cleanser into a rich lather by massaging in a circular motion. Rinse thoroughly and pat dry with a soft cloth.

Caution: Avoid contact with eyes. For external use only.

How Supplied: 8.75 oz. (NDC 0072-6420-08) plastic bottle with pump.
Shown in Product Identification Section, page 433

SEBULEX®
Antiseborrheic Treatment Shampoo

Active Ingredients: 2% sulfur and 2% salicylic acid. Also contains: D&C yellow #10, docusate sodium, EDTA, FD&C blue #1, fragrance, PEG-6 lauramide, PEG-14M, sodium dodecyl benzene sulfonate, sodium octoxynol-2 ethane sulfonate and water.

Action and Uses: A penetrating therapeutic shampoo for the temporary relief of itchy scalp and the scaling of dandruff. SEBULEX helps to relieve dandruff and itching, and removes excess oil. It penetrates and softens the crusty, matted layers of scales adhering to the scalp, and leaves the hair soft and manageable.

Administration and Dosage: SEBULEX liquid should be shaken before use. SEBULEX is massaged into wet scalp. Lather should be allowed to remain on scalp for about 5 minutes and then rinsed. Application is repeated, followed by a thorough rinse. Initially, SEBULEX can be used daily, or every other day, or as directed, depending on the condition. Once symptoms are under control, one or two treatments a week usually will maintain control of itching, oiliness and scaling.

Caution: If undue skin irritation develops or increases, discontinue use. For external use only. Contact with eyes should be avoided. In case of contact, flush eyes thoroughly with water. Keep this and all drugs out of reach of children.

How Supplied: SEBULEX in 4 oz. (NDC 0072-2700-04) and 8 oz. (NDC 0072-2700-08) plastic bottles.
Shown in Product Identification Section, page 433

SEBUTONE® and SEBUTONE® CREAM
Antiseborrheic Tar Shampoo

Active Ingredients: Coal tar 0.5%, salicylic acid 2%, sulfur 2%. SEBUTONE also contains: D&C yellow #10, docusate sodium, EDTA, FD&C blue #1, fragrance, lanolin oil, PEG-6 lauramide, PEG-90M, sodium dodecyl benzene sulfonate, sodium octoxynol-2 ethane sulfonate, titanium dioxide, and water. SEBUTONE CREAM also contains: Ceteareth-20, D&C yellow #10, dextrin, docusate sodium, EDTA, FD&C blue #1, fragrance, laureth-4, lanolin oil, magnesium aluminum silicate, PEG-6 lauramide, PEG-14 M, sodium dodecyl benzene sulfonate, sodium octoxynol-2 ethane sulfonate, stearyl alcohol, titanium dioxide and water.

Action and Uses: A surface-active, penetrating therapeutic shampoo for the temporary relief of itchy scalp and the scaling of stubborn dandruff and psoriasis. Provides prompt and prolonged relief of itching, helps control oiliness and rid the scalp of scales and crust. Tar ingredient is chemically and biologically standardized to produce uniform therapeutic activity. Wood's light demonstrates residual microfine particles of tar on the scalp several days after a course of SEBUTONE shampoo. In addition to its antipruritic and antiseborrheic actions, SEBUTONE also helps offset excessive scalp dryness with a special moisturizing emollient.

Administration and Dosage: SEBUTONE liquid should be well shaken before use. A liberal amount of SEBUTONE or SEBUTONE CREAM is massaged into the wet scalp for 5 minutes and the scalp is then rinsed. Application is repeated, followed by a thorough rinse. Use as often as necessary to keep the scalp free from itching and scaling or as directed. No other shampoo or soap washings are required.

Caution: If undue skin irritation develops or increases, discontinue use. In rare instances, temporary discoloration of white, blond, bleached or tinted hair may occur. Contact with the eyes is to be avoided. In case of contact flush eyes with water. For external use only. Keep this and all drugs out of reach of children.

How Supplied: SEBUTONE in 4 oz. (NDC 0072-5000-04) and 8 oz. (NDC 0072-5000-08) plastic bottles.
SEBUTONE CREAM in 4 oz. (NDC 0072-5100-01) tubes.
Shown in Product Identification Section, page 433

Whitby Pharmaceuticals, Inc.
1211 SHERWOOD AVENUE
P.O. BOX 85054
RICHMOND, VA 23261-5054

AMESEC®
[am'ah-sec]
Antiasthmatic

Description: Each capsule contains:
Aminophylline .... 130 mg
 (equivalent to 104 mg theophylline)
Ephedrine hydrochloride .... 25 mg
Each capsule also contains colloidal silicon dioxide, FD&C Blue No. 2, FD&C Red No. 3, FD&C Yellow No. 6, gelatin, iron oxide black, and starch.

Indications: For temporary relief of bronchial asthma.

Warnings: Do not take this product unless a diagnosis of asthma has been made by a physician.
As with any drug, if you are pregnant or nursing a baby, seek the advice of a health professional before using this product.
Keep this and all drugs out of the reach of children. In case of accidental overdose, seek professional assistance or contact a Poison Control Center immediately.

Drug Interaction Precaution: Do not take this product if you are presently taking a prescription antihypertensive or antidepressant drug containing a monoamine oxidase inhibitor.

Caution: Do not continue to take this product but seek medical assistance immediately if symptoms are not relieved within one hour or become worse. Do not take this product if you are presently

Continued on next page

Whitby Pharm.—Cont.

taking a prescription drug for asthma or give to children under 12 years or exceed recommended dosage except under the advice and supervision of a physician. Excessive use may cause toxic effects and even death in children. Do not take this product if you have heart disease, high blood pressure, thyroid disease, diabetes, or difficulty in urination due to enlargement of the prostate gland, or if nausea, vomiting, or restlessness occurs. Nervousness, tremor, sleeplessness, nausea, and loss of appetite may occur.

Usual Adult Dosage: One capsule every six hours not to exceed five capsules a day or as directed by a physician.

How Supplied: Bottles of 100 capsules.

CORTICAINE®
[kort'ah-kān ″]
(hydrocortisone acetate)
External Analgesic

Description: The active ingredient in Corticaine® is hydrocortisone acetate 0.5%. Corticaine also contains esters of mixed saturated fatty acids, stearyl alcohol, glycerin, polysorbate 40, menthol, BHA, BHT, disodium EDTA, and purified water with methylparaben and propylparaben as preservatives.
Store at controlled room temperature 15° to 30°C (59° to 86°F). Keep tube well closed.

Indications: For the temporary relief of itching associated with external anal inflammation.

Warnings: For external use only. Avoid contact with the eyes. If condition worsens, or symptoms persist for more than 7 days or clear up and occur again within a few days, stop use of this product and do not begin use of any other hydrocortisone product unless you have consulted a physician. Do not use for the treatment of diaper rash. Consult a physician. Do not exceed the recommended daily dosage unless directed by a physician. In case of bleeding, consult a physician promptly. Do not put this product into the rectum by using fingers or any mechanical device or applicator.

Dosage and Administration: For adults and children 2 years of age and older: apply to the affected area not more than three to four times daily. For children under 2 years of age: do not use, consult a physician. When practical, cleanse the affected area with mild soap and warm water and rinse thoroughly. Gently dry by patting or blotting with toilet tissue or a soft cloth before application of this product. For children under 12 years of age: consult a physician.

How Supplied: Corticaine® (hydrocortisone acetate) is supplied in 1 ounce tubes.
Shown in Product Identification Section, page 433

VICON-C® Capsules
[vī'kon]
(Therapeutic Vitamins and Minerals)

Description: Each yellow and orange capsule contains:
Ascorbic acid	300 mg
Niacinamide	100 mg
Zinc sulfate, USP*	80 mg
Magnesium sulfate, USP**	70 mg
Thiamine mononitrate	20 mg
d-Calcium pantothenate	20 mg
Riboflavin	10 mg
Pyridoxine hydrochloride	5 mg

*As 50 mg dried zinc sulfate.
**As 50 mg dried magnesium sulfate.

Each capsule also contains D&C Yellow No. 10, FD&C Yellow No. 6, gelatin, microcrystalline cellulose, soybean oil, stearic acid, talc, sodium propionate, and titanium dioxide.

Indications and Usage: VICON-C® is indicated in the treatment of patients with deficiencies of, or increased requirements for, Vitamin C, B-complex vitamins, zinc, and/or magnesium. The components of VICON-C have important roles in nutrition, tissue growth and repair, and the prevention of hemorrhage. Tissue injury resulting from trauma, burns, or surgery may rapidly deplete the body stores of Vitamin C, the B-Complex vitamins, and zinc. Patients maintained on parenteral fluids for extended periods or patients with burns, wounds, or diarrhea often develop deficiencies of Vitamin C, the B-Complex vitamins, and zinc.
VICON-C is recommended for deficiencies or the prevention of deficiencies of Vitamin C, the B-Complex vitamins, magnesium, and/or zinc in conditions such as febrile diseases, chronic or acute infections, burns, fractures, surgery, toxic conditions, physiologic stress, alcoholism, pregnancy, lactation, geriatrics, peptic ulcer, colitis, and in conditions involving special diets and weight-reduction diets. It is also recommended in dentistry for these deficiencies in conditions such as herpetic stomatitis, aphthous stomatitis, cheilosis, herpangina, gingivitis, and states involving oral surgery.

Dosage and Administration: One capsule two or three times daily or as directed by a physician for treatment of deficiencies.

How Supplied: Bottles of 60 capsules and unit dose pack of 100 capsules.
Shown in Product Identification Section, page 433

VICON® PLUS Capsules
[vī'kon]
(Therapeutic Vitamins and Minerals)

Description: Each red and beige capsule contains:
[See table top of next column]

Each capsule also contains D&C Yellow No. 10, FD&C Blue No. 1, FD&C Red No. 40, FD&C Yellow No. 6, gelatin, lactose, magnesium stearate, talc, and titanium dioxide.

Vitamin A	4,000 IU
Vitamin E	50 IU
Ascorbic Acid	150 mg
Zinc sulfate, USP*	80 mg
Magnesium sulfate, USP**	70 mg
Niacinamide	25 mg
Thiamine mononitrate	10 mg
d-Calcium pantothenate	10 mg
Riboflavin	5 mg
Manganese chloride	4 mg
Pyridoxine hydrochloride	2 mg

*As 50 mg dried zinc sulfate.
**As 50 mg dried magnesium sulfate.

VICON® PLUS is an extended range vitamin-mineral supplement formulated to aid patient recovery by helping to meet increased nutritional demands.

Indications and Usage: For nutritional supplementation of the patient undergoing physiologic stress due to surgery, burns, trauma, febrile illnesses, or poor nutrition.

Dosage and Administration: One capsule twice daily or as prescribed by a physician for treatment of deficiencies. Dosage should not exceed eight capsules daily due to the possible toxicity of large doses of vitamin A.

How Supplied: Bottles of 60 capsules.
Shown in Product Identification Section, page 433

VI-ZAC® Capsules
[vī-zak]
(Therapeutic Vitamin-Mineral)

Description: Each orange capsule contains:
Vitamin A	5,000 IU
Absorbic acid	500 mg
Vitamin E	50 IU
Zinc sulfate, USP*	80 mg

*As 50 mg dried zinc sulfate

Each capsule also contains methylcellulose, FD&C Yellow No. 6, FD&C Yellow No. 10, gelatin, lactose, magnesium stearate, and titanium dioxide.

Indications and Usage: VI-ZAC® is indicated in the treatment of patients with deficiencies of, or increased requirements for, Vitamins A, C, and E and zinc. The VI-ZAC formulation is a limited vitamin-mineral formulation designed to meet special needs. It is particularly indicated where there is no requirement for supplemental amounts of the B-Complex vitamins and their attendant appetite stimulation. The formulation is also designed for patients who cannot tolerate magnesium supplements but do need supplemental amounts of zinc.

Precautions: Although rarely encountered, vitamin A in large doses daily for several months or longer may cause toxicity.

Dosage and Administration: One or two capsules daily or as directed by the physician for the treatment of deficiencies.

How Supplied: Bottles of 60.
Shown in Product Identification Section, page 433

Whitehall Laboratories Inc.

Division of American Home Products Corporation
685 THIRD AVENUE
NEW YORK, NY 10017

ADVIL®
[ad 'vil]
Ibuprofen Tablets, USP
Ibuprofen Caplets
Pain Reliever/Fever Reducer

WARNING: ASPIRIN-SENSITIVE PATIENTS. Do not take this product if you have had a severe allergic reaction to aspirin, e.g.—asthma, swelling, shock or hives, because even though this product contains no aspirin or salicylates, cross-reactions may occur in patients allergic to aspirin.

Active Ingredient: Each tablet contains Ibuprofen 200 mg.

Inactive Ingredients: Acacia, Acetylated Monoglycerides, Beeswax or Carnauba Wax, Calcium Sulfate, Colloidal Silicon Dioxide, Dimethicone, Iron Oxide, Lecithin, Pharmaceutical Glaze, Povidone, Sodium Benzoate, Sodium Carboxymethylcellulose, Starch, Stearic Acid, Sucrose, Titanium Dioxide.

Indications: For the temporary relief of minor aches and pains associated with the common cold, headache, toothache, muscular aches, backache, for the minor pain of arthritis, for the pain of menstrual cramps and for reduction of fever.

Dosage and Administration: Adults: Take one tablet every 4 to 6 hours while symptoms persist. If pain or fever does not respond to one tablet, two tablets may be used but do not exceed six tablets in 24 hours unless directed by a doctor. The smallest effective dose should be used. Take with food or milk if occasional and mild heartburn, upset stomach, or stomach pain occurs with use. Consult a doctor if these symptoms are more than mild or if they persist. Children: Do not give this product to children under 12 except under the advice and supervision of a doctor.

Warnings: Do not take for pain for more than 10 days or for fever for more than 3 days unless directed by a doctor. If pain or fever persists or gets worse, if new symptoms occur, or if the painful area is red or swollen, consult a doctor. These could be signs of serious illness. If you are under a doctor's care for any serious condition, consult a doctor before taking this product. As with aspirin and acetaminophen, if you have any condition which requires you to take prescription drugs or if you have had any problems or serious side effects from taking any nonprescription pain reliever, do not take this product without first discussing it with your doctor. IF YOU EXPERI-ENCE ANY SYMPTOMS WHICH ARE UNUSUAL OR SEEM UNRELATED TO THE CONDITION FOR WHICH YOU TOOK IBUPROFEN, CONSULT A DOCTOR BEFORE TAKING ANY MORE OF IT. Although ibuprofen is indicated for the same conditions as aspirin and acetaminophen, it should not be taken with them except under a doctor's direction. Do not combine this product with any other ibuprofen-containing product. As with any drug, if you are pregnant or nursing a baby, seek the advice of a health professional before using this product. **IT IS ESPECIALLY IMPORTANT NOT TO USE IBUPROFEN DURING THE LAST 3 MONTHS OF PREGNANCY UNLESS SPECIFICALLY DIRECTED TO DO SO BY A DOCTOR BECAUSE IT MAY CAUSE PROBLEMS IN THE UNBORN CHILD OR COMPLICATIONS DURING DELIVERY. Keep this and all drugs out of the reach of children. In case of accidental overdose, seek professional assistance or contact a poison control center immediately.**

How Supplied: Coated tablets in bottles of 8, 24, 50, 100, 165 and 250. Coated caplets in bottles of 24, 50, 100, 165, and 250.

Storage: Store at room temperature; avoid excessive heat 40°C (104°F).
Shown in Product Identification Section, page 434

ADVIL® Cold and Sinus
(formerly CoADVIL®)
Ibuprofen/Pseudoephedrine Caplets*
Pain Reliever/Fever Reducer/Nasal Decongestant

WARNING: ASPIRIN-SENSITIVE PATIENTS. Do not take this product if you have had a severe allergic reaction to aspirin, eg, asthma, swelling, shock or hives, because even though this product contains no aspirin or salicylates, cross-reactions may occur in patients allergic to aspirin.

Indications: For temporary relief of symptoms associated with the common cold, sinusitis or flu, including nasal congestion, headache, fever, body aches, and pains.

Directions: *Adults:* Take 1 caplet every 4 to 6 hours while symptoms persist. If symptoms do not respond to 1 caplet, 2 caplets may be used, but do not exceed 6 caplets in 24 hours unless directed by a doctor. The smallest effective dose should be used. Take with food or milk if occasional and mild heartburn, upset stomach, or stomach pain occurs with use. Consult a doctor if these symptoms are more than mild or if they persist. *Children:* Do not give this product to children under 12 years of age except under the advice and supervision of a doctor.

Warnings: Do not take for colds for more than 7 days or for fever for more than 3 days unless directed by a doctor. If the cold or fever persists or gets worse, or if new symptoms occur, consult a doctor. These could be signs of serious illness. As with aspirin and acetaminophen, if you have any condition which requires you to take prescription drugs or if you have had any problems or serious side effects from taking any nonprescription pain reliever, do not take this product without first discussing it with your doctor. IF YOU EXPERIENCE ANY SYMPTOMS WHICH ARE UNUSUAL OR SEEM UNRELATED TO THE CONDITION FOR WHICH YOU TOOK THIS PRODUCT, CONSULT A DOCTOR BEFORE TAKING ANY MORE OF IT. If you are under a doctor's care for any serious condition, consult a doctor before taking this product.
Do not exceed recommended dosage because at higher doses nervousness, dizziness, or sleeplessness may occur. Do not take this product if you have high blood pressure, heart disease, diabetes, thyroid disease or difficulty in urination due to enlargement of the prostate gland, except under the advice and supervision of a doctor.

Drug Interaction Precaution: Do not take this product if you are presently taking a prescription drug for high blood pressure or depression without first consulting your doctor. Do not combine this product with other nonprescription pain relievers. Do not combine this product with any other ibuprofen-containing product. As with any drug, if you are pregnant or nursing a baby, seek the advice of a health professional before using this product.
IT IS ESPECIALLY IMPORTANT NOT TO USE THIS PRODUCT DURING THE LAST 3 MONTHS OF PREGNANCY UNLESS SPECIFICALLY DIRECTED TO DO SO BY A DOCTOR BECAUSE IT MAY CAUSE PROBLEMS IN THE UNBORN CHILD OR COMPLICATIONS DURING DELIVERY. Keep this and all drugs out of the reach of children. In case of accidental overdose, seek professional assistance or contact a poison control center immediately.

Active Ingredients: Each caplet contains Ibuprofen 200 mg and Pseudoephedrine HCl 30 mg.

Inactive Ingredients: Carnauba or Equivalent Wax, Croscarmellose Sodium, Iron Oxides, Methylparaben, Microcrystalline Cellulose, Propylparaben, Silicon Dioxide, Sodium Benzoate, Sodium Lauryl Sulfate, Starch, Stearic Acid, Sucrose, Titanium Dioxide.

How Supplied: Advil® Cold and Sinus is an oval-shaped tan-colored caplet supplied in consumer bottles of 40 and blister packs of 20. Medical samples are available in a 2's pouch dispenser.

Storage: Store at room temperature; avoid excessive heat (40°C, 104°F).
Shown in Product Identification Section, page 434

---

*Oval-Shaped tablets

Continued on next page

Whitehall—Cont.

ANACIN®
[an 'a-sin]
Coated Analgesic Tablets
Coated Analgesic Caplets

Description: Each tablet or caplet contains: Aspirin 400 mg, Caffeine 32 mg. Anacin® has a special protective coating that makes each tablet or caplet easy to swallow.

Indications and Usage: Anacin provides fast relief from the pain of headache, sprains, muscular aches, sinus pressure ... discomforts and fever of colds ... pain caused by tooth extraction and toothache ... menstrual cramps. Anacin also temporarily relieves the minor aches and pains of arthritis and rheumatism.

Warnings: Children and teenagers should not use this medicine for chicken pox or flu symptoms before a doctor is consulted about Reye Syndrome, a rare but serious illness reported to be associated with aspirin. If pain persists for more than 10 days, or redness is present, or in arthritic or rheumatic conditions affecting children under 12 years of age, consult a physician immediately. As with any drug, if you are pregnant or nursing a baby, seek the advice of a health professional before using this product. **IT IS ESPECIALLY IMPORTANT NOT TO USE ASPIRIN DURING THE LAST 3 MONTHS OF PREGNANCY UNLESS SPECIFICALLY DIRECTED TO DO SO BY A DOCTOR BECAUSE IT MAY CAUSE PROBLEMS IN THE UNBORN CHILD OR COMPLICATIONS DURING DELIVERY.** Keep this and all drugs out of the reach of children. In case of accidental overdose, seek professional assistance or contact a poison control center immediately.

Dosage and Administration: Adults: 2 tablets or caplets with water every 4 hours, as needed. Do not exceed 10 tablets or 10 caplets daily. **Children** 6–12 years of age: half the adult dosage.

Inactive Ingredients: Tablets contain Hydroxypropyl Methylcellulose, Microcrystalline Cellulose, Polyethylene Glycol, Starch, Surfactant.
Caplets contain Hydroxypropyl Methylcellulose, Iron Oxide, Microcrystalline Cellulose, Polyethylene Glycol, Starch, Surfactant.

How Supplied: Tablets: In tins of 12's and bottles of 30's, 50's, 100's, 200's and 300's. Caplets: In bottles of 30's, 50's and 100's.
Shown in Product Identification Section, page 434

ASPIRIN FREE ANACIN®
[an 'a-sin]
Film Coated Acetaminophen Tablets
Film Coated Acetaminophen Caplets

Description: Aspirin Free Tablets and Caplets: Each film coated tablet or caplet contains acetaminophen 500 mg.

Indications and Actions: Aspirin Free Anacin provides safe, fast, temporary relief from pain of headache, colds, flu, muscle aches, backache, toothache, menstrual cramps, reduction of fever, and temporary relief of minor arthritis pain.

Warnings: If pain persists for more than 10 days or redness is present or in arthritic or rheumatic conditions affecting children under 12, consult a physician immediately. Keep this and all drugs out of the reach of children. In case of accidental overdose, seek professional assistance or contact a poison control center immediately. Prompt medical attention is critical for adults as well as for children, even if you do not notice any signs or symptoms. As with any drug, if you are pregnant or nursing a baby, seek the advice of a health professional before using this product.

Dosage and Administration: Adults: 2 tablets or caplets 3 or 4 times a day. Do not exceed 8 tablets or caplets in any 24-hour period.

Overdosage: Acetaminophen in massive overdosage may cause hepatic toxicity in some patients. In all cases of suspected overdose, immediately call your regional poison control center or the Rocky Mountain Poison Control Center for assistance in diagnosis and for directions in the use of N-acetylcysteine as an antidote. In adults, hepatic toxicity has rarely been reported with acute overdoses of less than 10 grams and fatalities with less than 15 grams. Importantly, young children seem to be more resistant than adults to the hepatotoxic effect of an acetaminophen overdose. Despite this, the measures outined below should be initiated in any adult or child suspected of having ingested an acetaminophen overdose.
Early symptoms following a potentially hepatoxic overdose may include: nausea, vomiting, diaphoresis, and general malaise. Clinical and laboratory evidence of hepatic toxicity may not be apparent until 48 to 72 hours post-ingestion. The stomach should be emptied promptly by lavage or by induction of emesis with syrup of ipecac. Patients' estimates of the quantity of a drug ingested are notoriously unreliable. Therefore, if an acetaminophen overdose is suspected, a serum acetaminophen assay should be obtained as early as possible, but no sooner than four hours following ingestion. Liver function studies should be obtained initially and at 24-hour intervals. The antidote, N-acetylcysteine, should be administered as early as possible and within 16 hours of the overdose ingestion for optimal results. Following recovery,

there are no residual structural or functional hepatic abnormalities.

Inactive Ingredients:
Maximum Strength Tablets:
Croscarmellose Sodium, FD&C Blue No. 1 Lake, Hydroxypropyl Methylcellulose, Polyethylene Glycol, Povidone, Propylene Gylcol, Starch, Stearic Acid, Titanium Dioxide.
Maximum Strength Caplets:
Calcium Stearate, Croscarmellose Sodium, D&C Red No. 7 Lake, FD&C Blue No. 1 Lake, Hydroxypropyl Methylcellulose, Polyethylene Glycol, Povidone, Propylene Glycol, Starch, Stearic Acid, Titanium Dioxide.

How Supplied: Maximum Strength Film Coated — Tablets (colored white, imprinted $_{AF}^{A}$ and "500") — tins of 12 and bottles of 30, 60, and 100. Caplets (colored white, imprinted "AF ANACIN")—bottles of 30, 60 and 100.
Shown in Product Identification Section, page 434

MAXIMUM STRENGTH ANACIN®
[an 'a-sin]
Coated Analgesic Tablets

Description: Each tablet contains: Aspirin 500 mg, Caffeine 32 mg. Maximum Strength Anacin has a special protective coating that makes each tablet easy to swallow.

Indications and Usage: Maximum Strength Anacin provides fast relief from the pain of headache, sprains, muscular aches, sinus pressure ... discomforts and fever of colds ... pain caused by tooth extraction and toothache ... menstrual cramps. Maximum Strength Anacin also temporarily relieves the minor aches and pains of arthritis and rheumatism.

Warnings: Children and teenagers should not use this medicine for chicken pox or flu symptoms before a doctor is consulted about Reye Syndrome, a rare but serious illness reported to be associated with aspirin. If pain persists for more than 10 days, or redness is present, or in arthritic or rheumatic conditions affecting children under 12 years of age, consult a physician immediately. As with any drug, if you are pregnant or nursing a baby, seek the advice of a health professional before using this product. **IT IS ESPECIALLY IMPORTANT NOT TO USE ASPIRIN DURING THE LAST 3 MONTHS OF PREGNANCY UNLESS SPECIFICALLY DIRECTED TO DO SO BY A DOCTOR BECAUSE IT MAY CAUSE PROBLEMS IN THE UNBORN CHILD OR COMPLICATIONS DURING DELIVERY.** Keep this and all drugs out of the reach of children. In case of accidental overdose, seek professional assistance or contact a poison control center immediately.

Dosage and Administration: Adults: 2 tablets with water 3 or 4 times a day. Do not exceed 8 tablets in any 24-hour period. Not recommended for children under 12 years of age.

Inactive Ingredients: Hydroxypropyl Methylcellulose, Microcrystalline Cellulose, Polyethylene Glycol, Starch, Surfactant.

How Supplied: Tablets: Tins of 12's and bottles of 20's, 40's, 75's, and 150's.
Shown in Product Identification Section, page 434

Maximum Strength
ANBESOL® Gel and Liquid
[an 'ba-sol ″]
Antiseptic-Anesthetic
Regular Strength
ANBESOL® Gel and Liquid
Antiseptic-Anesthetic
BABY ANBESOL®
Anesthetic Gel

Description: Anbesol is an antiseptic-anesthetic which is available in a Maximum Strength and Regular Strength gel and liquid. Baby Anbesol, available in gel, is an anesthetic only and is alcohol-free.
The Maximum Strength formulations contain Benzocaine 20% and Alcohol 60%.
The Regular Strength formulations contain Benzocaine 6.3%, Phenol 0.5% and Alcohol 70%.
The Baby Anbesol Gel contains Benzocaine 7.5%.

Indications: Maximum Strength and Regular Strength Anbesol are indicated for the fast temporary relief of pain due to toothache, braces, denture and orthodontic irritation, sore gums, cold and canker sores, and fever blisters. Regular Strength Anbesol and Baby Anbesol Gel are also indicated for the fast temporary relief of teething pain.

Actions: Temporarily deadens sensations of nerve endings to provide relief of pain and discomfort; reduces oral bacterial flora temporarily as an aid in oral hygiene (Regular and Maximum Strengths only).

Warnings: Flammable. Keep away from fire or flame. Avoid smoking during application and until product has dried. Do not use near eyes. For persistent or excessive teething pain, consult a physician or dentist. Localized allergic reactions may occur after prolonged or repeated use. Keep this and all drugs out of the reach of children.

Precautions: Not for prolonged use. If the condition persists or irritation develops, discontinue use and consult your physician or dentist. FOR GEL ONLY: NOT FOR USE UNDER DENTURES OR OTHER DENTAL WORK.

Dosage and Administration: Apply topically to the affected area on or around the lips, or within the mouth.
FOR DENTURE IRRITATION: Apply thin layer of gel to affected area and do not reinsert dental work until irritation/pain is relieved. Rinse mouth before reinserting dentures. If irritation/pain persists, contact a dentist.

Inactive Ingredients:
Maximum Strength Gel: Carbomer 934P, D&C Yellow #10, FD&C Blue #1, FD&C Red #40, Flavor, Polyethylene Glycol, Saccharin.
Maximum Strength Liquid: D&C Yellow #10, FD&C Blue #1, FD&C Red #40, Flavor, Polyethylene Glycol, Saccharin.
Regular Gel: Carbomer 934P, D&C Red #33 and Yellow #10, FD&C Blue #1 and Yellow #6, Flavor, Glycerin.
Regular Liquid: Camphor, Glycerin, Menthol, Potassium Iodide, Povidone Iodine.
Baby Gel: Carbomer 934P, D&C Red #33, Disodium Edetate, Flavor, Glycerin, Polyethylene Glycol, Saccharin, Water.

How Supplied: Maximum Strength Gel in .25 oz (7.2 g) tube, Maximum Strength Liquid in .31 oz (9 mL) bottle. Gel and Baby Gel in .25 oz (7.2 g) tubes. Regular Liquid in two sizes— .31 fl. oz. (9 mL) and .74 fl. oz. (22 mL) bottles.
Shown in Product Identification Section, page 434

Maximum Strength
ARTHRITIS PAIN FORMULA™
[är 'thrīt-is ' pān ' for-mye-la]
By the Makers of Anacin® Analgesic Tablets and Caplets

Description: Each caplet contains 500 mg microfined aspirin and two buffers, 27 mg Aluminum Hydroxide and 100 mg Magnesium Hydroxide.
Arthritis Pain Formula is a buffered analgesic and antipyretic with microfined aspirin.

Indications and Actions: Arthritis Pain Formula provides hours of relief from minor aches and pains of arthritis and rheumatism and low back pain. Also relieves the pain of headache, neuralgia, neuritis, sprains, muscular aches, discomforts and fever of colds, pain caused by tooth extraction and toothache, and menstrual discomfort.

Warnings: Children and teenagers should not use this medicine for chicken pox or flu symptoms before a doctor is consulted about Reye syndrome, a rare but serious illness reported to be associated with aspirin. As with any drug, if you are pregnant or nursing a baby, seek the advice of a health professional before using this product. **IT IS ESPECIALLY IMPORTANT NOT TO USE ASPIRIN DURING THE LAST 3 MONTHS OF PREGNANCY UNLESS SPECIFICALLY DIRECTED TO DO SO BY A DOCTOR BECAUSE IT MAY CAUSE PROBLEMS IN THE UNBORN CHILD OR COMPLICATIONS DURING DELIVERY.** Keep this and all medications out of children's reach. In case of accidental overdose, contact a physician immediately.

Precautions: If pain persists for more than 10 days, or redness is present, or in arthritic or rheumatic conditions affecting children under 12 years of age, consult a physician immediately.

Dosage and Administration: Adults: 2 caplets, 3 or 4 times a day. Do not exceed 8 caplets in any 24-hour period. For children under 12 years of age, consult a physician.

Inactive Ingredients: Hydrogenated Vegetable Oil, Microcrystalline Cellulose, Starch, Surfactant.

How Supplied: In plastic bottles of 40 (non-child-resistant size), 100 and 175 caplets.

COMPOUND W®
['käm-pound W]
Liquid and Gel

Description: Compound W is a salicylic acid (17% w/w) preparation available as a liquid or gel.

Indication: Compound W is indicated for the removal of common warts. The common wart is easily recognized by the rough "cauliflower-like" appearance of the surface.

Actions: Warts are common benign skin lesions which appear mainly on the back of hands and on fingers, but can also appear on other parts of the body. They are caused by an infectious virus which stimulates mitosis in the basal cell layer of the skin, resulting in the production of elevated epithelial growths. The keratolytic action of salicylic acid in a flexible collodion vehicle causes the cornified epithelium to swell, soften, macerate and then desquamate.

Warnings: For external use only. Do not use this product on irritated skin, on any area that is infected or reddened, if you are a diabetic, or if you have poor blood circulation. If discomfort persists, see your doctor. Do not use on moles, birthmarks, warts with hair growing from them, genital warts, or warts on the face, near the eyes or on mucous membranes (inside mouth, nose, anus, genitals, or on lips). Flammable. Keep away from fire or flame. Cap bottle or tube tightly and store at room temperature away from heat. Avoid smoking during application and until product has dried. If product gets into the eye, flush with water for 15 minutes. Avoid inhaling vapors. Keep this and all drugs out of the reach of children. In case of accidental ingestion, seek professional assistance or contact a poison control center immediately.

Precautions: If redness or irritation occurs, discontinue product for 2 days and then reapply. Should stinging or irritation recur, discontinue use. Covering the treated wart with a bandage will increase effectiveness, but may also increase the chance of irritation. If a bandage is used, first allow the liquid or gel to dry thoroughly.

Dosage and Administration: Wash affected area. The wart may be soaked in warm water for 5 minutes. Dry area thoroughly. Apply one drop at a time to suffi-

Continued on next page

Whitehall—Cont.

ciently cover each wart by using the plastic rod provided with the liquid or by squeezing the tube. Let dry. Repeat this procedure once or twice daily as needed (until wart is removed) for up to 12 weeks.

Inactive Ingredients: Liquid: Acetone Collodion, Alcohol 1.83% w/w, Camphor, Castor Oil, Ether 63.5%, Menthol, Polysorbate 80. Gel: Alcohol 67.5% by vol., Camphor, Castor Oil, Collodion, Colloidal Silicon Dioxide, Hydroxypropyl Cellulose, Hypophosphorous Acid, Polysorbate 80.

How Supplied: Compound W is available in .31 fluid oz. clear bottles with plastic applicators. Compound W Gel is available in .25 oz. tubes. Store at room temperature.

DENOREX®
[děn 'ō-reks]
Medicated Shampoo
DENOREX®
Mountain Fresh Herbal Scent
Medicated Shampoo
DENOREX®
Medicated Shampoo and Conditioner
DENOREX®
Extra Strength Medicated Shampoo
DENOREX®
Extra Strength Medicated Shampoo with Conditioners

Description: The Shampoo (Regular and Mountain Fresh Herbal) and the Shampoo and Conditioner contain Coal Tar Solution 9.0%, Menthol 1.5%. The Extra Strength Shampoo and the Extra Strength Shampoo with Conditioners contain Coal Tar Solution 12.5% and Menthol 1.5%.

Indications: Relieves scaling, itching, flaking of dandruff, seborrhea and psoriasis. Regular use promotes cleaner, healthier hair and scalp.

Actions: Denorex Shampoo is an antiseborrheic and antipruritic which loosens and softens scales and crusts. Coal tar helps correct abnormalities of keratinization by decreasing epidermal proliferation and dermal infiltration. Denorex also contains the antipruritic agent, menthol.

Warnings: For external use only. Discontinue treatment if irritation develops. Avoid contact with eyes. Keep this and all medicines out of children's reach.

Directions: For best results use regularly, but at least every other day. For severe scalp problems use daily. Wet hair thoroughly and briskly massage until you obtain a rich lather. Rinse thoroughly and repeat. Your scalp may tingle slightly during treatment.

Inactive Ingredients:
Shampoo: Also contains Chloroxylenol, Lauramide DEA, Stearic Acid, TEA-Lauryl Sulfate, Water (plus Fragrance and Hydroxypropyl Methylcellulose in the Mountain Fresh Herbal scent formula), and Alcohol 7.5%.
Shampoo and Conditioner: Chloroxylenol, Citric Acid, Fragrance, Hydroxypropyl Methylcellulose, Lauramide DEA, PEG-27 Lanolin, Polyquaternium-11, TEA-Lauryl Sulfate, Water, and Alcohol 7.5%.
Extra Strength: Chloroxylenol, FD&C Red #40, Fragrance, Glycol Distearate, Lauramide DEA, Methylcellulose, TEA-Lauryl Sulfate, Water, and Alcohol 10.4%.
Extra Strength With Conditioners: Chloroxylenol, Citric Acid, Cocodimonium Hydrolyzed Protein, FD&C Red #40, Fragrance, Glycol Distearate, Lauramide DEA, Methylcellulose, PEG-27 Lanolin, Polyquaternium-6, TEA-Lauryl Sulfate, Water, and Alcohol 10.4%.

How Supplied:
Lotion: 4 oz., 8 oz. and 12 oz. bottles in Regular Scent, Mountain Fresh Herbal Scent, Shampoo and Conditioner, Extra Strength Shampoo, and Extra Strength Shampoo With Conditioners.
Shown in Product Identification Section, page 434

DERMOPLAST®
[der 'mō-plăst]
Anesthetic Pain Relief Lotion

Description: DERMOPLAST Lotion contains Benzocaine 8% and Menthol 0.5%.

Actions: DERMOPLAST is a topical anesthetic and antipruritic.

Indications: DERMOPLAST is indicated for the fast, temporary relief of skin pain and itching due to sunburn, minor cuts, insect bites, abrasions, minor burns, and minor skin irritations.

Warnings: FOR EXTERNAL USE ONLY.
In case of accidental ingestion, seek professional assistance or contact a poison control center. Avoid contact with eyes. Not for prolonged use. If the condition for which this preparation is used persists or if rash or irritation develops, discontinue use and consult physician. Keep this and all drugs out of the reach of children.

Directions: Apply freely over sunburned or irritated skin. Repeat three or four times daily, as needed.

Inactive Ingredients: Aloe Vera Gel, Carbomer 934P, Ceteth-16, Glycerin, Glyceryl Stearate, Laneth-16, Methylparaben, Oleth-16, Propylparaben, Simethicone, Steareth-16, Triethanolamine, Water.

How Supplied: DERMOPLAST Anesthetic Pain Relief Lotion, in Net Wt. 3 fl. oz.

DERMOPLAST®
[der 'mō-plăst]
Anesthetic Pain Relief Spray

Description: DERMOPLAST is an aerosol containing Benzocaine 20% and Menthol 0.5%.

Indications: DERMOPLAST is indicated for the fast, temporary relief of skin pain and itching due to sunburn, minor cuts, insect bites, abrasions, minor burns, and minor skin irritations. May be applied without touching sensitive affected areas. Widely used in hospitals for pain and itch of episiotomy, pruritus vulvae, and postpartum hemorrhoids.

Warnings: FOR EXTERNAL USE ONLY. Avoid spraying in eyes. Contents under pressure. Do not puncture or incinerate. Do not use near open flame. Use only as directed. Intentional misuse by deliberately concentrating and inhaling the contents can be harmful or fatal. Do not take orally. Not for prolonged use. If the condition for which this preparation is used persists, or if a rash or irritation develops, discontinue use and consult physician.

Directions for Use: Hold can in a comfortable position 6–12 inches away from affected area. Point spray nozzle and press button. To apply to face, spray in palm of hand. May be administered three or four times daily, or as directed by physician.

Inactive Ingredients: Acetylated Lanolin Alcohol, *Aloe vera* Oil, Butane, Cetyl Acetate, Chlorofluorocarbon, Methylparaben, PEG-8 Laurate, Polysorbate 85.

How Supplied: DERMOPLAST Anesthetic Pain Relief Spray, in Net Wt 2 oz (57 g) and in Net Wt 2¾ oz (78 g). Do not expose to heat or temperatures above 120° F.

DRISTAN®
[drĭs 'tăn]
Nasal Spray
Menthol Nasal Spray

Description: Dristan Nasal Spray contains Phenylephrine HCl 0.5%, Pheniramine Maleate 0.2%.

Actions: Phenylephrine HCl is a sympathomimetic agent that constricts the smaller arterioles of the nasal passages producing a gentle and predictable decongesting effect.

Indications: Dristan Nasal Spray provides prompt temporary relief of nasal congestion due to colds, sinusitis, hay fever or other upper respiratory allergies.

Warnings: Do not exceed recommended dosage because symptoms may occur such as burning, stinging, sneezing, or increase of nasal discharge. Do not use this product for more than 3 days. If symptoms persist, consult a physician. The use of the dispenser by more than one person may spread infection. For adult use only. Do not give this product to children under 12 years except under the advice and supervision of a physician.

Keep these and all medicines out of the reach of children. In case of accidental ingestion, seek professional assistance or contact a Poison Control Center immediately.

Dosage and Administration: Squeeze Bottle—With head upright, insert nozzle in nostril. Spray quickly, firmly and sniff deeply.
Metered Dose Pump—Prime the metered dose pump by depressing pump firmly several times. With head upright, insert nozzle in nostril. Depress pump 2 or 3 times, all the way down, with a firm, even stroke and sniff deeply.
Adults: Spray 2 or 3 times into each nostril. Repeat every 4 hours as needed. Children under 12 years of age: As directed by a physician.

Inactive Ingredients: Dristan Nasal Spray and Dristan Nasal Spray Metered Dose Pump: Alcohol 0.4%, Benzalkonium Chloride 1:5000 in buffered isotonic aqueous solution, Eucalyptol, Hydroxypropyl Methylcellulose, Menthol, Sodium Chloride, Sodium Phosphate, Thimerosal Preservative 0.002%, and Water.
Dristan Menthol Nasal Spray: Benzalkonium Chloride 1:5000 in buffered isotonic aqueous solution, Camphor, Eucalyptol, Hydroxypropyl Methylcellulose, Menthol, Methyl Salicylate, Polysorbate 80, Sodium Chloride, Sodium Phosphate, Thimerosal Preservative 0.002%, and Water.

How Supplied: Dristan Nasal Spray: 15 mL and 30 mL plastic squeeze bottles, and 15 mL metered dose pumps.
Dristan Menthol Nasal Spray: 15 mL and 30 mL plastic squeeze bottles.

DRISTAN® ALLERGY
Nasal Decongestant/Antihistamine Caplets

Description: Each Dristan Allergy Coated Caplet contains: Pseudoephedrine Hydrochloride 60 mg and Brompheniramine Maleate 4 mg.

Actions: Pseudoephedrine HCl is an oral nasal decongestant and is effective in reducing nasal/sinus congestion. Brompheniramine maleate is an antihistamine effective in the control of the runny nose, sneezing, and watery eyes associated with elevated histamine levels in disorders of the respiratory tract.

Indications: DRISTAN ALLERGY CAPLETS provide hours of effective relief of symptoms associated with allergies, hay fever or other upper respiratory problems. DRISTAN ALLERGY CAPLETS are indicated for relief of nasal congestion, sinus pressure, swollen nasal passages, sneezing, runny nose, and itchy/watery eyes. Each caplet is coated for easy swallowing.

Directions: ADULTS and CHILDREN over 12 years of age: 1 caplet every 4 to 6 hours, not to exceed 4 caplets in 24 hours.

Warnings: Avoid alcoholic beverages and driving a motor vehicle or operating heavy machinery while taking this product. May cause drowsiness or excitability especially in children. Persons with asthma, glaucoma, high blood pressure, diabetes, heart or thyroid disease, difficulty in urination due to an enlarged prostate gland, or taking an antidepressant drug, should use only as directed by a physician. Do not exceed recommended dosage because at higher doses nervousness, dizziness, or sleeplessness may occur.
If symptoms do not improve within 7 days or are accompanied by high fever, discontinue use and see a physician.
As with any drug, if you are pregnant or nursing a baby, seek the advice of a health professional before using this product. Do not give to children under 12 years of age. Keep this and all drugs out of the reach of children. In case of accidental overdose, seek professional assistance or contact a poison control center immediately. Store at room temperature.

Active Ingredients: Each caplet contains Pseudoephedrine Hydrochloride 60 mg and Brompheniramine Maleate 4 mg.

Inactive Ingredients: Ammonium Hydroxide, Calcium Stearate, D&C Yellow #10 Lake, FD&C Blue #1 Lake, Hydrogenated Vegetable Oil, Hydroxypropyl Methylcellulose, Iron Oxide, Microcrystalline Cellulose, Pharmaceutical Glaze, Polyethylene Glycol, Polysorbate 80, Potassium Hydroxide, Propylene Glycol, Silica and Titanium Dioxide.

How Supplied: Green coated caplets in blister packs of 20 and bottles of 40.
Shown in Product Identification Section, page 434

DRISTAN® COLD
[drĭs 'tăn]
Nasal Decongestant/Antihistamine/Analgesic Coated Tablets

Description: Each Dristan Cold Coated Tablet contains: Phenylephrine HCl 5 mg, Chlorpheniramine Maleate 2 mg, Acetaminophen 325 mg.

Actions: Acetaminophen is both an analgesic and an antipyretic. Therapeutic doses of acetaminophen will effectively reduce an elevated body temperature. Also, acetaminophen is effective in relieving headache, body aches, and minor sore throat pain. Phenylephrine HCl is an oral nasal decongestant (sympathomimetic amine) effective as a vasoconstrictor to help reduce nasal congestion, sinus pressure, and swollen nasal passages. Phenylephrine produces little or no central nervous system stimulation. Chlorpheniramine maleate is an antihistamine effective in the control of runny nose, sneezing, and watery eyes associated with elevated histamine levels in disorders of the respiratory tract.

Indications: Dristan Cold is indicated for effective multi-symptom relief of colds, sinusitis, flu, hay fever, or other upper respiratory allergies: nasal congestion, sneezing, runny nose, fever, headache and minor aches and pains.

Warnings: Avoid alcoholic beverages and driving a motor vehicle or operating heavy machinery while taking this product. May cause drowsiness or excitability, especially in children. Persons with asthma, glaucoma, high blood pressure, diabetes, heart or thyroid disease, difficulty in urination due to enlarged prostate gland, or taking an antidepressant drug, should use only as directed by a physician. Do not exceed recommended dosage because at higher doses nervousness, dizziness, or sleeplessness may occur. If symptoms do not improve within 7 days or are accompanied by high fever, discontinue use and see a physician. As with any drug, if you are pregnant or nursing a baby, seek the advice of a health professional before using this product.
Do not give to children under 6 years of age. Keep this and all drugs out of the reach of children. In case of accidental overdose seek professional assistance or contact a poison control center immediately.

Dosage and Administration: Adults: Two tablets every four hours, not to exceed 12 tablets in 24 hours. Children 6–12 years of age: One tablet every four hours, not to exceed six tablets in 24 hours.

Inactive Ingredients: Calcium Stearate, Croscarmellose Sodium, D&C Yellow #10 Lake, FD&C Yellow #6 Lake, Hydroxypropyl Methylcellulose, Microcrystalline Cellulose, Polyethylene Glycol, Povidone, Starch, Stearic Acid.

How Supplied: Yellow/White coated tablets in tins of 12 and blister packages of 20 and bottles of 40 and 75.
Shown in Product Identification Section, page 434

Maximum Strength
DRISTAN® COLD
[drĭs 'tăn]
Nasal Decongestant/Analgesic Coated Caplets

Description: Each Maximum Strength Dristan Cold Coated Caplet contains: Pseudoephedrine HCl 30 mg and Acetaminophen 500 mg.

Actions: Pseudoephedrine HCl is an oral nasal decongestant and is effective in reducing nasal congestion, sinus pressure, and swollen nasal passages. Acetaminophen is both an analgesic and an antipyretic. This maximum strength nonaspirin pain reliever effectively reduces headache pain and the body aches associated with a cold. Acetaminophen also reduces an elevated body temperature.

Indications: Maximum Strength Dristan Cold is indicated for effective relief without drowsiness from nasal and sinus congestion, headache, fever, and minor

Continued on next page

Whitehall—Cont.

aches and pains due to colds, sinusitis, flu, and upper respiratory allergies.

Warnings: Persons with asthma, glaucoma, high blood pressure, heart disease, diabetes, thyroid disease, difficulty in urination due to an enlarged prostate gland, or taking an antidepressant drug should use only as directed by a physician. Do not exceed recommended dosage because at higher doses nervousness, dizziness, or sleeplessness may occur. If symptoms do not improve within 7 days, or are accompanied by high fever, discontinue use and see a physician. Do not give to children under 12 years of age. As with any drug, if you are pregnant or nursing a baby, seek the advice of a health professional before using this product. Keep this and all drugs out of the reach of children. In case of accidental overdose, seek professional assistance or contact a poison control center immediately.

Dosage and Administration: Adults and children over 12 years of age: Two caplets every 6 hours, not to exceed 8 caplets in any 24-hour period. Children under 12 should use only as directed by a physician.

Inactive Ingredients: Calcium Stearate, Croscarmellose Sodium, D&C Red #7 Lake, D&C Yellow #10 Lake, FD&C Yellow #6 Lake, Hydrogenated Vegetable Oil, Hydroxypropyl Methylcellulose, Microcrystalline Cellulose, Pharmaceutical Glaze, Polyethylene Glycol, Povidone, Starch, Stearic Acid, Titanium Dioxide.

How Supplied: Yellow coated caplets in blister packages of 20 and bottles of 40.
*Shown in Product Identification
Section, page 434*

DRISTAN® COLD & FLU

Description: A lemon flavored hot drink mix containing Acetaminophen 500 mg, Pseudoephedrine HCl 60 mg, Chlorpheniramine Maleate 4 mg, and Dextromethorphan HBr 20 mg.

Actions: Acetaminophen is both an analgesic and an antipyretic. Pseudoephedrine HCl is an oral nasal decongestant. Chlorpheniramine Maleate is an antihistamine effective in the control of symptoms caused by elevated histamine levels in disorders of the respiratory tract. Dextromethorphan HBr is a cough suppressant that provides temporary relief of cough due to colds.

Indications: DRISTAN COLD & FLU provides soothing hot liquid medication for hours of effective relief of cold and flu symptoms. DRISTAN COLD & FLU contains a **cough suppressant** to relieve irritating coughs; a **decongestant** to relieve nasal congestion, sinus pressure and reduce swollen nasal passages; an **antihistamine** to relieve sneezing, runny nose, and watery eyes; and an an-**algesic** to relieve headache, body aches, minor sore throat pain and reduce fever.

Directions: Adults and children 12 years of age: Dissolve one packet in 6 oz. cup of hot water. Sip while hot. Sweeten to taste if desired. May repeat every 4 hours, not to exceed 4 doses in 24 hours. Children under 12 years should use only as directed by a physician.

**Warnings: AVOID alcoholic beverages and driving a motor vehicle or operating heavy machinery while taking this product. May cause drowsiness or excitability especially in children. Do not take this product for persistent cough such as occurs with smoking, asthma or emphysema, or if cough is accompanied by excessive secretions (mucus), unless directed by a physician. A persistent cough may be a sign of a serious condition. If cough persists for more than 1 week, recurs, or if accompanied by fever, rash or persistent headache, consult a physician. Persons with asthma, glaucoma, high blood pressure, diabetes, heart or thyroid disease, difficulty in urination due to an enlarged prostate gland, or taking an antidepressant drug, should use only as directed by a physician.
Do not exceed recommended dosage because at higher doses nervousness, dizziness, or sleeplessness may occur. If symptoms do not improve within 7 days or are accompanied by high fever, discontinue use and see a physician. As with any drug, if you are pregnant or nursing a baby, seek the advice of a health professional before using this product. Do not give to children under 12 years of age. Keep this and all drugs out of the reach of children. In case of accidental overdose, seek professional assistance or contact a poison control center immediately.**

Active Ingredients: Each packet contains Acetaminophen 500 mg, Pseudoephedrine HCl 60 mg, Chlorpheniramine Maleate 4 mg, and Dextromethorphan HBr 20 mg.

Inactive Ingredients: Ascorbic Acid, Citric Acid, Corn Syrup, D&C Yellow #10 Lake, FD&C Yellow #6 Lake, Flavor, Sodium Citrate, Starch, Sucrose, Titanium Dioxide, Tricalcium Phosphate.

How Supplied: Dristan Cold and Flu is supplied as boxes of 6 or 12 individual use packets.
Store at room temperature.
*Shown in Product Identification
Section, page 434*

DRISTAN® SINUS
Ibuprofen/Pseudoephedrine Caplets*
Pain Reliever/Nasal Decongestant
WARNING: ASPIRIN-SENSITIVE PATIENTS. Do not take this product if you have had a severe allergic reaction to aspirin, eg, asthma, swelling, shock or hives, because even though this product contains no aspirin or salicylates, cross-reactions may oc-
***Oval-shaped tablets**

cur in patients allergic to aspirin. Use other Dristan formulas.

Indications: For temporary relief of symptoms associated with the common cold, sinusitis or flu, including nasal congestion, headache, fever, body aches, and pains.

Directions: *Adults:* Take 1 caplet every 4 to 6 hours while symptoms persist. If symptoms do not respond to 1 caplet, 2 caplets may be used, but do not exceed 6 caplets in 24 hours unless directed by a doctor. The smallest effective dose should be used. Take with food or milk if occasional and mild heartburn, upset stomach, or stomach pain occurs with use. Consult a doctor if these symptoms are more than mild or if they persist. *Children:* Do not give this product to children under 12 years of age except under the advice and supervision of a doctor.

Warnings: Do not take for colds for more than 7 days or for fever for more than 3 days unless directed by a doctor. If the cold or fever persists or gets worse, or if new symptoms occur, consult a doctor. These could be signs of serious illness. As with aspirin and acetaminophen, if you have any condition which requires you to take prescription drugs or if you have had any problems or serious side effects from taking any nonprescription pain reliever, do not take this product without first discussing it with your doctor.
IF YOU EXPERIENCE ANY SYMPTOMS WHICH ARE UNUSUAL OR SEEM UNRELATED TO THE CONDITION FOR WHICH YOU TOOK THIS PRODUCT, CONSULT A DOCTOR BEFORE TAKING ANY MORE OF IT. If you are under a doctor's care for any serious condition, consult a doctor before taking this product.
Do not exceed recommended dosage because at higher doses nervousness, dizziness or sleeplessness may occur. Do not take this product if you have high blood pressure, heart disease, diabetes, thyroid disease or difficulty in urination due to enlargement of the prostate gland, except under the advice and supervision of a doctor.
Drug Interaction Precaution: Do not take this product if you are presently taking a prescription drug for high blood pressure or depression without first consulting your doctor. Do not combine this product with other nonprescription pain relievers. Do not combine this product with any other ibuprofen-containing product. As with any drug, if you are pregnant or nursing a baby, seek the advice of a health professional before using this product. IT IS ESPECIALLY IMPORTANT NOT TO USE THIS PRODUCT DURING THE LAST 3 MONTHS OF PREGNANCY UNLESS SPECIFICALLY DIRECTED TO DO SO BY A DOCTOR BECAUSE IT MAY CAUSE PROBLEMS IN THE UNBORN CHILD OR COMPLICATIONS DURING DELIVERY. Keep this and all drugs out of the reach of children. In case of accidental overdose, seek professional assistance or contact a poison control center imme-

diately. Store at room temperature; avoid excessive heat (40°C, 104°F).

Active Ingredients: Each caplet contains Ibuprofen 200 mg and Pseudoephedrine HCl 30 mg.

Inactive Ingredients: Carnauba or Equivalent Wax, Croscarmellose Sodium, Iron Oxide, Methylparaben, Microcrystalline Cellulose, Propylparaben, Silicon Dioxide, Sodium Benzoate, Sodium Lauryl Sulfate, Starch, Stearic Acid, Sucrose, Titanium Dioxide.

How Supplied: Dristan Sinus is an oval-shaped white-colored caplet supplied in consumer blister packs of 20 and bottles of 40.

Shown in Product Identification Section, page 434

DRISTAN®
[drĭs'tăn]
12-hr Nasal Spray
12-hr Menthol Nasal Spray

Description: Dristan 12-hr Nasal Spray contains Oxymetazoline HCl 0.05%.

Actions: The sympathomimetic action of Dristan 12-hr Nasal Spray and Dristan 12-hr Menthol Nasal Spray constricts the smaller arterioles of the nasal passages, producing a prolonged (up to 12 hours), gentle and predictable decongesting effect.

Indications: Dristan 12-hr Nasal Spray and Dristan 12-hr Menthol Nasal Spray provide prompt temporary relief of nasal congestion due to colds, sinusitis, hay fever, or other upper respiratory allergies for up to 12 hours.

Warnings: Do not exceed recommended dosage because symptoms may occur such as burning, stinging, sneezing, or increase of nasal discharge. Do not use this product for more than 3 days. If symptoms persist, consult a physician. The use of the dispenser by more than one person may spread infection. Keep these and all medicines out of the reach of children. In case of accidental ingestion, seek professional assistance or contact a poison control center immediately.

Dosage and Administration: Squeeze Bottle—With head upright, insert nozzle in nostril. Spray quickly, firmly and sniff deeply.
Metered Dose Pump—Prime the metered dose pump by depressing pump firmly several times. With head upright, insert nozzle in nostril. Depress pump 2 or 3 times, all the way down, with a firm even stroke and sniff deeply.
Adults and children 6 years of age and over, spray 2 or 3 times into each nostril. Repeat twice daily—morning and evening. Not recommended for children under six years of age.

Inactive Ingredients: Dristan 12-hr Nasal Spray and Dristan 12-hr Nasal Spray Metered Dose Pump: Benzalkonium Chloride 1:5000 in buffered iso-

tonic aqueous solution, Hydroxypropyl Methylcellulose, Potassium Phosphate, Sodium Chloride, Sodium Phosphate, Thimerosal Preservative 0.002%, and Water.
Dristan 12-hr Menthol Nasal Spray: Benzalkonium Chloride 1:5000 in buffered isotonic aqueous solution, Camphor, Eucalyptol, Hydroxypropyl Methylcellulose, Menthol, Potassium Phosphate, Sodium Chloride, Sodium Phosphate, Thimerosal Preservative 0.002%, Water, and Alcohol 0.4%.

How Supplied: Dristan 12-hr Nasal Spray: 15 mL and 30 mL plastic squeeze bottles and 15 mL metered dose pump.
Dristan 12-hr Menthol Nasal Spray: 15 mL plastic squeeze bottle.

FREEZONE®
['frēz-ōn]
Solution

Description: Freezone is a solution which contains Salicylic Acid 13.6% w/w in a collodion vehicle.

Indications: Freezone is indicated for removal of corns and calluses. Relieves pain by removing corns and calluses.

Actions: Freezone penetrates corns and calluses painlessly, layer by layer, loosening and softening the corn or callus so that the whole corn or callus can be lifted off or peeled away in just a few days.

Warnings: For external use only. Do not use this product on irritated skin, on an area that is infected or reddened, if you are a diabetic, or if you have poor blood circulation. If discomfort persists, see your doctor or podiatrist. Flammable. Keep away from fire or flame. Cap bottle tightly and store at room temperature away from heat. If the product gets into eye, flush with water for 15 minutes. Avoid inhaling vapors. Keep this and all drugs out of reach of children. In case of accidental ingestion, seek the advice of a physician or contact a poison control center immediately.

Dosage and Administration: Wash affected area and dry thoroughly. Apply one drop at a time to sufficiently cover each corn/callus. Let dry. Repeat this procedure once or twice daily as needed for up to 14 days (until corn/callus is removed). May soak corn/callus in warm water for 5 minutes to assist in removal.

Inactive Ingredients: Alcohol (20.5%), Balsam Oregon, Castor Oil, Ether (64.8%), Hypophosphorous Acid and Zinc Chloride.

How Supplied: Available in a .31 fl. oz. glass bottle.
Store at room temperature away from heat.

MOMENTUM®
[mō-měn'tum]
Muscular Backache Formula

Description: Momentum contains Aspirin 500 mg, Phenyltoloxamine Citrate 15 mg, per caplet.

Indications: Momentum is indicated for the relief of pain caused by contracted muscles.

Actions: Momentum acts to relieve the pain of tense, contracted muscles. As pain subsides, muscles often relax, allowing an increased range of motion.

Warnings: Children and teenagers should not use this medicine for chicken pox or flu symptoms before a doctor is consulted about Reye Syndrome, a rare but serious illness reported to be associated with aspirin. Do not drive a car or operate machinery while taking this medication as this preparation may cause drowsiness in some persons. As with any drug, if you are pregnant or nursing a baby, seek the advice of a health professional before using this product. **IT IS ESPECIALLY IMPORTANT NOT TO USE ASPIRIN DURING THE LAST 3 MONTHS OF PREGNANCY UNLESS SPECIFICALLY DIRECTED TO DO SO BY A DOCTOR BECAUSE IT MAY CAUSE PROBLEMS IN THE UNBORN CHILD OR COMPLICATIONS DURING DELIVERY.** Keep this and all medicines out of children's reach. In case of accidental overdose, contact a physician immediately.

Precaution: If pain persists for more than 10 days or if redness is present, consult a physician immediately.

Dosage and Administration: Adults: Two caplets upon rising, then two caplets as needed at lunch, dinner, and bedtime. Dosage should not exceed 8 caplets in any 24-hour period. Not recommended for children.

Inactive Ingredients: Alginic Acid, Citric Acid, Colloidal Silicon Dioxide, Hydrogenated Vegetable Oil, Microcrystalline Cellulose, Starch and Surfactant.

How Supplied: Bottles of 24 and 48 white, uncoated caplets.

OUTGRO®
['aut-grō]
Solution

Description: Outgro solution contains Tannic Acid 25%, Chlorobutanol 5%.

Indications: Outgro provides fast, temporary pain relief of ingrown toenails.

Actions: Outgro temporarily relieves pain, reduces swelling and eases inflammation accompanying ingrown toenails. Daily use of Outgro toughens tender skin—allowing the nail to be cut and thus preventing further pain and discomfort. Outgro does not affect the growth, shape or position of the nail.

Continued on next page

Whitehall—Cont.

Warnings: For external use only. Do not use Outgro solution for more than 7 days unless directed by a doctor. Consult a doctor if no improvement is seen after 7 days. IF YOU HAVE DIABETES OR POOR CIRCULATION, SEE A DOCTOR FOR TREATMENT OF INGROWN TOENAIL. DO NOT APPLY THIS PRODUCT TO OPEN SORES. IF REDNESS AND SWELLING OF YOUR TOE INCREASES, OR IF A DISCHARGE IS PRESENT AROUND THE NAIL, STOP USING THIS PRODUCT AND SEE YOUR DOCTOR IMMEDIATELY. Flammable. Keep away from fire or flame. Avoid smoking during use and until product has dried. In case of accidental ingestion, seek professional assistance or call a poison control center immediately. KEEP THIS AND ALL DRUGS OUT OF THE REACH OF CHILDREN.

Directions: Cleanse affected toes thoroughly. Using rod in cap, either apply Outgro Solution in the crevice where the nail is growing into the flesh or place a small piece of cotton in the nail groove (the side of the nail where the pain is) and wet cotton thoroughly with Outgro solution several times daily until nail discomfort is relieved. Change cotton at least once daily. Do not use product for more than 7 days unless directed by a doctor (podiatrist or physician). In some instances, temporary discoloration of the nail and surrounding skin may occur.

Inactive Ingredients: Ethylcellulose, Isopropyl Alcohol 83% (by volume).

How Supplied: Available in .31 fl. oz. glass bottles.

OXIPOR VHC®
['äk-si-pōr VHC]
Lotion for Psoriasis

Description: OXIPOR VHC lotion for psoriasis contains Coal Tar Solution 48.5%, Salicylic Acid 1.0%, Benzocaine 2.0%.

Actions: Coal tar solution helps control cell growth and therefore prevents formation of new scales. Salicylic acid has a keratolytic action which helps peel off and dissolve away scales. Benzocaine is a local anesthetic that gives prompt relief from pain and itching. Alcohol is the solvent vehicle.

Indications: OXIPOR VHC has been clinically proven to relieve itching, redness and help dissolve and clear away the scales and crusts of psoriasis.

Warnings: For external use only. Avoid contact with eyes or mucous membranes. Use caution in exposing skin to sunlight after applying product. It may increase your tendency to sunburn for up to 24 hours after application. DO NOT USE in or around rectum or in genital area or groin except on advice of a doctor. Flammable. Keep away from fire or

flame. Avoid smoking during application and until product has dried. Do not chill. Not for prolonged use. If condition persists or if rash or irritation develops, discontinue use and consult physician. Keep out of children's reach.

Dosage and Administration: Shake bottle well before each application. SKIN: Wash affected area before applying to remove loose scales. With a small wad of cotton, apply twice daily. Allow to dry before contact with clothing. SCALP: Apply to scalp with fingertips making sure to get down to the skin itself. Leave on for as long as possible, even overnight. Shampoo. Then remove all loose scales with a fine comb. This product may temporarily discolor light-colored hair. Discoloration can be prevented by reducing the time the product is left on the scalp. Also be sure to rinse product out of hair thoroughly.

Inactive Ingredients: Alcohol 81% by volume, water.

How Supplied: Available in 1.9 oz. and 4.0 oz. bottles. Store at room temperature.

POSTURE®
[pos 'tūr]
600 mg
High Potency Calcium Supplement

Description: Each film-coated tablet of POSTURE® contains Tribasic Calcium Phosphate 1565.2 mg, which provides 600 mg of elemental calcium. POSTURE® is specially formulated not to produce gas.

	For Adults—
Two tablets contain:	% U.S. RDA*
Elemental Calcium .... 1200 mg ...120% (as calcium phosphate)	

*Percentage of U.S. Recommended Daily Allowance

Indication: POSTURE® Tablets provide a daily source of calcium to help maintain healthy bones or to supplement dietary calcium intake when directed by a physician.

Directions for Use: One or two tablets daily, or as recommended by a physician. Keep Out of Reach of Children.

Inactive Ingredients: Croscarmellose Sodium, Ethylcellulose, Magnesium Stearate, Microcrystalline Cellulose, Polyethylene Glycol, Povidone, Sodium Lauryl Sulfate.

How Supplied: In bottles of 60 scored tablets.

POSTURE®-D
600 mg
High Potency Calcium Supplement
with Vitamin D

Description: Each film-coated tablet of POSTURE®-D contains Tribasic Calcium Phosphate 1565.2 mg, which provides 600 mg of elemental calcium and

125 IU of Vitamin D. POSTURE®-D is specially formulated not to produce gas.

	For Adults—
Two tablets contain:	% U.S. RDA*
Elemental Calcium .... 1200 mg ...120% (as calcium phosphate)	
Vitamin D .... 250 IU 63%	

*Percentage of U.S. Recommended Daily Allowance.

Indication: POSTURE®-D Tablets provide a daily source of calcium and Vitamin D to help maintain healthy bones or to supplement dietary intake of calcium and Vitamin D when directed by a physician.

Directions for Use: One or two tablets daily, or as recommended by a physician. Keep Out of Reach of Children.

Inactive Ingredients: Croscarmellose Sodium, Ethylcellulose, Magnesium Stearate, Microcrystalline Cellulose, Polyethylene Glycol, Povidone, Sodium Lauryl Sulfate.

How Supplied: In bottles of 60 scored tablets.

PREPARATION H®
[prep-e 'rā-shen-āch]
Hemorrhoidal Ointment and Cream
PREPARATION H®
Hemorrhoidal Suppositories

Description: Preparation H is available in ointment, cream and suppository product forms. The **Ointment** contains Live Yeast Cell Derivative supplying 2,000 units Skin Respiratory Factor per ounce of Ointment, and Shark Liver Oil 3.0% in a specially prepared Rectal Petrolatum Base.
The **Cream** contains Live Yeast Cell Derivative supplying 2,000 units Skin Respiratory Factor per ounce of Cream and Shark Liver Oil 3.0% in a specially prepared Rectal Cream Base containing Petrolatum.
The **Suppositories** contain Live Yeast Cell Derivative, supplying 2,000 units Skin Respiratory Factor per ounce of Cocoa Butter Suppository Base and Shark Liver Oil 3.0%.

Actions: Live Yeast Cell Derivative acts by increasing the oxygen uptake of dermal tissues and facilitating collagen formation. Shark Liver Oil has been incorporated to act as a protectant which softens and soothes the tissues. Preparation H also lubricates inflamed, irritated surfaces to help make bowel movements less painful.

Indications: Preparation H helps shrink swelling of hemorrhoidal tissues caused by inflammation and gives prompt, temporary relief in many cases from pain and itch in tissues.

Precautions: In case of bleeding, or if your condition persists, a physician should be consulted. Keep this and all drugs out of the reach of children. In case of accidental ingestion, seek professional assistance or contact a poison control center immediately.

Dosage and Administration: Ointment/Cream: Before applying, remove protective cover from applicator. Lubricate applicator before each application and thoroughly cleanse after use. It is recommended that Preparation H Hemorrhoidal ointment/cream be applied freely to the affected rectal area whenever symptoms occur, from three to five times per day, especially at night, in the morning, and after each bowel movement. Frequent application with Preparation H ointment/cream provides continual therapy which leads to more rapid improvement of rectal conditions.

Suppositories: Whenever symptoms occur, remove wrapper, insert one suppository rectally from three to five times per day, especially at night, in the morning, and after each bowel movement. Frequent application with Preparation H suppositories provides continual therapy which leads to more rapid improvement of rectal conditions .

Inactive Ingredients: Ointment— Beeswax, Glycerin, Lanolin, Lanolin Alcohol, Mineral Oil, Paraffin, Phenylmercuric Nitrate 1:10,000 (as a preservative), Thyme Oil.
Cream—BHA, Cellulose Gum, Cetyl Alcohol, Citric Acid, Disodium EDTA, Glycerin, Glyceryl Stearate, Lanolin, Methylparaben, Phenylmercuric Nitrate, 1:10,000 (as a preservative), Propyl Gallate, Propylene Glycol, Propylparaben, Simethicone, Sodium Lauryl Sulfate, Stearyl Alcohol, Water, Xanthan Gum. May also contain Glyceryl Oleate and/or Polysorbate 80.
Suppositories — Beeswax, Glycerin, Phenylmercuric Nitrate 1:10,000 (as a preservative), Polyethylene Glycol 600 Dilaurate.

How Supplied: Ointment: Net Wt. 1 oz. and 2 oz. **Cream:** Net wt. 0.9 oz. and 1.8 oz. **Suppositories:** 12's, 24's, 36's and 48's.
Store at controlled room temperature in cool place but not over 80° F.
Shown in Product Identification Section, page 434

PREPARATION H®Cleansing Tissues
[prep-e 'rā-shen-āch]

Description: Preparation H Cleansing Tissues are alcohol-free, nonburning, pre-moistened tissues that soothe, clean, and freshen.

Indications and Use: Preparation H Cleansing Tissues are formulated to moisturize and cleanse rectal or vaginal skin that is itching, burning, or irritated due to hemorrhoids, diarrhea, rashes, or rectal/vaginal surgery. FOR HYGIENE, use Preparation H cleansing tissues after each bowel movement in place of, or in conjunction with, ordinary toilet tissue. FOR MAXIMUM HEMORRHOIDAL CARE, cleanse hemorrhoidal area with Preparation H Cleansing Tissues before

using Preparation H Suppositories, Ointment or Cream. TO USE AS A COMPRESS, fold Preparation H Cleansing Tissues and apply to irritated skin for 5 to 15 minutes. Preparation H Cleansing Tissues are safe and comfortable to use as often as you wish.

Directions: Gently apply Preparation H Cleansing Tissues as needed, particularly after each bowel movement, tampon change, or prior to use of Preparation H Suppositories, Ointment, or Cream.

Caution: In case of rectal bleeding or continued irritation, discontinue use and consult a physician promptly.

Ingredients: Purified Water, Propylene Glycol, Phenoxyethanol, Methylparaben, Propylparaben, Butylparaben and Citric Acid.

How Supplied: Preparation H Cleansing tissues are supplied in a portable, reusable, resealable package of 15 or a resealable package of 40 tissues.
Shown in Product Identification Section, page 434

PRIMATENE®
[prīm 'a-tēn]
Mist
(Epinephrine Inhalation Aerosol Bronchodilator)

Description: Primatene Mist contains Epinephrine 5.5 mg/mL.

Action: Epinephrine is a sympathomimetic agent which relaxes bronchial smooth muscle during an acute asthma attack.

Indications: Primatene Mist is indicated for temporary relief of shortness of breath, tightness of chest, and wheezing due to bronchial asthma. It eases breathing for asthma patients by reducing spasms of bronchial muscles.

Dosage and Administration: Inhalation dosage for adults and children 4 years of age and older: Start with one inhalation, then wait at least 1 minute. If not relieved, use once more. Do not use again for at least 3 hours. The use of this product by children should be supervised by an adult. Children under 4 years of age: Consult a physician. Each inhalation delivers 0.22 mg. of epinephrine.

Warnings: Do not use this product unless a diagnosis of asthma has been made by a physician. Do not use this product if you have heart disease, high blood pressure, thyroid disease, diabetes, or difficulty in urination due to enlargement of the prostate gland unless directed by a physician. As with any drug, if you are pregnant or nursing a baby, seek the advice of a health professional before using this product. Do not use this product if you have ever been hospitalized for asthma or if you are taking any prescription drug for asthma unless directed by a physician. Keep this and all drugs out of the reach of children. In case of accidental overdose, seek professional assistance

or contact a poison control center immediately. DO NOT CONTINUE TO USE THIS PRODUCT, BUT SEEK MEDICAL ASSISTANCE IMMEDIATELY IF SYMPTOMS ARE NOT RELIEVED WITHIN 20 MINUTES OR BECOME WORSE. DO NOT USE THIS PRODUCT MORE FREQUENTLY OR AT HIGHER DOSES THAN RECOMMENDED UNLESS DIRECTED BY A PHYSICIAN. EXCESSIVE USE MAY CAUSE NERVOUSNESS AND RAPID HEART BEAT AND POSSIBLY, ADVERSE EFFECTS ON THE HEART. **Drug Interaction Precaution:** Do not use this product if you are presently taking a prescription drug for high blood pressure or depression, without first consulting your physician.

Precautions: Contents under pressure. Do not puncture or throw container into incinerator. Using or storing near open flame or heating above 120° F (49° C) may cause bursting. Store at room temperature 59° F–86° F (15° C–30° C).

Directions For Use of The Mouthpiece:
The Primatene Mist mouthpiece, which is enclosed in the Primatene Mist 15mL size (not the refill size), should be used for inhalation only with Primatene Mist.
1. Take plastic cap off mouthpiece. (For refills, use mouthpiece from previous purchase.)
2. Take plastic mouthpiece off bottle.
3. Place other end of mouthpiece on bottle.
4. Turn bottle upside down. Place thumb on bottom of mouthpiece over circular button and forefinger on top of vial. Empty the lungs as completely as possible by exhaling.
5. Place mouthpiece in mouth with lips closed around opening. Inhale deeply while squeezing mouthpiece and bottle together. Release immediately and remove unit from mouth. Complete taking the deep breath, drawing the medication into your lungs and holding breath as long as comfortable.
6. Then exhale slowly keeping lips nearly closed. This distributes the medication in the lungs.
7. Replace plastic cap on mouthpiece.
8. The Primatene Mist mouthpiece should be washed once daily with soap and hot water, and rinsed thoroughly. Then it should be dried with a clean, lint-free cloth.

Inactive Ingredients: Alcohol 34%, Ascorbic Acid, Fluorocarbons (Propellant), Water. Contains No Sulfites.

How Supplied:
½ Fl. oz. (15mL) With Mouthpiece.
½ Fl. oz. (15mL) Refill
¾ Fl. oz. (22.5mL) Refill
Shown in Product Identification Section, page 435

Continued on next page

Whitehall—Cont.

PRIMATENE®
[prīm 'a-tēn]
Mist Suspension
(Epinephrine Bitartrate Inhalation Aerosol Bronchodilator)

Description: Primatene Mist Suspension contains Epinephrine Bitartrate 7.0 mg/mL.

Action: Epinephrine is a sympathomimetic agent which eases breathing for asthma patients by reducing spasms of bronchial muscles.

Indications: Primatene Mist Suspension is indicated for temporary relief of shortness of breath, tightness of chest, and wheezing due to bronchial asthma.

Dosage and Administration: Shake before using. Inhalation dosage for adults and children 4 years of age and older: Start with one inhalation, then wait at least 1 minute. If not relieved, use once more. Do not use again for at least 3 hours. The use of this product by children should be supervised by an adult. Children under 4 years of age: Consult a physician. Each inhalation delivers 0.3 mg. Epinephrine Bitartrate equivalent to 0.16 mg. Epinephrine Base.

Warnings: Do not use this product unless a diagnosis of asthma has been made by a physician. Do not use this product if you have heart disease, high blood pressure, thyroid disease, diabetes, or difficulty in urination due to enlargement of the prostate gland unless directed by a physician. As with any drug, if you are pregnant or nursing a baby, seek the advice of a health professional before using this product. Do not use this product if you have ever been hospitalized for asthma or if you are taking any prescription drug for asthma unless directed by a physician. Keep this and all drugs out of the reach of children. In case of accidental overdose, seek professional assistance or contact a poison control center immediately.
DO NOT CONTINUE TO USE THIS PRODUCT, BUT SEEK MEDICAL ASSISTANCE IMMEDIATELY IF SYMPTOMS ARE NOT RELIEVED WITHIN 20 MINUTES OR BECOME WORSE. DO NOT USE THIS PRODUCT MORE FREQUENTLY OR AT HIGHER DOSES THAN RECOMMENDED UNLESS DIRECTED BY A PHYSICIAN. EXCESSIVE USE MAY CAUSE NERVOUSNESS AND RAPID HEART BEAT AND POSSIBLY, ADVERSE EFFECTS ON THE HEART. DRUG INTERACTION PRECAUTION: Do not use this product if you are presently taking a prescription drug for high blood pressure or depression, without first consulting your physician.

Precautions: Contents under pressure. Do not puncture or throw container into incinerator. Using or storing near open flame or heating above 120° F (49° C) may cause bursting. Store at room temperature 59° F–86° F (15° C–30° C).

Directions For Use of The Inhaler:
1. SHAKE BEFORE USING.
2. HOLD INHALER WITH NOZZLE DOWN WHILE USING. Empty the lungs as completely as possible by exhaling.
3. Purse the lips as in saying "O" and hold the nozzle up to the lips keeping the tongue flat. As you start to take a deep breath, squeeze nozzle and can together, releasing one full application. Complete taking a deep breath, drawing medication into your lungs.
4. Hold breath for as long as comfortable. Then exhale slowly, keeping the lips nearly closed. This distributes the medication in the lungs.
5. The Primatene Mist Suspension nozzle should be washed once daily. After removing the nozzle from the vial, wash it with soap and hot water, and rinse thoroughly. Then it should be dried with a clean, lint-free cloth.

Inactive Ingredients: Fluorocarbons (Propellant), Sorbitan Trioleate. Contains No Sulfites.

How Supplied: ⅓ Fl. oz. (10mL) pocket-size aerosol inhaler.
Shown in Product Identification Section, page 435

PRIMATENE®
[prīm 'a-tēn]
Tablets

Description: Depending upon the state (see How Supplied), Primatene Tablets are available in 3 formulations:
Regular Formula: Theophylline Anhydrous 130 mg, Ephedrine Hydrochloride 24 mg.
P Formula: Theophylline Hydrous 130 mg, Ephedrine Hydrochloride 24 mg, Phenobarbital 8 mg (⅛ gr) per tablet. (Warning: May be habit forming.)
M Formula: Theophylline Anhydrous 130 mg, Ephedrine Hydrochloride 24 mg, Pyrilamine Maleate 16.6 mg per tablet.

Actions: Primatene Tablets contain two bronchodilators, theophylline, a methylxanthine, and ephedrine, a sympathomimetic amine. The pharmacologic action of theophylline may be mediated through inhibition of phosphodiesterase with a resulting increase in intracellular cyclic AMP. The β-adrenergic ephedrine acts by a different mechanism to produce cyclic AMP. The combination of a xanthine and a sympathomimetic appears to produce more smooth muscle relaxation than when either drug is used alone. Phenobarbital (present in the P formula) helps counteract the possible stimulation produced by ephedrine and acts as a mild sedative. Pyrilamine maleate (present in the M formula) is an antihistamine with a mild sedating action. Used at the start of an asthma attack, Primatene acts to (1) open bronchial tubes so breathing is natural, (2) relax bronchial muscles, (3) reduce congestion. Primatene helps relieve the asthma spasms, thus permit-

ting sleep at night and freedom from associated anxiety by day.

Indications: Primatene Tablets are indicated for relief and control of attacks of bronchial asthma.

Warnings: If symptoms persist, consult your physician. Some people are sensitive to ephedrine and, in such cases, temporary sleeplessness and nervousness may occur. These reactions will disappear if the use of the medication is discontinued. Do not exceed recommended dosage.
People who have heart disease, high blood pressure, diabetes or thyroid trouble or difficulty in urination due to enlargement of the prostate gland should take this preparation only on the advice of a physician. Both the "M" and "P" formulae may cause drowsiness. People taking the "M" or "P" formula should not drive or operate machinery.
As with any drug, if you are pregnant or nursing a baby, seek the advice of a health professional before using this product. Keep this and all drugs out of the reach of children.

Dosage and Administration: Adults: 1 or 2 tablets initially and then one every 4 hours, as needed, not to exceed 6 tablets in 24 hours. Children (6–12 years of age): One half adult dose. For children under 6, consult a physician.

Inactive Ingredients:
Regular Formula: Croscarmellose Sodium, D&C Yellow No. 10 Lake, FD&C Yellow No. 6 Lake, Magnesium Stearate, Microcrystalline Cellulose, Silica, Starch, Stearic Acid.
P Formula (Phenobarbital): Colloidal Silicon Dioxide, D&C Yellow No. 10, FD&C Yellow No. 6, Magnesium Stearate, Microcrystalline Cellulose, Sodium Starch Glycolate, Starch, Surfactant.
M Formula (Pyrilamine Maleate): D&C Yellow No. 10 Lake, FD&C Yellow No. 6 Lake, Hydrogenated Vegetable Oil, Magnesium Stearate, Microcrystalline Cellulose, Sodium Starch Glycolate, Surfactant, Talc.
Contains No Sulfites.

How Supplied: Available in three Primatene Tablet forms, Regular Formula, "M" Formula, and "P" Formula. "P" Formula, containing phenobarbital, is available in most states. In those states where phenobarbital is Rx only, "M" Formula, containing pyrilamine maleate, is available. Both "M" and "P" formulas are supplied in glass bottles of 24 and 60 tablets. Regular Primatene Tablets are supplied in 24 and 60 tablet thermoform blister cartons.
Shown in Product Identification Section, page 435

RIOPAN®
[rī 'opan]
magaldrate
Antacid

Description: RIOPAN is a buffer antacid containing the unique chemical entity Magaldrate. Each teaspoonful (5 mL) of suspension contains Magaldrate, 540 mg. Each Swallow Tablet contains Magaldrate, 480 mg. RIOPAN is considered dietetically sodium-free [containing not more than 0.013 mEq (0.3 mg) sodium per teaspoonful or 0.004 mEq (0.1 mg) sodium per tablet].

Actions: The active ingredient in RIOPAN, Magaldrate, demonstrates a rapid and uniform buffering action. The acid-neutralizing capacity of RIOPAN is 15.0 mEq/5mL and 13.5 mEq/tablet. RIOPAN does not produce acid rebound or alkalinization.

Indications: Riopan is indicated for the relief of heartburn, sour stomach, and acid indigestion. For symptomatic relief of hyperacidity associated with the diagnosis of peptic ulcer, gastritis, peptic esophagitis, gastric hyperacidity, and hiatal hernia.

Dosage and Administration: RIOPAN (magaldrate) Antacid *Suspension* —Take one or two teaspoonfuls, between meals and at bedtime, or as directed by the physician. RIOPAN Antacid *Swallow Tablets* —Take one or two tablets, between meals and at bedtime, or as directed by the physician. Take with enough water to swallow promptly.

Warnings: Patients should not take more than 18 teaspoonfuls (or 20 tablets) in a 24-hour period or use the maximum dosage for more than two weeks, or use if they have kidney disease except under the advice and supervision of a physician.

Drug Interaction Precaution: Do not use in patients taking a prescription antibiotic drug containing any form of tetracycline.

Inactive Ingredients: Suspension: Flavor, Glycerin, Potassium Citrate, Saccharin, Sorbitol, Xanthan Gum, Water. Swallow Tablets: Flavor, Magnesium Stearate, Menthol, Microcrystalline Cellulose, Polyethylene Glycol, Starch, Talc, Titanium Dioxide.

How Supplied: RIOPAN Antacid *Suspension* —in 12 fl. oz. (355 mL) plastic bottles. Individual Cups, 1 fl. oz. (30 mL) ea., tray of 10—10 trays per packer. Store at room temperature (approximately 25°C or 77°F). Avoid freezing. RIOPAN Antacid *Swallow Tablets* —Boxes of 60 and 100 in individual film strips (6 x 10 and 10 x 10, respectively).

RIOPAN PLUS®
[rī'opan plŭs]
magaldrate and simethicone
Antacid plus Anti-Gas

Description: RIOPAN PLUS is a buffer antacid plus anti-gas combination product containing the unique chemical entity Magaldrate. Each teaspoonful (5 mL) of suspension contains Magaldrate, 540 mg and Simethicone, 40 mg. Each Chew Tablet contains Magaldrate, 480 mg and Simethicone, 20 mg. RIOPAN PLUS is considered dietetically sodium-free, containing not more

than 0.013 mEq (0.3 mg) sodium per teaspoonful or 0.004 mEq (0.1 mg) sodium per tablet.

Actions: The active antacid ingredient in RIOPAN PLUS, Magaldrate, provides a rapid and uniform buffering action. The acid-neutralizing capacity of RIOPAN PLUS is 15.0 mEq/5mL and 13.5 mEq/tablet. RIOPAN PLUS does not produce acid rebound or alkalinization. Simethicone reduces the surface tension of gas bubbles so that the gas is more easily eliminated.

Indications: RIOPAN PLUS is indicated for the relief of heartburn, sour stomach and acid indigestion accompanied by the symptoms of gas. For symptomatic relief of hyperacidity associated with the diagnosis of peptic ulcer, gastritis, peptic esophagitis, gastric hyperacidity, and hiatal hernia. For postoperative gas pain.

Dosage and Administration: RIOPAN PLUS (magaldrate and simethicone) Antacid plus Anti-Gas *Suspension* —Take one or two teaspoonfuls between meals and at bedtime, or as directed by the physician. RIOPAN PLUS Antacid plus Anti-Gas *Chew Tablets* —Chew one or two tablets, between meals and at bedtime, or as directed by the physician.

Warnings: Patients should not take more than 12 teaspoonfuls (or 25 tablets) in a 24-hour period, or use the maximum dosage for more than two weeks, or use if they have kidney disease, except under the advice and supervision of a physician.

Drug Interaction Precaution: Do not use in patients taking a prescription antibiotic drug containing any form of tetracycline.

Inactive Ingredients: Chew Tablets: Flavor, Magnesium Stearate, Methylcellulose, Polyethylene Glycol, Silica, Sorbitol, Starch, Sucrose, Titanium Dioxide. Suspension: Flavor, Glycerin, PEG-8 Stearate, Potassium Citrate, Saccharin, Sorbitan Stearate, Sorbitol, Xanthan Gum, Water.

How Supplied: RIOPAN PLUS Antacid plus Anti-Gas *Suspension* —in 12 fl. oz. (355 mL) plastic bottles. Individual Cups, 1 fl. oz. (30 mL) ea., tray of 10— 10 trays per packer. Store at room temperature (approximately 25°C or 77°F). Avoid freezing. RIOPAN PLUS Antacid plus Anti-Gas *Chew Tablets* —in bottles of 60 and 100. Also, single rollpacks of 12 tablets and 3-roll rollpacks of 36 tablets.

RIOPAN PLUS® 2
[rī'opan plus 2]
magaldrate and simethicone
Double Strength
Antacid plus Anti-Gas

Description: RIOPAN PLUS 2 is a double strength buffer antacid plus anti-gas combination product containing the unique chemical entity Magaldrate.

Each teaspoonful (5 mL) of suspension contains Magaldrate, 1080 mg and Simethicone, 40 mg. Each Chew Tablet contains Magaldrate, 1080 mg and Simethicone, 20 mg. RIOPAN PLUS 2 is considered dietetically sodium-free [containing not more than 0.013 mEq (0.3 mg) sodium per teaspoonful or 0.021 mEq (0.5 mg) sodium per tablet].

Actions: Magaldrate, the active antacid ingredient in RIOPAN PLUS 2, provides a rapid and uniform buffering action. The acid-neutralizing capacity of Double Strength RIOPAN PLUS 2 is 30 mEq/5 mL and 30.0 mEq/tablet. RIOPAN PLUS 2 does not produce acid rebound or alkalinization. Simethicone reduces the surface tension of gas bubbles so that the gas is more easily eliminated.

Indications: RIOPAN PLUS 2 is indicated for the relief of heartburn, sour stomach and acid indigestion accompanied by the symptoms of gas. For symptomatic relief of hyperacidity associated with the diagnosis of peptic ulcer, gastritis, peptic esophagitis, gastric hyperacidity, and hiatal hernia. For postoperative gas pain.

Dosage and Administration: RIOPAN PLUS 2 (magaldrate and simethicone) *Suspension* —Take one or two teaspoonfuls between meals and at bedtime, or as directed by the physician. RIOPAN PLUS 2 Chew Tablets—Chew one or two tablets, between meals and at bedtime, or as directed by the physician.

Warnings: Patients should not take more than 12 teaspoonfuls (or 25 tablets) in a 24-hour period, or use the maximum dosage for more than two weeks, or use if they have kidney disease, except under the advice and supervision of a physician.

Drug Interaction Precaution: Do not use in patients taking a prescription antibiotic drug containing any form of tetracycline.

Inactive Ingredients: Chew Tablets: Flavor, Magnesium Stearate, Methylcellulose, Polyethylene Glycol, Saccharin, Silica, Sorbitol, Starch, Sucrose, Titanium Dioxide. Suspension: Flavor, Glycerin, PEG-8 Stearate, Potassium Citrate, Saccharin, Sorbitan Stearate, Sorbitol, Xanthan Gum, Water.

How Supplied: RIOPAN PLUS 2 *Suspension* —in 12 fl. oz. (355 mL) and 6 fl. oz. plastic bottles. Available in mint and cherry vanilla flavors. RIOPAN PLUS 2 Chew Tablets—in bottles of 60. Available in mint and cherry vanilla flavors. Store at room temperature (approximately 25°C or 77°F). Avoid freezing.

Shown in Product Identification Section, page 435

Continued on next page

Whitehall—Cont.

SEMICID®
[sĕm´ē-sĭd]
Vaginal Contraceptive Inserts

Description: Semicid is a safe and effective, nonsystemic, reversible method of birth control. Each vaginal contraceptive insert contains 100 mg of the spermicide nonoxynol-9. It contains no hormones and is odorless and nonmessy.
When used consistently and according to directions, the effectiveness of Semicid is approximately equal to other vaginal spermicides, but is less than oral contraceptives.

Actions: Semicid dissolves in the vagina and blends with natural vaginal secretions to provide effective spermicidal action.
Semicid requires no applicator and has no unpleasant taste. Unlike foams, creams and jellies, Semicid does not drip or run, and Semicid inserts are easier to use than the diaphragm. Also, Semicid does not effervesce like some inserts, so it is not as likely to cause a burning feeling. Semicid provides effective contraceptive protection when used properly. However, no contraceptive method or product can provide an absolute guarantee against becoming pregnant.

Indication: For the prevention of pregnancy.

Warnings: Do not insert in urinary opening (urethra). Do not take orally. If irritation occurs, discontinue use. If irritation persists, consult a physician. Keep this and all contraceptives out of the reach of children.

Precautions: As with all spermicides, some Semicid users may experience irritation, however, most women use Semicid safely and without irritation. If douching is desired, one should wait at least six hours after intercourse before douching. If either partner experiences irritation, discontinue use. If irritation persists, consult a physician.
If your doctor has told you that it is dangerous to become pregnant, ask your doctor if you can use Semicid.
If menstrual period is missed, a physician should be consulted.

Dosage and Administration: To use, unwrap one insert and insert it deeply into the vagina. It is essential that Semicid be inserted at least 15 minutes before intercourse. However, Semicid is also effective when inserted up to 1 hour before intercourse. If intercourse is delayed for more than 1 hour after Semicid is inserted, or if intercourse is repeated, then another insert must be inserted. Semicid can be used as frequently as needed.

Inactive Ingredients: Benzethonium Chloride, Citric Acid, D&C Red #21 Lake, D&C Red #33 Lake, Methylparaben, Polyethylene Glycol, Water.

How Supplied: Strip Packaging of 10's and 20's.

Keep Semicid at room temperature (not over 86°F or 30°C).

SLEEP–EZE 3®
[slēp-ēz]
**Nighttime Sleep Aid Tablets
Diphenhydramine Hydrochloride**

Description: Sleep-eze 3 is a nighttime sleep-aid that contains Diphenhydramine Hydrochloride, 25 mg per tablet.

Indication: Sleep-eze 3 helps to reduce difficulty in falling asleep.

Action: Sleep-eze 3 contains diphenhydramine, an antihistamine with anticholinergic and sedative action.

Warnings: Do not give to children under 12 years of age. Insomnia may be a symptom of serious underlying medical illness. If sleeplessness persists continuously for more than 2 weeks, consult your physician. As with any drug, if you are pregnant or nursing a baby, seek the advice of a health professional before using this product.
Do not take this product if you have asthma, glaucoma, emphysema, chronic pulmonary disease, shortness of breath, difficulty breathing or difficulty in urination due to enlargement of the prostate gland except under the advice and supervision of a physician.
In case of accidental ingestion or overdose, contact a physician or poison control center immediately. Keep this and all drugs out of the reach of children.

Drug Interaction: Avoid alcoholic beverages while taking this product. Do not take this product if you are taking sedatives or tranquilizers, without first consulting your doctor.

Precaution: This product contains an antihistamine and will cause drowsiness. It should be used only at bedtime.

Dosage and Administration: Take 2 tablets 20 minutes before going to bed.

Inactive Ingredients: Croscarmellose Sodium, Dicalcium Phosphate, D&C Yellow No. 10, FD&C Yellow No. 6, Magnesium Stearate, Microcrystalline Cellulose, Stearic Acid.

How Supplied: Packages of 12's, 24's, and 48's.

TODAY®
[tü-dā]
Vaginal Contraceptive Sponge

Description: Today Vaginal Contraceptive Sponge is a soft polyurethane foam sponge containing nonoxynol-9, a spermicide used by millions of women for over 25 years.
Today Sponge is Effective, Safe, and Convenient. Today Sponge provides 24-hour contraceptive protection without hormones, allowing spontaneity. Today Sponge is easy to use, nonmessy and disposable.

Active Ingredient: Each Today Sponge contains nonoxynol-9, one gram.

Inactive Ingredients: Benzoic acid, citric acid, sodium dihydrogen citrate, sodium metabisulfite, sorbic acid, water in a polyurethane foam sponge.

Indication: For the prevention of pregnancy.

Actions: Used as directed, Today Vaginal Contraceptive Sponge prevents pregnancy in three ways: 1) the spermicide nonoxynol-9 kills sperm before they can reach the egg; 2) Today Sponge traps and absorbs sperm; 3) Today Sponge blocks the cervix so that sperm cannot enter. Today Sponge is designed for easy insertion into the vagina. It is positioned against the cervix, and while in place provides protection against pregnancy for 24 hours. The soft polyurethane foam sponge is formulated to feel like normal vaginal tissue and has a specially designed ribbon loop attached to an interior web for maximum strength.
In clinical trials of Today Sponge in over 1,800 women worldwide who completed over 12,000 cycles of use, the method-effectiveness, i.e., the level of effectiveness seen in women who followed the printed instructions exactly and who used Today Sponge every time that they had intercourse, was 89 to 91%.

Instructions: Remove one Today Sponge from airtight inner pack, wet thoroughly with clean tap water, and squeeze gently several times until it becomes very sudsy. The water activates the spermicide. Fold the sides of Today Sponge upward until it looks long and narrow and then insert it deeply into the vagina with the string loop dangling below. Protection begins immediately and continues for 24 hours. It is not necessary to add creams, jellies, foams, or any other additional spermicide as long as Today Sponge is in place, no matter how many acts of intercourse may occur during a 24-hour period. Always wait 6 hours after your last act of intercourse before removing Today Sponge. If you have intercourse when Today Sponge has been in place for 24 hours, it must be left in place an additional 6 hours after intercourse before removing it. It is unlikely that Today Sponge will fall out. During a bowel movement or other form of internal straining, it may be pushed down to the opening of the vagina and perhaps fall out. If you suspect this is happening, simply insert a finger into your vagina and push the sponge back. If it should fall into the toilet, moisten a new sponge and insert it immediately.
To remove Today Sponge, place a finger in the vagina and reach up and back to find the string loop. Hook a finger around the loop. Slowly and gently pull the Sponge out. Some women, especially first-time users, may have difficulty removing the Sponge. This situation may be due to tension or unusually strong muscular pressure. Simple relaxation of the vaginal muscles and bearing down should make it possible to remove the Sponge without difficulty. See User Instruction Booklet (Section 7) for details

on removing Today Sponge or call the Today TalkLine 1-800-223-2329.

Warnings: Some cases of Toxic Shock Syndrome (TSS) have been reported in women using barrier contraceptives including Today Sponge. Although the occurrence of TSS is uncommon, some studies indicate that there is an increased risk of non-menstrual TSS with the use of barrier contraceptives, including Today Sponge. Today Sponge should not be left in place for more than 30 hours after insertion. If you experience two or more of the warning signs of TSS including fever, vomiting, diarrhea, muscular pain, dizziness, and rash similar to sunburn, consult your physician or clinic immediately. If you have difficulty removing the sponge from your vagina or you remove only a portion of the sponge, contact the Today Talk Line or consult your physician or clinic immediately. Today Sponge should not be used during the menstrual period. After childbirth, miscarriage or other termination of pregnancy, it is important to consult your physician or clinic before using this product. If you have ever had Toxic Shock Syndrome do not use Today Sponge.

A small number of men and women may be sensitive to the spermicide in this product (nonoxynol-9) and should not use this product if irritation occurs and persists. If you or your partner have ever experienced an allergic reaction to the spermicide used in this product, it is best to consult a physician before using Today Vaginal Contraceptive Sponge. If either you or your partner develops burning or itching in the genital area, stop using this product and contact your physician. A higher degree of protection against pregnancy will be afforded by using another method of contraception in addition to a spermicidal contraceptive. This is especially true during the first few months, until you become familiar with the method. In our clinical studies, approximately one-half of all accidental pregnancies occurred during the first three months of use. Where avoidance of pregnancy is essential, the choice of contraceptive should be made in consultation with a doctor or a family planning clinic. Any delay in your menstrual period may be an early sign of pregnancy. If this happens, consult your physician or clinic as soon as possible. Keep this and all drugs out of reach of children. In case of accidental ingestion of Today Sponge, call a poison control center, emergency medical facility or doctor. (For most people ingestion of small amounts of the spermicide alone should not be harmful.) As with any drug, if you are pregnant or nursing a baby, seek professional advice before using this product.

How To Store: Store at normal room temperature.

How Supplied: Packages of 1s, 3s, 6s, and 12s.

Shown in Product Indentification Section, page 435

Wyeth-Ayerst Laboratories
Division of American Home Products Corporation
P.O. BOX 8299
PHILADELPHIA, PA 19101

Wyeth-Ayerst Tamper-Resistant/Evident Packaging

Statements alerting consumers to the specific type of Tamper-Resistant/Evident Packaging appear on the bottle labels and cartons of all Wyeth-Ayerst over-the-counter products. This includes plastic cap seals on bottles, individually wrapped tablets or suppositories, and sealed cartons. This packaging has been developed to better protect the consumer.

ALUDROX®
[al 'ū-drox]
Antacid
(alumina and magnesia)
ORAL SUSPENSION

Composition: *Suspension* —each 5 ml teaspoonful contains 307 mg aluminum hydroxide [Al(OH)$_3$] as a gel and 103 mg of magnesium hydroxide. The inactive ingredients present are artificial and natural flavors, benzoic acid, butylparaben, glycerin, hydroxypropyl methylcellulose, methylparaben, propylparaben, saccharin, simethicone, sorbitol solution, and water. Sodium content is 0.10 mEq per 5 ml suspension.

Indications: For temporary relief of heartburn, upset stomach, sour stomach, and/or acid indigestion.

Directions: *Suspension* —Two teaspoonfuls (10 ml) every 4 hours or as directed by a physician. Medication may be followed by a sip of water if desired.

Warnings: Do not take more than 12 teaspoonfuls (60 ml) of suspension in a 24-hour period or use maximum dosage for more than two weeks except under the advice and supervision of a physician. Prolonged use of aluminum-containing antacids in patients with renal failure may result in or worsen dialysis osteomalacia. Elevated tissue aluminum levels contribute to the development of dialysis encephalopathy and osteomalacia syndromes. Also, a number of cases of dialysis encephalopathy have been associated with elevated aluminum levels in the dialysate water. Small amounts of aluminum are absorbed from the gastrointestinal tract and renal excretion of aluminum is impaired in renal failure. Prolonged use of aluminum-containing antacids in such patients may contribute to increased plasma levels of aluminum. Aluminum is not well removed by dialysis because it is bound to albumin and transferrin, which do not cross dialysis membranes. As a result, aluminum is deposited in bone, and dialysis osteomalacia may develop when large amounts of aluminum are ingested orally by pa-

---

tients with impaired renal function. As with any drug, if you are pregnant or nursing a baby, seek the advice of a health professional before using this product.

Drug Interaction Precautions: Do not take this product if you are presently taking a prescription antibiotic drug containing any form of tetracycline.
Keep at Room Temperature, Approx. 77°F (25°C).
Suspension should be kept tightly closed and shaken well before use. Avoid freezing.
Keep this and all drugs out of the reach of children.

How Supplied: *Oral Suspension* —bottles of 12 fluidounces.
Shown in Product Identification Section, page 435

Professional Labeling: Consult *1992 Physicians' Desk Reference.*

AMPHOJEL®
[am 'fo-jel]
Antacid
(aluminum hydroxide gel)
ORAL SUSPENSION • TABLETS

Composition: *Suspension* —Each 5 ml teaspoonful contains 320 mg aluminum hydroxide [Al(OH)$_3$] as a gel, and not more than 0.10 mEq of sodium. The inactive ingredients present are artificial and natural flavors, butylparaben, calcium benzoate, glycerin, hydroxypropyl methylcellulose, methylparaben, propylparaben, saccharin, simethicone, sorbitol solution, and water. *Tablets* are available in 0.3 and 0.6 g strengths. Each contains, respectively, the equivalent of 300 mg and 600 mg aluminum hydroxide as a dried gel. The 0.3 g (5 grain) tablet is equivalent to about 1 teaspoonful of the suspension and the 0.6 g (10 grain) tablet is equivalent to about 2 teaspoonfuls. Each 0.3 g tablet contains 0.08 mEq of sodium and each 0.6 g tablet contains 0.13 mEq of sodium.

Indications: For temporary relief of heartburn, upset stomach, sour stomach, and/or acid indigestion.

Directions: *Suspension* —Two teaspoonfuls (10 ml) to be taken five or six times daily, between meals and at bedtime or as directed by a physician. Medication may be followed by a sip of water if desired. *Tablets* —Two tablets of the 0.3 g strength, or one tablet of the 0.6 g strength, five or six times daily, between meals and at bedtime or as directed by a physician. It is unnecessary to chew the 0.3 g tablet before swallowing.

Warnings: Do not take more than 12 teaspoonfuls (60 ml) of suspension, or more than twelve 0.3 g tablets, or more than six 0.6 g tablets in a 24-hour period or use this maximum dosage for more than two weeks except under the advice and supervision of a physician. May cause constipation. Prolonged use of aluminum-containing antacids in patients

Continued on next page

Wyeth-Ayerst—Cont.

with renal failure may result in or worsen dialysis osteomalacia. Elevated tissue aluminum levels contribute to the development of dialysis encephalopathy and osteomalacia syndromes. Also, a number of cases of dialysis encephalopathy have been associated with elevated aluminum levels in the dialysate water. Small amounts of aluminum are absorbed from the gastrointestinal tract and renal excretion of aluminum is impaired in renal failure. Prolonged use of aluminum-containing antacids in such patients may contribute to increased plasma levels of aluminum. Aluminum is not well removed by dialysis because it is bound to albumin and transferrin, which do not cross dialysis membranes. As a result, aluminum is deposited in bone, and dialysis osteomalacia may develop when large amounts of aluminum are ingested orally by patients with impaired renal function. As with any drug, if you are pregnant or nursing a baby, seek the advice of a health professional before using this product.

Drug Interaction Precautions: Do not use this product if you are presently taking a prescription antibiotic containing any form of tetracycline.
Keep tightly closed and store at room temperature, Approx. 77°F (25°C).
Suspension should be shaken well before use. Avoid freezing.
Keep this and all drugs out of the reach of children.

How Supplied: *Suspension* —Peppermint flavored; without flavor—bottles of 12 fluidounces. *Tablets* —a convenient auxiliary dosage form—0.3 g (5 grain) bottles of 100; 0.6 g (10 grain), boxes of 100.

Shown in Product Identification Section, page 435

Professional Labeling: Consult *1992 Physicians' Desk Reference.*

BASALJEL®
[bā 'sel-jel]
(basic aluminum carbonate gel)
ORAL SUSPENSION ●CAPSULES ●TABLETS

Composition: *Suspension* —each 5 ml teaspoonful contains basic aluminum carbonate gel equivalent to 400 mg aluminum hydroxide [Al(OH)₃]. The inactive ingredients present are artificial and natural flavors, butylparaben, calcium benzoate, glycerin, hydroxypropyl methylcellulose, methylparaben, mineral oil, propylparaben, saccharin, simethicone, sorbitol solution, and water. *Capsule* contains dried basic aluminum carbonate gel equivalent to 608 mg of dried aluminum hydroxide gel or 500 mg aluminum hydroxide [Al(OH)₃]. The inactive ingredients present are D&C Yellow 10, FD&C Blue 1, FD&C Red 40, FD&C Yellow 6, gelatin, polacrilin potassium, polyethylene glycol, talc, and titanium dioxide. *Tablet* contains dried basic

aluminum carbonate gel equivalent to 608 mg of dried aluminum hydroxide gel or 500 mg aluminum hydroxide. The inactive ingredients present are cellulose, hydrogenated vegetable oil, magnesium stearate, polacrilin potassium, starch, and talc.

Indications: For the symptomatic relief of hyperacidity, associated with the diagnosis of peptic ulcer, gastritis, peptic esophagitis, gastric hyperacidity, and hiatal hernia.

Warnings: Do not take more than 24 tablets/capsules/teaspoonfuls of BASALJEL in a 24-hour period, or use this maximum dosage for more than two weeks except under the advice and supervision of a physician. Dosage should be carefully supervised since continued overdosage, in conjunction with restriction of dietary phosphorus and calcium, may produce a persistently lowered serum phosphate and a mildly elevated alkaline phosphatase. A usually transient hypercalciuria of mild degree may be associated with the early weeks of therapy. Prolonged use of aluminum-containing antacids in patients with renal failure may result in or worsen dialysis osteomalacia. Elevated tissue aluminum levels contribute to the development of dialysis encephalopathy and osteomalacia syndromes. Also, a number of cases of dialysis encephalopathy have been associated with elevated aluminum levels in the dialysate water. Small amounts of aluminum are absorbed from the gastrointestinal tract and renal excretion of aluminum is impaired in renal failure. Prolonged use of aluminum-containing antacids in such patients may contribute to increased plasma levels of aluminum. Aluminum is not well removed by dialysis because it is bound to albumin and transferrin, which do not cross dialysis membranes. As a result, aluminum is deposited in bone, and dialysis osteomalacia may develop when large amounts of aluminum are ingested orally by patients with impaired renal function. As with any drug, if you are pregnant or nursing a baby, seek the advice of a health professional before using this product.

Dosage and Administration: *Suspension* —two teaspoonfuls (10 ml) in water or fruit juice taken as often as every two hours up to twelve times daily. Two teaspoonfuls have the capacity to neutralize 23 mEq of acid. *Capsules* —two capsules as often as every two hours up to twelve times daily. Two capsules have the capacity to neutralize 24 mEq of acid. *Tablets* —two tablets as often as every two hours up to twelve times daily. Two tablets have the capacity to neutralize 25 mEq of acid. The sodium content of each dosage form is as follows: 0.13 mEq/5 ml for the suspension, 0.12 mEq per capsule, and 0.12 mEq per tablet.

Precautions: May cause constipation. Adequate fluid intake should be maintained in addition to the specific medical or surgical management indicated by the patient's condition.

Drug Interaction Precautions: Alumina-containing antacids should not be used concomitantly with any form of tetracycline therapy.

How Supplied: Suspension—bottles of 12 fluidounces.
Capsules—bottles of 100 and 500.
Tablets (scored)—bottles of 100.
Shown in Product Identification Section, page 435

Professional Labeling: Consult *1992 Physicians' Desk Reference.*

CEROSE–DM®
[se-ros 'DM]
Antihistamine/Nasal Decongestant/ Cough Suppressant

Description: Each teaspoonful (5 mL) contains 15 mg dextromethorphan hydrobromide, 4 mg chlorpheniramine maleate, and 10 mg phenylephrine hydrochloride. Alcohol 2.4%. The inactive ingredients present are artificial flavors, citric acid, edetate disodium, FD&C Yellow 6, glycerin, saccharin sodium, sodium benzoate, sodium citrate, sodium propionate, and water.

Indications: For the temporary relief of cough due to minor throat and bronchial irritation as may occur with the common cold or with inhaled irritants. Temporarily relieves nasal congestion, runny nose, and sneezing due to the common cold, hay fever, or other upper respiratory allergies.

Directions: Adults and children 12 years of age and over: One teaspoonful every four hours as needed. Children 6 to under 12 years of age: One-half teaspoonful every four hours as needed. Do not exceed six doses in a 24-hour period. For children under 6 years, consult a doctor.

Drug Interaction Precaution: Do not take this product if you are presently taking a prescription drug for high blood pressure or depression without first consulting your doctor.

Warnings: May cause marked drowsiness; alcohol may increase the drowsiness effect. Avoid alcoholic beverages while taking this product. Use caution when driving a motor vehicle or operating machinery. Do not take this product if you have heart disease, high blood pressure, thyroid disease, diabetes, asthma, glaucoma, emphysema, chronic pulmonary disease, shortness of breath, difficulty in breathing, or difficulty in urination due to enlargement of the prostate gland unless directed by a doctor. This product may cause excitability, especially in children. Do not exceed recommended dosage because at higher doses nervousness, dizziness, or sleeplessness may occur. Do not take this product for more than 7 days. A persistent cough may be a sign of a serious condition. If symptoms persist for more than one week, tend to recur, or are accompanied by fever, rash, or persistent headache, consult a doctor. Do not take this product

for persistent or chronic cough such as occurs with smoking, or if cough is accompanied by excessive phlegm (mucus) unless directed by a doctor. As with any drug, if you are pregnant or nursing a baby, seek the advice of a health professional before using this product.
Keep this and all drugs out of the reach of children. In case of accidental overdose, seek professional assistance or contact a Poison Control Center immediately.
Keep tightly closed—below 77° F (25° C).

How Supplied: Cases of 12 bottles of 4 fl. oz.; bottles of 1 pint.
Shown in Product Identification Section, page 435

COLLYRIUM for FRESH EYES
[ko-lir'e-um]
a neutral borate solution
EYE WASH

Description: Soothing Collyrium Eye Wash for Fresh Eyes is specially formulated to soothe, refresh, and cleanse irritated eyes. Collyrium Eye Wash is a neutral borate solution that contains boric acid, sodium borate and water.

Indications: To cleanse the eye, loosen foreign material, air pollutants or chlorinated water.

Recommended Uses:
Home—For emergency flushing of foreign bodies or whenever a soothing eye rinse is necessary.
Hospitals, dispensaries and clinics— For emergency flushing of chemicals or foreign bodies from the eye.

Directions: Puncture bottle by twisting clear cap fully down onto bottle; then remove clear cap from bottle and discard. Remove the eyecup from plastic bag. Rinse blue eyecup with clear water immediately before and after each use. Avoid contamination of rim and interior surfaces of eyecup. Fill blue eyecup one-half full with Collyrium Eye Wash. Apply cup tightly to the affected eye to prevent the escape of the liquid and tilt head backward. Open eyelid wide and rotate eyeball to thoroughly wash eye. Recap by twisting blue eyecup fully onto bottle for storage and subsequent use.

Warnings: Do not use if solution changes color or becomes cloudy, or with a wetting solution for contact lenses or other eye care products containing polyvinyl alcohol.
To avoid contamination do not touch tip of container to any surface. Replace cap after using. If you experience eye pain, changes in vision, continued redness, irritation of the eye, or if the condition worsens or persists, consult a doctor. Obtain immediate medical treatment for all open wounds in or near the eye.
The Collyrium for Fresh Eyes bottle is sealed for your protection. Prior to first use, remove cap and squeeze bottle. If bottle leaks, do not use.
Keep this and all medication out of the reach of children.

Keep bottle tightly closed at Room Temperature, Approx. 77°F (25°C).

How Supplied: Bottles of 4 fl. oz. (118 ml) with eyecup.
Shown in Product Identification Section, page 435

COLLYRIUM FRESH™
[ko-lir'e-um]
Sterile Eye Drops
Lubricant
Redness Reliever

Description: Collyrium Fresh is a specially formulated sterile eye drop which can be used, up to 4 times daily, to relieve redness and discomfort due to minor eye irritations caused by dust, smoke, smog, swimming, or sun glare.
The active ingredients are tetrahydrozoline HCl (0.05%) and glycerin (1.0%). Other ingredients include benzalkonium chloride (0.01%) and edetate disodium (0.1%) as preservatives, boric acid, hydrochloric acid and sodium borate.

Indications: For the temporary relief of redness due to minor eye irritations or discomfort due to burning or exposure to wind or sun.

Directions: Tilt head back and squeeze 1 to 2 drops into each eye up to 4 times daily, or as directed by a physician.

Warnings: Do not use if solution changes color or becomes cloudy. Remove contact lenses before using. If you have glaucoma, do not use this product except under the advice and supervision of a physician. Overuse of this product may produce increased redness of the eye. To avoid contamination, do not touch tip of container to any surface. Replace cap after using. If you experience eye pain, changes in vision, continued redness or irritation of the eye, or if the condition worsens or persists for more than 72 hours, discontinue use and consult a physician.
Keep this and all medication out of the reach of children.
Retain carton for complete product information.
Keep bottle tightly closed at Room Temperature, Approx. 77°F (25°C).

How Supplied: Bottles of ½ fl. oz. (15 ml) with built-in eye dropper.
Shown in Product Identification Section, page 435

NURSOY®
[nur-soy]
Soy protein isolate formula
READY–TO–FEED
CONCENTRATED LIQUID
POWDER

Breast milk is preferred feeding for newborns. NURSOY® milk-free formula is intended to meet the nutritional needs of infants and children who are not breast-fed and are allergic to cow's milk protein and/or intolerant to lactose. NURSOY Ready-to-Feed and Concentrated Liquid contain sucrose as their carbohydrate.

NURSOY Powder contains corn syrup solids and sucrose as its carbohydrate. Professional advice should be followed.

Ingredients (in normal dilution supplying 20 calories per fluidounce): 87% water; 6.7% sucrose; 3.4% oleo, coconut, oleic (safflower) and soybean oils; 2.0% soy protein isolate; and less than 1% of each of the following: potassium citrate; monobasic sodium phosphate; calcium carbonate; dibasic calcium phosphate; magnesium chloride; calcium chloride; soy lecithin; calcium carrageenan; calcium hydroxide; L-methionine; sodium chloride; potassium bicarbonate; taurine; ferrous, zinc, and cupric sulfates; L-carnitine; potassium iodide; ascorbic acid; choline chloride; alpha-tocopheryl acetate; niacinamide; calcium pantothenate; riboflavin; vitamin A palmitate; thiamine hydrochloride; pyridoxine hydrochloride; beta-carotene; phytonadione; folic acid; biotin; cholecalciferol; cyanocobalamin.
NURSOY Powder contains corn syrup solids and sucrose. NURSOY Ready-to-Feed and Concentrated Liquids contain only sucrose.

PROXIMATE ANALYSIS
at 20 calories per fluidounce
READY-TO-FEED, CONCENTRATED LIQUID, and POWDER

	(W/V)
Protein	1.8 %
Fat	3.6 %
Carbohydrate	6.9 %
Ash	0.27 %
Water	87.0 %
Crude fiber not more than	0.01 %
Calories/fl. oz.	20

Vitamins, Minerals: In normal dilution, each liter contains:

A	2,000	IU
D$_3$	400	IU
E	9.5	IU
K$_1$	100	mcg
C (ascorbic acid)	55	mg
B$_1$ (thiamine)	670	mcg
B$_2$ (riboflavin)	1000	mcg
B$_6$	420	mcg
B$_{12}$	2	mcg
Niacin	5000	mcg
Pantothenic acid	3000	mcg
Folic acid (folacin)	50	mcg
Choline	85	mg
Inositol	27	mg
Biotin	35	mcg
Calcium	600	mg
Phosphorus	420	mg
Sodium	200	mg
Potassium	700	mg
Chloride	375	mg
Magnesium	67	mg
Manganese	200	mcg
Iron	12.0	mg
Copper	470	mcg
Zinc	5	mg
Iodine	60	mcg

Preparation: *Ready-to-Feed* (32 fl. oz. cans of 20 calories per fluidounce formula)—shake can, open and pour into previously sterilized nursing bottle; attach nipple and feed. Cover opened can and immediately store in refrigerator.

Continued on next page

Wyeth-Ayerst—Cont.

Use contents of can within 48 hours of opening.

Prolonged storage of can at excessive temperatures should be avoided.

Expiration date is on top of can.

WARNING: DO NOT USE A MICROWAVE TO PREPARE OR WARM FORMULA. SERIOUS BURNS MAY OCCUR.

Concentrated Liquid —For normal dilution supplying 20 calories per fluidounce, use equal amounts of NURSOY® liquid and cooled, previously boiled water.

Note: Prepared formula should be used within 24 hours.

Prolonged storage of can at excessive temperatures should be avoided.

Expiration date is on top of can.

WARNING: DO NOT USE A MICROWAVE TO PREPARE OR WARM FORMULA. SERIOUS BURNS MAY OCCUR.

Powder —For normal dilution supplying 20 calories per fluidounce, add 1 scoop (8.9 grams or 1 standard tablespoonful) of NURSOY POWDER, packed and leveled, to 2 fluidounces of cooled, previously boiled water. For larger amounts of formula, add ¼ standard measuring cup of powder (35.5 grams), packed and leveled, to 8 fluidounces (1 standard measuring cup) of water.

Note: Prepared formula should be used within 24 hours.

Prolonged storage of can at excessive temperatures should be avoided.

Expiration date is on bottom of can.

WARNING: DO NOT USE A MICROWAVE TO PREPARE OR WARM FORMULA. SERIOUS BURNS MAY OCCUR.

How Supplied: *Ready-to-Feed* —presterilized and premixed, 32 fluidounce (1 quart) cans, cases of 6 cans; *Concentrated Liquid* —13 fluidounce cans, cases of 12 cans; *Powder* —1 pound cans, cases of 6 cans.

Questions or Comments regarding NURSOY: 1-800-99-WYETH.

Shown in Product Identification Section, page 435

SMA®
Iron fortified
Infant formula
READY–TO–FEED
CONCENTRATED LIQUID
POWDER

Breast milk is the preferred feeding for newborns. Infant formula is intended to replace or supplement breast milk when breast feeding is not possible or is insufficient, or when mothers elect not to breast feed.

Good maternal nutrition is important for the preparation and maintenance of breast feeding. Extensive or prolonged use of partial bottle feeding, before breast feeding has been well established, could make breast feeding difficult to maintain. A decision not to breast feed could be difficult to reverse.

Professional advice should be followed on all matters of infant feeding. Infant formula should always be prepared and used as directed. Unnecessary or improper use of infant formula could present a health hazard. Social and financial implications should be considered when selecting the method of infant feeding.

SMA® is closest in nutrient composition to human milk among prepared formulas with its physiologic fat blend, whey-dominated protein composition, amino acid pattern, mineral content and inclusion of beta-carotene and nucleotides. SMA, utilizing a hybridized safflower (oleic) oil, became the first infant formula offering fat and calcium absorption closest to that of human milk, with physiologic levels of linoleic acid and linolenic acid. Thus, the fat blend in SMA provides a ready source of energy, helps protect infants against neonatal tetany and produces a ratio of vitamin E to polyunsaturated fatty acids (linoleic acid) more than adequate to prevent hemolytic anemia and yields a serum lipid profile close to that of the breast-fed infant.

By combining reduced minerals whey with skimmed cow's milk, SMA reduces the protein content to fall within the range of human milk, adjusts the whey-protein to casein ratio to that of human milk, and subsequently reduces the mineral content to a physiologic level.

The resultant 60:40 whey-protein to casein ratio provides protein nutrition superior to a casein-dominated formula. In addition, the essential amino acids, including cystine, are present in amounts close to those of human milk. So the protein in SMA is of high biologic value.

Five nucleotides found in higher amounts in human milk compared to infant formula have been added to SMA at the levels found in breast milk. Laboratory studies have demonstrated benefits to the immunological system.

The physiologic mineral content makes possible a low renal solute load which helps protect the functionally immature infant kidney, increases expendable water reserves and helps protect against dehydration.

Use of lactose as the carbohydrate results in a physiologic stool flora and a low stool pH, decreasing the incidence of perianal dermatitis.

Ingredients: SMA Concentrated Liquid or Ready-to-Feed. Water; nonfat milk; reduced minerals whey; oleo, coconut, oleic (safflower or sunflower), and soybean oils; lactose; soy lecithin; taurine; cytidine-5'-monophosphate; calcium carrageenan; adenosine-5'-monophosphate; disodium uridine-5'-monophosphate; disodium inosine-5'-monophosphate; disodium guanosine-5'-monophosphate; *Minerals:* Potassium bicarbonate and chloride; calcium chloride and citrate; sodium bicarbonate and citrate; ferrous, zinc, cupric, and manganese sulfates. *Vitamins:* ascorbic acid, alpha tocopheryl acetate, niacinamide, vitamin A palmitate, calcium pantothenate, thiamine hydrochloride, riboflavin, pyridoxine hydrochloride, beta-carotene, folic acid, phytonadione, biotin, cholecalciferol, cyanocobalamin.

SMA Powder. Lactose; oleo, coconut, oleic (safflower or sunflower), and soybean oils; nonfat milk; whey protein concentrate; soy lecithin; taurine; cytidine-5'-monophosphate; adenosine-5'-monophosphate; disodium uridine-5'-monophosphate; disodium inosine-5'-monophosphate; disodium guanosine-5'-monophosphate. *Minerals:* Potassium phosphate; calcium hydroxide; magnesium chloride; calcium chloride; sodium bicarbonate; ferrous sulfate; potassium hydroxide; potassium bicarbonate; zinc, cupric, and manganese sulfates; potassium iodide. *Vitamins:* Ascorbic acid, choline chloride, inositol, alpha tocopheryl acetate, niacinamide, calcium pantothenate, vitamin A palmitate, riboflavin, thiamine hydrochloride, pyridoxine hydrochloride, beta-carotene, folic acid, phytonadione, biotin, cholecalciferol, cyanocobalamin.

PROXIMATE ANALYSIS
at 20 calories per fluidounce
READY-TO-FEED, POWDER, and
CONCENTRATED LIQUID:

	(W/V)
Fat	3.6 %
Carbohydrate	7.2 %
Protein	1.5 %
60% Lactalbumin (whey protein)	0.9 %
40% Casein	0.6 %
Ash	0.25%
Crude Fiber	None
Total Solids	12.6 %
Calories/fl. oz.	20

Vitamins, Minerals: In normal dilution, each liter contains:

A	2000	IU
D 3	400	IU
E	9.5	IU
K 1	55	mcg
C (ascorbic acid)	55	mg
B 1 (thiamine)	670	mcg
B 2 (riboflavin)	1000	mcg
B 6 (pyridoxine hydrochloride)	420	mcg
B 12	1.3	mcg
Niacin	5000	mcg
Pantothenic Acid	2100	mcg
Folic Acid (folacin)	50	mcg
Choline	100	mg
Biotin	15	mcg
Calcium	420	mg
Phosphorus	280	mg
Sodium	150	mg
Potassium	560	mg
Chloride	375	mg
Magnesium	45	mg
Manganese	100	mcg
Iron	12	mg
Copper	470	mcg
Zinc	5	mg
Iodine	60	mcg

Preparation: *Ready-to-Feed* (8 and 32 fl. oz. cans of 20 calories per fluidounce formula)—shake can, open and pour into previously sterilized nursing bottle; attach nipple and feed immediately. Cover opened can and immediately store in refrigerator. Use contents of can within 48 hours of opening.

Prolonged storage of can at excessive temperatures should be avoided. Expiration date is on top of can. WARNING: DO NOT USE A MICROWAVE TO PREPARE OR WARM FORMULA. SERIOUS BURNS MAY OCCUR.

Powder —(1 pound can)—For normal dilution supplying 20 calories per fluidounce, use 1 scoop (8.3 grams or 1 standard tablespoonful) of powder, packed and leveled, to 2 fluidounces of cooled, previously boiled water. For larger amount of formula, use ¼ standard measuring cup of powder (33.2 grams), packed and leveled, to 8 fluidounces (1 standard measuring cup) of water. Three of these portions make 26 fluidounces of formula.

Prolonged storage of can of powder at excessive temperatures should be avoided. Expiration date is on bottom of can. WARNING: DO NOT USE A MICROWAVE TO PREPARE OR WARM FORMULA. SERIOUS BURNS MAY OCCUR.

Concentrated Liquid —For normal dilution supplying 20 calories per fluidounce, use equal amounts of SMA® liquid and cooled, previously boiled water.

Prolonged storage of can at excessive temperatures should be avoided. Expiration date is on top of can. WARNING: DO NOT USE A MICROWAVE TO PREPARE OR WARM FORMULA. SERIOUS BURNS MAY OCCUR.

Note: Prepared formula should be used within 24 hours.

How Supplied: *Ready-to-Feed* —presterilized and premixed, 32 fluidounce (1 quart) cans, cases of 6 cans; 8 fluidounce cans, cases of 24 (4 carriers of 6 cans). *Powder* —1 pound cans with measuring scoop, cases of 6 cans. *Concentrated Liquid* —13 fluidounce cans, cases of 24 cans.

Also Available: SMA® lo-iron. For those who appreciate the particular advantages of SMA®, the infant formula closest in composition nutritionally to mother's milk, but who sometimes need or wish to recommend a formula that does not contain a high level of iron, there is SMA® lo-iron with all the benefits of regular SMA® but with a reduced level of iron of 1.4 mg per quart. Infants should receive supplemental dietary iron from an outside source to meet daily requirements.

Concentrated Liquid —13 fl. oz. cans, cases of 24 cans. *Powder* —1 pound cans with measuring scoop, cases of 6 cans. *Ready-to-Feed* —32 fl. oz. cans, cases of 6 cans.

Preparation of the standard 20 calories per fluidounce formula of SMA® lo-iron is the same as SMA® iron fortified given above.

Questions or Comments regarding SMA: 1-800-99-WYETH.

Shown in Product Identification Section, page 435

WYANOIDS® Relief Factor
[*wi 'a-noids*]
Hemorrhoidal Suppositories

Description: Active Ingredients: Live Yeast Cell Derivative, Supplying 2,000 units Skin Respiratory Factor Per Ounce of Cocoa Butter Suppository Base and Shark Liver Oil 3%. **Inactive Ingredients:** Beeswax, Glycerin, Phenylmercuric Nitrate 1:10,000 (as a preservative), Polyethylene Glycol 600 Dilaurate.

Indications: To help shrink swelling of hemorrhoidal tissues and provide prompt, temporary relief from pain and itching.

Usual Dosage: Use one suppository up to five times daily, especially in the morning, at night, and after bowel movements, or as directed by a physician.

Directions: Remove wrapper and insert one suppository rectally using gentle pressure. Frequent application and lubrication with Wyanoids® Relief Factor provide continual therapy which will lead to more rapid improvement of rectal conditions.

Caution: In case of bleeding or if the condition persists, the patient should consult a physician. Keep this and all medicines out of the reach of children. Do not store above 80°F.

How Supplied: Boxes of 12 and 24.
Shown in Product Identification Section, page 435

EDUCATIONAL MATERIAL

Audiovisual Programs
The **Wyeth-Ayerst Audiovisual Catalog,** listing audiovisual programs available through the Wyeth-Ayerst Audiovisual Library or on loan through the local Wyeth-Ayerst representative, can be obtained by writing Professional Service, Wyeth-Ayerst Laboratories, P.O. Box 8299, Philadelphia, PA 19101.

IDENTIFICATION PROBLEM?
Consult the
Product Identification Section
where you'll find
products pictured
in full color.

Zila Pharmaceuticals, Inc.
5227 NORTH 7th STREET
PHOENIX, AZ 85014

ZILACTIN® Medicated Gel
ZILADENT™ Oral Analgesic Gel
ZILACTOL™ Medicated Liquid

Description: **Zilactin** Medicated Gel stops pain and speeds healing of canker sores, fever blisters and cold sores. **ZilaDent** Oral Analgesic Gel contains a topical anesthetic and provides fast, long lasting relief from cuts and sores caused by braces, dentures, other dental appliances, bites, toothbrushes, etc. Both **Zilactin and ZilaDent** form a tenacious, occlusive film which holds the medication in place while controlling pain. Intra-orally, the film can last up to eight hours, usually allowing pain-free eating and drinking. Extra-orally, the film can last much longer.

Zilactol is a non film-forming medicated liquid that can often prevent developing cold sores or fever blisters from breaking out. Zilactol is specially formulated for treating the initial signs of tingling, itching or burning that signal an oncoming cold sore or fever blister. If a lesion does occur, Zilactol will significantly reduce the size of the outbreak.

Several clinical studies on the effectiveness of Zila's products are available on request.

Active Ingredients: Zilactin—Tannic Acid (7%); **ZilaDent**—Benzocaine (6%); **Zilactol**—Tannic Acid (7%)

Application: Zilactin and ZilaDent: Apply four times a day for the first three days and then as needed. Dry the affected area with a gauze pad, tissue or cotton swab. Apply a thin coat of Zilactin or ZilaDent and allow 30–60 seconds for the gel to dry into a film. Outside the mouth, Zilactin forms a transparent film. Inside the mouth, the film is white. ZilaDent forms a flesh colored film and is recommended for intra-oral use only. Replace dentures and other dental appliances only after film has dried completely.

Zilactol: Apply every 1–2 hours for the first three days and then as needed. For maximum effectiveness use at first signs of tingling or itching. Moisten a cotton swab with several drops of Zilactol. Apply directly on the developing cold sore or fever blister and allow to dry for 15 seconds.

Warning: A mild, temporary stinging sensation may be experienced when applying Zilactin, ZilaDent or Zilactol to an open cut, sore or blister. Stinging may be reduced or eliminated by applying ice before drying. DO NOT USE IN OR NEAR EYES. In the event of accidental contact with the eye, flush immediately and continuously for ten minutes. Seek immediate medical attention if pain or

Continued on next page

Zila—Cont.

irritation persists. For temporary relief only. As with all medications, keep out of the reach of children.

How Supplied: Zila products are nonprescription and carried by most drug wholesalers, major retail chains and independent pharmacies. Each product is available to physicians and dentists directly from Zila in full sized and single use packages. For further information call or write:

Zila Pharmaceuticals, Inc.
5227 N. 7th Street, Phoenix, AZ 85014,
(602) 266-6700

*U.S. patent numbers 4,285,934 and 4,381,296

Shown in Product Identification Section, page 435

EDUCATIONAL MATERIAL

Samples and literature are available to physicians and dentists on request.

Products are indexed by
generic and chemical names in the
YELLOW SECTION

Diagnostics Devices and Medical Aids

This section is intended to present product information on Diagnostics, Devices and Medical Aids designed for home use by patients. The information concerning each product has been prepared, edited and approved by the manufacturer.

The Publisher has emphasized to manufacturers the necessity of describing products comprehensively so that all information essential for intelligent and informed use is available. In organizing and presenting the material in this edition the Publisher is providing all the information made available by manufacturers.

In presenting the following material to the medical profession, the Publisher is not necessarily advocating the use of any product.

Lavoptik Company, Inc.
661 WESTERN AVENUE N.
ST. PAUL, MN 55103

LAVOPTIK® Eye Cups

Description: Device—Sterile disposable eye cups.

How Supplied: Individually bagged eye cups are packed 12 per box, NDC 10651-01004.

Ortho Pharmaceutical Corporation
Advanced Care Products
RARITAN, NJ 08869

ADVANCE®
Pregnancy Test

Active Ingredients: Human Chorionic Gonadotropin (HCG) alpha chain specific monoclonal antibody HCG, beta-chain specific antibody/enzyme conjugate, chromogenic substrate solution, and buffer solution.

Indications: An in-vitro pregnancy test for use in the home that can detect the presence of HCG in the urine as early as one (1) day past last missed period.

Actions: ADVANCE will accurately detect the presence or absence of HCG in urine in just thirty minutes. It is as accurate as pregnancy test methods used in many hospitals.

Dosage and Administration: Perform the test according to instructions. If, after thirty minutes, a blue color appears on the rounded end of the COLOR-STICK, the patient can assume she is pregnant. If the rounded end of the COLORSTICK remains white, and no blue color can be seen, no pregnancy hormone has been detected and the patient is probably not pregnant. The test results may be affected by certain health conditions such as an ovarian cyst or ectopic pregnancy and by certain medications such as thiazide diuretics, plurothiazine, hormones, steroids, chemotherapeutics, and thyroid drugs. For additional reassurance, a toll-free telephone number is included in each package insert. This service is staffed by Registered Nurses who can answer any questions the patient may have about her results, or how she performed the test.

How Supplied: Each ADVANCE test contains a plastic COLORSTICK, a plastic vial containing buffer solution, a glass tube containing dried test chemicals, a glass tube containing color developing solution, a test stand with urine collection and instructions for use.

Storage: Store at room temperature (59°–86°F). Do not freeze.
Shown in Product Identification Section, page 418

FACT PLUS™
Pregnancy Test

Active Ingredients: Human Chorionic Gonadotropin (HCG) antibody, HCG antibody/colored conjugate.

Indications: An in-vitro pregnancy test for use in the home that can detect the presence of HCG in the urine as early as the first day of a missed period.

Actions: FACT PLUS will accurately detect the presence or absence of HCG in urine in as soon as 5 minutes using urine collected at any time of day. One step FACT PLUS is the same pregnancy test method used in many hospitals.

Dosage and Administration: Using the urine dropper, drop five drops of urine in the Urine Well of the test disk. Wait for red to appear in End of Test Window (may take about 5 minutes). If, after the End of Test Window has turned red, a plus (+) sign has formed in the center of the test disk, the patient is probably pregnant. If a minus (−) sign appears, no pregnancy hormone has been detected and the patient is probably not pregnant. In the unlikely event that neither sign appears the test system has not worked properly and the patient should call the toll free number included in the package insert. This toll free number is staffed by Registered Nurses who can answer any questions the patient may have about her results, or how she performed the test. The test results may be affected by various other factors and medications such as thiazide diuretics, plurothiazine, hormones, steroids, chemotherapeutics, and thyroid drugs.

How Supplied: Each FACT PLUS kit contains a plastic test disk, a urine collection cup, a urine dropper, and complete instructions for use.

Storage: Store at room temperature (59–86°F). Do not freeze.
Shown in Product Identification Section, page 418

Parke-Davis
Consumer Health Products Group
Division of Warner-Lambert Company
201 TABOR ROAD
MORRIS PLAINS, NJ 07950

e·p·t® STICK TEST
Early Pregnancy Test

BEFORE YOU BEGIN THE e·p·t TEST:
- CAREFULLY READ THROUGH THIS ENTIRE INSERT.
- YOU CAN USE THIS TEST ANY TIME OF THE DAY.
- IF YOU HAVE ANY QUESTIONS, CALL TOLL-FREE 1-800-562-0266.
- REGISTERED NURSES ARE AVAILABLE TO ANSWER YOUR CALLS CONFIDENTIALLY.
- e·p·t IS VIRTUALLY 100% ACCURATE IN LABORATORY TESTS.

HOW e·p·t WORKS:
When a woman becomes pregnant, her body produces a special hormone known as hCG (Human Chorionic Gonadotropin), which appears in the urine. e·p·t can detect this hormone as early as the first day you miss your period.

If you test positive, you can assume you are pregnant and should see your doctor. A negative result means that no hCG has been detected and you can assume that you are not pregnant.

WHEN TO USE e·p·t:
e·p·t can detect hCG hormone levels in your urine as early as the day your period should have started. e·p·t can be used on the day of missed period as well as any day thereafter.

THE e·p·t TEST CONTAINS:
A. A pouch containing the test stick. The test stick has a small round window, a larger oval window, and an opening in the tip which is covered.
(A small paper packet (desiccant), helps keep the test fresh. Throw this away. It is NOT part of the test.)
B. A urine collection cap.
C. A tray that holds the test contents, with a built-in holder for the test stick.

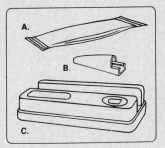

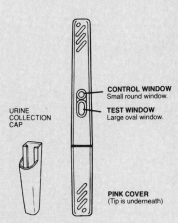

URINE COLLECTION CAP

CONTROL WINDOW
Small round window.

TEST WINDOW
Large oval window.

PINK COVER
(Tip is underneath)

The e·p·t test is easy to perform. SIMPLY DO THE FOLLOWING:
- REMOVE THE TEST STICK FROM THE POUCH.
Tear by the small notch on the end of the pouch.

Continued on next page

Parke-Davis—Cont.

- **PULL PINK COVER OFF TIP OF STICK.**
- **SLIDE THE TIP OF THE TEST STICK INTO THE URINE COLLECTION CAP.**

Make sure that the opening in the tip faces the cap area (see illustration). The cap should fit easily on the stick. <u>Make sure that the ridges on the cap and the test stick are both on the same side.</u>

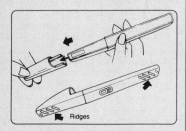

Ridges

- **COLLECT URINE.**

With the urine collection cap facing you, and pointing in a downward direction, hold the test stick in your urine stream until the cap is filled with urine. The test and control windows should be facing away from you. Do not let urine splash the test and control windows on the test stick.

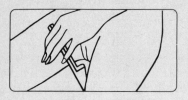

- **PLACE THE TEST STICK INTO THE HOLDER ON THE TRAY.** (Optional)

The test stick should fit easily into the built-in holder in the tray.

- **WAIT 4 MINUTES.**
<u>**DO NOT READ THE TEST RESULTS UNTIL AFTER 4 MINUTES.**</u>
(Earlier results may be invalid.)
NOTE: As the urine moves up the test stick, a dark pink or purple color will move across both windows. This color will fade after a few minutes. This is the normal way the test works.

READING THE e·p·t TEST RESULTS:

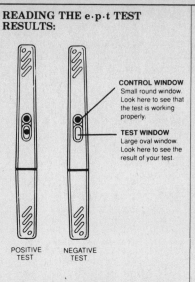

CONTROL WINDOW
Small round window. Look here to see that the test is working properly.

TEST WINDOW
Large oval window. Look here to see the result of your test.

POSITIVE TEST   NEGATIVE TEST

- **READ THE CONTROL WINDOW.**

After you have completed the test, a pink or purple circle will appear in the Control Window whether you are pregnant or not. This tells you that the e·p·t test is working properly. Now you can read your results in the Test Window.

IMPORTANT: If there is no color in the Control Window, call the toll-free number and DO NOT read the result in the Test Window since the result may be incorrect.

- **READ THE TEST WINDOW.**

POSITIVE– After the test stick has been in the urine for <u>four</u> minutes, you can assume you ARE PREGNANT if a circle of ANY SHADE of pink or purple remains in the Test Window.

NEGATIVE–  You can assume you ARE NOT PREGNANT if after four minutes NO CIRCLE is seen in the Test Window.

NOTE: EVEN IF A VERY FAINT PINK OR PURPLE CIRCLE IS VISIBLE IN THE TEST WINDOW, THE RESULT IS POSITIVE.

(The color of the circle in the Test Window DOES NOT HAVE to match the color of the circle in the Control Window).

INGREDIENTS:*
Test stick containing gold sol particles coated with hCG antibodies and anti-hCG antibodies.
* Not to be taken internally.
For in-vitro diagnostic use.
Store at 59°–86°F.

If this is a 2 kit package, save the tray for use with the second test stick.

QUESTIONS YOU MAY HAVE ABOUT e·p·t:

When can I do the test?
e·p·t can detect hCG levels as early as the first day of your missed period. You can perform the test at any time of the day.

Can I collect my urine in a cup instead of in the urine collection cap?
Yes. If you collect urine in a cup, place the urine collection cap on the test stick. Then dip the cap side into the cup to fill the cap with urine. Continue the test as instructed.

What if the test changes color, but the color isn't the same as the picture in the brochure?
If the test is positive, the Test Window will retain a circle of some shade of pink or purple color after the 4 minutes the test stick was in the urine. The color can be ANY SHADE of pink or purple and DOES NOT HAVE TO MATCH the color pictured or the color present in the Control Window.

NOTE: A positive test can result in a range of pink or purple shades. e·p·t is so sensitive that it can detect pregnancy as early as the day of a missed period. However, during pregnancy, each day after a missed period results in higher levels of hCG (the pregnancy hormone) in the urine. This is why testing a few days or a week after a missed period will result in a darker test result than the first day of a missed period.

What do I do if the test result is positive?
If the test result is positive, you should see a doctor to discuss your pregnancy and next steps. Early prenatal care is important to ensure the health of you and your baby.

What do I do if the test result is negative?
If the test result is negative, no pregnancy hormone (hCG) has been detected and you are probably not pregnant. However, you may have miscalculated when your period was due. If your period does not start within a week, repeat the test. If you still get a negative result after the second test, and your period still has not started, you should see a doctor.

What if I don't wait the full 4 minutes before reading the test result?
If you read the test result before the full 4 minutes have passed, you may not give the test enough time to work, and the results may be inaccurate.

What if I don't think the results of the test are correct?
If you follow the instructions carefully, you should not get a false result. Certain drugs and rare medical conditions may give a false result. Analgesics, antibiotics, and birth control pills should not affect the test result. If you repeat the test and continue to get an unexpected result, contact your doctor.

IF YOU HAVE FURTHER QUESTIONS ABOUT **e·p·t** CALL TOLL-FREE 1-800-562-0266 WEEKDAYS 9 AM to 5 PM EST.

Marketed by
PARKE-DAVIS Consumer Health Products Group
© 1991 Warner-Lambert Company
Morris Plains, NJ 07950 USA
Shown in Product Identification Section, page 419

Whitehall Laboratories Inc.

Division of American Home Products Corporation
685 THIRD AVENUE
NEW YORK, NY 10017

CLEARBLUE EASY™
Pregnancy Test Kit

Clearblue Easy is the easiest and one of the fastest pregnancy tests available because all you have to do is hold the absorbent tip in your urine stream, replace the cap, and in 3 minutes you'll know the test is complete when a blue line appears in the small window. The large window shows the test result. If there is a blue line in the large window, you are pregnant. If there is no line, you are not pregnant.

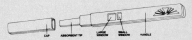

Clearblue Easy is a rapid, one-step pregnancy test for home use which detects tiny amounts of the pregnancy hormone HCG (human chorionic gonadotropin) in the urine. This hormone is produced in increasing amounts during the first part of pregnancy. Clearblue Easy uses sensitive monoclonal antibodies to detect the presence of the hormone from the first day of a missed period.

The pregnancy hormone, HCG, is most concentrated in your first morning urine, so it is recommended that you use this urine, particularly if you test on the day of your missed period.

A negative result means that no pregnancy hormone was detected and you are probably not pregnant. If your period does not start within a week, you may have miscalculated the day your period was due. Repeat the test using another Clearblue Easy test. If the second test still gives a negative result and you still have not menstruated, you should see your doctor.

Clearblue Easy is specially designed for easy use at home. However, if you do have questions about the test or results, give the Clearblue Easy TalkLine a call at 1-800-223-2329. A specially trained staff of advisors is available 24 hours a day to answer your questions.

Manufactured by Unipath Ltd.; Bedford, U.K. Unipath, Clearblue Easy and the fan device are trademarks.

Distributed by Whitehall Laboratories, New York, NY 10017.

Shown in Product Identification Section, page 434

CLEARPLAN EASY™
One-Step Ovulation Predictor

CLEARPLAN EASY is the easiest home ovulation predictor test to use because of its unique technological design. It consists of just one piece and involves only one step to get the results. To use CLEARPLAN EASY, a woman simply holds the absorbent tip in her urine stream (a woman can test any time of day) for 5 seconds, and after 5 minutes, she can read the results. A blue line will appear in the small window to show her that the test has worked correctly. The large window indicates the presence of luteinizing hormone (LH) in her urine. If there is a line in the large window which is similar to or darker than the line in the small window, she has detected her LH surge.

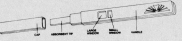

Laboratory tests confirm that CLEARPLAN EASY is over 98% accurate in detecting the LH surge as shown by radioimmunoassay (RIA).

CLEARPLAN EASY employs highly sensitive monoclonal antibody technology to accurately predict the onset of ovulation, and, consequently, the best time each month for a woman to try to become pregnant. The test monitors the amount of LH in a woman's urine. Small amounts of LH are present during most of the menstrual cycle, but the level normally rises sharply about 24 to 36 hours before ovulation (which is when an egg is released from the ovary). CLEARPLAN EASY detects this LH surge which precedes ovulation so that a woman knows 24–36 hours beforehand the time she is most able to become pregnant.

A woman will be most fertile during the 2 to 3 days after an LH surge is detected. Sperm can fertilize an egg for many hours after sexual intercourse. So, if sexual intercourse occurs during the 2–3 days after a similar or darker line appears in the large window, the chances of getting pregnant are maximized.

CLEARPLAN EASY contains 5 days of tests. If, because a woman's cycles are irregular or if for any other reason a woman does not detect her LH surge after 5 days of testing, she should continue testing with a second CLEARPLAN EASY kit. CLEARPLAN EASY offers users the support of a 24-hour TalkLine (1-800-223-2329). This service is operated by trained advisors who are available to answer any questions about using the test or reading the results.

Produced by Unipath Ltd., Bedford, U.K. Unipath, CLEARPLAN EASY and the fan device are trademarks.

Distributed by Whitehall Laboratories, New York, NY 10017.

Shown in Product Identification Section, page 434

Certified
Poison Control Centers

The poison control centers in the following list are certified by the American Association of Poison Control Centers. To receive certification, each center must meet certain criteria. It must, for example, serve a large geographics area; it must be open 24 hours a day and provide direct dialing or toll-free access; it must be supervised by a medical director; and it must have registered pharmacists or nurses available to answer questions from the public.

Staff members of these centers are trained to resolve toxicity situations in the home of the caller, but, in some instances, hospital referrals are given.

The centers have a wide variety of toxicology resources, including a computer capability covering some 350,000 substances that are updated quarterly. They also offer a range of educational services to the public as well as to the health-care professional. In some states, these large centers exist side by side with smaller poison control centers that provide more limited information.

AMERICAN ASSOCIATION OF POISON CONTROL CENTERS

ALABAMA

Children's Hospital of Alabama — Regional Poison Control Center

1600 Seventh Avenue, South
Birmingham, AL 35233-1711
Emergency Numbers:
(205) 939-9201; (205) 933-4050;
(800) 292-6678

ARIZONA

Arizona Poison & Drug Information Center

Arizona Health Sciences Center
Room 3204K
1501 N. Campbell Ave.
Tucson, AZ 85724
Emergency Numbers:
(602) 626-6016; (800) 362-0101
(AZ only)

Samaritan Regional Poison Center

Good Samaritan Medical Center
1130 East McDowell Road,
Suite A-5
Phoenix, AZ 85006
Emergency Number:
(602) 253-3334

CALIFORNIA

Fresno Regional Poison Control Center of Fresno Community Hospital and Medical Center

P.O. Box 1232
2823 Fresno Street
Fresno, CA 93715
Emergency Number:
(800) 346-5922 (CA only)

Los Angeles County Medical Association Regional Poison Control Center

1925 Wilshire Boulevard
Los Angeles, CA 90057
Emergency Number:
(213) 484-5151

San Diego Regional Poison Center

UCSD Medical Center,
225 Dickinson Street
San Diego, CA 92103
Emergency Numbers:
(619) 543-6000; (800) 876-4766
(619 area code only)

Santa Clara Valley Medical Center Regional Poison Center

751 South Bascom Ave.
San Jose, CA 95128
Emergency Numbers:
(408) 299-5112; (800) 662-9886

UCDMC Regional Poison Control Center

2315 Stockton Boulevard
Sacramento, CA 95817
Emergency Numbers:
(916) 453-3414; (800) 342-9293
(CA only)

COLORADO

Rocky Mountain Poison and Drug Center
645 Bannock Street
Denver, CO 80204-4507
Emergency Numbers:
(303) 629-1123; (800) 332-3073
(CO only)

D.C.

National Capital Poison Center
Georgetown University Hospital
3800 Reservoir Rd., NW
Washington, DC 20007
Emergency Numbers:
(202) 625-3333; (202) 784-4660
(TTY)

FLORIDA

Florida Poison Information Center at the Tampa General Hospital
P.O. Box 1289
Tampa, FL 33601
Emergency Numabers:
(813) 253-4444; (800) 282-3171
(FL only)

GEORGIA

Georgia Poison Control Center
Grady Memorial Hospital
Box 26066
80 Butler Street, SE
Atlanta, GA 30335-3801
Emergency Numbers:
(404) 589-4400; (800) 282-5846
(GA only);
(404) 525-3323 (TTY)

INDIANA

Indiana Poison Center
Methodist Hospital of Indiana, Inc.
P.O. Box 1367
1701 North Senate Blvd.
Indianapolis, IN 46206
Emergency Numbers:
(800) 382-9097; (317) 929-2323

KENTUCKY

Kentucky Regional Poison Center of Kosair
Children's Hospital
P.O. Box 35070
Louisville, KY 40232-5070
Emergency Numbers:
(502) 629-7275; (800) 722-5725
(KY only)

MARYLAND

Maryland Poison Center
20 North Pine Street
Baltimore, MD 21201
Emergency Numbers:
(301) 528-7701; (800) 492-2414
(MD only)

National Capital Poison Center (D.C. suburbs only)
Georgetown University Hospital
380 Reservoir Rd., NW
Washington, DC 20007

MASSACHUSETTS

Massachusetts Poison Control System
300 Longwood Avenue
Boston, MA 02115
Emergency Numbers:
(617) 232-2120; (800) 682-9211
(MA only)

MICHIGAN

Blodgett Regional Poison Center
1840 Wealthy SE
Grand Rapids, MI 49506
Emergency Numbers:
(800) 632-2727 (MI only)
(800) 356-3232 (TTY)

Poison Control Center, Children's Hospital of Michigan
3901 Beaubien Boulevard
Detroit, MI 48201
Emergency Numbrs:
(313) 745-5711; (800) 462-6642
(MI only)

MINNESOTA

Hennepin Regional Poison Center
Hennepin County Medical Center
701 Park Avenue
Minneapolis, MN 55415
Emergency Numbers:
(612) 347-3141; (612) 337-7474
(TTY)

Minnesota Regional Poison Center
St. Paul-Ramsey Medical Center
640 Jackson Street
St. Paul, MN 55101
Emergency Number:
(612) 221-2113

MISSOURI

**Cardinal Glennon Children's
Hospital Regional Poison Center**
1645 South Grand Boulevard
St. Louis, MO 63104
Emergency Numbers:
(314) 772-5200: (800) 366-8888

MONTANA

**Rocky Mountain Poison and
Drug Center**
645 Bannock Street
Denver, CO 80204-4507
Emergency Number:
(800) 525-5042 (MT only)

NEBRASKA

The Poison Center
8301 Dodge Street
Omaha, NE 68114
Emergency Numbers:
(402) 390-5400: (800) 642-9999
(NE only): (800) 228-9515
(Surrounding states)

NEW JERSEY

**New Jersey Poison
Information and Education
System**
201 Lyons Avenue
Newark, NJ 07112
Emergency Number:
(800) 962-1253 (NJ only)

NEW MEXICO

**New Mexico Poison and Drug
Information Center**
University of New Mexico
Albuquerque, NM 87131
Emergency Numbers:
(505) 843-2551: (800) 432-6866
(NM only)

NEW YORK

**Long Island Regional Poison
Control Center**
Nassau County Medical Center
2201 Hempstead Turnpike
East Meadow, NY 11554
Emergency Number:
(516) 542-2323

**New York City Poison Control
Center**
455 First Avenue, Room 123
New York, NY 10016
Emergency Numbers:
(212) 340-4494:
(212) POISONS

OHIO

Central Ohio Poison Center
Columbus Children's Hospital
700 Children's Drive
Columbus, OH 43205
Emergency Numbers:
(614) 228-1323: (800) 682-7625
(OH only): (614) 228-2272 (TTY)

**Regional Poison Control
System, Cincinnati Drug and
Poison Information Center**
231 Bethesda Avenue, M.L.
#144
Cincinnati, OH 45267-0144
Emergency Numbers:
(513) 558-5111: (800) 872-5111

OREGON

Oregon Poison Center
Oregon Health Sciences
University
3181 SW Sam Jackson Park
Road
Portland, OR 97201
Emergency Numbers:
(503) 494-8968 (local):
(800) 452-7165
(OR only)

PENNSYLVANIA

**The Poison Control Center
serving the greater Philadelphia
metropolitan area**
One Children's Center
34th & Civic Center Boulevard
Philadelphia, PA 19104
Emergency Number:
(215) 386-2100

Pittsburgh Poison Center
3705 Fifth Avenue at DeSoto
Street
Pittsburgh, PA 15213
Emergency Number:
(412) 681-6669

RHODE ISLAND

**Rhode Island Poison Center—
Rhode Island Hospital**
593 Eddy Street
Providence, RI 02902
Emergency Numbers:
(401) 277-5727

TEXAS

North Texas Poison Center
P.O. Box 35926
Dallas, TX 75235
Emergency Numbers:
(214) 590-5000: (800) 441-0040
(TX only)

UTAH

Intermountain Regional Poison Control Center
50 North Medical Drive
Building 428
Salt Lake City. UT 84132
Emergency Numbers:
(801) 581-2151: (800) 456-7707
(UT only)

VIRGINIA

National Capital Poison Center (Northern VA only)
Georgetown University Hospital
3800 Reservoir Rd.. NW
Washington. DC 20007
Emergency Numbers:
(202) 625-3333: (202) 84-4660
(TTY)

WEST VIRGINIA

West Virginia Poison Center
West Virginia University Health Sciences Center Charleston Division
3110 MacCorkle Avenue. SE
Charleston. WV 25304
Emergency Numbers:
(304) 348-4211: (800) 642-3625
(WV only)

WYOMING

Rocky Mountain Poison and Drug Center
645 Bannock Street
Denver. CO 80204-4507
Emergency Number:
(800) 442-2702 (WY only)